PCF8

PALLIATIVE CARE FORMULARY

Published by Pharmaceutical Press

Published by the Pharmaceutical Press
66-68 East Smithfield, London E1W 1AW, UK

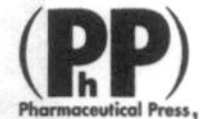, PhP, Palliative Care Formulary, PCF and 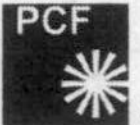 are trademarks of The Royal Pharmaceutical Society of Great Britain trading as Pharmaceutical Press.

Pharmaceutical Press is the publishing division of the Royal Pharmaceutical Society.

PCF8 2022
PCF7 2020, reprinted 2021
PCF6 2017, reprinted 2018
PCF5+ PDF 2016
PCF5+ PDF 2015
PCF5 2014, reprinted 2015
PCF4+ PDF 2013
PCF4+ PDF 2012
PCF4 2011, reprinted 2012 (twice), 2013
PCF3 2007, reprinted 2008, 2009
PCF2 2002, reprinted 2003
PCF1 1998

Typeset by Anytime Publishing Services, Derbyshire, UK
Printed in Italy by LEGO S.p.A.
ISBN 9780857114372

A catalogue record for this book is available from the British Library.

DISCLAIMER

Every effort has been made to ensure the accuracy of this text and that the best information available has been used. However, the Royal Pharmaceutical Society of Great Britain trading as Pharmaceutical Press makes no representations, warranties or guarantees, whether express or implied, that the content is accurate, complete or up to date and neither represents nor guarantees that the practices described herein will, if followed, ensure safe and effective patient care. The recommendations contained in this book reflect the editors' judgement regarding the state of general knowledge and practice in the field as of the date of publication. Information in a book of this type can never be all-inclusive, and therefore will not cover every eventuality.

This text is aimed at healthcare professionals and assumes a level of professional training to interpret the information herein. Information on the selection and clinical use of medicines is designed for prescribers, pharmacists and other healthcare professionals and is not suitable for patients or the general public. All information should be interpreted in light of professional knowledge and supplemented as necessary with additional specialist publications, and all users are responsible for ensuring appropriate use or reliance on such information. Those who use this book must make their own determinations regarding specific safe and appropriate patient-care practices, taking into account the personnel, equipment and practices available at the hospital or other facility at which they are located. So far as permitted by law, neither the Royal Pharmaceutical Society of Great Britain trading as Pharmaceutical Press nor the editors can be held responsible for or will accept any liability for damages, in any form, arising from or in relation to this text or incurred as a consequence of the use or application of any of the contents of this book. Mention of specific product brands does not imply endorsement.

Particularly when prescribing a drug for the first time, a doctor (or other independent prescriber) should study the contents of the manufacturer's summary of product characteristics (SPC), paying particular attention to indications, contra-indications, cautions, drug interactions and undesirable effects.

EDITORIAL STAFF

Editorial Board

Editors-in-Chief

Andrew Wilcock DM, FRCP
Consultant Physician, Hayward House, Nottingham University Hospitals NHS Trust, UK
Honorary Associate Professor in Palliative Medicine, Nottingham University, UK

Paul Howard BMedSci, MRCP
Consultant in Palliative Medicine, Isle of Wight Mountbatten Hospice and Isle of Wight NHS Trust, UK

Specialist Pharmacist Editor

Sarah Charlesworth BPharm, DipClinPharm, MRPharmS
Expert Clinical Writer (Palliative Care), Pharmaceutical Press, UK

Editor

Claire Stark Toller MA, MA, MRCP
Consultant in Palliative Medicine, Mountbatten Hampshire and University Hospital Southampton NHS Foundation Trust, UK

Editorial Advisory Board Members

Joanne Droney PhD, MRCPI
Consultant in Palliative Medicine, The Royal Marsden NHS Foundation Trust, London, UK

Stephen Oxberry PhD, FRCP
Medical Director and Consultant in Palliative Medicine, The Kirkwood, Huddersfield and Specialist Palliative Care Team, Calderdale and Huddersfield Foundation NHS Trust, UK

Anna Spathis MD, FRCP, MRCGP, FHEA
Assistant Professor, Cambridge University and Honorary Consultant in Palliative Medicine, Cambridge University Hospitals NHS Foundation Trust, UK

Honorary Editorial Consultant

Robert Twycross DM, FRCP
Emeritus Clinical Reader in Palliative Medicine, Oxford University, UK (Founding Editor-in-Chief)

Current and Previous Contributors

Robert Brodrick MA, MRCP
Consultant in Palliative Medicine, Cambridge University Hospitals NHS Foundation Trust, UK

Matthew Brown MD(Res), MRCS, FRCA, FFPMRCA
Consultant in Pain Medicine, The Royal Marsden NHS Foundation Trust, London, UK
Honorary Associate Faculty, The Institute of Cancer Research, UK

Alpna Chauhan FRCP
Consultant in Palliative Medicine, John Eastwood Hospice, Sutton-in-Ashfield, UK

Vincent Crosby FRCP
Consultant in Palliative Medicine, Hayward House Specialist Palliative Care Unit, Nottingham University Hospitals NHS Trust, UK

Laura Daly BDS, BSc, MFDS, RCS Ed
Community Dental Officer, Derbyshire Community Health Services NHS Foundation Trust, UK

Andrew Davies MSc, MD, FRCP
Professor of Palliative Medicine, Trinity College Dublin, University College Dublin and Our Lady's Hospice Dublin, Ireland

Joanne Droney PhD, MRCPI
Consultant in Palliative Medicine, The Royal Marsden NHS Foundation Trust, London, UK

Joanna Elverson MA(Ed), MRCP
Consultant in Palliative Medicine, St Oswald's Hospice, Newcastle Upon Tyne, UK

Ruth England FRCP
Consultant in Palliative Medicine, University Hospitals of Derby and Burton NHS Foundation Trust, UK

Caroline Facey FRCP
Consultant in Palliative Medicine, Chesterfield Royal Hospital NHS Foundation Trust, UK

Catherine Gwilt MA, BSc, MRCP
Consultant in Palliative Medicine, Kingston Hospital NHS Foundation Trust, UK

Emily Harrop BSc, DCH, FRCPCH, PhD, DipPallMed
Medical Director, Helen and Douglas House Hospices for Children and Young Adults, Oxford, UK

Jonathan Hindmarsh MPharm, MRPharmS, IP, MSc
Advanced Clinical Pharmacist in Palliative Care, St Benedict's Hospice and Specialist Palliative Care Centre, Sunderland, UK

Andrew Hughes MRCGP
Consultant in Palliative Medicine, St Oswald's Hospice, Newcastle Upon Tyne, UK

Vanessa Jackson MRCP
Specialist Registrar in Palliative Medicine, Hayward House, Nottingham University Hospitals NHS Trust, UK

Aleksandra Kotlińska-Lemieszek MD, PhD
Associate Professor in Palliative Medicine, Poznan University of Medical Sciences, Poznan, Poland

Susie Lapwood MA, DFSRH, DipPallMed, MRCGP
Emeritus Senior Associate Specialist, Helen and Douglas House Hospices for Children and Young Adults, Oxford, UK

Mark Lee MD, MRCP
Consultant in Palliative Medicine, St Benedict's Hospice and Specialist Palliative Care Centre, Sunderland, UK

Aoife Lowney
Consultant in Palliative Medicine, Cork University Hospital and Marymount University Hospital and Hospice, Ireland; Clinical Senior Lecturer University College Cork, Ireland

Staffan Lundstrom MD, PhD
Associate Professor in Palliative Medicine, Karolinska Institutet and Stockholms Sjukhem, Stockholm, Sweden

Laura Miller MSc, PgDip Dietetics
Team Lead Dietitian, Nottingham University Hospitals NHS Trust, UK

Simon Noble MD, DipPallMed, FRCP
Clinical Professor in Palliative Medicine, Cardiff University, UK

Mary Jane O'Leary MB BCh BAO, BMedSc, MMedSc, MRCPI
Consultant in Palliative Medicine, Cork University Hospital and Marymount University Hospital and Hospice, Ireland; Clinical Senior Lecturer, University College Cork, Ireland

Stephen Oxberry PhD, FRCP
Medical Director and Consultant in Palliative Medicine, The Kirkwood, Huddersfield and Specialist Palliative Care Team, Calderdale and Huddersfield Foundation NHS Trust, UK

Filipa Palma dos Reis MD
Specialist Registrar in Medical Oncology, Centro Hospitalar Lisboa Central, Lisbon, Portugal

Rachel Quibell MRCGP, FRCP
Consultant in Palliative Medicine, Newcastle upon Tyne Hospitals NHS Foundation Trust, UK

Rebecca Robinson MRCP
Consultant in Palliative Medicine, Hayward House, Nottingham University Hospitals NHS Trust, UK

Maulina Sharma MMedSci, FRCP
Consultant Dermatologist, University Hospitals of Derby & Burton NHS Foundation Trust, UK

Anna Spathis MD, FRCP, MRCGP, FHEA
Assistant Professor, Cambridge University and Honorary Consultant in Palliative Medicine, Cambridge University Hospitals NHS Foundation Trust, UK

Ana Sofia Spencer MD
Consultant in Medical Oncology, Centro Hospitalar Universitário de Lisboa Central, Lisbon, Portugal

Emma Tregenna MA Hons, MRCP
Specialist Registrar in Palliative Medicine, Cynthia Spencer Hospice, Northampton, UK

Cathrine Vincent MRCGP
Consultant in Palliative Medicine, Hayward House, Nottingham University Hospitals NHS Trust, UK

Farzana Virani MRCP
Consultant in Palliative Medicine, Oxford University Hospitals NHS Trust, UK

Jillian Wall MRCP
Consultant in Palliative Medicine, Royal Derby Hospital, University Hospitals of Derby and Burton NHS Foundation Trust, UK

Pharmaceutical Press Editorial Team

Managing Director

Karen Baxter *BSc, MSc, MRPharmS*

Content Director

Andrea Naylor *MA*

Senior Editorial Staff

Kiri Aikman *BPharm (NZ), PGDipClinPharm (NZ), ARPharmS*
Rebecca Luckhurst *BSc (Hons), MSc*

PCF Editorial Team

Julia H Carretero *BSc, MSc*
Sarah Charlesworth *BPharm, DipClinPharm, MRPharmS*
Harriet Fiddimore-Hicks *BSc (Hons), MSc*
Ibrahim Mohammed-Ali *BSc, MSc*
Louise Symmons *BSc (Hons), MSc*

Additional PCF Support

Libby Achilles *BSc (Hons)*
Sophia Aldwinckle *BSc (Hons)*
Allegra Chan *BSc (Hons)*
Darren Chan *BSc, MSc*
Carina de Campos
Zunera Dildar
Rebecca Harwood *BSc (Hons)*
Aoife Healy
Nick Judd *BA (Hons), MA*
Olivia Maskill *BSc (Hons)*
Anna McLachlan *BPharm, PGCertClinPharm*
Hang Nguyen *BSc (Hons)*
Jannah Ryan *BSc (Hons)*
Maleeha Sohaib
Elisabetta Stramiglio *BSc, MSc*

Acknowledgements

We acknowledge with thanks the help provided by various advisors and previous contributors, including: Peter Armstrong, Sabrina Bajwah, Kirsty Bannister, Claudia Bausewein, James Beattie, Jenny Beavis, Sarah Bell, Jason Boland, Sara Booth, Virginia Bray, Andrew Broadbent, Sandra Clawson, Aisling Considine, Brian Creedon, Sarah Cripps, Helen Crispin, Anthony Dickenson, Josle Drew, Magnus Ekström, Ronald Elin, Marie Fallon, Louise Free, Janet Hardy, Philippa Hawley, Miriam Johnson, Vaughan Keeley, Bruce Kennedy, Emma Kidd, Samuel King, Malgorzata Krajnik, Michael Lucey, Louise Lynch, Gurminder Mann, Laura McGeeney, Maria McKenna, Mary Mihalyo, Julie Mortimer, Fliss Murtagh, Katie O'Brien, Alison Orr, Victor Pace, Sean Parker, Mayank Patel, Russell Portenoy, Wendy Prentice, Maggie Presswood, Constanze Rémi, Jan Rémi, Victoria Revell, Graeme Rocker, Joy Ross, Aidan Ryan, Paul Selby, Wunna Swe, Mark Taubert, Jeremy Turner, Anne Waddington, Rebecca White, Sarah Williams, Olivia Worthington, Mark Wright, and by medical information departments in the pharmaceutical industry.

We are grateful to Karen Isaac for support and Sarah Keeling for typesetting. We are also grateful to our freelance colleagues in the production of PCF with special thanks to Chandni Halai, Bryony Jordan, Christopher J Lam, Penny Lyons, Harriet Pike, Melinda Presland, Sandy Sutton, Hannah Tan, Mary White, and Miguel Zalacain.

CONTENTS

PREFACE TO EIGHTH EDITION

Welcome to the eighth edition of the *Palliative Care Formulary* (*PCF8*). One third of the content has been fully updated, with additional minor updates also published for this new edition. *PCF8* consists of 35 chapters and appendices; of the monographs, one has been renamed (Tricyclic antidepressants, formerly Amitriptyline) and two have been discontinued (Carbamazepine, Danazol). This print edition reflects the online content on MedicinesComplete as of August 2022, where regular updating of *PCF* continues.

The target audience for *PCF* comprises doctors, nurses and pharmacists involved in the care of patients receiving palliative/hospice care. *PCF* is a core textbook for registrars in palliative medicine in the UK. It is referred to in many official healthcare documents, e.g. NICE clinical knowledge summaries.

Although written primarily with cancer patients in mind, *PCF* contains specific material relating to a number of other life-limiting diseases, e.g. COPD, end-stage heart failure, renal failure, hepatic failure, and Parkinson's disease. However, in relation to the use of strong opioids for analgesia, the focus in *PCF* is on cancer pain. Because the use of strong opioids for chronic *non-cancer* pain is generally associated with lower benefits and higher risks, specialist advice should be followed and/or sought from chronic pain teams.

PCF also includes a number of *Quick Clinical Guides* (listed inside the back cover and in the topic index). To enhance user-friendliness, each *Quick Clinical Guide* is generally limited to no more than two pages, and references are not included. We welcome the donation of clinical guidance from other sources for posting on our website (e-mail copies to hq@palliativedrugs.com).

The original inspiration for *PCF* came from a local formulary written by Dr Robert Twycross in Oxford over 30 years ago. He and Dr Andrew Wilcock became the founding editors-in-chief of *PCF* and worked together on six UK print editions, several country-specific editions, translations, spin-off publications and the website www.palliativedrugs.com. Sarah Charlesworth and Dr Paul Howard have been key contributors since the second and third editions, respectively. *PCF* was acquired by Pharmaceutical Press in August 2018 and the on-line *PCF* moved to the MedicinesComplete digital platform in January 2019. Dr Twycross remains an Honorary Editorial Consultant in recognition of his immeasurable contribution to the *PCF* and inspirational devotion to the specialty of palliative medicine.

The production of a book of this nature depends on the help and advice of numerous colleagues, both past and present. We acknowledge with gratitude the support of clinical colleagues, and of members of the palliativedrugs.com community who have provided feedback, particularly via surveys, by contributing to the *Syringe Driver Survey Database*, or by postings on the Bulletin Board.

Andrew Wilcock
Paul Howard
Editors-in-chief
August 2022

HOW PCF IS CONSTRUCTED

There is continual review and updating of the contents of *PCF*. Updates are published monthly on-line on MedicinesComplete; please refer here for the most up-to-date content.

The *Palliative Care Formulary* (*PCF*) is a unique independent professional publication which provides essential information for prescribers and health professionals involved in palliative and hospice care. *PCF* contains authoritative independent guidance on best practice and helps to ensure that drugs are used appropriately, safely and optimally.

Recommended International Non-proprietary Names (rINN) are used for drugs. The chapter order in Part 1 broadly follows that of the print edition of the *British National Formulary* (*BNF*).

Editorial board

The *PCF* editorial board is co-ordinated by Pharmaceutical Press. The board includes two medically qualified editors-in-chief who are accredited specialists in palliative medicine. The rest of the board comprises other members working in palliative medicine, and staff from Pharmaceutical Press, including a specialist palliative care pharmacist. The board meets regularly to discuss editorial policy, governance, ways of working, publishing schedules, content updates and new content. Contributors and expert advisors are identified to assist in the preparation of new content or the review and updating of current content.

Contributors

Contributors comprise palliative care health professionals appointed on the basis of their clinical knowledge and expertise. They have committed to reviewing one or more drug monographs or chapters, and work in liaison with the editorial board. Responsibilities include scrutinizing literature databases such as PubMed and accessing and studying relevant new publications in order to provide appropriate and accurate content.

Advisors

Advisors are drawn from a range of medical specialties, and include doctors, pharmacists, nurses and other health professionals. These advisors review the text by:

- checking amendments for scientific accuracy and to enhance clarity
- providing additional expert opinion in areas of controversy or when reliable evidence is lacking
- advising on areas where the *PCF* diverges from a manufacturer's summary of product characteristics (SPC)
- providing additional validation and clinical evidence about unauthorized (off-label) use.

Sources of *PCF* information

PCF uses various sources for its information, including:

Summary of product characteristics (SPC)

The SPCs are the principal source of product information. Manufacturers are contacted directly when further information is required.

Literature

Research papers and reviews relating to the drugs featured in *PCF* are carefully processed. When a difference between the advice in the *PCF* and a paper is noted, the new information is evaluated for reliability and relevance to UK clinical practice. If necessary, new text is drafted and thoroughly reviewed by the editors with support, as needed, from the editorial board and/or advisors.

PCF also accesses many on-line information resources (see p.xvii). For example, www.crediblemeds.org is used to flag drugs that have the potential to prolong QT interval to a clinically relevant degree.

Systematic reviews

PCF monitors various databases of systematic reviews, including the *Cochrane Library* and several other web-based resources.

Consensus guidelines

The advice in *PCF* is checked against consensus guidelines produced by expert bodies including the National Institute for Health and Care Excellence (NICE), the Scottish Medicines Consortium (SMC), and the Scottish Intercollegiate Guidelines Network (SIGN).

PCF also takes note of other expert bodies which produce clinical guidelines relevant to palliative care, e.g. Association for Palliative Medicine, British Lymphology Society.

Statutory information

PCF routinely processes relevant information from various government bodies, including statutory instruments and regulations affecting the Prescription Only Medicines order, controlled drugs and from the Medicines and Healthcare products Regulatory Agency (MHRA). Safety warnings issued by the Commission on Human Medicines (CHM) and guidelines on drug use issued by the UK health departments are routinely processed.

Relevant professional statements issued by the Royal Pharmaceutical Society (RPS), Nursing and Midwifery Council (NMC) and General Medical Council (GMC) are included in *PCF* as are guidelines from the medical Royal Colleges.

Pricing information

Drug prices are obtained from the on-line edition of the *BNF*. When available, the NHS indicative price is used. For non-proprietary (generic) products, the lowest NHS indicative price is used; if that is unavailable, the price listed in the Drug Tariff is used. Note. Prices for broken bulk, dispensing/sourcing fees and delivery charges are *not* included.

For special order or imported products, prices are obtained from Part VIIIB of the Drug Tariff (if listed); for products not listed in that section, the price can vary significantly and *PCF* may be unable to provide a useful price.

For information on how prices are used, see p.xvii.

Updated (minor change) March 2022

GETTING THE MOST OUT OF PCF

Information in a book of this type can never be all-inclusive, and thus will not cover every eventuality. Readers should satisfy themselves as to the appropriateness of the information before applying it in practice.

Particularly when prescribing a drug for the first time, a doctor (or other independent prescriber) should study the contents of the manufacturer's summary of product characteristics (SPC), paying particular attention to indications, contra-indications, cautions, drug interactions and undesirable effects (also see the respective sections below and on p.xvi).

PCF often refers to the use of medicinal products beyond the scope of their marketing authorization, e.g. in relation to indication, dose or route of administration. Such use has implications for the prescriber (see p.xix).

A cautious approach is always necessary when prescribing for children, the frail and the elderly, and for those with renal impairment, hepatic impairment or respiratory insufficiency (see the relevant chapters in Part 2). Further, if caring for a woman who is pregnant or breast-feeding, or for someone with porphyria, it is crucial to check a drug's suitability in the *BNF*, the SPC and other specialist resources.

The literature on the pharmacology of pain and symptom management in end-stage disease is growing continually, and it is impossible for anyone to be familiar with all of it. This is where a book like *PCF* comes into its own as a major accessible resource for prescribing clinicians involved in palliative care.

PCF is not an easy read; indeed, it was never intended that it would be read from cover to cover. It is essentially a reference book in which to study the monograph of an individual drug, or class of drugs, with specific questions in mind.

Part 1 comprises 139 drug monographs, some covering a class of drugs (e.g. antimuscarinics, bronchodilators, strong opioids) and others restricted to an individual drug (e.g. morphine, fentanyl, ketamine). Drugs marked with an asterisk (*) should generally be used only by, or after consultation with, a specialist palliative care service. A selection of Quick Clinical Guides cover key topics (see the inside back cover for index). These are purposefully brief to facilitate everyday use. Before use, it is important to study the associated text in order to fully understand their rationale.

Parts 2 and 3 and the appendices deal with themes which transcend the drug monographs, e.g. general advice about prescribing in palliative care, anticipatory prescribing in the community, administering drugs to patients with swallowing difficulties or enteral feeding tubes, the use of nebulized drugs, and continuous subcutaneous infusions.

Indications

In *PCF*, generally only those indications relevant to palliative care are listed. The use of medicinal products for indications beyond their marketing authorization (MA), i.e. off-label, has implications for the prescriber (see p.xx), and *PCF* attempts to highlight such use, applying the following convention:

- the symbol † highlights off-label use when no UK medicinal product containing that drug has an MA for that indication
- the statement 'Authorized indications vary between products; consult SPC for details' is used when variation exists between drugs within a particular class, e.g. bisphosphonates.

However, it is impractical for *PCF* to highlight all cases of off-label use, because an MA applies to a specific medicinal product (not the drug *per se*) and is based on what the manufacturer applied for. Thus, there can be variations in the individual SPCs of different medicinal products containing the same drug, i.e. variations in the indications can occur between different:

- manufacturers
- routes of administration
- formulations
- pack sizes.

Pharmacology

The information in the Pharmacology sections is derived from many sources (see How *PCF* is constructed, p.xii).

Reliable knowledge, levels of evidence and strength of recommendations

Research is the pursuit of reliable knowledge. The gold standard for drug treatment is the randomized controlled trial (RCT) or, better, a systematic review of homogeneous RCTs.

Over the last 20–30 years, numerous systems have been published for categorizing levels of evidence and the strength of the derived recommendations. Box A reproduces the system used by the *British Medical Journal*. This checklist is based on material published by three main sources, namely the US Agency for Health Care Policy and Research, the NHS Management Executive, and the North of England Guidelines Group.[1-3]

Box A A scheme for categorizing evidence and grading recommendations[4]

Category	*Level of evidence*	*Grade*	*Strength of recommendations*
Ia	Evidence obtained from a meta-analysis of RCTs	A	Directly based on Category I evidence without extrapolation
Ib	Evidence from at least one RCT		
IIa	Evidence obtained from at least one well-designed controlled study without randomization	B	Directly based on Category II evidence or by extrapolation from Category I evidence
IIb	Evidence obtained from at least one other well-designed quasi-experimental study		
III	Evidence obtained from well-designed non-experimental descriptive studies, such as comparative studies, correlation studies and case studies	C	Directly based on Category III evidence or by extrapolation from Category I or II evidence
IV	Evidence obtained from expert committee reports or opinions and/or clinical experiences of respected authorities	D	Directly based on category IV evidence or by extrapolation from Category I, II, or III evidence This grading indicates that directly applicable clinical studies of good quality are absent or not readily available

However, it is important to recognize that an RCT is *not* the only source of reliable knowledge. Broadly speaking, sources of knowledge can be conveniently grouped under three headings:

- *instrumental;* includes RCT data and data from other high-quality studies
- *interactive;* refers to anecdotal data (shared clinical experience), including retrospective and prospective surveys
- *critical;* data unique to the individual in question (e.g. personal choice) and societal/cultural factors (e.g. financial and logistic considerations).[5]

Relying on one type of knowledge alone is *not* good practice. All three sources must be exploited in the process of therapeutic decision-making. This is reflected in the Pharmacology sections.

Pharmaceutical company information

Although the manufacturer's SPC is an important source of information about a drug, it is important to remember that many published studies are sponsored by the drug company in question. This can lead to a conflict of interest between the desire for objective data and the need to make one's own drug as attractive as possible.[6] It is thus best to treat information from company representatives as inevitably biased. The information provided by *PCF* is commercially independent and should serve as a counterbalance to manufacturer bias.

Remember: it is often safer to stick with an 'old favourite' and not seek to be among the first to prescribe a newly released product which may simply be a 'me-too' drug rather than true innovation.[6]

Pharmacokinetics

Generally, pharmacokinetic data are taken from *Martindale: The Complete Drug Reference*[7] or from a manufacturer's SPC. Other sources are referenced in the text.

Contra-indications and cautions

> Contra-indications and cautions listed in SPCs sometimes vary between different manufacturers of products containing the same drug. Thus, a contra-indication in one SPC may be styled a caution in another, and vice versa. *PCF* attempts to collate and standardize contra-indications and cautions between products for individual monographs and across a class of drugs for class monographs.

PCF does *not* include universal contra-indications (e.g. history of hypersensitivity to the drug) and generally does *not* include a contra-indication from the SPC if the use of the drug in the stated circumstance is accepted prescribing practice in palliative care, e.g. use of oral morphine as an analgesic in a patient with obstructive airway disease.

As always, a cautious approach is necessary when prescribing for children, the frail, the elderly, and patients with organ impairment or respiratory insufficiency (see the relevant chapters in Part 2). If caring for a woman who is pregnant or breast-feeding, or for someone with porphyria, it is crucial to check a drug's suitability in both the *BNF* and SPC, or with a specialist medical information pharmacist.

The effect of sedative drugs on driving ability is covered in Chapter 22, p.809.

Drug interactions

Generally, information on drug interactions is taken from *Stockley's Drug Interactions*[8] or from a manufacturer's SPC. Other sources are referenced in the text.

It is assumed that clinicians are aware of the risk of common-sense pharmacodynamic interactions, e.g. that the concurrent prescription of two or more drugs with sedative properties is likely to result in more sedation than if each drug were prescribed alone. Likewise, two drugs with antimuscarinic properties prescribed concurrently will have an additive antimuscarinic effect. However, where specific MHRA warnings have been issued, these have been included.

On the other hand, clinically important pharmacokinetic interactions (leading to either increased or reduced effect) most likely to be encountered in palliative care are covered in individual drug monographs and in Chapter 19, p.781. However, it is not an exhaustive list and excludes anticancer, antiviral, HIV and immunosuppressive drugs (seek specialist advice).

Undesirable effects of drugs

As recommended by the European Commission, the term 'undesirable effect' is used rather than 'side effect' or 'adverse drug reaction'. Wherever possible, undesirable effects are categorized as:

- very common (>10%)
- common (<10%, >1%)
- uncommon (<1%, >0.1%)
- rare (<0.1%, >0.01%)
- very rare (<0.01%).

PCF generally includes information on the very common and common undesirable effects. Selected other undesirable effects are also included, e.g. uncommon or rare ones which may have serious consequences. The manufacturer's SPC should be consulted for a full list of undesirable effects.

Dose and use

PCF often highlights doses, routes or use in patient populations not covered by the MA of the authorized medicinal products available (off-label use) with the symbol †. However, as with indications (see p.xiv), it is impractical for *PCF* to highlight all cases of off-label use, and health professionals must be familiar with the specific SPC of the product they are using and implications for off-label use.

Further, unauthorized medicinal products may feature in this section, e.g. the use of special order or imported products, or the mixing of medicinal products together for administration via CSCI (see p.xix).

Generic and brand prescribing

Generally, *PCF* encourages generic prescribing on the basis of pharmaco-economics.[9] In most instances, branded and generic versions of the same drug will not differ significantly in terms of bio-availability and efficacy. However, there are some important exceptions (see below).[10] Further, in some circumstances, continuity of the same brand is important for patient safety, by reducing the risk of confusion and thereby a dispensing or administration error.[9,11,12] Thus, *PCF* recommends brand prescribing when:

- bio-availability differs significantly between brands, particularly for drugs with a narrow therapeutic index, e.g. some anti-epileptics, m/r formulations of diltiazem, LMWH, nifedipine, theophylline
- the product range is complex and there is a high risk of error which could be fatal, e.g. m/r opioid analgesics, TD opioid patches[11,12]
- formulation differs significantly between brands, resulting in them not being interchangeable, e.g. some inhaled corticosteroids, transmucosal fentanyl products
- products contain multiple ingredients, and brand name prescribing aids identification, e.g. antacids, compound alginates, macrogols, pancreatin supplements, topical skin products
- administration devices have different instructions for use and patient familiarity with one product is important, e.g. dry powder inhalers or self-injection devices.

Supply

Generally, the list of products indicates the range of formulations and strengths available, but is *not* an exhaustive list. Whenever possible, generic products are included; selected brands feature when either a generic product is unavailable or brand prescribing is important (see above).

Generally, costs reflect a 28 day supply, based on the most convenient strength and cheapest pack size. For short-course treatments, p.r.n. or parenteral formulations, costs may be listed either as per course, per dose or per ampoule/vial, as appropriate.

Costs are for indicative purposes only, to give a general comparison between available therapeutic options. Generally, costs:

- less than £5 have been rounded to the nearest 25p
- between £5–£10 have been rounded to the nearest 50p
- more than £10 have been rounded to the nearest full pound.

In some cases, e.g. TM fentanyl, to aid closer comparison, exact prices for individual dose units are used.

PCF recognizes that pharmaco-economics is a complicated area, that is constantly changing in response to various factors, including market demands, hospital and local contracts, and marketing tactics. Costs can also be vastly different in the community compared with in hospital, particularly regarding special order products not covered by Part VIIIB of the Drug Tariff. Thus, local circumstances need to be taken into account when cost is a particular consideration.

Reference Sources

Literature references

In choosing references, articles in hospice and palliative care journals have frequently been selected preferentially. Such journals are likely to be more readily available to our readers, and often contain detailed discussion.

It is not feasible to reference every statement in *PCF*. However, readers are invited to enter into constructive dialogue with the editors via the Bulletin Board at www.palliativedrugs.com. This is currently accessed by >30,000 health professionals in >160 countries.

On-line sources of information

Website references are not routinely given for articles available in traditionally published journals.

References to SPCs and PILs are generally *not* included. However, most can be freely accessed at www.medicines.org.uk or obtained directly from the manufacturer.

On-line sources of information are referenced when this is the usual route of publication and access is freely available, e.g. UK Department of Health guidelines, MHRA Drug Safety Updates, NICE guidance, SIGN guidance. The website address quoted is for the homepage or the page from which the guidance can be found and downloaded.

Information from the *BNF* and *BNF for Children* is available in multiple formats, including via an app and websites (via MedicinesComplete, NICE).

Whenever possible, subscription websites have been avoided. However, to ensure that the most current information is included when revising *PCF*, the following standard reference texts are consulted from subscribed access to Medicines Complete (www.medicinescomplete.com):

- *American Hospital Formulary Service (AHFS)*
- *Handbook of Drug Administration via Enteral Feeding Tubes*
- *Handbook on Injectable Drugs*
- *Martindale: The Complete Drug Reference*
- *Stockley's Drug Interactions.*

1 Eccles M et *al.* (1996) North of England evidence based guidelines development project: methods of guideline development. *British Medical Journal.* **312**: 760–762.
2 Department of Health (1996) *Clinical Guidelines: Using Clinical Guidelines to Improve Patient Care Within the NHS.* Department of Health: NHS Executive, Leeds.
3 Agency for Health Care Policy and Research (1992) Acute pain management, operative or medical procedures and trauma 92-0032. In: *Clinical Practice Guideline Quick Ref Guide for Clinicians.* AHCPR Publications, Rockville, Maryland, USA, pp. 1–22.
4 BMJ Publishing Group (2009) Resources for authors. Checklists and forms: clinical management guidelines. http://www.bmj.com/about-bmj/resources-authors
5 Aoun SM and Kristjanson LJ (2005) Challenging the framework for evidence in palliative care research. *Palliative Medicine.* **19**: 461–465.
6 Angell M (2004) *The Truth About the Drug Companies: how they deceive us and what to do about it.* Random House, New York.
7 Buckingham R (ed) *Martindale: The Complete Drug Reference.* London: Pharmaceutical Press www.medicinescomplete.com
8 Preston CL (ed) *Stockley's Drug Interactions.* London: Pharmaceutical Press www.medicinescomplete.com
9 UK Medicines Information (2017) Which medicines should be considered for brand-name prescribing in primary care? *Medicines Q&A.* www.evidence.nhs.uk
10 National Prescribing Centre (2000) Modified-release preparations. *MeReC Bulletin.* **11**: 13–16.
11 Smith J (2004) Building a Safer NHS for Patients - Improving Medication Safety. pp.105–111. Department of Health, London. Available from: www.dh.gov.uk (archived)
12 Care Quality Commission and NHS England (2013) Safer use of controlled drugs - preventing harms from fentanyl and buprenorphine transdermal patches. *Use of controlled drugs supporting information.* www.cqc.org.uk.

Updated (minor change) March 2022

THE USE OF MEDICINAL PRODUCTS BEYOND (OFF-LABEL) AND WITHOUT (UNAUTHORIZED) MARKETING AUTHORIZATION

The use of medicinal products off-label is widespread. Surveys suggest that up to one third of all prescriptions in palliative care come into this category.[1] *PCF* attempts to highlight such use, applying the following convention:

- the symbol † highlights off-label use when no UK medicinal product containing that drug has a marketing authorization (MA) for that indication
- the statement 'Authorized indications vary between products; consult SPC for details' is used when such variation exists between drugs within a particular class, e.g. bisphosphonates.

However, it is impractical for *PCF* to highlight all cases of off-label use, e.g. where the indication varies between different brands or formulations of the same drug, or where the medicinal product is being used in a dose, route or patient population not covered by the MA.

It is important for prescribers to understand that the MA regulates the specific medicinal product (not the drug *per se*) and the *marketing activities* of pharmaceutical companies, and not the prescriber's clinical practice. Even so, off-label use does have implications for health professionals, and these are discussed in this section.

Definitions

Marketing authorization (licence)

A marketing authorization (MA), previously called a product licence, is granted by a regulatory body to a pharmaceutical company for a specific medicinal product. It specifies the terms of use, including the indications, doses, routes and patient populations for which it can be marketed. *PCF* uses the term 'authorized' in preference to 'licensed'.

Off-label use

Although there is no official definition, generally 'off-label' describes the use of a medicinal product *beyond the specifications of its MA*, e.g. for an indication or in a dose, route or patient population not covered by the MA.

Unauthorized (unlicensed) medicinal product

PCF uses the term 'unauthorized' in preference to 'unlicensed'. There is no simple definition of an unauthorized medicinal product. Essentially, an unauthorized medicinal product is a product that does not have an MA for medicinal use in humans. Unauthorized medicinal products include:

- authorized medicinal products that have been manipulated, thus rendering them unauthorized, e.g. two or more medicinal products mixed together for administration in a syringe for CSCI (see Box A below and p.887)
- 'specials', e.g. special-order manufactured formulations made in the UK by a manufacturer with a specials manufacturing licence (MS) and medicinal products that require importation; for full details, see p.817
- medicinal products made in a local pharmacy (extemporaneously prepared) at the request of a prescriber for an individual patient, e.g. dilution of a cream
- new medicinal products undergoing clinical trials or awaiting an MA, e.g. if a patient wishes to continue an investigational product after a clinical trial.

The authorization (licensing) process

The UK left the European Union (EU) in January 2021. As a consequence:[2,3]

- in Great Britain (England, Wales and Scotland):
  - ▷ MA issued before this date remain valid but are now referred to as converted EU MA
  - ▷ for an initial two-year period, the MHRA will accept new applications already approved by the European Commission (EC) centralized process (see below). The manufacturer submits to the MHRA the same information as presented to the EC, along with other key documents and pays the required fee
- in Northern Ireland, which remains aligned to EU MA regulations and legislation, there are no changes.

Before a medicinal product can be marketed in the UK, it requires an MA (previously 'product licence'). There are four application procedures in the EU:

- *centralized* – application evaluated by the European Medicines Agency (EMA); the EC grants a single MA valid for the whole EU (also see above)
- *decentralized* – simultaneous application made by several member states, with one taking the lead; if successful, a national MA is then granted in each state
- *mutual recognition* – application for authorization in a member state when an MA exists in another member state; the new member state relies on the original member state's evaluation as a basis for its decision
- *national* – application for an MA in only one member state; in the UK, the application is evaluated by the Medicines and Healthcare products Regulatory Agency (MHRA) on behalf of the licensing authority, a body consisting of UK health ministers.[4]

Certain products, e.g. for HIV/AIDS, cancer and neurodegenerative diseases, must be authorized through the centralized procedure (EU) or internationally via the MHRA through Project Orbis (Great Britain).[5] The UK parallel import licensing scheme also allows a product authorized in other EU states to be imported and marketed in the UK if it has labels and a patient information leaflet (PIL) in English.[6]

In the UK, the MHRA evaluation comprises an evaluation of the efficacy, safety and quality of the product from a medical, pharmaceutical and scientific viewpoint to ensure that it satisfies predefined criteria. Advice is sought from the Commission on Human Medicines (CHM), an independent advisory body, which in turn is assisted by specialist expert advisory groups.

At a European level, the Committee for Medicinal Products for Human Use (CHMP) fulfils a similar role to the CHM. New products will have relatively limited safety information, and the pharmaceutical company is generally required to outline a risk management plan.

Restrictions are imposed if evidence of safety and efficacy is unavailable in specific patient groups, e.g. children. An MA is granted for up to 5 years and then renewed following re-evaluation of the risks and benefits.[4]

Thus, the process ensures that in relation to the product's authorized uses, there has been due consideration of its efficacy, safety and quality, that the benefits outweigh the potential risks, and that there is appropriate accompanying product information and labelling.[7] The MA defines the conditions and patient groups for which a pharmaceutical company can market and supply the product, with more information about the authorized uses provided by the manufacturer in the summary of product characteristics (SPC).

However, the MA regulates the marketing activities of the pharmaceutical industry, not the activities of the prescriber, and clinical experience may reveal other indications (i.e. off-label use). For these to be added to the existing MA, additional evidence would need to be gathered and submitted. The considerable expense of this, perhaps coupled with a small market for a new indication, dose or route, often means that a revised application is not made.

Prescribing for off-label use or unauthorized medicinal products

In the UK, the following may legally prescribe for off-label use or unauthorized medicinal products:[8]

- doctors and dentists (specifically safeguarded in the UK Medicines Act 1968)
- nurses, midwives or pharmacists who are registered as *independent prescribers*, if this is accepted clinical practice and within their clinical competence; chiropodist, optometrist, paramedic, physiotherapist, podiatrist and radiographer *independent prescribers* may only prescribe for off-label use (for conditions within their clinical competence)
- chiropodists, dieticians, nurses, optometrists, paramedics, pharmacists, podiatrists, physiotherapists, midwives and radiographers who are registered as *supplementary prescribers*, provided the prescribing is done within the framework of an agreed clinical management plan for a specific patient in partnership with a doctor or dentist.

These prescriptions can be dispensed by pharmacists;[9] local organizational policies should cover the administration of off-label or unauthorized medicinal products.[10]

The responsibility for the consequences of prescribing under such circumstances lies with the prescriber, who must be competent and must operate within the professional codes and ethics of their statutory bodies and the prescribing practices of their employers.[7,9,11–13] The prescriber must be fully informed about the actions and uses of the medicinal product, be assured of the quality of the particular product, and in the light of published evidence, balance both the potential good and the potential harm which might ensue.[13]

In addition to clinical trials, such prescriptions may be justified:

- when prescribing generic formulations for which indications are not described
- with established medicinal products for proven but unauthorized indications
- for conditions for which there are no other treatments (even in the absence of strong evidence)
- when using medicinal products in individuals not covered by the MA, e.g. children
- when mixing medicinal products before administration, e.g. two or more injections in a syringe for administration by CSCI (Box A).[14,15]

For information relating to the prescription and supply of a special, see p.817.

Box A Legislation surrounding the mixing of medicinal products[14]

Any *independent prescribers*, including non-medical prescribers, can mix medicinal products (including those that contain controlled drugs) and direct others to mix, as can *supplementary prescribers* when the preparation is part of the clinical management plan for an individual patient.

Existing good practice recommendations should be followed in relation to mixing all medicinal products.

Preparations resulting from mixing, other than when one product is a vehicle for the administration of the other, cannot be supplied or administered under patient group direction arrangements.

It is possible to draw a hierarchy of degrees of reasonableness relating to off-label and unauthorized use (Figure 1).[16] The more dangerous the medicinal product and the more flimsy the evidence, the more difficult it is to justify its prescription.

The General Medical Council (GMC) recommends that when prescribing off-label or prescribing an unauthorized medicinal product, doctors should:

- be satisfied that such use would better serve the patient's needs than an authorized alternative (if one exists)
- be satisfied that there is sufficient evidence/experience of using the medicinal product to show its safety and efficacy, seeking the necessary information from appropriate sources
- record in the patient's clinical notes the medicinal product prescribed and, when not following common practice, the reasons for the choice
- take responsibility for prescribing the medicinal product and for overseeing the patient's care, including monitoring the clinical effects, or arrange for another suitable doctor to do so.[11]

Prescribers should ensure they are familiar with the joint competency framework for *all* prescribers, produced by the Royal Pharmaceutical Society, which broadly reflects the advice of the GMC.[12]

Providing patient information

Prescribers (or those authorizing treatment on their behalf) should provide sufficient information to patients about the expected benefits and potential risks (undesirable effects, drug interactions, etc.) to enable them to make an informed decision (Box B). The PIL supplied by the manufacturer will not contain information about off-label use and may confuse patients.

In palliative care, off-label use is so widespread that concerns have been expressed that a detailed explanation on every occasion is impractical, would be burdensome for the patient and increase anxiety, and could result in the refusal of beneficial treatment.[17] A UK survey of over 220 palliative medicine doctors showed that, when using a drug for a routine off-label indication, <5% *always* mention this to their patients, and 20% *never* do. However, in situations where there is little evidence and limited clinical experience to support a drug's off-label use, these figures change to 75% and 5% respectively.[18]

This is a grey area and each clinician must decide how explicit to be; an appropriate level of counselling and a sensitive approach is essential. Some NHS trusts and other institutions have policies in place and have produced information cards or leaflets for patients and caregivers (Box C).

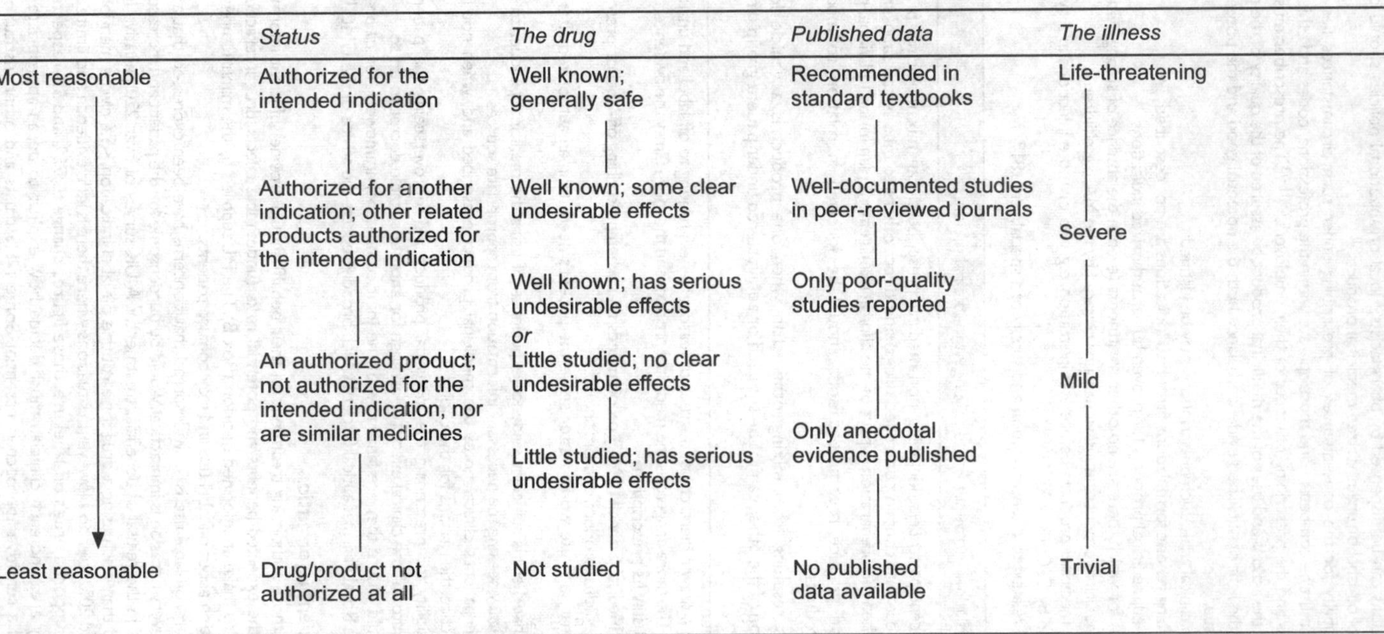

Status
The drug
Published data
The illness
Most reasonable
Least reasonable
Authorized for the intended indication
Authorized for another indication; other related products authorized for the intended indication
An authorized product; not authorized for the intended indication, nor are similar medicines
Drug/product not authorized at all
Well known; generally safe
Well known; some clear undesirable effects
Well known; has serious undesirable effects
or
Little studied; no clear undesirable effects
Little studied; has serious undesirable effects
Not studied
Recommended in standard textbooks
Well-documented studies in peer-reviewed journals
Only poor-quality studies reported
Only anecdotal evidence published
No published data available
Life-threatening
Severe
Mild
Trivial

Figure 1 Factors influencing the reasonableness of prescribing decisions.

Box B Providing information for patients about off-label use and medicinal products without a Marketing authorization[11]

Patients (or their proxies) should be given sufficient information about any proposed treatment to allow them to make an informed decision. Questions must be answered fully and honestly.

Some medicinal products are routinely used beyond their MA, e.g. when treating children and in palliative care.

In emergencies, or when there is no realistic alternative treatment and such information is likely to cause distress, it may not be practical or necessary to draw attention to the MA.

In other situations, when the prescription of an unauthorized medicinal product is supported by authoritative clinical guidance, it may be sufficient to describe in general terms why it is not authorized for the proposed use.

When prescribing a medicinal product which is unauthorized or off-label in a non-routine way, or when suitable authorized alternatives exist, the reason for this should be explained to the patient.

Box C Example of a patient information leaflet about off-label use

Use of medicines beyond their licence (off-label)

This leaflet contains important information about your medicines, so please read it carefully.

Generally, medicines prescribed by your doctor or bought over the counter from a pharmacist are licensed for use by the Medicines and Healthcare products Regulatory Agency (MHRA).

The licence (or marketing authorization) specifies the conditions and patient groups for which the medicine should be used, and how it should be given.

Patient information leaflets (PILs) supplied with medicines reflect the licensed uses. When a medicine is used beyond its licence, the information in the PIL may not be relevant to your circumstances.

In palliative care, medicines are commonly used for conditions or in ways that are not specified on the licence.

Your doctor will use medicines beyond the licence only when there is research and experience to back up such use.

Medicines used very successfully beyond the licence include some antidepressants and anti-epileptics (anti-seizure drugs) when given to relieve some types of pain. Also, instead of injecting into a vein or muscle, medicines are often given subcutaneously (under the skin), because this is more comfortable and convenient.

If you would like more information, please ask your doctor or pharmacist.

Alternatively, contact:

Dr/nurse ....

Hospital ....

....

....

Tel ....

A joint position statement has also been produced by the British Pain Society and the Association for Palliative Medicine (Box D),[19] together with a patient information booklet.[20]

Box D Recommendations of the British Pain Society and Association for Palliative Medicine of Great Britain and Ireland[19]

Use of medicines beyond (off-label) and without (unlicensed) Marketing Authorization (MA) in palliative care and pain medicine

1 This statement should be seen as reflecting the views of a responsible body of opinion within the clinical specialties of palliative medicine and pain medicine.

2 The use of medicines beyond and without an MA in palliative care and pain medicine practice is both necessary and common and should be seen as a legitimate aspect of clinical practice.

3 Organizations providing palliative care and pain medicine services should support therapeutic practices that are underpinned by evidence and advocated by a responsible body of professional opinion.

4 Health professionals involved in prescribing medicines beyond or without MA should select those medicines that offer the best balance of benefit against harm for any given patient.

5 Choice of treatment requires partnership between patients and health professionals, and informed consent should be obtained, whenever possible, before prescribing any medicine.

6 Patients should be offered accurate, clear and specific information that meets their needs about the use of medicines beyond or without an MA in accordance with professional regulatory body guidance. The information needs of carers and other health professionals involved in the care of the patient should also be considered and met as appropriate. The use of information cards or leaflets may help with this. It is often unnecessary to take additional steps when recommending medicines beyond or without MA.

7 Health professionals should inform, change and monitor their practice with regard to medicines beyond or without MA in the light of evidence from audit and published research.

8 The Department of Health should work with health professionals and the pharmaceutical industry to enable and encourage the extension of product licences where there is evidence of benefit in circumstances of defined clinical need.

1 Hagemann V *et al.* (2019) Drug use beyond the licence in palliative care: a systematic review and narrative synthesis. *Palliative Medicine.* **33**: 650–662.
2 MHRA (2021) European Commission (EC) Decision reliance procedure. www.gov.uk (accessed February 2022).
3 MHRA (2021) Great Britain Marketing Authorisations (MAs) for Centrally Authorised Products (CAPs) www.gov.uk (accessed February 2022).
4 Anonymous (2009) The licensing of medicines in the UK. *Drug and Therapeutics Bulletin.* **47**: 45–48.
5 MHRA (2020) Project Orbis. www.gov.uk (accessed February 2022).
6 MHRA (2015) Medicines: apply for a parallel import licence www.gov.uk (accessed February 2022)..
7 MHRA (2009) Off-label or unlicensed medicines: prescribers' responsibilities. *Drug Safety Update*. www.gov.uk.
8 Royal Pharmaceutical Society (2021) The professional guide for pharmacists. *Medicines, Ethics and Practice* (44e). www.rpharms.com.
9 Royal Pharmaceutical Society (2015) Professional guidance for the procurement and supply of specials. www.rpharms.com.
10 Royal Pharmaceutical Society and Royal College of Nursing (2019) Professional Guidance on the Administration of Medicines in Healthcare Settings. www.rpharms.com.
11 General Medical Council (2021) Good practice in prescribing and managing medicines and devices. www.gmc-uk.org.
12 Royal Pharmaceutical Society (2021) A competency framework for all prescribers. www.rpharms.com.
13 Royal Pharmaceutical Society (2016) Prescribing specials. Guidance for the prescribers of specials. www.rpharms.com.
14 Department of Health (2010) Mixing of medicines prior to administration in clinical practice: medical and non-medical prescribing. HMSO, London. www.gov.uk
15 Home Office (2012) Nurse and pharmacist independent prescribing, 'mixing of medicines', possession authorities under patient group directions and personal exemption provisions for schedule 4 Part II drugs. Circular 009/2012. www.gov.uk.
16 MHRA (2014) The supply of unlicensed medicinal products ("specials"). MHRA Guidance Note 14. Available from: www.gov.uk.
17 Pavis H and Wilcock A (2001) Prescribing of drugs for use outside their licence in palliative care: survey of specialists in the United Kingdom. *British Medical Journal.* **323**: 484–485.
18 Culshaw J *et al.* (2013) Off-label prescribing in palliative care: a survey of independent prescribers. *Palliative Medicine.* **27**: 314–319.
19 British Pain Society (2012) Use of medicines outside of their UK Marketing Authorisation in pain management and palliative care. www.britishpainsociety.org.
20 British Pain Society (2012) Use of medicines outside of their UK Marketing Authorisation in pain management and palliative medicine – information for patients. www.britishpainsociety.org.

Updated (minor change) February 2022

DRUG NAMES

All pharmaceuticals (i.e. drugs and biological therapies) marketed in Europe and the UK are known by their unique WHO International Nonproprietary (generic) Names (r**INN**) for active pharmaceutical substances.[1] Prior to the switch to rINN in 2003, most publications in the UK used the British Approved Name (**BAN**).

In the USA, United States Adopted Names (**USAN**s) are assigned to active drug ingredients and are used in place of rINNs. For most active ingredients the rINN, BAN, and USAN names are the same and this helps safe prescribing and dispensing of pharmaceuticals, as well as clear communication and exchange of information among health professionals around the world.

To aid understanding of the older literature and literature from the USA, Table 1 lists some examples where the names have differed or may still differ significantly from each other. Minor differences, e.g. 'f' instead of 'ph', 'e' instead of 'oe', 't' instead of 'th', have *not* been included.

In the UK, the BANs **adrenaline** and **noradrenaline** are still used in conjunction with the corresponding rINNs, i.e. **adrenaline (epinephrine)** and **noradrenaline (norepinephrine)**.

Care should be taken with proprietary drug (brand) names in different countries. Some proprietary names are identical or similar in spelling or pronunciation but contain different drugs, e.g. Urex® in the USA contains **methenamine**, but, in Australia, **furosemide**.[2]

The naming of combination products in different countries may also vary, e.g. in the UK the prefix co- is traditionally used for some combination products e.g. co-codamol, co-dydramol, and co-codaprin for codeine with paracetamol, dihydrocodeine with paracetamol, and codeine with aspirin, respectively.

Table 1 Drug names relevant to palliative care for which the rINN, the historical BAN and/or current USAN differ

rINN	*BAN*[a]	*USAN*
Alimemazine	Trimeprazine	Trimeprazine
Amobarbital	Amylobarbitone	
Bendroflumethiazide	Bendrofluazide	Bendroflumethiazide
Benzylpenicillin		Penicillin G
Calcitonin (salmon)	Salcatonin	Calcitonin
Carmellose		Carboxymethylcellulose
Chlorphenamine	Chlorpheniramine	Chlorpheniramine
Clomethiazole	Chlormethiazole	
Dexamfetamine	Dexamphetamine	Dextroamphetamine
Dextropropoxyphene		Propoxyphene
Dicycloverine	Dicyclomine	Dicyclomine
Diethylstilbestrol	Stilboestrol	Diethylstilbestrol
Dosulepin	Dothiepin	Dothiepin
Epinephrine	Adrenaline[b]	Epinephrine
Glibenclamide		Glyburide
Glycerol	Glycerine	Glycerin
Glyceryl trinitrate		Nitroglycerin
Hyoscine		Scopolamine
Isoprenaline		Isoproterenol
	Ispaghula	Psyllium
Levomepromazine	Methotrimeprazine	

continued

Table 1 Continued

rINN	*BAN*[a]	*USAN*
Levothyroxine	Thyroxine	
Liquid paraffin		Mineral oil
Macrogols	Macrogols	Polyethylene glycols
Methenamine hippurate	Hexamine hippurate	
Norepinephrine	Noradrenaline[b]	Norepinephrine
Paracetamol		Acetaminophen
Pethidine		Meperidine
Phenobarbital	Phenobarbitone	
Phenoxymethylpenicillin		Penicillin V
Phytomenadione		Phytonadione
Retinol	Vitamin A	Vitamin A
Rifampicin		Rifampin
Salbutamol		Albuterol
Simeticone	Simethicone	Simethicone
Sodium cromoglicate	Sodium cromoglycate	Cromolyn sodium
Tetracaine	Amethocaine	
Torasemide	Torasemide	Torsemide
Trihexyphenidyl	Benzhexol	Trihexyphenidyl

a. historical list to aid understanding of the older literature; all pharmaceuticals marketed in the UK are now known by rINN
b. in the UK, the BANs are still used in conjunction with the corresponding rINNs, i.e. adrenaline (epinephrine) and noradrenaline (norepinephrine).

1 World Health Organisation (2017) Guidance on the use of International Nonproprietary Names (INNs) for pharmaceutical substances. Geneva: World Health Organisation. www.who.int.
2 Merchant L *et al.* (2020) Identical or similar brand names used in different countries for medications with different active ingredients: a descriptive analysis. *BMJ Quality and Safety*. **29**: 988–991.

Updated August 2021

ABBREVIATIONS

Drug administration

In 2005, the Joint Commission on Accreditation of Healthcare Organizations (JCAHO) in the USA published National Patient Safety Goals. These include a series of recommendations about ways in which confusion (and thus errors) can be reduced by avoiding the use of certain abbreviations on prescriptions. The full set of recommendations is available at http://www.jointcommission.org/standards/national-patient-safety-goals.

Although some traditional abbreviations remain acceptable (Table 1), others are not. Thus, it is recommended that, as in *PCF*, the following are written in full:

- at bedtime
- once daily
- each morning
- every other day
- before food
- after food
- units (i.e. *not* U or IU).

Table 1 Abbreviations in *PCF* for drug administration times

Times	*UK*	*Latin*
Twice per day	b.d.	*bis die*
Three times per day	t.d.s.	*ter die sumendus*
Four times per day	q.d.s.	*quarter die sumendus*
Every 4 hours etc.	q4h	*quaque quarta hora*
Rescue medication (as needed/required)	p.r.n.	*pro re nata*
Give immediately	stat	*stat*

Because of widespread usage, the term 'immediate-release' is now used (without abbreviation) in *PCF*, rather than 'normal-release'. For 'slow-release', 'extended-release' etc., 'm/r' (modified-release) is used generically.

Although the following conventions have *not* been adopted in *PCF*, readers should be aware of the following recommendations for handwritten and printed prescriptions, and other printed medical matter, e.g. packaging, patient records:

- include a space between the drug dose and the unit of measure, e.g. 25 mg, not 25mg
- write 'per' instead of an oblique (mistaken for a figure 1), e.g. 200 mg per day, not 200mg/day
- use 'subcut' or 'subcutaneous' instead of SC (mistaken for SL)
- write 'less than' or 'greater than' instead of < and > (mistaken for a letter L or number 7; or written the wrong way around and thus signifying the opposite of the intended meaning).

amp	ampoule containing a single dose (cf. vial)
CD	controlled drug; preparation subject to prescription requirements under the Misuse of Drugs Act (UK); for regulations see *BNF*
CIVI	continuous intravenous infusion
CSCI	continuous subcutaneous infusion
e/c	enteric-coated (gastro-resistant)
ED	epidural
IM	intramuscular
IT	intrathecal
IV	intravenous
IVI	intravenous infusion
m/r	modified-release; alternatives, controlled-release, extended-release, prolonged-release, slow-release, sustained-release

OTC	over the counter (i.e. can be obtained without a prescription)
PO	*per os*, by mouth
POM	prescription-only medicine
PR	*per rectum*
PV	*per vaginam*
SC	subcutaneous
SL	sublingual
TD	transdermal
TM	transmucosal
vial	sterile container with a rubber bung containing either a single or multiple doses (cf. amp)
WFI	water for injections

General

*	specialist use only
†	unauthorized (unlicensed) use
ACBS	Advisory Committee on Borderline Substances
AHFS	American Hospital Formulary Service
AKPS	Australia-modified Karnofsky Performance Status Scale
BNF	*British National Formulary*
BP	*British Pharmacopoeia*
CHM	Commission on Human Medicines
CI	confidence interval
CSM	Committee on Safety of Medicines (now part of CHM)
DH	Department of Health (UK)
ECOG	Eastern Cooperative Oncology Group
EMA	European Medicines Agency
EORTC	European Organisation for Research and Treatment of Cancer
ESRF	end-stage renal failure
FDA	Food and Drug Administration (USA)
HR	hazard ratio
IASP	International Association for the Study of Pain
ICU	intensive care unit
MHRA	Medicines and Healthcare products Regulatory Agency
MRC	Medical Research Council
N/A	not applicable
NICE	National Institute for Health and Care Excellence
(not UK)	not commercially available in the UK
(not USA)	not commercially available in the USA
NPF	*Nurse Prescribers' Formulary*
NPSA	National Patient Safety Association
NRS	numerical rating scale
NYHA	New York Heart Association
OR	odds ratio
PCF	Palliative Care Formulary
PCS/PCU	palliative care service/unit
PI	package insert (USA), equivalent to SPC
PIL	patient information leaflet (UK)
QCG	Quick Clinical Guide
rINN	recommended International Nonproprietary Name
RPS	Royal Pharmaceutical Society
SD	standard deviation
SIGN	Scottish Intercollegiate Guidelines Network
SMC	Scottish Medicines Consortium
SPC	summary of product characteristics (UK)
UK	United Kingdom
UKMi	UK Medicines Information
USA	United States of America

USP	*United States Pharmacopeia*
VAS	visual analogue scale, 0–100mm
WHO	World Health Organization

Receptor types

α_1, α_2	alpha-adrenergic type 1, 2
β_2	beta-adrenergic type 2
δ	delta-opioid
κ	kappa-opioid
μ	mu-opioid
$5HT_{1A}, 5HT_{2A}$	5-hydroxytryptamine (serotonin) type 1A, 2A etc.
A_1, A_2, A_{2A}	adenosine type 1, 2, 2A
CB_1, CB_2	cannabinoid type 1, 2
D_2	dopamine type 2
$GABA_A, GABA_B$	gamma-aminobutyric acid type A, B
H_1, H_2	histamine type 1, 2
M_1, M_2	muscarinic acetylcholine type 1, 2 etc.
MT_1, MT_2	melatonin type 1, 2
NOP	nociceptin opioid peptide
SST_1, SST_2	somatostatin type 1,2 etc.

Chemical symbols

Ca^{2+}	calcium
Cl^-	chloride
K^+	potassium
Mg^{2+}	magnesium
Na^+	sodium

Ion channels

Ca_v	calcium (voltage-gated)
K_v	potassium (voltage-gated)
Na_v	sodium (voltage-gated)
TRP, $TRPV_1$	transient receptor potential (vanilloid type 1)

Medical

5HT	5-hydroxytryptamine (serotonin)
ACE	angiotensin-converting enzyme
ACTH	adrenocorticotropic hormone
ADH	antidiuretic hormone (vasopressin)
ALS	amyotrophic lateral sclerosis
ALT	alanine aminotransferase
AMPA	α-amino-3-hydroxy-5-methylisoxazole-4-propionic acid
APTT	activated partial thromboplastin time
AST	aspartate aminotransferase
ATP	adenosine triphosphate
AUC	area under the plasma concentration–time curve
AV	atrioventricular
BP	blood pressure
CHF	congestive heart failure
CKD	chronic kidney disease
C_{max}	maximum plasma drug concentration
CNS	central nervous system
COPD	chronic obstructive pulmonary disease
COX	cyclo-oxygenase; alternative, prostaglandin synthase
Coxibs	selective COX-2 inhibitors
CrCl	creatinine clearance
CRP	C-reactive protein

CSF	cerebrospinal fluid
CT	computed tomography
CVA	cerebrovascular accident
CVS	cardiovascular system
CYP450	cytochrome P450
DIC	disseminated intravascular coagulation
DOAC	direct oral anticoagulant
DVT	deep vein thrombosis
ECG (EKG)	electrocardiogram
EFT	enteral feeding tube
eGFR	formula-based estimation of glomerular filtration rate
ERCP	endoscopic retrograde cholangiopancreatography
FBC	full blood count
FEV_1	forced expiratory volume in 1 second
FRC	functional residual capacity
FSH	follicle-stimulating hormone
FVC	forced vital capacity of lungs
GABA	gamma-aminobutyric acid
GI	gastro-intestinal
GFR	glomerular filtration rate
GnRH	gonadotropin-releasing hormone
Hb	haemoglobin
HIV	human immunodeficiency virus
HLA	human leukocyte antigen
Ig	immunoglobulin
IL-6	interleukin 6
INR	international normalized ratio
LABA	long-acting β_2-adrenergic receptor agonist
LFTs	liver function tests
LH	luteinizing hormone
LMWH	low molecular weight heparin
MAOI	monoamine oxidase inhibitor
MARI	monoamine re-uptake inhibitor
MND	motor neurone disease
MRI	magnetic resonance imaging
MSU	mid-stream specimen of urine
NaSSA	noradrenergic and specific serotoninergic antidepressant
NDRI	noradrenaline (norepinephrine) and dopamine re-uptake inhibitor
NG	nasogastric
NJ	nasojejunal
NMDA	N-methyl D-aspartate
NNH	number needed to harm, i.e. the number of patients needed to be treated in order to harm one patient sufficiently to cause withdrawal from a drug trial
NNT	number needed to treat, i.e. the number of patients needed to be treated in order to achieve 50% improvement in one patient compared with placebo
NO	nitric oxide
NRI	noradrenaline (norepinephrine) re-uptake inhibitor
NSAID	non-steroidal anti-inflammatory drug
NSCLC	non-small-cell lung carcinoma
$PaCO_2$	arterial partial pressure of carbon dioxide
PaO_2	arterial partial pressure of oxygen
PCA	patient-controlled analgesia
PE	pulmonary embolus/embolism
PEF	peak expiratory flow
PEG	percutaneous endoscopic gastrostomy
PG	prostaglandin
PPI	proton pump inhibitor
PT	prothrombin time

RCT	randomized controlled trial
RIMA	reversible inhibitor of monoamine oxidase type A
RTI	respiratory tract infection
SaO_2	oxygen saturation
SCLC	small cell lung cancer
SIADH	syndrome of inappropriate secretion of antidiuretic hormone
SLE	systemic lupus erythematosus
SNRI	serotonin and noradrenaline (norepinephrine) re-uptake inhibitor
SpO_2	peripheral capillary oxygen saturation
SRE	skeletal-related events
SSRI	selective serotonin re-uptake inhibitor
TCA	tricyclic antidepressant
TIBC	total iron-binding capacity; alternative, plasma transferrin concentration
Tl_{CO}	transfer factor of the lung for carbon monoxide
T_{max}	time to reach C_{max}
TNFα	tumour necrosis factor alpha
TSH	thyroid-stimulating hormone
U&E	urea and electrolytes
UTI	urinary tract infection
VEGF	vascular endothelial growth factor
VIP	vasoactive intestinal polypeptide
VTE	venous thromboembolism
WBC	white blood cell
w/v	weight of solute (g) per 100mL

Units

cm	centimetre(s)
cps	cycles per sec
dL	decilitre(s)
g	gram(s)
Gy	gray(s)
h	hour(s)
Hg	mercury
kcal	kilocalories
kg	kilogram(s)
L	litre(s)
mg	milligram(s)
microL	microlitre(s)
micromol	micromole(s)
min	minute(s)
mL	millilitre(s)
mm	millimetre(s)
mmHg	millimetre(s) of mercury
mmol	millimole(s)
mosmol	milli-osmole(s)
msec	millisecond(s)
nm	nanometre(s)
nmol	nanomole(s)
sec	second(s)

Updated (minor change) February 2022

1: GASTRO-INTESTINAL SYSTEM

ANTACIDS AND ANTIFLATULENTS

Indications: Occasional dyspepsia and/or acid reflux, gassy dyspepsia, †hiccup (if associated with gastric distension).

Note. PPIs (see p.31) are generally used when continuous gastric acid reduction is indicated.[1]

Pharmacology

Antacids generally contain one or more of the following, which neutralize gastric acid:

- magnesium salts
- aluminium hydroxide
- sodium bicarbonate
- calcium carbonate.

***Magnesium salts** are laxative and can cause diarrhoea*; ***aluminium salts** constipate*. Thus, most proprietary antacids contain a mixture of both so as to have a neutral impact on intestinal transit, e.g. **co-magaldrox**. With doses of 100–200mL/24h or more, the effect of **magnesium salts** tends to override the constipating effect of **aluminium**.[2]

Other ingredients may be combined with antacids to relieve the symptoms of dyspepsia, e.g.:

- oxetacaine
- hydrotalcite (aluminium magnesium carbonate hydroxide hydrate)
- sodium alginate
- peppermint oil
- simeticone (silica-activated dimeticone).

In post-radiation oesophagitis and candidosis which is causing painful swallowing, an **aluminium hydroxide–magnesium hydroxide** suspension containing **oxetacaine**, a local anaesthetic, can be helpful. It is only available as a special order product in the UK. Give 5–10mL (without fluid) 15min before meals and at bedtime, and p.r.n. before drinks. This should be regarded as short-term symptomatic treatment while time and specific treatment of the underlying condition permits healing of the damaged mucosa.

Hydrotalcite, an **aluminium–magnesium** complex, binds bile salts and is of specific benefit in patients with bile salt reflux, e.g. after certain forms of gastroduodenal surgery. It is available only in combination with **simeticone** in the UK.

Sodium alginate prevents oesophageal reflux pain by forming an inert low-density raft on the top of the acidic stomach contents. Both acid and air bubbles are necessary to produce the raft. Commercially available products combine **sodium alginate** with weak antacids, e.g. Gaviscon®, Peptac®; most of the antacid content adheres to the alginate raft. This neutralizes acid which seeps into the oesophagus around the raft.

Peppermint oil and **simeticone** are antiflatulents and are available alone or in combination products. They facilitate belching, easing flatulence, distension and postprandial gastric discomfort. They may help hiccup associated with gastric distension (see Prokinetics, Table 2, p.25). **Peppermint oil** acts by decreasing the tone of the lower oesophageal sphincter; this can result in gastro-oesophageal reflux. **Simeticone** (silica-activated dimeticone or dimethylpolysiloxane) is a mixture of liquid dimeticones with silicon dioxide. It acts as an antifoaming agent and alters the surface tension of bubbles, causing them to coalesce. This facilitates their removal by belching. **Simeticone** is inert and is not absorbed. The onset of action is <5min, and duration of action is approximately 1–2h.

Cautions

Risk of hypermagnesaemia with **magnesium**-containing antacids in renal impairment; **calcium carbonate** is preferable.

The relatively high sodium content (e.g. 4–6mmol/10mL) of some antacids and alginate products may be detrimental to patients on salt-restricted diets, e.g. those with hypertension, heart failure or renal impairment; low-sodium alternatives (e.g. <1mmol/10mL) are preferable (see Supply).

Sodium bicarbonate: risk of sodium loading and metabolic alkalosis; do not use as a single-product antacid. **Calcium carbonate**: rebound acid secretion, about 2h after a dose; also hypercalcaemia, particularly when taken with **sodium bicarbonate**.

Drug interactions

Antacids can impact on the absorption of other PO drugs by:

- temporarily increasing the pH of the stomach contents
- delaying gastric emptying
- forming insoluble complexes in the GI tract
- damaging enteric coating, resulting in exposure of the drug to gastric acid, and of the stomach mucosa to the drug.

Selected interactions where additional caution may be necessary are listed in Box A. Generally, these can be avoided by separating administration of the antacid and the affected drug by ≥2h.

Box A Interactions between antacids and other PO drugs[a,3]

All e/c or gastroresistant formulations
Bisphosphonates
Dexamethasone[b]
Fexofenadine
Gabapentin
Itraconazole *capsules*
Nitrofurantoin[b]
Quinolones, e.g. ciprofloxacin
Rifampicin
Tetracyclines, e.g. demeclocycline

a. *not* an exhaustive list; limited to drugs most likely to be encountered in palliative care and *excludes* anticancer, HIV and immunosuppressive drugs (seek specialist advice)

b. magnesium trisilicate can reduce absorption by 50–75%.

Antacids should not be administered by enteral feeding tube as they can cause the feed to coagulate and block the tube (see Chapter 28, Table 2, p.863).

Large doses of antacids may lead to alkalization of the urine and thereby affect the action of other drugs, e.g.:

- **methenamine** action is inhibited at urinary pH >5.5
- the excretion of round-the-clock anti-inflammatory doses of **aspirin** is increased. Occasional doses of **aspirin** are not affected.[3]

Dose and use

Generally, antacids should be taken PO p.r.n. after meals and at bedtime. The dose of liquid formulations is generally 10mL. If symptoms persist and/or regular use is required, consider a PPI (p.31) and testing for *Helicobacter pylori*.[1]

†Hiccup associated with gastric distension

For **peppermint oil**:

- one to two capsules PO p.r.n. up to t.d.s.

For **simeticone**:

- start with 100–125mg PO p.r.n. or after meals and at bedtime
- maximum daily dose 800mg/24h.

Supply

Note. Low Na^+ is defined as <1mmol/tablet or 10mL dose.

Magnesium trisilicate mixture BP (generic)
Oral suspension (**magnesium trisilicate** 250mg, **magnesium carbonate** 250mg and **sodium bicarbonate** 250mg/5mL), 28 days @ 10mL t.d.s. & at bedtime = £9; *peppermint flavour, 6mmol Na^+/10mL.*

Co-magaldrox
Maalox® (Sanofi-Aventis)
Oral suspension (sugar-free) **co-magaldrox** 175/200 (**aluminium hydroxide** 175mg/5mL, **magnesium hydroxide** 200mg/5mL), 28 days @ 10mL t.d.s. & at bedtime = £10.50; *low Na^+.*

Mucogel® (Chemidex)
Oral suspension (sugar-free) **co-magaldrox** 220/195 (**aluminium hydroxide** 220mg/5mL, **magnesium hydroxide** 195mg), 28 days @ 10mL t.d.s. & at bedtime = £7; *low Na^+.*

Antacid with **oxetacaine**
Oral suspension **oxetacaine** 10mg, **aluminium hydroxide** 200mg, **magnesium hydroxide** 100mg/5mL, 28 days @ 10mL t.d.s. *before* meals & at bedtime = £153; *low Na^+* (unauthorized product, available as a special order from Rosemont; see Chapter 24, p.817). *Available as Mucaine® suspension (Wyeth) in some countries.*

Antacid with **sodium alginate**
Alginate raft-forming oral suspension (generic)
Oral suspension (sugar-free) **calcium carbonate** 80mg, **sodium alginate** 250mg, **sodium bicarbonate** 133.5mg/5mL, 28 days @ 10mL t.d.s. & at bedtime = £4.50; *peppermint or aniseed flavour also available.*
Brands include Acidex®, Gaviscon® and Peptac®. Other compound alginate products are available, e.g. with ***potassium bicarbonate****, and many products are available OTC.*

Hydrotalcite with **simeticone**
Altacite Plus® (Peckforton)
Oral suspension (sugar-free) simeticone 125mg, **hydrotalcite** 500mg/5mL, 28 days @ 10mL q.d.s. = £12; *low Na^+.*

Peppermint oil (generic)
Capsules 0.2mL, 28 days @ 1 capsule t.d.s. = £7.

Simeticone
Wind-eze® (Teva)
Capsules 125mg, 28 days @ 125mg q.d.s. = £12.
Tablets chewable 125mg, 28 days @ 125mg q.d.s. = £8.

WindSetlers® (Thornton & Ross)
Capsules 100mg, 28 days @ 100mg q.d.s. = £11.

1 NICE (2014) Dyspepsia and gastro-oesophageal reflux disease. *Clinical Guideline* CG184. www.nice.org.uk
2 Morrissey J and Barreras R (1974) Antacid therapy. *New England Journal of Medicine*. **290**: 550–554.
3 Baxter K and Preston CL. *Stockley's Drug Interactions*. London: Pharmaceutical Press. www.medicinescomplete.com (accessed December 2017).

Updated March 2018

ANTIMUSCARINICS

Indications: Smooth muscle spasm (e.g. bladder, intestine), motion sickness (**hyoscine *hydrobromide***), drying secretions (including surgical premedication, †sialorrhoea (**glycopyrronium** PO authorized in children; see SPC), †drooling, †death rattle/noisy rattling breathing, and †inoperable bowel obstruction), †paraneoplastic pyrexia and sweating.

Contra-indications: Narrow-angle glaucoma (unless moribund), tachycardia (heart rate >100 beats/min); see Cautions and **hyoscine *butylbromide*** (p.16), bowel obstruction (unless part of medical management), paralytic ileus, toxic megacolon, prostatic enlargement with urinary retention, myasthenia gravis (unless moribund).

Note. Contra-indications vary between different antimuscarinic drugs (see individual SPCs). When possible, *PCF* collates and standardizes contra-indications across a class of drugs; the above are applicable for antimuscarinics given parenterally, SL, TD and PO. The exception is PO **hyoscine *butylbromide*** (p.15), where low bio-availability reduces the likelihood of systemic antimuscarinic effects.

Pharmacology

Chemically, antimuscarinics are classified as tertiary amines or quaternary ammonium compounds (Box A).

Box A Chemical classification of antimuscarinics

Tertiary amines	**Quaternary ammonium compounds**
Naturally occurring (belladonna alkaloids)	***Synthetic/semisynthetic***
Atropine	Glycopyrronium
Hyoscine *hydrobromide*	Hyoscine *butylbromide*
Hyoscyamine (l-atropine; not UK)[a]	Ipratropium bromide
	Propantheline
Synthetic/semisynthetic	Tiotropium bromide
Dicycloverine	Trospium
Orphenadrine	
Oxybutynin	**Other**
Tolterodine	Darifenacin
	Fesoterodine
	Solifenacin

a. because the d-isomer is virtually inactive, hyoscyamine is twice as potent as racemic atropine.

Numerous other drugs have antimuscarinic effects (Box B). In addition, some drugs generally not considered antimuscarinic have been shown to have detectable antimuscarinic activity by means of a radioreceptor assay, including **codeine, digoxin, dipyridamole, isosorbide, loperamide, nifedipine, prednisolone, ranitidine, theophylline, warfarin.**[1] Thus, potentially, multiple drugs can contribute to the total 'antimuscarinic burden' and thereby exacerbate toxicity, particularly in the frail elderly.[2]

Box B Drugs with antimuscarinic effects used in palliative care

Antimuscarinics (see Box A)	Antiparkinsonians, e.g.
Analgesics	orphenadrine
pethidine (*not* recommended)	procyclidine
nefopam (mostly postoperative)	Antipsychotics (atypical)
Antidepressants	clozapine
TCAs, e.g. amitriptyline, imipramine	olanzapine
paroxetine (SSRI)	Antipsychotics (typical)
Antihistamines, e.g.	phenothiazines, e.g.
chlorphenamine	chlorpromazine
cyclizine	levomepromazine
dimenhydrinate (not UK)	prochlorperazine
promethazine	

At least five different types of muscarinic receptors have been identified (M_1–M_5).[3] They are widely distributed, but their expression and functional relevance varies between tissues. Most antimuscarinic drugs act as non-selective antagonists, e.g. **atropine, glycopyrronium, hyoscine *hydrobromide*, hyoscine *butylbromide*.** Newer drugs have aimed to be more selective in their actions; e.g. **oxybutynin** and **tolterodine** are *relatively* selective for M_3 receptors, which predominate in the bladder (see Urinary antimuscarinics, p.611). Nonetheless, undesirable effects are unavoidable because M_3 receptors are also important in other tissues of the body, e.g. salivary gland and bowel, resulting in dry mouth and constipation.

Within the heart, M_2 receptors are mostly responsible for conveying parasympathetic effects on pacemaker activity, atrioventricular conduction and force of contraction. Other subtypes are also present (M_1, M_3, M_5) but their functional significance is uncertain. Further, cardiac disease can alter receptor expression, e.g. the density of M_2 decreases and M_3 increases in chronic atrial fibrillation.[3] Within the coronary arteries in mice, M_3 receptors are the most important in mediating acetylcholine-induced vasodilation; it is not known if this is true in humans, although the genes for M_2 and M_3 receptors are expressed.[3] Thus, although the cardiac toxicity of **hyoscine *butylbromide*** has been the recent focus of attention (see p.16), all antimuscarinics have this potential. This is particularly so in patients with cardiac disease associated with a detrimental autonomic nervous system imbalance (increased sympathetic and decreased parasympathetic (vagal) activity).[4] Indeed, increasing vagal activity appears beneficial in cardiac disease, and there is growing interest in the use of electrical stimulation or drugs to augment vagal function, e.g. in heart failure.[4,5]

Antimuscarinic effects can be divided into central and peripheral (Box C); undesirable central and peripheral effects have been summarized as:

> *'Dry as a bone, blind as a bat, red as a beet, hot as a hare, mad as a hatter.'*

Box C Antimuscarinic effects

CNS effects

Drowsiness
Cognitive impairment } increased risk of falls and fracture[6]
Delirium
Restlessness
Agitation

Peripheral effects

Visual

Mydriasis
Loss of accommodation } blurred vision (and thus may impair driving ability)

Cardiovascular

Tachycardia, palpitations
Extrasystoles } also related to noradrenaline (norepinephrine) potentiation and a quinidine-like action
Arrhythmias

Gastro-intestinal

Dry mouth (inhibition of salivation)
Heartburn (relaxation of lower oesophageal sphincter)
Constipation (decreased intestinal motility → ileus)

Urinary tract

Hesitancy of micturition
Retention of urine

Skin

Reduced sweating
Flushing

At *toxic* doses, all the tertiary amines, including **hyoscine *hydrobromide***, cause CNS stimulation resulting in mild central vagal excitation, respiratory stimulation, agitation and delirium. However, at typical *therapeutic* doses, **hyoscine *hydrobromide*** (but *not* **atropine**) causes CNS depression.

Synthetic tertiary amines generally cause less central stimulation than the naturally occurring alkaloids. Quaternary ammonium compounds do not cross the blood–brain barrier in any significant amount, and accordingly have only peripheral effects (Box C).[7] They are also less well absorbed from the GI tract.

The muscarinic receptors in salivary glands are very responsive to antimuscarinics, and inhibition of salivation occurs at lower doses than required for other antimuscarinic effects.[8] In some patients, a reduction in excess saliva results in improved speech.[9]

In the UK, parenteral antimuscarinics are widely used to reduce death rattle (noisy rattling breathing) which occurs in about 1/3 of patients close to death (see QCG: Death rattle (noisy rattling breathing), p.11).[10] Although the use of antimuscarinics for this purpose has been questioned,[10–12] secretions are often, but not always, reduced.[13–15] For example, a prospective clinical survey concluded that antimuscarinics reduce death rattle in 1/2–2/3 of patients.[16]

Antimuscarinics are generally given as soon as death rattle becomes evident. In an RCT, the *prophylactic* use of **hyoscine *butylbromide*** 20mg SC q.d.s. halved the number of patients developing death rattle (27%→13%).[17] However, for the majority of dying patients who do *not* develop death rattle (about two-thirds[10]), it could be argued that the prophylactic approach represents an unnecessary overtreatment and risk of undesirable effects. It is too soon to gauge how these findings may influence practice.

In relation to death rattle, belladonna alkaloids are generally equally effective,[13,14] and **glycopyrronium** may sometimes be effective when the alkaloids have not been.[18] Although one study reported that **hyoscine *hydrobromide*** acts faster than **glycopyrronium**, there is no detectable difference between the two drugs after 1h.[19] In practice, undesirable effects, availability, fashion, familiarity and cost are probably the main influences in choice of drug.

Antimuscarinic drugs differ in their pharmacokinetic characteristics (Table 1).

Table 1 Pharmacokinetic details of selected antimuscarinic drugs[8]

	Bio-availability	*Plasma halflife*	*Duration of action (antisecretory)*
CNS + peripheral effects			
Atropine	50% PO	2–2.5h[a]	no data
Hyoscine *hydrobromide*	60–80% SL	1–4h[a]	1–9h
Peripheral effects only			
Glycopyrronium	<5% PO	1–1.5h[a]	7h
Hyoscine *butylbromide*	<1% PO[20]	1–5h[20]	<2h[b,21]
Propantheline	<50% PO	2–3h	4–6h

a. after IM injection into deltoid muscle
b. in volunteers; possibly longer in moribund patients.

Cautions

After the sudden death of a patient with cardiac disease given an IV bolus of **hyoscine *butylbromide*** at colonoscopy, the MHRA issued a warning highlighting its cardiac toxicity (see p.16).[22]

Cardiac disease, e.g. myocardial infarction, ischaemia, arrhythmia, heart failure, hypertension; other conditions predisposing to tachycardia, e.g. thyrotoxicosis, ß agonist use. Bladder outflow obstruction (prostatism). Likely to exacerbate acid reflux. Ulcerative colitis. Narrow-angle glaucoma may be precipitated in those at risk, particularly the elderly. Use in hot weather or pyrexia may lead to heatstroke. Frail elderly patients are particularly susceptible to cognitive impairment/delirium with centrally acting antimuscarinics.

Use in renal or hepatic impairment

In end-stage renal or hepatic failure, do not use **hyoscine *hydrobromide*** for death rattle, because of an increased risk of delirium. Use **hyoscine *butylbromide*** (dose unchanged) or, if unavailable, **glycopyrronium** instead (lower doses may be sufficient).

Antimuscarinics differ in their potential to cause toxicity when renal or hepatic function is impaired; see Chapters 17 (p.746) and 18 (p.776) for general information on the choice of antimuscarinic and use in ESRF and severe hepatic impairment.

Drug interactions

Concurrent treatment with ≥2 antimuscarinic drugs (including antihistamines, phenothiazines and TCAs; see Box B) will increase the likelihood of undesirable effects and (when centrally acting) of central toxicity, e.g. restlessness, agitation, delirium (see Box C). Children, the elderly and patients with renal or hepatic impairment are more susceptible to the central effects of non-quaternary antimuscarinics.

Because antimuscarinics competitively block the final common (cholinergic) pathway through which prokinetics act,[23] concurrent prescription with **metoclopramide** and **domperidone** should be avoided as far as possible.

The increased GI transit time produced by antimuscarinics may allow increased drug absorption from some formulations, e.g. **digoxin** and **nitrofurantoin** tablets and **potassium** m/r tablets, but reduced absorption from others, e.g. **paracetamol** tablets. Dissolution and absorption of SL tablets (e.g. **glyceryl trinitrate**) may be reduced because of decreased saliva production.

Both antimuscarinics and opioids cause constipation (by different mechanisms) and, if used together, will result in an increased need for laxatives, and may even result in paralytic ileus. On the other hand, morphine and **hyoscine *butylbromide*** or **glycopyrronium** are sometimes purposely combined in terminally ill patients with inoperable bowel obstruction in order to prevent colic and to reduce vomiting.

Undesirable effects

What is a desired effect becomes an undesirable effect in different circumstances (see Box C). Thus, dry mouth is an almost universal *undesirable* effect of antimuscarinics except when a reduction of oropharyngeal secretions is intended, as in death rattle.

Dose and use

In palliative care patients, there is an association between the number of antimuscarinic drugs used and worsening fatigue and quality of life.[2] Other undesirable effects (e.g. delirium, constipation) are hard to distinguish from symptoms of underlying disease. Thus, careful monitoring is essential and, when possible, drugs with antimuscarinic effects should be avoided or discontinued.

By injection, there is no good evidence to recommend one antimuscarinic in preference to another.[14] However, because **atropine** and **hyoscyamine** (not UK) tend to stimulate the CNS rather than sedate, concurrent prescription of **midazolam** or **haloperidol** is more likely to be necessary. In the UK, **glycopyrronium, hyoscine *butylbromide*** and **hyoscine *hydrobromide*** are used in preference to **atropine.** Generally, *PCF* favours **hyoscine *butylbromide*,** based on its lack of central effects and lower cost.

When given IM, **atropine**, **hyoscine *hydrobromide*** and **glycopyrronium** are all absorbed faster from the deltoid muscle than from the gluteal muscles.[8]

Urinary antispasmodic

Antimuscarinics are used to relieve smooth muscle spasm in the bladder (see p.611).

Intestinal antispasmodic and antisecretory

Antimuscarinics are used to reduce intestinal colic and intestinal secretions, particularly gastric, associated with †inoperable organic bowel obstruction in terminally ill patients (Table 2). Also see QCG: Inoperable bowel obstruction, p.266.

Table 2 Antispasmodic and antisecretory drugs: typical SC doses

Drug	*Stat and p.r.n. doses*	*CSCI dose/24h*
Glycopyrronium	200microgram	600–1,200microgram
Hyoscine *butylbromide*	20mg	60–300mg
Hyoscine *hydrobromide*[a]	400microgram	1,200–2,000microgram

a. atropine doses are generally the same as for hyoscine *hydrobromide*.

†*Death rattle (noisy rattling breathing)*

Treatment regimens are based mostly on local clinical experience. In the UK, antimuscarinic drugs for death rattle are generally given SC/CSCI as soon as death rattle becomes evident.[24] See QCG: Death rattle (noisy rattling breathing), p.11.

In some countries the SL route is preferred, particularly in home care, because it circumvents the need for injections; e.g. **glycopyrronium**, see p.12).

†*Drooling (and sialorrhoea)*

Seen particularly in patients with ALS/MND, advanced Parkinson's disease and with various disorders of the head and neck. A survey of UK neurologists[25] with a special interest in MND/ALS showed that their preferred first-line drugs for sialorrhoea are:

- **hyoscine *hydrobromide***, e.g. 1mg/3 days TD[26]
- **amitriptyline**, e.g. 10–25mg PO at bedtime
- **atropine,** e.g. 1% ophthalmic solution, 4 drops on the tongue or SL q4h p.r.n.

In relation to the latter, drop size varies with applicator and technique. *Thus, the dose varies from 200–500microgram per drop (800microgram–2mg/dose).* It is important to titrate the dose upwards until there is an adequate effect; in an RCT, 500microgram q.d.s. was no better than placebo.[27]

Glycopyrronium is the most popular second-line drug, typically PO or SL.[25] It is recommended for first-line use in patients with cognitive impairment.[28] **Glycopyrronium** is also used for drooling in other conditions, e.g. PO solutions are authorized in children >3 years and adolescents with chronic neurological disorders (see p.12).

In patients in whom antimuscarinics are contra-indicated, ineffective or not tolerated, the parotid ± submandibular glands can be injected with **botulinum toxin.**[25] Injections are generally effective within 2 weeks, and benefit lasts 3–4 months.[29–33] In patients with a relatively long prognosis (years rather than months), radiotherapy and surgery are further options.[25]

Conversely, some patients have tenacious salivary secretions that are difficult/distressing to clear. This is caused by an increase in viscosity of saliva as the water content decreases. Whenever possible, drugs that cause dry mouth (particularly antimuscarinic drugs) should be stopped. There are case reports of benefit from the use of a β-blocker in this setting (Box D).

Box D β-blockers for tenacious salivary secretions[25,34–39]

Blockade of the β_1-adrenoceptor in salivary glands reduces mucin secretion and thereby decreases the viscosity of saliva, aiding its clearance.

The optimal β-blocker and dose is not known. Compared to other (more lipophilic) β-blockers used in this setting, atenolol has the advantage of lower penetration of the blood-brain barrier and, thus, less likelihood of undesirable CNS effects. It is also available in an oral solution:

- start with †atenolol 25mg PO once daily
- if necessary, increase in 25mg increments
- maximum dose 100mg once daily (reduced in severe renal impairment).

Monitor heart rate and BP. If poorly tolerated, e.g. bradycardia, cold peripheries, Raynaud's phenomenon, consider switching to a β_1-partial agonist, e.g. celiprolol.

†*Paraneoplastic pyrexia and sweating*

Antimuscarinic drugs are used in the treatment of paraneoplastic pyrexia (Box E).

Box E Symptomatic drug treatment of paraneoplastic pyrexia and sweating

Prescribe an antipyretic:

- paracetamol 500–1,000mg PO q.d.s. or p.r.n. (generally less toxic than an NSAID) *or*
- NSAID, e.g. ibuprofen 200–400mg PO t.d.s. or p.r.n. (or the locally preferred alternative).

If the sweating does not respond to an NSAID, prescribe an antimuscarinic drug, e.g.:

- amitriptyline 25–50mg PO at bedtime
- propantheline 15–30mg PO b.d.–t.d.s. on an empty stomach
- hyoscine *hydrobromide* 1mg/3 days TD[40]
- glycopyrronium 200microgram–2mg PO t.d.s.[41]

If an antimuscarinic fails, other PO options include:

- gabapentin, see p.297
- H_2-receptor antagonist, see p.27
- olanzapine 5mg b.d.[42]
- propranolol 10–20mg b.d.–t.d.s.
- thalidomide 100mg at bedtime.[43,44]

Thalidomide is generally seen as the last resort, even though the response rate appears to be high.[44] This is mostly because it can cause an irreversible painful peripheral neuropathy and other undesirable effects (see p.603).

Overdose

In the past, **physostigmine** (not UK), a cholinesterase inhibitor, was sometimes administered to correct antimuscarinic toxicity/poisoning. This is no longer recommended, because **physostigmine** itself can cause serious toxic effects, including cardiac arrhythmias and seizures.[45–47]

A benzodiazepine can be given to control marked agitation and seizures. Phenothiazines should *not* be given, because they will exacerbate the antimuscarinic effects and could precipitate an acute dystonia (see Drug-induced movement disorders, p.805).

Anti-arrhythmics are *not* advisable if an arrhythmia develops, but hypoxia and acidosis should be corrected.

1 Tune I *et al.* (1992) Anticholinergic effects of drugs commonly prescribed for the elderly; potential means of assessing risk of delirium. *American Journal of Psychiatry.* **149:** 1393–1394.

2 Hochman MJ *et al.* (2016) Anticholinergic drug burden in noncancer versus cancer patients near the end of life. *Journal of Pain and Symptom Management.* **52:** 737–743.e733.

3 Abrams P *et al.* (2006) Muscarinic receptors: their distribution and function in body systems, and the implications for treating overactive bladder. *British Journal of Pharmacology.* **148**: 565–578.

4 He X *et al.* (2015) Novel strategies and underlying protective mechanisms of modulation of vagal activity in cardiovascular diseases. *British Journal of Pharmacology.* **172**: 5489–5500.

5 He B *et al.* (2016) Autonomic modulation by electrical stimulation of the parasympathetic nervous system: an emerging intervention for cardiovascular diseases. *Cardiovascular Therapeutics.* **34**: 167–171.

6 Suehs BT *et al.* (2019): The relationship between anticholinergic exposure and falls, fractures, and mortality in patients with overactive bladder. *Drugs & Aging.* **36**: 957–967.

7 Sweetman SC, (ed) (2005) Martindale: The Complete Drug Reference. (34e) Pharmaceutical Press, London, pp. 475.

8 Ali-Melkkila T *et al.* (1993) Pharmacokinetics and related pharmacodynamics of anticholinergic drugs. *Acta Anaesthesiologica Scandinavica.* **37**: 633–642.

9 Rashid H *et al. (1997) Management of secretions in esophageal cancer patients with glycopyrrolate. Annals of Oncology.* **8:** 198–199.

10 Lokker ME *et al.* (2014) Prevalence, impact, and treatment of death rattle: a systematic review. *Journal of Pain and Symptom Management.* **47**: 105–122.

11 Wee B and Hillier R (2012) Interventions for noisy breathing in patients near to death. *Cochrane Database of Systematic Reviews.* **1**: CD005177. www.cochranelibrary.com.

12 Boland JW and Boland EG (2019) Noisy upper respiratory tract secretions: pharmacological management. *BMJ Supportive & Palliative Care.* doi: 10.1136/bmjspcare-2019-001791.

13 Likar R *et al.* (2008) Efficacy of glycopyrronium bromide and scopolamine hydrobromide in patients with death rattle: a randomized controlled study. *Wiener Klinische Wochenschrift.* **120**: 679–683.

14 Wildiers H *et al.* (2009) Atropine, hyoscine butylbromide, or scopolamine are equally effective for the treatment of death rattle in terminal care. *Journal of Pain and Symptom Management.* **38**: 124–133.

15 Hugel H *et al.* (2006) Respiratory tract secretions in the dying patient: a comparison between glycopyrronium and hyoscine hydrobromide. *Journal of Palliative Medicine.* **9**: 279–284.

16 Hughes A *et al.* (2000) Audit of three antimuscarinic drugs for managing retained secretions. *Palliative Medicine.* **14**: 221–222.

17 van Esch HJ *et al.* (2021) Effect of prophylactic subcutaneous scopolamine butylbromide on death rattle in patients at the end of life: the SILENCE *randomized clinical trial. JAMA.* **326**: 1268–1276.

18 Mirakhur R and Dundee J (1980) A comparison of the effects of atropine and glycopyrollate on various end organs. *Journal of the Royal Society of Medicine*. **73**: 727–730.
19 Back I *et al.* (2001) A study comparing hyoscine hydrobromide and glycopyrrolate in the treatment of death rattle. *Palliative Medicine*. **15**: 329–336.
20 Boehringer Ingelheim GmbH. Data on file.
21 Herxheimer A and Haefeli L (1966) Human pharmacology of hyoscine butylbromide. *Lancet*. **ii**: 418–421.
22 MHRA (2017) Hyoscine butylbromide (Buscopan) injection: risk of serious adverse effects in patients with underlying cardiac disease. *Drug Safety Update*. www.gov.uk/drug-safety-update.
23 Schuurkes JAJ *et al.* (1986) Stimulation of gastroduodenal motor activity: dopaminergic and cholinergic modulation. *Drug Development Research*. **8**: 233–241.
24 Bennett M *et al.* (2002) Using anti-muscarinic drugs in the management of death rattle: evidence based guidelines for palliative care. *Palliative Medicine*. **16**: 369–374.
25 Hobson EV *et al.* (2013) Management of sialorrhoea in motor neuron disease: a survey of current UK practice. *Amyotrophic Lateral Sclerosis Frontotemporal Degeneration*. **14**: 521–527.
26 Talmi YP *et al.* (1990) Reduction of salivary flow with transdermal scopolamine: a four-year experience. *Otolaryngology Head and Neck Surgery*. **103**: 615–618.
27 De Simone GG *et al.* (2006) Atropine drops for drooling: a randomized controlled trial. *Palliative medicine*. **20**: 665–671.
28 NICE (2016) Motor neurone disease: assessment and management. *NICE Guideline NG42*. www.nice.org.uk.
29 Ondo WG *et al. (2004)* A double-blind placebo-controlled trial of botulinum toxin B for sialorrhea in Parkinson's disease. *Neurology*. **62**: 37–40.
30 Jongerius P *et al.* (2004) Effect of botulinum toxin in the treatment of drooling: a controlled clinical trial. *Pediatrics*. **114**: 620–627.
31 Mancini F *et al.* (2003) Double-blind, placebo-controlled study to evaluate the efficacy and safety of botulinum toxin type A in the treatment of drooling in parkinsonism. *Movement Disorders*. **18**: 685–688.
32 Lipp A *et al.* (2003) A randomized trial of botulinum toxin A for treatment of drooling. *Neurology*. **61**: 1279–1281.
33 Ellies M *et al.* (2004) Reduction of salivary flow with botulinum toxin: extended report on 33 patients with drooling, salivary fistulas, and sialadenitis. *Laryngoscope*. **114**: 1856–1860.
34 Proctor GB and Carpenter GH (2014) Salivary secretion: mechanism and neural regulation. *Monographs in Oral Science*. **24**: 14–29.
35 Nederfors T *et al.* (1994) Effects of the beta-adrenoceptor antagonists atenolol and propranolol on human unstimulated whole saliva flow rate and protein composition. *Scandinavian Journal of Dental Research*. **102**: 235–237.
36 Westerlund A *et al.* (1985) Central nervous system side-effects with hydrophilic and lipophilic beta-blockers. *European Journal of Clinical Pharmacology*. **28(Suppl)**: 73–76.
37 MND Info sheet. https://www.mndassociation.org/app/uploads/information-sheet-p3-managing-saliva-problems.pdf
38 Newall AR *et al.* (1996) The control of oral secretions in bulbar ALS/MND. *Journal of Neurological Sciences*. **139 (Suppl)**: 43–44.
39 Woodman MJ and Howard P Beta-blockers for tenacious saliva: a case report. *BMJ Supportive & Palliative Care*. 2022 March 24. Online ahead of print.
40 Mercadante S (1998) Hyoscine in opioid-induced sweating. *Journal of Pain and Symptom Management*. **15**: 214–215.
41 Klaber M and Catterall M (2000) Treating hyperhidrosis. *British Medical Journal*. **321**: 703.
42 Zylicz Z and Krajnik M (2003) Flushing and sweating in an advanced breast cancer patient relieved by olanzapine. *Journal of Pain and Symptom Management*. **25**: 494–495.
43 Deaner P (2000) The use of thalidomide in the management of severe sweating in patients with advanced malignancy: trial report. *Palliative medicine*. **14**: 429–431.
44 Calder K and Bruera E (2000) Thalidomide for night sweats in patients with advanced cancer. *Palliative medicine*. **14**: 77–78.
45 Aquilonius SM and Hedstrand U (1978) The use of physostigmine as an antidote in tricyclic anti-depressant intoxication. *Acta Anaesthesiologica Scandinavica*. **22**: 40–45.
46 Caine ED (1979) Anticholinergic toxicity. *New England Journal of Medicine*. **300**: 1278.
47 Newton RW (1975) Physostigmine salicylate in the treatment of tricyclic antidepressant overdosage. *Journal of the American Medical Association*. **231**: 941–943.

Updated (minor change) February 2022

Quick Clinical Guide: Death rattle (noisy rattling breathing)

Death rattle occurs in about one third of dying patients. It is caused by fluid collecting in the upper airway, arising from one or more sources

- saliva (most common)
- bronchial mucosa (e.g. inflammation/infection)
- pulmonary oedema
- gastric reflux.

Rattling breathing can also occur in patients with a tracheostomy.

Non-drug treatment

- if the patient is unconscious, ease the family's distress by explaining that the rattle is not distressing to the patient
- position the patient semi-prone to encourage postural drainage, but upright or semi-recumbent if the cause is pulmonary oedema or gastric reflux
- suction the upper airway but, because it can be distressing, generally restrict use to unconscious patients.

Drug treatment

If the rattle is associated with distressing breathlessness in a semi-conscious patient, supplement the recommendations below with an opioid (e.g. morphine) and an anxiolytic sedative (e.g. midazolam).

Saliva

Because they do not affect existing secretions, an antimuscarinic drug should be given SC as soon as the rattle begins (Table 1). Hyoscine *butylbromide* is widely used, because it is the cheapest and is free of CNS effects.

CSCI treatment is generally started at the same time as the first or second SC dose; increase the dose if ≥ 2 p.r.n. doses/day are needed.

Table 1 Antimuscarinic drugs for death rattle

Drug	*Stat and p.r.n. SC dose*	*CSCI dose/24h*
Hyoscine *butylbromide*	20mg	20–120mg
Hyoscine *hydrobromide*	400microgram	1,200–1,600microgram
Glycopyrronium	200microgram	600–1,200microgram

In end-stage renal or hepatic failure, do *not* use hyoscine *hydrobromide*, because of an increased risk of delirium. Use hyoscine *butylbromide* (dose unchanged) or, if unavailable, glycopyrronium (lower doses may be sufficient).

Respiratory tract infection

Generally, it is *not* appropriate to prescribe an antibacterial in an imminently dying patient. Rarely, one may be indicated if death rattle is caused by profuse purulent sputum in a semi-conscious patient.

Pulmonary oedema

Consider furosemide 20–40mg SC/IM/IV q2h p.r.n. Beware precipitating urinary retention.

Gastric reflux

Consider metoclopramide 10mg SC/IV q2h p.r.n. ± antacid, e.g. omeprazole 40mg by IV/SC infusion once daily.

Antimuscarinics block the prokinetic effect of metoclopramide; avoid concurrent use if possible.

Updated (minor change) February 2022

GLYCOPYRRONIUM

Class: Antimuscarinic.

Indications: Drying secretions (including surgical premedication, control of upper airway secretions (injection), COPD (inhalers), †sialorrhoea (PO solution authorized in children; see Dose and use), †drooling, †death rattle (noisy rattling breathing), †smooth muscle spasm (e.g. intestine, bladder), †inoperable intestinal obstruction), †paraneoplastic pyrexia and sweating, †hyperhidrosis.[1,2]

Contra-indications: See Antimuscarinics (p.4). For tachycardia (heart rate >100 beats/min), also see Pharmacology, and **hyoscine *butylbromide*** (p.16).

Pharmacology

Glycopyrronium is a synthetic ionized quaternary ammonium antimuscarinic which penetrates biological membranes slowly and erratically.[3] In consequence it rarely causes sedation or delirium.[4,5] Absorption PO is poor, and IV it is about 35 times more potent than PO.[6] Even so, glycopyrronium 200–400microgram PO t.d.s. produces plasma concentrations associated with an antisialagogic effect lasting up to 8h.[7-9]

By injection, glycopyrronium is 2–5 times more potent than **hyoscine *hydrobromide*** as an antisecretory drug,[6] and may be effective in some patients who fail to respond to **hyoscine**. However, the efficacy of parenteral **hyoscine *hydrobromide***, **hyoscine *butylbromide*** and glycopyrronium as antisialagogues is generally similar, with death rattle reduced in 1/2–2/3 of patients.[10] Further, provided that time is taken to explain the cause of the rattle to the relatives and there is ongoing support, relatives' distress is relieved in >90% of cases.[11]

Parenterally, the optimal single dose of glycopyrronium is 200microgram;[12,13] this appears less likely to increase heart rate and cause tachycardia compared with parenteral doses of other antimuscarinic drugs, e.g. **atropine**, **hyoscine *butylbromide*** (see p.15).[14,15] Nonetheless, comparative patient safety data are lacking and, even in young healthy volunteers, changes in cardiac conduction are seen after 200microgram IV.[14] Thus, particularly in those with cardiovascular disease, it would seem appropriate to consider applying similar contra-indications and cautions as for other antimuscarinics (p.6).

Although at standard doses glycopyrronium does not change ocular pressures or pupil size, it can precipitate narrow-angle glaucoma. It is excreted unchanged by the kidneys and lower doses may be sufficient in patients with severe renal impairment (see Chapter 17, p.746).[3,16]

Glycopyrronium can also be used in other situations where an antimuscarinic effect is needed, e.g. paraneoplastic pyrexia and sweating (see Antimuscarinics, Box E, p.9), hyperhidrosis, sialorrhoea and drooling.

Glycopyrronium PO or SL has been used to reduce drooling in adults with various conditions, e.g. MND/ALS, Parkinson's disease, cancers of the head and neck or oesophagus.[17-19] PO solutions authorized for drooling in children and adolescents ≥3 years with chronic neurological disorders are available (see Dose and use).[20] Glycopyrronium has also been given by nebulizer.[19] It is also used as a bronchodilator (inhaled or nebulized) in asthma and COPD.[21,22]

Bio-availability <5% PO.

Onset of action 1min IV; 30–40min SC, PO.

Time to peak plasma concentration immediate IV; no data SC, PO.

Plasma halflife 1–1.5h.

Duration of action 7h.

Cautions

See Antimuscarinics (p.6); renal impairment (lower doses may be sufficient; also see Chapter 17, p.746).

Drug interactions

Concurrent treatment with ≥2 antimuscarinic drugs (including antihistamines, phenothiazines and TCAs; see Antimuscarinics, Box B, p.4) will increase the likelihood of undesirable effects (see Antimuscarinics, Box C, p.5).

See Antimuscarinics (p.7).

Undesirable effects

Peripheral antimuscarinic effects (see Antimuscarinics, Box C, p.5). The US Product Information lists the following effects, which are not included in the UK SPC:
Very common (>10%): inflammation at the injection site.
Common (<10%, >1%): dysphagia, photosensitivity.

Dose and use

Glycopyrronium is an alternative to **hyoscine *hydrobromide***, **hyoscine *butylbromide*** and **atropine**.[18,23,24] For indications where a parenteral antimuscarinic is required, *PCF* generally prefers **hyoscine *butylbromide***; it is unlikely to cause CNS effects and is cheaper than glycopyrronium.

For CSCI, dilute with WFI, sodium chloride 0.9% or glucose 5%.

CSCI compatibility with other drugs: There are 2-drug compatibility data for glycopyrronium in WFI with **alfentanil**, **clonazepam**, **diamorphine**, **haloperidol**, **hydromorphone**, **levomepromazine**, **metoclopramide**, **midazolam**, **morphine sulfate** and **oxycodone**.

Glycopyrronium is *incompatible* with **dexamethasone** and **ketorolac**. For more details and 3-drug compatibility data, see Appendix 3 (p.933).

Compatibility charts for mixing drugs in sodium chloride 0.9% can be found in the extended appendix section of the on-line *PCF* on www.medicinescomplete.com.

†Antispasmodic and inoperable intestinal obstruction

- start with 200microgram SC stat
- continue with 600–1,200microgram/24h CSCI *and/or* 200microgram SC q2h p.r.n.

†Death rattle (noisy rattling breathing)[25]

See QCG: Death rattle (noisy rattling breathing), p.11:
- start with 200microgram SC stat
- continue with 600–1,200microgram/24h CSCI *and/or* 200microgram SC q1h p.r.n.
- alternatively, the SL route can be used: 100microgram SL q6h p.r.n.

†Drooling

Administer PO as an oral solution/suspension. Tablets are expensive and only available in higher doses. Various products are available (see Supply). The authorized PO solutions are indicated for severe sialorrhoea in children >3years and adolescents with chronic neurological disorders. Thus, use in adults is off-label. When considering an unauthorized product, cost, suitability and availability, particularly in a non-hospital setting, need to be considered (see Chapter 24, p.817).
- start with 200microgram PO stat and q8h
- if necessary, increase dose progressively every 2–3 days to 1mg q8h[26]
- occasionally doses of ≤2mg q8h are needed.

A subsequent reduction in dose may be possible, particularly when initial dose escalation has been rapid. Oral solutions/suspensions can be given by enteral feeding tube (also see Chapter 28, p.853).[9,18]

†Paraneoplastic pyrexia and sweating

- start with 200microgram PO t.d.s.
- if necessary, increase progressively to 2mg PO t.d.s. (also see Antimuscarinics, Box E, p.9).

†Localized hyperhidrosis

- apply topically as a 0.5–4% cream or aqueous solution once daily–b.d., avoiding the nose, mouth and particularly the eyes; do not wash treated skin for 3–4h[2,27]
- if severe, or if alternative treatments fail, use 1–2mg PO b.d.–t.d.s., titrated to response (see above and Supply for products available).[1]

Supply

Glycopyrronium *bromide* (generic)
Oral solution 1mg/5mL, 28 days @ 1mg t.d.s. = £255.
Tablets 1mg, 2mg, 28 days @ 1mg t.d.s. = £647. *Authorized as add-on therapy in treatment of peptic ulcer.*
Injection 200microgram/mL, 1mL or 3mL amp = £1.50.

Sialanar® (Proveca)
Oral solution 320microgram/mL glycopyrronium base (equivalent to 400microgram/mL (2mg/5mL) glycopyrronium *bromide*), 28 days @ 1mg t.d.s = £270.

Unauthorized oral products
Glycopyrronium *bromide*
Oral solution or oral suspension 200microgram/5mL, 500microgram/5mL, 2.5mg/5mL and 5mg/5mL, 28 days @ 1mg t.d.s. = £40; (available as a special order; see Chapter 24, p.817) *price based on 5mg/5mL oral solution specials tariff in community; prices vary significantly between formulations and quantities ordered.*
For locally prepared formulations, see Box A.

Box A Examples of locally prepared glycopyrronium formulations for PO use

From glycopyrronium powder[28]

Glycopyrronium oral solution 100microgram/mL
Dissolve 100mg of glycopyrronium powder (obtainable from AMCo) in 100mL of sterile or distilled water to produce a 1mg/mL concentrate. This is stable for about 28 days if stored in a refrigerator.

Dilute the required volume of the concentrate 1 part with 9 parts sterile or distilled water (i.e. for every 1mL of concentrate, add 9mL of water) to give a *glycopyrronium oral solution 100microgram/mL*.

To avoid microbial contamination, store in a refrigerator and discard any unused diluted solution after 1 week.

Cost: 28 days @ 1mg (10mL) t.d.s. = £11 worth of glycopyrronium powder (but need to buy 3g = £327).

Glycopyrronium oral suspension 500microgram/mL[29]
Add 5mL of glycerol to 50mg of glycopyrronium powder and mix to form a smooth paste. Add 50mL of Ora-Plus® in portions and mix well. Add sufficient Ora-Sweet® or Ora-Sweet SF® to make a total volume of 100mL.
This suspension is stable for 90 days at room temperature or in a refrigerator.
Cost: 28 days @ 1mg (2mL) t.d.s. = £9 worth of glycopyrronium powder (but need to buy 3g = £327).

From glycopyrronium injection

Glycopyrronium oral suspension 100microgram/mL[30]
Combine 25mL of Ora-Plus® and 25mL of Ora-Sweet®; add to 50mL of preservative-free glycopyrronium injection 200microgram/mL to make up to 100mL, and mix well.

Stable for 35 days at room temperature or in a refrigerator (refrigeration minimizes risk of microbial contamination).

In a taste test, this formulation masked the bitter taste of glycopyrronium better than water or syrup-based vehicles, and was preferred by most patients.

Cost: 28 days @ 1mg (10mL) t.d.s. = £210 worth of glycopyrronium injection.

Unauthorized topical products
Glycopyrronium *bromide*
Cream 2% (20mg/mL) in Cetomacrogol cream (Formula A) 30g = £180; (available as a special order; see Chapter 24, p.817).
For a locally prepared cream, see Box B.

Box B Example of locally prepared glycopyrronium cream 10mg/mL (1%)[31]

Mix 1g of glycopyrronium powder with propylene glycol to make a paste. Incorporate into a water-washable cream base until smooth, making a total of 100g. Refrigerate after preparation. Stable for 60 days.

Cost: 100g = £109 worth of glycopyrronium *powder* (but need to buy 3g = £327).

1 Solish N *et al.* (2007) A comprehensive approach to the recognition, diagnosis, and severity-based treatment of focal hyperhidrosis: recommendations of the Canadian Hyperhidrosis Advisory Committee. *Dermatologic Surgery*. **33**: 908–923.
2 Kim WO *et al.* (2008) Topical glycopyrrolate for patients with facial hyperhidrosis. *British Journal of Dermatology*. **158**: 1094–1097.
3 Mirakhur R and Dundee J (1983) Glycopyrrolate pharmacology and clinical use. *Anaesthesia*. **38**: 1195–1204.
4 Gram D *et al.* (1991) Central anticholinergic syndrome following glycopyrrolate. *Anesthesiology*. **74**: 191–193.
5 Wigard D (1991) Glycopyrrolate and the central anticholinergic syndrome (letter). *Anesthesiology*. **75**: 1125.
6 Mirakhur R and Dundee J (1980) A comparison of the effects of atropine and glycopyrollate on various end organs. *Journal of the Royal Society of Medicine*. **73**: 727–730.
7 Ali-Melkkila T *et al.* (1989) Glycopyrrolate; pharmacokinetics and some pharmacodynamics findings. *Acta Anaesthesiologica Scandinavica*. **33**: 513–517.
8 Blasco P (1996) Glycopyrrolate treatment of chronic drooling. *Archives of Paediatric and Adolescent Medicine*. **150**: 932–935.
9 Olsen A and Sjogren P (1999) Oral glycopyrrolate alleviates drooling in a patient with tongue cancer. *Journal of Pain and Symptom Management*. **18**: 300–302.
10 Hughes A *et al.* (2000) Audit of three antimuscarinic drugs for managing retained secretions. *Palliative medicine*. **14**: 221–222.
11 Hughes A *et al.* (1997) Management of 'death rattle'. *Palliative Medicine*. **11**: 80–81.
12 Mirakhur R *et al.* (1978) Evaluation of the anticholinergic actions of glycopyrronium bromide. *British Journal of Clinical Pharmacology*. **5**: 77–84.
13 Back I *et al.* (2001) A study comparing hyoscine hydrobromide and glycopyrrolate in the treatment of death rattle. *Palliative Medicine*. **15**: 329–336.
14 Mirakhur RK (1979) Intravenous administration of glycopyrronium: effects on cardiac rate and rhythm. *Anaesthesia*. **34**: 458–462.
15 Mirakhur R *et al.* (1978) Atropine and glycopyrronium premedication. A comparison of the effects on cardiac rate and rhythm during induction of anaesthesia. *Anaesthesia*. **33**: 906–912.
16 Ali-Melkkila T *et al.* (1993) Pharmacokinetics and related pharmacodynamics of anticholinergic drugs. *Acta Anaesthesiologica Scandinavica*. **37**: 633–642.
17 Hobson EV *et al.* (2013) Management of sialorrhoea in motor neuron disease: a survey of current UK practice. *Amyotrophic Lateral Sclerosis Frontotemporal Degeneration*. **14**: 521–527.
18 Rashid H *et al.* (1997) Management of secretions in esophageal cancer patients with glycopyrrolate. *Annals of Oncology*. **8**: 198–199.
19 UK Medicines Information (2017) Hypersalivation – can glycopyrronium be used to treat it? *Medicines Q&A*. www.evidence.nhs.uk.
20 NICE (2017) Severe sialorrhoea (drooling) in children and young people with chronic neurological disorders: oral glycopyrronium bromide. *Evidence summary*. www.nice.org.uk.
21 Hansel TT *et al.* (2005) Glycopyrrolate causes prolonged bronchoprotection and bronchodilatation in patients with asthma. *Chest*. **128**: 1974–1979.
22 Buhl R and Banerji D (2012) Profile of glycopyrronium for once-daily treatment of moderate-to-severe COPD. *International Journal of Chronic Obstructive Pulmonary Disease*. **7**: 729–741.
23 Lucas V and Amass C (1998) Use of enteral glycopyrrolate in the management of drooling. *Palliative Medicine*. **12**: 207.
24 Davis M and Furste A (1999) Glycopyrrolate: a useful drug in the palliation of mechanical bowel obstruction. *Journal of Pain and Symptom Management*. **18**: 153–154.
25 Bennett M *et al.* (2002) Using anti-muscarinic drugs in the management of death rattle: evidence based guidelines for palliative care. *Palliative Medicine*. **16**: 369–374.
26 Arbouw ME *et al.* (2010) Glycopyrrolate for sialorrhea in Parkinson disease: a randomized, double-blind, crossover trial. *Neurology*. **74**: 1203–1207.
27 Kavanagh GM *et al.* (2006) Topical glycopyrrolate should not be overlooked in treatment of focal hyperhidrosis. *British Journal of Dermatology*. **155**: 477–500.
28 Amass C (2007) Personal communication. Pharmacist, East and North Hertfordshire NHS Trust.
29 Anonymous (2004) Glycopyrrolate 0.5mg/mL oral liquid. *International Journal of Pharmaceutical Compounding*. **8**: 218.
30 Landry C *et al.* (2005) Stability and subjective taste acceptability of four glycopyrrolate solutions for oral administration. *International Journal of Pharmaceutical Compounding*. **9**: 396–398.
31 Glasnapp A and Schroeder BJ (2001) Topical therapy for localized hyperhidrosis. *International Journal of Pharmaceutical Compounding*. **5**: 28–29.

Updated September 2019

HYOSCINE BUTYLBROMIDE

Class: Antimuscarinic.

Indications: Smooth muscle spasm (e.g. bladder, GI tract), †drying secretions (e.g. †death rattle (noisy rattling breathing), †inoperable bowel obstruction).

Contra-indications: ***Parenteral:*** See Antimuscarinics (p.4). For tachycardia (heart rate >100 beats/min), also see Cautions below.

Pharmacology

Hyoscine *butylbromide* is an antimuscarinic (see p.4) and has both smooth muscle relaxant (antispasmodic) and antisecretory properties. It is a quaternary compound and, unlike **hyoscine *hydrobromide*** (p.18), it does not cross the blood-brain barrier. Consequently, it does not have a central anti-emetic effect or cause drowsiness.

Oral bio-availability, based on urinary excretion, is <1%.[1] Thus, any antispasmodic effect reported after PO administration probably relates to a local contact effect on the GI mucosa.[2] In an RCT, hyoscine *butylbromide* 10mg t.d.s. PO and **paracetamol** 500mg t.d.s. both significantly reduced the severity of intestinal colic by >50%.[3] However, the difference between the benefit from these two drugs (both given in suboptimal doses) and placebo was only 0.5cm on a 10cm scale of pain intensity. This is of dubious clinical importance.[4] Thus, the therapeutic value of PO hyoscine *butylbromide* for intestinal colic remains debatable.[5]

The main uses for hyoscine *butylbromide* in palliative care are as an antispasmodic and antisecretory drug in inoperable bowel obstruction, and as an antisecretory drug for death rattle (noisy rattling breathing). In bowel obstruction, in comparison with hyoscine *butylbromide* (60–80mg/24h CSCI), **octreotide** (300–800microgram/24h CSCI; see p.591) provides more effective and rapid improvements in nausea and vomiting and reduction in NG tube output.[6,7] However, in those patients responding to either drug, after about 3–6 days, overall symptom relief is similar, and NG tube removal is possible with both.[6,7] Further, the presence of colic would favour the use of hyoscine *butylbromide over* **octreotide**. For a suggested management approach, see QCG: Inoperable bowel obstruction (p.266).

In healthy volunteers, hyoscine *butylbromide* 20mg SC has a maximum antisecretory duration of action of 2h.[8] On the other hand, the same dose by CSCI is often effective for 1 day in death rattle. Hyoscine *butylbromide and* **hyoscine *hydrobromide*** act faster than **glycopyrronium** (p.12) for this indication,[9,10] but the overall efficacy is generally the same,[11] with death rattle reduced in 1/2–2/3 of patients. However, provided that time is taken to explain the cause of the rattle to the relatives and there is ongoing support, relatives' distress is relieved in >90% of cases.[12]

Bio-availability <1% PO.[1]

Onset of action <10min SC/IM/IV; 1–2h PO.[13]

Time to peak plasma concentration 15min–2h PO.1

Plasma halflife 5–10h.

Duration of action <2h in volunteers,[8] but possibly longer in moribund patients.

Cautions

The MHRA has issued a warning highlighting the risk of serious undesirable effects with hyoscine *butylbromide* injection in patients with underlying cardiac disease.[14] This followed the death of a patient in 2016 from cardiac arrest after IV hyoscine *butylbromide* during colonoscopy, and the coroner's recommendation to the MHRA to clarify the cautions in the SPC, emphasizing that 'additional caution should be exercised when administering IV hyoscine *butylbromide* to patients with ischaemic heart disease'.

In its own review, the MHRA identified reports of eight deaths over 16 years associated with the use of IV/IM hyoscine *butylbromide*, and published the following advice:

- hyoscine *butylbromide* injection can cause serious undesirable effects including tachycardia, hypotension and anaphylaxis
- these undesirable effects can result in a fatal outcome in patients with underlying cardiac disease, e.g. heart failure, coronary heart disease, cardiac arrhythmia, hypertension
- hyoscine *butylbromide* injection should be used with caution in patients with cardiac disease
- monitor these patients, and ensure that resuscitation equipment, and personnel who are trained to use this equipment, are readily available
- hyoscine *butylbromide* injection is contra-indicated in patients with tachycardia.

However, full data are not available, and it is difficult to interpret the specific relevance of the reports to use in a palliative care setting, where the SC/CSCI route of administration is more likely than IV/IM.

Nonetheless, in healthy volunteers, an increase in heart rate of ~15bpm is evident 5min after hyoscine *butylbromide* 20mg SC, which lasts about 1h. On the other hand, no effect on heart rate was observed with doses <0.4mg/min CIVI.[8] This equates to <575mg/24h, well above typical doses given CSCI in palliative care.

PCF advises clinicians to remind themselves of the long-standing cautions relating to the use of any antimuscarinic, particularly in patients with cardiovascular disease, and to continue to balance the potential for benefit and harm for each patient individually.

See Antimuscarinics (p.6). PO **hyoscine *butylbromide*** has a low bio-availability, reducing the likelihood of systemic antimuscarinic effects.

Drug interactions

Concurrent treatment with ≥2 antimuscarinic drugs (including antihistamines, phenothiazines and TCAs; see Antimuscarinics, Box B, p.4) will increase the likelihood of undesirable effects (see Antimuscarinics, Box C, p.5).

See Antimuscarinics (p.7).

Undesirable effects

Common (<10%,>1%): peripheral antimuscarinic effects (see Antimuscarinics, Box C, p.5).
Unknown: hypotension (IV), anaphylactic shock (see Cautions).

Dose and use

Hyoscine *butylbromide* is generally used SC/CSCI in palliative care because of poor PO bio-availability ± unsuitability of the PO route. For CSCI dilute with WFI, sodium chloride 0.9% or glucose 5%.

CSCI compatibility with other drugs: There are 2-drug compatibility data for hyoscine *butylbromide* in WFI with **alfentanil**, **clonazepam**, **dexamethasone**, **diamorphine**, **haloperidol**, **hydromorphone**, **levomepromazine**, **midazolam**, **morphine sulfate**, **octreotide** and **oxycodone**.

Incompatibility may occur with **cyclizine**. For more details and 3-drug compatibility data, see Appendix 3 (p.933).

Compatibility charts for mixing drugs in sodium chloride 0.9% can be found in the extended appendix of the on-line *PCF* on www.medicinescomplete.com.

Inoperable intestinal obstruction with colic

- start with 20mg SC stat and 60mg/24h CSCI and 20mg SC q1h p.r.n.
- if necessary, increase to 120mg/24h
- maximum reported dose 300mg/24h.

Note. The maximum benefit from hyoscine *butylbromide* may be seen only after about 3 days.[6,7] Some centres add **octreotide** 500microgram/24h CSCI if hyoscine *butylbromide* 120mg/24h fails to relieve symptoms adequately, see QCG: Inoperable bowel obstruction (p.266).[15,16]

For patients with obstructive symptoms without colic, **metoclopramide** (see p.268) should be tried before an antimuscarinic drug, because the obstruction is often more functional than organic. See QCG: Inoperable bowel obstruction (p.266).

Death rattle (noisy rattling breathing)

See QCG: Death rattle (noisy rattling breathing), p.11:

- start with 20mg SC stat
- continue with 20–60mg/24h CSCI, and/or 20mg SC q1h p.r.n.
- some centres use higher doses, namely 60–120mg/24h CSCI.[10]

Bladder spasm

Use only when more specific bladder antispasmodics (see p.611) are inappropriate, e.g. when PO route unavailable.

- start with 20mg SC stat
- continue with 60–120mg/24h CSCI, and/or 20mg SC q1h p.r.n.

Supply

Buscopan® (Sanofi)

Tablets 10mg, 28 days @ 20mg q.d.s. = £12. *Also available OTC as Buscopan® IBS Relief and Buscopan® Cramps.*

Injection 20mg/mL, 1mL amp = £0.25.

1 Boehringer Ingelheim GmbH *Data on file.*

2 Tytgat GN (2007) Hyoscine butylbromide: a review of its use in the treatment of abdominal cramping and pain. *Drugs.* **67**: 1343-1357.

3 Mueller-Lissner S *et al.* (2006) Placebo- and paracetamol-controlled study on the efficacy and tolerability of hyoscine butylbromide in the treatment of patients with recurrent crampy abdominal pain. *Alimentary Pharmacology & Therapeutics.* **23**: 1741-1748.

4 Farrar JT *et al.* (2000) Defining the clinically important difference in pain outcome measures. *Pain.* **88**: 287-294.

5 Thompson DG and Wingate DL (1981) Oral hyoscine butylbromide does not alter the pattern of small intestinal motor activity. *British Journal of Pharmacology.* **72**: 685-687.

6 Mystakidou K et *al.* (2002) Comparison of octreotide administration vs conservative treatment in the management of inoperable bowel obstruction in patients with far advanced cancer: a randomized, double-blind, controlled clinical trial. *Anticancer Research.* **22**: 1187-1192.

7 Peng X et *al.* (2015) Randomized clinical trial comparing octreotide and scopolamine butylbromide in symptom control of patients with inoperable bowel obstruction due to advanced ovarian cancer. *World Journal of Surgical Oncology.* **13**: 50.

8 Herxheimer A and Haefeli L (1966) Human pharmacology of hyoscine butylbromide. *Lancet.* **ii**: 418–421.

9 Back I *et al.* (2001) A study comparing hyoscine hydrobromide and glycopyrrolate in the treatment of death rattle. *Palliative Medicine.* **15**: 329–336.

10 Bennett M *et al.* (2002) Using anti-muscarinic drugs in the management of death rattle: evidence based guidelines for palliative care. *Palliative Medicine.* **16**: 369–374.

11 Hughes A *et al.* (2000) Audit of three antimuscarinic drugs for managing retained secretions. *Palliative Medicine.* **14**: 221–222.

12 Hughes A *et al.* (1997) Management of 'death rattle'. *Palliative Medicine.* **11**: 80–81.

13 Sanches Martinez J *et al.* (1988) Clinical assessment of the tolerability and the effect of IK-19 in tablet form on pain of spastic origin. *Investigacion Medica International.* **15**: 63-65.

14 MHRA (2017) Hyoscine butylbromide (Buscopan) injection: risk of serious adverse effects in patients with underlying cardiac disease. *Drug Safety Update.* www.gov.uk/drug-safety-update

15 Ripamonti CI *et al.* (2008) Management of malignant bowel obstruction. *European Journal of Cancer.* **44**: 1105-1115.

16 Ripamonti C and Mercadante S (2004) How to use octreotide for malignant bowel obstruction. *Journal of Supportive Oncology.* **2**: 357-364.

Updated September 2019

HYOSCINE HYDROBROMIDE

Class: Antimuscarinic.

Indications: Prevention of motion sickness, drying secretions (including surgical premedication, †sialorrhoea, †drooling, †death rattle (noisy rattling breathing) and †inoperable intestinal obstruction), †paraneoplastic pyrexia and sweating, †smooth muscle spasm (e.g. intestine, bladder).

Contra-indications: See Antimuscarinics (p.4). For tachycardia (heart rate >100 beats/min), also see **hyoscine *butylbromide*** (p.16).

Pharmacology

Hyoscine *hydrobromide* is a naturally occurring belladonna alkaloid with smooth muscle relaxant (antispasmodic) and antisecretory properties. Unlike **hyoscine *butylbromide***, hyoscine *hydrobromide* crosses the blood-brain barrier, and repeated administration SC q4h will result in accumulation and may lead to sedation and delirium. On the other hand, a small number of patients are stimulated rather than sedated by hyoscine *hydrobromide* (also see Antimuscarinics, p.4). For this reason, *PCF* generally prefers **hyoscine *butylbromide***; it is also cheaper.

Hyoscine *hydrobromide* is almost completely hepatically metabolized, and the metabolites are excreted in the urine. Despite hyoscine *hydrobromide* having a plasma halflife of several hours, the duration of the antisecretory effect in volunteers after a single dose is only about 2h.[1] On the other hand, particularly after repeated injections in moribund patients, a duration of effect of up to 9h has been observed.[2] Hyoscine *hydrobromide* relieves death rattle in 1/2–2/3 of patients.[3]

However, provided that time is taken to explain the cause of the rattle to the relatives and there is ongoing support, relatives' distress is relieved in >90% of cases.[2]

Hyoscine *hydrobromide* can also be used in other situations where an antimuscarinic effect is needed, e.g. sialorrhoea, drooling, paraneoplastic pyrexia and sweating (see Antimuscarinics, Box E, p.9), and smooth muscle spasm (e.g. intestine, bladder).

Hyoscine *hydrobromide* has anti-emetic properties (see p.258). However, generally it is only used as prophylactic treatment for motion sickness PO or by TD patch.[4] The TD patch:

- comprises a reservoir containing hyoscine 1.5mg
- the average amount of hyoscine absorbed *over 3 days* is 1mg
- because of an initial priming dose released from the patch, steady state is reached after about 6h and maintained for 3 days
- after a single application of two patches, the average elimination halflife is 9.5h
- after patch removal, because hyoscine continues to be absorbed from the skin, the plasma concentration only decreases to about one third over the next 24h
- absorption is best when the patch is applied on hairless skin behind the ear.[4]

The patch has also been used to control opioid-induced nausea and also oesophageal spasm.[5-7] Other off-label uses include the management of drooling and sialorrhoea in children and adults with various conditions, including disorders of the head and neck.[8-10]

Bio-availability 60–80% SL.

Onset of action 3–5min IM, 10–15min SL.

Time to peak effect 20–60min SL/SC, 24h TD.

Plasma halflife 1–4h IM.[11]

Duration of action IM 15min (spasmolytic), 1–9h (antisecretory).[11]

Cautions

See Antimuscarinics (p.4); renal and hepatic impairment (see Dose and use; also see Chapters 17 and 18, p.746 and p.776).

Drug interactions

Concurrent treatment with ≥2 antimuscarinic drugs (including antihistamines, phenothiazines and TCAs; see Antimuscarinics, Box B, p.4) will increase the likelihood of undesirable effects, and (when centrally acting) of central toxicity, e.g. restlessness, agitation, delirium (see Antimuscarinics, Box C, p.5). Children, the elderly, and patients with renal or hepatic impairment are more susceptible to the central effects of antimuscarinics.

See Antimuscarinics (p.7).

Undesirable effects

Antimuscarinic effects (see Box C, p.5), including central antimuscarinic syndrome, e.g. hyperactive delirium, drowsiness, ataxia.

TD patch: despite the relatively small dose, delirium has been reported;[12] local irritation ± rash occasionally occurs.

Dose and use

†*Death rattle (noisy rattling breathing)*

See QCG: Death rattle (noisy rattling breathing), p.11:

- start with 400microgram SC stat
- continue with 1,200microgram/24h CSCI, and/or 400microgram SC q1h p.r.n.
- if necessary, increase to 1,600microgram/24h CSCI
- avoid in patients with end-stage renal or hepatic failure because of an increased risk of delirium.

For CSCI dilute with WFI, sodium chloride 0.9% or glucose 5%.

CSCI compatibility with other drugs: There are 2-drug compatibility data for hyoscine *hydrobromide* in WFI with **clonazepam, cyclizine, dexamethasone, diamorphine, haloperidol, hydromorphone, levomepromazine, midazolam, morphine sulfate** and **oxycodone.**

For more details and 3-drug compatibility data, see Appendix 3 (p.933).

Compatibility charts for mixing drugs in sodium chloride 0.9% can be found in the extended appendix of the on-line *PCF* on www.medicinescomplete.com.

Note. *PCF* favours **hyoscine *butylbromide*** (p.15); it is cheaper and is free of CNS effects. Other options include **glycopyrronium** (p.12) and **atropine** (see Antimuscarinics, p.4).

†Drooling and sialorrhoea

TD patches contain metal and must be removed before MRI to avoid burns (see Chapter 30, p.901).
Wash hands after handling the TD patch (and wash the application site after removing the patch) to avoid transferring hyoscine *hydrobromide* into the eyes (may cause mydriasis and exacerbate narrow-angle glaucoma).
Also see general use of TD patches, Chapter 30, p.901.

- hyoscine *hydrobromide* 1.5mg TD patch applied behind the ear; remove after 3 days, applying the new patch behind the alternate ear
- behind the ear is the authorized site of application, but other areas, e.g. the back, have been used[13]
- one patch delivers 1mg over 3 days, i.e. approximately 300microgram/24h; if necessary, two patches can be used concurrently.[14,15]

Note. An alternative drug PO with antimuscarinic effects may be preferable in some patients because of convenience or concurrent symptom management, e.g. **amitriptyline** (see p.228).

Supply

Kwells® (Bayer Plc)
Tablets chewable 150microgram, 300microgram, 12 tablets = £2; *also available OTC.*

Scopoderm® (GlaxoSmithKline Consumer Health)
TD (post-auricular) patch 1.5mg (releasing 1mg over 3 days), 1 patch = £6.50; *also available OTC.*

Hyoscine *hydrobromide* (generic)
Injection 400microgram/mL, 1mL amp = £4.75; 600microgram/mL, 1mL amp = £5.50.

1 Herxheimer A and Haefeli L (1966) Human pharmacology of hyoscine butylbromide. *Lancet*. **ii**: 418–421.
2 Hughes A *et al.* (1997) Management of 'death rattle'. *Palliative Medicine*. **11**: 80–81.
3 Hughes A *et al.* (2000) Audit of three antimuscarinic drugs for managing retained secretions. *Palliative Medicine*. **14**: 221–222.
4 Clissold S and Heel R (1985) Transdermal hyoscine (scopolamine). A preliminary review of its pharmacodynamic properties and therapeutic efficacy. *Drugs*. **29**: 189–207.
5 Ferris FD *et al.* (1991) Transdermal scopolamine use in the control of narcotic-induced nausea. *Journal of Pain and Symptom Management*. **6**: 289-393.
6 Harris SN *et al.* (1991) Nausea prophylaxis using transdermal scopolamine in the setting of patient-controlled analgesia. *Obstetrics and Gynecology*. **78**: 673-677.
7 Murray-Brown F and Davies IL (2016) Oesophageal spasm, vomiting and hyoscine hydrobromide patch. *BMJ Supportive and Palliative Care*. **6**: 125-127.
8 Gordon C *et al.* (1985) Effect of transdermal scopolamine on salivation. *Journal of Clinical Pharmacology*. **25**: 407–412.
9 Becelli R *et al.* (2014) Use of scopolamine patches in patients treated with parotidectomy. *Journal of Craniofacial Surgery*. **25**: e88-89.
10 UK Medicines Information (2017) Hypersalivation - can hyoscine hydrobromide be used to treat it? *Medcines Q&A*. www.evidence.nhs.uk.
11 Ali-Melkkila T *et al.* (1993) Pharmacokinetics and related pharmacodynamics of anticholinergic drugs. *Acta Anaesthesiologica Scandinavica*. **37**: 633–642.
12 Wilkinson J (1987) Side-effects of transdermal scopolamine. *Journal of Emergency Medicine*. **5**: 389–392.
13 Lewis DW *et al.* (1994) Transdermal scopolamine for reduction of drooling in developmentally delayed children. *Developmental Medicine & Child Neurology*. **36**: 484–486.

14 Dreyfuss P *et al.* (1991) The use of transdermal scopolamine to control drooling. A case report. *American Journal of Physical Medicine and Rehabilitation*. **70**: 220–222.
15 Talmi YP *et al.* (1990) Reduction of salivary flow with transdermal scopolamine: a four-year experience. *Otolaryngology – Head and Neck Surgery*. **103**: 615–618.

Updated September 2019

PROPANTHELINE

Class: Antimuscarinic.

Indications: Smooth muscle spasm (e.g. bladder, intestine), urinary frequency and incontinence, hyperhidrosis, †gustatory sweating in diabetic neuropathy, †paraneoplastic sweating, †drooling and sialorrhoea.

Contra-indications: See Antimuscarinics (p.4). In addition, hiatus hernia associated with reflux oesophagitis; severe ulcerative colitis.

Pharmacology

Propantheline is a quaternary antimuscarinic (see p.4); it does not cross the blood-brain barrier and thus does *not* cause central effects. It doubles gastric half-emptying time[1] and slows GI transit generally. It has variable effects on drug absorption (see Drug interactions). Propantheline is extensively metabolized in the small intestine before absorption. *If taken with food, the effect of propantheline by mouth is almost abolished.*[2]
Bio-availability <50% PO (much reduced if taken after food).
Onset of action 30–60min.
Time to peak plasma concentration 2h.
Plasma halflife 2–3h.
Duration of action 4–6h.

Cautions

See Antimuscarinics (p.6).

Drug interactions

Concurrent treatment with ≥2 antimuscarinic drugs (including antihistamines, phenothiazines and TCAs; see Antimuscarinics, Box B, p.4) will increase the likelihood of undesirable effects (see Antimuscarinics, Box C, p.5).

See Antimuscarinics (p.7).

Undesirable effects

Peripheral antimuscarinic effects (see Antimuscarinics, Box C, p.5).

Dose and use

Intestinal colic

- start with 15mg t.d.s. *1h before meals* and 30mg at bedtime
- maximum dose 30mg q.d.s.

Urinary frequency

- same as for colic, but largely replaced by urinary antimuscarinics (see p.611), **amitriptyline** (see p.228) or **imipramine**.

Sweating

- same as for colic.

Also one of several alternatives to reduce †paraneoplastic sweating (for other options, see Antimuscarinics, Box D, p.8):

- give 15–30mg b.d.–t.d.s. *on an empty stomach*.

Has also been used for hyperhydrosis associated with spinal cord injury.[3]

†*Drooling and sialorrhoea*

Has been used in MND/ALS:

- give 15mg t.d.s.[4] *on an empty stomach*.

However, other options are generally preferred; see p.8.

Supply

Pro-Banthine® (Kyowa Kirin)

Tablets 15mg, 28 days @ 15mg t.d.s. and 30mg at bedtime = £26.

1 Hurwitz A *et al.* (1977) Prolongation of gastric emptying by oral propantheline. *Clinical Pharmacology and Therapeutics.* **22**: 206–210.

2 Ekenved G *et al.* (1977) Influence of food on the effect of propantheline and L-hyoscyamine on salivation. *Scandinavian Journal of Gastroenterology.* **12**: 963–966.

3 Canaday BR and Stanford RH (1995) Propantheline bromide in the management of hyperhidrosis associated with spinal cord injury. *The Annals of Pharmacotherapy.* **29**: 489–492.

4 Norris FH *et al.* (1985) Motor neurone disease: towards better care. *British Medical Journal.* **291**: 259–262.

Updated September 2019

PROKINETICS

Indications: See Box A.

Pharmacology

Prokinetics accelerate GI transit and include:

- D_2 antagonists, e.g. **domperidone** (p.271), **metoclopramide** (p.268)
- $5HT_4$ agonists, e.g. **metoclopramide**, **prucalopride**
- motilin agonists, e.g. **erythromycin**.

For drugs in development, RCTs of non-antibacterial motilin agonists have been disappointing, with more promising results seen with ghrelin agonists and acetylcholinesterase antagonists.[1]

Drugs that enhance intestinal transit indirectly are not considered prokinetics (e.g. bulk-forming agents; other laxatives; drugs that cause diarrhoea by increasing GI secretions, such as **misoprostol**). Some drugs increase contractile motor activity but not in a co-ordinated fashion, so do not reduce transit time, e.g. **bethanechol**. Such drugs are not prokinetic.[2]

D_2 antagonists and $5HT_4$ agonists act by triggering a cholinergic system in the wall of the GI tract (Table 1 and Figure 1).[3] This action is impeded by opioids. Further, antimuscarinic drugs competitively block cholinergic receptors on the intestinal muscle fibres (and elsewhere).[4] Thus, all drugs with antimuscarinic properties reduce the impact of prokinetic drugs. The extent of this depends on several factors, including the respective doses of the interacting drugs and times of administration. Thus, the concurrent administration of prokinetics and antimuscarinic drugs is generally best avoided. On the other hand, even if the peripheral prokinetic effect is completely blocked, **domperidone** and **metoclopramide** will still exert an anti-emetic effect at the dopamine receptors in the area postrema (see p.258).

Erythromycin is reported to improve symptoms in about half of patients. A review suggested that, overall, its prokinetic effect was greater than that of **metoclopramide** (Table 1). However, the studies, mainly in diabetic gastroparesis, were small and open to bias.[7] Further, **erythromycin** can cause intestinal colic and diarrhoea. There are concerns about the possible development of bacterial resistance or tolerance to the prokinetic effects of **erythromycin**, although there are reports of **erythromycin** 250mg b.d. given for over a year without apparent loss of efficacy.[8-10] Thus, **erythromycin** is generally used second-line when **metoclopramide** and **domperidone** have been ineffective. Although **azithromycin** and **clarithromycin** are also reported to improve gastric emptying, benefit has not been confirmed in an RCT.[11]

Table 1 Comparison of gastric prokinetic drugs[5]

Drug	*Erythromycin*	*Domperidone*	*Metoclopramide*
Mechanism of action			
Motilin agonist	+	–	–
D_2 antagonist	–	+	+
$5HT_4$ agonist	–	–	+
Response to treatment[a,b]			
Gastric emptying (mean % acceleration)	45	30	20
Symptom relief (mean % improvement)	50	50	40

a. all percentages rounded to nearest 5%

b. although acceleration in gastric emptying is a useful indicator of the efficacy of a prokinetic drug, it correlates poorly with symptom relief in gastroparesis and functional dyspepsia; this may be partly due to the frequent co-existence of impaired gastric accommodation and visceral hypersensitivity.[6]

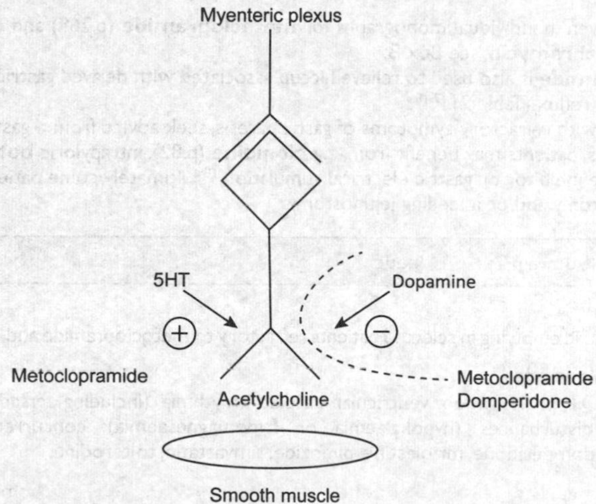

Figure 1 Schematic representation of drug effects on antroduodenal co-ordination via a postganglionic effect on the cholinergic nerves from the myenteric plexus.
⊕ stimulatory effect of 5HT triggered by metoclopramide;
⊖ inhibitory effect of dopamine;
– – – blockade of dopamine inhibition by metoclopramide and domperidone.

Prucalopride, a $5HT_4$ agonist that exerts mostly lower GI effects, is authorized for adults with chronic constipation that is failing to respond to laxatives (see p.40). RCT data also suggest **prucalopride** 2–4mg/24h PO may be of benefit in gastroparesis and GI pseudo-obstruction.[12,13] **Prucalopride** may have a role in treating constipation in patients with parkinsonism (see Laxatives, p.40).[14]

Use of prokinetics in palliative care

Prokinetics are used in various situations in palliative care, mostly off-label (Box A). D_2 antagonists block the dopaminergic 'brake' on gastric emptying induced by stress, anxiety and nausea from any cause. In contrast, $5HT_4$ agonists have a direct excitatory effect. However, when used for functional dyspepsia, dual-action **metoclopramide** is no more potent than **domperidone** in standard doses.[15,16]

Box A Indications for prokinetics in palliative care[a]

Functional dyspepsia (with delayed gastric emptying)

Gastro-oesophageal reflux disease

Gastroparesis (delayed gastric emptying)
- autonomic neuropathy, e.g. diabetic, paraneoplastic
- cancer, e.g. head of pancreas
- drug-induced, e.g. opioids
- post-surgical
- spinal cord compression/injury

Functional GI obstruction (peristaltic failure)
- cancer, e.g. linitis plastica (locally diffuse mural infiltration)
- drug-induced, e.g. opioids

Hiccup (Table 2)

a. mostly off-label; individual monographs list authorized indications.

Doses are given in individual monographs for **metoclopramide** (p.268) and **domperidone** (p.271); for **erythromycin**, see Box B.

Metoclopramide is also used to relieve hiccup associated with delayed gastric emptying and/or oesophageal reflux (Table 2).[17,18]

For patients with refractory symptoms of gastroparesis, seek advice from a gastroenterologist. In some settings, patients may benefit from, e.g. **clonidine** (p.82), intrapyloric **botulinum toxin**, a cholinesterase inhibitor or gastric electrical stimulation.[19] Ultimately, some patients may need a venting gastrostomy and/or a feeding jejunostomy.

Box B Erythromycin as a prokinetic

Indications

†Delayed gastric emptying in selected patients refractory to metoclopramide and domperidone.

Contra-indications

History of QT prolongation, ventricular cardiac arrythmia (including *torsade de pointes*), electrolyte disturbances (hypokalaemia or hypomagnesaemia); concurrent use with amisulpride, domperidone, mizolastine, pimozide, simvastatin, tolterodine.

Cautions

Coronary artery disease, severe cardiac insufficiency, conduction disturbances. Risk factors for QT interval prolongation (see Chapter 20, Box C p.800); known, or risk factors for, *Clostridium difficile* colonization.

Drug interactions

Concurrent use with other drugs that increase the QT interval should be avoided. Erythromycin is a moderately potent inhibitor of CYP3A4 and P-glycoprotein and can increase the plasma levels of drugs that are substrates of these, e.g. alfentanil, apixaban, carbamazepine, edoxaban, dabigatran, midazolam, rivaroxaban, statins, theophylline, warfarin (see Chapter 19, Table 8, p.790).

Dose

The optimal dose and frequency of administration is unknown, but benefit is seen below erythromycin's antibacterial dose.[20] Because of concern about tachyphylaxis, some also suggest starting with low doses, e.g.:[3]

- start with 50–100mg PO q.d.s. (use suspension) 30min before meals and at bedtime
- if necessary, increase every few days by 25–50mg/24h to 250mg q.d.s.
- maximum reported dose 500mg q.d.s.[20]

Others have started with higher doses (e.g. 250mg b.d.) and have seen prolonged benefit.[10]

Table 2 Drug treatment of hiccup (PO unless stated otherwise)[a]

Class of drug	*Drug*	*Acute relief*	*Maintenance regimen*
Reduce gastric distension ± gastro-oesophageal reflux			
Antiflatulent (carminative)	Peppermint oil[b,c]	One or two capsules	Probably best used p.r.n. only, see p.1
Antiflatulent (defoaming agent)	Simeticone	100–25mg	See p.1
Prokinetic	Metoclopramide[c,d]	10mg	10mg t.d.s.[21]
PPI	Lansoprazole	30mg	30mg each morning
Central suppression of the hiccup reflex			
First-line options			
$GABA_B$ agonist	Baclofen	5mg	5–10mg t.d.s., occasionally more[22-24]
Anti-epileptic	Pregabalin	25–75mg b.d. for 3 days[e] Also see p.302	25–75mg b.d.
	Gabapentin	100–400mg t.d.s. for 3 days[e] Also see p.302	≤400mg t.d.s.
Second-line options			
Dopamine antagonist	Metoclopramide	As above	As above
Third-line options			
L-type calcium-channel blocker	Nifedipine	10mg PO/SL	10–20mg t.d.s., occasionally more[25,26]
Anti-epileptic	Valproate	200–500mg	15mg/kg/24h in divided doses[27]
Dopamine antagonist	Haloperidol	1.5–3mg b.d.–t.d.s. (≤5mg t.d.s. if severe)	500microgram–1mg t.d.s. (≤3mg t.d.s. if severe)
Benzodiazepine	Midazolam	2mg IV, followed by 1–2mg increments every 3–5min	10–60mg/24h by CSCI if patient in last days of life[28]

a. mostly off-label; individual monographs list authorized indications
b. an old-fashioned remedy that facilitates belching by relaxing the lower oesophageal sphincter; can result in gastro-oesophageal reflux
c. peppermint oil and metoclopramide should not be used concurrently, because of their opposing actions on the gastro-oesophageal sphincter
d. tightens the lower oesophageal sphincter and hastens gastric emptying
e. use the lowest dose initially in elderly, frail patients and those with renal impairment.

Supply

For **metoclopramide**, **domperidone** and drugs in Table 2, see the respective individual drug monographs.

Erythromycin (generic)
Tablets e/c 250mg, 28 days @ 250mg q.d.s. = £5.50.
Oral suspension (as ethyl succinate) 125mg/5mL, 250mg/5mL, 500mg/5mL, 28 days @ 250mg q.d.s. = £48.

Prucalopride
Resolor® (Shire)
Tablets 1mg, 2mg, 28 days @ 2mg once daily = £60.

1 Vijayvargiya P *et al.* (2019) Effects of promotility agents on gastric emptying and symptoms: A systematic review and meta-analysis. *Gastroenterology*. **156**: 1650–1660.
2 Rayner CK and Horowitz M (2005) New management approaches for gastroparesis. *Nature Clinical Practice Gastroenterology and Hepatology*. **2**: 454-462.
3 Patrick A and Epstein O (2008) Review article: gastroparesis. *Alimentary Pharmacology and Therapeutics*. **27**: 724-740.
4 Schuurkes JAJ *et al.* (1986) Stimulation of gastroduodenal motor activity: dopaminergic and cholinergic modulation. *Drug Development Research*. **8**: 233–241.
5 Sturm A *et al.* (1999) Prokinetics in patients with gastroparesis: a systematic analysis. *Digestion*. **60**: 422–427.
6 Tack J and Camilleri M (2018) New developments in the treatment of gastroparesis and functional dyspepsia. *Current Opinion in Pharmacology*. **43**: 111–117.
7 Maganti K *et al.* (2003) Oral erythromycin and symptomatic relief of gastroparesis: a systematic review. *American Journal of Gastroenterology*. **98**: 259-263.
8 Dhir R and Richter JE (2004) Erythromycin in the short- and long-term control of dyspepsia symptoms in patients with gastroparesis. *Journal of Clinical Gastroenterology*. **38**: 237–242.
9 Hunter A *et al.* (2005) The use of long-term, low-dose erythromycin in treating persistent gastric stasis. *Journal of Pain and Symptom Management*. **29**: 430–433.
10 Rea E and Husbands E (2017) Erythromycin: prophylaxis against recurrent small bowel obstruction. *BMJ supportive & palliative care*. **7**: 261–263.
11 Acosta A and Camilleri M (2015) Prokinetics in gastroparesis. *Gastroenterology Clinics of North America*. **44**: 97–111.
12 Vijayvargiya P and Camilleri M (2019) Use of prucalopride in adults with chronic idiopathic constipation. *Expert review of clinical pharmacology*. **12**: 579–589.
13 Carbone F *et al.* (2019) Prucalopride in Gastroparesis: A Randomized Placebo-Controlled Crossover Study. *The American Journal of Gastroenterology*. **114**: 1265–1274.
14 Doi H *et al.* (2012) Plasma levodopa peak delay and impaired gastric emptying in Parkinson's disease. *Journal of the Neurological Sciences*. **319**: 86–88.
15 Loose FD (1979) Domperidone in chronic dyspepsia: a pilot open study and a multicentre general practice crossover comparison with metoclopramide and placebo. *Pharmatheripeutica*. **2**: 140–146.
16 Moriga M.(1981) A multicentre double blind study of domperidone and metoclopramide in the symptomatic control of dyspepsia. In: Towse G, editor. *International congress and symposium series: Progress with Domperidone, a gastrokinetic and anti-emetic agent*. International Congress Symposium. London: Royal Society of Medicine. 77–79.
17 Twycross R and Wilcock A (2016) *Introducing Palliative Care* (5e). palliativedrugs.com, Nottingham, 166–170.
18 Jeon YS *et al.* (2018) Management of hiccups in palliative care patients. *BMJ supportive & palliative care*. **8**: 1–6.
19 Myint AS *et al.* (2018) Current and emerging therapeutic options for gastroparesis. *Gastroenterology & Hepatology*. **14**: 639–645.
20 UKMI (2018) What is the optimal prokinetic dose of erythromycin in adults? *Medicines Q&A*. www.sps.nhs.uk.
21 Wang T and Wang D (2014) Metoclopramide for patients with intractable hiccups: a multicentre, randomised, controlled pilot study. *Internal Medicine Journal*. **44**: 1205-1209.
22 Ramirez FC and Graham DY (1992) Treatment of intractable hiccup with baclofen: results of a double-blind randomized, controlled, crossover study. *American Journal of Gastroenterology*. **87**: 1789–1791.
23 Guelaud C *et al.* (1995) Baclofen therapy for chronic hiccup. *European Respiratory Journal*. **8**: 235–237.
24 Zhang C *et al.* (2014) Baclofen for stroke patients with persistent hiccups: a randomized, double-blind, placebo-controlled trial. *Trials*. **15**: 295.
25 Lipps DC *et al.* (1990) Nifedipine for intractable hiccups. *Neurology*. **40**: 531–532.
26 Brigham B and Bolin T (1992) High dose nifedipine and fludrocortisone for intractable hiccups. *Medical Journal of Australia*. **157**: 70.
27 Jacobson P *et al.* (1981) Treatment of intractable hiccups with valproic acid. *Neurology*. **31**: 1458–1460.
28 Wilcock A and Twycross R (1996) Case report: midazolam for intractable hiccup. *Journal of Pain and Symptom Management*. **12**: 59–61.

Updated (minor change) April 2021

H_2-RECEPTOR ANTAGONISTS

In 2019, the manufacture of all **ranitidine** formulations stopped because of concerns about a carcinogenic contaminant (N-nitrosodimethylamine, NDMA).[1] Currently, it is unclear if **ranitidine** will be manufactured again.

In the absence of oral **ranitidine**, oral **famotidine** or nizatidine are suitable alternatives, given a similar lack of drug interactions. Local costs may influence the choice of one over another. *PCF* features **ranitidine** (until its ultimate fate is known) and **famotidine**.

The loss of injectable **ranitidine** is of greater relevance to palliative care practice, given its use in the medical management of malignant bowel obstruction. In the UK, parenteral **famotidine** is not available but may be imported (see below); experience of its use SC/CSCI is limited. Parenteral PPIs are a more readily available alternative (see p.31).

Class: Gastroprotective drugs.

Indications: Chronic episodic dyspepsia, acid reflux, prevention and treatment of peptic ulceration (including NSAID-related ulceration), reduction of malabsorption and fluid loss in short bowel syndrome (**cimetidine**), prevention of degradation of pancreatin supplements (**cimetidine**), †reduction of gastric secretions in bowel obstruction, †paraneoplastic sweating.

Pharmacology

Cimetidine, alone among H_2 antagonists, can cause serious CYP450-related drug interactions (see Drug interactions and Chapter 19, Table 8, p.790) and is best avoided.

H_2-receptor antagonists (H_2 antagonists) include **cimetidine**, **famotidine**, **nizatidine** and **ranitidine**. All are equally effective at gastric acid suppression.[2] However, because of their greater acid suppression and/or tolerability, PPIs (p.31) are generally preferred over H2 antagonists and **misoprostol**, which is now rarely used.[3] Other effects include increasing lower oesophageal sphincter pressure and reducing the volume of gastric secretions.[4,5] H_2 antagonists are more effective than PPIs in reducing the volume of gastric secretions, which has led some to recommend the use of **ranitidine** in patients with bowel obstruction.[5,6] Further, injection formulations of **ranitidine** (unlike PPIs) can be mixed with other drugs, making administration by CSCI more convenient (see Dose and use).

Anecdotally, H_2 antagonists are of benefit in paraneoplastic sweating.[7] The mechanism is unknown. An early therapeutic trial of an H_2 antagonist is reasonable on the basis that it is likely to be better tolerated than the other drugs used in this setting (see Antimuscarinics, Box E, p.9).

Pharmacokinetic data are shown in Table 1.

Table 1 Pharmacokinetic details for ranitidine and famotidine

	Ranitidine	*Famotidine*
Bio-availability	50% PO	40–45% PO
Onset of action	<1h	1h
Time to peak plasma concentration	2–3h PO 15min IM	1–3h PO
Plasma halflife	2–3h	3h
Duration of action	8–12h	6–10h (after single doses)

Cautions

Hepatic impairment, renal impairment (dose reduction required; see individual SPCs and Dose and use).

Gastric acid suppression is associated with an increased risk of *Clostridium difficile* infection; H_2 antagonists have a lower risk than PPIs (p.31).[8]

Drug interactions

H_2 antagonists increase gastric pH, and this reduces the absorption of some drugs and formulations. Clinically important examples include **itraconazole** (capsules only), **posaconazole**, antivirals and protein kinase inhibitors (seek specialist advice); see respective SPCs for full details. Rarely, absorption is increased, e.g. **saquinavir**.[9]

Cimetidine is the only H_2 antagonist that affects the CYP450 enzyme system. It is classified as a weak inhibitor of multiple CYP enzymes involved in drug metabolism (CYP1A2, CYP2D6, CYP2C19, CYP3A4/5). Thus, caution is required with concurrent use of drugs that are metabolized by these enzymes (see Chapter 19, Table 8, p.790). Table 2 lists interactions where close monitoring ± dose adjustment are required.

Table 2 Clinically important CYP450-related interactions with cimetidine[a,9]

Drug group	*Drug effect increased by cimetidine*[b]
Anticoagulants	Warfarin and other coumarins
Anti-epileptics	Carbamazepine (transient), phenytoin
Benzodiazepines	Alprazolam, diazepam, chlordiazepoxide, flurazepam, midazolam[c], nitrazepam, triazolam (not UK)
Calcium antagonists	Potentially all, including diltiazem and nifedipine
Local anaesthetics	Flecainide, lidocaine (IV), procainamide
Opioids	Alfentanil, fentanyl, methadone
SSRIs	All
TCAs	Potentially all
Xanthines	Aminophylline, theophylline
Miscellaneous	Erythromycin, mirtazapine, moclobemide, quinine, quinidine (not UK), zaleplon, zolmitriptan

a. *not* an exhaustive list; limited to drugs most likely to be encountered in palliative care and *excludes* anticancer, antiviral, HIV and immunosuppressive drugs (seek specialist advice)
b. either specifically reported or likely based on pharmacokinetic studies
c. midazolam reports inconsistent.

Undesirable effects

Cimetidine occasionally causes gynaecomastia.

Possible increased risk of pneumonia (gastric acid suppression leads to bacterial overgrowth in the upper-GI and respiratory tracts); association stronger for PPIs (p.31).[10]

Dose and use

NICE guidance: in the treatment of uninvestigated dyspepsia or proven gastro-oesophageal reflux disease, H_2 antagonists are a second-line option after PPIs (p.31). In all other acid-related disorders where efficacy may be similar, PPIs remain generally preferable to H_2 antagonists.[3]

Uninvestigated dyspepsia or reflux-like symptoms

For ≤6 weeks:
- **ranitidine** 150mg PO b.d. or 300mg at bedtime *or*
- **famotidine** 10mg PO b.d.

Proven gastro-oesophageal reflux disease

Initial treatment for 8–12 weeks:
- **ranitidine** 150mg PO b.d. or 300mg at bedtime *or*
- **famotidine** 20mg PO b.d.

Proven severe oesophagitis

Initial treatment for 8–12 weeks:
- **ranitidine** 150mg PO q.d.s. or 300mg b.d. *or*
- **famotidine** 40mg PO b.d.

Peptic ulcer (including NSAID-related)

- stop the NSAID; if continuation is necessary, use long-term gastric protection after ulcer healing (see below)
- test for *Helicobacter pylori:*
  - ▷ if negative, use an H_2 antagonist for 4–8 weeks (8 weeks if continuing an NSAID)
  - ▷ if positive, and the ulcer is NSAID-related, use an H2 antagonist for 8 weeks, followed by eradication therapy (see *BNF*) *or*
  - ▷ if positive, and the ulcer is *not* NSAID-related, use eradication therapy first and then review (see *BNF*)
- where indicated, use:
  - ▷ **ranitidine** 150mg PO b.d. or 300mg at bedtime (for NSAID-related *duodenal* ulcer give 300mg PO b.d for 4 weeks) *or*
  - ▷ **famotidine** 40mg PO at bedtime (unauthorized for NSAID-related ulcers)
- if symptoms recur, use the lowest effective dose either as long-term maintenance or, when symptoms are infrequent, p.r.n.

Gastric protection in patients taking an NSAID who are at high risk of peptic ulcer disease

- **ranitidine** 300mg PO b.d. *or* †**famotidine** 20mg PO b.d.
- *in addition,* consider switching the NSAID to a COX-2 selective NSAID, e.g. **celecoxib;**[3] also see NSAIDs, p.352.

Non-variceal upper-GI haemorrhage

See PPIs, p.31.

Bowel obstruction

See parenteral administration.

†Paraneoplastic sweating

- **ranitidine** 150mg PO b.d. *or*
- **famotidine** 20–40mg PO once daily.

Benefit is generally seen within 2–3 days.[7] Also see Antimuscarinics, Box E, p.9.

Parenteral administration

Ranitidine

Ranitidine 50mg can be given IM/IV t.d.s.–q.d.s. Although unauthorized, it is also given SC/CSCI:

- **ranitidine** 50mg SC b.d.–q.d.s. *or*
- **ranitidine** 150–200mg/24h CSCI, using WFI or sodium chloride 0.9% as diluent.

CSCI compatibility with other drugs: limited *clinical experience* suggests that **ranitidine** is compatible with **diamorphine, fentanyl, haloperidol, hydromorphone, hyoscine *butylbromide,* methadone, metoclopramide, morphine sulfate, octreotide** and **oxycodone.**

There are mixed reports of *incompatibility* with **levomepromazine** and **midazolam.** Successful combinations at lower concentrations are reported; to minimize the risk of precipitation, **ranitidine** should always be the last drug added to an already diluted combination of drugs.

For more information, see the www.palliativedrugs.com Syringe Driver Survey Database; we encourage members to submit combinations containing **ranitidine.**

Famotidine

Famotidine 20mg can be given IV b.d. diluted to 5mL with sodium chloride 0.9% and given over 2min (not UK; may be imported as a special order product).

SC/CSCI use is unauthorized and there is a lack of published information on such use. However, a reasonable approach may be:

- **famotidine** 20mg SC b.d. (case series poster, n=35)[11] *or*
- **famotidine** 40mg/24h CSCI, using WFI or sodium chloride 0.9% as diluent.[12]

CSCI compatibility with other drugs: limited *laboratory stability data* suggest that **famotidine** is compatible with **haloperidol**, **hydromorphone**, **metoclopramide**, **midazolam** and **morphine sulfate** at similar concentrations to those found in palliative care.[13] **Famotidine** appears compatible with **ketorolac** or **octreotide** at very low concentrations.[14,15]

We encourage members to submit combinations containing **famotidine** to the www.palliativedrugs.com Syringe Driver Survey Database.

Renal or hepatic impairment

- **ranitidine**: if CrCl <50mL/min, reduce PO dose to 150mg at bedtime; it can be increased to 150mg b.d. if an ulcer fails to respond; parenteral doses should be halved
- **famotidine**: if CrCl <50mL/min or patient is undergoing dialysis, halve the PO or parenteral dose.

In hepatic impairment, dose adjustment is not generally required for either **ranitidine** or **famotidine**.

Supply

Ranitidine (generic)

Tablets 150mg, 300mg, 28 days @ 150mg b.d. or 300mg at bedtime = £0.75.

Tablets effervescent 150mg, 300mg, 28 days @ 150mg b.d. or 300mg at bedtime = £35; *may contain Na⁺.*

Oral solution 75mg/5mL, 28 days @ 150mg b.d. or 300mg at bedtime = £15; *may contain alcohol. Sugar-free versions available.*

Injection 25mg/mL, 2mL amp = £0.50.

*Note. All **ranitidine** prices listed here are pre-discontinuation costs.*

Famotidine (generic)

Tablets 20mg, 40mg, 28 days @ 20mg b.d. or 40mg at bedtime = £24 or £38 respectively.

Injection 10mg/mL, 2mL vial = £3 (not UK; available to import, see Chapter 24, p.817). *Store in a fridge. Multidose vial may also be available.*

Ranitidine and **famotidine** tablets are available as an OTC measure for acid dyspepsia and heartburn.

1 Department of health and social care (2020) Ranitidine: all formulations update to SDA/2019/005. *Medicine supply notification. MSN/2020/025*. www.npa.co.uk.

2 Tougas G and Armstrong D (1997) Efficacy of H2 receptor antagonists in the treatment of gastroesophageal reflux disease and its symptoms. *Canadian Journal of Gastroenterology*. **11** (Suppl B): 51B–54B.

3 NICE (2014) Dyspepsia and gastro-oesophageal reflux disease. *Clinical Guideline*. CG184 (updated 2019). www.nice.org.uk.

4 Iwakiri K *et al.* (2011) The effects of nizatidine on transient lower esophageal sphincter relaxations (TLESRs) and acid reflux in healthy subjects. *Journal of Smooth Muscle Research*. **47**: 157–166.

5 Clark K *et al.* (2009) Reducing gastric secretions–a role for histamine 2 antagonists or proton pump inhibitors in malignant bowel obstruction? *Supportive Care in Cancer*. **17**: 1463–1468.

6 Currow DC *et al.* (2015) Double-blind, placebo-controlled, randomized trial of octreotide in malignant bowel obstruction. *Journal of Pain and Symptom Management*. **49**: 814–821.

7 Howard P (2022) Personal communication.

8 Tleyjeh IM *et al.* (2013) The association between histamine 2 receptor antagonist use and Clostridium difficile infection: a systematic review and meta-analysis. *PLoS One*. **8**: e56498.

9 Baxter K and Preston CL *Stockley's Drug Interactions*. London: Pharmaceutical Press. www.medicinescomplete.com (accessed May 2015).

10 Fohl AL and Regal RE (2011) Proton pump inhibitor-associated pneumonia: not a breath of fresh air after all? *World Journal of Gastrointestinal Pharmacology and Therapeutics*. **2**: 17–26.

11 Fang *et al.* (2012). Subcutaneous Administration of Famotidine Evaluation (SAFE). A retrospective study in palliative patients. [Case Series Poster].

12 Palliativedrugs.com Bulletin board (2020) Famotidine. Bulletin board thread (28 May 2020). *Royal Pharmaceutical Society*. www.palliativedrugs.com.

13 Keyi X *et al.* (1993). Stability of famotidine in polyvinyl chloride minibags and polypropylene syringes and compatibility of famotidine with selected drugs. *Annals of Pharmacotherapy*. **27**: 422–426.

14 Nassr S *et al.* (2001). HPLC-DAD method for studying the stability of solutions containing morphine, dexamethasone, haloperidol, midazolam, famotidine, metoclopramide, and dimenhydrinate. *Journal of Liquid Chromatography and Related Technologies*. **24**: 265–281.

15 Nassr S *et al.* (2003). HPLC-DAD methods for studying the stability of solutions containing hydromorphone, ketorolac, haloperidol, midazolam, *famotidine, metoclopramide, dimenhydrinate, and scopolamine. Journal of Liquid Chromatography and Related Technologies*. **26**: 2909–2929.

Updated (minor change) January 2022

PROTON PUMP INHIBITORS

Class: Gastroprotective drugs.

Indications: Authorized indications vary between products; consult the manufacturers' SPCs for details. They include acid dyspepsia, acid reflux, peptic ulceration, prevention and treatment of NSAID-related ulceration and eradication of *Helicobacter pylori* (with antibacterials), †prevention of degradation of pancreatin supplements (see p.63).

Pharmacology

Proton pump inhibitors (PPIs) include **esomeprazole** (the *S*-enantiomer of **omeprazole**), **lansoprazole**, **omeprazole**, **pantoprazole** and **rabeprazole**. Following absorption they are selectively taken up by gastric parietal cells and converted into active metabolites which irreversibly inhibit the proton pump (H^+/K^+-ATPase), thereby blocking gastric acid secretion.

PPIs provide symptomatic relief of acid dyspepsia and acid reflux, help prevent and heal peptic ulcers (including those associated with NSAIDs), and reduce the risk of recurrent ulceration and rebleeding.[1-3] Because of their greater acid suppression and/or tolerability, PPIs are generally preferred over H_2 antagonists (p.27) and **misoprostol**, which is now rarely used.[4] However, H_2 antagonists are more effective than PPIs in reducing the volume of gastric secretions, which may be an advantage in some situations, e.g. bowel obstruction (see p.27).

There is relatively little comparative data to guide the choice of one PPI over another on the basis of efficacy, and thus factors such as patient preference, risk of drug interaction, cost, and local guidelines will determine choice.[4]

Because PPIs are rapidly degraded by acid, they are formulated as e/c granules or tablets. These dissolve in the duodenum, where the drug is rapidly absorbed. The bio-availability of **lansoprazole** is reduced by food, and the manufacturer recommends that it should be given ≥30min before food. However, the reduced bio-availability appears not to reduce efficacy.[5-7]

The plasma halflives of PPIs are mostly <2h but, because they irreversibly inhibit the proton pump, the antisecretory activity continues for several days until new proton pumps are synthesized.

Elimination is predominantly by metabolism in the liver to inactive derivatives excreted mostly in the urine. Most PPIs are metabolized via CYP2C19 and to a variable extent CYP3A4; the exception is **rabeprazole**, which mostly undergoes non-enzymatic metabolism. CYP2C19 is subject to genetic polymorphism (see Chapter 19, p.783), with higher levels of activity associated with lower plasma concentrations of **omeprazole**, **lansoprazole** and **pantoprazole**, and higher rates of treatment failure, e.g. in *Helicobacter pylori* eradication.[8,9]

Pharmacokinetic data are shown in Table 1.

Onset of action <2h.

Duration of action >24h.

Table 1 Pharmacokinetic details of PPIs given PO

	Bio-availability (%)	*Time to peak plasma concentration (h)*	*Plasma halflife (h)*
Esomeprazole	68 (20mg dose) 89 (40mg dose)	1–2	1.3
Lansoprazole	80–90	1.5–2	1–2
Omeprazole	60	3–6	0.5–3
Pantoprazole	77	2–2.5	1
Rabeprazole	52	1.6–5	1

Cautions

The maximum daily dose should be reduced in severe hepatic impairment (see Dose and use, individual SPCs and Chapter 18, p.776). Rebound acid hypersecretion and dyspepsia can occur after stopping long-term PPI use.

Drug interactions

PPIs increase gastric pH, and this can affect the absorption of some drugs and formulations; generally, absorption is reduced, e.g. **itraconazole** (capsules only), **posaconazole**, antivirals and protein kinase inhibitors (seek specialist advice). However, rarely absorption can be increased, e.g. **digoxin** (high dose PPIs in the elderly) and **saquinavir**;[9] see respective SPCs for full details.

Esomeprazole and **omeprazole** are weak–moderate inhibitors of CYP2C19 (see Chapter 19, p.781). Important interactions include:

- inhibition of the metabolism of **citalopram** and **escitalopram**, increasing the risk of QT interval prolongation (see SSRIs, p.232, and Chapter 20, p.797); the maximum daily dose should be reduced (see SPC)[10]
- a reduction in the antithrombotic effect of **clopidogrel** (a pro-drug activated by CYP2C19); avoid concurrent use with any PPI, use an H_2 antagonist instead[11]
- inhibition of the metabolism of **diazepam**
- inhibition of the metabolism of **warfarin**; isolated reports of raised INR with all PPIs.[9]

Undesirable effects

Common (<10%, >1%): headache, abdominal pain, nausea, vomiting, diarrhoea or constipation, flatulence.

Clostridium difficile infection

PPI use about doubles the risk of *Clostridium difficile* infection;[12] this is about 40% higher than the risk associated with H_2-receptor antagonists.[13] PPIs also increase the risk of recurrent *Clostridium difficile* infection (OR 1.7).[12] Counts of *Clostridium difficile* organisms, which cannot survive at normal stomach pH, increase when the pH is >5 and go on to infect the bowel. Further, the spores can live for up to 6h on moist surfaces, long enough to allow transmission between patients.[14] The concomitant use of PPIs and antibacterials further increases the risk of *Clostridium difficile* infection (OR 3.5–4).[15]

Hypomagnesaemia

Severe hypomagnesaemia is rare and generally with prolonged use, i.e. >1 year. The measurement of serum magnesium before starting a PPI and periodically thereafter has been suggested for patients using a PPI long-term.[16] However, a routine annual measurement in every patient appears unnecessary and should be reserved for older patients, particularly those taking **digoxin** or drugs that can cause hypomagnesaemia, e.g. diuretics (also see Magnesium, p.638).[17]

Vitamin B_{12} deficiency

Gastric acid helps release vitamin B_{12} from dietary proteins, allowing its absorption. Thus, the risk of vitamin B_{12} deficiency increases with long-term PPI use.

Other toxicities

Renal toxicity: PPI use is associated with an increased risk of acute kidney injury and of developing chronic kidney disease. An acute interstitial nephritis may be responsible in some cases.[18] However, NSAID use is a common confounding variable, and definite causality is not established.[19]

Fracture: Observational studies suggest that PPIs are associated with a modest increase in the risk of hip, vertebral and any-site fracture with both short (<1 year) and long-term use.[20] Reduced GI absorption of calcium may contribute, but the exact mechanism is unclear; long-term PPI use does not appear to change bone structure or the rate at which bone mineral density is lost.[18] Those at risk of osteoporosis are recommended to ensure an adequate intake of vitamin D and calcium, using supplements if necessary.[21]

Pneumonia: PPI use is associated with an increased risk of community-acquired pneumonia, possibly via acid suppression leading to bacterial overgrowth in the upper GI and respiratory tracts. The increased risk is present in patients receiving PPIs for gastro-oesophageal reflux (also an independent risk factor for pneumonia), but not prophylactic PPIs taken because of NSAID use.[22,23]

Ocular damage: This has been reported, mostly with IV **omeprazole**.[24,25] PPIs possibly cause vasoconstriction by blocking H^+/K^+-ATPase. Because the retinal artery is an end-artery, anterior ischaemic optic neuropathy may result. If the PPI is stopped, visual acuity may improve, but some patients have become permanently blind, in some instances after only 3 days. Impaired hearing and deafness have also been reported, again mostly with IV **omeprazole.**

Hyponatraemia: The frequency of this is uncertain but PPIs may cause SIADH (see **Demeclocycline,** p.568). If no other cause for hyponatraemia is found, consider stopping PPI or switching to an H_2 antagonist.
Subacute cutaneous lupus erythematosus (SCLE): Reported very rarely in patients, weeks, months or even years after starting PPIs.[26]

Dose and use

In severe hepatic impairment both PO and parenteral doses may need to be reduced. See individual SPCs and Chapter 18, p.776.

PO dose recommendations are limited to **lansoprazole** and **omeprazole** (**esomeprazole, pantoprazole** and **rabeprazole** are more expensive) and are mostly based on NICE guidance (see Table 2), which can differ from the SPC and *BNF.*[4] In non-erosive reflux disease or mild oesophagitis, long-term maintenance treatment appears to provide better symptom control than p.r.n. use;[27] thus, the latter is best reserved for when symptoms are infrequent.

The SPC for **lansoprazole** states that administration should be ≥30min before food in order to achieve optimal acid inhibition. However, this precaution is unnecessary (see Pharmacology).

Table 2 NICE dose recommendations[4]

	Low dose	*Standard dose*	*Double dose*[a]
Lansoprazole	15mg once daily	30mg once daily	30mg b.d.
Omeprazole	10mg once daily	20mg once daily	40mg once daily

a. in severe hepatic impairment, do not exceed the standard dose.

Uninvestigated dyspepsia or reflux-like symptoms

- use standard dose PPI for 4 weeks; consider testing for *Helicobacter pylori* in patients with dyspepsia
- subsequently, use the lowest effective dose either as long-term maintenance or, when symptoms infrequent, p.r.n.
- if there is an inadequate response to a PPI, switch to an H_2 antagonist.

Proven gastro-oesophageal reflux disease

- use standard dose PPI for 4–8 weeks
- subsequently, use the lowest effective dose either as long-term maintenance or, when symptoms infrequent, p.r.n.
- if there is an inadequate response to a PPI, switch to an H_2 antagonist.

Proven severe oesophagitis

- use **lansoprazole** 30mg PO or **omeprazole** 40mg once daily for 8 weeks
- if inadequate, increase the dose to b.d. or switch to an alternate PPI
- subsequently, use the lowest effective dose as long-term maintenance as necessary.

Peptic ulcer (including NSAID-related)

- stop any NSAIDs; if continuation is necessary, use long-term gastric protection after ulcer healing (see below)
- test for *Helicobacter pylori:*
  - ▷ if negative, use standard dose PPI (or H_2 antagonist) for 4–8 weeks (8 weeks if continuing an NSAID)
  - ▷ if positive, and the ulcer is NSAID-related, use standard dose PPI (or H_2 antagonist) for 8 weeks, followed by eradication therapy (see *BNF*) *or*
  - ▷ if positive, and the ulcer is *not* NSAID-related, use eradication therapy first and then review (see *BNF*)
- if symptoms recur, use the lowest effective dose either as long-term maintenance or, when symptoms infrequent, p.r.n.

Gastric protection in patients taking an NSAID who are at high risk of peptic ulcer disease

- use standard dose PPI (or double-dose H_2 antagonist) *and*
- consider use of a COX-2 selective NSAID (continue gastric protection[4]) (see NSAIDs, p.352).

Non-variceal upper-GI haemorrhage

Ideally, an endoscopy should first confirm bleeding or stigmata of recent bleeding. A typical regimen is:[28]

- give an initial high dose of parenteral PPI, e.g. **esomeprazole** 80mg IVI in ≤100mL sodium chloride 0.9% over 30min
- continue parenteral administration for 72h, e.g. **esomeprazole** 40mg IV b.d.
- switch to PO administration, e.g. **omeprazole** 40mg PO once daily for 4 weeks.

Note. Although IV **omeprazole** can be used in identical doses to IV **esomeprazole**, it is unauthorized for this indication, the high-dose infusion takes longer (40–60min), and costs more. Conversely, PO **omeprazole** is cheaper than PO **esomeprazole.**

For patients with swallowing difficulties, **lansoprazole** and **omeprazole** can be given as orodispersible or dispersible tablets respectively (Note. There is *no* SL absorption from orodispersible tablets). Oral suspensions are available, but expensive (see Supply). Some *capsules* containing e/c granules can be opened and the e/c granules swallowed with water or fruit juice, or mixed with apple sauce or yoghurt; check the specific manufacturer's SPC. *Care must be taken not to crush or chew the e/c granules* (see Chapter 28, p.854).

Specific procedures are available from the manufacturers for administration by enteral feeding tubes (see Chapter 28, p.860). For patients with obstructive dysphagia and acid dyspepsia, or with severe gastritis and vomiting, the rectal route has also been used.[29]

Parenteral administration

IV **omeprazole** (**esomeprazole** and **pantoprazole**) are used in palliative care to treat painful reflux oesophagitis or upper-GI haemorrhage in patients unable to take PO medication.

Although PPIs are unauthorized for administration subcutaneously, there are case reports and small case series (largest **esomeprazole** CSCI in 7 patients over 17 days[30]) reporting such use:

- **esomeprazole:**
  - ▷ 40mg diluted in 50mL sodium chloride 0.9% and given by subcutaneous infusion over 20min–1h as a single daily dose[31]
  - ▷ 20mg diluted to a total volume of 33mL (*or* 40mg to 66mL) using sodium chloride 0.9% and given by CSCI over 24h[30]
- **omeprazole** 40mg diluted in 100mL sodium chloride 0.9% and given by subcutaneous infusion over 3–4h as a single daily dose[32]
- **pantoprazole** 40mg diluted in 10mL sodium chloride 0.9% and given by subcutaneous bolus over 2 minutes as a single daily dose;[33] this volume may be better tolerated given by subcutaneous infusion over 20min.

After reconstitution, PPI injections/infusions are alkaline (pH 8.6–11.5) and should not be mixed with other drugs. Note. **Esomeprazole** infusion may appear yellow.

Famotidine (not UK), a H_2-receptor antagonist, given IV, SC or CSCI is an alternative, see p.29.

Supply

Esomeprazole (generic)

Capsules enclosing e/c granules or hard e/c capsule 20mg, 40mg, 28 days @ 20mg each morning = £2.50.

Tablets e/c 20mg, 40mg, 28 days @ 20mg each morning = £2.50.

Sachets (containing e/c granules; Nexium®) 10mg, 28 days @ 20mg each morning = £50.

Injection (powder for reconstitution) 40mg vial = £2.50. Reconstitute with 5mL sodium chloride 0.9%. Doses ≤40mg can be given by IV bolus injection over 3min; or for IVI, further dilute in 500–100mL sodium chloride 0.9% and give over 10–30min.

Lansoprazole (generic)

Capsules enclosing e/c granules 15mg, 30mg, 28 days @ 30mg each morning = £0.75.

Tablets orodispersible 15mg, 30mg, 28 days @ 30mg each morning = £3.50.

Oral suspension 5mg/5mL, 15mg/5mL, 30mg/5mL, 28 days @ 30mg each morning = £27 (unauthorized products, available as a special order, p.817). Price based on Specials tariff in community.

Omeprazole (generic)
Capsules enclosing e/c granules or hard e/c capsules 10mg, 20mg, 40mg, 28 days @ 20mg each morning = £0.75.
Tablets e/c 10mg, 20mg, 40mg, 28 days @ 20mg each morning = £6.50.
Tablets dispersible enclosing e/c pellets 10mg, 20mg, 40mg, 28 days @ 20mg each morning = £10.
Oral suspension (sugar-free) 10mg/5mL, 20mg/5mL, 28 days @ 20mg each morning = £366.
Infusion (powder for reconstitution) 40mg vial = £5.00. Reconstitute with 5mL sodium chloride 0.9% and further dilute to 100mL. Doses ≤40mg can be given IVI over at least 20–30min. *The diluted solution is stable for 12h.*

Pantoprazole (generic)
Tablets e/c 20mg, 40mg, 28 days @ 40mg each morning = £1.
Injection (powder for reconstitution) 40mg vial = £4.50. Reconstitute with 10mL sodium chloride 0.9%. Doses ≤40mg can be administered by IV bolus or by IVI further diluted with 100mL sodium chloride 0.9% or glucose 5%, over 2–15 minutes. *The diluted solution is stable for 12h.*

Omeprazole and **esomeprazole** e/c tablets are available as an OTC measure for heartburn.

*For details of **rabeprazole**, see BNF; Combination products of **omeprazole** with **ketoprofen**, and **esomeprazole** with **naproxen** are also available.*

1 Frech EJ and Go MF (2009) Treatment and chemoprevention of NSAID-associated gastrointestinal complications. *Therapeutics and Clinical Risk Management.* **5**: 65–73.
2 Leontiadis GI *et al.* (2007) Systematic reviews of the clinical effectiveness and cost-effectiveness of proton pump inhibitors in acute upper gastrointestinal bleeding. *Health Technology Assessment.* **11**: iii–iv, 1–164.
3 Leontiadis GI *et al.* (2005) Systematic review and meta-analysis of proton pump inhibitor therapy in peptic ulcer bleeding. *British Medical Journal.* **330**: 568.
4 NICE (2014) Dyspepsia and gastro-oesophageal reflux disease. *Clinical Guideline.* CG184. www.nice.org.uk.
5 Moules I *et al.* (1993) Gastric acid inhibition by the proton pump inhibitor lansoprazole is unaffected by food. *British Journal of Clinical Research.* **4**: 153–161.
6 Delhotal-Landes B *et al.* (1991) The effect of food and antacids on lansoprazole absorption and disposition. *European Journal of Drug Metabolism and Pharmacokinetics.* **3**: 315–320.
7 Andersson T (1990) Bioavailability of omeprazole as enteric coated (ec) granules in conjunction with food on the first and seventh days of treatment. *Drug Investigations.* **2**: 184–188.
8 Shi S and Klotz U (2008) Proton pump inhibitors: An update of their clinical use and pharmacokinetics. *European Journal of Clinical Pharmacology.* **64**: 935–951.
9 Baxter K and Preston CL *Stockley's Drug Interactions.* London: Pharmaceutical Press www.medicinescomplete.com (accessed December 2017).
10 MHRA (2011) Citalopram and escitalopram: QT interval prolongation – new maximum daily dose restrictions (including in elderly patients), contraindications, and warnings. *Drug Safety Update.* **5**. www.gov.uk/drug-safety-update.
11 MHRA (2010) Clopidogrel and proton pump inhibitors: Interaction – updated advice. *Drug Safety Update.* **3**: www.gov.uk/drug-safety-update.
12 Oshima T *et al.* (2018) Magnitude and direction of the association between clostridium difficile infection and proton pump inhibitors in adults and pediatric patients: A systematic review and meta-analysis. *Journal of Gastroenterology.* **53**: 84–94.
13 Azab M *et al.* (2017) Comparison of the hospital-acquired clostridium difficile infection risk of using proton pump inhibitors versus histamine-2 receptor antagonists for prophylaxis and treatment of stress ulcers: A systematic review and meta-analysis. *Gut and Liver.* **11**: 781–788.
14 Jump RL *et al.* (2007) Vegetative clostridium difficile survives in room air on moist surfaces and in gastric contents with reduced acidity: A potential mechanism to explain the association between proton pump inhibitors and C. difficile-associated diarrhea? *Antimicrobial Agents and Chemotherapy.* **51**: 2883–2887.
15 Kwok CS *et al.* (2012) Risk of clostridium difficile infection with acid suppressing drugs and antibiotics: Meta-analysis. *American Journal of Gastroenterology.* **107**: 1011–1019.
16 MHRA (2012) Proton pump inhibitors in long term use: Reports of hypomagnesaemia. *Drug Safety Update.* **5**: www.gov.uk/drug-safety-update.
17 Begley J *et al.* (2016) Proton pump inhibitor associated hypomagnasaemia - a cause for concern? *British Journal of Clinical Pharmacology.* **81**: 753–758.
18 Nehra AK *et al.* (2018) Proton pump inhibitors: Review of emerging concerns. *Mayo Clinic Proceedings.* **93**: 240–246.
19 Kamal F *et al.* (2018) The association between proton pump inhibitor use with acute kidney injury and chronic kidney disease. *Journal of Clinical Gastroenterology.* **52**: 468–476.
20 Zhou B *et al.* (2016) Proton-pump inhibitors and risk of fractures: An update meta-analysis. *Osteoporosis International.* **27**: 339–347.
21 MHRA (2012) Proton pump inhibitors in long-term use: Recent epidemiological evidence of increased risk of bone fracture *Drug Safety Update.* **5**: www.gov.uk/drug-safety-update.
22 Hsu W-T *et al.* (2017) Risk of pneumonia in patients with gastroesophageal reflux disease: A population-based cohort study. *PLoS One.* **12**: e0183808.
23 Filion KB *et al.* (2014) Proton pump inhibitors and the risk of hospitalisation for community-acquired pneumonia: Replicated cohort studies with meta-analysis. *Gut.* **63**: 552–558.
24 Schonhofer P (1994) Intravenous omeprazole and blindness. *Lancet.* **343**: 665.

25 Schonhofer P et al. (1997) Ocular damage associated with proton pump inhibitors. *British Medical Journal.* **314**: 1805.
26 MHRA (2015) Proton pump inhibitors: Very low risk of subacute cutaneous lupus erythematosus. *Drug Safety Update.* **9**: www.gov.uk/drug-safety-update.
27 Boghossian TA et al. (2017) Deprescribing versus continuation of chronic proton pump inhibitor use in adults. *Cochrane Database of Systematic Reviews.* **3**: CD011969. www.cochranelibrary.com.
28 NICE (2016) Acute upper gastrointestinal bleeding in over 16s: Management. *Clinical Guideline* CG141. www.nice.org.uk.
29 Zylicz Z and van Sorge A (1998) Rectal omeprazole in the treatment of reflux pain in esophageal cancer. *Journal of Pain and Symptom Management.* **15**: 144–145.
30 Hindmarsh J et al. Administering esomeprazole subcutaneously via a syringe driver in the palliative demographic: A case series. *Journal of Clinical Pharmacy and Therapeutics.* 2021 December 27. Online ahead of print.
31 Desmidts T and Constans T (2009) Subcutaneous infusion of esomeprazole in elderly patients in palliative care: A report of two cases. *Journal of the American Geriatrics Society.* **57**: 1724–1725.
32 Agar M et al. (2004) The use of subcutaneous omeprazole in the treatment of dyspepsia in palliative care patients. *Journal of Pain and Symptom Management.* **28**: 529–531.
33 Michelon H et al. Subcutaneous pantoprazole in an elderly, palliative care patient. *BMJ Supportive & Palliative Care.* 2019 August 28. Online ahead of print.

Updated (minor change) February 2022

LOPERAMIDE

Class: Antimotility drug.

Indications: Acute and chronic diarrhoea, †ileostomy (to improve faecal consistency).[1]

Contra-indications: Colitis (ulcerative, infective or antibiotic-associated); acute dysentery; conditions where inhibition of peristalsis should be avoided because of a risk of ileus, megacolon or toxic megacolon.

Pharmacology

Loperamide is a potent μ-opioid receptor agonist (μ agonist).[2] Although well absorbed from the GI tract, loperamide is almost completely extracted and metabolized by cytochrome P450 (particularly CYP3A4) in the liver, where it is conjugated, and the conjugates excreted in the bile. Because of this extensive first-pass metabolism, in normal circumstances little loperamide reaches the systemic circulation.

The antidiarrhoeal action of loperamide results from direct absorption into the gut wall. Like **morphine** and other μ agonists, loperamide increases intestinal transit time by decreasing propulsive activity and increasing non-propulsive activity via its effect on the myenteric plexus in the longitudinal muscle layer.[3,4] Loperamide also increases anal sphincter tone and improves night-time continence in patients with ileo-anal pouches.[5]

Loperamide also modifies the intestinal transport of water and electrolytes by stimulating absorption[6] and by an anti-secretory action mediated by calmodulin antagonism, a property not shared by other opioids.[7-9]

Paradoxically, loperamide reduces the sodium-dependent uptake of glucose and other nutrients from the small bowel.[10] The development of tolerance to the GI effects of loperamide has been shown in animal studies.[11] However, loperamide has been successfully used in patients with chronic diarrhoea for several years without evidence of tolerance.[12]

Loperamide is a substrate for P-glycoprotein, the efflux membrane transporter in the blood-brain barrier, and, although highly lipophilic,[4] loperamide is actively excluded from the CNS.[13,14] Consequently, unlike **morphine**, which has both central and peripheral constipating effects, loperamide generally acts only peripherally when used within the recommended dose range.[2] Note. Higher levels of loperamide, e.g. associated with abuse, can overwhelm the P-glycoprotein pump and thereby produce CNS opioid effects (also see Undesirable effects).

Unlike other drugs used for diarrhoea, e.g. **diphenoxylate** (in **co-phenotrope**) and **codeine**, loperamide has no analgesic effect in therapeutic or supratherapeutic doses. The lack of CNS effects is one reason why loperamide is a popular first-line choice for the control of diarrhoea. This includes diarrhoea associated with chemotherapy or radiotherapy, although when severe and/or complicated loperamide is combined with **octreotide** (see Dose and use).[15]

As an antidiarrhoeal, loperamide is about 3 times more potent mg for mg than **diphenoxylate** and 50 times more potent than **codeine**.[16] It is longer acting and, if used regularly, generally needs to be given only b.d. However, its maximum therapeutic impact may not manifest for 16–24h; this has implications for initial dosing.[14] The following regimens are approximately equivalent:

- loperamide 2mg b.d.
- **diphenoxylate** 2.5mg q.d.s. (in **co-phenotrope**)
- **codeine phosphate** 60mg q.d.s.

Loperamide is available in a range of formulations. Orodispersible tablets (Imodium® Instants), which melt on the tongue, are bio-equivalent to the capsules and are preferred by some patients. A combination product with **simeticone** provides more rapid relief of diarrhoea and abdominal discomfort from bloating in acute non-specific diarrhoea than either loperamide or **simeticone** alone.[17,18] One suggested explanation is that the surfactant effect of **simeticone** enhances the contact of loperamide with the gut mucosa. However, both these products are relatively expensive (see Supply).

Bio-availability ~0.3%.

Onset of action about 1h; maximum effect 16–24h.[19]

Time to peak plasma concentration 2.5h (oral solution); 5h (capsules).[20]

Plasma halflife 11h,[20] but up to 41h with doses of ≥16mg/24h.[21]

Duration of action up to 3 days.[12]

Cautions

Loperamide should be used with caution in patients who are at risk of *torsade de pointes* or other cardiac arrhythmias (see Undesirable effects) and in patients who are using drugs that can alter the absorption or metabolism of loperamide (see Drug interactions).

Patients with AIDS are at risk of toxic megacolon if loperamide is used in viral or bacterial colitis.

Severe hepatic impairment (see Chapter 18, p.776, and Undesirable effects below).

Loperamide has become a drug of abuse, both to prevent withdrawal from other opioids and also to bring about euphoria in high doses.[22] High doses are associated with QT prolongation and potentially fatal cardiac arrhythmias, e.g. *torsade de pointes* (see Undesirable effects and Chapter 20, p.797).

Drug interactions

A patient on **clozapine** (an atypical antipsychotic) died of toxic megacolon after taking loperamide during an episode of food poisoning; additive inhibition of intestinal motility was considered the precipitating cause.[23]

Loperamide triples the PO bio-availability of **desmopressin**, possibly by both reducing GI enzymic degradation and slowing GI motility.[24]

Some CYP3A4 and P-glycoprotein inhibitors, e.g. **itraconazole**, increase plasma concentrations of loperamide significantly. Generally, these increases have not been associated with significant CNS effects. However, because of the risk of cardiac arrhythmia with high loperamide plasma concentrations, caution should be taken with potent CYP3A4 or P-glycoprotein inhibitors (see Chapter 19, Table 8, p.790).

Undesirable effects

Common (<10%, >1%): headache, dizziness, nausea, flatulence, constipation.

Uncommon (<1%, >0.1%): drowsiness, dry mouth, dyspepsia, vomiting, abdominal pain or discomfort, rash.

Rare (<0.1%, >0.01%): fatigue, depression of consciousness, incoordination, hypertonia, abdominal distension, ileus, faecal impaction, megacolon, urinary retention, angioedema, pruritus, urticaria, bullous skin eruptions.

CNS effects

Severe hepatic impairment can increase plasma concentrations of loperamide and the risk of undesirable effects, including suppression of consciousness ± respiration.[25] This may also occur in children, particularly <2 years, who receive excessive doses and in those who abuse loperamide in high doses (e.g. 100–400mg).[26-29] If **naloxone** is considered necessary, repeated doses may be needed because loperamide has a longer duration of action than **naloxone** (see Opioid antagonists (Therapeutic target within the CNS), p.490).

Cardiac arrythmias

Many of the reports of loperamide-induced cardiac arrhythmias occurred when loperamide was taken in higher than recommended doses (range 40–1600mg/24h), either for the treatment of diarrhoea or as a drug of abuse.[30-32]

Cardiac arrhythmias may occur if absorption is enhanced or metabolism inhibited (see Drug interactions). *Loperamide should be considered in any case of unexplained cardiac arrhythmia.* Plasma concentrations can be measured (normal therapeutic range 0.24–1.2mg/mL).[21,32]

Dose and use

Confirm that the diarrhoea is not secondary to a colitis (see Contra-indications) or faecal impaction.
In severe diarrhoea, ensure adequate fluid and electrolyte replacement is given, e.g. by using oral rehydration salts or IV fluids.

Note. For patients on a sodium-restricted diet, Imodium® *oral solution* contains Na^+ 4.85mg/5mL.

Acute diarrhoea

- start with 4mg PO stat
- continue with 2mg after each loose stool for up to 5 days
- maximum recommended dose 16mg/24h.

Chemotherapy- or radiotherapy-induced diarrhoea[15]

Seek specialist advice. A complicating feature is any one of the following: moderate–severe cramping, nausea and vomiting, fever, sepsis, neutropenia, bleeding, dehydration.

Mild–moderate and no complicating features

Increase in stools <7/day (or only moderate increase in stoma output):

- give 4mg PO stat
- continue with 2mg q4h or after each loose stool
- maximum recommended dose 16mg/24h.

Severe and/or any complicating feature (needs inpatient care)

Increase in stools ≥7/day (or severe increase in stoma output) and/or any complicating feature (see above): combine the above with **octreotide** (see p.591) and IV fluids. An exception is neutropenic enterocolitis, when antidiarrhoeal drugs should be avoided because of their potential to exacerbate ileus.

Note. Immunotherapy-related diarrhoea needs a different approach; loperamide should *not* be used other than when diarrhoea is mild (increase in stools <4/day, mild increase in stoma output).[33]

Chronic diarrhoea

If symptomatic treatment is appropriate, the same initial approach as for acute diarrhoea is used for 2–3 days, after which a prophylactic b.d. regimen is instituted based on the needs of the patient during the previous 24h, plus 2mg after each loose stool. The effective dose varies widely. It is sometimes necessary to increase the dose to 32mg/24h; *this is twice the recommended maximum dose/24h.* Such doses should *not* be used with a CYP3A4 inhibitor (see Drug interactions) or in someone at risk of a cardiac arrhythmia. Some recommend ECG monitoring when going above recommended doses (see below).

†High-output stoma/ileostomy or intestinal fistula

Very high doses of loperamide may be necessary to reduce life-threatening stoma or fistula output to safer/manageable volumes. Specialist guidelines in the UK regard 80mg/24h as the usual maximum dose.[32] Because of concerns over prolonged QT, an ECG should be done before increasing the dose above 16mg/24h, after any dose increase (time to steady state is 2–8 days) and every 3 years if remaining on a high dose. For doses >80mg/24h, additional monitoring of loperamide plasma concentrations is recommended; these should also be measured if cardiac concerns arise.[32]

Such doses should *not* be used with a CYP3A4 inhibitor (see Drug interactions) or in someone at risk of a cardiac arrhythmia. However, **octreotide** (± lower-dose loperamide) is probably a better option (see p.591).

Supply

Loperamide (generic)
Capsules 2mg, 5 days @ 2mg p.r.n., max 16mg/24h = £1.
Tablets 2mg, 5 days @ 2mg p.r.n., max 16mg/24h = £2.

Imodium® (Janssen)
Orodispersible tablets 2mg, 5 days @ 2mg p.r.n., max 16mg/24h = £13.
Oral solution (sugar-free) 1mg/5mL, 5 days @ 2mg p.r.n., max 16mg/24h = £4.75; *contains alcohol; also contains* Na^+ *4.85mg/5mL*.

With **simeticone**
Imodium® Plus (McNeil)
Caplets (capsule-shaped tablets) containing loperamide 2mg, **simeticone** 125mg, 5 days @ 1 p.r.n., max 4 caplets/24h = £7.

Loperamide capsules are available to purchase OTC for acute diarrhoea.

1 UK Medicines Information (2019) Can high dose loperamide be used to reduce stoma output? *Medicines Q&A*. www.evidence.nhs.uk.
2 Shannon H and Lutz E (2002) Comparison of the peripheral and central effects of the opioid agonists loperamide and morphine in the formalin test in rats. *Neuropharmacology*. **42**: 253–261.
3 Van Nueten JM *et al.* (1979) Distribution of loperamide in the intestinal wall. *Biochemical Pharmacology*. **28**: 1433-1434.
4 Ooms L *et al.* (1984) Mechanisms of action of loperamide. *Scandinavian Journal of Gastroenterology*. **19 (suppl 96)**: 145–155.
5 Hallgren T *et al.* (1994) Loperamide improves anal sphincter function and continence after restorative proctocolectomy. *Digestive Diseases and Sciences*. **39**: 2612-2618.
6 Dashwood MR *et al.* (1990) Autoradiographic demonstration of [3H] loperamide binding to opioid receptors in rat and human small intestine. *Progress in Clinical and Biological Research*. **328**: 165-169.
7 Merritt J *et al.* (1982) Loperamide and calmodulin. *Lancet*. **1**: 283.
8 Zavecz J *et al.* (1982) Relationship between anti-diarrheal activity and binding to calmodulin. *European Journal of Pharmacology*. **78**: 375–377.
9 Daly J and Harper J (2000) Loperamide: novel effects on capacitative calcium influx. *Celluar and Molecular Life Sciences*. **57**: 149–157.
10 Klaren P *et al.* (2000) Effect of loperamide on Na+/D-glucose cotransporter activity in mouse small intestine. *Journal of Pharmacy and Pharmacology*. **52**: 679–686.
11 Tan-No K *et al.* (2003) Development of tolerance to the inhibitory effect of loperamide on gastrointestinal transit in mice. *European Journal of Pharmaceutical Sciences*. **20**: 357-363.
12 Heel R *et al.* (1978) Loperamide: A review of its pharmacological properties and therapeutic efficacy in diarrhoea. *Drugs*. **15**: 33–52.
13 Heykants J *et al.* (1974) Loperamide (R 18553), a novel type of antidiarrheal agent. Part 5: The pharmacokinetics of loperamide in rats and man. *Arzneimittel-Forschung Drug Research*. **24**: 1649–1653.
14 Sadeque A *et al.* (2000) Increased drug delivery to the brain by P-glycoprotein inhibition. *Clinical Pharmacology and Therapeutics*. **68**: 231–237.
15 Bossi P *et al.* (2018) Diarrhoea in adult cancer patients: ESMO Clinical Practice Guidelines. *Annals of Oncology*. **29**: 126–142.
16 Schuermans V *et al.* (1974) Loperamide (R18553), a novel type of antidiarrhoeal agent. Part 6: clinical pharmacology. Placebo-controlled comparison of the constipating activity and safety of loperamide, diphenoxylate and codeine in normal volunteers. *Arzneimittel-Forschung Drug Research*. **24**: 1653–1657.
17 Kaplan MA *et al.* (1999) Loperamide-simethicone vs loperamide alone, simethicone alone, and placebo in the treatment of acute diarrhea with gas-related abdominal discomfort. A randomized controlled trial. *Archives of Family Medicine*. **8**: 243-248.
18 Hanauer SB *et al.* (2007) Randomized, double-blind, placebo-controlled clinical trial of loperamide plus simethicone versus loperamide alone and simethicone alone in the treatment of acute diarrhea with gas-related abdominal discomfort. *Current Medical Research Opinion*. **23**: 1033-1043.
19 Dreverman JWM and van der Poel AJ (1995) Loperamide oxide in acute diarrhoea: a double-blind placebo-controlled trial. *Alimentary Pharmacology and Therapeutics*. **9**: 441–446.
20 Killinger J *et al.* (1979) Human pharmacokinetics and comparative bioavailability of loperamide hydrochloride. *Journal of Clinical Pharmacology*. **19**: 211–218.
21 FDA (2016) Drug safety communication: FDS warns about serious heart problems with high doses of the antidiarrheal medicine loperamide (Imodium), including from abuse and misuse. Available from: https://www.fda.gov/Drugs/DrugSafety/ucm504617.htm.
22 Vakkalanka JP *et al.* (2017) Epidemiologic trends in loperamide abuse and misuse. *Annals of Emergency Medicine*. **69**: 73-78.
23 Eronen M *et al.* (2003) Lethal gastroenteritis associated with clozapine and loperamide. *American Journal of Psychiatry*. **160**: 2242–2243.
24 Callreus T *et al.* (1999) Changes in gastrointestinal motility influence the absorption of desmopressin. *European Journal of Clinical Pharmacology*. **55**: 305–309.
25 Baker DE (2007) Loperamide: a pharmacological review. *Reviews in Gastroenterological Disorders*. **7 (Suppl 3)**: S11-18.
26 Friedli G and Haenggeli CA (1980) Loperamide overdose managed by naloxone. *Lancet*. **1**: 1413.
27 Minton N and Smith P (1987) Loperamide toxicity in a child after a single dose. *BMJ*. **294**: 1383.
28 Litovitz T *et al.* (1997) Surveillance of loperamide ingestions: an analysis of 216 poison center reports. *Journal of Toxicology and Clinical Toxicology*. **35**: 11-19.
29 Bhatti Z *et al.* (2017) Loperamide metabolite-induced cardiomyopathy and QTc prolongation. *Clinical Toxicology*. **55**: 659–661.
30 Swank KA *et al.* (2017) Adverse event detection using the FDA post-marketing drug safety surveillance system: Cardiotoxicity associated with loperamide abuse and misuse. *Journal of the American Pharmacists Association*. **57 (Supp 2)**: S63–S67.
31 MHRA (2017) Loperamide (Imodium): reports of serious cardiac adverse reactions with high doses of loperamide associated with abuse or misuse. *Drug Safety Update*. www.gov.uk.

32 British Intestinal Failure Alliance (2018) Position statement: The use of high dose loperamide in patients with intestinal failure. www.bapen.org.uk.
33 Le Haanen JB et al. (2017) Management of toxicities from immunotherapy: ESMO Clinical Practice Guidelines for diagnosis, treatment and follow-up. *Annals of Oncology*. **28 (Suppl 4)**: 119–142.

Updated October 2019

LAXATIVES

There is limited RCT evidence about laxative use in palliative care patients.[1] Consequently, guidelines for the management of constipation in palliative care are based largely on consensus best practice and expert opinion.[1-5]

Constipation is common in advanced cancer,[6] and is generally caused by multiple factors, e.g. poor diet, weakness, the underlying disease, drugs (particularly opioids). It can be defined as the passage of small, hard faeces infrequently and with difficulty,[2] and is characterized by:

- *slow GI transit:* prolonged transit time allows more absorption of water from the faeces by the GI tract, manifesting as decreased frequency of bowel movements and small, hard faeces[7,8]
- *disordered rectal evacuation:* the need to strain when defaecating.[7]

The aims of drug management of constipation are:

- to restore the amount of water in the faeces by:
  - ▷ reducing GI tract transit time
  - ▷ increasing faecal water
  - ▷ increasing the ability of the faeces to retain water
- to improve rectal evacuation by improving faecal consistency and promoting peristalsis.

There are two broad classes of laxatives: those acting predominantly as *faecal softeners* and those acting predominantly as *stimulant laxatives* (Table 1).

Table 1 Classification of commonly used laxatives

Class of laxative	*General mode of action*	*Common laxatives*
Faecal softeners		
Surface-wetting agents	Act as a detergent, lowering surface tension, thereby allowing water and fats to penetrate hard, dry faeces	Docusate sodium[a] Poloxamer 188 (in co-danthramer)
Osmotic laxatives	Water is retained in the gut lumen, with a subsequent increase in faecal volume	Lactulose syrup Macrogols (e.g. Movicol®) Magnesium hydroxide suspension (e.g. Phillips' Milk of Magnesia®), sometimes combined with liquid paraffin (a lubricant), e.g. Mil-Par® Magnesium sulfate (Epsom salts)
Stimulant laxatives	Act via direct contact with the submucosal and myenteric plexus in the large bowel, resulting in rhythmic muscle contractions and improved intestinal motility. Also increase water secretion into the bowel lumen, thereby adding a degree of softening	Bisacodyl Dantron Senna Sodium picosulfate
Lubricants	Coat the surface of the stool to make it more slippery and easier to pass	Liquid paraffin[b] Arachis oil
Bulk-forming agents (fibre)	Increase faecal bulk through water-binding and increasing bacterial cell mass. This causes intestinal distension and thereby stimulates peristalsis; only a limited role in palliative care	Ispaghula (psyllium) husk (e.g. Fybogel®) Methylcellulose (e.g. Celevac®) Sterculia (e.g. Normacol®)

a. reflects predominant action; at doses >400mg/24h also has a stimulant effect
b. limited role in palliative care due to potentially serious undesirable effects.

Faecal softeners also increase faecal mass and can thereby stimulate peristalsis. Further, **lactulose** (an osmotic laxative) is converted by colonic fermentation to organic acids that act as contact stimulants in the large bowel (see p.54).[9] Conversely, stimulant laxatives reduce water absorption from the faeces and thus have a softening action (see p.49).

At doses commonly used, **docusate sodium** (≤400mg/24h) acts mainly by lowering surface tension (enabling water and fats to penetrate into the substance of the faeces), but at higher doses it also acts as a stimulant laxative (see p.52).

To date, RCTs of laxatives in palliative care patients have failed to show clinically meaningful differences (Table 2). A Cochrane review has concluded that there is inadequate experimental evidence to guide the optimal treatment of constipation with laxatives.[1]

There is evidence for the benefit of some laxatives, e.g. **bisacodyl**, **sodium picosulfate**, **macrogols**, compared with placebo. However, these laxatives are rarely used as the comparator arm in RCTs of new medications.[10]

Table 2 RCTs of laxatives in palliative care patients

Interventions	*Sample size and setting*	*Outcome*
Senna and lactulose vs. co-danthramer (dantron and poloxamer)[11]	51 hospice inpatients	Participants on high-dose strong opioids; those receiving senna and lactulose had more bowel evacuations compared with those receiving co-danthramer, but there was no difference in patient preference
Senna and lactulose vs. magnesium hydroxide and liquid paraffin (unpublished data)[12]	118 hospice inpatients	No significant difference in efficacy outcomes between interventions
Senna vs. lactulose[13]	75 hospice inpatients	No significant difference in efficacy outcomes between interventions
Senna vs. misrakasneham (Ayurvedic herbal remedy)[14]	36 outpatients	No significant difference in efficacy outcomes between interventions
Senna vs. senna and docusate[15]	74 hospice inpatients	No significant difference between the groups, suggesting no benefit in routinely adding docusate. Although the dose of senna could be titrated to response, the dose of docusate was fixed and thus may not always have been optimal[16]
Senna vs. macrogol 3350[17]	70 outpatients	Both titrated to response. No significant difference in efficacy, tolerability or patient preference. High attrition rate resulted in an underpowered study

Given the limited RCT evidence, the following should be noted:

- an appreciation of the pathophysiology of constipation (particularly opioid-induced)[2,18] and of how different laxatives work, as well as their cost, will guide laxative choice
- generally, all laxatives given in sufficient quantities are capable of normalizing GI tract function in constipated patients[19,20]
- compliance with laxative treatment may be limited in individual patients by palatability, undesirable effects (e.g. colic, flatulence), volume needed and polypharmacy. Patient preference and drug tolerability should be taken into account
- the concurrent prescription of several different laxatives should be avoided
- laxative doses should be titrated every 1–2 days according to response, up to the maximum recommended or tolerable dose, before changing to an alternative
- immobile patients with faecal incontinence are at risk of perineal skin irritation from **dantron**-containing laxatives

- anal seepage with associated irritation can be problematic with **liquid paraffin**. Absorption of **liquid paraffin** can also cause a foreign-body granulomatous reaction. Absorption is enhanced by concurrent use of **docusate sodium**
- traditionally, a combination of a stimulant laxative with a faecal softener has been recommended in palliative care patients.[2,21] However, the results of the RCT that compared **senna** alone with **senna** and **docusate** in hospice patients (see Table 2)[15,16] and comparable results from a non-randomized, non-blinded sequential cohort study in cancer inpatients[21] suggest that it is reasonable to prescribe a stimulant laxative alone, at least initially[16]
- if an adequate result is not achieved after 3–4 days using a stimulant laxative alone despite dose titration, consider adding a faecal softener
- if colic occurs, a softener should be added
- if faecal leakage occurs, reduce the dose of the faecal softener.[2,3]

Rectal interventions

Rectal products available for the management of constipation include suppositories and enemas (see Rectal products, p.59). As far as possible, rectal interventions should be avoided in patients who are neutropenic or thrombocytopenic, because of the risk, respectively, of infection or bleeding.

About one third of palliative care patients need rectal measures,[22,23] either because of failed oral treatment or electively, e.g. in bedbound frail elderly patients, patients with paralysis (see QCG: Bowel management in paraplegia and tetraplegia, p.47).

A Cochrane review of the management of constipation and faecal incontinence in patients with central neurological disease included 22 trials and 902 patients with diagnoses such as Parkinson's disease, multiple sclerosis and spinal cord injuries. The review concluded that there was limited evidence supporting bulk-forming laxatives (**ispaghula**) or **macrogols** (and also for abdominal massage and transanal irrigation).[24]

Opioid-induced constipation

Opioids are a major contributory factor for constipation in palliative care patients, reducing quality of life and sometimes resulting in opioid discontinuation.[25-27] Opioids cause constipation by increasing ring contractions, decreasing propulsive intestinal activity and by enhancing the resorption of fluid and electrolytes.[28,29] Tolerance does not develop to these effects.[30] Although some strong opioids are possibly less constipating than **morphine** (e.g. **buprenorphine**, **fentanyl**, **methadone**), most patients receiving any opioid regularly will need a laxative concurrently.[31] Thus, as a general rule, all patients prescribed **morphine** (or another opioid) should also be prescribed a laxative (see QCG: Opioid-induced constipation, p.45).

Peripherally acting opioid antagonists represent an additional approach to the management of opioid-induced constipation (see p.45 and Opioid antagonists (Therapeutic target outside the CNS), p.500). There is moderate-quality evidence to suggest that, compared with placebo, both SC **methylnaltrexone** (in palliative care inpatients with advanced disease; 60% with cancer) and PO **naldemedine** (in outpatients with cancer) are effective in opioid-induced constipation in those who have not had a good response with conventional laxatives.[32]

Other approaches

Several other drugs are authorized for chronic idiopathic constipation and/or more specific circumstances (Table 3). Generally, their use is reserved for patients failing to respond to conventional laxatives.

A case series reported benefit from **linaclotide** 145–290microgram/24h PO or **prucalopride** 1–4mg/24h PO for constipation in patients with neurodegenerative parkinsonism.[33] **Prucalopride** may have a particular role for patients experiencing a delay in the onset of benefit from **levodopa** due to impaired gastric emptying (also see Prokinetics, p.22).[34]

For opioid-induced constipation in non-cancer pain, although improvements are seen compared with placebo, they are of uncertain clinical significance (**lubiprostone**), not always sustained (**prucalopride**),[35,36] or similar to those of **senna** (**lubiprostone**).[37] Consequently, specialist guidelines do not recommend their use.[38] An expert consensus statement considers them third-line drugs, for use only when laxatives (stimulant + faecal softener) and a peripherally acting opioid antagonist (see p.500) are inadequate.[39]

Table 3 Other drugs authorized for chronic idiopathic constipation

Drug	*Mode of action*	*Comments*
Linaclotide	Guanylate cyclase-C agonist ↑ secretion of ions and water into GI tract	In UK, only authorized for moderate–severe irritable bowel syndrome with constipation
Lubiprostone (not UK[a])	Chloride channel activator ↑ secretion of ions and water into GI tract	Also authorized for irritable bowel syndrome with constipation in women, and opioid-induced constipation
Prucalopride	$5HT_4$ agonist with mostly lower GI prokinetic effects	Also see Prokinetics (p.22). Dose 2mg PO once daily; use 1mg once daily in those >65 years and/or when eGFR <30mL/min/m^2

a. discontinued in the UK for commercial reasons.

1 Candy B *et al.* (2015) Laxatives for the management of constipation in people receiving palliative care. *Cochrane Database of Systematic Reviews*. **19**: CD003448. www.thecochranelibrary.com.

2 Larkin PJ *et al.* (2018) Diagnosis, assessment and management of constipation in advanced cancer: ESMO Clinical Practice Guidelines. *Annals of Oncology*. **29 (Suppl 4)**: 111–125.

3 NICE (2013) Palliative cancer care - constipation. Clinical Knowledge Summaries. http://cks.nice.org.uk.

4 Librach SL *et al.* (2010) Consensus recommendations for the management of constipation in patients with advanced, progressive illness. *Journal of Pain and Symptom Management*. **40**: 761–773.

5 Davies A *et al.* (2020) MASCC recommendations on the management of constipation in patients with advanced cancer. *Supportive Care in Cancer*. **28**: 23–33.

6 Droney J *et al.* (2008) Constipation in cancer patients on morphine. *Supportive Care in Cancer*. **16**: 453–459.

7 Soligo M *et al.* (2006) Patterns of constipation in urogynecology: clinical importance and pathophysiologic insights. *American Journal of Obstetrics and Gynecology*. **195**: 50–55.

8 Lewis SJ and Heaton KW (1997) Stool form scale as a useful guide to intestinal transit time. *Scandinavian Journal of Gastroenterology*. **32**: 920–924.

9 Jouet P *et al.* (2008) Effects of therapeutic doses of lactulose vs. polyethylene glycol on isotopic colonic transit. *Alimentary Pharmacology and Therapeutics*. **27**: 988–993.

10 Ford AC (2013) Death knell for placebo-controlled trials in chronic idiopathic constipation? *Gastroenterology*. **145**: 897–898.

11 Sykes N (1991) A clinical comparison of laxatives in a hospice. *Palliative Medicine*. **5**: 307–314.

12 Sykes N (1991) A clinical comparison of lactulose and senna with magnesium hydroxide and liquid paraffin emulsion in a palliative care population. [cited in Candy B et *al.* (2011) Laxatives or methylnaltrexone for the management of constipation in palliative care patients. *Cochrane Database of Systematic Reviews*. CD003448. www.thecochranelibrary.com.

13 Agra Y *et al.* (1998) Efficacy of senna versus lactulose in terminal cancer patients treatment with opioids. *Journal of Pain and Symptom Management*. **15**: 1–7.

14 Ramesh P *et al.* (1998) Managing morphine-induced constipation: a controlled comparison of an Ayurvedic formulation and senna. *Journal of Pain and Symptom Management*. **16**: 240–244.

15 Tarumi Y *et al.* (2013) Randomized, double-blind, placebo-controlled trial of oral docusate in the management of constipation in hospice patients. *Journal of Pain and Symptom Management*. **45**: 2–13.

16 Sykes N (2013) Emerging evidence on docusate: commentary on Tarumi et al. *Journal of Pain Symptom Management*. **45**: 1.

17 Hawley P *et al.* (2020) PEG vs. sennosides for opioid-induced constipation in cancer care. *Support Care Cancer*. **28**: 1775–1782.

18 Fallon M and Hanks G (1999) Morphine, constipation and performace status in advanced cancer patients. *Palliative Medicine*. **13**: 159–160.

19 Sykes NP (1996) A volunteer model for the comparison of laxatives in opioid-related constipation. *Journal of Pain and Symptom Management*. **11**: 363–369.

20 Portenoy RK (1987) Constipation in the cancer patient: causes and management. *Medical Clinics of North America*. **71**: 303–311.

21 Hawley PH and Byeon JJ (2008) A comparison of sennosides-based bowel protocols with and without docusate in hospitalized patients with cancer. *Journal of Palliative Medicine*. **11**: 575–581.

22 Twycross RG and Lack SA (1986) Control of Alimentary Symptoms in Far Advanced Cancer. Churchill Livingstone, Edinburgh, p. 173–174.

23 Twycross RG and Harcourt JMV (1991) The use of laxatives at a palliative care centre. *Palliative Medicine*. **5**: 27–33.

24 Coggrave M *et al.* (2014) Management of faecal incontinence and constipation in adults with central neurological diseases. *Cochrane Database of Systematic Reviews*. **13**: CD002115. www.thecochranelibrary.com.

25 Sykes N (1998) The relationship between opioid use and laxative use in terminally ill cancer patients. *Palliative Medicine*. **12**: 375–382.

26 Bell T *et al.* (2009) Opioid-induced constipation negatively impacts pain management, productivity, and health-related quality of life: findings from the National Health and Wellness Survey. *Journal of Opioid Management*. **5**: 137–144.

27 Candrilli SD *et al.* (2009) Impact of constipation on opioid use patterns, health care resource utilization, and costs in cancer patients on opioid therapy. *Journal of Pain and Palliative Care Pharmacotherapy*. **23**: 231–241.

28 Beubler E. Opiates and intestinal transport: in vivo studies. In: Turnberg LA, editor. *Intestinal secretion*. Hertfordshire: Smith Kline and French; 1983. p. 53–55.

29 Kurz A and Sessler DI (2003) Opioid-induced bowel dysfunction: pathophysiology and potential new therapies. *Drugs*. **63**: 649–671.

30 Ross GR *et al.* (2008) Morphine tolerance in the mouse ileum and colon. *Journal of Pharmacology and Experimental Therapeutics.* **327**: 561–572.
31 Radbruch L *et al.* (2000) Constipation and the use of laxatives: a comparison between transdermal fentanyl and oral morphine. *Palliative Medicine.* **14**: 111–119.
32 Candy B *et al.* (2018) Mu-opioid antagonists for opioid-induced bowel dysfunction in people with cancer and people receiving palliative care. *Cochrane Database of Systematic Reviews.* **6**: CD006332.
33 Freitas ME AA, Lang AE, Liu LWC (2018) Linaclotide and prucalopride for management of constipation in patients with parkinsonism. *Movement Disorders Clinical Practice.* **5**: 218–220.
34 Doi H *et al.* (2012) Plasma levodopa peak delay and impaired gastric emptying in Parkinson's disease. *Journal of the Neurological Sciences.* **319**: 86–88.
35 Wald A (2016) Constipation: Advances in Diagnosis and Treatment. *JAMA.* **315**: 185–191.
36 Vijayvargiya P and Camilleri M (2019) Use of prucalopride in adults with chronic idiopathic constipation. *Expert review of clinical pharmacology.* **12**: 579–589.
37 Marciniak CM *et al.* (2014) Lubiprostone vs Senna in postoperative orthopedic surgery patients with opioid-induced constipation: a double-blind, active-comparator trial. *World Journal of Gastroenterology.* **20**: 16323–16333.
38 Crockett SD *et al.* (2019) American Gastroenterological Association Institute Guideline on the Medical Management of Opioid-Induced Constipation. *Gastroenterology.* **156**: 218–226.
39 Farmer AD *et al.* (2019) Pathophysiology and management of opioid-induced constipation: European expert consensus statement. *United European gastroenterology journal.* **7**: 7–20.

Updated (minor change) January 2020

Quick Clinical Guide: Opioid-induced constipation

Generally, all patients prescribed an opioid should also be prescribed a laxative, with the aim of achieving bowel movement without straining every 1–3 days. A standardized protocol aids management.

Although all laxatives given in sufficient quantities are capable of normalizing bowel function in constipated patients, *PCF* favours a stimulant laxative based on efficacy, convenience and cost.

Sometimes, rather than automatically changing to the local standard laxative, it may be more appropriate to optimize a patient's existing regimen.

These guidelines can also be followed in patients who are not on opioids, although smaller doses may well suffice.

1 Ask about the patient's past and present bowel habit and use of laxatives; record the date of last bowel action.

2 Palpate for faecal masses in the line of the colon; examine the rectum digitally if the bowels have not been open for ≥3 days or if the patient reports rectal discomfort or has diarrhoea suggestive of faecal impaction with overflow.

3 For inpatients, keep a daily record of bowel actions.

4 Encourage fluids generally, and fruit juice and fruit specifically.

5 When an opioid is prescribed, prescribe bisacodyl or senna and titrate the dose according to response:

Bisacodyl

If *not* constipated:

- generally start with 5mg at bedtime
- if no response after 24–48h, increase to 10mg at bedtime.

If already constipated:

- generally start with 10mg at bedtime
- if no response after 24–48h, increase to 20mg at bedtime
- if no response after a further 24–48h, consider adding a second daytime dose
- if necessary, consider increasing to a maximum of 20mg t.d.s.

Senna

If *not* constipated:

- generally start with 15mg at bedtime
- if no response after 24–48h, increase to 15mg at bedtime and each morning.

If already constipated:

- generally start with 15mg at bedtime and each morning
- if no response after 24–48h, increase to 22.5mg at bedtime and each morning
- if no response after a further 24–48h, consider adding a third daytime dose
- if necessary, consider increasing to a maximum of 30mg t.d.s.

An oral solution (7.5mg/5mL) is an alternative to tablets; it is tasteless and odourless.

6 During dose titration and subsequently, if ≥3 days since last bowel action, and there are faeces in the rectum, give suppositories, e.g. bisacodyl 10mg and glycerol 4g, or a micro-enema. If these are ineffective, administer a phosphate enema and possibly repeat the next day.

7 If the maximum dose of the stimulant laxative is ineffective and/or there has been no bowel evacuation within 3–4 days of commencing a stimulant, add a faecal softener laxative and titrate as necessary, e.g:

- macrogols (e.g. Movicol®) 1 sachet each morning *or*
- lactulose 15mL once daily–b.d.

8 In a patient receiving opioids, if adequately titrated oral laxatives + rectal interventions fail to produce the desired response, consider SC methylnaltrexone.

Methylnaltrexone
Methylnaltrexone is a peripherally acting opioid antagonist administered as an SC injection. It is relatively expensive and should be considered in patients with opioid-induced constipation only when the optimum use of laxatives is ineffective. In patients with advanced disease, because constipation is generally multifactorial in origin, methylnaltrexone is added to the existing laxative regimen.
• dose recommendations: ▷ for patients weighing 38-61kg, start with 8mg on alternate days ▷ for patients weighing 62–114kg, start with 12mg on alternate days ▷ outside this range, give 150microgram/kg on alternate days ▷ dose frequency can be varied as necessary; maximum use, once daily • in severe renal impairment (creatinine clearance <30mL/min), reduce the dose: ▷ for patients weighing 62–114kg, reduce to 8mg ▷ outside this range, reduce to *75microgram/kg*, rounding up the dose volume to the nearest 0.1mL • methylnaltrexone is contra-indicated in cases of known or suspected bowel obstruction. It should be used with caution in patients with conditions that may predispose to perforation • common undesirable effects include abdominal pain/colic, diarrhoea, flatulence, and nausea and vomiting; these generally resolve after a bowel movement; postural hypotension can also occur • about 1/3–1/2 of patients given methylnaltrexone have a bowel movement within 4h. The bowel movement can occur rapidly; consider having pads and a commode in place, particularly for those with poor mobility.

Note. An alternative is naldemedine 200microgram PO once daily. No dose adjustment is needed in renal or hepatic impairment.

9 If the stimulant laxative causes bowel colic, divide the total daily dose into smaller more frequent doses or use a faecal softener alone (see 7), and titrate as necessary.

10 As initial treatment, a faecal softener is preferable in patients with a history of colic with stimulant laxatives.

Updated January 2020

Quick Clinical Guide: Bowel management in paraplegia and tetraplegia

Introduction

This Quick Clinical Guide is informed by guidelines developed by the Multidisciplinary Association for Spinal Cord Injury Professionals (www.mascip.co.uk) but has a bias towards patients with cancer-related spinal cord compression.

The level and completeness of the spinal cord lesion determines the impact on bowel function and thereby the management approach. In all, there may be impaired/lost perception of the need to defaecate.

Level of spinal cord lesion	*Impact on bowel function*
Above T12–L1 (cauda equina and anal reflex intact)	*Reflex (spastic) bowel:* increased tone in colon and external anal sphincter results in constipation and faecal retention; loss of rectal sensation and voluntary control of the external anal sphincter can lead to reflex uncontrolled evacuation. *Generally responds to rectal stimulation (suppository, digital).*
Below T12–L1 (cauda equina involved, no anal reflex)	*Areflexic (flaccid) bowel:* flaccid colon and external anal sphincter results in constipation and a risk of faecal incontinence. *Generally needs digital removal of faeces.*
Conus medullaris (the distal end of the spinal cord, surrounded by the sacral nerves)	May manifest a mixture of the above features. *May need a mixed approach.*

Aims

An individualized bowel management programme has two broad aims.

1 To achieve the controlled regular evacuation of faeces:
- *reflex bowel:* aim for Bristol scale 4 faeces (smooth, soft, sausage-like) every day or alternate days
- *flaccid bowel:* aim for Bristol scale 3 faeces (sausage-like with surface cracks) to facilitate digital removal once or twice daily, occasionally more.

2 To prevent complications of constipation and incontinence, e.g. anal fissure, haemorrhoids, megacolon, megarectum, perineal skin ulceration.

Oral measures

3 When possible (may be difficult when appetite poor):
- maintain a high fluid intake
- encourage a well-balanced diet containing fruit, vegetables and whole grains.

4 If necessary, prescribe a stimulant laxative, e.g. senna 15mg PO, 8–12h before the bowel intervention; for those having intervention daily, and in those taking morphine or another constipating drug, this will equate to a regular bedtime dose. The dose should be carefully titrated to achieve the type of faeces required (see Aims), but without causing an uncontrolled evacuation or faecal incontinence.

5 Having something to eat or drink 15–30min before the bowel intervention may aid the movement of stool into the rectum (via the gastrocolic reflex).

Rectal and other measures

6 Initially, if impacted with faeces, empty the rectum digitally. Then develop a regular bowel intervention routine.

7 For *reflex bowel:*
- insert a stimulant suppository (e.g. bisacodyl 10mg) or an osmotic micro-enema into the rectum and wait for 30min
- abdominal massage may be of benefit, e.g.:
  - ▷ using the heel of the hand, apply gentle but firm pressure in one continuous movement clockwise along the lie of the colon
  - ▷ as above, but with lighter stroking movements
- the above measures may result in faeces being expelled
- to ensure complete evacuation of the rectum and sigmoid colon, digitally stimulate the rectum:
  - ▷ insert a double-gloved and lubricated finger
  - ▷ slowly rotate finger 3–4 times, maintaining contact with the rectal mucosa; generally within 15–20 seconds relaxation of the external sphincter is felt, flatus or faeces are passed, or the internal sphincter contracts (indicating colonic activity)
  - ▷ withdraw finger and wait 5min to allow for reflex passage of faeces; replace soiled outer glove with a clean one
  - ▷ if necessary, repeat the stimulation 3–4 times until rectum is fully empty
- if the above measures do not achieve complete evacuation of the rectum, proceed to digital removal of faeces:
  - ▷ insert a gloved and lubricated finger
  - ▷ gently remove small amounts of faeces at a time, avoiding using a hooked finger.

  Note. Autonomic dysreflexia (see below) can also occur in response to rectal stimulation caused by bowel intervention; instilling lidocaine 2% gel 5–10min before any rectal intervention may reduce the risk of a recurrence.

8 For *flaccid bowel:*
- consider following step 5 with abdominal massage (see step 7)
- if this fails, use digital removal of faeces.

9 Patients who are unable to transfer to the toilet or a commode will need nursing assistance. Sometimes it is easiest for a patient to defaecate onto a pad while in bed in a lateral position, with knees flexed.

10 A pattern will emerge for each patient, allowing the rectal measures to be adjusted to the individual patient's needs and response.

Autonomic dysreflexia in spinal cord transection (mostly T6 and above)

This potentially life-threatening overactivity of the autonomic nervous system can occur in response to noxious stimuli originating below the level of injury. Clinical features include: sudden uncontrolled rise in blood pressure (systolic ≥25mmHg above baseline) risking cerebral haemorrhage; pounding headache; flushing and sweating (above the level of the injury); cold with goose pimples (below the level of injury); nasal congestion; blurred vision; anxiety and breathlessness.

When possible and if the spine is stable, sit the patient up with legs down, and remove any tight clothing, e.g. socks and shoes. A distended rectum (or bladder) is a common cause and the immediate removal of faeces may be necessary using a gloved finger lubricated with lidocaine 2% gel. Similarly, if urinary catheterization is required, first instil lidocaine 2% gel into the urethra.

For persistent symptoms (and/or systolic blood pressure >150mmHg) give a vasodilator. If the patient has not used a phosphodiesterase type-5 inhibitor within the last 48h, use glyceryl trinitrate 400microgram spray (1–2 sprays) SL, repeat every 20–30min until resolved. If blood pressure remains high (or if the patient has used a phosphodiesterase type-5 inhibitor), options include nifedipine 10mg PO (bite into and swallow the liquid contents of an immediate-release capsule).

Seek specialist advice, e.g. from a spinal cord injury centre; hospital admission and management in a high-dependency unit may be required.

Updated (minor change) October 2021

ISPAGHULA (PSYLLIUM) HUSK

Ispaghula husk is *not recommended* for patients taking constipating drugs, and in those with decreasing dietary intake and activity. However, it can be helpful in regulating the consistency of faeces (making them more formed) in patients with faecal incontinence and those with a colostomy/distal ileostomy.

Class: Bulk-forming laxative.

Indications: Colostomy/ileostomy regulation, faecal incontinence, anal fissure, haemorrhoids, diverticular disease, irritable bowel syndrome, ulcerative colitis.

Contra-indications: Dysphagia, bowel obstruction, colonic atony, faecal impaction.

Pharmacology

Ispaghula (psyllium) is derived from the husks of an Asian plant, *Plantago ovata*. It has very high water-binding capacity, is partly fermented in the colon, and increases bacterial cell mass, thereby further increasing faecal bulk. Like other bulk-forming laxatives, ispaghula stimulates peristalsis by increasing faecal mass. Its water-binding capacity also helps to make loose faeces more formed in some patients with a colostomy/distal ileostomy.

Onset of action full effect obtained only after several days.

Duration of action best taken regularly to obtain a consistent ongoing effect; may continue to act for 2–3 days after the last dose.

Cautions

Adequate fluid intake should be maintained to avoid bowel obstruction.

Undesirable effects

Flatulence, abdominal distension, faecal impaction, bowel obstruction.

Hypersensitivity reactions in patients or carers as a result of ingestion, inhalation or skin contact with the powder.

Dose and use

Ispaghula swells in contact with fluid and needs to be drunk quickly before it absorbs water. Stir the granules or powder briskly in 150mL of water and swallow immediately; carbonated water can be used if preferred.

- give 1 sachet each morning–t.d.s., preferably after meals; not immediately before going to bed.

Supply

Ispaghula husk (generic)

Oral granules 3.5g/sachet, 28 days @ 1 sachet b.d. = £5; *sugar- and gluten-free, plain, lemon or orange flavour available.*

Updated October 2019

STIMULANT LAXATIVES

Indications: Prevention and treatment of constipation.

Contra-indications: Severe dehydration, acute inflammatory bowel disease, large bowel obstruction.

Pharmacology

Stimulant laxatives act through direct contact with the submucosal (Meissner's) plexus and the deeper myenteric (Auerbach's) plexus, resulting in both a motor and a secretory effect in the large intestine. The motor effect precedes the secretory effect and is the more important laxative action. There is a decrease in segmenting muscular activity and an increase in propulsive waves.

Senna (sennoside) is a naturally occurring plant-derived anthranoid and a pro-drug. It passes unabsorbed and unchanged through the small intestine as an inactive glycoside and is hydrolyzed by *bacterial glycosidases* in the large intestine to yield active compounds.[1] Thus, **senna** has no effect on the small intestine but becomes active in the large intestine. Differences in bacterial flora may be partly responsible for differences in individual responses.

Dantron is a synthetic anthranoid. It is not a glycoside and has a direct action on the large intestine.[2] Whereas systemic absorption of **senna** or its metabolites is small, **dantron** is absorbed to some extent from the small intestine with subsequent significant urinary excretion.

Bisacodyl and **sodium picosulfate** are phenolics and are both pro-drugs. They are hydrolyzed to the same active metabolite, bis-(p-hydroxyphenyl)-pyridyl-2-methane (BHPM), which stimulates propulsive motor activity and ion secretion into the GI tract.[1,3,4] **Bisacodyl** is hydrolyzed to BHPM by *intestinal enzymes* and, to ensure a laxative effect in the colon after oral intake, **bisacodyl** is formulated as an e/c tablet. **Sodium picosulfate** is hydrolyzed by *colonic bacteria* and thus potentially has a more uncertain action because of its dependence on bacterial flora. RCTs support the efficacy and safety of **bisacodyl** versus placebo and **sodium picosulfate** versus placebo in patients with chronic constipation.[5]

Bisacodyl is often given by suppository. The laxative effect is the result of local direct contact with the rectal mucosa after dissolution of the suppository and after activation by hydrolysis. Thus, the minimum time for response is generally >20min.[6]

Phenolphthalein (not UK) is a stimulant laxative that is present in some proprietary laxatives, e.g. Fam-Lax®. It is generally *not* recommended for use in palliative care, because it can cause a drug rash or photosensitivity. Rarely, it causes encephalitis, which can be fatal. It is also associated with increased risk of developing cancer. Laxatives containing **phenolphthalein** are prohibited in many countries.[7]

To date, RCTs of stimulant laxatives in palliative care patients have failed to show clinically meaningful differences (see Laxatives, Table 2, p.41). A small, non-blinded dose-ranging study in palliative care patients with opioid-induced constipation showed that **sodium picosulfate** alone yielded a satisfactory result in 15/20 patients (normal stool consistency, no need for enemas, suppositories or manual evacuation, and no noteworthy undesirable effects).[8]

In the past, a combination of a stimulant laxative with a faecal softener was often prescribed routinely in palliative care patients.[9,10] However, the results of an RCT that compared **senna** alone with **senna** and **docusate** in hospice patients (see Laxatives, Table 2, p.41)[11] and comparable results from a non-randomized, non-blinded, sequential cohort study in cancer inpatients suggest that *generally a stimulant laxative alone will be satisfactory*.[12,13] In countries where combined products are not available, this will also reduce the patient's tablet load.

If a stimulant laxative is used alone but a satisfactory result is not achieved despite dose titration within a week, consider adding a faecal softener. If faecal leakage occurs, the dose of this will need to be reduced.[9,14]

However, generally, all laxatives given in sufficient quantities are capable of normalizing bowel function in constipated patients (see p.40), and a small RCT suggests that in outpatients with cancer and opioid-induced constipation, bowel protocols based on **macrogol 3350** or **senna** appear similar in regards to efficacy, tolerability and patient preference (see Macrogols (polyethylene glycols), p.55).[15]

Nonetheless, because **senna** is cheaper, *PCF* continues to favour it as a reasonable first-line choice.

Onset of action

Bisacodyl tablets 6–12h;[6] suppositories 10–45min.[1]
Dantron 6–12h.
Senna 8–12h.
Sodium picosulfate 6–24h (median 12h).[8]

Cautions

Because very high doses in rodents revealed a carcinogenic risk,[16-18] UK marketing authorizations for laxatives containing **dantron** are limited to constipation in terminally ill patients.

Undesirable effects

Intestinal colic, diarrhoea. **Bisacodyl** suppositories may cause local rectal inflammation. **Dantron** discolours urine, typically red, but sometimes green or bluish. It may also stain the peri-anal skin. Prolonged contact with skin (e.g. in urinary or faecally incontinent patients) may cause a **dantron** burn (a red erythematous rash with a definite edge); if ignored, this may cause painful excoriation.

Dose and use

The doses recommended here for opioid-induced constipation are often higher than those featured in the *BNF* and SPCs. For frail patients not receiving opioids or other constipating drugs, the PO starting doses of a stimulant laxative will generally be lower.

Because round-the-clock opioids constipate, b.d. or t.d.s. laxatives may be necessary rather than the traditional once daily dose (at bedtime or each morning). Requirements do not correlate closely with the opioid dose; individual titration is necessary.

All palliative care services should have a protocol for the management of opioid-induced constipation (see QCG: Opioid-induced constipation, p.45).[19-21] Likewise, there is need for a protocol for patients with paraplegia and tetraplegia (see QCG: Bowel management in paraplegia and tetraplegia, p.47).

Bisacodyl

If *not* constipated:

- generally start with 5mg PO at bedtime
- if no response after 24–48h, increase to 10mg at bedtime.

If already constipated:

- generally start with 10mg PO at bedtime
- if no response after 24–48h, increase to 20mg at bedtime
- if no response after a further 24–48h, consider adding a second daytime dose
- if necessary, consider increasing to a maximum of 20mg t.d.s.

By suppository: give 10–20mg PR once daily. For an optimal result, it is best to give **bisacodyl** suppositories *30min after breakfast* and thereby co-ordinate the drug response with the gastrocolonic reflex.[22]

Dantron

Because of the undesirable effects and cost of **dantron**, other stimulant laxatives are preferred.

Senna

If *not* constipated:

- generally start with 15mg PO at bedtime
- if no response after 24–48h, increase to 15mg at bedtime and each morning.

If already constipated:

- generally start with 15mg PO at bedtime and each morning
- if no response after 24–48h, increase to 22.5mg at bedtime and each morning
- if no response after a further 24–48h, consider adding a third daytime dose
- if necessary, consider increasing to a maximum of 30mg t.d.s.

Senna oral solution (7.5mg/5mL) can be used instead of tablets; it is tasteless and odourless.

Sodium picosulfate

- start with 5–10mg (5–10mL of oral solution) at bedtime; 10mg if taking regular opioids
- if necessary, increase by 5mg/24h until a satisfactory result is achieved
- median satisfactory dose = 15mg at bedtime
- typical maximum dose = 30mg at bedtime.[8]

Consider a lower dose b.d. in the frail elderly.

Supply

Bisacodyl (generic)

Tablets e/c 5mg, 28 days @ 10mg at bedtime = £5.

Suppositories 5mg, 10mg, 28 days @ 10mg once daily = £8.

Senna (generic)
Tablets total **sennosides**/tablet 7.5mg, 28 days @ 15mg b.d. = £3.50.

Senokot® (Reckitt Benckiser)
Oral solution (sugar-free) total **sennosides** 7.5mg/5mL, 28 days @ 10mL b.d. = £5.50.

Sodium picosulfate (generic)
Oral solution (elixir) 5mg/5mL, 28 days @ 10mL at bedtime = £7; *may contain alcohol.*

Note. **Sodium picosulfate** oral solution 5mg/5mL is available as Dulcolax® Pico liquid. The proprietary name Dulcolax® (not prescribable on NHS prescriptions) is also used for **bisacodyl** tablets and suppositories.

1 Jauch R *et al.* (1975) Bis-(p-hydroxyphenyl)-pyridyl-2-methane: the common laxative principle of bisacodyl and sodium picosulfate. *Arzneimittel-Forschung Drug Research.* **25**: 1796–1800.
2 Lennard-Jones J. (1994) Clinical aspects of laxatives, enemas and suppositories. In: Kamm M, Lennard-Jones J, editors. *Constipation.* Petersfield: Wrightson Biomedical Publishing. p. 327–341.
3 De Schryver AM *et al.* (2003) Effects of a meal and bisacodyl on colonic motility in healthy volunteers and patients with slow-transit constipation. *Digestive Diseases Sciences.* **48**: 1206–1212.
4 Krueger D *et al.* (2018) bis-(p-hydroxyphenyl)-pyridyl-2-methane (BHPM) – the active metabolite of the laxatives bisacodyl and sodium picosulfate – enhances contractility and secretion in human intestine in vitro. *Neurogastroenterology & Motility.* **30**: e13311.
5 Noergaard M *et al.* (2019) Long term treatment with stimulant laxatives – clinical evidence for effectiveness and safety? *Scandinavian Journal of Gastroenterology.* **54**: 27–34.
6 Flig E *et al.* (2000) Is bisacodyl absorbed at all from suppositories in man? *International Journal of Pharmaceutics.* **196**: 11–20.
7 Cooper GS *et al.* (2000) Risk of ovarian cancer in relation to use of phenolphthalein-containing laxatives. *British Journal of Cancer.* **83**: 404–406.
8 Twycross RG *et al.* (2006) Sodium picosulfate in opioid-induced constipation: results of an open-label, prospective, dose-ranging study. *Palliative Medicine.* **20**: 419–423.
9 Larkin PJ *et al.* (2008) The management of constipation in palliative care: clinical practice recommendations. *Palliative Medicine.* **22**: 796–807.
10 Portenoy RK (1987) Constipation in the cancer patient: causes and management. *Medical Clinics of North America.* **71**: 303–311.
11 Tarumi Y *et al.* (2013) Randomized, double-blind, placebo-controlled trial of oral docusate in the management of constipation in hospice patients. *Journal of Pain and Symptom Management.* **45**: 2–13.
12 Sykes N (2013) Emerging evidence on docusate: commentary on Tarumi et al. *Journal of Pain Symptom Management.* **45**: 1.
13 Hawley PH and Byeon JJ (2008) A comparison of sennosides-based bowel protocols with and without docusate in hospitalized patients with cancer. *Journal of Palliative Medicine.* **11**: 575–581.
14 NICE (2013) Palliative care - constipation. *Clinical Knowledge Summaries.* http://cks.nice.org.uk
15 Hawley P *et al.* (2019) PEG vs. sennosides for opioid-induced constipation in cancer care. *Supportive Care in Cancer.* (epub ahead of print).
16 Mori H *et al.* (1985) Induction of intestinal tumours in rats by chrysazin. *British Journal of Cancer.* **52**: 781–783.
17 Mori H *et al.* (1986) Carcinogenicity of chrysazin in large intestine and liver of mice. *Japanese Journal of Cancer Research (Gann).* **77**: 871–876.
18 CSM (Committee on Safety of Medicines and Medicines Control Agency) (2000) Danthron restricted to constipation in the terminally ill. *Current Problems in Pharmacovigilance.* **26 (May)**: 4.
19 Larkin PJ *et al.* (2018) Diagnosis, assessment and management of constipation in advanced cancer: ESMO Clinical Practice Guidelines. *Annals of Oncology.* **29**: **(Suppl 4)** 111–125.
20 Farmer AD *et al.* (2019) Pathophysiology and management of opioid-induced constipation: European expert consensus statement. *United European Gastroenterology Journal.* **7**: 7–20.
21 Crockett SD *et al.* (2019) American Gastroenterological Association Institute Guideline on the Medical Management of Opioid-Induced Constipation. *Gastroenterology.* **156**: 218–226.
22 Bharucha AE *et al.* (2013) American Gastroenterological Association Technical Review on Constipation. *Gastroenterology.* **144**: 218–238.

Updated October 2019

DOCUSATE SODIUM

Class: Surface-wetting agent (faecal softener).

Indications: Constipation, haemorrhoids, anal fissure, bowel preparation before abdominal radiography, †partial bowel obstruction.

Pharmacology

Although sometimes classified as a stimulant laxative, docusate sodium is principally an emulsifying and wetting agent. In most patients, it has a relatively weak effect on GI transit at doses commonly used (≤400mg/24h). Other wetting agents include **poloxamer 188** (in **co-danthramer**).

Docusate lowers surface tension, thereby allowing water and fats to penetrate hard, dry faeces. It also stimulates fluid secretion by the small and large intestines.[1,2] Docusate does not interfere with protein or fat absorption.[3]

Systematic reviews highlight a lack of high quality studies exploring docusate either alone or in combination with a stimulant laxative.[4,5] Of two small studies involving hospice or hospital inpatients with cancer, the combined use of **senna** (p.41) and docusate appeared no more effective than **senna** alone.[6,7]

In palliative care, docusate is generally *not* recommended as the sole laxative for opioid-induced constipation. The exception is patients with partial bowel obstruction, where the aim is to prevent constipation from aggravating the situation, using a laxative with a low risk of exacerbating bowel colic. However, such use has not been formally examined. The routine use of docusate alongside a stimulant laxative is also generally *not* recommended; *PCF* favours the initial use of a stimulant laxative alone and titrating this to effect, reserving the use of a faecal softer to when there is a lack of response or bowel colic (see QCG: Opioid-induced constipation, p.45).[8]

Onset of action 1–2 days.

Cautions

Docusate enhances the absorption of **liquid paraffin**;[9] combined preparations of these substances are prohibited in some countries.

Undesirable effects

Diarrhoea, nausea, abdominal cramp, rashes.

Docusate oral solution may cause a bitter aftertaste or burning sensation, minimized by drinking plenty of water after taking the solution.

Dose and use

Despite evidence suggesting it is generally unnecessary, many centres still routinely use docusate in combination with a stimulant laxative, e.g. **senna**, or **bisacodyl** (see p.49). Docusate is often used alone for patients with persistent partial bowel obstruction. Dose varies according to individual need:

- generally start with 100mg PO b.d.
- if necessary, increase to 200mg b.d.–t.d.s.; *the latter is higher than the authorized maximum dose of 500mg/day.*

Docusate can also be used as an enema (see Rectal products, p.59).

Supply

Docusate sodium (generic)

Capsules 100mg, 28 days @ 100mg b.d. = £4.

Oral solution (sugar-free) 12.5mg/5mL, 50mg/5mL, 28 days @ 100mg b.d. = £17.

1 Donowitz M and Binder H (1975) Effect of dioctyl sodium sulfosuccinate on colonic fluid and electrolyte movement. *Gastroenterology*. **69**: 941–950.

2 Moriarty K *et al.* (1985) Studies on the mechanism of action of dioctyl sodium sulphosuccinate in the human jejunum. *Gut.* **26**: 1008–1013.

3 Wilson J and Dickinson D (1955) Use of dioctyl sodium sulfosuccinate (aerosol O.T.) for severe constipation. *Journal of the American Medical Association*. **158**: 261–263.

4 Hurdon V *et al.* (2000) How useful is docusate in patients at risk for constipation? A systematic review of the evidence in the chronically ill. *Journal of Pain and Symptom Management*. **19**: 130–136.

5 Canadian Agency for Drugs and Technologies in Health (2014) Dioctyl Sulfosuccinate or Docusate (Calcium or Sodium) for the prevention or management of constipation: a review of the clinical effectiveness. www.cadth.ca.

6 Hawley PH and Byeon JJ (2008) A comparison of sennosides-based bowel protocols with and without docusate in hospitalized patients with cancer. *Journal of Palliative Medicine*. **11**: 575–581.

7 Tarumi Y *et al.* (2013) Randomized, double-blind, placebo-controlled trial of oral docusate in the management of constipation in hospice patients. *Journal of Pain and Symptom Management*. **45**: 2–13.

8 Sykes N (2013) Emerging evidence on docusate: commentary on Tarumi et al. *Journal of Pain Symptom Management*. **45**: 1.

9 Godfrey H (1971) Dangers of dioctyl sodium sulfosuccinate in mixtures. *Journal of the American Medical Association*. **215**: 643.

Updated September 2019

LACTULOSE

Class: Osmotic laxative.

Indications: Constipation, hepatic encephalopathy.

Contra-indications: Intestinal obstruction, galactosaemia.

Pharmacology

Lactulose is a synthetic disaccharide, a combination of galactose and fructose, which is not absorbed by the small intestine.[1] It is a 'small bowel flusher', i.e. through an osmotic effect lactulose deposits a large volume of fluid into the large intestine. Lactulose is fermented by colonic bacteria to short-chain fatty acids which act as contact stimulants and acidify the contents of the ascending colon.

Lactulose (unlike **macrogols**) is a prebiotic, stimulating the growth of beneficial colonic bacteria, e.g. bifidobacteria.[2] Consequently, the bacterial uptake of ammonia is increased (± production inhibited) and the systemic absorption of ammonia is reduced.[3] Thus, lactulose is used in cirrhotic patients for both the prevention and treatment of encephalopathy; associated benefits include a reduction in mortality and serious morbidity, e.g. hepatorenal syndrome, and variceal bleeding.[4]

Lactulose has been shown to be more effective than increasing dietary fibre.[5] It does not affect the management of diabetes mellitus; because bio-availability is negligible, the number of calories absorbed is negligible. (Note. Generic products may differ.)

There are limited data to guide laxative use in a palliative care population (see Laxatives, Table 2, p.41). In a small RCT in palliative care patients receiving high-dose strong opioids, those given a combination of lactulose and **senna** had more bowel evacuations compared with those given **co-danthramer**, but there was no difference in patient preference.[6] In healthy volunteers, lactulose alone was effective in opioid-induced constipation, but the volume required (mean 55mL b.d.) is likely to preclude widespread use.[7]

A Cochrane review of lactulose and **macrogols** for chronic constipation concluded that **macrogols** are better than lactulose in terms of bowel movements per week, faecal consistency, relief of abdominal pain, and the need for additional products.[8] This review included 10 trials with a total of nearly 900 patients aged 3 months to 70 years. However, the volume per dose of **macrogols** is 5–10 times greater than that of lactulose (see p.55), which will be unacceptable to many patients.

Bio-availability <1%.

Onset of action up to 48h.

Cautions

Lactose intolerance.

Undesirable effects

Abdominal bloating, flatulence (generally only in the first few days of treatment), nausea (may be reduced if lactulose is diluted with water or fruit juice, or taken with meals), intestinal colic.

Dose and use

Lactulose can be used in patients who experience intestinal colic with stimulant laxatives, or who fail to respond to stimulant laxatives alone:

- start with 15mL PO once daily–b.d. and adjust according to need; can be diluted with water or fruit juice.

Hepatic encephalopathy

- start with 30–50mL PO t.d.s. and adjust the dose to produce 2–3 soft evacuations per day.

Supply

Lactulose (generic)

Oral solution 10g/15mL, 28 days @ 15mL b.d. = £5.

Oral solution (sachets) 10g/15mL sachet, 28 days @ 1 sachet b.d. = £14.

1 Schumann C (2002) Medical, nutritional and technological properties of lactulose. An update. *European Journal of Nutrition*. **41 (Suppl 1):**117–25.
2 Bouhnik Y *et al.* (2004) Prospective, randomized, parallel-group trial to evaluate the effects of lactulose and polyethylene glycol-4000 on colonic flora in chronic idiopathic constipation. *Alimentary Pharmacology and Therapeutics*. **19:** 889–899.
3 Ruszkowski J and Witkowski JM (2019) Lactulose: patient- and dose-dependent prebiotic properties in humans. *Anaerobe*. **59:** 100–106.
4 Gluud LL *et al.* (2016) Non-absorbable disaccharides versus placebo/no intervention and lactulose versus lactitol for the prevention and treatment of hepatic encephalopathy in people with cirrhosis. *Cochrane Database of Systematic Reviews*. **4:** CD003044. www.thecochranelibrary.com
5 Quah HM *et al.* (2006) Prospective randomized crossover trial comparing fibre with lactulose in the treatment of idiopathic chronic constipation. *Techniques in Coloproctology*. **10:** 111–114.
6 Sykes N (1991) A clinical comparison of laxatives in a hospice. *Palliative Medicine*. **5:** 307–314.
7 Sykes NP (1996) A volunteer model for the comparison of laxatives in opioid-related constipation. *Journal of Pain and Symptom Management*. **11:** 363–369.
8 Lee-Robichaud H *et al.* (2010) Lactulose versus polyethylene glycol for chronic constipation. *Cochrane Database of Systematic Reviews*. **7:** CD007570. www.thecochranelibrary.com

Updated (minor change) February 2021

MACROGOLS (POLYETHYLENE GLYCOLS)

Class: Osmotic laxative.

Indications: Constipation, faecal impaction.

Contra-indications: Acute inflammatory bowel disease, bowel obstruction, paralytic ileus.

Pharmacology

Macrogols are large, inert, biologically inactive polymers that bind water molecules. The resultant macrogol solution is retained within the gut lumen, softening faeces and, by increasing faecal volume, stimulating peristalsis. Unlike **lactulose** (p.54), they are not probiotic. Macrogol 3350 is available in the UK, with the number referring to the molecular weight.

Macrogols are unchanged in the GI tract. There is negligible absorption and no known systemic pharmacological activity. No dose reduction is needed in renal impairment. However, in severe renal impairment, the use of high-dose macrogols, e.g. to prepare for bowel colonoscopy, requires caution because of the risk of electrolyte imbalance (also see below).

To minimize the risk of water and electrolyte imbalance, electrolytes (potassium chloride, sodium bicarbonate, sodium chloride) are generally added to macrogols to make an isotonic solution. Observation of their use for 6 months in elderly patients (n=118) found no increased risk of electrolyte abnormalities.[1] Nonetheless, there are rare reports of hypokalaemia and hyperkalaemia with macrogols, the former due to GI loss of potassium and the latter because of the added potassium, generally in patients with other predisposing factors, e.g. severe renal impairment.

When used at high dose to prepare for bowel colonoscopy, e.g. 4L macrogol 3350 solution over 1 or 2 doses, there are rare reports of renal failure or hyponatraemia, possibly due to an inadequate or excessive water intake respectively (although in one patient with severe hyponatraemia, biochemical findings were consistent with SIADH, see p.568).[2-4] Patients should be counselled on maintaining an appropriate fluid intake (see Dose and use).

Although macrogols are generally well tolerated, some patients struggle with the volume of fluid needed, particularly in the presence of other symptoms limiting intake, e.g. anorexia, nausea, delayed gastric emptying.

In opioid-induced constipation, two small RCTs have compared macrogols with **lactulose** (p.54) or **senna** (p.49).[5,6] Both RCTs have methodological limitations. In patients on **methadone** maintenance treatment, there were no significant differences between macrogol 3350 (about 1 sachet at night) and **lactulose** (30mL at night) in reducing the frequency of hard stools.[5] In outpatients with cancer, macrogol 3350 or **senna** titrated to effect (up to about 1 sachet t.d.s. or 22.5mg t.d.s. respectively) appeared similar in regards to efficacy, tolerability and patient preference.[6]

In chronic constipation, there are no studies comparing macrogols with stimulant laxatives. On the other hand, a Cochrane review of macrogols and **lactulose** for chronic constipation in adults and in children concluded that macrogols are better than **lactulose** in terms of bowel movements per week, faecal consistency, relief of abdominal pain (children only) and the need for additional products.[7] However, the volume per dose of macrogols is 5–10 times greater than that of **lactulose** (see p.54); this will be unacceptable to many patients.

A systematic review in children suggested that macrogols may be better than other treatments, but the evidence is poor.[8] However, in faecal impaction in children, macrogols are no better than enemas and cause more faecal incontinence.[9] Children also find macrogols less palatable than **lactulose**.[10]

Onset of action 1–2 days for constipation; 1–3 days for faecal impaction.

Drug interactions

There are isolated reports of decreased effect of other drugs, e.g. anti-epileptics, when taken at the same time as macrogols. Consequently, some SPCs recommend that other drugs should not be taken within 1 hour of taking a macrogol.[11]

Undesirable effects

Uncommon (<1%, >0.1%): abdominal bloating, discomfort, borborygmi, hyponatraemia (when used as a hypotonic solution), nausea.

Very rare (<0.01%): severe electrolyte shift (oedema, shortness of breath, heart failure, dehydration).

Frequency unknown: hyper- or hypokalaemia (macrogol 3350 with electrolytes).

Dose and use

Patients should maintain their usual fluid intake; the fluid content of the macrogol solution is in addition to this.

Stop treatment if symptoms of fluid and electrolyte shift occur (see Undesirable effects).

Macrogol 3350 *concentrated oral liquid* contains ethanol and a large amount of benzyl alcohol. This product is not authorized for faecal impaction, because the dose needed would exceed the maximum acceptable daily intake of benzyl alcohol. The manufacturer's maximum recommended dose for constipation is 25mL (diluted with 100mL of water) t.d.s.

Macrogol 3350 is available as an oral powder sachet, a concentrated oral liquid and an oral solution sachet. The powder and concentrated liquid products need to be dissolved or diluted in water:

- dissolve 1 sachet (13.125g/sachet) of oral powder in half a glass of water (about 125mL) *or*
- dilute 25mL of the concentrated oral liquid with 100mL water (total volume 125mL).

The solution is generally used immediately after reconstitution or dilution. However, reconstituted powder sachets can be kept (covered) for up to 6h in a refrigerator, and the diluted oral liquid can be kept (covered) for 24h at room temperature.

Note. Although the 25mL oral solution sachet (Movicol® Ready to Take) does not need further dilution, it is recommended that patients drink 2–2.5L fluid/24h to maintain good health.

Constipation

- start with 1 sachet (13.125g/sachet) or 125mL of *diluted* oral liquid concentrate PO once daily
- if necessary, increase to b.d. or t.d.s. (maximum daily dose if using the oral liquid concentrate, see above).

Faecal impaction

The concentrated oral liquid is not authorized for faecal impaction (see above). When there is a large mass of hard faeces within the rectum, remove this first using digital fragmentation followed by suppository or enema (see p.59).[12]

- start with 8 sachets (13.125g/sachet) PO on day 1, taken in <6h
- patients with cardiovascular impairment should restrict the rate of intake to 2 sachets/h
- if necessary, repeat on days 2 and 3; most patients do not need the full dose on the second day.

For convenience, all 8 oral powder sachets can be made up together in 1L of water and kept in a refrigerator for a maximum of 6h, after which any remaining solution should be discarded.

Note. For Movicol® Ready to Take sachets, although the product itself does not need diluting, patients are recommended to take an additional 1L fluid/24h.

Supply

Macrogol 3350 with electrolytes: sodium bicarbonate, sodium chloride and potassium chloride, *(containing per sachet or 25mL dose of oral liquid: Na^+ = 8mmol, K^+ = 0.7mmol, Cl^- = 7mmol and bicarbonate = 2mmol).*

Oral powder (sachet) macrogol 3350 = 13.125g, 28 days @ 1 sachet once daily = £3.75; *available as sugar-free and in a range of flavours. Brands include CosmoCol®, Laxido®, Molaxole®, Movicol®; not all have the full range of flavours available.*

Oral liquid (concentrate) macrogol 3350 = 13.125g/25mL, 28 days @ 25mL (diluted with 100mL water) once daily = £7.50; *orange flavour, contains ethanol and benzyl alcohol.*

Oral solution (sachet) macrogol 3350 = 13.125g, 25mL sachet, 28 days @ 1 sachet once daily = £7.50

Macrogol 3350 with electrolytes: sodium bicarbonate, sodium chloride and potassium chloride, *(containing per sachet: Na^+ = 4mmol, K^+ = 0.35mmol, Cl^- = 3.5mmol and bicarbonate = 1mmol).*

Oral powder (half-strength/paediatric sachet) macrogol 3350 = 6.563g, 28 days @ 1 sachet once daily = £4: *available as sugar-free and in a range of flavours.*

Brands include CosmoCol-Half®, CosmoCol Paediatric®, Laxido Paediatric®, Movicol Half®, Movicol Paediatric®; not all have the full range of flavours available.

Note. Macrogol 3350 (with other salts and electrolytes) is available in products containing larger doses, e.g. Moviprep® (100g), Klean-prep® (69g); authorized for bowel cleansing before radiological examination, colonoscopy or surgery.

1 Chassagne P *et al.* (2017) Tolerance and long-term efficacy of polyethylene glycol 4000 (Forlax®) compared to lactulose in elderly patients with chronic constipation. *The Journal of Nutrition, Health and Aging*. **21:** 429–439.

2 Choi NK *et al.* (2013) Polyethylene glycol bowel preparation does not eliminate the risk of acute renal failure: a population-based case-crossover study. *Endoscopy*. **45:** 208–213.

3 Connor A *et al.* (2012) Consensus guidelines for the safe prescription and administration of oral bowel-cleansing agents. *Gut*. **61:** 1525–1532.

4 Ko SH *et al.* (2014) Case of inappropriate ADH syndrome: hyponatremia due to polyethylene glycol bowel preparation. *World Journal of Gastroenterology*. **20:** 12350–12354.

5 Freedman MD *et al.* (1997) Tolerance and efficacy of polyethylene glycol 3350/electrolyte solution versus lactulose in relieving opiate induced constipation: a double-blinded placebo-controlled trial. *Journal of Clinical Pharmacology*. **37:** 904–907.

6 Hawley P *et al.* (2019) PEG vs. sennosides for opioid-induced constipation in cancer care. *Supportive Care in Cancer*. (epub ahead of print)

7 Lee-Robichaud H *et al.* (2010) Lactulose versus polyethylene glycol for chronic constipation. *Cochrane Database of Systematic Reviews*. **7:** CD007570. www.thecochranelibaray.com

8 Gordon M *et al.* (2016) Osmotic and stimulant laxatives for the management of childhood constipation. *Cochrane Database of Systematic Reviews*. **8:** CD009118. www.thecochranelibaray.com

9 Bekkali NL *et al.* (2009) Rectal fecal impaction treatment in childhood constipation: enemas versus high doses oral PEG. *Pediatrics*. **124:** e1108–1115.

10 Voskuijl W *et al.* (2004) PEG 3350 (Transipeg) versus lactulose in the treatment of childhood functional constipation: a double blind, randomised, controlled, multicentre trial. *Gut*. **53:** 1590–1594.

11 Galen (2015) Laxido orange, powder for oral solution. *SPC*. www.medicines.org.uk

12 Larkin PJ *et al.* (2018) Diagnosis, assessment and management of constipation in advanced cancer: ESMO Clinical Practice Guidelines. *Annals of Oncology*. **29 (Suppl 4):** 111–125.

Updated October 2019

MAGNESIUM SALTS

Class: Osmotic laxative.

Indications: Constipation, particularly in patients who experience intestinal colic with stimulant laxatives or who fail to respond to the latter.

Contra-indications: Severe renal impairment.

Pharmacology

Magnesium ions are poorly absorbed from the gut. Their action is mainly osmotic, but other factors may be important, e.g. the release of cholecystokinin, or nitric oxide.[1] Magnesium ions also decrease absorption or increase secretion in the small bowel.

Magnesium salts are generally not used first line in palliative care patients, as they may be unpredictably effective. Magnesium *sulfate* is more potent than magnesium *hydroxide* and tends to produce a large volume of liquid faeces. In patients with idiopathic constipation, magnesium salts often lead to a sense of distension and the sudden passage of offensive liquid faeces which is socially inconvenient; it is difficult to adjust the dose to produce a normal soft result. However, when magnesium *hydroxide* is used as an osmotic laxative in conjunction with a stimulant laxative in opioid-induced constipation, this is not generally a problem.

An RCT of magnesium hydroxide and **liquid paraffin** vs. **senna** and **lactulose** failed to differentiate between the two combination treatments.[2]

Cautions

Renal impairment (risk of hypermagnesaemia; see Magnesium, Box A, p.640).

Drug interactions

Oral magnesium salts act as antacids, and the resulting increase in gastric pH may affect the absorption of several drugs if taken concurrently (see p.1).

Dose and use

For the treatment of hypomagnesaemia, see p.638.
For use of magnesium in antacids, see p.1.

Magnesium hydroxide

For opioid-induced constipation, as an alternative to **lactulose** or **macrogols** when an osmotic laxative is indicated (see QCG: Opioid-induced constipation, p.45):

- if the maximum dose of a stimulant laxative (e.g. **bisacodyl**, **senna**) is ineffective, halve the dose and add magnesium hydroxide 15–30mL b.d., and titrate as necessary; mix with water before administration
- alternatively, switch completely to magnesium hydroxide 15–60mL b.d.

Magnesium sulfate

A typical dose is 5–10g of crystals/powder (one or two 5mL spoonfuls) once daily *before breakfast*; dissolve in about 250mL of warm water.

Supply

All the preparations below are available OTC.

Magnesium hydroxide

Oral suspension hydrated magnesium oxide 415mg (7.1mmol elemental magnesium)/5mL, 28 days @ 15mL b.d. = £14; available OTC as Phillips' Milk of Magnesia®; *do not store in a cold place.*

Magnesium sulfate

Oral powder (Epsom salts) 4mmol/g elemental magnesium, 28 days @ 5g once daily = £1.

1 Izzo AA *et al.* (1994) Nitric oxide as a mediator of the laxative action of magnesium sulphate. *British Journal of Pharmacology.* **113:** 228–232.

2 Sykes N (1991) A clinical comparison of lactulose and senna with magnesium hydroxide and liquid paraffin emulsion in a palliative care population. [cited in Candy B et *al.* (2011) Laxatives or methylnaltrexone for the management of constipation in palliative care patients. *Cochrane Database of Systematic Reviews.* CD003448. www.thecochranelibrary.com

Updated October 2019

RECTAL PRODUCTS FOR CONSTIPATION

Indications: Constipation (oral laxatives ineffective or not feasible), faecal impaction (preferred initial treatment when hard faecal mass in rectum).

Contra-indications: Neutropenia, thrombocytopenia (risk of infection or bleeding from digital rectal examination ± interventions), undiagnosed abdominal pain, severe colitis, inflammation or infection of the abdomen, toxic megacolon, bowel obstruction, paralytic ileus, recent anorectal or gynaecological surgery, radiotherapy to the pelvic area or anorectal trauma.[1]
Arachis (peanut) oil: patients with peanut allergy.
Phosphates enema: CHF, dehydration, severe renal impairment.

Pharmacology

Rectal measures include suppositories and enemas. These soften the faeces and stimulate anorectal motility, either directly and/or by distending the rectum (Table 1). They act more quickly than PO laxatives to clear a full rectum or faecal impaction.[1] The evidence base for laxative suppositories and enemas in palliative care is generally limited to clinical experience and retrospective studies. Survey data indicate that about one third of palliative care patients receiving opioids need rectal measures (laxative suppositories, enemas and/or digital fragmentation ± evacuation) either regularly and electively, or intermittently and p.r.n., generally in addition to PO laxatives.[2]

There is evidence supporting the use of **bisacodyl** suppositories in postoperative ileus[3] and in pre-colonoscopy preparations[4] and of **docusate sodium** enemas in spinal injury patients.[5] In practice, for soft faeces, a **bisacodyl** suppository is given on its own; for hard faeces, **glycerol** alone or **glycerol** plus **bisacodyl** is used.

The laxative effect of **bisacodyl** is the result of local direct contact with the rectal mucosa after dissolution of the suppository and after activation by enteric enzymes (see Stimulant laxatives, p.49). The minimum time for response is thus generally >15min and may be up to 3h.[6] Defaecation a few minutes after the insertion of a **bisacodyl** suppository is the result of anorectal stimulation. **Bisacodyl** suppositories occasionally cause faecal leakage, even after a successful evacuation.

Osmotic *micro-enemas* contain **sodium citrate** and **sodium lauryl sulfoacetate** with several excipients, including **glycerol** and **sorbitol**. **Sodium lauryl sulfoacetate** is a faecal softener (surface-wetting agent) similar to **docusate sodium** (p.52), whereas **sodium citrate** draws fluid into the GI tract by osmosis, an action enhanced by **sorbitol**.

Osmotic *standard enemas* are larger volume and should be given by an experienced health professional. They contain phosphates and should be used with caution in elderly patients because of a risk of serious electrolyte disturbances. Fatalities have been reported from hyperphosphataemia and phosphate nephropathy.[7]

When treating a hard faecal impaction, a **docusate sodium** micro-enema will help to soften the faecal mass. This should be instilled into the rectum and retained overnight before giving a stimulant suppository (**bisacodyl**) or an osmotic enema (Table 1).

An **arachis (peanut) oil** retention enema is sometimes used in patients with a hard faecal impaction; instil and leave overnight before giving a stimulant laxative suppository or an osmotic enema.

Cautions

Cautions vary according to the individual products and circumstances of use.

Therapeutic or prophylactic anticoagulation, coagulation and platelet disorders (risk of bleeding/intramural haematoma).[1]

Undesirable effects

Abdominal discomfort, anorectal irritation, diarrhoea, rectal mucosal injury, perforation of the bowel, electrolyte disturbances (phosphate containing enemas, particularly in the elderly with renal impairment or ACE inhibitor use), bacteraemia.

Dose and use

A digital rectal examination should be undertaken to determine the most appropriate rectal intervention. When there are faeces in the rectum, suppositories or micro-enemas are used; if the rectum is empty, use standard phosphate or overnight retention enemas. Note. Findings on digital rectal examination relate poorly to the degree of faecal loading in the distal large bowel; e.g. in one case series, 30% of those with an empty rectum on digital examination had a large amount of faeces in the higher rectum/sigmoid colon on abdominal radiograph.[8]

When faecal impaction presents as a large mass of hard faeces within the rectum, the mass should first be removed by digital fragmentation followed by suppository or enema (see below); high-dose PO **macrogol** can then be used to clear the remaining large bowel (see p.55).[1] Digital evacuation is the final approach to faecal impaction, but is a distressing procedure and the patient may need sedation. Distress can be reduced by explaining the procedure, using plenty of lubrication and encouraging the patient to respond to any urge to defaecate.

Suppositories and enemas can also be given via a stoma (off-label).

Table 1 Rectal products for the relief of constipation or faecal impaction[a]

Rectal laxative	*Dose/volume*	*Predominant mode of action*	*Time to effect*[b]	*Cost per dose*
Suppositories[c]				
Bisacodyl	10mg	Stimulates propulsive activity after hydrolysis by enteric enzymes[9]	15–60min	10mg = £0.25
Glycerol[d]	4g	Hygroscopic; softens and lubricates	15–30min	4g = £0.25
Enemas[e]				
Docusate sodium micro-enema[c]	120mg in 10g	Faecal softener (surface-wetting agent); some direct stimulant action	5–20min	£4.75
Sodium citrate micro-enema[c]	5–10mL	Osmotic effect; other excipients may also soften the faeces (see text)	5–15min	5mL = £0.50
Phosphates enema[f]	118–128mL	Osmotic effect	2–5min	£2 Long tube = £28
Arachis (peanut) oil retention enema	130mL	Faecal softener	Overnight retention enema	130mL = £48

a. digital rectal examination will indicate the most appropriate intervention (see Dose and use)

b. as stated in SPC

c. suppositories and osmotic micro-enemas should be administered only if there are faeces in the rectum; place suppository in contact with the rectal mucosa

d. dip suppositories in water before administration

e. warm enemas to room temperature before use

f. avoid use in dehydrated patients (particularly those taking, e.g. diuretics, ACE inhibitors, NSAIDs); serious electrolyte disturbances may occur, e.g. hyperphosphataemia, particularly with prolonged retention (i.e. no bowel evacuation within 10min).

1 Larkin PJ *et al.* (2018) Diagnosis, assessment and management of constipation in advanced cancer: ESMO Clinical Practice Guidelines. *Annals of Oncology*. **29 (Suppl 4)**: 111–125.

2 Twycross RG and Harcourt JMV (1991) The use of laxatives at a palliative care centre. *Palliative Medicine*. **5**: 27–33.

3 Wiriyakosol S *et al.* (2007) Randomized controlled trial of bisacodyl suppository versus placebo for postoperative ileus after elective colectomy for colon cancer. *Asian Journal of Surgery*. **30**: 167–172.

4 Rapier R and Houston C (2006) A prospective study to assess the efficacy and patient tolerance of three bowel preparations for colonoscopy. *Gastroenterology Nursing*. **29**: 305–308.
5 Amir I *et al.* (1998) Bowel care for individuals with spinal cord injury: comparison of four approaches. *Journal of Spinal Cord Medicine*. **21**: 21–24.
6 Flig E *et al.* (2000) Is bisacodyl absorbed at all from suppositories in man? *International Journal of Pharmaceutics*. **196**: 11–20.
7 Niv G *et al.* (2013) Perforation and mortality after cleansing enema for acute constipation are not rare but are preventable. *International Journal of Geriatric Medicine*. **6**: 323–328.
8 Smith RG and Lewis S (1990) The relationship between digital rectal examination and abdominal radiographs in elderly patients. *Age and Ageing*. **19**: 142–143.
9 von Roth W and von Beschke K (1988) Pharmakokinetik und laxierende wirkung von bisacodyl nach gabe verschiedener zubereitungsformen. *Arzneimittel Forschung Drug Research*. **38**: 570–574.

Updated October 2019

TOPICAL PRODUCTS FOR HAEMORRHOIDS

Indications: Pain ± pruritus ani from haemorrhoids.

Introduction

Haemorrhoids are the symptomatic enlargement ± distal displacement of the vascular-rich connective tissue anal cushions. Generally, they present with painless rectal bleeding during defaecation ± prolapse beyond the anal canal, although they can also cause perianal pruritus and, when acutely thrombosed, sudden onset pain. They are associated with chronic straining because of, e.g. constipation, coughing, heavy lifting. The classification of haemorrhoids is based on their position relative to the dentate line (Box A).

Box A Classification of haemorrhoids

The dentate line divides the upper two-thirds and lower third of the anal canal.

Internal

Haemorrhoids originate above the dentate line. They are generally painless unless prolapse leads to incarceration and strangulation → anal sphincter spasm → ischaemia and necrosis of the haemorrhoid → further spasm ± painful thrombosis. They are graded I–IV:

- low-grade: do not prolapse (I), or only on straining, reducing spontaneously (II)
- high-grade: prolapsed, only reducing manually (III) or irreducible ± complications, e.g. incarcerated, acutely thrombosed (IV).

External

Haemorrhoids originate below the dentate line. Generally require no specific treatment unless uncomfortable. Can acutely thrombose causing pain that is maximal for 1–3 days and resolves over 1–2 weeks. The clot can be excised within the first 72h, otherwise treat with simple analgesia and warm bath soaks. There may be a residual perianal skin tag.

Mixed

Haemorrhoids originate both above and below the dentate line.

Management strategy

This includes:

- relieving exacerbating factors, e.g. constipation (see p.40)
- good anal hygiene; use soft, moist toilet wipes after defaecation, avoiding excessive wiping
- simple analgesia, e.g. **paracetamol** (p.331); warm baths may be soothing
- topical products for symptom relief (see below)
- non-operative measures, e.g. rubber band ligation, injection sclerotherapy.

More invasive surgical approaches are reserved for when the above fail or complications occur, and for high-grade internal hemorrhoids.

Topical products for symptom relief

Topical products, (e.g. creams, ointments, suppositories) generally contain one or more of the following:

- mild astringents, e.g. aluminium acetate, bismuth subgallate/oxide, hamamelis (witch hazel), zinc oxide
- mild antiseptics, e.g. benzyl benzoate, Peru balsam
- lubricants/emollients, e.g. white soft paraffin, lanolin
- corticosteroids, e.g. **hydrocortisone, prednisolone**
- local anaesthetics, e.g. **lidocaine, pramocaine** (pramoxine), **cinchocaine** (dibucaine).

Note. Some products, not featured here, also contain vasoconstrictors.

There is no evidence that any topical product is superior to another in terms of efficacy or tolerability. Internal haemorrhoids may be treated with suppositories, but these are not always effective because they are inserted into the rectum, bypassing the anal canal where the medication is needed. External haemorrhoids are generally best treated with a cream or ointment.

Creams or ointments containing mild astringents, mild antiseptics or lubricants can provide symptomatic relief of perianal pruritus, soreness and excoriation.

Topical products containing corticosteroids may be helpful if local inflammation is exacerbating discomfort ± pruritus. Infection (bacterial, viral, e.g. *Herpes simplex*, or fungal, e.g. candidosis) must first be excluded, and treatment generally limited to a maximum of 7 days, because prolonged use with excessive amounts can lead to atrophy of the anal skin. However, this is unlikely with low concentration hydrocortisone.

Topical products containing local anaesthetics are mostly used to relieve pain associated with an anal fissure (also see topical **glyceryl trinitrate** ointment, p.88), but will also relieve pruritus ani. They should be used for only a few days, because they can rarely cause local irritation from contact dermatitis.

Undesirable effects

Contact dermatitis may occur with products containing lanolin, corticosteroids or local anaesthetics. Skin sensitization or allergic reactions to Peru balsam may be an issue in susceptible patients.

Dose and use

Topical products containing mild astringents ± antiseptics ± lubricants

- apply cream/ointment or insert suppositories morning and night and after each bowel evacuation until symptoms have cleared
- a rectal nozzle (provided) can be used for internal haemorrhoids.

Topical products containing corticosteroids ± local anaesthetics

- apply cream/ointment or insert suppositories morning and night and after each bowel evacuation up to a maximum of 4 applications of cream/ointment or 3 suppositories/24h
- generally, a maximum treatment duration of 7 days is advised; however, this can be extended to ≤3 weeks, provided the corticosteroid ± local anaesthetic does not cause local irritation.

Note. Products containing a local anaesthetic to ease painful defaecation are best applied 15–20min *before* defaecation and p.r.n. to the maximum amount and duration above.

Supply

The following list is highly selective. Other OTC products are also available.

Topical products containing mild astringents ± antiseptics ± lubricants
Anusol® (Church & Dwight)
Cream zinc oxide, bismuth oxide, Peru balsam, 23g, 43g = £2.50 and £3.75.
Ointment zinc oxide, bismuth subgallate, Peru balsam, bismuth oxide, 25g = £2.50.
Suppositories zinc oxide, bismuth subgallate, Peru balsam, bismuth oxide, 24 = £4.

Topical products containing corticosteroids
Anusol HC® (Church & Dwight)
***Ointment* hydrocortisone** 0.25%, benzyl benzoate, bismuth subgallate, bismuth oxide, Peru balsam, zinc oxide, 30g = £2.50.
***Suppositories* hydrocortisone** 10mg, bismuth subgallate, bismuth oxide, Peru balsam, benzyl benzoate, zinc oxide, 12 = £1.75.

Topical products containing local anaesthetics
Germoloids® (Bayer)
***Cream* lidocaine** 0.7%, zinc oxide 25g, 55g = £2.50 and £4.75.
***Ointment* lidocaine** 0.7%, zinc oxide 25g, 55g = £2.75 and £4.50.
***Suppositories* lidocaine** 13.2mg, zinc oxide, 24 =£4.50.

Lidocaine (generic)
***Ointment* lidocaine** 5%,15g = £6.

Topical products containing both corticosteroids and local anaesthetics
Germoloids® HC (Bayer)
***Spray* hydrocortisone** 0.2% and **lidocaine** 1%, 30mL = £5.50.

Xyloproct® (Aspen)
***Ointment* hydrocortisone** 0.275%, **lidocaine** 5%, aluminium acetate, zinc oxide, 20g = £4.25.

Scheriproct® (Bayer)
***Ointment* prednisolone** 0.19%, **cinchocaine** 0.5%, 30g = £3.25
***Suppositories* prednisolone** 1.3mg, **cinchocaine** 1mg, 12 = £1.50.

Updated April 2019

PANCREATIN

Class: Enzyme supplement.

Indications: Pancreatic exocrine insufficiency.

Pharmacology

Pancreatic exocrine insufficiency occurs when there is insufficient production or delivery of pancreatic enzymes required for the digestion and absorption of food. Common causes are cancer of the head/body of the pancreas, chronic pancreatitis, pancreatic resection and cystic fibrosis. It can also occur following duodenectomy, gastrectomy or untreated coeliac disease, via a reduction in cholecystokinin and thereby post-prandial pancreatic stimulation. It is increasingly recognized as a complication of diabetes mellitus.[1] Its presence is associated with poorer outcomes, including reduced quality of life and survival.[2]

Pancreatic exocrine insufficiency results in undigested dietary carbohydrate, protein and fat. Stools containing large amounts of fat (steatorrhoea) are pale, bulky, offensive, frothy, greasy and difficult to flush away. There can be abdominal pain and distension, increased flatus, weight loss, and mineral and vitamin deficiency (A, D, E and K). However, malnutrition may not be immediately obvious and *malabsorption is common even in patients without overt steatorrhoea*.[3,4] A low faecal elastase (<200microgram/g) helps to confirm the diagnosis of pancreatic exocrine deficiency when there is clinical uncertainty. While awaiting the results of this, the response to a therapeutic trial of pancreatin can also be evaluated (the monoclonal faecal elastase test is not affected by pancreatin).[3]

Pancreatin is a preparation of porcine lipase, proteases and amylase. Pancreatin hydrolyzes fats to glycerol and fatty acids, degrades protein into amino acids, and converts starch into dextrin and sugars. Pancreatin should be offered to all patients with pancreatic exocrine deficiency to reduce malabsorption and thereby improve nutrition ± symptoms of steatorrhoea. Because most patients with cancer of the pancreas have malabsorption at diagnosis, pancreatin is considered a routine supportive therapy.[5] Retrospective data suggest that pancreatin may improve survival in this group, particularly in patients with >10% body weight loss at diagnosis, possibly because this indicates greater levels of (correctable) pancreatic exocrine insufficiency/malabsorption.[6]

Pancreatin is inactivated by gastric acid and formulations containing pancreatin in gastro-resistant granules are generally used. An alkaline pH (>5.5) is required for optimal disintegration of the e/c coating in the duodenum. Thus, acid suppression, e.g. with a PPI, improves their efficacy. Nonetheless, guidelines generally recommend the addition of a PPI only when there are persistent symptoms despite reasonable doses of pancreatin, i.e. 75,000 units of lipase/meal, with higher doses of pancreatin reserved for if this strategy fails.[2,7] However, some centres routinely prescribe a PPI when there is a likely complete/significant loss of pancreatic bicarbonate excretion, because of its important contribution to duodenal alkalinity; this would include patients with pancreatic cancer.[6]

Pancreatin has been used to clear feed-related blockages in enteral feeding tubes. However, this should only be considered when other options have failed (see Chapter 28).[8]

Although the use of pancreatin was considered potentially helpful for pancreatic pain in chronic pancreatitis, a meta-analysis of RCTs has found no overall benefit.[9]

Undesirable effects

Very common (>10%): abdominal pain.
Common (<10%, >1%): nausea and vomiting, constipation or diarrhoea.
If abdominal symptoms worsen after starting Creon®, anecdotally, tolerability can be improved by switching to another product, e.g. Nutrizym 22®.

Irritation of the anal canal can occur when active enzymes reach the rectum because of, e.g. excess dose, rapid GI transit.

Very rarely, strictures of the ileo-caecum and proximal colon (fibrosing colonopathy) have been linked with very high doses of pancreatin (i.e. >10,000 units of lipase/*kg*/24h). Although most reports involve children with cystic fibrosis, it has also occurred in adults with and without cystic fibrosis.[10,11]

Dose and use

Pancreatin should be offered to all patients with pancreatic exocrine deficiency to reduce malabsorption and thereby improve nutrition ± symptoms of steatorrhoea. This includes those with no/minimal symptoms of steatorrhoea, because underlying malabsorption is common. Apart from enzyme replacement, other nutritional support may be required; seek advice from a dietitian.

There are several different pancreatin products, all derived from pigs. Jewish and Muslim faith leaders have considered their use acceptable because of the lack of an alternative.[12,13]

Gastro-resistant pancreatin formulations should be used, except for a few specific situations, e.g. patients with enteral feeding tubes, rapid gastrojejunal transit; seek advice from a specialist dietitian. Several products are available, but Creon® is a good choice in terms of cost and range of strengths available, starting with Creon® 25,000 (Table 1).[14-16]

Table 1 Starting dose recommendations for Creon®

Dietary intake	*Number of Creon® 25,000 capsules*[a,b]
Snack/milky drink	1–2
Normal meal	2–3
Large meal/fatty food/takeaways	3–4

a. the number of capsules varies with the size and the fat, carbohydrate or protein content of the snack/meal
b. or of other products containing similar amounts of enzymes, e.g. Nutrizym 22®, Pancrease® HL.

If necessary, further dose increases are made every 3–4 days to normalize faecal size, consistency and frequency. There is no maximum dose. However, if there is a lack of progressive improvement, other causes of malabsorption should be considered, e.g. bacterial overgrowth, bile salt malabsorption, coeliac disease.

If symptoms of steatorrhea are not adequately controlled despite reasonable doses of pancreatin, i.e. 75,000 units of lipase/meal, consider adding a PPI before further increasing the dose of pancreatin. Note. Some centres add a PPI routinely in patients with unresectable pancreatic cancer (see Pharmacology).

A reduction in malabsorption should lead to improvements in the patient's nutritional status and weight; in some patients, e.g. those with advanced pancreatic cancer, only a slowing of the rate of weight loss is possible.

Patients should also be advised:

- that pancreatin is required for all meals, snacks, milky drinks and oral nutritional supplement drinks, except for:
  - ▷ small amounts of vegetables (except potatoes, beans and pulses)
  - ▷ small amounts of fruit (except avocado) or dried fruit
  - ▷ sugary sweets
  - ▷ drinks containing only a small amount of milk, fruit squashes or fizzy drinks
- to swallow the capsules whole with sips of a cold (≤ room temperature) drink, after the first few mouthfuls of food
- *not to crush/chew or hold the capsule in the mouth*; this can cause stomatitis
- when taking more than one capsule, eating a large meal, or one that lasts >30min, to spread out the taking of the capsules across the meal's duration
- to increase the dose to control symptoms, rather than restrict their diet (Note. A low-fat diet is *not* indicated.)
- that if a dose is missed, not to try and make up by taking it later; resume the correct dose with the next snack/milky drink/meal
- *not* to store capsules in hot places, e.g. direct sunlight, car glove box, trouser pocket
- to treat constipation with laxatives, and *not* by reducing pancreatin
- to report any irritation of the anal passage; this suggests active enzymes are reaching the lower bowel. Prescribe a barrier cream and add a PPI (to enhance enzyme release in the duodenum) before making a dose reduction
- to report any symptoms suggestive of diabetes mellitus (e.g. thirst, polyuria), because pancreatin, by improving the absorption of carbohydrates, occasionally unmasks an underlying diabetic state.

Because of the size of the capsules, some patients may have difficulty swallowing them. Smaller capsules are available (e.g. Creon® 10,000), but the larger number required for an effective dose may be impractical, particularly for those with more complex swallowing difficulties. If necessary, the capsules can be opened and the granules sprinkled on a teaspoon of cold (≤ room temperature) acidic soft food, e.g. jam, yoghurt, apple sauce, tomato sauce. This must be taken immediately (the gastro-resistant enteric coating starts to dissolve if left to stand) and the mouth rinsed with a cold drink to ensure no granules remain, particularly between teeth or under dentures.

The granules must not be crushed, chewed or added to alkaline drinks or foods, e.g. milk, because this destroys the gastro-resistant coating. This causes the release of the enzymes in the mouth and thereby a loss of efficacy and stomatitis. Further, because heat inactivates pancreatin, the granules must not be mixed with hot drinks or food, and the capsules stored appropriately (i.e. <25°C).

Supply

Creon® (Mylan)

Capsules (enclosing gastro-resistant granules) Creon® 10,000, lipase 10,000 units, amylase 8,000 units, protease 600 units, 28 days @ 2 t.d.s. = £22.

Higher strength capsules (enclosing gastro-resistant granules)

Creon® 25,000, lipase 25,000 units, amylase 18,000 units, protease 1,000 units, 28 days @ 2 t.d.s. = £47.

Pancrease® HL

Higher strength capsules (enclosing gastro-resistant granules) lipase 25,000 units, amylase 22,500 units, protease 1,250 units, 28 days @ 2 t.d.s. = £63.

Nutrizym 22®

Higher strength capsules (enclosing gastro-resistant granules) lipase 22,000 units, amylase 19,800 units, protease 1,100 units, 28 days @ 2 t.d.s. = £52.

1 Ewald N *et al.* (2007) Pancreatin therapy in patients with insulin-treated diabetes mellitus and exocrine pancreatic insufficiency according to low fecal elastase 1 concentrations. Results of a prospective multi-centre trial. *Diabetes Metabolism Research Reviews.* **23**: 386–391.
2 Dominguez-Munoz JE (2018) Diagnosis and treatment of pancreatic exocrine insufficiency. *Current Opinion Gastroenterology Journal.* **34**: 349–354.
3 Imrie CW *et al.* (2010) Review article: Enzyme supplementation in cystic fibrosis, chronic pancreatitis, pancreatic and periampullary cancer. *Alimentary Pharmacology & Therapeutics.* **32** (Suppl 1): 1–25.
4 Dominguez-Munoz JE and Iglesias-Garcia J (2010) Oral pancreatic enzyme substitution therapy in chronic pancreatitis: Is clinical response an appropriate marker for evaluation of therapeutic efficacy? *Journal of the Pancreas.* **11**: 158–162.
5 NICE (2018) Pancreatic cancer in adults: Diagnosis and management. *Clinical Guidelines* (NG85). www.nice.org.uk
6 Dominguez-Munoz JE *et al.* (2018) Impact of the treatment of pancreatic exocrine insufficiency on survival of patients with unresectable pancreatic cancer: A retrospective analysis. *BMC Cancer.* **18**: 534.
7 Löhr JM *et al.* (2017) United European Gastroenterology evidence-based guidelines for the diagnosis and therapy of chronic pancreatitis. *United European Gastroenterology Journal.* **5**: 153–199.
8 White R and Bradnam V (2015) *Handbook of Drug Administration via Enteral Feeding Tubes.* London: Pharmaceutical Press. www.medicinescomplete.com (accessed June 2015).
9 Yaghoobi M *et al.* (2016) Pancreatic enzyme supplements are not effective for relieving abdominal pain in patients with chronic pancreatitis: Meta-analysis and systematic review of randomized controlled trials. *Canadian Journal Gastroenterology and Hepatology.* 8541839.
10 Hausler M *et al.* (1998) First adult patient with fibrosing colonopathy. *American Journal of Gastroenterology.* **93**: 1171–1172.
11 Bansi DS *et al.* (2000) Fibrosing colonopathy in an adult owing to over use of pancreatic enzyme supplements. *Gut.* **46**: 283–285.
12 UKMI (2018) What factors to consider when advising on medicines suitable for a halal diet. *Medicines Q&As.* www.sps.nhs.uk
13 Pancreatic Cancer Action My religion restricts me from eating pork, so can I still take pancreatic enzymes? *Pancreatic enzyme replacement therapy (PERT)* www.pancreaticcanceraction.org (accessed February 2019).
14 Bruno MJ *et al.* (1998) Placebo controlled trial of enteric coated pancreatin microsphere treatment in patients with unresectable cancer of the pancreatic head region. *Gut.* **42**: 92–96.
15 Thorat V *et al.* (2012) Randomised clinical trial: The efficacy and safety of pancreatin enteric-coated minimicrospheres (Creon 40000 MMS) in patients with pancreatic exocrine insufficiency due to chronic pancreatitis--a double-blind, placebo-controlled study. *Alimentary Pharmacology Therapeutics.* **36**: 426–436.
16 Seiler CM *et al.* (2013) Randomised clinical trial: A 1-week, double-blind, placebo-controlled study of pancreatin 25 000 ph. Eur. Minimicrospheres (Creon 25000 MMS) for pancreatic exocrine insufficiency after pancreatic surgery, with a 1-year open-label extension. *Alimentary Pharmacology & Therapeutics.* **37**: 691–702.

Updated (minor change) January 2020

2: CARDIOVASCULAR SYSTEM

FUROSEMIDE

Class: Loop diuretic.

Indications: Oedema, hypertension (unresponsive to usual treatments), †malignant ascites associated with portal hypertension and hyperaldosteronism (with **spironolactone**).

Contra-indications: Hepatic encephalopathy, anuric renal failure.

Pharmacology

Loop diuretics inhibit Na^+ (and hence water) resorption from the ascending limb of the loop of Henle in the renal tubule. They also increase urinary excretion of K^+, Mg^{2+}, H^+ and Cl^-. Loop diuretics, of which furosemide is the most commonly prescribed, are used to treat fluid overload in chronic heart failure and ESRF in order to improve symptoms of breathlessness and oedema.[1-4]

A diuretic-induced reduction in plasma volume can activate several neurohumoral systems, e.g. renin–angiotensin–aldosterone, resulting in impaired renal perfusion and increased Na+ and water resorption. These changes contribute towards a reduced effect of the diuretic ('diuretic resistance') and also renal impairment. Strategies to overcome 'resistance' to furosemide include:

- a progressive increase in dose and b.d. administration
- switching to a loop diuretic with a higher/more consistent bio-availability
- adding a thiazide diuretic
- switching to parenteral administration.

Other loop diuretics include **bumetanide** and **torasemide**, with respective PO doses of 1mg and 10mg equivalent to 40mg of furosemide.[5-7] Compared with furosemide they are more expensive, but they have a higher (≥80%) and more consistent PO bio-availability.[5,6] Thus, some patients may have improved diuresis when switched to them from furosemide.

In the UK, furosemide is the only loop diuretic available in a parenteral formulation. When switching from PO to IV because of fluid overload, a 1:1 conversion is generally used.[8] Based on bio-availability, this represents an increase in dose. Thus, although some use the same PO:IV conversion ratio in patients with *controlled oedema* no longer able to take drugs PO at the end of life, a conversion ratio of 2:1 may be sufficient. *Whatever the circumstance and dose used, patients receiving parenteral furosemide require close monitoring.*

Thiazide-type diuretics, e.g. **bendroflumethiazide, indapamide, metolazone** (not UK, but see Supply), block distal tubule Na^+ resorption and thereby antagonize part of the renal adaptations to a loop diuretic. All thiazides are equally effective when added to a PO/IV loop diuretic, and the combination can avoid the need for parenteral administration of a loop diuretic in both chronic heart failure and ESRF.[4,9] Close monitoring of plasma electrolytes and renal function is required, particularly because of the increased risk of hypokalaemia ± hypomagnesaemia. Initially, when diuresis is likely to be at its greatest, daily monitoring may be necessary. An aldosterone antagonist, e.g. **spironolactone**, is sometimes also added to augment the diuresis and conserve K^+.[9]

Compared with bolus IV doses, furosemide by CIVI appears to provide a greater diuresis with a similar or better safety profile.[10] However, the data are inconsistent and insufficiently robust to specifically recommend one approach rather than the other.[11]

Furosemide is effective when given by SC injection (off-label). However, because the concentration of the injection is 10mg/mL, volume considerations may limit feasibility. Diuresis reaches a maximum 2–3h after the SC injection is administered and lasts for about 4h.[12,13] Furosemide has been successfully given SC/CSCI as a means of avoiding hospital admission, and for when oral medication becomes problematic in the last days of life.[14-16] In a report of 47 episodes of the use of furosemide CSCI in 37 patients with end-stage chronic heart failure, the majority benefited (>80%), with a mild or severe site reaction seen in one quarter and one episode, respectively.[14]

Nebulized furosemide has been used in a patient at home with decompensated CHF as a temporary measure when IV access could not be established. A dose of 80mg resulted in a rapid improvement in pulmonary oedema and breathlessness, diuresis, and a weight loss of 1kg. However, despite repeated daily doses, overall there was insufficient diuresis to prevent admission for central line insertion and IV furosemide.[17]

Ascites

When caused by a *transudate* associated with portal hypertension from, e.g. cirrhosis or extensive liver metastases, furosemide alone has little effect, even when total daily doses of 100–200mg PO are used.[18,19] Thus, furosemide in ascites is best limited to concurrent use with **spironolactone** when the latter alone is insufficient (see p.73).

Octreotide 300microgram SC b.d. (see p.593) can suppress the diuretic-induced activation of the renin–angiotensin–aldosterone system, and its addition has improved renal function and Na^+ and water excretion in patients with cirrhosis and ascites receiving furosemide and **spironolactone.**[20,21]

Breathlessness

There is current interest in the use of *nebulized* furosemide for the treatment of breathlessness (Box A). However, a review of 42 trials concluded that there was currently insufficient evidence to support its routine use.[22] Further, in one study,[23] five out of seven patients reported a deterioration in their breathing after furosemide. Thus, ideally, nebulized furosemide should be used only in a clinical trial.

Box A Nebulized furosemide and breathlessness

Experimentally induced cough and breathlessness

Nebulized furosemide 20–40mg attenuates cough and breathlessness,[24-27] possibly via an effect on vagal sensory nerve endings.

The reduction in breathlessness may result from increasing sensory traffic to the brain stem from sensitized slowly adapting pulmonary stretch receptors. However, the effect:

- has not been demonstrated consistently (e.g. a dose of 120mg had no effect)
- shows wide interindividual variability
- is of short duration (generally <2h).

Further, systemic absorption can be sufficient to induce a diuresis.[28-31]

COPD

Compared with placebo in moderate–severe COPD, nebulized furosemide has reduced breathlessness ± increased exercise time during endurance testing[32,33] but *not* incremental exercise testing.

The mechanism underlying the benefit is unclear, but improvements are seen in airway function (e.g. slow vital capacity at rest) and dynamic ventilatory mechanics (e.g. inspiratory capacity and breathing pattern).[33] Although small but significant bronchodilation was seen in one study,[32] this is unlikely to be a direct effect of nebulized furosemide.

When given alongside initial 'standard' treatment for an exacerbation of COPD, nebulized furosemide results in additional improvement in breathlessness and various respiratory parameters.[34] However, it does not have an established role in this setting.

Cancer

In patients with cancer, nebulized furosemide has been used to relieve severe breathlessness.[35,36] However, RCTs have failed to show benefit.[23,37]

Pharmacokinetic data are summarized in Table 1.

Table 1 Pharmacokinetic details[38-40]

Drug	*Bumetanide*	*Furosemide*	*Torasemide*
Bio-availability PO (%)	80–95	60–70[a]	~80
Onset of action (min)	30–60 PO ≤2 IV (not UK)	30–60 PO 30 SC 2–5 IV	≤60 PO ≤10 IV (not UK)
T_{max} (h)	0.5–2 PO	1.5 PO	≤1 PO
Plasma halflife (h)	1–2	0.5–2[b]	3.5
Duration of action (h)	4–6 PO 2 IV	4–6 PO 4 SC 2 IV	≤8 PO/IV

a. varies widely due to erratic absorption and can be as low as 10%
b. longer in chronic heart failure (1–6h) and in ESRF (10h).

Cautions

Severe electrolyte disturbances (correct before treatment and monitor during use); elderly (lower doses); renal impairment (monitor during use); hepatic impairment; diabetes, hypoproteinaemia.

Some patients receive long-term diuretic therapy for hypertension or non-heart failure ankle oedema. This often becomes inappropriate as physical deterioration progresses, and may lead to postural hypotension and prerenal failure. In these circumstances, the dose of furosemide should be reduced and possibly discontinued altogether. However, the withdrawal of diuretics requires careful monitoring to prevent the subsequent insidious onset of chronic heart failure.[41]

Drug interactions

Serious drug interactions: Furosemide-induced electrolyte disturbances, particularly hypokalaemia, can increase the risk of:

- cardiac arrhythmia and death with drugs known to prolong the QT interval, e.g. **citalopram**, **methadone** (see Chapter 20, p.797)
- **digoxin** toxicity
- **lithium** toxicity (possibly).[42]

Plasma electrolytes, drug concentrations and the patient's clinical condition should be monitored closely.

Concurrent use of furosemide with **risperidone** is associated with an increased risk of death in elderly patients with dementia. The reason is unclear, but the manufacturer advises avoiding this combination unless the benefits clearly outweigh the risks.

Furosemide can *decrease* **vancomycin** levels by up to 50%.

Aliskiren, **indometacin**, **phenytoin** and possibly other NSAIDs can reduce the diuretic effect of furosemide (up to 50% reduction with **phenytoin**); a larger dose of furosemide may be required.

Additive pharmacodynamic interactions with furosemide increase the risk of:

- hypokalaemia with other K^+ depleting drugs, e.g. corticosteroids, β_2 agonists, **theophylline**
- hyponatraemia with other Na^+ depleting drugs, e.g. **carbamazepine**
- hypotension with other drugs that lower blood pressure, e.g. ACE inhibitors, angiotensin II receptor antagonists, TCAs
- nephrotoxicity with other renally toxic drugs, e.g. NSAIDs, aminoglycosides
- ototoxicity with other ototoxic drugs, e.g. aminoglycosides, **vancomycin.**

Colestyramine, **colestipol** and **sucralfate** decrease absorption of furosemide; give furosemide 2–3h before these drugs.

Undesirable effects

Transient pain at the site of SC injection.[40]
Frequency not stated: dyspepsia, thirst, dizziness, dehydration, drowsiness, weakness, muscle cramps.
Rare: tinnitus and deafness (generally after rapid injection; may be permanent).
Biochemical disturbances: hyperglycaemia, hyperuricaemia, hypocalcaemia, hypokalaemia, hypomagnesaemia, hyponatraemia, metabolic alkalosis.

Dose and use

Ascites

Use only as a supplement to **spironolactone** (p.73):
- start with 40mg PO each morning
- increase in steps of 40mg each morning every 3–5 days
- maximum dose 160mg each morning.

Symptomatic relief of fluid overload in chronic heart failure and ESRF

- start with 40mg PO each morning
- if necessary, increase the dose progressively in 40mg increments
- usual maximum dose 160mg/24h, generally given as 80mg each morning and noon
- in patients admitted to hospital with decompensated chronic heart failure, much higher doses are sometimes used, e.g. ≤600mg/24h.[7]

The Frusol® brand of furosemide oral solution is authorized for administration via NG or PEG tubes, see SPC and also Chapter 28, p.853.

Once the excess fluid has been cleared, attempts can be made to reduce the furosemide to the lowest effective maintenance dose. Excessive diuresis is generally indicated by worsening renal function. Conversely, weight gain is an early indicator of fluid overload. Some patients are taught to adjust their diuretic dose according to changes in body weight.

Addition of a thiazide diuretic

Seek specialist advice: When there is an inadequate response to an optimally titrated dose of furosemide PO/IV, benefit may be obtained from the addition of a thiazide diuretic (see Pharmacology). A typical starting dose for **bendroflumethiazide, indapamide** and **metolazone** is 2.5mg PO given each morning or less frequently (see below); other thiazide diuretics can also be used.[9]

Close monitoring of plasma electrolytes, renal function and clinical response (e.g. blood pressure, body weight, diuresis) is generally required when a thiazide diuretic is added to furosemide. Particularly for outpatients, or with ongoing use, alternate day or even less frequent dosing is preferable, e.g. 1–2 times weekly.[7]

In ESRF, prolonged benefit has been obtained from short courses, e.g. **metolazone** 2.5–5mg once daily for 2–5 days.[4]

Parenteral administration

Parenteral administration may be necessary when the response to PO diuretics is inadequate in a patient with fluid overload, or when a patient is no longer able to take PO diuretics, e.g. at the end of life.

Patients with fluid overload

When switching from furosemide PO to IV, a 1:1 conversion is generally used. Although data are mixed, the largest study to date suggests bolus IV and CIVI administration result in similar changes in patients' symptoms and renal function, and guidelines recommend either.[10,11] However, many centres only switch to CIVI when the maximum dose of bolus IV is insufficient, e.g.:
- start with *bolus IV:* 40–80mg b.d. (morning and noon); dilute with sodium chloride 0.9% to a suitable volume, e.g. 20mL, and give at a maximum rate of 4mg/min (2.5mg/min in severe renal impairment)
- if insufficient, switch to *CIVI:* 200–250mg/24h; dilute in a convenient volume of sodium chloride 0.9%
- generally, the fluid overload takes 3–5 days to clear; a switch back to the patient's usual PO maintenance dose of furosemide is then attempted.

Some palliative care services have used CSCI furosemide as a way of managing decompensated chronic heart failure in the hospice or community setting:

- start with the same dose CSCI as the patient's current PO total daily dose
- weigh the patient daily
- after 48h, if the daily weight loss is not ≥1kg/day, consider obtaining cardiologist/heart failure nurse specialist advice; options include:
  - ▷ increasing the furosemide dose by 50%
  - ▷ adding a thiazide diuretic PO (see above)
  - ▷ adding or increasing the dose of an aldosterone antagonist, e.g. PO **spironolactone**
- because furosemide injection is 10mg/mL, practical dose limits for a CME T34 syringe driver are 200mg/24h and 300mg/24h for a 30mL and 50mL syringe respectively
- if CSCI furosemide fails to provide the necessary weight loss, admission to hospital/hospice for IV furosemide may be unavoidable.

Patients unable to take PO furosemide

For patients with chronic heart failure in the last days of life, unless they are anuric or clinically hypovolaemic, a loop diuretic should generally be continued for symptom management. Once unable to take furosemide PO:

- *if fluid overloaded*, switch to IV bolus or CSCI furosemide using a PO to IV conversion of 1:1 (this represents an increase in dose; see Pharmacology)
- if *not* fluid overloaded, although some use a 1:1 conversion, using half the PO dose IV may suffice.

Alternatively, in a patient without fluid overload, some clinicians will monitor the situation *daily* and only commence parenteral furosemide if fluid overload develops. *This approach requires the whole team to have the necessary expertise to monitor for symptoms and signs of pulmonary oedema.*

Incompatibility: Furosemide injection is alkaline, and there is a high risk of *incompatibility* when mixed with acidic drugs. Because of this and the lack of compatibility data, *furosemide should not be mixed in the same syringe with any other drugs* (see Chapter 29, p.892).[43]

If further dilution is required, sodium chloride 0.9% is recommended; do *not* mix or dilute with glucose solutions or other acidic fluids.

Supply

Furosemide (generic)

Tablets 20mg, 40mg, 500mg, 28 days @ 40mg each morning = £0.75.

Oral solution (sugar-free) 20mg/5mL, 40mg/5mL, 50mg/5mL, 28 days @ 40mg each morning = £17; *some formulations may contain alcohol.*

Injection 10mg/mL, 2mL amp = £0.25, 5mL amp = £0.75, 25mL amp = £3.

For other loop diuretics (e.g. **bumetanide, torasemide**) and thiazide diuretics (e.g. **bendroflumethiazide, indapamide, metolazone**), see the *BNF*.

Note. Although there is no authorized **metolazone** product available in the UK, it is widely used and obtained via import as a special order product (see Chapter 24, p.817); it costs more than other thiazides, particularly the 2.5mg tablet.

1 NICE (2018) Chronic heart failure in adults: diagnosis and management. *NICE Guideline*. NG106. www.nice.org.uk

2 Ponikowski P *et al.* (2016) 2016 ESC Guidelines for the diagnosis and treatment of acute and chronic heart failure: the Task Force for the diagnosis and treatment of acute and chronic heart failure of the European Society of Cardiology (ESC). Developed with the special contribution of the Heart Failure Association (HFA) of the ESC. *European Heart Journal.* **37**: 2129–2200.

3 Yancy CW *et al.* (2017) 2017 ACC/AHA/HFSA focused update of the 2013 ACCF/AHA guideline for the management of heart failure: a report of the American College of Cardiology/American Heart Association Task Force on clinical practice guidelines and the Heart Failure Society of America. *Circulation.* **136**: e137–e161.

4 Cheng HW *et al.* (2014) Combination therapy with low-dose metolazone and furosemide: a "needleless" approach in managing refractory fluid overload in elderly renal failure patients under palliative care. *International Urology and Nephrology.* **46**: 1809–1813.

5 Ward A and Heel RC (1984) Bumetanide. A review of its pharmacodynamic and pharmacokinetic properties and therapeutic use. *Drugs.* **28**: 426–464.

6 Vargo DL *et al.* (1995) Bioavailability, pharmacokinetics, and pharmacodynamics of torsemide and furosemide in patients with congestive heart failure. *Clinical Pharmacology and Therapeutics*. **57**: 601–609.

7 Heart Failure Society of America (2010) Comprehensive heart failure practice guideline. *Journal of Cardiac Failure*. **16**: e1–e194.

8 Felker GM *et al.* (2011) Diuretic strategies in patients with acute decompensated heart failure. *New England Journal of Medicine*. **364**: 797–805.

9 Jentzer JC *et al.* (2010) Combination of loop diuretics with thiazide-type diuretics in heart failure. *Journal of the American College of Cardiology*. **56**: 1527–1534.

10 Amer M *et al.* (2012) Continuous infusion versus intermittent bolus furosemide in ADHF: an updated meta-analysis of randomized control trials. *Journal of Hospital Medicine*. **7**: 270–275.

11 Yancy CW *et al.* (2013) 2013 ACCF/AHA guideline for the management of heart failure: a report of the American College of Cardiology Foundation/American Heart Association Task Force on practice guidelines. *Circulation*. **128**: e240–e327.

12 Goenaga MA *et al.* (2004) Subcutaneous furosemide. *Annals of Pharmacotherpy*. **38**: 1751.

13 Farless LB *et al.* (2012) Intermittent subcutaneous furosemide: parenteral diuretic rescue for hospice patients with congestive heart failure resistant to oral diuretic. *American Journal of Hospice and Palliative Care*. **30**: 791–792.

14 Zacharias H *et al.* (2011) Is there a role for subcutaneous furosemide in the community and hospice management of end-stage heart failure? *Palliative Medicine*. **26**: 658–663.

15 Galindo-Ocana J *et al.* (2013) Subcutaneous furosemide as palliative treatment in patients with advanced and terminal-phase heart failure. *BMJ Supportive and Palliative Care*. **3**: 7–8.

16 Bahamonde AL *et al.* (2018) Subcutaneous furosemide in patients with refractory heart failure. *BMJ Supportive and Palliative Care*. **8**: 354–355.

17 Towers KA *et al.* (2010) Nebulised frusemide for the symptomatic treatment of end-stage congestive heart failure. *Medical journal of Australia*. **193**: 555.

18 Amiel S *et al.* (1984) Intravenous infusion of frusemide as treatment for ascites in malignant disease. *British Medical Journal*. **288**: 1041.

19 Fogel M *et al.* (1981) Diuresis in the ascitic patient: a randomized controlled trial of three regimens. *Journal of Clinical Gastroenterology*. **3**: 73–80.

20 Kalambokis G *et al.* (2006) The effects of treatment with octreotide, diuretics, or both on portal hemodynamics in nonazotemic cirrhotic patients with ascites. *Journal of Clinical Gastroenterology*. **40**: 342–346.

21 Kalambokis G *et al.* (2005) Renal effects of treatment with diuretics, octreotide or both, in non-azotemic cirrhotic patients with ascites. *Nephrology, Dialysis, Transplantation*. **20**: 1623–1629.

22 Newton PJ *et al.* (2008) Nebulized furosemide for the management of dyspnea: does the evidence support its use? *Journal of Pain and Symptom Management*. **36:** 424-441.

23 Stone P *et al.* (2002) Re: nebulized furosemide for dyspnea in terminal cancer patients. *Journal of Pain and Symptom Management*. **24**: 274–275; author reply 275–276.

24 Ventresca P *et al.* (1990) Inhaled furosemide inhibits cough induced by low-chloride solutions but not by capsaicin. *American Review of Respiratory Disease*. **142**: 143–146.

25 Bianco S *et al.* (1989) Protective effect of inhaled furosemide on allergen-induced early and late asthmatic reactions. *New England Journal of Medicine*. **321**: 1069–1073.

26 Nishino T *et al.* (2000) Inhaled furosemide greatly alleviates the sensation of experimentally induced dyspnea. *American Journal of Respiratory and Critical Care Medicine*. **161**: 1963–1967.

27 Grogono JC *et al.* (2018) Inhaled furosemide for relief of air hunger versus sense of breathing effort: a randomized controlled trial. *Respiratory research*. **19**: 181.

28 Waskiw-Ford M *et al.* (2018) Effect of inhaled nebulized furosemide (40 and 120 mg) on breathlessness during exercise in the presence of external thoracic restriction in healthy men. *Frontiers in Physiology*. **9**: 86.

29 Laveneziana P *et al.* (2008) Inhaled furosemide does not alleviate respiratory effort during flow-limited exercise in healthy subjects. *Pulmonary Pharmacology and Therapeutics*. **21**: 196–200.

30 Newton PJ *et al.* (2012) The acute haemodynamic effect of nebulised frusemide in stable, advanced heart failure. *Heart Lung Circulation*. **21**: 260–266.

31 Moosavi SH *et al.* (2006) Effect of inhaled furosemide on air hunger induced in healthy humans. *Respiritory Physiology and Neurobiology*. **156**: 1–8.

32 Ong KC *et al.* (2004) Effects of inhaled furosemide on exertional dyspnea in chronic obstructive pulmonary disease. *American Journal of Respiratory and Critical Care Medicine*. **169:** 1028–1033.

33 Jensen D *et al.* (2008) Mechanisms of dyspnoea relief and improved exercise endurance after furosemide inhalation in COPD. *Thorax*. **63**: 606–613.

34 Sheikh Motahar Vahedi H *et al.* (2013) The adjunctive effect of nebulized furosemide in acute treatment of patients with chronic obstructive pulmonary disease exacerbation: a randomized controlled clinical trial. *Respiratory Care*. **58**: 1873–1877.

35 Shimoyama N and Shimoyama M (2002) Nebulized furosemide as a novel treatment for dyspnea in terminal cancer patients. *Journal of Pain and Symptom Management*. **23**: 73–76.

36 Kohara H *et al.* (2003) Effect of nebulized furosemide in terminally ill cancer patients with dyspnea. *Journal of Pain and Symptom Management*. 26: 962–967.

37 Wilcock A *et al.* (2008) Randomised, placebo-controlled trial of nebulised furosemide for breathlessness in patients with cancer. *Thorax*. **63**: 872-875.

38 Haegeli L *et al.* (2007) Sublingual administration of furosemide: new application of an old drug. *British Journal of Clinical Pharmacology*. **64**: 804–809.

39 Murray MD *et al.* (1997) Variable furosemide absorption and poor predictability of response in elderly patients. *Pharmacotherapy*. **17**: 98-106.

40 Verma AK *et al.* (2004) Diuretic effects of subcutaneous furosemide in human volunteers: a randomized pilot study. *Annals of Pharmacotherapy*. **38**: 544–549.

41 Walma E *et al.* (1997) Withdrawal of long term diuretic medication in elderly patients: a double blind randomised trial. *British Medical Journal*. **315**: 464–468.

42 Baxter K and Preston CL *Stockley's Drug Interactions. London: Pharmaceutical Press* www.medicinescomplete.com (accessed December 2017).

43 Trissel LA *Handbook on Injectable Drugs. Maryland, USA: American Society of Health-System Pharmacists* www.medicinescomplete.com (accessed October 2013).

Updated May 2019

SPIRONOLACTONE

Class: Potassium-sparing diuretic; mineralocorticoid (aldosterone) receptor antagonist (MRA).

Indications: Ascites and peripheral oedema associated with portal hypertension and hyperaldosteronism (i.e. as seen in cirrhosis, hepatocellular cancer, extensive hepatic metastases), chronic heart failure, nephrotic syndrome, primary hyperaldosteronism, resistant hypertension.

Contra-indications: Hyperkalaemia, Addison's disease, anuria, severe renal impairment, concurrent use with potassium supplements or potassium-sparing diuretics.

Pharmacology

Spironolactone and two metabolites (7α-thiomethyl-spironolactone and canrenone) bind to cytoplasmic mineralocorticoid receptors and function as aldosterone antagonists. This results in a potassium-sparing diuretic effect in the distal tubules of the kidney.

A diuretic-induced reduction in plasma volume can activate several neurohumoral systems, e.g. the renin–angiotensin–aldosterone system, sympathetic nervous system, ADH secretion, resulting in impaired renal perfusion and increased Na^+ and water resorption. These changes contribute towards a reduced effect of the diuretic ('diuretic resistance') and also renal impairment.

In patients with cirrhosis receiving spironolactone ± **furosemide**, improved renal function and diuresis is seen with co-administration of **octreotide** 300microgram SC b.d. (see p.593) or **clonidine** 75microgram PO b.d. (see p.83) due to inhibition of the renin–angiotensin–aldosterone (**octreotide** and **clonidine**) and sympathetic nervous (**clonidine**) systems.[1-3] Note. Patients in the **clonidine** study were considered to have an overactive sympathetic nervous system based on a higher than normal serum noradrenaline (norepinephrine) level.[3]

Spironolactone also binds to the androgen receptor and to a lesser extent to oestrogen and progesterone receptors. The resultant anti-androgenic effect is used to treat acne and hirsutism in women, particularly when associated with polycystic ovary syndrome. However, it can also result in undesirable effects such as menstrual disorders and, in men, gynaecomastia, breast pain or impotence. **Eplerenone**, an aldosterone antagonist with greater selectively for the mineralocorticoid receptor, has been used as an alternative in these circumstances;[4,5] it is substituted for spironolactone on a 1:1 basis.[6]

Caution is required when using spironolactone in patients with prostate cancer. Although there are reports of cancer regression in keeping with an androgen-blocking effect, disease progression has also been reported.[7] It is suggested that spironolactone acts as an androgen receptor modulator and thus can exert both anti- and pro-androgenic effects.

Aldosterone binds to the mineralocorticoid receptor and activates pro-inflammatory and other cell pathways.[8-11] Thus, by preventing the binding of aldosterone, spironolactone has anti-inflammatory and other effects. Although the full therapeutic potential of this remains to be determined, benefit is seen with spironolactone in various experimental and clinical settings, with reductions in cancer growth, cancer cachexia and insulin resistance, for example.[12-14]

Ascites

Hyperaldosteronism is a concomitant of ascites associated with portal hypertension (a *transudate* with a relatively low albumin concentration, best indicated by a serum–ascites albumin gradient of ≥11g/L) as seen in cirrhosis, hepatocellular cancer and extensive hepatic metastases.[15,16] Most evidence comes from cirrhosis, but spironolactone in a median total daily dose of 200–300mg/24h is successful in most patients with these conditions (90% in cirrhosis).[15-20]

In patients with cirrhosis, the combined use of spironolactone + **furosemide** provides a more rapid effect than spironolactone alone, but requires closer monitoring and more frequent dose adjustments.[18] Thus, particularly in outpatients, the initial use of spironolactone alone may be preferable.[20] In contrast, treatment with even large PO doses of a loop diuretic alone, e.g. **furosemide** 200mg, generally fails to reduce ascites.[21]

Note. Paracentesis is used for patients failing to respond to or tolerate diuretic therapy. Paracentesis is also preferable for patients with predominantly peritoneal ascites (an *exudate* with relatively high albumin concentration, best indicated by a serum–ascites albumin gradient of ≤11g/L) or chylous ascites, because these are unlikely to respond to diuretics,[17,19] and also for patients with a tense distended abdomen in need of rapid relief.

For patients requiring frequent paracentesis and with a prognosis of >1 month, an indwelling tunnelled drain can be considered, e.g. Pleurx® catheter. Patients are taught to drain off fluid using special drainage sets with vacuum bottles, initially up to 2L every day for 1–2 weeks, and then as needed, generally every other day.

Chronic heart failure

Spironolactone improves morbidity and mortality in patients with chronic heart failure and a reduced left ventricular ejection fraction. It is added in low dose (e.g. 12.5–25mg) to standard treatment.[6,22,23] Its aldosterone antagonist action helps reduce vascular and myocardial fibrosis, sympathetic nervous system activation, baroreceptor dysfunction and K^+ and Mg^{2+} depletion.

Hypertension

Aldosterone antagonists are used as a fourth-line add-on therapy in patients with hypertension failing to respond to more usual antihypertensives.[24,25]

Spironolactone is extensively metabolized. The 7α-thiomethyl-spironolactone and canrenone metabolites have long halflives and are excreted in the urine. Consequently, because of their accumulation and the increased risk of hyperkalaemia, the use of spironolactone requires caution in mild–moderate renal impairment and is generally contra-indicated in severe renal impairment.
Bio-availability 60–90%.
Onset of action 2–4h.
Maximum effect 7h (single dose), 2–3 days (multiple doses).
Time to peak plasma concentration 2–3h; active metabolites 3–4.5h PO.
Plasma halflife 1–1.5h; active metabolites 14–17h (multiple doses).
Duration of action >24h (single dose), 2–3 days (multiple doses).

Cautions

Prostate cancer (see Pharmacology); elderly; hepatic impairment, may induce reversible hyperchloraemic metabolic acidosis in patients with decompensated hepatic cirrhosis; renal impairment (see Dose and use).

Drug interactions

Serious drug interactions: *Hyperkalaemia* with potassium supplements (avoid concurrent use), table salt substitutes (contain both potassium and sodium chlorides), potassium-sparing diuretics, ACE inhibitors, angiotensin II receptor antagonists, certain antimicrobials (**trimethoprim**, **nitrofurantoin**), **ciclosporin**, LMWH and **tacrolimus**, particularly if other risk factors also present, e.g. elderly, renal impairment, diabetes.[26-28]

May induce *hyponatraemia*, particularly if used with other diuretics. Natriuretic effect reduced by **aspirin**, **indometacin** and possibly other NSAIDs.

Spironolactone increases the plasma concentration of digoxin by up to 25% and can interfere with digoxin plasma concentration assays; measure free digoxin levels using a chemiluminescent assay.[27]

Undesirable effects

Very common (>10%): CNS disturbances (drowsiness, dizziness, confusion, headache, fever, ataxia, fatigue), GI disturbances (anorexia, dyspepsia, nausea, vomiting, peptic ulceration, colic).
Common (<10%, >1%): gastritis, hyperkalaemia, gynaecomastia, breast pain.[29]

Dose and use

To reduce the risk of gastric irritation, advise patient to take with food. If, despite this, once daily spironolactone causes nausea and vomiting, try giving in divided doses.

For patients with swallowing difficulties, although an unauthorized oral suspension is available, it is expensive. A cheaper (and authorized) alternative is to disperse generic spironolactone tablets in water (also see Chapter 28, p.854).

In patients with ascites and moderate renal impairment (e.g. eGFR 30–59mL/min/1.73m^2), halve the recommended dose.

Cirrhotic or malignant ascites associated with portal hypertension

Most experience comes from cirrhotic ascites.[15,16,18,20,21,30] Elimination of ascites may take 10–28 days:

- when close monitoring is possible (e.g. inpatients):
  - ▷ start spironolactone 100mg PO and **furosemide** 40mg PO each morning
  - ▷ if necessary, increase both every 3–5 days, maintaining the 100mg:40mg ratio, up to a usual maximum of 400mg/24h and 160mg/24h respectively
- when close monitoring is *not* possible (e.g. outpatients) or when minimal fluid overload:
  - ▷ start spironolactone alone 100mg PO each morning
  - ▷ if necessary, increase by 100mg every 3–5 days
  - ▷ typical maintenance dose 200–300mg/24h; maximum dose 400mg/24h
  - ▷ if not achieving the desired weight loss with spironolactone, consider adding **furosemide** 40mg each morning; if necessary, increase to a maximum of 160mg/24h.

Monitor body weight and renal function:

- adjust doses to achieve a weight loss of 0.5–1kg/24h (<0.5kg/24h when peripheral oedema absent)
- once ascites has resolved, reduce dose of diuretics to the lowest effective maintenance dose
- if Na^+ falls to <125mmol/L, temporarily stop all diuretics
- if K^+ falls to <3.5mmol/L, temporarily stop or decrease the dose of **furosemide**
- if K^+ rises to >5.5mmol/L, halve the dose of spironolactone; if >6mmol/L, temporarily stop spironolactone
- if creatinine rises to >150micromol/L, temporarily stop all diuretics
- if hepatic encephalopathy or muscle cramps develop, temporarily stop all diuretics.

Even if paracentesis becomes necessary, diuretics should be continued because they reduce the rate of recurrence. Note. When >5L are to be removed, stop diuretics 2 days before paracentesis and start again 1–2 days afterwards.[31]

Severe chronic heart failure (NYHA class III or IV disease)

Seek specialist advice. Spironolactone is used in patients with a reduced left ventricular ejection fraction who remain symptomatic despite an ACE inhibitor + ß-blocker. The following is based on several sets of published guidelines:

- do *not* prescribe spironolactone unless serum K^+ <5mmol/L and creatinine <200micromol/L or eGFR >30mL/min/1.73m^2
- start with 12.5–25mg PO once daily; check serum K^+ and creatinine after 4–7 days
- if necessary, *after 1 month*, increase to 25–50mg once daily; check serum K^+ and creatinine after 1 week
- if K^+ rises to >5mmol/L, halve the dose; if >5.5mmol/L, stop spironolactone completely
- occasionally, higher doses are used
- it is particularly important to monitor potassium levels when spironolactone and an ACE inhibitor are prescribed concurrently.[6,22,28,32]

Resistant hypertension

Seek specialist advice. Spironolactone is used as a fourth-line add-on therapy for hypertension not responding to a combination of three more usual antihypertensives:

- do not prescribe if serum K^+ is >4.5mmol/L
- start with 25mg PO once daily; check serum Na^+, K^+ and creatinine within 1 month and repeat at intervals thereafter
- typical dose 25–50mg once daily, maximum dose 100mg/24h.[24,33]

Supply

Spironolactone (generic)

Tablets 25mg, 50mg, 100mg, 28 days @ 200mg each morning = £4.25.

Oral suspension (sugar-free) 5mg/5mL, 10mg/5mL, 25mg/5mL, 50mg/5mL, 100mg/5mL, 28 days @ 200mg each morning = £93 (unauthorized products, available as a special order; see Chapter 24, p.817.) *Price based on Specials tariff in community.*

Spironolactone oral suspension can also be prepared locally for individual patients.[34]

Spironolactone is also available in fixed dose combinations with **hydroflumethiazide** or **furosemide**. However, these are more expensive and do not allow titration of the individual drugs.

1 Kalambokis G *et al.* (2005) Renal effects of treatment with diuretics, octreotide or both, in non-azotemic cirrhotic patients with ascites. *Nephrology, Dialysis, Transplantation*. **20**: 1623–1629.

2 Kalambokis G *et al.* (2006) The effects of treatment with octreotide, diuretics, or both on portal hemodynamics in nonazotemic cirrhotic patients with ascites. *Journal of Clinical Gastroenterology*. **40**: 342–346.

3 Lenaerts A *et al.* (2006) Effects of clonidine on diuretic response in ascitic patients with cirrhosis and activation of sympathetic nervous system. *Hepatology*. **44**: 844–849.

4 Barnes BJ and Howard PA (2005) Eplerenone: a selective aldosterone receptor antagonist for patients with heart failure. *Annals of Pharmacotherapy*. **39**: 68–76.

5 Dimitriadis G *et al.* (2011) Eplerenone reverses spironolactone-induced painful gynaecomastia in cirrhotics. *Hepatology International*. **5**: 738–739.

6 Ponikowski P *et al.* (2016) ESC guidelines for the diagnosis and treatment of acute and chronic heart failure: the Task Force for the diagnosis and treatment of acute and chronic heart failure of the European Society of Cardiology (ESC) developed with the special contribution of the Heart Failure Association (HFA) of the ESC. *European Heart Journal*. **37**: 2129–2200.

7 Sundar S and Dickinson PD (2012) Spironolactone, a possible selective androgen receptor modulator, should be used with caution in patients with metastatic carcinoma of the prostate. *BMJ Case Reports*. doi:10.1136/bcr.11.2011.5238.

8 Chantong B *et al.* (2012) Mineralocorticoid and glucocorticoid receptors differentially regulate NF-kappaB activity and pro-inflammatory cytokine production in murine bv-2 microglial cells. *Journal of Neuroinflammation*. **9**: 260.

9 Syngle A *et al.* (2009) Effect of spironolactone on endothelial dysfunction in rheumatoid arthritis. *Scandinavian Journal of Rheumatology*. **38**: 15–22.

10 Syngle A *et al.* (2013) Spironolactone improves endothelial dysfunction in ankylosing spondylitis. *Clinical Rheumatology*. **32**: 1029–1036.

11 Sun YE *et al.* (2012) Intrathecal injection of spironolactone attenuates radicular pain by inhibition of spinal microglia activation in a rat model. *PLoS One*. **7**: e39897.

12 King S *et al.* (2014) Evidence for aldosterone-dependent growth of renal cell carcinoma. *International Journal of Experimental Pathology*. **95**: 244–250.

13 Springer J *et al.* (2014) Prevention of liver cancer cachexia-induced cardiac wasting and heart failure. *European Heart Journal*. **35**: 932–941.

14 Ogino K *et al.* (2014) Spironolactone, not furosemide, improved insulin resistance in patients with chronic heart failure. *International Journal of Cardiology*. **171**: 398–403.

15 Greenway B *et al.* (1982) Control of malignant ascites with spironolactone. *British Journal of Surgery*. **69**: 441–442.

16 Fernandez-Esparrach G *et al.* (1997) Diuretic requirements after therapeutic paracentesis in non-azotemic patients with cirrhosis. A randomized double-blind trial of spironolactone versus placebo. *Journal of Hepatology*. **26**: 614–620.

17 Pockros P *et al.* (1992) Mobilization of malignant ascites with diuretics is dependent on ascitic fluid characteristics. *Gastroenterology*. **103**: 1302–1306.

18 Moore KP *et al.* (2003) The management of ascites in cirrhosis: report on the consensus conference of the International Ascites Club. *Hepatology*. **38**: 258–266.

19 Becker G *et al.* (2006) Malignant ascites: systematic review and guideline for treatment. *European Journal of Cancer*. **42**: 589–597.

20 Runyon BA (2012) Management of adult patients with ascites due to cirrhosis: update 2012. *American Association for the Study of Liver Diseases*. www.aasld.org

21 Fogel M *et al.* (1981) Diuresis in the ascitic patient: a randomized controlled trial of three regimens. *Journal of Clinical Gastroenterology*. **3**: 73–80.

22 NICE (2018) Chronic heart failure in adults: diagnosis and management. *NICE Guideline*. NG106. www.nice.org.uk

23 Yancy CW *et al.* (2017) 2017 ACC/AHA/HFSA focused update of the 2013 ACCF/AHA guideline for the management of heart failure: a report of the American College of Cardiology/American Heart Association Task Force on clinical practice guidelines and the Heart Failure Society of America. *Circulation*. **136**: e137–e161.

24 NICE (2011) Hypertension in adults: diagnosis and management. *Clinical Guideline*. CG127. www.nice.org.uk

25 Wang C *et al.* (2016) Efficacy and safety of spironolactone in patients with resistant hypertension: a meta-analysis of randomised controlled trials. *Heart Lung and Circulation*. **25**: 1021–1030.

26 Antoniou T *et al.* (2015) Trimethoprim-sulfamethoxazole and risk of sudden death among patients taking spironolactone. *Canadian Medical Association Journal*. **187**: e138–e143.

27 Baxter K and Preston CL Stockley's drug interactions: London: Pharmaceutical Press www.medicinescomplete.com (accessed July 2018).

28 MHRA (2016) Spironolactone and renin-angiotensin system drugs in heart failure: risk of potentially fatal hyperkalaemia. *Drug Safety Update*. www.gov.uk/drug-safety-update

29 Williams EM *et al.* (2006) Use and side-effect profile of spironolactone in a private cardiologist's practice. *Clinical Cardiology*. **29**: 149–153.

30 Sharma S and Walsh D (1995) Management of symptomatic malignant ascites with diuretics: two case reports and a review of the literature. *Journal of Pain and Symptom Management*. **10**: 237–242.

31 Twycross R and Wilcock A (2016) Introducing palliative care (5e). Palliativedrugs.com Ltd. Nottingham. UK. 138–142.

32 Shchekochikhin D *et al.* (2013) Increased spironolactone in advanced heart failure: effect of doses greater than 25 mg/day on plasma potassium concentration. *Cardiorenal Medicine*. **3**: 1–6.

33 Dahal K *et al.* (2015) The effects of aldosterone antagonists in patients with resistant hypertension: a meta-analysis of randomized and nonrandomized studies. *American Journal of Hypertension*. **28**: 1376–1385.

34 Allen LV Jr and Erickson MA 3rd (1996) Stability of ketoconazole, metolazone, metronidazole, procainamide hydrochloride, and spironolactone in extemporaneously compounded oral liquids. *American Journal of Health System Pharmacy*. **53**: 2073–2078.

Updated (minor change) March 2021

SYSTEMIC LOCAL ANAESTHETICS

Local anaesthetics and their orally administered congeners are sometimes useful as third- or fourth-line drugs in the treatment of neuropathic pain. An analgesic effect has been reported when the following drugs have been administered systemically:[1]

- **lidocaine** IV, SC (and also TD)[2,3]
- **flecainide** PO
- **mexiletine** PO
- **tocainide** PO (not UK).

The mechanism by which they provide relief is not fully understood, but probably includes blockade of sodium channels that accumulate at sites of nerve injury (also see Anti-epileptics, p.280). This stabilizes the nerve membrane and thus suppresses injury-induced hyperexcitability in the peripheral and central nervous systems. Some antidepressants and anti-epileptics that benefit neuropathic pain also have membrane-stabilizing properties, e.g. **amitriptyline**, **carbamazepine**.[4]

Other actions may be relevant and can occur at lower concentrations than necessary for sodium channel blockade. These include anti-inflammatory effects, interaction with other receptors (e.g. NMDA-receptor channel complex) and increased inhibitory neurotransmission (e.g. a **lidocaine** metabolite increases glycine levels).[5]

A systematic review of 32 RCTs, mostly of IV **lidocaine** and PO **mexiletine**, found benefit for various neuropathic pains, e.g. diabetic neuropathy, trigeminal neuralgia, post-herpetic neuralgia and post-stroke neuropathic pain.[1] However, benefit was inconsistent in some pains, e.g. diabetic neuropathy, and absent in others, e.g. cancer-related neuropathic pain. Most of the studies had methodological weaknesses, e.g. those reporting efficacy comparable to **amantadine**, **carbamazepine**, **gabapentin** and **morphine** were generally underpowered.

Thus, the place, if any, of systemic local anaesthetics for neuropathic pain is uncertain. If used in cancer-related neuropathic pain, they should be considered for use only when the combination of a strong opioid + NSAID + antidepressant + anti-epileptic is ineffective or poorly tolerated (also see Adjuvant analgesics, p.325).

The use of systemic **lidocaine** has been explored in various other pains, e.g. postoperative, critical limb ischaemia, colic (renal, bowel),[6-9] as well as persistent hiccup and status epilepticus.[10,11] Although benefit is reported, the evidence is insufficient to support the routine use of systemic **lidocaine** in these settings.

*Systemic lidocaine

*The use of systemic **lidocaine** is limited to specialist palliative care or pain services. There should be an agreed protocol to ensure appropriate safety considerations are followed, including patient monitoring and staff training to manage toxicity.*[12]

Lidocaine has a narrow therapeutic index, and there are important contra-indications and cautions to be observed (see manufacturer's SPC). Contra-indications include patients at greater risk of cardiac arrhythmias, e.g. those with any type of cardiac disease, electrolyte abnormalities, and those already taking an anti-arrhythmic. Cautions include factors that increase the risk of toxicity, e.g. patients who are elderly, cachectic, or have renal or hepatic impairment.

A normal 12-lead ECG is a mandatory prerequisite. When administering IV **lidocaine** in a day case setting, particularly in non-cancer pain, some services monitor heart rhythm continuously and blood pressure/SpO_2 frequently, e.g. every 8 minutes, and ensure immediate access to resuscitation equipment. However, because of limited access to heart rhythm monitors, some palliative care centres follow IV **lidocaine** protocols that do not require intense monitoring.[13]

Non-cancer pain

In non-cancer pain, improvement lasting 4–20 weeks after a single dose of IV **lidocaine** has been reported in patients with, e.g. central pain syndrome, diabetic neuropathy.[14,15] However, benefit is mostly limited to a few hours or days.[14,16] Some services repeat the dose weekly for as long as it is beneficial.[17] Alternatively, ongoing relief will necessitate CIVI or CSCI **lidocaine** or the use of an oral analogue, e.g. **flecainide**, **mexiletine**. However, the response to IV **lidocaine** does not reliably predict subsequent benefit from PO **mexiletine**, and undesirable effects can limit its chronic use.[15,18] For example, in a cohort of patients with non-cancer neuropathic pain treated with **mexiletine**, the median time to discontinuation (for any reason) was 6 weeks, with only

20% persisting with its use >1 year.[19] Further, recent specialist guidelines were strongly against the use of **mexiletine**, because of a lack of evidence.[20] Finally, although a **mexiletine** product is again available in the UK, its authorization is limited to relief of myotonia in non-dystrophic myotonic disorders, and its cost prohibitive (~£50 per 167mg capsule).

Cancer pain

Subsequent to the two negative RCTs of cancer-related neuropathic pain included in the large systematic review,[1] there have been four further small RCTs of IV/SC **lidocaine** (n≤50).[21,22] Three were negative (two in neuropathic pain, one in bone pain) and one positive (opioid-refractory pain, mostly neuropathic).[23] In the latter, compared with placebo, pain relief with IV **lidocaine** was faster (40 vs. 75min), of greater magnitude (75 vs. 25% reduction) and duration (9 vs. 4 days). Otherwise, reports of benefit are limited to case reports/series. Various regimens are used (Box A). There is limited published experience in children.[24-26]

Box A Examples of systemic lidocaine regimens for cancer-related neuropathic pain

Various approaches have been described.

Intermittent IVI ± an initial loading dose

- IVI 2mg/kg over 20*min* loading dose, followed immediately by 2mg/kg over 1h (used in the positive RCT)[23] *or*
- IVI 5mg/kg over 1–2h; subsequent infusions can be progressively increased to a maximum dose of 10mg/kg (or 900mg).[13]

When providing benefit of several days or more, the above is repeated p.r.n.

Initial IVI to identify responders followed by CIVI

- IVI 1–2mg/kg over 15–20*min*; followed by CIVI 1mg/kg/h if initial IVI was of benefit.[27]

CSCI

- CSCI 0.5mg/kg/h increasing to a maximum of 1.5mg/kg/h (maximum dose limited to 80–120mg/h by some).[28]

Generally, continuous infusions are given for days–weeks, although up to 8 months is reported.[29] Accumulation resulting in toxicity can occur (see Monitoring use).

Example guidelines/protocols are available from the Document library on www.palliativedrugs.com.

Monitoring use

*When receiving IVI, CIVI or CSCI **lidocaine**, patients should always be monitored closely for initial signs of toxicity:*

- metallic taste
- circumoral numbness or tingling
- light-headedness, dizziness, drowsiness
- tinnitus.

If any of these occur, stop the **lidocaine** until resolved and subsequently restart at a lower dose. Worsening toxicity is indicated by the progressive appearance of:

- visual changes
- muscle twitching
- seizures
- ECG changes (see below)
- coma
- cardiorespiratory depression and arrest.

Cardiovascular toxicity is more likely to lead to serious harm or death. Generally, it appears after neurotoxicity and is suggested by changes in heart rate, blood pressure, ECG (widening of QRS complex, ST segment changes, ventricular ectopics) and cardiac arrhythmia. Successful treatment of severe toxicity with a lipid emulsion has been reported.[30]

With CIVI/CSCI, accumulation of **lidocaine** and its active metabolites, e.g. monoethylglycinexylidide, glycinexylidide, can occur and lead to toxicity. Particular caution is needed in the elderly, in whom clearance is already reduced.[31-33] For example, two elderly patients (≥70 years), despite normal renal/liver function and receiving a relatively small dose of **lidocaine** (200–300mg/24h), developed severe drowsiness after 10 days.[34]

Thus, some suggest that with continuous infusions, serum levels should be monitored, e.g. 1–3 days after starting treatment/any dose increase, or when toxicity is suspected.[29] Analgesia is generally seen with serum levels of 1.5–5microgram/mL (and severe neurotoxicity with levels ≥10microgram/mL).[2,35] However, there is large interindividual variation, and the beneficial/toxic effect relates more to the amount of free **lidocaine** (unbound to protein), rather than the total serum level (bound plus unbound).[31]

However, because the monitoring of serum levels is not always readily available, some palliative care centres follow **lidocaine** continuous infusion protocols that do not require it.[28]

Lidocaine medicated plasters

These are authorized for post-herpetic neuralgia (Box B). Sufficient high-quality data are lacking to recommend them for first-line use in this setting.[3,20,36] Indeed, NICE considers the data insufficient to make any recommendations on their use.[37] Thus, in post-herpetic neuralgia, the plasters are best reserved for situations where antidepressants (e.g. **amitriptyline**, **duloxetine**) and anti-epileptics (e.g. **gabapentin**) are contra-indicated, ineffective or poorly tolerated. Further, in 2017, the NHS limited its prescribing in primary care to post-herpetic neuralgia (essentially third-line after an antidepressant and a gabapentinoid), unless advised by specialist pain teams.[38]

The analgesic effect of the **lidocaine** plasters is considered to be local via a non-selective block of peripheral sodium channels on sensory afferents in the epidermis.[39] However, neither the density of epidermal nerve fibres nor the results of quantitative sensory testing/nerve conduction studies predict pain relief from the plasters.[40,41] Indeed, some patients with a complete loss of epidermal nerve fibres report benefit. Thus, the exact mechanism of effect is unclear.[40,42]

There is also a strong placebo effect. In chronic back pain, active and placebo plasters provide similar reductions in pain intensity, sensory and affective scores and pain-related brain activity (functional MRI).[43] If the main effect of the **lidocaine** plasters is physical protection in patients with allodynia, they are an unnecessarily expensive form of plaster.

Box B Use of lidocaine 5% medicated plasters

Each plaster contains 700mg lidocaine. *Only about 5% of the plaster dose is absorbed.* Steady-state is achieved after 3 days. Maximum concentrations (0.07–0.19microgram/mL) are well below systemic analgesic levels (1.5–5microgram/mL) and serious toxic levels (≥10microgram/mL).

Caution is needed in patients with severe cardiac, severe hepatic or severe renal impairment. Accumulation of lidocaine and its active metabolites can occur in severe renal impairment, and CNS toxicity has been reported, e.g. delirium.[60]

A recommended maximum of three plasters are applied to cover the painful area on a 12h on, 12h off basis. If necessary, the plasters can be cut, but they must not be applied close to the eyes or mouth, or on inflamed/broken skin or wounds.

Similar considerations apply as for other medical transdermal products, e.g. skin hair should be clipped rather than shaved; fold plasters in half and dispose of safely (>660mg remains in the plasters); remove before MRI scans (see Chapter 30, p.901).

The 12h off periods are to help reduce the risk of skin reactions, but these still occur in about 15% of patients. The skin on the head and neck appears most susceptible.[61] The skin can be rested for longer when necessary, but up to 5% of patients have to discontinue.

Generally, high-quality data are lacking. Experience with post-herpetic neuralgia suggests that overall <50% of patients will obtain sufficient benefit to warrant continuing with the plasters,[62] that a 2-week trial may be needed to identify responders,[63] and, for those who respond, sustained benefit (≥4 years) has been reported.[64] The magnitude of the benefit appears similar to that obtained with pregabalin (p.297), but the plasters are better tolerated.[44]

Anaphylaxis is a very rare complication (≤1:10,000).

Situations in which **lidocaine** plasters have been used include:

- diabetic polyneuropathy[44]
- post-surgical neuropathic pain[41,45]
- post-traumatic neuropathic pain[41]
- osteoarthritis[46]
- carpal tunnel syndrome[47]
- erythromelalgia[48]
- myofascial pain[49]
- cancer-related neuropathic pain[50,51]
- back pain[52]
- trigeminal neuralgia.[53]

Most evidence of benefit comes from low-quality open studies or case reports/series. RCTs have shown mixed benefit in peripheral neuropathic pain (mostly post-surgical/post-traumatic)[41,45,54] and traumatic rib fracture,[55,56] and no benefit in post-herniorrhaphy or back pain.[43,45,57] Even when **lidocaine** plasters are beneficial, the treatment effect size is small–medium (0.3–0.4) and the NNT for 50% pain relief ranges from 4–20.[41,58]

A survey showed that, in palliative care, the main use of the plasters is for neuropathic pain associated with invasion of the chest wall by mesothelioma, breast or lung cancer. They were considered acceptable, well tolerated and beneficial to most patients. On the other hand, there were concerns about an unpredictable or variable response and high cost.[59]

*Flecainide

*The use of **flecainide** is limited to specialist palliative care or pain services.*

Flecainide is a class 1C anti-arrhythmic authorized for use primarily in the prevention and treatment of supraventricular and ventricular arrhythmias. Rarely, it is used to treat nerve injury pain. There are important contra-indications and cautions to be observed (see manufacturer's SPC). **Flecainide** has a narrow therapeutic index, and some patients experience psychoneurological and cardiac toxicity within the recommended therapeutic range (also see **lidocaine** above).[65,66] Flecainide is both metabolized by and inhibits CYP2D6 (see Chapter 19, Table 8, p.791).

Response rates for neuropathic pain in non-controlled studies in cancer and AIDS patients vary from 30–60%.[67-70] Generally, tricyclic antidepressants should be stopped at least 48h before starting **flecainide**. Initial doses are comparable to those used in cardiology:

- start with 50mg PO b.d.
- usual dose 100mg b.d.
- maximum dose 200mg b.d.[67,70]

See SPC for circumstances requiring dose adjustment.

Supply

Lidocaine hydrochloride (generic)
Medicated plaster 5%, 30 = £72.
Injection solution (preservative free) 5mg/mL (0.5%), 10mg/mL (1%), 20mg/mL (2%) 2mL, 5mL, 10mL and 20mL = £1.

Versatis® (Grunenthal)
Medicated plaster 5%, 30 = £72.

For topical use of **lidocaine** in oral inflammation and ulceration or in wound care, see p.669 and p.688 respectively.

Flecainide (generic)
Tablets 50mg, 100mg, 28 days @100mg b.d. = £5.

1 Challapalli V *et al.* (2005) Systemic administration of local anesthetic agents to relieve neuropathic pain. *Cochrane Database of Systematic Reviews*. CD003345. www.thecochranelibrary.com (Last reviewed 2017).
2 Devulder J *et al.* (1993) Neuropathic pain in a cancer patient responding to subcutaneously administered lignocaine. *Clinical Journal of Pain*. **9**: 220–223.
3 Derry S *et al.* (2014) Topical lidocaine for neuropathic pain in adults. *Cochrane Database of Systematic Reviews*. CD010958. www.thecochranelibrary.com (Last reviewed 2016).

4 Devor M (2006) Sodium channels and mechanisms of neuropathic pain. *Journal of Pain*. **7**: S3–S12.
5 van der Wal SE *et al.* (2016) The *in vitro* mechanisms and *in vivo* efficacy of intravenous lidocaine on the neuroinflammatory response in acute and chronic pain. *European Journal of Pain*. **20**: 655–674.
6 Weibel S *et al.* (2018) Continuous intravenous perioperative lidocaine infusion for postoperative pain and recovery in adults. *Cochrane Database of Systematic Reviews*. CD009642. www.thecochranelibrary.com
7 Vahidi E *et al.* (2015) Comparison of intravenous lidocaine versus morphine in alleviating pain in patients with critical limb ischaemia. *Emergency Medical Journal*. **32**: 516–519.
8 Firouzian A *et al.* (2016) Does lidocaine as an adjuvant to morphine improve pain relief in patients presenting to the ED with acute renal colic? A double-blind, randomized controlled trial. *American Journal of Emergency Medicine*. **34**: 443–448.
9 Bafuma PJ *et al.* (2015) Opiate refractory pain from an intestinal obstruction responsive to an intravenous lidocaine infusion. *American Journal of Emergency Medicine*. **33**: 1544.e3–1544.e4.
10 Kaneishi K and Kawabata M (2013) Continuous subcutaneous infusion of lidocaine for persistent hiccup in advanced cancer. *Palliative Medicine*. **27**: 284–285.
11 Zeiler FA *et al.* (2015) Lidocaine for status epilepticus in adults. *Seizure*. **31**: 41–48.
12 Dickerson DM and Apfelbaum JL (2014) Local anesthetic systemic toxicity. *Aesthetic Surgery Journal*. **34**: 1111–1119.
13 Peixoto RD and Hawley P (2015) Intravenous lidocaine for cancer pain without electrocardiographic monitoring: a retrospective review. *Journal of Palliative Medicine*. **18**: 373–377.
14 Backonja M and Gombar KA (1992) Response of central pain syndromes to intravenous lidocaine. *Journal of Pain and Symptom Management*. **7**: 172–178.
15 Viola V *et al.* (2006) Treatment of intractable painful diabetic neuropathy with intravenous lignocaine. *Journal of Diabetes and its Complications*. **20**: 34–39.
16 Kosharskyy B *et al.* (2013) Intravenous infusions in chronic pain management. *Pain Physician*. **16**: 231–249.
17 Przeklasa-Muszynska A *et al.* (2016) Intravenous lidocaine infusions in a multidirectional model of treatment of neuropathic pain patients. *Pharmacological Reports*. **68**: 1069–1075.
18 Attal N *et al.* (2000) Intravenous lidocaine in central pain: a double-blind, placebo-controlled, psychophysical study. *Neurology*. **54**: 564–574.
19 Carroll IR *et al.* (2008) Mexiletine therapy for chronic pain: survival analysis identifies factors predicting clinical success. *Journal of Pain and Symptom Management*. **35**: 321–326.
20 Finnerup NB *et al.* (2015) Pharmacotherapy for neuropathic pain in adults: a systematic review and meta-analysis. *Lancet Neurology*. **14**: 162–173.
21 Lee JT *et al.* (2019) Lidocaine for cancer pain in adults: a systematic review and meta-analysis. *Journal of Palliative Medicine*. **22**: 326–334.
22 Hawley P (2019) Personal communication.
23 Sharma S *et al.* (2009) A phase II pilot study to evaluate use of intravenous lidocaine for opioid-refractory pain in cancer patients. *Journal of Pain and Symptom Management*. **37**: 85–93.
24 Berde C *et al.* (2016) Lidocaine infusions and other options for opioid-resistant pain due to pediatric advanced cancer. *Pediatric Blood and Cancer*. **63**: 1141–1143.
25 Gibbons K *et al.* (2016) Continuous lidocaine infusions to manage opioid-refractory pain in a series of cancer patients in a pediatric hospital. *Pediatric Blood and Cancer*. **63**: 1168–1174.
26 Massey GV *et al.* (2002) Continuous lidocaine infusion for the relief of refractory malignant pain in a terminally ill pediatric cancer patient. *Journal of Pediatric Hematology/Oncology*. **24**: 566–568.
27 Thomas J *et al.* (2004) Intravenous lidocaine relieves severe pain: results of an inpatient hospice chart review. *Journal of Palliative Medicine*. **7**: 660–667.
28 Seah DS *et al.* (2017) Subcutaneous lidocaine infusion for pain in patients with cancer. *Journal of Palliative Medicine*. **20**: 667–671.
29 Ferrini R (2000) Parenteral lidocaine for severe intractable pain in six hospice patients continued at home. *Journal of Palliative Medicine*. **3**: 193–200.
30 Cao D *et al.* (2015) Intravenous lipid emulsion in the emergency department: a systematic review of recent literature. *Journal of Emergency Medicine*. **48**: 387–397.
31 Rosenberg PH *et al.* (2004) Maximum recommended doses of local anesthetics: a multifactorial concept. *Regional Anesthesia and Pain Medicine*. **29**: 564–575; discussion 524.
32 Brose W and Cousins M (1991) Subcutaneous lidocaine for treatment of neuropathic pain. *Pain*. **45**: 145–148.
33 Yamashita S *et al.* (2002) Lidocaine toxicity during frequent viscous lidocaine use for painful tongue ulcer. *Journal of Pain and Symptom Management*. **24**: 543–545.
34 Tei Y *et al.* (2005) Lidocaine intoxication at very small doses in terminally ill cancer patients. *Journal of Pain and Symptom Management*. **30**: 6–7.
35 Ferrante FM *et al.* (1996) The analgesic response to intravenous lidocaine in the treatment of neuropathic pain. *Anesthesia and Analgesia*. **82**: 91–97.
36 Scottish Medicines Consortium (2008) Lidocaine 5% medicated plaster (Versatis). 334/06. www.scottishmedicines.org.uk
37 NICE (2013) Pharmacological management of neuropathic pain in adults in non-specialist setting. *Clinical Guideline* CG173. www.nice.org.uk
38 NHS England (2017) Items which should not routinely be prescribed in primary care: guidance for CCGs. *NHS England Gateway Publication 07448*. www.england.nhs.uk
39 Madsen CS *et al.* (2013) Differential effects of a 5% lidocaine medicated patch in peripheral nerve injury. *Muscle Nerve*. **48**: 265–271.
40 Herrmann DN *et al.* (2006) Skin biopsy and quantitative sensory testing do not predict response to lidocaine patch in painful neuropathies. *Muscle Nerve*. **33**: 42–48.
41 Demant DT *et al.* (2015) Pain relief with lidocaine 5% patch in localized peripheral neuropathic pain in relation to pain phenotype: a randomised, double-blind, and placebo-controlled, phenotype panel study. *Pain*. **156**: 2234–2244.
42 Campbell JN (2012) How does topical lidocaine relieve pain? *Pain*. **153**: 255–256.
43 Hashmi JA *et al.* (2012) Lidocaine patch (5%) is no more potent than placebo in treating chronic back pain when tested in a randomised double blind placebo controlled brain imaging study. *Molecular Pain*. **8**: 29.
44 Baron R *et al.* (2009) 5% lidocaine medicated plaster versus pregabalin in post-herpetic neuralgia and diabetic polyneuropathy: an open-label, non-inferiority two-stage RCT study. *Current Medical Research and Opinion*. **25**: 1663–1676.
45 Cheville AL *et al.* (2009) Use of a lidocaine patch in the management of postsurgical neuropathic pain in patients with cancer: a phase III double-blind crossover study (N01CB). *Supportive Care in Cancer*. **17**: 451–460.
46 Burch F *et al.* (2004) Lidocaine patch 5% improves pain, stiffness, and physical function in osteoarthritis pain patients. A prospective, multicenter, open-label effectiveness trial. *Osteoarthritis and Cartilage*. **12**: 253–255.

47 Nalamachu S *et al.* (2006) A comparison of the lidocaine patch 5% vs naproxen 500 mg twice daily for the relief of pain associated with carpal tunnel syndrome: a 6-week, randomized, parallel-group study. *Medscape General Medicine*. **8**: 33.

48 Davis MD and Sandroni P (2005) Lidocaine patch for pain of erythromelalgia: follow-up of 34 patients. *Archives of Dermatology*. **141**: 1320–1321.

49 Lin YC *et al.* (2012) Therapeutic effects of lidocaine patch on myofascial pain syndrome of the upper trapezius: a randomized, double-blind, placebo-controlled study. *American Journal of Physical Medicine and Rehabilitation*. **91**: 871–882.

50 Fleming JA and O'Connor BD (2009) Use of lidocaine patches for neuropathic pain in a comprehensive cancer centre. *Pain Research and Management*. **14**: 381–388.

51 Garzon-Rodriguez C *et al.* (2013) Lidocaine 5% patches as an effective short-term co-analgesic in cancer pain. Preliminary results. *Supportive Care in Cancer*. **21**: 3153–3158.

52 Likar R *et al.* (2015) Treatment of localized neuropathic pain of different etiologies with the 5% lidocaine medicated plaster — a case series. *International Journal of General Medicine*. **8**: 9–14.

53 Tamburin S *et al.* (2014) Effect of 5% lidocaine medicated plaster on pain intensity and paroxysms in classical trigeminal neuralgia. *Annals of Pharmacotherpy*. **48**: 1521–1524.

54 Sansone P *et al.* (2017) Efficacy of the topical 5% lidocaine medicated plaster in the treatment of chronic post-thoracotomy neuropathic pain. *Pain Management*. **7**: 189–196.

55 Ingalls NK *et al.* (2010) Randomized, double-blind, placebo-controlled trial using lidocaine patch 5% in traumatic rib fractures. *Journal of the American College of Surgeons*. **210**: 205–209.

56 Cheng YJ (2016) Lidocaine skin patch (Lidopat(R) 5%) is effective in the treatment of traumatic rib fractures: a prospective double-blinded and vehicle-controlled study. *Medical Principles and Practice*. **25**: 36–39.

57 Bischoff JM *et al.* (2013) Lidocaine patch (5%) in treatment of persistent inguinal postherniorrhaphy pain: a randomized, double-blind, placebo-controlled, crossover trial. *Anesthesiology*. **119**: 1444–1452.

58 Meier T *et al.* (2003) Efficacy of lidocaine patch 5% in the treatment of focal peripheral neuropathic pain syndromes: a randomized, double-blind, placebo-controlled study. *Pain*. **106**: 151–158.

59 Palliativedrugs.com Ltd Lidocaine 5% medicated plasters — what is your experience? *Latest additions: Survey results (October 2012)*. www.palliativedrugs.com

60 Byun EK *et al.* (2016) Delirium associated with lidocaine patch administration: a case presentation. *Physical Medicine and Rehabilitation*. **8**: 597–601.

61 Nalamachu S *et al.* (2013) Influence of anatomic location of lidocaine patch 5% on effectiveness and tolerability for postherpetic neuralgia. *Patient Preference and Adherence*. **7**: 551–557.

62 Binder A *et al.* (2009) Topical 5% lidocaine (lignocaine) medicated plaster treatment for post-herpetic neuralgia: results of a double-blind, placebo-controlled, multinational efficacy and safety trial. *Clinical Drug Investigation*. **29**: 393–408.

63 Katz NP *et al.* (2002) Lidocaine patch 5% reduces pain intensity and interference with quality of life in patients with postherpetic neuralgia: an effectiveness trial. *Pain Medicine*. **3**: 324–332.

64 Sabatowski R *et al.* (2012) Safety and efficacy outcomes of long-term treatment up to 4 years with 5% lidocaine medicated plaster in patients with post-herpetic neuralgia. *Current Medical Research and Opinion*. **28**: 1337–1346.

65 Nestico PF *et al.* (1988) New antiarrhythmic drugs. *Drugs*. **35**: 286–319.

66 Bennett M (1997) Paranoid psychosis due to flecainide toxicity in malignant neuropathic pain. *Pain*. **70**: 93–94.

67 von Gunten CF *et al.* (2007) Flecainide for the treatment of chronic neuropathic pain: a phase II trial. *Palliative Medicine*. **21**: 667–672.

68 Chong S *et al.* (1997) Pilot study evaluating local anesthetics administered systemically for treatment of pain in patients with advanced cancer. *Journal of Pain and Symptom Management*. **13**: 112–117.

69 Sinnott C *et al.* (1991) Flecainide in cancer nerve pain. *Lancet*. **337**: 1347.

70 Dunlop R *et al.* (1988) Analgesic effects of oral flecainide. *Lancet*. **1**: 420–421.

Updated July 2019

*CLONIDINE

Class: α_2-Adrenergic receptor agonist (α_2 agonist).

Indications: Hypertension, migraine prophylaxis, menopausal flushing, †pain unresponsive to standard treatments, †refractory agitation in the imminently dying, †spasticity, †diarrhoea or †gastroparesis related to autonomic dysfunction in diabetes mellitus, †sweats and hot flushes, †ascites, †opioid withdrawal.

Contra-indications: Cardiac conduction defects.

Pharmacology

Clonidine is a potent α_2 and imidazoline receptor agonist. It also binds to α_1-receptors.[1] The net effect of clonidine on noradrenergic transmission is probably dependent on the background activity of the pathway. In 'overactive' pathways (e.g. causing agitation), it *reduces* transmission by binding to *presynaptic* α_2-autoreceptors. Conversely, in 'underactive' pathways (e.g. descending pain-inhibitory pathways), the predominant effect is agonism of *post*-synaptic α_2-receptors, *increasing* overall transmission.[2] In relation to the antihypertensive effect of clonidine, imidazoline agonism is probably the most important mode of action. Indeed, this use of clonidine has been eclipsed by the development of less sedating imidazoline-selective antihypertensives (e.g. **moxonidine**).[1]

Analgesia: Spinal clonidine reduces pain transmission through activation of spinal α_2-receptors.[3] The site(s) of action of systemically administered (PO/SC/IV) α_2 agonists are unclear but may include spinal α_2-receptors, reduced peripheral sympathetic activity and/or altered limbic noradrenergic transmission.

Postoperatively, clonidine given IV or IT augments the analgesic effects of opioids.[4,5] Clonidine also enhances the analgesic effects of local anaesthetics administered ED, IT or peripherally (e.g. single nerve or plexus blocks or applied directly to the wound).[6–12] Further, treatment with high-dose ED clonidine alone (a bolus of 10microgram/kg followed by an infusion of 6microgram/kg/h) can provide effective postoperative analgesia.[13] Compared with ED clonidine, IV clonidine is less potent and more sedating, but achieves comparable analgesia.[14]

In neuropathic pain, clonidine provides reproducible pain relief in some patients, particularly when given via the ED or IT routes.[15–22] There is limited evidence to suggest clonidine (0.1%) gel applied topically improves painful diabetic neuropathy.[23]

ED clonidine is effective in cancer-related neuropathic pain, generally as an 'add-on' drug to spinal **morphine** plus **bupivacaine** (see Spinal analgesia, p.908).[24,25] A typical dose is 150–300microgram/24h ED, but benefit has been reported in some patients on higher IT doses, up to 1mg/24h.[21]

ED clonidine is absorbed into the systemic circulation producing significant plasma concentrations (reflected clinically by drowsiness and cardiovascular effects), reaching a peak after 20min. IT clonidine produces similar effects; sedation occurs within 15–30min and lasts 1–2h.[21,26,27] The analgesic effect of clonidine can be reversed by α antagonists but not by **naloxone**.[15] Clonidine can thus be used in the management of unexpected acute pain in addicts receiving **naltrexone**.

Although most experience with clonidine for analgesia is with spinal use, some centres report benefit with clonidine SC or CSCI for opioid poorly-responsive pain, (e.g. neuropathic, muscle spasm) in the setting of a pain crisis and/or a patient in the last weeks of life, particularly if there is concurrent hyperactive delirium.[28]

An alternative to clonidine in some settings is **dexmedetomidine**, a more selective α_2 agonist. When given with local anaesthetics IT, **dexmedetomidine** provides a more rapid onset and prolonged sensory block than clonidine.[29] There are some reports of the use of **dexmedetomidine** as an analgesic in a palliative care setting (Box A).

Refractory agitation in the imminently dying: Clonidine (and **dexmedetomidine**) has sedative and anxiolytic effects and is used in ICUs for rousable sedation, particularly in patients with delirium. Some PCUs use clonidine SC/CSCI for refractory agitation in the imminently dying as an alternative to **phenobarbital** (p.315), or when dopaminergic drugs are best avoided, e.g. **haloperidol** in a patient with Parkinson's disease.[28] The use of **dexmedetomidine** is also reported in this setting (Box A).

Spasticity: In patients with spinal cord injury, the addition of TD clonidine reduces muscle spasticity that has failed to respond to maximal doses of **baclofen**.[30,31] In healthy volunteers, clonidine induces muscular relaxation and reduces pain caused by distension in the stomach, colon and rectum.[32,33] **Tizanidine** (p.662), also an α_2 agonist, causes less hypotension than clonidine.

Diabetic GI autonomic neuropathy: Clonidine improves symptoms of gastroparesis and chronic diarrhoea.[34,35] The improvement in diarrhoea is due partly to the stimulation of α_2-adrenergic receptors on enterocytes, which promotes intestinal fluid and electrolyte absorption, inhibits anion secretion and increases bowel transit time. Benefit is also reported for other causes of intractable diarrhoea, e.g. neuroendocrine tumours, short bowel syndrome.[35]

Sweats and hot flushes: There is RCT evidence that clonidine relieves sweating and hot flushes resulting from hormonal manipulation in women with breast cancer, but not in men with prostate cancer.[36,37] More recent trials in patients with breast cancer and hot flushes have found benefit from various antidepressants (see p.223) and **gabapentin** (p.297).[38] Comparative trials suggest **venlafaxine** works faster than clonidine, and participants prefer **venlafaxine** over **gabapentin**.[38] There is RCT evidence of benefit from **gabapentin** in men with hot flushes resulting from medical or surgical castration;[39] **venlafaxine** and SSRIs are also reported to be of benefit, see p.223.

Ascites: In patients with cirrhosis and ascites refractory to **spironolactone** ± **furosemide**, the addition of clonidine 75–100microgram PO b.d. can improve the response to diuretic therapy by inhibiting the renin–angiotensin–aldosterone and sympathetic nervous systems (see p.73).[40,41]

Opioid withdrawal: Increased sympathetic (noradrenergic) activity has been implicated in various symptoms of opioid withdrawal, e.g. shivering, sweating, anxiety, diarrhoea. Clonidine reduces these symptoms and has been used alone to manage opioid withdrawal. However, although as effective as reducing doses of **methadone**, clonidine is associated with more undesirable effects, e.g. hypotension.[42]

Nausea and vomiting: Premedication with clonidine (IV, PO) can reduce postoperative nausea and vomiting. This may relate to a reduced sympathetic outflow or analgesic requirement, or general sedative effect.[4,43] However, the effect is inconsistent and inferior to more standard approaches, e.g. $5HT_3$ antagonists.[44]

Other uses: Clonidine is used in dystonia[45] and also to reduce symptoms in several psychiatric conditions, e.g. attention deficit hyperactivity disorder, post-traumatic stress disorder and autism.[46]

About half of a dose of clonidine is excreted unchanged by the kidneys, and most of the remainder is metabolized by the liver to inactive metabolites. Accumulation occurs in renal impairment, extending its halflife up to 40h.

Bio-availability 75–100% PO; 60% TD.[47]

Onset of action 30–60min IV, PO; 2–3 days TD.

Time to peak plasma concentration 1.5–5h PO; 20min ED; 2 days TD.

Plasma halflife 12–16h.

Duration of action 8–24h PO; 24h TD.

Cautions

Severe coronary insufficiency, recent myocardial infarction, stroke, peripheral vascular disease, renal impairment, constipation. May precipitate depression in susceptible patients; occasionally precipitates delirium.[48]

Abrupt curtailment of long-term treatment likely to cause agitation, sympathetic overactivity, rebound hypertension (worsened if also taking a β-blocker); withdraw treatment progressively, e.g. over 2–4 days (ED or SC/CSCI) or 1 week (PO). Discontinue any β-blocker several days before discontinuing clonidine.

Drug interactions

Effects reduced or abolished by drugs with α antagonist activity, e.g. **mirtazapine**, TCAs and antipsychotic drugs, although the hypotensive effects of the phenothiazines can be additive. Concerns regarding serious undesirable effects with concurrent use of **methylphenidate** (see SPC) appear unfounded.[49]

Undesirable effects

Very common (>10%): sedation and dry mouth (initially), dizziness, orthostatic hypotension, transient pruritus and erythema (TD route).

Common (<10%, >1%): headache, fatigue, depression (long-term use), disturbed sleep, nausea, vomiting, constipation, erectile dysfunction, salivary gland pain, local reactions with TD route (e.g. rash, hyperpigmentation, excoriation).

Rare (<0.1%, ≥0.01%): decreased lacrimation.

α_2 agonists (clonidine and **dexmedetomidine**) promote breast cancer cell growth and spread *in vitro* and in animal models;[50] the clinical relevance of this is unknown.

Dose and use

> Sedation and hypotension can occur; patients who are mobile should be warned/monitored appropriately.

Clonidine can be given PO, SC/CSCI, spinally, intranasally and TD (not UK, but can be imported; see Supply).[20,51,52]

†*Spinal analgesia*

ED clonidine is generally given with **diamorphine/morphine** and **bupivacaine** (see p.908). A typical ED regimen would be:

- a test bolus dose of 50–150microgram in 5mL sodium chloride 0.9% injection over 5min
- if relief obtained, 150–300microgram/24h by infusion.

Clonidine is also used IT. A typical IT regimen would be:

- a test bolus dose of 50microgram in 5mL sodium chloride 0.9% injection over 5min
- if relief obtained, 50–150microgram/24h by infusion.

†*Pain unresponsive to standard treatments*[28]

For opioid poorly-responsive pain, e.g. neuropathic pain, in the setting of a pain crisis and/or a patient in the last weeks of life, particularly if there is concurrent hyperactive delirium:

- start with clonidine 150microgram/24h CSCI and/or 75–150microgram SC q8h p.r.n.
- if necessary, increase the CSCI by 150microgram daily
- in renal impairment (CrCl <30mL/min), consider halving the above doses
- typically effective dose 300–600microgram/24h
- maximum reported dose ≤1,500microgram/24h.[53]

Continue prior treatments if partially effective; consider gradual reduction if ineffective or poorly tolerated.

For CSCI, sodium chloride 0.9% is used as a diluent.

CSCI compatibility with other drugs: limited clinical experience suggests that clonidine is compatible with **fentanyl, haloperidol, hyoscine *butylbromide*, ketamine, levomepromazine, methadone, metoclopramide, midazolam, morphine sulfate** and **oxycodone.**[28]

For more information, see the www.palliativedrugs.com Syringe Driver Survey Database; we encourage members to submit combinations containing clonidine.

No effective PO regimen has been described for pain management, but the PO bio-availability suggests a PO:SC dose ratio of 1:1.

†*Refractory agitation in the imminently dying*[28,53]

Generally, clonidine is used SC/CSCI as an alternative to **phenobarbital** (p.315) or when dopaminergic drugs are best avoided, e.g. **haloperidol** in a patient with Parkinson's disease. Follow the same approach as for pain unresponsive to standard treatments above.

†*Spasticity*

PO **tizanidine** (p.662) causes less hypotension and has generally replaced the use of PO clonidine for spasticity.

However, clonidine CSCI is an option for patients no longer able to take PO **tizanidine** (and/or PO **baclofen**). Follow the same approach as for pain unresponsive to standard treatments above.

†*Gastroparesis or diarrhoea related to autonomic dysfunction in diabetes mellitus*

- start with 50microgram PO b.d.
- if necessary, increase by 50microgram every 24h
- usual maintenance dose 150microgram b.d.
- usual maximum dose for diabetic gastroparesis 300microgram b.d.
- usual maximum dose for diabetic diarrhoea 600microgram b.d.

For other causes of intractable diarrhoea, use similar doses.

†*Sweats and hot flushes*

- start with 50microgram PO b.d.
- after 2 weeks, if necessary, increase to 75microgram b.d.
- for some patients, the optimum dose is 100microgram b.d.

†*TD*

TD patches (not UK) contain metal and must be removed before MRI to avoid burns (see Chapter 30, p.901).

TD is generally better tolerated than PO, but the relationship between effective doses of PO and TD clonidine is not predictable.

- start with a patch delivering 100microgram/24h applied once every 7 days and review.

Box A Dexmedetomidine

Dexmedetomidine is a more highly selective α_2 adrenergic agonist than clonidine. It is mostly used for 'conscious sedation' (e.g. remaining responsive to verbal stimulation) in adult ICU patients and non-intubated adult patients undergoing diagnostic or surgical procedures. Off-label uses include the treatment of delirium, insomnia and as an adjuvant analgesic, mostly within the ICU setting. It is expensive.

Although a potential role for dexmedetomidine in palliative care has long been recognised,[54] published experience is mostly limited to case series and reports.[54–59] In the largest study, improvements in pain and agitation were reported in nine children and adolescents, mostly in the last days of life, although in two use exceeded 2 weeks, and in one 4 months.[55] Benefit was similarly reported in eight adult patients, mostly for delirium ± pain in the last days of life, but also intractable pain (used for 11 weeks) and opioid-induced hyperalgesia.[59] The most robust prospective data comes from an open-label pilot study of 22 adults with hyperactive delirium in the last week of life. Although delirium improved in all, only half of patients remained on dexmedetomidine until death; the commonest reason for stopping was a request for deeper sedation by the patient or family.[60]

Dexmedetomidine is generally administered CIVI but has been given alone by CSCI, with dose adjustments generally made on a daily basis. Although sources state that it appears compatible with fentanyl, glycopyrronium, midazolam and morphine, these data are mostly limited to mixing at a Y-site connection immediately before infusion.

The degree of monitoring of vital signs (e.g. heart rate, blood pressure) when used in a PCU setting varies from none to initial close monitoring when starting or increasing a dose.[61] Caution is required as, apart from cardiovascular effects (e.g. bradycardia, hypotension), opioid-related respiratory depression has occurred as a consequence of a rapid reduction in pain ± improved opioid sensitivity.[58]

Thus, the exact role of dexmedetomidine in palliative care is yet to be determined. Quite possibly, dexmedetomidine will be eclipsed by an increasing use of the much cheaper alternative clonidine in such settings.

Supply

Clonidine (generic)
Tablets 25microgram, 28 days @ 50microgram b.d. = £4.
Oral solution (sugar-free) 50microgram/5mL, 28 days @ 50microgram b.d. = £190.
Note. See Chapter 28, Table 2, p.863 for alternative and cheaper off-label options.

Catapres® (Glenwood)
Tablets (scored) 100microgram, 28 days @ 50microgram b.d. = £2.25.
Injection 150microgram/mL, 1mL amp = £0.50. *Available but not listed in the* BNF, *as no longer recommended for use in hypertensive crisis.*

Catapres® TTS
Transdermal patch 100microgram/24h, 200microgram/24h, 300microgram/24h, 1 patch (7 days' treatment) = price unavailable (not UK; obtainable via import; see Chapter 24, p.817).

Dexmedetomidine (generic)
Injection (concentrate for dilution and infusion) 100microgram/mL, 2mL amp, 4mL and 10mL vial = £16, £31 and £78 respectively.

1 Bousquet P *et al.* (2020) Imidazoline receptor system: the past, the present, and the future. *Pharmacological Reviews.* **72**: 50–79.
2 Erdozain AM *et al.* (2019) Differential α_{2A}- and α_{2C}-adrenoceptor protein expression in presynaptic and postsynaptic density fractions of postmortem human prefrontal cortex. *Journal of Psychopharmacology.* **33**: 244–249.
3 Bahari Z and Meftahi GH (2019) Spinal α_2-adrenoceptors and neuropathic pain modulation; therapeutic target. *British Journal of Pharmacology.* **176**: 2366–2381.

4 Engelman E and Marsala C (2013) Efficacy of adding clonidine to intrathecal morphine in acute postoperative pain: meta-analysis. *British Journal of Anaesthesia*. **110**: 21–27.

5 Sanchez Munoz MC *et al.* (2017) What is the place of clonidine in anesthesia? Systematic review and meta-analyses of randomized controlled trials. *Journal of Clinical Anesthesia*. **38**: 140–153.

6 Elia N *et al.* (2008) Clonidine as an adjuvant to intrathecal local anesthetics for surgery: systematic review of randomized trials. *Regional Anesthesia and Pain Medicine*. **33**: 159–167.

7 Popping DM *et al.* (2009) Clonidine as an adjuvant to local anesthetics for peripheral nerve and plexus blocks: a meta-analysis of randomized trials. *Anesthesiology*. **111**: 406–415.

8 Ya Deau JT *et al.* (2008) Clonidine and analgesic duration after popliteal fossa nerve blockade: Randomized, double-blind, placebo-controlled study. *Anesthesia and Analgesia*. **106**: 1916–1920.

9 Schnabel A *et al.* (2011) Efficacy and safety of clonidine as additive for caudal regional anesthesia: a quantitative systematic review of randomized controlled trials. *Paediatric Anaesthesia*. **21**: 1219–1230.

10 Mohamed SA and Abdel-Ghaffar HS (2013) Effect of the addition of clonidine to locally administered bupivacaine on acute and chronic postmastectomy pain. *Journal of Clinical Anesthesia*. **25**: 20–27.

11 Bharti N *et al.* (2013) Postoperative analgesic effect of intravenous (i.v.) clonidine compared with clonidine administration in wound infiltration for open cholecystectomy. *British Journal of Anaesthesia*. **111**: 656–661.

12 Mohammad W *et al.* (2015) A randomized double-blind study to evaluate efficacy and safety of epidural magnesium sulfate and clonidine as adjuvants to bupivacaine for postthoracotomy pain relief. *Anesthesia Essays and Researches*. **9**: 15–20.

13 Abd-Elsayed AA *et al.* (2015) A double-blind randomized controlled trial comparing epidural clonidine vs bupivacaine for pain control during and after lower abdominal surgery. *Ochsner Journal*. **15**: 133–142.

14 Bernard JM *et al.* (1995) Comparison of intravenous and epidural clonidine for postoperative patient-controlled analgesia. *Anesthesia and Analgesia*. **81**: 706–712.

15 Quan D *et al.* (1993) Clonidine in pain management. *Annals of Pharmacotherapy*. **27**: 313–315.

16 Siddall PJ *et al.* (2000) The efficacy of intrathecal morphine and clonidine in the treatment of pain after spinal cord injury. *Anesthesia and Analgesia*. **91**: 1493–1498.

17 Walters JL *et al.* (2012) Idiopathic peripheral neuropathy responsive to sympathetic nerve blockade and oral clonidine. *Case Reports in Anesthesiology*. Article ID 407539.

18 Glynn C *et al.* (1988) A double-blind comparison between epidural morphine and epidural clonidine in patients with chronic noncancer pain. *Pain*. **34**: 123–128.

19 Max MB *et al.* (1988) Association of pain relief with drug side effects in postherpetic neuralgia: a single-dose study of clonidine, codeine, ibuprofen and placebo. *Clinical Pharmacology and Therapeutics*. **43**: 363–371.

20 Zeigler D *et al.* (1992) Transdermal clonidine versus placebo in painful diabetic neuropathy. *Pain*. **48**: 403–408.

21 Ackerman LL *et al.* (2003) Long-term outcomes during treatment of chronic pain with intrathecal clonidine or clonidine/opioid combinations. *Journal of Pain and Symptom Management*. **26**: 668–677.

22 Rauck RL *et al.* (2015) Intrathecal clonidine and adenosine: effects on pain and sensory processing in patients with chronic regional pain syndrome. *Pain*. **156**: 88–95.

23 Wrzosek A *et al.* (2015) Topical clonidine for neuropathic pain. *Cochrane Database of Systematic Reviews*. **8**: CD010967. www.cochranelibrary.com.

24 Eisenach JC *et al.* (1995) Epidural clonidine analgesia for intractable cancer pain. The Epidural Clonidine Study Group. *Pain*. **61**: 391–399.

25 Chen H *et al.* (2004) Contemporary management of neuropathic pain for the primary care physician. *Mayo Clinic Proceedings*. **79**: 1533–1545.

26 Wells J and Hardy P (1987) Epidural clonidine. *Lancet*. **i**: 108.

27 Malinovsky JM *et al.* (2003) Sedation caused by clonidine in patients with spinal cord injury. *British Journal of Anaesthesia*. **90**: 742–745.

28 Personal Communication (2021) Paul Howard, Mountbatten Hospice, Isle of Wight.

29 Zhang C *et al.* (2016) Comparison of dexmedetomidine and clonidine as adjuvants to local anesthetics for intrathecal anesthesia: a meta-analysis of randomized controlled trials. *Journal of Clinical Pharmacology*. **56**: 827–834.

30 Weingarden S and Belen J (1992) Clonidine transdermal system for treatment of spasticity in spinal cord injury. *Archives of Physical Medicine and Rehabilitation*. **73**: 876–877.

31 Yablon S and Sipski M (1993) Effect of transdermal clonidine on spinal spasticity: a case series. *American Journal of Physical Medicine and Rehabilitation*. **72**: 154–156.

32 Thumshirn M *et al.* (1999) Modulation of gastric sensory and motor functions by nitrergic and alpha2-adrenergic agents in humans. *Gastroenterology*. **116**: 573–585.

33 Viramontes BE *et al.* (2001) Effects of an alpha(2)-adrenergic agonist on gastrointestinal transit, colonic motility, and sensation in humans. *American Journal of Physiology Gastrointestinal and Liver Physiology*. **281**: G1468–G1476.

34 Rosa-Silva L *et al.* (1995) Treatment of diabetic gastroparesis with oral clonidine. *Alimentary Pharmacology and Therapeutics*. **9**: 179–183.

35 Fragkos KC *et al.* (2016) What about clonidine for diarrhoea? A systematic review and meta-analysis of its effect in humans. *Therapeutic Advances in Gastroenterology*. **9**: 282–301.

36 Frisk J (2010) Managing hot flushes in men after prostate cancer--a systematic review. *Maturitas*. **65**: 15–22.

37 Rada G (2010) Non-hormonal interventions for hot flashes in women with a history of breast cancer. *Cochrane Database of Systematic Reviews*. **2**: CD004923. www.cochranelibrary.com.

38 Johns C *et al.* (2016) Informing hot flash treatment decisions for breast cancer survivors: a systematic review of randomized trials comparing active interventions. *Breast Cancer Research and Treatment*. **156**: 415–426.

39 Loprinzi CL *et al.* (2009) A phase III randomized, double-blind, placebo-controlled trial of gabapentin in the management of hot flashes in men (N00CB). *Annals of Oncology*. **20**: 542–549.

40 Yang YY *et al.* (2010) Association of the G-protein and alpha2-adrenergic receptor gene and plasma norepinephrine level with clonidine improvement of the effects of diuretics in patients with cirrhosis with refractory ascites: a randomised clinical trial. *Gut*. **59**: 1545–1553.

41 Singh V *et al.* (2013) Midodrine and clonidine in patients with cirrhosis and refractory or recurrent ascites: a randomized pilot study. *American Journal Gastroenterology*. **108**: 560–567.

42 Gowing L *et al.* (2016) Alpha2-adrenergic agonists for the management of opioid withdrawal. *Cochrane Database of Systematic Reviews*. CD002024. www.cochranelibrary.com.

43 Yadav G *et al.* (2013) A prospective, randomized, double blind and placebo-control study comparing the additive effect of oral midazolam and clonidine for postoperative nausea and vomiting prophylaxis in granisetron premedicated patients undergoing laparoscopic cholecystecomy. *Journal of Anaesthesiology, Clinical Pharmacology*. **29**: 61–65.

44 Shilpa SN *et al.* (2015) Comparison of efficacy of clonidine versus ondansetron for prevention of nausea and vomiting post thyroidectomy: a double blind randomized controlled trial. *Journal of Clinical and Diagnostic Research*. **9**: UC01–UC03.
45 McCluggage HL (2016) Changing from continuous SC to transdermal clonidine to treat dystonia in a teenage boy with end-stage leucodystrophy. *BMJ Supportive and Palliative Care*. **8**: 433–435.
46 Dowben JS *et al.* (2011) Clonidine: diverse use in pharmacologic management. *Perspectives in Psychiatric Care*. **47**: 105–108.
47 Toon S *et al.* (1989) Rate and extent of absorption of clonidine from a transdermal therapeutic system. *Journal of Pharmacy and Pharmacology*. **41**: 17–21.
48 Delaney J *et al.* (2006) Clonidine-induced delirium. *International Journal of Cardiology*. **113**: 276–278.
49 Preston CL *Stockley's Drug Interactions*. London: Pharmaceutical Press www.medicinescomplete.com (accessed December 2021)
50 Xia M *et al.* (2016) Dexmedetomidine regulate the malignancy of breast cancer cells by activating alpha2-adrenoceptor/ERK signaling pathway. *European Review for Medical and Pharmacological Sciences*. **20**: 3500–3506.
51 Davis K *et al.* (1991) Topical application of clonidine relieves hyperalgesia in patients with sympathetically maintained pain. *Pain*. **47**: 309–317.
52 Mitra S *et al.* (2013) Intranasal clonidine vs. midazolam as premedication in children: a randomized controlled trial. *Indian Pediatrics*. **51**: 113–118.
53 Glynn C. Personal communication. 1997.
54 Soares LG *et al.* (2002) Dexmedetomidine: a new option for intractable distress in the dying. *Journal of Pain and Symptom Management*. **24**: 6–8.
55 Burns J *et al.* (2017) The use of dexmedetomidine in pediatric care: a preliminary study. *Journal of Palliative Medicine*. **20**: 779–783.
56 Roberts SB *et al.* (2011) Dexmedetomidine as an adjuvant analgesic for intractable cancer pain. *Journal of Palliative Medicine*. **14**: 371–373.
57 Hilliard N *et al.* (2015) A case report of dexmedetomidine used to treat intractable pain and delirium in a tertiary palliative care unit. *Palliative Medicine*. **29**: 278–281.
58 Ferguson L and Hooper S (2020) Dexmedetomidine withdrawal syndrome and opioid sensitivity. *BMJ Supportive & Palliative Care*. 2020 December 22. Online ahead of print.
59 Hofherr ML *et al.* (2020) Dexmedetomidine: a novel strategy for patients with intractable pain, opioid-induced hyperalgesia, or delirium at the end of life. *Journal of Palliative Medicine*. **23**: 1515–1517.
60 Thomas B *et al.* (2021) Dexmedetomidine for hyperactive delirium at the end of life: an open-label single arm pilot study with dose escalation in adult patients admitted to an inpatient palliative care unit. *Palliative Medicine*. **35**: 729–737.
61 Coyne PJ *et al.* (2010) Dexmedetomidine: exploring its potential role and dosing guideline for its use in intractable pain in the palliative care setting. *Journal of Pain & Palliative Care Pharmacotherapy*. **24**: 384–386.

Updated (minor change) December 2021

GLYCERYL TRINITRATE

Class: Nitrate.

Indications: Angina, left ventricular failure, anal fissure, †smooth muscle spasm pain (particularly of the oesophagus, rectum and anus or cutaneous leiomyomas),[1] †biliary and †renal colic, †painful diabetic neuropathy,[2,3] †symptomatic relief of breathlessness in acute *cardiogenic* pulmonary oedema (in conjunction with diuretics)[4] or paroxysmal nocturnal dyspnoea. ***TD patch (selected brands and strengths):*** maintenance of venous patency, prevention of phlebitis, treatment of drug extravasation.

Contra-indications: Severe hypotension (systolic <90mmHg), severe aortic or mitral stenosis, cardiac tamponade, constrictive pericarditis, hypertrophic obstructive cardiomyopathy, non-cardiac pulmonary oedema, marked anaemia, severe hypovolaemia, raised intracranial pressure, narrow-angle glaucoma. Concurrent use of **avanafil**, **sildenafil**, **tadalafil** and **vardenafil** (may precipitate hypotension and myocardial infarction).[5]

Pharmacology

Glyceryl trinitrate (GTN) relaxes smooth muscle in blood vessels and the GI tract. This effect is mediated via its metabolism to nitric oxide (NO), which stimulates guanylate cyclase. This leads to an increase in cyclic guanosine monophosphate, which reduces the amount of intracellular calcium available for muscle contraction.[6]

Endogenous NO is produced when the NMDA-receptor is stimulated by excitatory amino acids (see **Ketamine**, p.691), and NO synthase inhibitors attenuate the development of opioid tolerance.[7] This points to a wider role of NO in pain modulation. GTN has a range of clinical effects:

Smooth muscle relaxant/antispasmodic: NO is involved in the regulation of distal oesophageal peristalsis and relaxation of the lower oesophageal sphincter. Thus, GTN can improve dysphagia and odynophagia associated with oesophagitis and oesophageal spasm.[8-10]

NO is also the major inhibitory neurotransmitter in the internal anal sphincter. In patients with acute anal fissure, GTN ointment 0.2–0.4% applied b.d. to the anal canal relieves painful spasm, improves quality of life and aids healing.[11] However, 30% of patients experience headache which, although transient, can be severe enough to discontinue treatment. **Diltiazem** 2% cream is an alternative; it is as effective as GTN ointment but causes less headache and less anal irritation.[12] Injections of **botulinum toxin** into the internal sphincter have also been used, but their exact role remains to be clarified. About 90% of acute anal fissures resolve with non-surgical approaches. However, for chronic fissures, i.e. those persisting >6 weeks, surgery is the most effective approach.[11]

Analgesic: GTN administered systemically using a TD patch enhances pain relief in cancer patients; when applied directly as a gel or TD patch, it also reduces local pain and inflammation, e.g. from thrombophlebitis, tendinopathies.[13-18] In an RCT for diabetic neuropathic pain affecting the feet, locally applied GTN spray reduced mean pain scores significantly from 7.5 to 4.6 (NNT = 4).[2] In a second RCT, the concurrent use of PO **valproate** provided no additional benefit.[3]

Vasodilator: Nitrates cause venous then arterial dilation in a dose-related manner. They have been given by IVI in *acute* heart failure to reduce pre- and after-load, which helps to relieve breathlessness. Generally, they were used in conjunction with diuretics, but alone when hypertension was the cause of the acute heart failure.[4] However, the role of nitrates in acute heart failure has been questioned; they do not appear to provide any survival advantage and their routine use is no longer recommended.[19] Nitrates are not suitable for patients with hypotension (systolic <90mmHg), severe obstructive valvular disease, or long-term use (nitrate tolerance generally develops after 24–48h).

Short-acting nitrates such as GTN and **isosorbide dinitrate** are used SL to treat or prevent angina episodes.[20] Because of tolerance, the chronic use of nitrates in cardiovascular disease is best reserved for specific circumstances, such as nocturnal angina or paroxysmal nocturnal dyspnoea. In these settings, p.r.n. GTN spray SL may be helpful or, if a frequent occurrence, a regular bedtime dose of a longer-acting nitrate PO. In those unable to swallow tablets, a bedtime application of TD GTN can be used. All these approaches permit a daily nitrate-free period of ≥10h.

TD GTN appears to improve outcomes in acute stroke, potentially via its vasodilator effects improving peri-lesional perfusion along with lowering and stabilization of systolic blood pressure.[21]

In cancer, the use of TD GTN could potentially improve perfusion of the tumour, thereby increasing anticancer drug delivery or decreasing hypoxia, which is associated with invasion, metastasis and drug resistance.[22] Studies in various settings are ongoing; however, initial findings of benefit from TD GTN alongside chemotherapy in patients with lung cancer have not been replicated.[23,24] Use of a low dose (i.e. application of one sixth of a 5mg TD patch daily) in patients with prostate cancer and an increasing PSA after surgery or radiotherapy increased the PSA doubling time from 13 to 32 months.[25]

GTN is rapidly absorbed through the buccal mucosa, but orally it is inactivated by extensive first-pass metabolism in the GI mucosa and liver. Many patients on long-acting or TD nitrates develop tolerance, i.e. experience a reduced therapeutic effect. Tolerance is generally prevented if nitrate levels are allowed to fall for ≥10h in every 24h (a 'nitrate holiday'). This may not be possible for patients with persistent pain. If tolerance develops, it will be necessary to increase the dose to restore efficacy.

Bio-availability 40% SL.

Onset of action 1–3min SL; 30–60min ointment or TD patch.

Time to peak plasma concentration 3–6min SL; 2h TD.

Plasma halflife 1–3min SL; 2–4min TD.

Duration of action 30–60min SL; 8h ointment; 24h TD patch.

Cautions

Severe hepatic or renal impairment, hypothyroidism, hypovolaemia, hypoxaemia, hypothermia, recent myocardial infarction. Topically applied GTN can be absorbed in sufficient quantities to cause undesirable systemic effects.

Drug interactions

Serious drug interactions: Concurrent use of **avanafil**, **sildenafil**, **tadalafil** and **vardenafil** may precipitate profound hypotension and myocardial infarction and is contra-indicated.

Exacerbates the hypotensive effect of other drugs. Drugs causing dry mouth may reduce the effect of sublingual nitrates.

Undesirable effects

Very common (>10%): headache (sometimes severe).
Common (<10%, >1%): flushing, dizziness, nausea.
Uncommon (<1%, >0.1%): local stinging, itching or burning sensation after SL spray, TD or rectal administration.
Rare (<0.1%, >0.01%): postural hypotension, tachycardia (paradoxical bradycardia also reported); may be more frequent with IV use.
These effects generally settle with continued use.

Dose and use

TD patches: some contain metal and must be removed before MRI to avoid burns (see Chapter 30, p.901).
Injection: glass, polyethylene or polypropylene apparatus should be used with parenteral GTN, as loss of potency will occur if PVC is used.

If necessary, **paracetamol** can be used for headache.

†Intermittent dysphagia and/or odynophagia

- start with 400–500microgram SL 5–15min before eating
- if necessary, increase to a maximum single dose of 1mg
- instruct the patient to swallow or spit out tablet once pain relief is obtained (or if headache develops)
- repeat p.r.n.

†Persistent smooth muscle spasm

Consider:

- GTN TD patches, starting with 5mg/24h *or*
- orally active nitrates, e.g. **isosorbide mononitrate**, start with 20mg PO b.d. (8am and 3pm).

If a 'nitrate holiday' is not possible, a TD patch may have to remain in place for 24h, or m/r **isosorbide mononitrate** considered instead (see Pharmacology).

Anal fissure pain

- use 0.2–0.4% rectal ointment
- using a covered finger, gently insert a 2.5cm length (or pea-sized quantity) of ointment about 1cm into the anal canal b.d. for 6–8 weeks.[26]

†Painful diabetic neuropathy

- apply GTN spray locally to the painful extremity: 1 spray/sole of foot/day.

Angina on effort

The patient should stop and rest sitting down; tablets/spray are placed/directed under the tongue and should not be swallowed:

- start with one SL tablet (300 or 600microgram) or spray (400microgram)
- the dose is repeated every 5min until the pain goes or the maximum dose is reached (1,200microgram/15min)
- if there is no relief, immediate medical attention should be sought.

For prophylactic use, take immediately before the activity known to cause angina.

†Acute cardiogenic pulmonary oedema in conjunction with diuretics

Use under the guidance of a cardiologist:

- start with 10–20microgram/min IVI, titrate every 3–5min as needed in 5–10microgram/min increments, up to a maximum of 200microgram/min.

Supply

Because GTN is an explosive substance, spray formulations contain additives (e.g. medium-chain partial glycerides or alcohol) to stabilize the solution and minimize the potential for explosion.

Glyceryl trinitrate (generic)
Tablets SL 300microgram, 500microgram, 100 = £2.75 and £2.25 respectively; *store in the original glass container; because of degradation, unused tablets should be discarded after 8 weeks.*
Aerosol SL spray 400microgram/metered dose, 200-dose unit = £3.50, *contains alcohol.*
Pump SL spray 400microgram/metered dose, 180-dose unit = £2.75, 200-dose unit = £3, *contains alcohol.*
Injection 1mg/mL, 50mL vial = £16.
Injection 5mg/mL, 5mL and 10mL amps = £6.50 and £13 respectively; *must be diluted before use. Contains propylene glycol; maximum recommended use of 3 days.*

Nitrocine (UCB Pharma)
Injection 1mg/mL, 10mL amp = £6.

Nitronal (Merck Serono)
Injection 1mg/mL, 5mL amp and 50mL vial = £2 and £15 respectively.

TD products
Minitran® (Mylan)
TD patch 5mg/24h, 10mg/24h, 15mg/24h, 28 days @ 1 patch daily = £11, £12 and £13 respectively.

Topical products
Ointment 0.2%, 30g = £23 (unauthorized product, available as a special order; see Chapter 24, p.817). *Note. Price based on Specials tariff in community.*

Rectogesic® (Kyowa Kirin Ltd)
Rectal ointment 0.4%, 30g = £40. *Discard 8 weeks after opening. Contains propylene glycol and lanolin (irritants).*

This is not a complete list; see BNF *for more information.*

Diltiazem
Ointment or cream 2%, 30g = £15 or £28 respectively (unauthorized products, available as a special order; see Chapter 24, p.817). *Note. Price based on Specials tariff in community.*

Isosorbide mononitrate
Tablets 10mg, 20mg, 40mg, 28 days@ 20mg b.d. = £0.75.
Tablets m/r 25mg, 40mg, 50mg, 60mg, 28 days @ 40mg once daily = £5.50.
Capsules m/r 25mg, 40mg, 50mg, 60mg, 28 days @ 40mg once daily = £6.50.

1 George S *et al.* (1997) Pain in multiple leiomyomas alleviated by nifedipine. *Pain.* **73**: 101–102.
2 Agrawal RP *et al.* (2007) Glyceryl trinitrate spray in the management of painful diabetic neuropathy: a randomized double blind placebo controlled cross-over study. *Diabetes Research and Clinical Practice.* **77**: 161–167.
3 Agrawal RP *et al.* (2009) Management of diabetic neuropathy by sodium valproate and glyceryl trinitrate spray: a prospective double-blind randomized placebo-controlled study. *Diabetes Research and Clinical Practice.* **83**: 371–378.
4 Ponikowski P *et al.* (2016) 2016 ESC Guidelines for the diagnosis and treatment of acute and chronic heart failure: The Task Force for the diagnosis and treatment of acute and chronic heart failure of the European Society of Cardiology (ESC). Developed with the special contribution of the Heart Failure Association (HFA) of the ESC. *European Journal of Heart Failure.* **18**: 891–975.
5 Baxter K and Preston CL *Stockley's Drug Interactions.* London: Pharmaceutical Press www.medicinescomplete.com (accessed May 2017).
6 Hashimoto S and Kobayashi A (2003) Clinical pharmacokinetics and pharmacodynamics of glyceryl trinitrate and its metabolites. *Clinical Pharmacokinetics.* **42**: 205–221.
7 Elliott K *et al.* (1994) The NMDA receptor antagonists, LY274614 and MK-801, and the nitric oxide synthase inhibitor, NG-nitro-L-arginine, attenuate analgesic tolerance to the mu-opioid morphine but not to kappa opioids. *Pain.* **56**: 69–75.
8 McDonnell F and Walsh D (1999) Treatment of odynophagia and dysphagia in advanced cancer with sublingual glyceryl trinitrate. *Palliative Medicine.* **13**: 251–252.
9 Tutuian R and Castell DO (2006) Review article: oesophageal spasm - diagnosis and management. *Alimentary Pharmacology and Therapeutics.* **23**: 1393–1402.
10 Maradey-Romero C *et al.* (2014) Treatment of esophageal motility disorders based on the chicago classification. *Current Treatment Options Gastroenterology.* **12**: 441–455.
11 Nelson RL *et al.* (2012) Non surgical therapy for anal fissure. *Cochrane Database of Systematic Reviews.* **2**: CD003431. www.thecochranelibrary.com
12 Sajid MS *et al.* (2013) Systematic review of the use of topical diltiazem compared with glyceryltrinitrate for the nonoperative management of chronic anal fissure. *Colorectal Disease.* **15**: 19–26.
13 Ferreira S *et al.* (1992) Blockade of hyperalgesia and neurogenic oedema by topical application of nitroglycerin. *European Journal of Pharmacology.* **217**: 207–209.

14 Berrazueta J *et al.* (1994) Local transdermal glyceryl trinitrate has an antiinflammatory action on thrombophlebitis induced by sclerosis of leg varicose veins. *Angiology*. **5**: 347–351.
15 Lauretti G *et al.* (1999) Oral ketamine and transdermal nitroglycerin as analgesic adjuvants to oral morphine therapy and amitriptyline for cancer pain management. *Anesthesiology*. **90**: 1528–1533.
16 Lauretti GR *et al.* (2002) Double-blind evaluation of transdermal nitroglycerine as adjuvant to oral morphine for cancer pain management. *Journal of Clinical Anesthesia*. **14**: 83–86.
17 El-Sheikh SM and El-Kest E (2004) Transdermal nitroglycerine enhanced fentanyl patch analgesia in cancer pain management. *Egyptian Journal of Anaesthesia*. **20**: 291–294.
18 Gambito ED *et al.* (2010) Evidence on the effectiveness of topical nitroglycerin in the treatment of tendinopathies: a systematic review and meta-analysis. *Archives of Physical Medicine and Rehabilitation*. **91**: 1291–1305.
19 Ho EC *et al.* (2016) Impact of nitrate use on survival in acute heart failure: A propensity-matched analysis. *Journal of the American Heart Association*. **5**: e002531.
20 Montalescot G *et al.* (2013) 2013 ESC guidelines on the management of stable coronary artery disease: the Task Force on the management of stable coronary artery disease of the European Society of Cardiology. *European Heart Journal*. **34**: 2949–3003.
21 Appleton JP *et al.* (2017) Therapeutic potential of transdermal glyceryl trinitrate in the management of acute stroke. *CNS Drugs*. **31**: 1–9.
22 Sukhatme V *et al.* (2015) Repurposing Drugs in Oncology (ReDO)-nitroglycerin as an anti-cancer agent. *Ecancermedicalscience*. **9**: 568.
23 Yasuda H *et al.* (2006) Randomized phase II trial comparing nitroglycerin plus vinorelbine and cisplatin with vinorelbine and cisplatin alone in previously untreated stage IIIB/IV non-small-cell lung cancer. *Journal of Clinical Oncology*. **24**: 688–694.
24 Davidson A *et al.* (2015) A phase III randomized trial of adding topical nitroglycerin to first-line chemotherapy for advanced nonsmall-cell lung cancer: the Australasian lung cancer trials group NITRO trial. *Annals of Oncology*. **26**: 2280–2286.
25 Siemens DR *et al.* (2009) Phase II study of nitric oxide donor for men with increasing prostate-specific antigen level after surgery or radiotherapy for prostate cancer. *Urology*. **74**: 878–883.
26 Gagliardi G *et al.* (2010) Optimal treatment duration of glyceryl trinitrate for chronic anal fissure: results of a prospective randomized multicenter trial. *Techniques in Coloproctology*. **14**: 241–248.

Updated December 2019

NIFEDIPINE

Class: Calcium-channel blocker.

Indications: Prophylaxis of stable angina, hypertension, Raynaud's phenomenon (immediate-release only authorized formulation), †severe smooth muscle spasm pain (particularly of the oesophagus, rectum and anus, cutaneous leiomyomas),[1-5] †intractable hiccup.[6]

Contra-indications: Cardiogenic shock, severe aortic stenosis, acute or unstable angina (may cause hypotension and reflex tachycardia precipitating myocardial or cerebrovascular ischaemia). *Do not use within 1 month of myocardial infarction.*
Modified-release 24-hourly oral products: hepatic impairment, previous or current GI obstruction or stenosis, inflammatory bowel disease.

Pharmacology

Nifedipine inhibits the influx of calcium through L-type channels into cells, thereby modifying cell function, e.g. smooth muscle contraction, neural transmission.[7] It has a range of clinical effects:
Smooth muscle relaxant/antispasmodic: Nifedipine is used to relieve dysphagia and chest pain associated with oesophageal spasm.[8-10] It also relieves painful spasm associated with an anal fissure. In this setting, topical application of nifedipine cream is more effective and better tolerated than PO administration.[11] However, topical treatment with either **glyceryl trinitrate** (p.88) or **diltiazem** is generally preferred in practice.

Nifedipine may help hiccup by relieving oesophageal spasm or by interference with nerve pathways involved in hiccup.[6,12] However, alternative treatments are generally tried before nifedipine (See Prokinetics, Table 2, p.25).
Analgesic: In animal studies, nifedipine and other calcium-channel blockers augment the analgesic effects of **paracetamol**, **morphine** and anti-epileptics.[13-15] The clinical relevance of this is uncertain; inconsistent benefit has been found from the addition of calcium-channel blockers to postoperative pain regimens.[16-18]
Vasodilator: Nifedipine is used to treat angina, hypertension and Raynaud's phenomenon; supporting evidence in Raynaud's phenomenon is low quality, with conflicting conclusions from systematic reviews.[19,20] It has a relatively greater effect on blood vessels than on the myocardium, and has no anti-arrhythmic activity. It rarely precipitates heart failure, because any negative inotropic effect is offset by a reduction in left ventricular work.

Nifedipine promotes cancer proliferation *in vitro* and in animal models of breast cancer, via activation of a cellular growth pathway.[21] The relevance of these findings to patients is unknown.

Nifedipine undergoes extensive first-pass metabolism in the liver to inactive metabolites that are excreted in the urine. Higher plasma concentrations are seen in slow metabolizers, which are more prevalent in South American, South Asian and black African populations.[22,23] Hepatic impairment increases bio-availability and halflife, and the dose may need to be reduced (modified-release 24-hourly oral products are contra-indicated in hepatic impairment, because of the duration of action). For pharmacokinetic data, see Table 1.

Table 1 Nifedipine PO pharmacokinetics

	Immediate-release capsules	*Modified-release 12-hourly product*[a]	*Modified-release 24-hourly product*[a]
Bio-availability	45–55%	45–55%	65–85%
Onset of action	15min	No data	No data
Time to peak plasma concentration	30–60min	No data	No data
Plasma halflife	2–3.5h	2–5h[b]	2–5h[b]
Duration of action	8h	12h	24h

a. illustrative values, based on Adipine® MR (12-hourly product) or Adalat® LA (24-hourly product); different products may not be bio-equivalent (see Supply)

b. after discontinuation.

Cautions

May exacerbate angina; discontinue nifedipine if angina occurs 30–60min after the first dose. Rarely, it may precipitate or worsen heart failure; avoid in patients with significantly impaired cardiac function or heart failure. Hepatic impairment. May impair glucose tolerance and worsen diabetes mellitus.

Drug interactions

Serious drug interactions: augments the hypotensive and negative inotropic effects of other drugs, e.g. α and β antagonists, **chlorpromazine.**[24]

Nifedipine is metabolized by and inhibits CYP3A4 and CYP2D6; it also inhibits CYP1A2 and CYP2C8/9. Caution is needed with concurrent use of drugs that inhibit or induce these enzymes, particularly in poor CYP2D6 metabolizers (see Chapter 19, Table 8, p.790).[24] Reports of interactions where dose adjustment or close monitoring are needed are listed in Table 2.

Table 2 CYP450 interactions with nifedipine that can alter drug plasma concentrations

Nifedipine plasma concentration		*Drug plasma concentration*	
increased by	*decreased by*	*increased by nifedipine*	*decreased by nifedipine*
Azole antifungals	Carbamazepine	Digoxin	Quinidine
Cimetidine[a]	Phenobarbital	Quinidine	
Fluoxetine	Phenytoin	Tacrolimus	
Grapefruit juice	Rifampicin[b]	Theophylline	
Macrolide antibacterials	St John's wort		
Protease inhibitors			

a. reduce nifedipine dose by 50%

b. manufacturer considers that rifampicin renders nifedipine ineffective.

Undesirable effects

Common (<10%, >1%): headache, dizziness, vasodilation, peripheral oedema, constipation.
Uncommon (<1%, >0.1%): asthenia, lethargy, malaise, agitation, nervousness, sleep disorder, tremor, vertigo, abnormal vision, chest pain, tachycardia, palpitations, postural hypotension, oedema, breathlessness, dry mouth, dyspepsia, abdominal pain, nausea, rash, pruritus, sweating, transient increase in liver enzymes.

Dose and use

Patients with angina should *not* bite into or use an immediate-release capsule SL, because of the risk of rapid-onset hypotension and reflex tachycardia, which could lead to myocardial or cerebrovascular ischaemia.

For SL administration, patients should bite into and use the liquid contents of the immediate-release capsules immediately (unauthorized use). *Modified-release formulations must* not *be used SL or chewed.*

- start with 10mg PO/SL stat and 10–20mg t.d.s. *or*
- m/r 20mg PO b.d. or m/r 30–60mg PO once daily (see Supply for 12-hourly or 24-hourly m/r oral products).

†Achalasia

- start with 10–20mg SL 30–45min before food; usual maximum dose 60–80mg/24h.

†Painful spasm associated with anal fissure

- m/r 20mg PO b.d.; *topical treatments preferred*, see Pharmacology.

† Intractable hiccup

- doses ≤160mg/24h PO have been used with concurrent **fludrocortisone** 0.5–1mg PO to overcome associated orthostatic hypotension;[6] generally a third-line option, see Prokinetics, Table 2, p.25.

Remains of some m/r tablets (e.g. Adalat® LA) may appear in the patient's faeces ('ghost tablets'), but these are inert residues and do not affect the efficacy of the products.

Supply

Immediate-release products
Nifedipine (generic)
Soft capsules (containing liquid) 5mg, 10mg, 28 days @ 10mg t.d.s. = £61.
Oral suspension 5mg/5mL, 10mg/5mL, 28 days @ 10mg t.d.s. = £66 (unauthorized product, available as a special order; see Chapter 24, p.817). *Price based on Specials tariff in community.*
Oral solution (drops) 20mg/mL, 30mL = £230 (unauthorized product, available as a special order; see Chapter 24, p.817). *Price based on Specials tariff in community.*

Modified-release products

Because of their different dosing regimens and concern over possible non-bio-equivalence, the *BNF* recommends that m/r formulations of nifedipine should be prescribed by brand name.[25]

Modified-release 12-hourly oral products
Adipine® MR (Chiesi)
Tablets m/r 10mg, 20mg, 28 days @ 20mg b.d. = £5.

Coracten® SR (UCB Pharma)
Capsules m/r 10mg, 20mg, 28 days @ 20mg b.d. = £5.

Modified-release 24-hourly oral products
Adalat® LA (Bayer)
Tablets m/r 30mg, 28 days @ 30mg once daily = £7.

Adipine® XL (Chiesi)
Tablets m/r 30mg, 60mg, 28 days @ 30mg once daily = £4.75.

Coracten® XL (UCB Pharma)
Capsules m/r 30mg, 60mg, 28 days @ 30mg once daily = £5.

This is not a complete list; see BNF for more information.

1 McLoughlin R and McQuillan R (1997) Using nifedipine to treat tenesmus. *Palliative Medicine*. **11**: 419–420.
2 George S *et al.* (1997) Pain in multiple leiomyomas alleviated by nifedipine. *Pain*. **73**: 101–102.
3 Cargill G *et al.* (1982) Nifedipine for relief of esophageal chest pain. *New England Journal of Medicine*. **307**: 187–188.
4 Al-Waili N (1990) Nifedipine for intestinal colic. *Journal of the American Medical Association*. **263**: 3258.
5 Celik A *et al.* (1995) Hereditary proctalgia fugax and constipation: report of a second family. *Gut*. **36**: 581–584.
6 Brigham B and Bolin T (1992) High dose nifedipine and fludrocortisone for intractable hiccups. *Medical Journal of Australia*. **157**: 70.
7 Castell DO (1985) Calcium-channel blocking agents for gastrointestinal disorders. *American Journal of Cardiology*. **55**: 210B–213B.
8 Achem SR and Gerson LB (2013) Distal esophageal spasm: an update. *Current Gastroenterology Reports*. **15**: 325.
9 Cross-Adame E *et al.* (2013) Treatment of esophageal (noncardiac) chest pain: Review. *Clinical Gastroenterology and Heptology*. **12**: 1224–1245.
10 Maradey-Romero C *et al.* (2014) Treatment of esophageal motility disorders based on the chicago classification. *Current Treatment Options Gastroenterology*. **12**: 441–455.
11 Golfam F *et al.* (2014) Comparison of topical nifedipine with oral nifedipine for treatment of anal fissure: a randomized controlled trial. *Iran Red Crescent Medical Journal*. **16**: e13592.
12 Steger M *et al.* (2015) Systemic review: the pathogenesis and pharmacological treatment of hiccups. *Alimentary Pharmacology and Therapeutics*. **42**: 1037–1050.
13 Koleva M and Dimova S (2000) Effects of nifedipine, verapamil, diltiazem and trifluoperazine on the antinociceptive activity of acetaminophen. *Methods and Findings in Experimental and Clinical Pharmacology*. **22**: 741–745.
14 Michaluk J *et al.* (1998) Effects of various Ca2+ channel antagonists on morphine analgesia, tolerance and dependence, and on blood pressure in the rat. *European Journal of Pharmacology*. **352**: 189–197.
15 El-Azab MF and Moustafa YM (2012) Influence of calcium channel blockers on anticonvulsant and antinociceptive activities of valproic acid in pentylenetetrazole-kindled mice. *Pharmacological Reports*. **64**: 305–314.
16 Carta F *et al.* (1990) Effect of nifedipine on morphine-induced analgesia. *Anesthesia and Analgesia*. **70**: 493–498.
17 Zarauza R *et al.* (2000) A comparative study with oral nifedipine, intravenous nimodipine, and magnesium sulfate in postoperative analgesia. *Anesthesia and Analgesia*. **91**: 938–943.
18 Casey G *et al.* (2006) Perioperative nimodipine and postoperative analgesia. *Anesthesia and Analgesia*. **102**: 504–508.
19 Ennis H *et al.* (2016) Calcium channel blockers for primary Raynaud's phenomenon. *Cochrane Database of Systematic Reviews*. **2**: CD002069. www.cochranelibrary.com.
20 Rirash F *et al.* (2017) Calcium channel blockers for primary and secondary Raynaud's phenomenon. *Cochrane Database of Systematic Reviews*. **12**: CD000467. www.cochranelibrary.com.
21 Guo DQ *et al.* (2014) Nifedipine promotes the proliferation and migration of breast cancer cells. *PLoS One*. **9**: e113649.
22 Sowunmi A *et al.* (1995) Ethnic differences in nifedipine kinetics: comparisons between Nigerians, Caucasians and South Asians. *British Journal of Clinical Pharmacology*. **40**: 489–493.
23 Castaneda-Hernandez G *et al.* (1996) Interethnic variability in nifedipine disposition: reduced systemic plasma clearance in Mexican subjects. *British Journal of Clinical Pharmacology*. **41**: 433–434.
24 Preston CL *Stockley's Drug Interactions (online edition)*. Pharmaceutical Press, London. www.medicinescomplete.com (accessed September 2019).
25 *British National Formulary* (online edition). London: BMJ Group and Pharmaceutical Press. www.bnf.org (accessed September 2019).

Updated (minor change) September 2021

ANTICOAGULANTS

Anticoagulants are used predominantly to prevent or treat venous thrombo-embolism (VTE). There are a range of drugs that act at various points in the coagulation cascade (Figure 1).

LMWH (derived from porcine heparin) and **fondaparinux** (a synthetic heparin pentasaccharide) both inhibit factor Xa.[2] **Fondaparinux** is an alternative for patients who need to avoid LMWH because of hypersensitivity, a history of heparin-induced thrombocytopenia, or for religious or cultural reasons.[3-5] The use of **unfractionated heparin** is limited to specific circumstances, e.g. renal impairment (CrCl <30mL/min), increased risk of bleeding.

For the treatment of VTE in patients without cancer, **warfarin** is being replaced by DOACs, e.g. **apixaban**, **edoxaban**, **rivaroxaban** (direct Xa inhibitors) or **dabigatran etexilate** (direct thrombin inhibitor). DOACs are non-inferior to **warfarin** with respect to recurrent

VTE and bleeding[6-9] and have the advantage of standard doses and no need to monitor levels of anticoagulation. All are authorized for both treatment of VTE and secondary prevention of recurrent VTE, and recommended by NICE.[10] However, only a minority of patients in the development studies had cancer-related VTE.

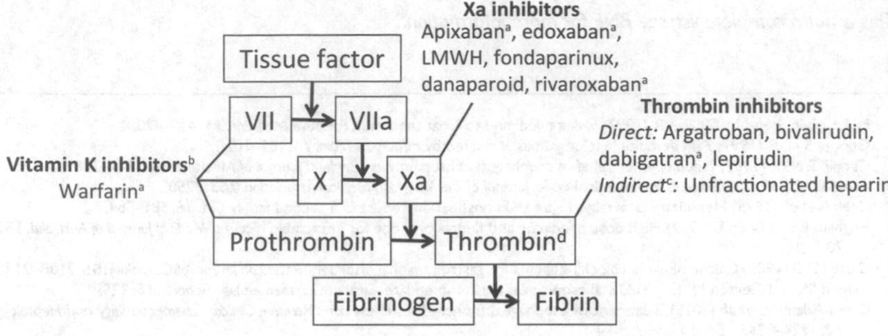

Figure 1 Sites of action of anticoagulants. Unless indicated otherwise, administration is parenteral, e.g. SC, IV, CIVI (see individual SPC). Heparins are antagonized by protamine sulfate, warfarin by vitamin K_1 (phytomenadione).[1] Specific antidotes are increasingly available for the direct oral anticoagulants (see text).

a. administered PO
b. vitamin K inhibitors also reduce factor IX synthesis, inhibiting coagulation amplification pathways
c. indirect thrombin inhibitors activate antithrombin III, a regulator of coagulation
d. thrombin also triggers several amplification pathways (factors V, VIII, IX and XI) that promote further factor X activation and thus further thrombin generation.

For the treatment of VTE in patients with cancer, LMWH has been considered the gold-standard anticoagulant because, compared with **warfarin**, it halved the rate of recurrent VTE (8% vs. 14%).[11,12] However, RCT data comparing DOACs with LMWH for cancer-related VTE has emerged, and the use of DOACs is increasing in this setting (Box A). Nonetheless, LMWH continues to be preferred in patients considered at high risk of bleeding and/or insufficiently robust to have been included in the DOAC RCTs (Box A).[13]

Because there are significant differences in pharmacology between DOACs (Table 1), follow local guidelines or seek advice from a haematologist about the most appropriate choice, and do so urgently if bleeding occurs during use (Box B).

If the need arises to switch from a DOAC to LMWH, stop the DOAC and give the first dose of LMWH at the same time as when the next dose of DOAC was due.

General considerations in patients with cancer

Compared with non-cancer patients, those with cancer are more likely to experience VTE and, despite anticoagulation, recurrent VTE. The increased risk results from a cancer-related pro-inflammatory state associated with:

- activation of the coagulation cascade by procoagulant proteins expressed by the cancer
- damage to blood vessel walls
- venous stasis
- other general risk factors (Box C).

In palliative care, LMWH will continue to be the most appropriate VTE treatment for many patients, given most will be considered at high risk of bleeding (Box A). In general, patients agreeing to the indefinite use of LMWH have found it acceptable and straightforward; no need to check INR and little need for dose adjustments.[35–38] However, compared with **warfarin** or a DOAC, treatment with LMWH is more expensive (Table 2). Note. The specific antidotes for DOACs are also expensive, e.g. one 200mg vial of **andexanet alfa** costs £2,775; low-dose and high-dose treatment requires 5 and 9 vials, respectively.

Box A Emerging use of DOACs in cancer-related VTE

Patients recruited to RCTs of DOACs had a good performance status (all ECOG 0–2, mostly ≤1) and only 50–70% metastatic disease; most presented with symptomatic VTE (50–80%) during anticancer treatment (60–70%; mostly chemotherapy). In addition to risk factors for bleeding (see below), exclusion criteria included concurrent use of NSAIDs, low haemoglobin (<100g/L), active liver disease and hepatic impairment (ALT/AST and bilirubin three times and twice the upper limit of normal respectively).

DOACs have been found to be non-inferior to LMWH in reducing recurrent VTE.[17–19] Conversely, rates of major bleeding and clinically relevant non-major bleeding (CRNMB), particularly in those with GI cancer, are significantly higher with some (edoxaban, rivaroxaban) [17,18,20] but not all (apixaban);[21,22] the absolute increase in major bleeding and CRNMB rates were 2–3% and 5–9% respectively.[17,18] There is no difference in mortality among treatments.

Consequently, recent guidelines of cancer-related VTE consider DOACs to be:[23]

- an alternative to LMWH for the initial treatment of VTE, specifically apixaban or rivaroxaban
- a preferred alternative to LMWH for the short-term (3–6 months) treatment of VTE, specifically apixaban, edoxaban or rivaroxaban
- an alternative to LMWH for long-term (>6 months) secondary thromboprophylaxis in those at high risk of recurrent VTE.

The following are considered contra-indications to DOACs.[24]

Absolute contra-indications (in addition to the usual general contra-indications for anticoagulation):

- concurrent drugs that risk a potentially serious drug interaction with a DOAC, e.g. potent inducers or inhibitors of:
  - ▷ CYP3A4 (apixaban, rivaroxaban) *and/or*
  - ▷ P-glycoprotein (apixaban, edoxaban, rivaroxaban)

Relative contra-indications (treat when the risk of harm from VTE exceeds the risk from bleeding; a lack of safety data means some also consider these absolute contra-indications):

- intracranial or spinal lesion at higher risk of bleeding, e.g. primary or secondary CNS cancer
- active GI ulceration at high risk of bleeding
- active but non-life-threatening bleeding, e.g. trace haematuria
- intracranial or CNS bleeding within past 4 weeks
- recent high-risk surgery or bleeding events
- thrombocytopenia (platelets ≤50 x 10^9/L).

Patients with any of the risk factors above are considered at high risk of bleeding, and LMWH is generally preferred. Other situations favouring LMWH include:

- actively progressing cancer
- poor performance status (ECOG ≥2) or prognosis (≤3 months) and other features that excluded participation in DOAC RCTs (see above)
- extremes of body weight (<50–60kg, >120kg)
- end-stage renal failure (CrCl <15mL/min)
- nephrostomy tubes
- impaired GI absorption.

An individualized approach based on patient involvement in decision-making is recommended, taking into account all potential benefits of DOACs (e.g. PO administration, similar efficacy) and harms (e.g. greater bleeding risk with some, potential drug–drug interactions, lack of ease of reversal). During use, patients and clinicians should remain vigilant for signs and symptoms of bleeding, particularly in those at increased risk, e.g. the elderly, those with renal impairment (monitor renal function to ensure dose remains appropriate).[15]

The pharmacology of DOACs differ (Table 1); follow local guidelines or seek advice from a haematologist about the most appropriate choice, and do so urgently if bleeding occurs during use (Box B).

Table 1 Selected characteristics and pharmacokinetic data for DOACs for the treatment of VTE;[13,14] also see individual SPCs. For additional considerations for cancer-related VTE, see Box A

	Apixaban	*Dabigatran etexilate*[a]	*Edoxaban*	*Rivaroxaban*
Site of action (Factor)	Xa	IIa	Xa	Xa
Prodrug	No	Yes	No	No
Bio-availability	50%	3–7%	60%	100% with food, ≥66% fasting
Time to peak plasma concentration	3–4h	0.5–2h	1–2h	2–4h
Plasma halflife	12h	12–14h	10–14h	5–13h
Elimination	25% renal; 75% biliary or GI	85% renal (unchanged)	35% renal (unchanged)	33% renal (unchanged); 66% hepatically metabolized
Formulation	2.5mg, 5mg tablets	75mg, 110mg, 150mg capsules	15mg, 30mg, 60mg tablets	2.5mg, 10mg, 15mg, 20mg tablets
Administration	Can be crushed and given in apple puree or dispersed in apple juice/water PO or dispersed in 60mL water via NG tube	Capsules must *not* be opened	Can be crushed and given in apple puree PO or dispersed in water PO or via NG tube	Take *with* food Can be crushed and given in apple puree or dispersed in water PO or via gastric tube
Treatment dose for VTE (for 6 months)	10mg b.d. for 1 week, then 5mg b.d.; if continued >6 months, 2.5mg b.d.	150mg b.d. after ≥5 days of parenteral anticoagulant	60mg once daily after ≥5 days of parenteral anticoagulant	15mg b.d. for 3 weeks, then 20mg once daily; if continued >6 months, 10mg or 20mg once daily when low or high risk of recurrent VTE respectively
Dose in renal impairment[b]				
CrCl 30–50mL/min	No adjustment	110mg or 150mg b.d. based on bleeding risk	30mg once daily	Consider reducing the 20mg once daily dose to 15mg once daily, based on bleeding risk
CrCl 15–29mL/min	Caution, but no adjustment	Contra-indicated	30mg once daily	Consider reducing the 20mg once daily dose to 15mg once daily, based on bleeding risk

continued

Table 1 Continued

	Apixaban	*Dabigatran etexilate*[a]	*Edoxaban*	*Rivaroxaban*
CrCl <15mL/min (ESRF)	Not recommended	Contra-indicated	Not recommended	Not recommended
Dose in hepatic impairment[c]				
'Mild' (Child-Pugh A)	Caution, but no adjustment[d]	Caution, but no adjustment[d]	Caution, but no adjustment[d]	Caution, but no adjustment
'Moderate' (Child-Pugh B)	Caution, but no adjustment[d]	Caution, but no adjustment[d]	Caution, but no adjustment[d]	Contra-indicated
'Severe' (Child-Pugh C)	Not recommended	Contra-indicated	Not recommended	Contra-indicated
Other factors	None	110mg b.d. if age >80 years, concurrent verapamil, or increased bleeding risk	30mg once daily if weight ≤60kg, or concurrent interacting drugs (see below)	None
Drug interactions[e]	CYP3A4 and P-glycoprotein potent inhibitors and inducers not recommended	P-glycoprotein potent inhibitors contra-indicated; potent inducers not recommended	Dose adjustment needed for P-glycoprotein potent inhibitors, caution with potent inducers[e]	CYP3A4 and P-glycoprotein potent inhibitors and inducers not recommended
Antidote	Andexanet alfa	Idarucizumab	†Andexanet alfa	Andexanet alfa
RCT in patients with cancer	Yes	No	Yes	Yes

a. *not* recommended for cancer-related VTE, see Box A

b. CrCl should be calculated; eGFR is not considered a suitable alternative (see p.734).[15] Discontinue DOAC if acute renal failure develops

c. liver disease with coagulopathy and clinically relevant bleeding risk is a contra-indication for all DOACs

d. SPCs advise either caution (apixaban, edoxaban) or do not recommend use (dabigatran etexilate) in patients with elevated LFTs (ALT/AST and bilirubin twice and ≥1.5 upper limit of normal respectively).

e. also see Chapter 19, Table 8, p.790; particular caution with drugs for short-term use, e.g. clarithromycin, erythromycin.[16] In patients with cancer-related VTE, a concurrent interacting drug is considered a contra-indication for all DOACs (see Box A).

Box B Management of bleeding in patients on DOACs[25,26]

General principles

For most bleeds, supportive care measures, e.g. local haemostatic control, haemodynamic support, blood transfusions, will be sufficient. Reversal strategies are reserved for severe or life-threatening bleeds and include:

- drug removal: activated charcoal, haemodialysis (dabigatran etexilate)
- specific antidotes: sequestering and neutralizing agents, i.e. andexanet alfa (apixaban, †edoxaban, rivaroxaban) or idarucizumab (dabigatran etexilate)
- non-specific antidotes: prohaemostatic agents, e.g. prothrombin complex concentrates.

Minor bleeding

- document the time of the most recent dose of DOAC
- apply local haemostatic measures, if feasible
- if bleeding continues, consider tranexamic acid (see below)
- delay next dose of DOAC or stop.

Major bleeding

- apply local haemostatic measures, if feasible
- give IV fluid replacement
- *obtain advice from haematologist urgently*
- stop DOAC
- document the time of the last dose; if taken <2h ago, consider giving activated charcoal PO
- arrange laboratory tests *as recommended by haematologist*, e.g. FBC, prothrombin time, APTT, renal function (to calculate CrCl)
- give tranexamic acid 15mg/kg IV t.d.s.–q.d.s. (or 25mg/kg PO t.d.s.); reduce dose in renal impairment (see Haemostatics, Table 2, p.116)
  - ▷ if feasible, apply topically to bleeding point, e.g. as a mouthwash, nasal drops
- consider also other possible causes of a coagulopathy, e.g. DIC
- give IV blood product support as indicated by Hb, other coagulopathy, platelets (if count <75 x 10^9/L).

If ongoing life- or limb-threatening bleeding

- *obtain further advice from haematologist urgently regarding use of specific or non-specific antidotes (see above).*

Box C Main risk factors for VTE in medical patients[4,27-34]

Age ≥40 years, particularly >60 years

Immobility

Dehydration

Obesity

Cancer, particularly metastatic, especially of the pancreas, stomach, bladder, ovary, uterus, kidney or lung; also haematological

Chronic respiratory or cardiac disease

Other serious medical conditions, e.g. sepsis, leg weakness (including spinal cord compression), inflammatory bowel disease, collagen disorder

Varicose veins/chronic venous insufficiency

Previous VTE

Cancer chemotherapy, e.g. platinum-based drugs, fluorouracil (5-FU), mitomycin-C, thalidomide

Growth factors, e.g. granulocyte colony stimulating factor, erythropoietin

Radiotherapy, e.g. to the pelvis

Hormone therapy, e.g. oral contraceptives, hormone replacement, tamoxifen, anastrozole, possibly progestins

Thrombophilia

The potential benefit vs. risk of indefinite anticoagulation should be continually reviewed. Nonetheless, anticoagulation is often continued until death or very close to death, despite the increasing risk of clinically relevant bleeding (8% of patients in the last week of life in one case series).[39] This suggests that it is appropriate to discontinue anticoagulation sooner, e.g. at the point where comfort measures only are indicated.

Table 2 Cost of anticoagulants

Drug	*Route*	*Example maintenance dose*[a]	*Approximate 28-day cost*
Apixaban	PO tablets	5mg b.d.	£53
Dabigatran etexilate	PO capsules	150mg b.d.	£48
Edoxaban	PO tablets	60mg once daily	£49
LMWH	SC injection	1 injection/24h	£150–£170
Rivaroxaban	PO tablets	20mg once daily	£50
Warfarin	PO tablets or suspension	3mg once daily	£1[b] or £70[b] respectively

a. actual dose can depend on age, weight ± renal impairment or for warfarin the INR; consult specific SPCs

b. does not include cost of checking INR.

Generally, patients with cancer admitted for surgical or medical reasons should be offered thromboprophylaxis, except where the probable benefit is outweighed by the associated bleeding risk (see p.104).[33] This would include patients admitted to a palliative care unit with a potentially reversible acute medical illness. Duration of treatment is generally about 2 weeks.[31]

If anticoagulation is contra-indicated, mechanical measures, e.g. graduated compression stockings, intermittent pneumatic compression, should be considered.[33] However, the evidence in medical patients is limited, and there have been reports of harm.[40,41]

However, thromboprophylaxis appears less relevant in patients receiving palliative care with a poor performance status in their last weeks of life, at a stage when managing any VTE symptomatically is appropriate.[42] National guidelines already state that patients in their last days of life should *not* be offered any form of thromboprophylaxis (also see p.104).[33]

1 Noble S and Johnson M (2012) Management of cancer associated thrombosis in people with advanced disease. *BMJ Supportive and Palliative Care*. **2**: 163–167.

2 Hoppensteadt D *et al.* (2003) Heparin, low-molecular-weight heparins, and heparin pentasaccharide: basic and clinical differentiation. *Hematology Oncology Clinics of North America*. **17**: 313–341.

3 Baglin T *et al.* (2006) Guidelines on the use and monitoring of heparin. *British Journal of Haematology*. **133**: 19–34.

4 Blann AD and Lip GY (2006) Venous thromboembolism. *British Medical Journal*. **332**: 215–219.

5 Cohen AT *et al.* (2006) Efficacy and safety of fondaparinux for the prevention of venous thromboembolism in older acute medical patients: randomised placebo controlled trial. *British Medical Journal*. **332**: 325–329.

6 Schulman S *et al.* (2009) Dabigatran versus warfarin in the treatment of acute venous thromboembolism. *New England Journal of Medicine*. **361**: 2342–2352.

7 Bauersachs R *et al.* (2010) Oral rivaroxaban for symptomatic venous thromboembolism. *New England Journal of Medicine*. **363**: 2499–2510.

8 Agnelli G *et al.* (2013) Oral apixaban for the treatment of acute venous thromboembolism. *New England Journal of Medicine*. **369**: 799–808.

9 Buller HR *et al.* (2013) Edoxaban versus warfarin for the treatment of symptomatic venous thromboembolism. *New England Journal of Medicine*. **369**: 1406–1415.

10 NICE (2019) Anticoagulants, including direct-acting oral anticoagulants (DOACs). *Key Therapeutic Topic KTT16*. www.nice.org.uk.

11 Kearon C *et al.* (2016) Antithrombotic therapy for VTE disease: chest guideline and expert panel report. *Chest*. **149**: 315–352.

12 Noble S and Sui J (2016) The treatment of cancer associated thrombosis: does one size fit all? Who should get LMWH/warfarin/DOACs? *Thrombosis Research*. **140 (Suppl 1)**: 154–159.

13 Farge D *et al.* (2019) 2019 international clinical practice guidelines for the treatment and prophylaxis of venous thromboembolism in patients with cancer. *Lancet Oncology*. **20**: e566–e581.

14 NHS Nottinghamshire Area Prescribing Committee (2021) Direct oral anticoagulants (DOACs) for the treatment of DVT or PE, or prevention against recurrent DVT or PE (in Adults). *Clinical Guidelines*. www.nottsapc.nhs.uk.

15 MHRA (2020) Direct-acting oral anticoagulants (DOACs): reminder of bleeding risk, including availability of reversal agents. *Drug Safety Update*. www.gov.uk/drug-safety-update.

16 MHRA (2020) Erythromycin: caution required due to cardiac risks (QT interval prolongation); drug interaction with rivaroxaban. *Drug Safety Update*. www.gov.uk/drug-safety-update.
17 Raskob GE *et al.* (2018) Edoxaban for the treatment of cancer-associated venous thromboembolism. *New England Journal of Medicine*. **378**: 615–624.
18 Young AM *et al.* (2018) Comparison of an oral Factor Xa inhibitor with low molecular weight heparin in patients with cancer with venous thromboembolism: results of a randomized trial (SELECT-D). *Journal of Clinical Oncology*. **36**: 2017–2023.
19 Agnelli G *et al.* (2020) Apixaban for the treatment of venous thromboembolism associated with cancer. *New England Journal of Medicine*. **382**: 1599–1607.
20 Li A *et al.* (2019) Direct oral anticoagulant (DOAC) versus low-molecular-weight heparin (LMWH) for treatment of cancer associated thrombosis (CAT): A systematic review and meta-analysis. *Thrombosis Research*. **173**: 158–163.
21 McBane R, 2nd *et al.* (2020) Apixaban and dalteparin in active malignancy associated venous thromboembolism: The ADAM VTE trial. *Journal of Thrombosis and Haemostasis*. **18**: 411–421.
22 Ageno W *et al.* (2021) Bleeding with apixaban and dalteparin in patients with cancer-associated venous thromboembolism: results from the Caravaggio study. *Thrombosis and Haemostasis*. **121**: 616–624.
23 Lyman GH *et al.* (2021) American Society of Haematology 2021 guidelines for management of venous thromboembolism: prevention and treatment in patients with cancer. *Blood Advances*. **5**: 927–974.
24 Key NS *et al.* (2020) Venous thromboembolism prophylaxis and treatment in patients with cancer: ASCO clinical practice guideline update. *Journal of Clinical Oncology*. **38**: 496–520.
25 NICE (2016) Reversal of the anticoagulant effect of dabigatran: idarucizumab. *Evidence Summary ESNM 73*. www.nice.org.uk.
26 Samuelson BT and Cuker A (2017) Measurement and reversal of the direct oral anticoagulants. *Blood Reviews*. **31**: 77–84.
27 Samama MM *et al.* (1999) A comparison of enoxaparin with placebo for the prevention of venous thromboembolism in acutely ill medical patients. Prophylaxis in medical patients with enoxaparin study group. *New England Journal of Medicine*. **341**: 793–800.
28 De Cicco M (2004) The prothrombotic state in cancer: pathogenic mechanisms. *Critical Reviews in Oncology Hematology*. **50**: 187–196.
29 Deitcher SR and Gomes MP (2004) The risk of venous thromboembolic disease associated with adjuvant hormone therapy for breast carcinoma: a systematic review. *Cancer*. **101**: 439–449.
30 Leizorovicz A *et al.* (2004) Randomized, placebo-controlled trial of dalteparin for the prevention of venous thromboembolism in acutely ill medical patients. *Circulation*. **110**: 874–879.
31 Leizorovicz A and Mismetti P (2004) Preventing venous thromboembolism in medical patients. *Circulation*. **110 (Suppl 1)**: 13–19.
32 Chew HK *et al.* (2006) Incidence of venous thromboembolism and its effect on survival among patients with common cancers. *Archives of Internal Medicine*. **166**: 458–464.
33 NICE (2019) Venous thromboembolism in over 16s: reducing the risk of hospital-acquired deep vein thrombosis or pulmonary embolism. *Clinical Guideline 89*. www.nice.org.uk.
34 Kahn SR *et al.* (2012) Prevention of VTE in nonsurgical patients: Antithrombotic therapy and prevention of thrombosis, 9th ed: American College of Chest Physicians Evidence-Based Clinical Practice Guidelines. *Chest*. **141 (Suppl)**: e195–e226.
35 Johnson M (1997) Problems of anticoagulation within a palliative care setting: an audit of hospice patients taking warfarin. *Palliative Medicine*. **11**: 306–312.
36 Johnson M and Sherry K (1997) How do palliative physicians manage venous thromboembolism? *Palliative Medicine*. **11**: 462–468.
37 Noble SI and Finlay IG (2005) Is long-term low-molecular-weight heparin acceptable to palliative care patients in the treatment of cancer related venous thromboembolism? A qualitative study. *Palliative Medicine*. **19**: 197–201.
38 Noble SI *et al.* (2006) Acceptability of low molecular weight heparin thromboprophylaxis for inpatients receiving palliative care: qualitative study. *British Medical Journal*. **332**: 577–580.
39 Noble S *et al.* (2019) Management of venous thromboembolism in far-advanced cancer: current practice. *BMJ Supportive and Palliative Care*. 2019 June 25. Online ahead of print.
40 Dennis M *et al.* (2009) Effectiveness of thigh-length graduated compression stockings to reduce the risk of deep vein thrombosis after stroke (CLOTS trial 1): a multicentre, randomised controlled trial. *Lancet*. **373**: 1958–1965.
41 Dennis M *et al.* (2013) Effectiveness of intermittent pneumatic compression in reduction of risk of deep vein thrombosis in patients who have had a stroke (CLOTS 3): a multicentre randomised controlled trial. *Lancet*. **382**: 516–524.
42 White C *et al.* (2019) Prevalence, symptom burden, and natural history of deep vein thrombosis in people with advanced cancer in specialist palliative care units (HIDDen): a prospective longitudinal observational study. *Lancet Haematology*. **6**: e79–e88.

Updated (minor change) January 2022

LOW MOLECULAR WEIGHT HEPARIN (LMWH)

Class: Parenteral anticoagulant.

Indications: Authorized indications vary between products; consult SPCs for details. Thromboprophylaxis, initial treatment of venous thrombo-embolism (VTE), treatment of cancer-associated thrombosis, †thrombophlebitis migrans, †disseminated intravascular coagulation (DIC).

Contra-indications: IM use (risk of injection-site haematoma); active major bleeding; suspected or confirmed heparin-induced thrombocytopenia (HIT) with LMWH; known bleeding diathesis (including bleeding peptic ulcer); severe uncontrolled hypertension; haemorrhagic stroke; diabetic or haemorrhagic retinopathy; bacterial endocarditis; injury or surgery to brain, spinal cord, eyes or ears.
Stated contra-indications and cautions vary; see individual SPCs.

Pharmacology

Four LMWHs are available in the UK, including **dalteparin**, **enoxaparin** and **tinzaparin** that feature in the *PCF*. All are derived from porcine heparin. Some patients need to avoid the use of LMWH because of known hypersensitivity or for religious or cultural reasons; the most appropriate parenteral alternative is **fondaparinux**, a non-porcine synthetic heparin pentasaccharide.

LMWH acts mainly by potentiating the inhibitory effect of antithrombin III on factor Xa. The dose of LMWH is determined by the patient's weight, and routine monitoring of an anticoagulant effect is not necessary. However, in cases where the patient is considered at risk of bleeding, has renal impairment (CrCl <30mL/min) or a history of recurrent thrombosis, anti-factor Xa activity levels can be measured.

LMWH is an established initial treatment for deep vein thrombosis (DVT) and pulmonary embolism (PE); it is more effective than unfractionated heparin (UFH), with the advantages of a longer duration of action permitting once daily administration, and a better safety profile (fewer major haemorrhages).[1]

In cancer patients, LMWH became the anticoagulant of choice for the treatment of VTE, as it is more effective than **warfarin**, with a similar or reduced risk of bleeding.[2–4] However, the efficacy of DOACs appears similar to that of LMWH in this setting, and DOACs are being increasingly used (see p.95).

Experimental models suggest that LMWH has an anticancer effect via the inhibition of metastatic spread.[5] However, clinical trials in a range of cancers have overall failed to demonstrate an improvement in survival ± time to disease progression.[5] Thus, LMWH is *not* recommended as routine adjunctive treatment.[3]

LMWHs are primarily renally excreted and can accumulate in renal impairment (see Dose and use below). For pharmacokinetic details, see Table 1.

Table 1 LMWH pharmacokinetics[6–10]

	Dalteparin	*Enoxaparin*	*Tinzaparin*
Bio-availability SC[a]	87%	100%	87%
Onset of action	3min IV 2–4h SC	5min IV 3h SC	5min IV 2–3h SC
Time to peak plasma activity[a]	4h SC	2–6h SC	4–5h SC
Plasma activity halflife[a]	2h IV 3–5h SC	2–4.5h IV 4.5–7h SC	1.5h IV 3–4h SC
Duration of action	10–24h SC	>24h SC	24h

a. based on anti-factor Xa activity.

Cautions

Contra-indications and cautions vary between manufacturers; see individual SPCs.

Risk factors for bleeding include serious concurrent illness, severe renal and hepatic impairment (see Dose and use below), chronic heavy consumption of alcohol, age, and possibly female sex.

Monitor closely if spinal analgesia is used in a patient receiving LMWH *thromboprophylaxis*; and, because of the risk of a spinal haematoma, spinal analgesia should be avoided in a patient receiving *therapeutic* doses of LMWH.

Drug interactions

Enhanced bleeding tendency with NSAIDs (particularly **ketorolac**) and other drugs with anticoagulant/antiplatelet effect.

Inhibition of aldosterone secretion by heparin/LMWH may cause hyperkalaemia. The risk appears to increase with duration of therapy and is higher in patients with diabetes mellitus, chronic renal failure, acidosis and those taking potassium supplements or potassium-sparing drugs. The CSM recommends measuring plasma potassium in such patients before starting heparin and regularly thereafter, particularly if heparin is to be continued for >1 week, although a specific frequency is not stated.

Undesirable effects

Common (<10%, >1%): headache, dizziness, pain at the injection site, minor bleeding (haematoma at the injection site), major bleeding in surgical patients receiving thromboprophylaxis and patients being treated for VTE, tachycardia, chest pain, oedema, hypotension, hypertension, anaemia, nausea, constipation, reversible increases in liver transaminases, back pain, haematuria.
Uncommon (<1%, >0.1%): major bleeding in patients receiving thromboprophylaxis, immune-mediated heparin-induced thrombocytopenia (see QCG: Heparin-induced thrombocytopenia, p.112),[11] abdominal pain, diarrhoea.

Dose and use

LMWH should be prescribed by brand name because they are not interchangeable.

Routine platelet count monitoring

All patients should have a baseline platelet count before starting LMWH (or any other heparin).
Postoperative patients receiving UFH (any surgery) or LMWH (cardiopulmonary bypass only) should have their platelet count checked every 2–3 days for 2 weeks or until heparin is stopped.

Postoperative patients and cardiopulmonary bypass patients receiving any type of heparin who have been exposed to heparin in the last 3 months should have a repeat platelet count after 24h to exclude rapid-onset HIT caused by pre-existing cross-reacting antibodies.

Medical and postoperative (other than cardiopulmonary bypass) patients receiving LMWH do not need routine platelet monitoring.[11]

Renal impairment

In severe renal impairment (creatinine clearance <30mL/min), accumulation of **dalteparin**, **enoxaparin** and **tinzaparin** occurs to a variable degree, increasing overall exposure and prolonging anti-factor Xa activity halflife. Monitoring of anti-factor Xa activity is advised to guide dosing, particularly in those at increased risk of bleeding (see specific SPCs). For example, the dose of **tinzaparin** should be reduced if anti-factor Xa activity exceeds 1.5 units/mL (usual range 0.5–1.5 units/mL). For **enoxaparin**, the manufacturer recommends specific dose reduction for both prophylaxis and treatment (see SPC).

Specialist guidelines consider UFH IV an alternative to LMWH in severe renal impairment. A thromboprophylaxis dose may need to be reduced (follow local guidance); monitoring of APTT is required to guide a treatment dose.[12,13]

Severe hepatic impairment

Reduced synthesis of clotting factors increases the risk of bleeding. Consider dose reduction for **dalteparin**, **enoxaparin** (also possible risk of accumulation) and **tinzaparin**.

SC injections

May cause transient stinging and local bruising.[14] Long-term treatment is not acceptable to some cancer patients (about 15%).[15]

Rotate injection sites daily, e.g. between different abdominal quadrants (see SPCs for the manufacturers' recommendations). Create a skin fold by squeezing the skin between thumb and forefinger and insert the total length of the needle vertically into the thickest part of the fold; do *not* rub the injection site.

Thromboprophylaxis in patients with cancer

Recommendations vary between guidelines.[16] *PCF* reflects NICE and British Committee for Standards in Haematology guidance.[3,13]

Generally, patients with cancer admitted for surgical or medical reasons should be offered thromboprophylaxis, except where the likely benefit is outweighed by the associated bleeding risk; standardized assessments help with this determination, e.g. Department of Health VTE risk assessment tool (this also applies to patients without cancer).[17]

Undergoing surgery

Patients with cancer undergoing major surgery are at high risk of VTE; they have twice the risk of developing a DVT and three times the risk of a fatal PE.[18] Abdominal and pelvic surgery is particularly high-risk.

Standard mechanical measures are recommended, e.g. graduated compression stockings, intermittent pneumatic compression, until mobility is regained.[13] They should not be used alone unless drug thromboprophylaxis treatment is contra-indicated.[19]

For those who have undergone major cancer surgery in the abdomen or pelvis, or hip surgery, an extended period of thromboprophylaxis is more effective than the usual ~1 week (Table 2).[13]

Table 2 Thromboprophylaxis with LMWH in patients with cancer[13]

	Dalteparin	*Enoxaparin*	*Tinzaparin*
Undergoing surgery involving the abdomen, pelvis or hip[a]	5,000 units SC once daily; start evening before surgery; continue for 4 weeks	4,000 units (40mg) SC once daily; start 12h before surgery; continue for 4 weeks	4,500 units 12h before surgery, then once daily; continue for 4 weeks
Reduced mobility because of an intercurrent illness[a]	5,000 units SC once daily	4,000 units (40mg) SC once daily	4,500 units SC once daily
Cost per dose (pre-filled syringe)	5,000 units/0.2mL = £2.75	4,000 units (40mg) /0.4mL = £2.25	4,500 units/0.45mL = £3.50

a. for other types of major surgery and in medical patients, thromboprophylaxis is continued until the patient no longer has significantly reduced mobility (generally 1–2 weeks).

Reduced mobility because of an intercurrent illness

Hospitalized cancer patients are at high risk of VTE. NICE guidelines recommend thromboprophylaxis is considered in patients who have ≥3 days reduced mobility relative to their normal state, when there is ≥1 risk factor such as cancer (see Anticoagulants, Box C, p.100).[20] Duration of treatment is generally ≤2 weeks (Table 2).[21]

In patients receiving palliative care who have a reasonable performance status and prognosis, thromboprophylaxis can be considered and is generally acceptable.[22] The decision to start should take into account temporary increases in thrombotic risk factors (e.g. due to reversible acute pathology) and risk of bleeding (consider using a standardized assessment to help evaluate these risks; see above), along with likely prognosis and the views of patients, family/informal carers and the multiprofessional team.[13] NICE guidance suggests reviewing the use of thromboprophylaxis daily, but this seems excessive and will often be impractical.

However, thromboprophylaxis appears less relevant in patients receiving palliative care who have a poor performance status in their last weeks of life, at a stage when symptom relief alone is more appropriate,[23] particularly as thromboprophylaxis is associated with an increased risk of clinically relevant bleeding.[24] Patients in their last days of life should *not* be offered any form of thromboprophylaxis.[13]

If anticoagulation is contra-indicated, mechanical measures, e.g. graduated compression stockings, intermittent pneumatic compression, should be considered.[13] However, the evidence in medical patients is limited, and there have been reports of harm.[25,26]

Outpatient chemotherapy

Thromboprophylaxis should *not* be offered routinely to mobile patients with cancer receiving chemotherapy or immunotherapy as outpatients. However, it may be considered in those at very high thrombotic risk, i.e. those with:[13]

- pancreatic cancer
- multiple myeloma receiving chemotherapy + **thalidomide** (p.603), **lenalidomide** or **pomalidomide**
- additional risk factors for VTE.

Generally, LMWH is used, although DOACs (specifically **apixaban**, **rivaroxaban**) may be an alternative in those at low risk of bleeding, given for 6 months from the start of chemotherapy.[19,27]

Indwelling venous catheters

The presence of a central (subclavian) or peripheral indwelling venous catheter can lead to catheter-related thrombosis. However, routine thromboprophylaxis with LMWH or **warfarin** does not reduce the risk of thrombosis and is *not* recommended.[19]

Long-distance air travel

The risk of DVT increases 2–3 times with long-haul flights ≥3h. The risk increases with journey duration and in travellers with pre-existing risk factors (see Anticoagulants, Box C, p.100). Generally, the VTE becomes evident 1–2 weeks after the flight.[28] Three levels of risk have been proposed, with management varying accordingly:

- *high risk*: those with active cancer, a previous travel-related or unprovoked DVT, major surgery within the previous 4 weeks (can be longer, e.g. no long-haul flights advised for 3 months after a hip replacement), or ≥2 other pre-existing risk factors. Advise general measures, graduated compression stockings and LMWH thromboprophylaxis according to local guidance
- *moderate risk*: one risk factor, not considered high risk. Advise general measures and graduated compression stockings
- *low risk*: no pre-existing risk factors. Advise general measures only.

General measures include:

- avoid prolonged immobility; stretch the calf muscles frequently by moving the feet up and down; walk around
- avoid constrictive clothing around the waist and lower limbs
- maintain a normal fluid intake, avoiding excessive alcohol
- highlight symptoms of VTE and need for urgent medical review.

Below-knee graduated (class 1) compression stockings should be properly fitted, providing 14–17mmHg of pressure at the ankle (unless contra-indicated, e.g. peripheral arterial disease). Proprietary flight socks providing equivalent compression are suitable alternatives.

If LMWH is used:

- prescribe 3 injections (1 each for the outward and return journeys, and 1 spare)
- provide a covering letter for the use of the injections (along with any other drugs required, see p.815) to ease passage through security, immigration and customs
- provide training in the correct administration of the injection (see the information on self-administration included in the patient information leaflet) and its disposal
- self-administer **dalteparin** 5,000 units, **enoxaparin** 4,000 units (40mg) or **tinzaparin** 4,500 units SC 2–4h before departure
- if there is a stop-over followed by another long flight, another injection is not necessary unless the second flight is more than 24h after the first.

Treatment

Recommendations vary between guidelines.[16] *PCF* generally reflects NICE and British Committee for Standards in Haematology guidance.[3,12]

DVT and PE in cancer patients: initial treatment

Confirm the diagnosis radiologically (e.g. ultrasound, CT pulmonary angiography). Treat DVT and PE presenting either symptomatically or as an incidental finding with LMWH for 6 months:

- **dalteparin** maximum daily dose 18,000 units/24h; give 200 units/kg SC once daily for the first month, followed by 150 units/kg SC once daily thereafter *or*
- **enoxaparin** 100 units/kg (1mg/kg) SC b.d. (see Box A) *or*
- **tinzaparin** 175 units/kg SC once daily.[12]

Note. In the UK, only **dalteparin** and **tinzaparin** are authorized for extended (6 months) treatment of cancer-associated VTE.

A DOAC is an alternative in patients at low risk of bleeding with no contra-indications or additional concerns limiting their use (see p.97).

Grade 2 compression stockings should *not* be used routinely to reduce post-thrombotic syndrome or recurrent DVT. However, they can be trialled in patients with symptomatic post-thrombotic syndrome.[12]

An inferior vena caval filter should only be used when there is a strong contra-indication to anticoagulation. It should be removed as soon as anticoagulation becomes possible.

DVT and PE cancer patients: ongoing treatment

Indefinite anticoagulation beyond 6 months should be considered for patients who have a DVT or PE and have an ongoing major risk factor for VTE, such as cancer (see Anticoagulants, Box C, p.100).[3,12]

In cancer patients, the evidence that LMWH is more effective than **warfarin** relates to the first 3–6 months of anticoagulation.[3] Although probable that LMWH would continue to remain more

Box A Enoxaparin dose for VTE[29-32]

Until 2017, two different dosing regimens for enoxaparin were authorized in different EU countries; in the UK this was 150 units/kg (1.5mg/kg) SC once daily.

The dosing for enoxaparin has been made consistent across the EU as either:

- a once daily injection of 150 units/kg (1.5mg/kg) for uncomplicated patients with low risk of VTE recurrence *or*
- twice daily injections of 100 units/kg (1mg/kg) for all other patients, i.e. those with obesity, symptomatic PE, cancer-related VTE, recurrent VTE or proximal (iliac vein) thrombosis.

Note. Dose adjustments may be required, e.g. in renal impairment; see SPC.

Robust evidence for the use of the b.d. regimen over the once daily regimen is limited. A meta-analysis of five studies (only one an RCT) found no significant difference in risk of recurrent VTE or major bleeding. Thus, despite the recommendation that cancer patients receive the b.d. regimen, the previous UK dose of 150 units/kg (1.5mg/kg) once daily may be preferable in terms of treatment burden and acceptability in palliative care patients.

effective than **warfarin**, efficacy and safety data are lacking to guide the choice of anticoagulant for indefinite use in this population. Thus, the practice had been to discuss this uncertainty with patients, along with the potential benefits and harms of continuing with LMWH vs. switching to **warfarin**.[4] However, as DOACs are used increasingly for initial treatment, so too they will be for ongoing treatment (see p.95).

When a switch to **warfarin** or a DOAC is considered in a patient with cancer that is stable or cured, LMWH should be continued until therapeutic levels are reached (for **warfarin** this equates to a therapeutic INR on 2 consecutive days; for DOAC, see individual SPCs).

VTE in a seemingly cured cancer patient may be an indication of occult recurrence. If truly idiopathic, a minimum of 6–12 months of anticoagulation is recommended, and indefinite anticoagulation should be considered.

Provided no contra-indications develop, indefinite anticoagulation is generally continued in patients with cancer until they reach the stage when symptom relief alone becomes more appropriate, e.g. in the last few weeks or days of life.

Special circumstances

There is no standard approach to the following circumstances; seek specialist advice.[3,4,33]

Recurrent VTE despite anticoagulation

Consider:

- is patient adhering to treatment?
- is the dose of anticoagulant correct? Measure anti-factor Xa activity levels (LMWH), INR (**warfarin**)
- excluding HIT, see QCG: Heparin-induced thrombocytopenia, p.112
- possible mechanical compression from tumour masses
- for those on LMWH:
  - ▷ ensure on full weight-based therapeutic dose
  - ▷ if necessary, make further increases guided by anti-factor Xa activity levels
  - ▷ for **enoxaparin**, if on a once daily dosing regimen, switch to 100 units/kg (1mg/kg) SC b.d.
- for those on **warfarin** or a DOAC, switch to LMWH.

Note. Insertion of an inferior vena caval filter is *not* recommended for recurrence alone.

Bleeding while anticoagulated

Consider:

- bleeding source, severity, impact and reversibility
- supportive measures, **tranexamic acid** (see Haemostatics, p.114), blood transfusion
- in a major or life-threatening bleed:
  - ▷ withholding anticoagulation and the use of reversal agents (also see Anticoagulants, Box B, p.100)
  - ▷ use of a retrievable inferior vena caval filter (in acute or subacute VTE only); remove when bleeding has stopped and recommencing anticoagulation is appropriate.

VTE in thrombocytopenia

- when platelet count >50 x 10^9/L, use normal LMWH dose
- when platelet count <50 x 10^9/L:
  - ▷ in acute VTE, during the highest risk of recurrence, use normal LMWH dose and give platelet transfusions to maintain platelet count >50 x 10^9/L; if persistent thrombocytopenia or other bleeding risk prevents anticoagulation, consider insertion of a temporary inferior vena caval filter
  - ▷ in subacute/chronic VTE, use half normal LMWH dose
  - ▷ omit LMWH if platelet count <25 x 10^9/L
- if thrombocytopenia develops during LMWH treatment, exclude HIT, see QCG: Heparin-induced thrombocytopenia, p.112.

†Thrombophlebitis migrans

- *do not use **warfarin**, because it is ineffective*
- generally responds rapidly to small doses of LMWH:
  - ▷ **dalteparin**: 2,500–5,000 units SC once daily; if necessary, titrate to maximum permitted dose, 200 units/kg once daily *or*
  - ▷ **enoxaparin**: ≤6,000 units (60mg) once daily; if necessary, titrate to 150 units/kg (1.5mg/kg) SC once daily.
- continue treatment indefinitely.[34]

†Disseminated intravascular coagulation (DIC)

Confirm the diagnosis

Diagnosis is made on the basis of the presence of a clinical condition known to be associated with DIC, together with various haematological indices:

- thrombocytopenia (platelet count <150 x 10^9/L in 98% of cases)
- elevated plasma D-dimer concentration, a fibrin degradation product (85% of cases)
- prolonged prothrombin time and/or partial thromboplastin time (50–60% of cases)
- decreased plasma fibrinogen concentration (40% of cases).

These can be scored to indicate the likelihood of overt DIC, with scores predictive of mortality (Box B).[35] Overt DIC represents a stressed and decompensated haemostatic system, generally resulting in clinical consequences. In non-overt DIC, the haemostatic system is under stress but compensated.

DIC is a dynamic state, and serial laboratory tests, e.g. daily, are required to fully evaluate the clinical situation.

Box B Diagnostic scoring system for DIC[35]

Risk assessment

If the patient has an underlying disorder known to be associated with DIC, proceed to measure and score the haematological indices below:

	Score			
	0	*1*	2	3
Platelets (x 10^9/L)	>100	<100	<50	
D-dimer increase (ng/mL)	none		moderate (250–5,000)	strong (>5,000)
Prolonged PT (sec)	<3	3–6	>6	
Fibrinogen (g/L)	>1	<1		

Calculate total score:

≥5 Compatible with overt DIC, repeat score daily

<5 Suggestive (not affirmative) for non-overt DIC; repeat score in 1–2 days

Management

When possible, correct the underlying cause, e.g. sepsis.

Seek specialist advice:

- on the use of platelet transfusions, fresh frozen plasma, other coagulation factors and **tranexamic acid** in patients actively bleeding, requiring an invasive procedure, or at risk of bleeding complications
- on the use of anticoagulants, e.g. UFH, LMWH, prophylactically in those not bleeding, or when thrombosis predominates.

Note. Generally, antifibrinolytic drugs, e.g. **tranexamic acid** and **aminocaproic acid** (not UK), should *not* be used in DIC, because they increase the risk of end-organ damage from microvascular thromboses.

LMWH is the anticoagulant of choice in the treatment of *chronic* DIC; this commonly presents as recurrent thromboses in both superficial and deep veins which do not respond to **warfarin**.

Overdose

See individual SPCs for details.

With recommended doses of LMWH, there should be no need for an antidote. However, an accidental overdose may result in haemorrhagic complications.

Protamine sulfate partially reverses the effects of LMWH on factor Xa (**dalteparin** 25%, **enoxaparin** 60%, **tinzaparin** 65–80%). It should be used only in an emergency and in accordance with the recommendations in the individual LMWH SPCs.[36] However, typically:

- for each 100 units (or 1mg **enoxaparin**) of LMWH, **protamine sulfate** 1mg is given
- a maximum of 50mg by slow IV injection is given *over 10min*.

Decisions regarding the necessity and dose of subsequent **protamine** injections are based on clinical response.

Alternatively, recombinant **activated factor VIIa concentrate** can be used. In three patients who bled after surgery or an invasive procedure, a single IV dose of 20–30microgram/kg successfully reversed anticoagulation from LMWH. It did not precipitate thrombosis, despite the patients all having a risk factor for hypercoagulation, e.g. cancer-related surgery.[37]

Supply

Dalteparin

Fragmin® (Pfizer)

Injection (single-dose graduated syringe for SC injection) 10,000 units/mL, 1mL syringe = £5.50.

Injection (single-dose syringe for SC injection) 2,500 units/0.2mL = £2.

Injection (single-dose syringe for SC injection) 5,000 units/0.2mL = £2.75, 7,500 units/0.3mL = £4.25, 10,000 units/0.4mL = £5.50, 12,500 units/0.5mL = £7, 15,000 units/0.6mL = £8.50, 18,000 units/0.72mL = £10.

Fragmin® (Pfizer)

Injection (single-dose ampoule for SC or IV injection) 10,000 units/4mL, 4mL amp = £5.

Injection (single-dose ampoule for SC or IV injection) 10,000 units/mL, 1mL amp = £5.

Injection (multiple-dose vial for SC injection) 100,000 units/4mL, 4mL vial = £49.

Enoxaparin

Arovi® (Rovi Biotech)

Injection (single-dose syringe for SC injection) 2,000 units (20mg)/0.2mL = £1.50, 4,000 units (40mg)/0.4mL = £2.25, 6,000 units (60mg)/0.6mL = £3, 8,000 units (80mg)/0.8mL = £4, 10,000 units (100mg)/1mL = £5.50.

Injection (single-dose syringe for SC injection) 12,000 units (120mg)/0.8mL = £6.50, 15,000 units (150mg)/1mL = £7.50.

Note. Enoxaparin 1mg = 100 units; other brands include Clexane®, Inhixa® Ledraxen®.

Clexane® (Sanofi)

Injection (Clexane® Multidose; multiple-dose vial for SC or IV injection) 30,000 units (300mg)/3mL, 3mL vial = £21.

Tinzaparin (generic)
Injection (single-dose syringe for SC injection) 2,500 units/0.25mL = £2, 3,500 units/0.35mL = £2.75, 4,500 units/0.45mL = £3.50.

Innohep® (Leo)
Injection (single-dose syringe for SC injection) 8,000 units/0.4mL = £4.75, 10,000 units/0.5mL = £6, 12,000 units/0.6mL = £7, 14,000 units/0.7mL = £8.50, 16,000 units/0.8mL = £9.50, 18,000 units/0.9mL = £11.

Innohep® (Leo)
Injection (multiple-dose vial for SC injection) 20,000 units/2mL, 2mL vial = £11.
Injection (multiple-dose vial for SC injection) 40,000 units/2mL, 2mL vial = £34.

Protamine sulfate (generic)
Injection 50mg/5mL, 5mL amp = £5.

1 Robertson L and Jones LE (2017) Fixed dose subcutaneous low molecular weight heparins versus adjusted dose unfractionated heparin for the initial treatment of venous thromboembolism. *Cochrane Database of Systematic Reviews*. **2**: CD001100. www.cochranelibrary.com.
2 Kearon C *et al.* (2016) Antithrombotic therapy for VTE disease: chest guideline and expert panel report. *Chest*. **149**: 315–352.
3 Watson HG *et al.* (2015) Guideline on aspects of cancer-related venous thrombosis. *British Journal of Haematology*. **170**: 640–648.
4 Noble S and Sui J (2016) The treatment of cancer associated thrombosis: does one size fit all? Who should get LMWH/warfarin/DOACs? *Thrombosis Research*. **140 (Suppl 1)**: 154–159.
5 Zhang N *et al.* (2016) Low molecular weight heparin and cancer survival: clinical trials and experimental mechanisms. *Journal of Cancer Research and Clinical Oncology*. **142**: 1807–1816.
6 Fossler MJ *et al.* (2001) Pharmacodynamics of intravenous and subcutaneous tinzaparin and heparin in healthy volunteers. *American Journal of Health System Pharmacy*. **58**: 1614–1621.
7 Fareed J *et al.* (1990) Pharmacologic profile of a low molecular weight heparin (enoxaparin): experimental and clinical validation of the prophylactic antithrombotic effects. *Acta Chirurgica Scandinavica Supplementum*. **556 (Suppl)**: 75–90.
8 Dawes J (1990) Comparison of the pharmacokinetics of enoxaparin (Clexane) and unfractionated heparin. *Acta Chirurgica Scandinavica Supplementum*. **556 (Suppl)**: 68–74.
9 Bara L and Samama M (1990) Pharmacokinetics of low molecular weight heparins. *Acta Chirurgica Scandinavica Supplementum*. **556 (Suppl)**: 57–61.
10 Hirsh J *et al.* (2001) Heparin and low-molecular-weight heparin: mechanisms of action, pharmacokinetics, dosing, monitoring, efficacy, and safety. *Chest*. **119 (Suppl)**: 64–94.
11 Watson H *et al.* (2012) Guidelines on the diagnosis and management of heparin-induced thrombocytopenia: second edition. *British Journal of Haematology*. **159**: 528–540.
12 NICE (2012) Venous thromboembolic diseases: the management of venous thromboembolic diseases and the role of thrombophilia testing. *Clinical Guideline*. CG144. www.nice.org.uk (updated 2015).
13 NICE (2019) Venous thromboembolism in over 16s: reducing the risk of hospital-acquired deep vein thrombosis or pulmonary embolism. *Clinical Guideline 89*. www.nice.org.uk.
14 Noble SI and Finlay IG (2005) Is long-term low-molecular-weight heparin acceptable to palliative care patients in the treatment of cancer related venous thromboembolism? A qualitative study. *Palliative Medicine*. **19**: 197–201.
15 Wittkowsky AK (2006) Barriers to the long-term use of low-molecular weight heparins for treatment of cancer-associated thrombosis. *Journal of Thrombosis and Haemostasis*. **4**: 2090–2091.
16 Ay C *et al.* (2017) Cancer-associated venous thromboembolism: burden, mechanisms, and management. *Thrombosis Haemostasis*. **117**: 219–230.
17 Department of Health (2010) VTE risk assessment tool. www.nice.org.uk/guidance/ng89/resources (accessed December 2019).
18 Kakkar AK and Williamson RC (1999) Prevention of venous thromboembolism in cancer patients. *Seminars in Thrombosis and Hemostasis*. **25**: 239–243.
19 Farge D *et al.* (2019) 2019 international clinical practice guidelines for the treatment and prophylaxis of venous thromboembolism in patients with cancer. *Lancet Oncology*. **20**: e566–e581.
20 Cunningham MS *et al.* (2006) Prevention and management of venous thromboembolism in people with cancer: a review of the evidence. *Clinical Oncology (Royal College of Radiologists)*. **18**: 145–151.
21 Leizorovicz A and Mismetti P (2004) Preventing venous thromboembolism in medical patients. *Circulation*. **110 (Suppl 1)**: 13–19.
22 Noble SI *et al.* (2006) Acceptability of low molecular weight heparin thromboprophylaxis for inpatients receiving palliative care: qualitative study. *British Medical Journal*. **332**: 577–580.
23 White C *et al.* (2019) Prevalence, symptom burden, and natural history of deep vein thrombosis in people with advanced cancer in specialist palliative care units (HIDDen): a prospective longitudinal observational study. *Lancet Haematology*. **6**: e79–e88.
24 Tardy B *et al.* (2017) Bleeding risk of terminally ill patients hospitalized in palliative care units: the RHESO study. *Journal of Thrombosis and Haemostasis*. **15**: 420–428.
25 Dennis M *et al.* (2013) Effectiveness of intermittent pneumatic compression in reduction of risk of deep vein thrombosis in patients who have had a stroke (CLOTS 3): a multicentre randomised controlled trial. *Lancet*. **382**: 516–524.
26 Dennis M *et al.* (2009) Effectiveness of thigh-length graduated compression stockings to reduce the risk of deep vein thrombosis after stroke (CLOTS trial 1): a multicentre, randomised controlled trial. *Lancet*. **373**: 1958–1965.
27 Wang TF *et al.* (2019) The use of direct oral anticoagulants for primary thromboprophylaxis in ambulatory cancer patients: guidance from the SSC of the ISTH. *Journal of Thrombosis and Haemostasis*. **17**: 1772–1778.
28 NICE (2013) DVT prevention for travellers. *Clinical Knowledge Summaries*. www.cks.nice.org.uk.

29 Sanofi (2017) Clexane (enoxaparin sodium): Updates to strength expression, dose regimens in DVT/PE, use in patients with severe renal impairment. *Direct Healthcare Professional Communication.* Available from www.gov.uk/drug-safety-update/letters-sent-to-healthcare-professionals-in-june-2017.

30 Diaz AH *et al.* (2012) Enoxaparin once daily vs. twice daily dosing for the treatment of venous thromboembolism in cancer patients: a literature summary. *Journal of Oncology Pharmacy Practice.* **18**: 264–270.

31 Bhutia S and Wong PF (2013) Once versus twice daily low molecular weight heparin for the initial treatment of venous thromboembolism. *Cochrane Database of Systematic Reviews.* CD003074. www.cochranelibrary.com.

32 Niu J *et al.* (2020) Once-daily vs. twice-daily dosing of enoxaparin for the management of venous thromboembolism: a systematic review and meta-analysis. *Experimental and Therapeutic Medicine.* **20**: 3084–3095.

33 Carrier M *et al.* (2013) Management of challenging cases of patients with cancer-associated thrombosis including recurrent thrombosis and bleeding: guidance from the SSC of the ISTH. *Journal of Thrombosis and Haemostasis.* **12**: 116–117.

34 Walsh-McMonagle D and Green D (1997) Low-molecular weight heparin in the management of Trousseau's syndrome. *Cancer.* **80**: 649–655.

35 British Committee for Standards in Haematology (2010) Guidelines for the diagnosis and management of disseminated intravascular coagulation. *British Journal of Haematology.* **145**: 24–33.

36 British National Formulary. Section 2.8.3 Protamine sulfate. London: BMJ Group and Pharmaceutical Press www.medicinescomplete.com (accessed August 2017).

37 Firozvi K *et al.* (2006) Reversal of low-molecular-weight heparin-induced bleeding in patients with pre-existing hypercoagulable states with human recombinant activated factor VII concentrate. *American Journal of Hematology.* **81**: 582–589.

Updated (minor change) February 2022

Quick Clinical Guide: Heparin-induced thrombocytopenia (HIT)

Consistent with the Guidelines of the Haemostasis and Thrombosis Task Force of the British Committee for Standards in Haematology

1 Both unfractionated heparin (UFH) and low molecular weight heparin (LMWH) can cause thrombocytopenia (platelet count <100 x 10^9/L).

2 An early mild fall in platelet count is often seen after starting heparin (<4 days), particularly postoperatively. This is asymptomatic and corrects spontaneously despite continuing heparin.

3 In <1% of patients, *immune* HIT develops 5–10 days after starting heparin. Can occur sooner or later; rarely, several days after heparin has been stopped.

4 If a patient has had treatment with heparin within the last 3 months, HIT can manifest <1 day after restarting treatment.

5 HIT is less common with:
- LMWH than UFH
- medical than surgical patients.

6 Heparin-dependent IgG antibody–platelet factor 4 complexes bind to the platelet surface, causing disruption and release of procoagulant material.

7 HIT manifests as *venous* or *arterial* thrombo-embolism and can be fatal.

8 **Diagnosis**

The probability of HIT is initially judged on clinical grounds, aided by a scoring system (Box A).

Box A '4Ts' score to predict probability of HIT

4Ts	*Clinical findings*			*Score*
Thrombocytopenia	Platelet count fall[a]		Platelet nadir[b]	
	<30%	*or*	<10 x 10^9/L	0
	30–50%	*or*	10–19 x 10^9/L	1
	>50%	*and*	≥20 x 10^9/L	2
Timing of platelet count fall or other sequelae[c]	≤4 days (without recent heparin exposure)			0
	Consistent with immunization but unclear (missing counts), or onset >10 days, or ≤1 day (if heparin exposure 30–100 days ago)			1
	Clear onset within 5–10 days, or ≤1 day (if heparin exposure within last 30 days)			2
Thrombosis or other sequelae	None			0
	Progressive or recurrent thrombosis; erythematous skin lesions; suspected thrombosis			1
	New thrombosis; skin necrosis; post-heparin bolus acute systemic reaction			2
Other cause for thrombocytopenia	Definite			0
	Possible			1
	None			2

a. to determine % fall, compare the highest platelet count with the lowest

b. severe thrombocytopenia (platelet count <15 x 10^9/L) is unusual in HIT

c. day 0 = first day of heparin exposure; the day the platelet count starts to fall is considered the day of onset of thrombocytopenia (it generally takes 1–3 days more until the arbitrary threshold defining thrombocytopenia is passed).

Box A Continued

Calculate total score (maximum 8):

Score	*Probability*	*Implications*
6–8	high	Stop heparin, commence alternative anticoagulant and perform further tests
4–5	intermediate	
0–3	low	HIT excluded, no need for further tests

9 Treatment

Stop heparin immediately if high or intermediate probability of HIT, and obtain advice from a haematologist urgently.

While awaiting laboratory results (e.g. platelet activation assay, antigen assay):

- prescribe a treatment dose of a non-heparin (e.g. argatroban, danaparoid) or synthetic heparin (e.g. fondaparinux) parenteral anticoagulant, whether or not there is clinical evidence of a DVT
- only when the platelet count has recovered to ≥150 x 10^9/L, prescribe warfarin
- continue the non-heparin anticoagulant until the INR reaches a therapeutic level, typically 5–7 days. Note. Argatroban can falsely increase the INR
- when a thrombotic complication has occurred, continue anticoagulation for 3 months; when no thrombosis, 1 month is sufficient.

Do *not* use warfarin alone (risk of skin necrosis and venous limb gangrene).
Consider platelet transfusion when there is bleeding, but *not* prophylactically.

10 Preventing recurrence

- record the diagnosis in the patient's notes as a serious allergy
- issue antibody card (but most patients are antibody negative after 3 months)
- if possible, avoid surgery for >3 months after HIT
- although cross-reactivity between UFH and LMWH is uncommon, advise the patient not to have injections of any type of heparin in the future
- if subsequent anticoagulation is required, a non-heparin (e.g. argatroban, danaparoid) or synthetic heparin (e.g. fondaparinux) parenteral anticoagulant should be used; in certain situations, a DOAC may be an option, e.g. orthopaedic surgery
- for patients with a history of HIT requiring renal dialysis or cardiac surgery, seek specialist advice.

Updated December 2019

HAEMOSTATICS

Indications: Prevention/treatment of bleeding (authorized indications vary between products; consult SPC for details), †subarachnoid haemorrhage, †surface bleeding including from, e.g. fungating tumours on the skin, nose, mouth, pharynx, and other hollow organs (lungs, stomach, rectum, bladder, uterus).

Contra-indications: Active thrombo-embolic disease, e.g. recent thrombo-embolism, DIC; history of convulsions.
Tranexamic acid: severe renal impairment (but see Dose and use).

Pharmacology

The most commonly used haemostatics are **tranexamic acid** and **aminocaproic acid** (not UK). These are synthetic antifibrinolytic drugs derived from lysine. They bind to plasminogen and prevent its interaction as plasmin with fibrin, thereby preventing dissolution of haemostatic plugs.[1] **Tranexamic acid** has a longer duration of action and causes fewer undesirable GI effects than **aminocaproic acid**.[2]

Systemic or topical use of antifibrinolytics reduces blood loss in various circumstances, e.g. epistaxis (topical/PO), menorrhagia (PO), major injury (IV) and peri-operatively (IV, topical).[3-7] Antifibrinolytics are used in patients with cancer to control surface bleeding. In patients with leukaemia and thrombocytopenia, antifibrinolytics appear to reduce bleeding and the need for platelet transfusions, but supporting data are too limited to recommend routine use.[8,9] Benefit from PO, IV or nebulized **tranexamic acid** is reported in patients with haemoptysis due to various causes, e.g. bronchiectasis, lung cancer. Supporting data are limited, but suggest bleeding is reduced in duration and severity.[10-12] A small RCT that compared nebulized **tranexamic acid** with sodium chloride 0.9% found significant improvements in blood volume expectorated, proportion achieving full resolution (92% vs. 50% at day 5), and the need for invasive intervention (0% vs. 18%).[13]

Antifibrinolytics do not reverse therapeutic anticoagulation but are used in the management of major bleeding in patients receiving a DOAC (see Anticoagulants, Box A, p.97). In patients on **warfarin** undergoing minor oral surgery or dental extraction, the application of topical **tranexamic acid** reduces the incidence of postoperative bleeding.[14,15]

For the management of severe surface bleeding associated with platelet dysfunction and non-variceal upper GI haemorrhage, see **Desmopressin**, p.572 and PPIs, p.31, respectively.

The evidence that antifibrinolytics may increase the risk of thrombosis is generally limited to case reports, with many RCTs identifying no such concerns.[5] However, this has not been well evaluated in patients potentially at higher risk because of an underlying prothrombotic tendency, e.g. those with cancer. On the other hand, it is suggested that **tranexamic acid** could be antithrombotic by inhibiting the wider effects of prothrombin and plasmin, which include promoting inflammation, platelet aggregation and coagulation.[16]

Antifibrinolytics are generally contra-indicated in DIC, even when haemorrhagic manifestations (ecchymoses, haematomas) are predominant. This is because clot formation is the trigger for further intravascular coagulation (and platelet consumption), and thereby end-organ damage from microvascular thromboses.[17] Rarely, antifibrinolytics have been used in DIC when there is severe bleeding due to a marked hyperfibrinolytic state;[17] *seek specialist advice.*

Etamsylate (not UK; see Supply) acts by increasing capillary vascular wall resistance and platelet adhesiveness in the presence of a vascular lesion. This is achieved by inhibiting the biosynthesis and actions of those PGs that cause platelet disaggregation, vasodilation and increased capillary permeability, thereby promoting platelet activation and aggregation, and also by increasing communication between platelets, leucocytes and endothelial cells via the cell adhesion molecule P-selectin.[18] Thus, **etamsylate** is of limited value in thrombocytopenia. It does not cause vasoconstriction, nor does it affect normal coagulation; it has no effect on prothrombin time, fibrinolysis or platelet count.

Studies have mainly explored the use of **etamsylate** for menorrhagia or for peri-ventricular haemorrhage in premature infants.[18] In palliative care, it is used for surface bleeding ± **tranexamic acid**. Rarely, parenteral use may be necessary, e.g. in patients with bleeding and complete dysphagia due to oesophageal cancer.

Tranexamic acid and **aminocaproic acid** are excreted in the urine mainly unchanged. Thus, dose reduction is necessary in renal impairment. Although the SPC gives severe renal impairment as a contra-indication to **tranexamic acid**, there are reports of its use in this circumstance in reduced doses (see Table 2).[19,20] **Etamsylate** is also excreted in the urine mainly unchanged, but generally no dose reduction is required even in severe renal impairment.[21] Pharmacokinetic details are listed in Table 1.

Table 1 Pharmacokinetics of antifibrinolytic and haemostatic drugs

	Tranexamic acid	*Aminocaproic acid*	*Etamsylate*
Bio-availability PO	30–50%[a]	100%	100%
Onset of action (route-dependent)	1–3h	1–3h	30min IV
Time to peak plasma concentration	3h PO	2h	4h PO; 1h IV
Plasma halflife	2–3h	2h	5–17h PO; 2–2.5h IM/IV
Duration of action	24h	12–18h	no data

a. systemic bio-availability minimal with oral rinse when not swallowed.

Cautions

History of thrombo-embolism, renal impairment.

In both microscopic and macroscopic haematuria, there is a risk of clot formation causing ureteric obstruction or urinary retention.[22]

Undesirable effects

Tranexamic acid and aminocaproic acid: possible increased risk of thrombosis; hypotension, bradycardia, arrhythmia (give slowly IV), nausea, vomiting, abdominal pain, diarrhoea (generally settles if the dose is reduced), muscle weakness, seizures (generally following high-dose IV use, e.g. 100mg/kg).[23]

Tranexamic acid: disturbances in colour vision (discontinue drug).

Etamsylate: fever, headache, rash.

Dose and use

Generally, antifibrinolytics should be used as one part of a multimodal approach to the management of surface bleeding (Box A).

Note. Haemostatic agents are generally not indicated for the treatment of catastrophic haemorrhage. Supportive non-drug measures should be used, with sedation for distress if needed, see p.171.

†Surface bleeding from any site

For haematuria, see below.

Tranexamic acid

- give 1.5g PO stat and 1g t.d.s.
- if the bleeding has not stopped after 3 days, increase dose to 1.5–2g t.d.s. (manufacturer's recommended maximum dose is 1.5g t.d.s., but doses of ≤2g q.d.s. have been used)
- discontinue 1 week after cessation of bleeding or reduce to 500mg t.d.s.
- restart if bleeding recurs, and possibly continue indefinitely.

IV use may be necessary, e.g. acute severe haemorrhage, patients with complete dysphagia; give 15mg/kg IV over 5–10min t.d.s.–q.d.s.

The dose should be reduced in renal impairment (Table 2).

Other than for bleeding fungating cancer in the skin and anterior epistaxis, topical **tranexamic acid** (see Box B) is generally used only if other options, including PO **tranexamic acid**, have failed.

Note. For bleeding wounds, consider antibiotics if there are signs or symptoms of infection, as infected wounds are more likely to bleed.

Box A Other measures to manage bleeding in addition to systemic tranexamic acid

Review drugs

- discontinue anticoagulants (e.g. LMWH, warfarin), anti-platelet drugs (e.g. aspirin, clopidogrel) and other drugs which impair platelet function (e.g. most NSAIDs, SSRIs)
- if analgesia is required, prescribe paracetamol or an NSAID that does *not* impair platelet function (see NSAIDs, Table 4, p.344).

Topical options

- *bleeding points (nose, mouth, wounds):* apply silver nitrate stick
- *mouth, rectum:* sucralfate suspension 2g in 10mL b.d.[24]
- *wounds:*
  - ▷ adrenaline (epinephrine) (1 in 1,000) 1mg in 1mL on gauze (short-term only because of the risk of ischaemic necrosis and rebound vasodilation)
  - ▷ sucralfate paste 2 x 1g tablets crushed in 5mL water-soluble gel, e.g. KY® Jelly[25]
  - ▷ sympathomimetic vasoconstrictors, e.g. xylometazoline nasal spray applied directly onto malignant wounds,[26] but short-term use only (risk of rebound vasodilation after several days' application)
- *fungating cancer in the skin:* alginate haemostatic dressings (e.g. Kaltostat®, Sorbsan®)
- *posterior epistaxis:* sympathomimetic vasoconstrictors, e.g. xylometazoline nasal spray (see above for wounds).[27]

Systemic drugs

- *second-line:* switch from first-line tranexamic acid/aminocaproic acid (not UK) to, or combine with, etamsylate (not UK) 500mg PO q.d.s. either indefinitely or until 1 week after cessation of bleeding; take after food if nausea, vomiting or diarrhoea is a problem
- *third-line:* desmopressin (p.572).

Note. Etamsylate and desmopressin augment platelet function, and thus are of limited value in thrombocytopenia.

Specialist measures

- radiotherapy, e.g. skin, lung, oesophagus, rectum, bladder, uterus, vagina[28]
- coagulation, e.g. diathermy, cryotherapy, LASER
- embolization.[29,30]

Table 2 Tranexamic acid doses in renal impairment

Plasma creatinine (micromol/L)	*Creatinine clearance (mL/min)*	*PO dose*	*IV dose*[a]
120–249	50–80	15mg/kg b.d.	10mg/kg b.d.
250–500	10–50	15mg/kg once daily	10mg/kg once daily
>500	<10	7.5mg/kg once daily or 15mg/kg every 2 days[4,5]	5mg/kg once daily or 10mg/kg every 2 days

a. CSCI dose/24h should be similarly adjusted.

†Subcutaneous administration

Some centres give **tranexamic acid** CSCI; typical doses are 1,500–2,000mg/24h, infused alone, using WFI as diluent when necessary.[35-37] In addition, loading and/or p.r.n. doses are sometimes given SC. **Tranexamic acid** ≤500mg can be given SC undiluted, but for comfort, larger volumes will need to be divided between sites. Alternatively, some centres infuse 500–1,000mg SC diluted in 50mL sodium chloride 0.9% over about 30min under gravity.[38]

Box B Topical tranexamic acid for surface bleeding

When using tranexamic acid 5% solutions, generally it is cheaper to dilute the contents of a standard 100mg/mL (10%) 5mL ampoule with 5mL water than to use special-order products (see Supply). Ideally, give instillations at body temperature.

The following recommendations are mostly from anecdotal reports:

- *fungating cancer in the skin (10% solution):* soak the undiluted contents of a 100mg/mL, 5mL ampoule into gauze and apply with pressure for 10min; leave *in situ* covered with a dressing[31]
- *anterior epistaxis (10% solution):* soak the undiluted contents of a 100mg/mL, 5mL ampoule into a cotton pledget/gauze and insert into the nostril for 10min[7,32]
- *mouth (5% solution):* use 500mg/10mL (dilute 1 x 100mg/mL, 5mL ampoule with 5mL water) as a mouthwash, q.d.s. and swallow after use;[14,15] alternatively, some centres disperse a 500mg tablet in 10mL of water
- *rectum (5% solution):* instil as an enema, 5,000mg/100mL (dilute 10 x 100mg/mL, 5mL ampoules with 50mL water) once daily or b.d.[33]
- *lungs (10% solution):*
  - ▷ haemoptysis: nebulize the undiluted contents of a 100mg/mL, 5mL ampoule t.d.s.–q.d.s.[11,13]
  - ▷ pleural haemorrhage: instil the undiluted contents of 10 x 100mg/mL, 5mL ampoules (50mL) intrapleurally via a thoracic drain once daily, clamping drain for 1h; benefit seen after 1–2 instillations[34]
- *bladder:* see Haematuria below.

Aminocaproic acid (not UK)

In oliguria or end-stage renal disease, give 15–25% of the normal dose.[20]

Acute bleeding syndromes due to elevated fibrinolytic activity[39]

- stat dose of 5g PO (or 4–5g IVI in 250mL of diluent) during the first hour of treatment, then 1.25g/h PO (or 1g/h IVI in 50mL of diluent) for 8h or until bleeding stops; suitable diluents for IVI are sodium chloride 0.9% or glucose 5%
- manufacturer's maximum recommended dose = 30g/24h PO/IV.

Chronic bleeding tendency

- give 5–30g PO daily in divided doses at 3–6h intervals
- when bleeding is controlled, adjust to the lowest effective dose.

Bleeding from oral cancers[40]

- give 500mg PO q.d.s. until bleeding stops
- then discontinue by tapering dose frequency every 2–3 days.

†Haematuria

Haematuria in advanced cancer is generally associated with urinary tract cancer, most commonly bladder cancer. It may also be caused by chronic radiation cystitis, which can develop several years after pelvic radiotherapy.[41] In many cases, haematuria is mild and no intervention is necessary. Seek urological advice to guide appropriate management.

Correct the correctable

- can the cancer be modified? If the patient is well enough, consider cystoscopy for resection/local control of bleeding, e.g. with diathermy
- can other factors be modified?
  - ▷ instead of a non-selective NSAID, prescribe **paracetamol** or an NSAID that does not impair platelet function (see NSAIDs, Table 4, p.344)
  - ▷ consider checking PT, APTT and FBC
  - ▷ culture urine; treat infection if present.

Non-drug treatment

When haematuria is associated with clot formation, there is a risk of obstruction and clots should be removed by irrigating the bladder with sodium chloride 0.9% via a three-way 22–24 French urinary catheter. Once *all* clots have been removed, for ongoing haematuria, start continuous irrigation with sodium chloride 0.9%. If this approach fails, cystoscopy for clot removal and/or local control of bleeding is indicated. Rarely, it may be necessary to consider:

- other bladder irrigations or instillations, e.g. **alum**, prostaglandin analogues
- arterial embolization
- urinary diversion, e.g. nephrostomy
- hyperbaric oxygen.[42]

Drug treatment

When the above approaches have failed or are inappropriate, **tranexamic acid** (PO, IV, or, if this fails, by a 5% intravesical instillation, 100mL once daily–b.d.) may be used, although there is a risk of clot retention until the bleeding has completely stopped, and this may necessitate clot removal under general anaesthetic. Although a reduction in/cessation of haematuria is reported following **tranexamic acid**, the full clinical relevance is unclear; supporting evidence is limited to a small uncontrolled case series in patients with polycystic kidney disease and a pilot RCT in patients with severe haematuria of unknown cause, which found no difference in RBC transfusion requirements.[43,44]

Supply

Tranexamic acid (generic)

Tablets 500mg, 28 days @ 1g t.d.s. = £18.

Oral solution or suspension 500mg/5mL (10%), 28 days @ 1g t.d.s. = £70 or £93 respectively (unauthorized products, available as a special order; see Chapter 24, p.817). *Prices based on Specials tariff in community.*

Mouthwash 500mg/10mL (5%), 28 days @ 10mL q.d.s. = £79 (unauthorized product, available as a special order; see Chapter 24, p.817). *Price based on Specials tariff in community.*

Injection 100mg/mL (10%), 5mL amp = £1.50.

Etamsylate

Tablets 500mg, 20 = £10–£50 (not UK, obtainable via import; see Chapter 24, p.817).

Injection 125mg/mL, 2mL amp = <£10 (not UK, obtainable via import; see Chapter 24, p.817).

Sucralfate

Antepsin® (Chugai)

Tablets 1g, 60 = £10–£50 (not UK, obtainable via import; see Chapter 24, p.817).

Oral suspension 1g/5mL, 28 days @ 2g b.d. = £202.

Enema 2g/20mL, 2g/50mL = £7 and £25 respectively (unauthorized products, available as a special order; see Chapter 24, p.817.). *Prices based on Specials tariff in community.*

---

1 Mannucci PM (1998) Hemostatic drugs. *New England Journal of Medicine*. **339**: 245–253.

2 Okamoto S *et al.* (1964) An active stereoisomer (trans form) of AMCHA and its antifibrinolytic (antiplasminic) action in vitro and in vivo. *Keio Journal of Medicine*. **13**: 177–185.

3 McCormack PL (2012) Tranexamic acid: a review of its use in the treatment of hyperfibrinolysis. *Drugs*. **72**: 585–617.

4 Ker K *et al.* (2012) Effect of tranexamic acid on surgical bleeding: systematic review and cumulative meta-analysis. *British Medical Journal*. **344**: e3054.

5 Roberts I *et al.* (2013) The CRASH-2 trial: a randomised controlled trial and economic evaluation of the effects of tranexamic acid on death, vascular occlusive events and transfusion requirement in bleeding trauma patients. *Health Technol Assess*. **17**: 1–79.

6 Shang J *et al.* (2016) Combined intravenous and topical tranexamic acid versus intravenous use alone in primary total knee and hip arthroplasty: A meta-analysis of randomized controlled trials. *International Journal of Surgery*. **36**: 324–329.

7 Joseph J *et al.* (2018) Tranexamic acid for patients with nasal haemorrhage (epistaxis)(Review). *Cochrane Database of Systematic Reviews*. **12**: CD004328. www.cochranelibrary.com.

8 Estcourt LJ *et al.* (2016) Antifibrinolytics (lysine analogues) for the prevention of bleeding in people with haematological disorders. *Cochrane Database Syst Rev*. **3**: CD009733. www.cochranelibrary.com.

9 Antun AG *et al.* (2013) Epsilon aminocaproic acid prevents bleeding in severely thrombocytopenic patients with hematological malignancies. *Cancer*. **119**: 3784-3787.

10 Prutsky G *et al.* (2016) Antifibrinolytic therapy to reduce haemoptysis from any cause. *Cochrane Database of Systematic Reviews*. **11**: CD008711. www.cochranelibrary.com.

11 Gadre A and Stoller JK (2017) Tranexamic acid for haemoptysis: A review. *Clinical Pulmonary Medicine*. **24**: 69–74.
12 Bellam BL *et al.* (2016) Efficacy of tranexamic acid in haemoptysis: A randomized, controlled pilot study. *Pulmonary Pharmacology and Therapeutics*. **40**: 80–83.
13 Wand O *et al.* (2018) Inhaled Tranexamic Acid for Hemoptysis Treatment: A Randomized Controlled Trial. *Chest*. **154**: 1379–1384.
14 Engelen ET *et al.* (2018) Antifibrinolytic therapy for preventing oral bleeding in people on anticoagulants undergoing minor oral surgery or dental extractions. *Cochrane Database of Systematic Reviews*. **7**: CD012293. www.cochranelibrary.com.
15 de Vasconcellos SJA *et al.* (2017) Topical application of tranexamic acid in anticoagulated patients undergoing minor oral surgery: A systematic review and meta-analysis of randomized clinical trials. *Journal of Cranio-Maxillofacial Surgery*. **45**: 20–26.
16 Godier A *et al.* (2012) Tranexamic acid: less bleeding and less thrombosis? *Critical Care*. **16**: 135.
17 Wada H *et al.* (2013) Guidance for diagnosis and treatment of DIC from harmonization of the recommendations from three guidelines. *Journal of Thrombosis and Haemostasis*. **11**: 761–767.
18 Garay RP *et al.* (2006) Therapeutic efficacy and mechanism of action of ethamsylate, a long-standing hemostatic agent. *American Journal of Therapeutics*. **13**: 236–247.
19 Andersson L *et al.* (1978) Special considerations with regard to the dosage of tranexamic acid in patients with chronic renal diseases. *Urological Research*. **6**: 83–88.
20 Lacy C *et al.*, (eds) (2003) Lexi-Comp's Drug Information Handbook. (11e) Lexi-Comp and the American Pharmaceutical Association, Hudson, Ohio.
21 Ashley C and Dunleavy A Ethamsylate monograph. *The Renal Drug Database*. CRC Press, Taylor & Francis group www.renaldrugdatabase.com.
22 Schultz M and van der Lelie H (1995) Microscopic haematuria as a relative contraindication for tranexamic acid. *British Journal of Haematology*. **89**: 663–664.
23 Murkin JM *et al.* (2010) High-dose tranexamic Acid is associated with nonischemic clinical seizures in cardiac surgical patients. *Anesthesia and Analgesia*. **110**: 350-353.
24 Kochhar R *et al.* (1988) Rectal sucralfate in radiation proctitis. *Lancet*. **332**: 400.
25 Regnard C and Makin W (1992) Management of bleeding in advanced cancer: a flow diagram. *Palliative Medicine*. **6**: 74–78.
26 Recka K *et al.* (2012) Management of bleeding associated with malignant wounds. *Journal Palliative of Medicine*. **15**: 952–954.
27 Krempl GA and Noorily AD (1995) Use of oxymetazoline in the management of epistaxis. *Annals of Otology, Rhinology, and Laryngology*. **104**: 704–706.
28 Cihoric N *et al.* (2012) Clinically significant bleeding in incurable cancer patients: effectiveness of hemostatic radiotherapy. *Radiation Oncololgy*. **7**: 132.
29 Rankin E *et al.* (1988) Transcatheter embolisation to control severe bleeding in fungating breast cancer. *European Journal of Surgical Oncology*. **14**: 27–32.
30 Broadley K *et al.* (1995) The role of embolization in palliative care. *Palliative Medicine*. **9**: 331–335.
31 Palliativedrugs.com (2013). Topical Tranexamic Acid - What do you do? *Survey*. March-April: Available from www.palliativedrugs.com.
32 Zahed R *et al.* (2013) A new and rapid method for epistaxis treatment using injectable form of tranexamic acid topically: a randomized controlled trial. *American Journal of Emergency Medicine*. **31**: 1389–1392.
33 McElligott E *et al.* (1991) Tranexamic acid and rectal bleeding. *Lancet*. **337**: 431.
34 deBoer W *et al.* (1991) Tranexamic acid treatment of haemothorax in two patients with malignant mesothelioma. *Chest*. **100**: 847–848.
35 Personal Communication (2017) Subcutaneous administration of tranexamic acid. St Christopher's Hospice. London, UK.
36 Sutherland A *et al.* (2021) Subcutaneous tranexamic acid: a novel approach to managing bleeding. *Annals of hematology and oncology*. **8**: 1356.
37 Palliativedrugs.com (2019) Haemostatics – What do you use? Survey (data on file). Available from www.palliativedrugs.com
38 Howard P and Curtin J (2022) Bleeding management in palliative medicine: subcutaneous tranexamic acid - retrospective chart review. *BMJ Supportive and Palliative Care*. (Epub ahead of print).
39 Roberts SB *et al.* (2010) Palliative use of aminocaproic acid to control upper gastrointestinal bleeding. *Journal of Pain and Symptom Management*. **40**: e1-e3.
40 Setla J (2004) Duration of aminocaproic acid therapy in bleeding for malignant wounds. *Palliativedrugs.com Ltd.* www.palliativedrugs.com.
41 Pascoe C *et al.* (2019) Current management of radiation cystitis: a review and practical guide to clinical management. *BJU International*. **123**: 585–594.
42 Cardinal J *et al.* (2018) Scoping review and meta-analysis of hyperbaric oxygen therapy for radiation-induced hemorrhagic cystitis. *Current Urology Reports*. **19**: 38.
43 Peces R *et al.* (2012) Medical therapy with tranexamic acid in autosomal dominant polycystic kidney disease patients with severe haematuria. *Nefrologia*. **32**: 160–165.
44 Moharamzadeh P *et al.* (2017) Effect of tranexamic acid on gross hematuria: A pilot randomized clinical trial study. *American Journal of Emergency Medicine*. **35**: 1922–1925.

Updated (minor change) February 2022

3: RESPIRATORY SYSTEM

BRONCHODILATORS

Palliative care clinicians caring for patients with end-stage COPD need to be aware of the latest management guidelines. Some patients with cancer also suffer from COPD or asthma, or occasionally both. Concurrent COPD can be a major cause of breathlessness, notably in lung cancer, but may be unrecognized and so go untreated.

The guidelines provided here (Box A–C, Table 1) for the use of bronchodilators in patients with asthma and COPD are based on the British Thoracic Society/Scottish Intercollegiate Guidelines Network guidelines on asthma[1] and the National Institute for Health and Care Excellence COPD guidelines.[2] These have much in common with international guidelines produced by the Global Initiative for Asthma (GINA) and the Global Initiative for Chronic Obstructive Lung Disease (GOLD), although there are some differences in emphasis.[3,4]

Generally, the guidelines should be followed. However, for patients in the last weeks or days of life, particularly those having difficulties with metered-dose inhalers, the regular use of short-acting nebulized bronchodilators may be preferable.

If a patient is receiving long-term PO corticosteroids for another indication (see p.556), it is often possible to discontinue inhaled corticosteroids.

In contrast to other drug delivery methods, inhalation delivers respiratory drugs directly to the bronchi and enables a smaller dose to work more quickly and with fewer undesirable systemic effects. β_2-Adrenergic receptor agonists (β_2 agonists), e.g. **salbutamol** (p.130), **salmeterol** (p.132), act directly on bronchial smooth muscle to cause bronchodilation, whereas antimuscarinics, e.g. **ipratropium** (p.127), **tiotropium** (p.128), act by reducing the vagal tone to the airways. Both classes of drug improve breathlessness by airway bronchodilation and/or reducing air-trapping at rest (static hyperinflation) and on exertion (dynamic hyperinflation). A reduction in hyperinflation probably explains why clinical benefit may be seen in patients with COPD with little or no change in the FEV_1.[5]

β_2 Agonists are used in both asthma and COPD; antimuscarinics in COPD and *acute* asthma. Their use is often combined in *acute* asthma and COPD (Table 1 and Box B). In asthma and severe COPD, bronchodilators are generally combined with inhaled corticosteroids (Box A, Box B; also see p.140).

In asthma and COPD, if optimal inhaled therapy provides inadequate relief, a third class of bronchodilator, the methylxanthines, is sometimes used systemically, e.g. PO **theophylline** m/r (p.137). Because of a narrow therapeutic index, their use requires careful monitoring to avoid toxicity.

β-Adrenergic receptor blocking drugs (β-blockers), both cardioselective and non-selective, are contra-indicated in patients with asthma. They should also be avoided in patients with COPD, unless there are compelling reasons for their use, e.g. severe glaucoma. In such circumstances, a cardioselective β-blocker should be used with extreme caution under specialist guidance.

Table 1 Summary of the immediate management of an acute asthma attack in adults[1,a]

	Severity of attack		
	Moderate	*Severe*	*Life-threatening*[b]
Evaluation		Any of the following:	
PEF[c]	>50–75%	33–50%	<33%
SpO_2 (pulse oximeter)		≥92%	<92%; check blood gases
General condition	No features of severe asthma	Unable to complete sentence in one breath; respirations ≥25/min, pulse ≥110/min	Silent chest, poor respiratory effort, cyanosis, PaO_2 <8kPa, normal or raised $PaCO_2$,[d] arrhythmia, hypotension, exhaustion, altered consciousness
Chest radiograph	Necessary if pneumothorax, pneumomediastinum or consolidation suspected, life-threatening asthma, failure to respond to treatment, or if ventilation required		
Place of care	Hospital if life-threatening or if moderate/severe with failure to respond to treatment or if psychosocial concerns Intensive care if life-threatening or if severe with failure to respond to treatment and ventilation required		
Treatment			
Oxygen	Not needed	Via face/venturi mask or nasal cannulae at flow rate that maintains SpO_2 94–98%	
Bronchodilators[e]	Salbutamol 100microgram (one puff) via a spacer; repeat every minute up to a maximum of 1mg (10 puffs) *or* Salbutamol 5mg or terbutaline 10mg via oxygen-driven nebulizer		Use nebulized β_2 agonist as for moderate–severe, but give with ipratropium 500microgram via an oxygen-driven nebulizer; use spacer only if nebulizer unavailable
	If inadequate response after 15min, give nebulized β_2 agonist		Repeat above
	If inadequate response after 15min:		
		Use nebulized β_2 agonist + ipratropium (if not already given) or consider continuous nebulization of salbutamol 5–10mg/h (requires specific nebulizer)	
Corticosteroid[f]	Prednisolone 40–50mg PO stat & once daily for 5 days or until recovery		
Other treatments[g]		Magnesium sulfate 1.2–2g IV over 20min	
		Aminophylline 5mg/kg IV over 20min, followed by 500–700microgram/kg/h[h]	

a. full guidance available from www.brit-thoracic.org.uk
b. obtain senior/intensive care unit help as soon as life-threatening asthma recognized
c. % of best peak expiratory flow (PEF) within past 2 years or, if unavailable, predicted PEF
d. termed near-fatal asthma when $PaCO_2$ is raised and/or mechanical ventilation is necessary with raised inflation pressures
e. IV β_2 agonists are reserved for patients in whom inhaled route unreliable (see full guidance)
f. the earlier corticosteroids are given, the better the outcome; where PO not possible, give hydrocortisone 100mg IV stat & q.d.s.
g. when poor response to standard bronchodilator therapies; requires guidance from senior/experienced staff (see full guidance)
h. monitor plasma levels daily (aim for 10–20mg/L or 55–110micromol/L); in patients already taking regular PO theophylline, omit loading dose and measure plasma level on admission.

Box A Summary of the management of chronic asthma in adults[1]

Start treatment at the level most appropriate to the initial severity of asthma. The aim is to achieve control as soon as possible, defined as:
- no daytime symptoms
- no night-time awakening due to asthma
- no need for rescue medication
- no asthma attacks
- no limitations on activity, including exercise
- normal lung function, i.e. FEV_1 ± PEF >80% predicted or best
- minimal undesirable effects from drugs.

Before initiating a new drug, check adherence and inhaler technique and eliminate trigger factors.

Intermittent reliever therapy
Inhaled short-acting β_2 agonist p.r.n., e.g. salbutamol.

Move to regular preventer therapy if:
- symptomatic/inhaler needed ≥3 times a week
- night-time symptoms ≥ once a week
- asthma attack requiring PO corticosteroids in the past 2 years.

Regular preventer therapy
Low-dose inhaled corticosteroid, e.g. beclometasone 400microgram/24h or equivalent[a]
+ inhaled short-acting β_2 agonist p.r.n.
If there is insufficient response, consider initial add-on therapy.

Initial add-on therapy
Inhaled long-acting β_2 agonist (LABA)[b], e.g. salmeterol 50microgram b.d. or formoterol 12microgram b.d.
+ low-dose inhaled corticosteroid[a]
+ inhaled short-acting β_2 agonist p.r.n.[c]

Additional add-on therapies
Either increase the inhaled corticosteroid to a medium dose or consider a therapeutic trial of a PO leukotriene receptor antagonist
+ inhaled LABA (when of known benefit)[b]
+ inhaled short-acting β_2 agonist p.r.n.[c]

High-dose therapies
If asthma not controlled, refer to specialist care.

Moving up or down treatment levels
Review treatment regularly, moving up a treatment level if control inadequate or use of ≥3 doses of short-acting β_2 agonist/week. Conversely, if control good, consider going down a level. The most appropriate drug to reduce first may be influenced by individual patient circumstances. Reduce dose of inhaled corticosteroid slowly, e.g. ≤50% every 3 months.

a. doses of inhaled corticosteroids are expressed as low, medium or high (see p.140); high doses are used only after specialist evaluation

b. inhaled LABAs should *not* be used without inhaled corticosteroids, because of concern over an increase in severe asthma exacerbations and asthma-related deaths; combination inhalers are thus recommended to ensure the LABA is taken with an inhaled corticosteroid and to improve adherence

c. formoterol, a LABA with a rapid onset of action, can be used as an alternative to a short-acting β_2 agonist (see p.132).

Box B Summary of palliative drug treatment in COPD[2]

Smoking and β-blockers may cause bronchoconstriction and should be avoided.

The choice of drug(s) is informed by the degree of benefit obtained from a therapeutic trial, patient preference, undesirable effects, potential to reduce exacerbations and cost. Evaluate benefit in terms of improvement in symptoms, activities of daily living, exercise capacity and rapidity of symptom relief; discontinue if ineffective.

Breathlessness and/or exercise limitation
Short-acting β_2 agonist, e.g. salbutamol, or short-acting antimuscarinic bronchodilator, e.g. ipratropium, p.r.n.

Exacerbations or persistent breathlessness
Management is influenced by the presence of features that suggest a likelihood of a response to a corticosteroid, e.g.:

- previous asthma or atopy
- eosinophilia
- substantial variation in FEV_1 over time (>400mL)
- substantial diurnal variation in peak expiratory flow (>20%).

Short-acting β_2 agonist p.r.n. +

- regular LABA and inhaled corticosteroid *(suggestive features present)*, *or*
- regular LABA and long-acting antimuscarinic bronchodilator *(no suggestive features)*.

Persistent exacerbations (two moderate or one severe within a year) or breathlessness (irrespective of FEV_1)
Exacerbations are moderate if they require PO corticosteroid ± antibacterial, and severe if hospital admission is necessary.

Short-acting β_2 agonist p.r.n. +

- regular LABA, long-acting antimuscarinic bronchodilator and inhaled corticosteroid.

Patients with distressing or disabling breathlessness despite maximal use of inhalers (with spacer if appropriate) should be considered for nebulizer therapy.

Other drugs
Reserved for patients with distressing symptoms despite maximal inhaled therapy:

- oral corticosteroids: when unavoidable in advanced COPD, keep dose to a minimum; in patients >65 years, provide routine osteoporosis prophylaxis; in those <65 years, monitor for osteoporosis and treat if necessary
- theophylline: requires caution, particularly in the elderly; monitor serum concentration and for risk of drug–drug interaction; can be used earlier in patients unable to use inhaled therapy
- mucolytics: can be considered in patients with chronic productive cough
- for the role of oxygen in COPD, see p.144
- for the role of opioids and benzodiazepines for breathlessness in advanced COPD and the last days of life, see p.412.

Diagnosing asthma and COPD

The diagnosis of asthma or COPD is based mainly on the history and examination, supported by objective tests and, ultimately, the response to treatment.

In asthma, there are recurrent episodes of respiratory symptoms (>1 of wheeze, cough, breathlessness, chest tightness) caused by variable airflow obstruction. Airflow should be compared objectively during both symptomatic and asymptomatic periods using spirometry preferably or peak expiratory flow rate. Patients with airflow obstruction and a high probability of asthma can start a trial of treatment (Box A).

3

Box C Summary of the initial management of exacerbations of COPD[2]

Diagnosis

A sustained worsening of symptoms of acute onset, beyond the normal day-to-day variation experienced by the patient. Commonly reported symptoms are:

- worsening breathlessness, cough
- increased sputum volume
- change in sputum colour.

Management

Optimize bronchodilator use (Box B). For patients with distressing or disabling breathlessness despite maximal use of inhalers:

- consider use of a nebulizer
- PO corticosteroid, e.g. prednisolone 30mg once daily for 5 days
- antibacterials if purulent sputum.

Admission to hospital should be considered if:

- rapid onset of symptoms
- acute confusion or impaired consciousness
- severe breathlessness, cyanosis, SpO_2 <90%, PaO_2 <7kPa, arterial pH <7.35
- already receiving long-term oxygen
- increasing peripheral oedema
- living alone or unable to cope at home
- poor ± deteriorating general condition and level of activity
- significant co-morbidity (particularly cardiac disease, insulin-dependent diabetes mellitus)
- changes on chest radiograph.

For those needing hospitalization, investigations will include:

- chest radiograph, ECG
- arterial blood gases
- serum theophylline concentration, if already taking theophylline
- if sputum purulent, sputum microscopy and culture
- if pyrexial, blood cultures.

For those needing hospitalization, management will also include:

- oxygen to keep SaO_2 within an individualized target range, according to local protocols
- consideration of the need for:
  - ▷ IV aminophylline if poor response to other bronchodilators
  - ▷ non-invasive ventilation (NIV)
  - ▷ a respiratory stimulant, e.g. doxapram (if NIV unavailable)
  - ▷ intubation.

Those with an intermediate probability should be further investigated, initially with reversibility testing using inhaled **salbutamol** 400microgram. In those with obstruction, an improvement in FEV_1 of ≥12% and ≥200mL is considered a positive result. An improvement in FEV_1 >400mL strongly suggests asthma.

If there is incomplete response, prescribe corticosteroids, generally inhaled, e.g. **beclometasone** 200microgram b.d. or equivalent for 6 weeks and re-evaluate degree of response.[1]

Further tests are recommended for patients without obstruction and an intermediate probability of asthma and when there is only a low probability of asthma.[1]

In suspected COPD, post-bronchodilator spirometry is generally sufficient to indicate the presence of airflow obstruction (FEV_1/FVC <0.7) and its severity. COPD is now classified as:

- stage 1 (mild; FEV_1 ≥80% of predicted)
- stage 2 (moderate; FEV_1 50–79%)
- stage 3 (severe; FEV_1 30–49%)
- stage 4 (very severe; FEV_1 <30%).[2]

In palliative care, when airflow obstruction is suspected, evaluating the impact on symptoms of a 1–2 week trial of a bronchodilator is probably the most pragmatic and relevant approach.

Delivery devices

Pressurized metered-dose inhalers (pMDIs) are the most commonly prescribed delivery device; the correct inhaler technique should be carefully explained to the patient and subsequently checked.[1,6] The patient should be instructed to inhale slowly and then, if possible, hold their breath for 10 seconds. Even with a good pMDI technique, 80% of the dose is deposited in the mouth and oropharynx.

If inhaler technique does not improve with training or in patients with poor respiratory effort, consider using a pMDI plus a large-volume (650–850mL) spacer device to deliver single-dose actuations. There should be minimal delay between actuation and inhalation, but normal (tidal) breathing is as effective as taking a single breath.

Build-up of static on plastic and polycarbonate spacers attracts drug particles and reduces drug delivery. To reduce static, spacers should be washed once a month with detergent, rinsed and left to dry without wiping.[1] Spacers should be replaced every 6–12 months.[1]

Dry powder inhalers, e.g. Turbohaler®, or breath-actuated metered-dose inhalers are other options, but they are no more effective than a pMDI ± a spacer.[1,7] Patients generally prefer dry powder inhalers over a pMDI ± a spacer, but they are not suited to patients with poor inspiratory effort. Compared with pMDIs, actuation of a dry powder inhaler causes less sensation in the oropharynx, and patients should be informed of this to avoid inadvertent overuse. Breath-actuated metered-dose inhalers are triggered at low inspiratory flow rates, are popular with patients and are the easiest to use correctly.[8]

Nebulizers are more expensive and less convenient than a pMDI but may be preferable in patients with a poor inhaler technique, e.g. children, the frail, patients with end-stage disease. Because of improved drug delivery, there may be better symptom relief in this group of patients.[9] However, the higher doses administered can increase the risk of undesirable effects, and their use should be carefully monitored (also see Nebulized drugs, p.904).

Overall, however, there is no evidence to suggest that a nebulizer is superior to any inhaler device for the delivery of a β_2 agonist or corticosteroid for the treatment of stable asthma, or to a pMDI + spacer in the initial treatment of acute asthma, unless there are life-threatening features. In patients with COPD and a good inhaler technique, nebulized bronchodilator therapy is indicated only in severe acute exacerbations or when there is distressing or disabling breathlessness despite maximal use of inhalers.[2]

In patients with lung cancer, concurrent COPD can be a major cause of breathlessness but may be unrecognized and so go untreated.[10] Breathlessness can be improved in most patients with lung cancer and COPD by a β_2 agonist together with an antimuscarinic bronchodilator; this is equally effective when given by a pMDI + a spacer or by nebulizer (see Nebulized drugs, p.904).[10]

Supply

Spacer devices are not interchangeable; prescribe a device that is compatible with the pMDI.

Inhaler and spacer devices
AeroChamber Plus® (Trudell Medical UK Ltd)
Spacer medium volume for use with all pMDIs; standard adult device = £5, with mask = £8.50.

Volumatic® (GlaxoSmithKline UK Ltd)
Spacer large volume for use with *Clenil Modulite®*, *Flixotide®*, *Seretide®*, *Serevent®* and *Ventolin®* pMDIs = £4, with paediatric mask = £7.

This is not a complete list; see BNF *for more information, including devices for paediatric use.*

1 BTS/SIGN (2019) British guideline on the management of asthma. A National Clinical Guideline. *British Thoracic Society and Scottish Intercollegiate Guidelines Network.* Available from: www.brit-thoracic.org.uk

2 NICE (2018) Chronic obstructive pulmonary disease in over 16s: diagnosis and management. *NICE Guideline* NG115. Updated July 2019. www.nice.org.uk

3 NHLBI/WHO (2019) Global Initiative for Asthma (GINA). Pocket guide for asthma management and prevention. www.ginasthma.com

4 NHLBI/WHO (2019) Global initiative for chronic obstructive lung disease. Global strategy for the diagnosis, management and prevention of chronic obstructive pulmonary disease. www.goldcopd.org

5 Laveneziana P *et al.* (2012) New physiological insights into dyspnea and exercise intolerance in chronic obstructive pulmonary disease patients. *Expert Reviews in Respiratory Medicine.* **6**: 651–662.

6 MHRA (2018) Pressurised metered dose inhalers (pMDI): risk of airway obstruction from aspiration of loose objects. *Drug Safety Update*. www.gov.uk
7 Anonymous (2003) Inhaler devices for the management of asthma and COPD. *Effective Health Care Bulletins*. **8**: 1–12.
8 Lenney J *et al.* (2000) Inappropriate inhaler use: assessment of use and patient preference of seven inhalation devices. *Respiratory Medicine*. **94**: 496–500.
9 Tashkin DP *et al.* (2007) Comparing COPD treatment: nebulizer, metered dose inhaler, and concomitant therapy. *American Journal of Medicine*. **120**: 435–441.
10 Congleton J and Muers MF (1995) The incidence of airflow obstruction in bronchial carcinoma, its relation to breathlessness, and response to bronchodilator therapy. *Respiratory Medicine*. **89**: 291–296.

Updated (minor update) September 2021

IPRATROPIUM BROMIDE

Class: Quaternary ammonium antimuscarinic bronchodilator.

Indications: Reversible airways obstruction, particularly in COPD.

Contra-indications: Hypersensitivity to **atropine** or its derivatives.

Pharmacology

Ipratropium is a short-acting antimuscarinic which blocks all muscarinic receptor subtypes with equal affinity. In patients with COPD, cholinergic vagal efferent nerves to the airways activate muscarinic receptors, resulting in increased resting bronchial tone and mucus secretion.[1] Antimuscarinics block these effects and cause bronchodilation. Short-acting antimuscarinics increase FEV_1 but have less consistent benefit on breathlessness, need for rescue medication, walking distance and quality of life.[2]

For patients with COPD-related breathlessness and exercise limitation, an inhaled short-acting antimuscarinic bronchodilator *or* a short-acting β_2 agonist are recommended as initial treatment on a p.r.n. basis. However, a short-acting β_2 agonist is generally preferred as it has a more rapid onset of action and, unlike a short-acting antimuscarinic bronchodilator, can also be prescribed concurrently with a long-acting antimuscarinic bronchodilator (e.g. **tiotropium**, p.128), which subsequently may be required (see Bronchodilators, Box B, p.124). For persistent symptoms, compared with the regular use of ipratropium, **tiotropium** is safer and more effective across a range of outcomes.[3]

In acute exacerbations of COPD when there is insufficient relief with an inhaled short-acting β_2 agonist, a short-acting antimuscarinic bronchodilator is often added, despite limited evidence to support this (also see Bronchodilators, Box C, p.125).[4]

In severe or life-threatening asthma attacks, nebulized ipratropium bromide is used (see Bronchodilators, Table 1, p.122).[5] However, in chronic asthma, the use of antimuscarinic bronchodilators are not recommended.[5]

Bio-availability most of the 10–30% of the inhaled dose which reaches the lower airways is absorbed.
Onset of action 3–30min asthma; 15min COPD.
Peak response 1.5–3h asthma; 1–2h COPD.
Plasma halflife 2.3–3.8h.
Duration of action 4–8h.

Cautions

Narrow-angle glaucoma (see below), bladder neck obstruction, prostatic hypertrophy.

Undesirable effects

A small increase in cardiovascular events (e.g. myocardial infarction, heart failure, cardiac arrhythmia, stroke) has been reported in patients with COPD using ipratropium regularly and requires further investigation.[6]

Common (<10%, >1%): headache, dizziness, dry mouth, oropharyngeal irritation, cough, bronchoconstriction, vomiting, GI motility changes.
Uncommon (<1%, >0.1%): visual accommodation changes, tachycardia.
Rare (<0.1%, >0.01%): cardiac arrhythmia, e.g. atrial fibrillation, laryngospasm, nausea, urinary retention.

Nebulized drug droplets may reach the eye, and there have been uncommon reports of precipitation of narrow-angle glaucoma and rare reports of eye pain, mydriasis and increased intra-ocular pressure.

Dose and use

In most patients, administration t.d.s. is sufficient.

Pressurized metered-dose inhaler

- give 20–40microgram (1–2 puffs) p.r.n. up to t.d.s.–q.d.s.

Nebulizer solution

- use with a mouthpiece to minimize any nebulized drug entering the eye
- give 250–500microgram p.r.n. up to t.d.s.–q.d.s in COPD; generally given q.d.s. in an exacerbation of COPD
- give 500microgram q4–6h in acute exacerbation of asthma (see Bronchodilators, Table 1, p.122).[5]

Also see Nebulized drugs, p.904.

Supply

Ipratropium bromide (generic)
Pressurized metered-dose inhaler 20microgram/puff, 28 days @ 40microgram (2 puffs) t.d.s. = £5.50.
Nebulizer solution (single-dose units) 250microgram/mL, 20 x 1mL (250microgram) = £4.50, 20 x 2mL (500microgram) = £3.25; *may be diluted with sterile sodium chloride 0.9%.*

With **salbutamol** (generic)
Nebulizer solution (single-dose units) ipratropium bromide 500microgram, **salbutamol** 2.5mg/2.5mL, 60 x 2.5mL = £24.

1 Gross NJ *et al.* (1989) Cholinergic bronchomotor tone in COPD. Estimates of its amount in comparison with that in normal subjects. *Chest.* **96**: 984–987.
2 NICE (2018) Chronic obstructive pulmonary disease in over 16s: diagnosis and management. *Clinical Guideline.* NG115. Updated July 2019. www.nice.org.uk
3 Cheyne L *et al.* (2016) Tiotropium versus ipratropium bromide for chronic obstructive pulmonary disease. *Cochrane Database of Systematic Reviews.* **9**: CD009552. www.thecochranelibrary.com
4 McCrory D and Brown CD (2008) Anticholinergic bronchodilators versus beta2-sympathomimetic agents for acute exacerbations of chronic obstructive pulmonary disease. *Cochrane Database of Systematic Reviews.* **4**: CD003900. www.thecochranelibrary.com
5 BTS/SIGN (2019) British guideline on the management of asthma. A National Clinical Guideline. Revised edition July 2019. *British Thoracic Society and Scottish Intercollegiate Guidelines Network.* Available from: www.brit-thoracic.org.uk
6 NHLBI/WHO (2019) Global initiative for chronic obstructive lung disease. Global strategy for the diagnosis, management and prevention of chronic obstructive pulmonary disease. www.goldcopd.com

Updated November 2019

TIOTROPIUM

Class: Quaternary ammonium antimuscarinic bronchodilator.

Indications: Maintenance treatment of airways obstruction in COPD; add-on therapy in severe chronic asthma (specialist use only; Spiriva® Respimat®).

Contra-indications: Hypersensitivity to **atropine** or its derivatives, including **ipratropium**; lactose intolerance (dry powder formulation).

Pharmacology

Tiotropium bromide is structurally related to **ipratropium bromide** but is longer acting and thus has the convenience of once daily administration.[1-3] Its main effect is to inhibit muscarinic M_3-receptors in airway smooth muscle and mucous glands, and M_1-receptors in parasympathetic ganglia. Because it is a quaternary compound, relatively little tiotropium is absorbed into the systemic circulation. However, a small amount of tiotropium is excreted renally unchanged and, theoretically, accumulation could occur in patients with moderate–severe renal impairment.

In patients with COPD, tiotropium is safer and more effective than the use of regular **ipratropium** in improving lung function, relieving breathlessness, reducing exacerbations and exacerbation-related hospitalizations, and improving quality of life.[4,5] Compared with **salmeterol**, tiotropium has similar efficacy but appears better tolerated.[6]

Tiotropium can be introduced in combination with a LABA in patients with breathlessness or experiencing exacerbations, when there are no features suggesting the likelihood of a response to a corticosteroid (see Bronchodilators, Box B, p.124).[7] The combination of tiotropium and a LABA leads to a small improvement in quality of life and spirometry, compared with either drug given alone.[8]

Alternative antimuscarinic bronchodilators authorized for maintenance treatment in COPD are **aclidinium**, **glycopyrronium** (p.12), **umeclidinium**.

In patients with asthma, tiotropium should *not* be used for an acute attack. Compared with a short-acting β_2 agonist, e.g. **salbutamol**, tiotropium-induced bronchodilation is relatively slow onset (≤30 vs. 5min).[9] Further, **ipratropium** should *not* be used as rescue medication in patients on regular tiotropium, because the muscarinic receptors will already be occupied.[10] In chronic asthma, the use of tiotropium should be on the advice of specialist asthma services.[11]

Bio-availability 20% dry powder inhalation, 33% solution for inhalation (soft mist inhaler).
Onset of action ≤30min.
Peak response 1–3h.
Plasma halflife 5–6 days.
Duration of action >24h.

Cautions

Powder or solution accidentally sprayed into the eye may precipitate narrow-angle glaucoma in susceptible patients; cardiac arrhythmia, bladder neck obstruction, prostatic hypertrophy, moderate–severe renal impairment (creatinine clearance ≤50mL/min).

Undesirable effects

Common (<10%, >1%): dry mouth (generally mild and improves with continued use).
Uncommon (<1%, >0.1%): dizziness, headache, cardiac arrhythmia (e.g. atrial fibrillation, tachycardia), epistaxis, oral candidosis, pharyngitis, cough, dysphagia, dysphonia, constipation, dysuria, urinary retention, pruritus, rash.
Rare (<0.1%, >0.01%): blurred vision, increased intra-ocular pressure, glaucoma, oropharyngeal irritation, bronchoconstriction, gastro-oesophageal reflux, dry skin.

Dose and use

Increased mortality from cardiovascular disease and from all causes has been reported with use of the Spiriva® Respimat® pressurized metered-dose inhaler (pMDI).[12] Data are mixed, with no excess deaths seen in a large study comparing the pMDI and dry powder inhalers.[13] However, because those with unstable cardiovascular disease (defined as myocardial infarction within 6 months, hospitalized for Class III or IV heart failure, or had unstable or life-threatening arrhythmia requiring new treatment within 12 months) or moderate–severe renal impairment were excluded, tiotropium is best avoided in these groups.

For maintenance treatment of COPD in combination with a LABA in patients with breathlessness or experiencing exacerbations, when there are no features suggesting the likelihood of a response to a corticosteroid (see Bronchodilators, Box B, p.124):

Dry powder inhaler

- give 1 capsule once daily via the dedicated inhalation device.

Note. In the UK there are two different brands of dry powder capsules, both delivering 10microgram, but differences in labelling may cause confusion (see Supply).

Pressurized metered-dose inhaler

- give 5microgram (2 puffs) once daily via the Spiriva® Respimat® inhalation device.

Supply

Spiriva® (Boehringer Ingelheim)

Dry powder inhaler capsules for use with the HandiHaler® device, 28 days @ 1 capsule (delivering 10microgram/inhalation) once daily = £35; *contains lactose. Note. Labelled as 18microgram capsules.*

Pressurized metered-dose inhaler (Spiriva® Respimat®) 2.5microgram/puff, 28 days @ 5microgram once daily = £23.

Braltus® (Teva)

Dry powder inhaler capsules for use with the Zonda® device, 28 days @ 1 capsule (delivering 10microgram/inhalation) once daily = £25; *contains lactose.*

1 Barnes PJ (2000) The pharmacological properties of tiotropium. *Chest.* **117 (suppl)**: 63s–66s.
2 Hvizdos KM and Goa KL (2002) Tiotropium bromide. *Drugs.* **62**: 1195–1203; discussion 1204–1195.
3 Gross NJ (2004) Tiotropium bromide. *Chest.* **126**: 1946–1953.
4 Cheyne L *et al.* (2016) Tiotropium versus ipratropium bromide for chronic obstructive pulmonary disease. *Cochrane Database of Systematic Reviews.* **9**: CD009552. www.thecochranelibrary.com
5 Barr RG *et al.* (2006) Tiotropium for stable chronic obstructive pulmonary disease: A meta-analysis. *Thorax.* **61**: 854–862.
6 Chong J *et al.* (2012) Tiotropium versus long-acting beta-agonists for stable chronic obstructive pulmonary disease. *Cochrane Database of Systematic Reviews.* **9**: CD009157. www.thecochranelibrary.com
7 NICE (2018) Chronic obstructive pulmonary disease in over 16s: diagnosis and management. *Clinical Guideline.* NG115. Updated July 2019. www.nice.org.uk
8 Farne HA and Cates CJ (2015) Long-acting beta2-agonist in addition to tiotropium versus either tiotropium or long-acting beta2-agonist alone for chronic obstructive pulmonary disease. *Cochrane Database of Systematic Reviews.* **10**: CD008989. www.thecochranelibrary.com
9 Calverley PMA (2000) The timing and dose pattern of bronchodilation with tiotropium in stable COPD [abstract P523]. *European Respiratory Journal.* **16 (suppl 31)**: 56s.
10 Sutherland ER and Cherniack RM (2004) Management of chronic obstructive pulmonary disease. *New England Journal of Medicine.* **350**: 2689–2697.
11 BTS/SIGN (2019) British guideline on the management of asthma. A National Clinical Guideline. Revised edition July 2019. *British Thoracic Society and Scottish Intercollegiate Guidelines Network.* Available from: www.brit-thoracic.org.uk
12 Jenkins CR and Beasley R (2013) Tiotropium Respimat increases the risk of mortality. *Thorax.* **68**: 5-7.
13 Wise RA *et al.* (2013) Tiotropium Respimat inhaler and the risk of death in COPD. *New England Journal of Medicine.* **369**: 1491-1501.

Updated November 2019

SALBUTAMOL

Class: β_2-Adrenergic receptor agonist (β_2 agonist, sympathomimetic).

Indications: Asthma and other conditions associated with reversible airways obstruction.

Contra-indications: Lactose intolerance (dry powder formulation).

Pharmacology

Short-acting β_2 agonists (salbutamol, **terbutaline**) have an important role in the management of chronic asthma and COPD and acute exacerbations of both (see Bronchodilators, p.121).[1,2] At low doses, they have predominantly a β_2 agonist bronchodilator effect and no major impact on the heart. However, with increasing dose, tachycardia can occur and rarely prolongation of the QT interval, which may predispose to *torsade de pointes*, a ventricular tachyarrhythmia (see Chapter 20, p.797).

In chronic asthma, short-acting β_2 agonists should be used only p.r.n.[1] They are not recommended for regular use, because little benefit has been shown in RCTs. Further, regular use has also been associated with poorer asthma control.[3] Thus, p.r.n. use ≥3 times a week is one indication for the need for prophylactic therapy with an inhaled corticosteroid (see Bronchodilators, Box A, p.123).[1]

In chronic COPD, for breathlessness and exercise limitation, either a short-acting β_2 agonist or a short-acting antimuscarinic bronchodilator can be used p.r.n. If symptoms persist, a regular long-acting bronchodilator is recommended (see Bronchodilators, Box B, p.124).[2] Thus, for p.r.n. symptom relief, a short-acting β_2 agonist is generally preferred; it has a more rapid onset of action and, unlike a short-acting antimuscarinic bronchodilator, can also be prescribed concurrently with a long-acting antimuscarinic bronchodilator (see **Tiotropium**, p.128).

Plasma potassium concentration should be monitored in severe asthma because β_2 agonists, particularly in combination with **theophylline** and inhaled corticosteroids, can cause *hypokalaemia*, which further increases the QT interval and risk of arrhythmia.

For details of the use of salbutamol in the treatment of *hyperkalaemia*, see **Potassium**, p.635.

Bio-availability 10–20% of the dose reaches the lower airways.
Onset of action 5min inhaled; 3–5min nebulized.
Peak response 0.5–2h inhaled; 1.2h nebulized.
Plasma halflife 4–6h inhaled and nebulized.
Duration of action 4–6h inhaled and nebulized.

Cautions

Hyperthyroidism, myocardial insufficiency, cardiac arrhythmia, susceptibility to QT prolongation, hypertension, diabetes mellitus (risk of ketoacidosis if given by CIVI).

Drug interactions

Serious drug interaction: increased risk of hypokalaemia with corticosteroids, diuretics, **theophylline.**[4]

Undesirable effects

Common (<10%, >1%): tremor, headaches, tachycardia.
Uncommon (<1%, >0.1%): mouth and throat irritation from dry powder inhalation.

Dose and use

Also see Nebulized drugs, p.904.

Asthma

In moderate–severe asthma attacks, β_2 agonists can be given by pressurized metered-dose inhaler (pMDI) + spacer or nebulizer and repeated until symptoms improve. In life-threatening asthma, they should be nebulized and combined with **ipratropium** (see Bronchodilators, Table 1, p.122).

Pressurized metered-dose inhaler or dry powder inhaler

Chronic asthma:

- give 100–200microgram p.r.n. up to q.d.s.
- give 200microgram before exercise in exercise-induced bronchoconstriction.

Acute asthma (see Bronchodilators, Table 1, p.122):

- give 100microgram via a spacer; repeat every minute up to a maximum of 1mg (10 puffs).[1]

Note. pMDIs deliver 100microgram/puff; dry powder inhalers deliver 100microgram or 200microgram/inhalation.

Nebulizer solution

Chronic asthma:

- give 2.5–5mg p.r.n. up to q.d.s. in patients for whom inhalers are unsuitable.

Acute asthma (see Bronchodilators, Table 1, p.122):

- give 5mg up to every 15–30min via an oxygen-driven nebulizer
- give 5–10mg/h by continuous nebulization (requires specific nebulizer).[1]

COPD

In acute exacerbations of COPD, bronchodilator use should be optimized (see Bronchodilators, Box B, p.124); both nebulizers and inhalers can be used to administer inhaled therapy during exacerbations (see Bronchodilators, Box B, p.124 and Box C, p.125).

In stable COPD, patients with distressing or disabling breathlessness despite maximal bronchodilator therapy using inhalers should be considered for nebulizer therapy (also see Delivery devices, p.126).[2]

Pressurized metered-dose inhaler or dry powder inhaler

- give 100–200microgram p.r.n. up to q.d.s.

Note. pMDIs deliver 100microgram/puff; dry powder inhalers deliver 100microgram or 200microgram/inhalation.

Nebulizer solution

- give 2.5–5mg p.r.n. up to q.d.s. via an oxygen-driven nebulizer unless the patient is hypercapnic or acidotic, when compressed air should be used. If oxygen therapy is required by such patients, administer simultaneously by nasal cannulae.

Supply

Salbutamol (generic)

Pressurized metered-dose inhaler 100microgram/puff, 28 days @ 200microgram p.r.n. up to q.d.s. = £1.50.

Nebulizer solution (single-dose units) 1mg/mL, 20 × 2.5mL (2.5mg) = £2.50; 2mg/mL, 20 × 2.5mL (5mg) = £4; *may be diluted with sterile sodium chloride 0.9%.*

Airomir® Autohaler® (Teva)

Breath-actuated metered-dose inhaler, 100microgram/puff, 28 days @ 200microgram p.r.n. up to q.d.s. = £6.

Easyhaler Salbutamol® (Orion)

Dry powder inhaler 100microgram/inhalation, 200microgram/inhalation, 28 days @ 200microgram p.r.n. up to q.d.s. = £3.50; *contains lactose.*

Ventolin® (GlaxoSmithKline UK)

Dry powder inhaler blisters for use with Accuhaler® device, 200microgram/blister, 28 days @ 200microgram p.r.n. up to q.d.s. = £7.

Nebulizer solution (multiple-dose bottle for use with a nebulizer or ventilator) 5mg/mL, 20mL = £2.25; *may be diluted with sterile sodium chloride 0.9%.*

With **ipratropium bromide**, see p.127.

For spacer devices, see p.126.

Note. See *BNF* for oral and parenteral formulations.

1 BTS/SIGN (2019) British guideline on the management of asthma. A National Clinical Guideline. Revised edition July 2019. *British Thoracic Society and Scottish Intercollegiate Guidelines Network.* Available from: www.brit-thoracic.org.uk

2 NICE (2018) Chronic obstructive pulmonary disease in over 16s: diagnosis and management. *Clinical Guideline.* NG115. Updated July 2019. www.nice.org.uk

3 Sears M (2000) Short-acting inhaled B-agonists: to be taken regularly or as needed? *Lancet.* **355**: 1658–1659.

4 Baxter K and Preston CL *Stockley's Drug Interactions.* London: Pharmaceutical Press. www.medicinescomplete.com (accessed December 2017).

Updated November 2019

INHALED LONG-ACTING β_2 AGONISTS (LABAS)

Class: β_2-Adrenergic receptor agonist (β_2 agonist, sympathomimetic).

Indications: Add-on therapy in asthma (including nocturnal asthma and exercise-induced symptoms) for those treated with inhaled corticosteroids (see Bronchodilators, Box A, p.123). Reversible airways obstruction in COPD in patients requiring long-term regular bronchodilator therapy (see Bronchodilators, Box B, p.124).

Contra-indications: Salmeterol should not be used for the relief of acute asthma, because of its slow onset of action.

Pharmacology

The selective LABAs **salmeterol** and **formoterol** have a bronchodilating effect which lasts for 12h. **Indacaterol**, authorized only for COPD, has a duration of action of 24h but is less well established than other LABAs. **Salmeterol** has a relatively slow onset of action; **formoterol** has an onset of action similar to **salbutamol**, and can be used *in addition to maintenance treatment* as a p.r.n. reliever inhaler in certain circumstances (see Dose and use).

In patients with asthma, inhaled LABAs are added when symptoms are inadequately relieved by a regular *low-dose* inhaled corticosteroid (see Bronchodilators, Box A, p.123).[1] The addition of inhaled LABAs to inhaled corticosteroids improves lung function and symptoms, and decreases asthma attacks more effectively than increasing the dose of inhaled corticosteroids alone.[1]

However, safety concerns have been identified when LABAs have been used *without* an inhaled corticosteroid, i.e. increased life-threatening and fatal exacerbations of asthma. *Thus, in patients with asthma, inhaled LABAs should not be used without inhaled corticosteroids* (see Cautions).[1]

Combined LABA + corticosteroid inhalers are recommended in asthma guidelines.[1] Although there is no difference in efficacy compared with separate inhalers, combination inhalers ensure that inhaled LABAs are not used without a corticosteroid, and may aid patient adherence.[1]

In patients with COPD, a LABA is introduced when symptoms are unrelieved by the use of a p.r.n. short-acting bronchodilator. It is used in combination either with an inhaled corticosteroid *or* with a long-acting muscarinic bronchodilator, depending on whether features suggesting the likelihood of benefit from an inhaled corticosteroid are present or absent (see Bronchodilators, Box B, p.124).[2]

Inhaled LABAs and long-acting antimuscarinic bronchodilators, e.g. **tiotropium** (p.128), have similar efficacy in terms of improving lung function, relieving breathlessness, reducing exacerbations and hospitalizations, and improving quality of life. Compared with **salmeterol**, **tiotropium** appears better tolerated.[2,3] The combination of **tiotropium** and a LABA leads to a small improvement in quality of life and spirometry compared with either drug given alone.[4] For pharmacokinetic details, see Table 1.

Table 1 Pharmacokinetics of inhaled LABAs

	Formoterol	*Salmeterol*
Bio-availability	30–50% of the delivered dose reaches the lungs (Turbohaler®)	Approximately 10% of the delivered dose reaches the lungs (aerosol)[5]
Onset of action	1–3min	10–20min
Peak response	5–10min	≤30min[5]
Plasma halflife	≤8h	≤8h (plasma concentration low or undetectable after therapeutic doses)[5]
Duration of action	About 12h	12–16h[5]

Cautions

In asthma, inhaled LABAs should *not* be used without inhaled corticosteroids, because of concern over an increase in life-threatening and fatal exacerbations. To ensure safe use, the MHRA/CHM advise that in chronic asthma LABAs should:[6]

- be added only if regular use of standard-dose inhaled corticosteroids has failed to control asthma adequately
- not be initiated in patients with rapidly deteriorating asthma
- be introduced at a low dose, titrated (up or down) appropriately, and be discontinued in the absence of benefit

Further, the use of a combination LABA + corticosteroid inhaler will aid adherence.

Hyperthyroidism, cardiovascular disease, arrhythmias, susceptibility to QT prolongation or concurrent use of drugs that prolong the QT interval (see Chapter 20, p.797), hypertension, paradoxical bronchoconstriction (discontinue and use alternative treatment), severe liver cirrhosis (**formoterol**), diabetes mellitus (may cause hyperglycaemia; monitor blood glucose).

Drug interactions

Serious drug interaction: increased risk of hypokalaemia with corticosteroids, diuretics, **theophylline**.

Undesirable effects

Common (<10%, >1%): headache, tremor, palpitations, muscle cramps.
Uncommon (<1%, >0.1%): tachycardia.
Rare (<0.1%) or very rare (<0.01%): arrhythmias, e.g. atrial fibrillation, supraventricular tachycardia, QT interval prolongation, paradoxical bronchoconstriction.

Dose and use

The dose varies for **formoterol** and **salmeterol** with formulation and indication (Table 2).

Asthma

An inhaled LABA should be added *only* if p.r.n. treatment with a short-acting β_2 agonist *and* regular prophylactic therapy with an inhaled corticosteroid is insufficient to control symptoms (see Bronchodilators, Box A, p.123). Use of a combination inhaler will help ensure the concurrent use of a LABA + a corticosteroid (Table 3 and Table 4).

Because **formoterol** has a fast onset of action, extra doses can be used on a p.r.n. basis to relieve bronchospasm instead of a short-acting β_2 agonist (see Tables 2 and 3 for authorized products). This approach is generally limited to those patients requiring initial (i.e. LABA + low-dose inhaled corticosteroid) or additional add-on therapies (see Bronchodilators, Box A, p.123).[1]

COPD

An inhaled LABA is used when exacerbations or persistent symptoms occur despite short-acting bronchodilators p.r.n. (Table 2), either in combination with inhaled corticosteroid (Table 3 and Table 4) or with a long-acting antimuscarinic bronchodilator (also see Bronchodilators, Box B, p.124).

Because **formoterol** has a fast onset of action, extra doses can be used on a p.r.n. basis *in addition to regular maintenance LABA* to relieve bronchospasm, instead of a short-acting β_2 agonist (see Table 2 for authorized products).

Supply

See Table 2, Table 3 and Table 4.

1 BTS/SIGN (2019) British guideline on the management of asthma. A National Clinical Guideline. Revised edition July 2019. *British Thoracic Society and Scottish Intercollegiate Guidelines Network*. Available from: www.brit-thoracic.org.uk
2 NICE (2018) Chronic obstructive pulmonary disease in over 16s: diagnosis and management. *Clinical Guideline*. NG115. Updated July 2019. www.nice.org.uk
3 Chong J *et al.* (2012) Tiotropium versus long-acting beta-agonists for stable chronic obstructive pulmonary disease. *Cochrane Database of Systematic Reviews*. **9**: CD009157. www.thecochranelibrary.com
4 Farne HA and Cates CJ (2015) Long-acting beta2-agonist in addition to tiotropium versus either tiotropium or long-acting beta2-agonist alone for chronic obstructive pulmonary disease. *Cochrane Database of Systematic Reviews*. **10**: CD008989. www.thecochranelibrary.com
5 Cazzola M *et al.* (2002) Clinical pharmacokinetics of salmeterol. *Clinical Pharmacokinetics*. **41**: 19–30.
6 MHRA (2014) Guidance: Asthma. Long-acting β2 agonists: use and safety. Available from: www.gov.uk/government/publications

Updated (minor change) August 2020

Table 2 Adult doses (as puffs) of LABA

Formulation	*Formoterol or Foradil® (DPI)*	*Atimos Modulite® (pMDI)*	*Oxis® Turbohaler® (DPI)*		*Salmeterol or Serevent® Evohaler® (pMDI)*	*Serevent® Accuhaler® (DPI)*
LABA	Formoterol	Formoterol	Formoterol	Formoterol	Salmeterol	Salmeterol
Labelled strength (microgram)	12	12	6	12	25	50
Asthma[a]						
Starting dose	1 b.d.	1 b.d.	1–2 daily–b.d.	1 daily–b.d.	2 b.d.	1 b.d.
Maximum dose	2 b.d.	2 b.d.	4 b.d.[b]	2 b.d.[b]	4 b.d.	2 b.d.
Reliever dose	n/a	n/a	1–2 p.r.n.	1 p.r.n.	n/a	n/a
COPD						
Starting dose	1 b.d.	1 b.d.[c]	2 daily–b.d.	1 daily–b.d.	2 b.d.	1 b.d.
Maximum dose	1 b.d.	1 b.d.[c]	2 b.d.[c]	1 b.d.[c]	2 b.d.	1 b.d.
Cost per 60 puffs	£12, £28	£18	£25	£25	£15	£35

DPI = dry powder inhaler; pMDI = pressurized metered-dose inhaler; n/a = not authorized

a. LABA must only be used in patients receiving an inhaled corticosteroid (see Cautions)

b. occasionally higher doses are used; seek specialist advice

c. additional doses above those prescribed for regular therapy may be used for relief of symptoms, see SPC for details.

3

Table 3 Adult doses (as puffs) of formoterol and corticosteroid combination inhalers (examples only; see *BNF* for all available products)

Brand	*Fostair®,[a] or Fostair® NEXThaler®,[a]*	*Fostair®,[a] or Fostair® NEXThaler®,[a]*	*Symbicort®*	*Symbicort® Turbohaler®*	*Symbicort® Turbohaler®*	*Flutiform®*
Formulation	pMDI or DPI	pMDI or DPI	pMDI	DPI	DPI	pMDI[c]
Corticosteroid	Beclometasone	Beclometasone	Budesonide	Budesonide	Budesonide	Fluticasone
LABA	Formoterol	Formoterol	Formoterol	Formoterol	Formoterol	Formoterol
Labelled strengths[b]	100/6	200/6	200/6	100/6, 200/6	400/12	50/5, 125/5, 250/10
Asthma maintenance						
Starting dose	1–2 b.d.	2 b.d.	n/a	1–2 b.d.	1 b.d.	2 b.d.
Maximum dose	2 b.d.	2 b.d.	n/a	4 b.d.	2 b.d.	2 b.d.
Asthma maintenance and reliever therapy						
Maintenance dose	1 b.d.	n/a	n/a	1 b.d. (or 2 daily)[d]	n/a	n/a
Reliever dose	1 p.r.n.	n/a	n/a	1 p.r.n. (maximum of 6 per episode)	n/a	n/a
Maximum reliever doses/24h	8	n/a	n/a	8[e]	n/a	n/a
COPD with features suggestive of the likelihood of a response to a corticosteroid						
Starting dose	2 b.d.	n/a	2 b.d.	2 b.d.[d]	1 b.d.	n/a
Maximum dose	2 b.d.	n/a	2 b.d.	2 b.d.[d]	1 b.d.	n/a
Cost per 60 puffs	£15, £15	£15, £15	£14	£14, £14	£28	£7, £14, £23

DPI = dry powder inhaler; pMDI = pressurized metered-dose inhaler; n/a = not authorized

a. contain extra-fine particles improving delivery and thereby about doubling the relative potency of the corticosteroid component (see Inhaled corticosteroids, p.140)

b. inhaled corticosteroid/LABA dose in microgram/metered inhalation

c. breath-actuated inhalers available for some strengths

d. Symbicort® Turbohaler® 200/6 only; for asthma maintenance and reliever use maximum dose 2 puffs b.d.

e. up to 12 puffs/24h for a limited time.

Table 4 Adult doses (as puffs) of salmeterol and corticosteroid combination inhalers (examples only; see *BNF* for all available products)

Brand	*Seretide® Evohaler®*	*Seretide® Accuhaler®*
Formulation	pMDI	DPI
Corticosteroid	Fluticasone	Fluticasone
LABA	Salmeterol	Salmeterol
Labelled strengths[a]	50/25, 125/25, 250/25	100/50, 250/50, 500/50
Asthma maintenance		
Starting dose	2 b.d.	1 b.d.
Maximum dose	2 b.d.	1 b.d.
COPD with features suggestive of the likelihood of a response to a corticosteroid		
Starting dose	n/a	1 b.d.
Maximum dose	n/a	1 b.d.
Cost per 60 puffs	£9, £12, £15	£18, £34, £33

DPI = dry powder inhaler; pMDI = pressurized metered-dose inhaler; n/a = not authorized

a. inhaled corticosteroid/LABA dose in microgram/metered inhalation.

THEOPHYLLINE

Class: Methylxanthine.

Indications: Reversible airways obstruction; given by injection as **aminophylline** for severe or life-threatening asthma attacks (see below).

Contra-indications: Uncontrolled arrhythmias, seizure disorders.

Pharmacology

Because of its inferior safety and efficacy compared with other alternatives, the use of theophylline in patients with asthma should be on the advice of specialist asthma services; in patients with COPD, it should be considered only after a trial of a LABA or in those unable to use inhaled therapy (see Bronchodilators, Box A, p.123 and Box B, p.124).[1,2]

Theophylline is given by injection as **aminophylline**, a mixture containing ethylenediamine to increase the solubility of theophylline. **Aminophylline** must be given by slow IV injection over 20–30min and/or CIVI (see Dose and use); it is too irritant for IM use and is a potent gastric irritant PO. **Aminophylline** should be used only with guidance from senior/experienced staff. It is generally reserved for use in severe or life-threatening asthma attacks or an exacerbation of COPD that does not respond to initial therapy (see Bronchodilators, Table 1, p.122 and Box C, p.125).[1,2]

Theophylline shares the actions of the other xanthine alkaloids (e.g. caffeine) on the CNS, myocardium, kidney and smooth muscle. It has a relatively weak CNS effect but a more powerful relaxant effect on bronchial smooth muscle. This is mainly by inhibiting phosphodiesterase 3 (PDE3). This leads to an accumulation of cyclic AMP, which, through various mechanisms (e.g. reduced intracellular calcium), leads to smooth muscle relaxation.

An anti-inflammatory effect in the airways through inhibition of PDE4 and activation of histone deacetylase-2 has been shown at plasma concentrations as low as 5mg/L.[3] Thus, there is interest in the use of low-dose theophylline alongside inhaled corticosteroids in patients with asthma and COPD, particularly as reduced histone deacetylase-2 activity is associated with corticosteroid resistance and reduced benefit.[3,4] However, in patients with COPD receiving LABA + an inhaled corticosteroid, the addition of low-dose theophylline in an RCT did not increase histone deacetylase-2 levels or reduce the number of exacerbations.[5]

Numerous other effects of theophylline have been described, but their benefit in relation to asthma or COPD is unclear. Some patients require plasma concentrations at the higher end of, or exceeding, the usual therapeutic range.[6] Theophylline is an adenosine receptor antagonist. Plasma adenosine levels are increased in situations where intra-abdominal pressure is pathologically increased, e.g. as a result of bowel obstruction, pancreatitis and peritonitis, resulting in tissue hypoxia. Early work suggests that infusions of theophylline reduce mortality in this situation, possibly by preventing the deleterious effect of adenosine on renal perfusion.[7] This may also explain why theophylline reduces the incidence of radiological contrast-induced acute kidney injury.[8] Conversely, an adenosine antagonist effect may account for some of the more serious undesirable effects of theophylline, e.g. cardiac arrhythmia, seizure.

Although theophylline inhibits proliferation and augments apoptosis of cancer cells, the clinical relevance of this remains to be determined.[9] An anti-inflammatory effect may also explain the benefit seen in an animal model of cancer cachexia.[10]

Theophylline is metabolized by the liver. Its therapeutic index is narrow, and some patients experience toxic effects even in the therapeutic range. Plasma concentrations of theophylline are influenced by infection, hypoxia, smoking, various drugs (see below), hepatic impairment, thyroid disorders and heart failure; all these can make the use of theophylline difficult. Steady-state theophylline levels are attained within 3–4 days of adjusting the dose of an m/r preparation. Blood for theophylline levels should be taken 4–6h after the last dose.

Bio-availability ≥90%; 80% m/r.

Onset of action 40–60min PO; immunomodulation ≤3 weeks.

Plasma halflife 6–12h, but wide interindividual variation.

Duration of action 12h m/r theophylline PO; immunomodulation several days.

Cautions

Elderly, cardiac disease, hypertension, hyperthyroidism and hypothyroidism, peptic ulcer, hepatic impairment, pyrexia.

Drug interactions

Theophylline may potentiate hypokalaemia associated with β_2 agonists, corticosteroids, diuretics and hypoxia.[11,12]

Theophylline is metabolized mainly by CYP1A2, and to some extent by CYP3A4 and CYP2E1. Caution is required with concurrent use of drugs that inhibit or induce these enzymes (see Chapter 19, Table 8, p.790). Reports of interactions where closer monitoring ± dose adjustment are required are listed in Box A.

Theophylline can reduce the plasma levels of **lithium** by 20–30%.

Box A Interactions between theophylline and other drugs involving CYP450[12]

Plasma concentrations of theophylline

Increased by	**Decreased by**
Aciclovir	Smoking
Allopurinol	Heavy alcohol intake
Cimetidine	Carbamazepine
Clarithromycin	Isoprenaline
Diltiazem	Phenobarbital and other barbiturates
Erythromycin	Phenytoin
Fluconazole	Rifampicin
Fluvoxamine[a]	Ritonavir
Mexiletine[b]	St John's wort
Oral contraceptives	Sulfinpyrazone
Quinolone antibacterials (ciprofloxacin, but not ofloxacin)	
Troleandomycin[b] (not UK)	
Verapamil	

a. avoid concurrent use; if unavoidable, reduce the dose of theophylline by 50% and monitor closely

b. reduce the dose of theophylline by 50%.

Undesirable effects

Common (<10%, >1%): headache, dyspepsia, nausea, vomiting; risk of seizures and arrhythmias increases as plasma levels increase; hyperpnoea (fast breathing) when given IV.

Dose and use

Because it is not possible to ensure bio-equivalence between different m/r theophylline products, they should be prescribed by brand name and not interchanged.

An m/r formulation should be used.[1] An unauthorized immediate-release oral liquid is available for patients who may require it, e.g. those with swallowing difficulties or being fed by enteral feeding tube; however, it is expensive (see Chapter 28, Table 2, p.863). For m/r products:

- starting dose varies between brands; see individual SPCs
- maintain on a single brand, because absorption rates vary between products
- titrate dose according to response and plasma theophylline level
- in patients whose symptoms manifest diurnal fluctuation, a larger evening or morning dose is appropriate to ensure maximum therapeutic benefit when symptoms are most severe
- begin monitoring 5 days after starting PO treatment and recheck levels at least 3 days after any dose adjustment; the sample for drug plasma concentration monitoring should be taken 4–6h after a PO dose of theophylline m/r
- for bronchodilation, the recommended therapeutic range is 10–20mg/L (55–110micromol/L).

However, some patients may experience unacceptable undesirable effects even within the recommended therapeutic range, and for them a lower range may suffice, e.g. 5–15mg/L (28–83micromol/L). This is also considered an appropriate range for the anti-inflammatory effects of theophylline.[3] Ultimately, the clinical response, rather than the plasma level, will determine the need for dose adjustment.

Give IV **aminophylline** in severe asthma attack or exacerbation of COPD only with guidance from senior/experienced staff:[1,2]

- loading dose 250–500mg (maximum 5mg/kg) IV over 20–30min; omit if already on regular PO theophylline and check theophylline levels stat
- maintenance dose 500–700microgram/kg/h CIVI (300microgram/kg/h in the elderly); check blood levels 4–6h after starting CIVI and then daily; adjust dose to achieve a level of 10–20mg/L (55–110micromol/L).

If converting a patient from IV **aminophylline** to PO theophylline, multiply the total daily dose of IV **aminophylline** by 0.8 (salt factor) to give the total daily dose of PO theophylline; this should be halved into a practical b.d. m/r dose and plasma levels monitored as above.[13]

Supply

Modified-release

Uniphyllin Continus® (Napp)

Tablets m/r 200mg, 300mg, 400mg, 28 days @ 200mg b.d. = £3.

Immediate-release

Oral solution or suspension 50mg/5mL, 28 days @ 125mg t.d.s. = £441 or £334 respectively (unauthorized products, available as a special order; see Chapter 24, p.817); *price based on specials tariff in community.*

Aminophylline (generic)

Injection 25mg/mL, 10mL amp = £0.75.

1 BTS/SIGN (2019) British guideline on the management of asthma. A National Clinical Guideline. Revised edition July 2019. *British Thoracic Society and Scottish Intercollegiate Guidelines Network.* Available from: www.brit-thoracic.org.uk

2 NICE (2018) Chronic obstructive pulmonary disease in over 16s: diagnosis and management. *Clinical Guideline.* NG115. Updated July 2019. www.nice.org.uk

3 Barnes PJ (2013) Theophylline. *American Journal of Respiratory and Critical Care Medicine.* **188**: 901–906.

4 Ford PA *et al.* (2010) Treatment effects of low-dose theophylline combined with an inhaled corticosteroid in COPD. *Chest.* **137**: 1338–1344.

5 Cosio BG *et al.* (2016) Oral low-dose theophylline on top of inhaled fluticasone-salmeterol does not reduce xxacerbations in patients with severe COPD. *Chest.* **150**: 123–130.

6 Mokry J and Mokra D (2013) Immunological aspects of phosphodiesterase inhibition in the respiratory system. *Respiratory Physiology and Neurobiology*. **187**: 11–17.
7 Bodnar Z *et al.* (2011) Beneficial effects of theophylline infusions in surgical patients with intra-abdominal hypertension. *Langenbecks Archive of Surgery*. **396**: 793–800.
8 Dai B *et al.* (2012) Effect of theophylline on prevention of contrast-induced acute kidney injury: a meta-analysis of randomized controlled trials. *American Journal of Kidney Disease*. **60**: 360–370.
9 Kapoor S (2016) Theophylline and its direct anti-neoplastic effects. *Respiratory Medicine*. **119**: e1.
10 Olivan M *et al.* (2012) Theophylline is able to partially revert cachexia in tumour-bearing rats. *Nutrition and Metabolism*. **9**: 76.
11 Sweetman S (2011) Martindale: the Complete Drug Reference (online edition). www.medicinescomplete.com/mc/martindale/current
12 Baxter K and Preston CL *Stockley's Drug Interactions*. London: Pharmaceutical Press. www.medicinescomplete.com (accessed May 2017).
13 UK Medicines Information (2017) How is an intravenous aminophylline dose converted to an oral aminophylline dose? *Medicines Q&A*. www.evidence.nhs.uk

Updated (minor change) April 2020

INHALED CORTICOSTEROIDS

Indications: Reversible and irreversible airways obstruction, †stridor, †lymphangitis carcinomatosa, †radiation pneumonitis, †cough after insertion of a bronchial stent (see Nebulized drugs, p.904).

Pharmacology

Inhaled corticosteroids reduce airway inflammation. **Fluticasone** is given in a smaller dose because it is twice as potent as **beclometasone** and **budesonide**, which are considered approximately equivalent. However, variations with different formulations can occur. For example, the **beclometasone** formulations Kelhale® and Qvar® deliver a greater fraction of smaller particles to the lung, approximately doubling their potency compared with other **beclometasone** formulations (see Dose and use, Table 2). This is also true for the combined **beclometasone** + **formoterol** formulations in Fostair® and Fostair® NEXThaler®.[1] **Ciclesonide** and **mometasone** are relatively new and less well-established inhaled corticosteroids.

Inhaled corticosteroids reach the systemic circulation via both the pulmonary circulation and the GI tract. Long-term high-dose inhaled corticosteroids have been associated with adrenal suppression, and deaths from Addisonian crisis (acute adrenal failure) have occurred rarely (see Cautions).[2,3] Daily doses of **beclometasone** ≤1,500microgram or equivalent do not generally lead to adrenal suppression.[4] However, there is significant variation among individuals, and formulation and duration of treatment are also important. Accordingly, systemic corticosteroids (p.556) should be considered to cover stressful periods (e.g. infection, surgery) in patients receiving long-term high-dose inhaled corticosteroids, i.e. **beclometasone** >1,000microgram/24h or equivalent (see Cautions).

In patients with asthma, inhaled corticosteroids are the most effective preventer drug, and there is a low threshold for their use (see Bronchodilators, Box A, p.123).[5] Improvement in symptoms generally occurs within 3–7 days, but maximal improvement in symptoms and lung function may take 1–2 months. If a low dose fails to improve symptoms, it is recommended that an inhaled long-acting β_2 agonist (LABA) (p.132), e.g. **salmeterol** or **formoterol**, is added before using higher doses of an inhaled corticosteroid (see Bronchodilators, Box A, p.123).[5] If medium-dose inhaled corticosteroids are subsequently used, they should be continued only if they have clear benefit over the lower dose. An alternative to increasing the dose of inhaled corticosteroid is the addition of a PO leukotriene-receptor antagonist (e.g. **montelukast**, **zafirlukast**), which complements the anti-inflammatory effect of the corticosteroid. The use of high-dose inhaled corticosteroids should be on the advice of specialist asthma services (see Bronchodilators, Box A, p.123).

In patients with COPD, inhaled corticosteroids are recommended in conjunction with an inhaled LABA for patients with exacerbations or persistent breathlessness and features suggestive of the likelihood of a response to a corticosteroid (see Bronchodilators, Box B, p.124).[6] It should be noted that studies in COPD have generally used high-dose inhaled corticosteroids, e.g. **fluticasone** 1,000microgram/24h. Despite this, the overall clinical benefit of inhaled corticosteroids is relatively small.[7] For example, the addition of an inhaled corticosteroid to a LABA reduces the proportion of people experiencing one or more exacerbations from 47% to 42% per annum.[7] Further, inhaled corticosteroids do not modify the long-term decline in FEV_1, nor mortality.[8] This relatively small benefit must be balanced on an individual patient basis against the undesirable effects of using inhaled corticosteroids. If the inhaled corticosteroid is ineffective or poorly tolerated, it can be safely stopped, provided the inhaled LABA is continued.[8]

The only evidence to support the other indications for inhaled or nebulized corticosteroids listed above is clinical experience.

For pharmacokinetic details, see Table 1.

Table 1 Pharmacokinetics of inhaled corticosteroids in asthma

	Beclometasone dipropionate[9-11]	*Budesonide*[a,12]	*Fluticasone propionate*[a,12]
Bio-availability	62%[b] pMDI	39% DPI 6% nebulizer solution	30% pMDI 14% DPI
Onset of action	Days to weeks	Days to weeks	Days to weeks
Time to peak plasma concentration	30–60min[b] pMDI	5–10min DPI 10–30min nebulizer solution	1–2h DPI
Plasma halflife	3h[b] pMDI	2–3h	8h

DPI = dry powder inhaler; pMDI = pressurized metered-dose inhaler

a. data from Micromedex

b. values for beclometasone *17-monopropionate*, the form to which most of the dipropionate is converted before reaching the circulation.

Cautions

Active or quiescent tuberculosis, mycetoma, immunosuppression.

Because of the risk of adrenal suppression, patients receiving the following should be warned not to abruptly stop treatment, and should be given both a steroid *treatment* and a steroid *emergency* card (see Systemic corticosteroids, p.562, Box G, p.563 and Box H, p.563):[3,13]

- long-term (≥4 weeks) high-dose inhaled corticosteroids, i.e. equivalent to:
  - ▷ **beclometasone** >1,000microgram/24h
  - ▷ **fluticasone** >500microgram/24h
- inhaled corticosteroids with drugs that may inhibit their metabolism by CYP3A4, e.g. azole antifungals, protease inhibitors (see below); patients have also become Cushingoid.

See national guidance for full details on dose adjustments required to cover sick days, surgery or invasive treatment.[3]

Drug interactions

Increased systemic exposure can occur when co-administered with strong CYP3A4 inhibitors, e.g. **clarithromycin**, **itraconazole** (see Chapter 19, Table 8, p.790).

Undesirable effects

Oral candidosis, sore throat, hoarse voice, cough, paradoxical bronchospasm, hypersensitivity reactions (e.g. rash), skin bruising. Rarely, psychiatric effects, including psychomotor hyperactivity, sleep disorders, anxiety, depression, aggression.[14]

Inhaled corticosteroids are associated with increased risk of cataract, which is dose and duration related.[15] There is a small increased risk of glaucoma with higher doses (i.e. **beclometasone** >1,600microgram/24h or equivalent).[16] Rarely, central serous chorioretinopathy.[17] Increased risk of onset and worsening of diabetes, particularly in patients receiving the equivalent of **fluticasone** ≥1,000microgram/24h.[18]

Data on the impact of inhaled corticosteroids on bone mineral density and risk of fracture are mixed; a recent meta-analysis found a small statistically significant, but clinically questionable, increase in risk of fracture.[19]

In COPD, inhaled corticosteroids (**budesonide**, **fluticasone**) are associated with a small increase in the frequency of non-fatal pneumonia (6–18 additional hospital admissions per 1,000 patients treated),[20] and it is recommended that patients are informed of this when inhaled corticosteroids are prescribed.[6] Data are mixed, but the risk appears similar for both **budesonide** and **fluticasone**.[20] An increased risk of infection may also exist in patients with asthma taking inhaled corticosteroids.[21] However, any such risk is far outweighed by their overall benefit in asthma.

Dose and use

Patients who are corticosteroid-dependent should be given both a steroid *treatment* and a steroid *emergency* card (see Cautions).

Because of their differing potency and doses (Table 2), inhalers containing **beclometasone** should be prescribed by brand name and not interchanged.[1]

Table 2 Categorization of doses (in microgram/24h) of inhaled corticosteroids in single or combination inhalers[a,5]

	Low-dose	*Medium-dose*	*High-dose*[b]
Pressurized metered-dose inhalers			
Beclometasone			
Clenil Modulite®, Soprobec®	400	800	1,000–2,000
Fostair®, Kelhale®, Qvar® (any)	200	400	800
Ciclesonide			
Alvesco®	160	320	640
Fluticasone propionate			
Flixotide Evohaler®, Flutiform®, Flutiform K-haler®, Seretide Evohaler®, generic combinations with salmeterol	200	500	1,000
Dry powder inhalers			
Beclometasone			
Beclometasone Easyhaler®	400	800	
Fostair NEXThaler®	200	400	800
Budesonide			
Budesonide Easyhaler®, Budelin Novolizer®, DuoResp Spiromax®, Fobumix Easyhaler®, Pulmicort Turbohaler®, Symbicort Turbohaler®	320–400	640–800	1,280–1,600
Fluticasone			
Flixotide Accuhaler®, AirFluSal Forspiro®, Fusacomb Easyhaler®, Seretide Accuhaler®, Stalpex Orbicel®	200	500	1,000
Relvar Ellipta®		92	184
Mometasone			
Asmanex Twisthaler®	400	800	

a. with a LABA (p.132); formoterol: DuoResp Spiromax®, Flutiform® (any), Fobumix® (any), Fostair® (any), Symbicort Turbohaler®; salmeterol: AirFluSal® (any), Combisal®, Fusacomb®, Sereflo®, Seretide® (any), Sirdupla®, Stalpex®; vilanterol: Relvar Ellipta®

b. in patients with asthma, high doses should be used only after referral to secondary care.

Pressurized metered-dose inhaler (pMDI) or dry powder inhaler

pMDIs are most commonly prescribed; alternatives include breath-actuated and dry powder inhalers.

- check the patient's inhaler technique
- use a large-volume spacer device if patient on a pMDI, particularly when they:
  - ▷ have a poor inhaler technique
  - ▷ are using a high dose (Table 2)
  - ▷ develop a hoarse voice, sore throat or oral candidosis
- instruct patient to rinse their mouth out after use to reduce systemic availability and oral candidosis

- in asthma, start with a dose appropriate to severity, e.g. **beclometasone** 100–400microgram b.d. or equivalent (Table 2), and titrate to the lowest dose effective against symptoms (see Bronchodilators, Box A, p.123); b.d. dosing is generally preferred (except for **ciclesonide** which is given once daily);[5] however, if subsequently the asthma is controlled on a low dose, e.g. 200–400microgram/24h, once daily administration could be considered[5]
- in COPD, inhaled corticosteroids, e.g. **fluticasone** 1,000microgram/24h, are used in conjunction with an inhaled LABA in patients with features that suggest a likelihood of a response to a corticosteroid (see Bronchodilators, Box B, p.124).[6]

Nebulizer solution

- **budesonide** 1–2mg b.d.; occasionally more or **fluticasone** 0.5–2mg b.d.
- use a mouthpiece to limit environmental contamination and/or contact with the patient's eyes. However, a mask may be unavoidable in those incapable of using a mouthpiece, e.g. when acutely ill, fatigued or very young.

Supply

Beclometasone (generic)
Dry powder inhaler 200microgram/inhalation, 28 days @ 200microgram b.d. = £4.25; *available as Beclometasone Easyhaler®.*

Clenil Modulite® (Chiesi)
Pressurized metered-dose inhaler 50microgram, 100microgram, 200microgram, 250microgram/puff, 28 days @ 200microgram b.d. = £4.50.

Soprobec® (Glenmark)
Pressurized metered-dose inhaler 50microgram, 100microgram, 200microgram, 250microgram/puff, 28 days @ 200microgram b.d. = £3.50. *Soprobec® is equivalent to Clenil Modulite® in potency.*

Kelhale® (Cipla)
Pressurized metered-dose inhaler 50microgram, 100microgram/puff, 28 days @ 100microgram b.d. = £1.50. *Kelhale® is approximately twice as potent as Clenil Modulite® and Soprobec®.*

Qvar® (Teva)
Pressurized metered-dose inhaler 50microgram, 100microgram/puff, 28 days @ 100microgram b.d. = £4.75; *also available as Qvar® Easi-Breathe®.*
Breath-actuated inhaler Autohaler®, 50microgram, 100microgram/puff, 28 days @ 100microgram b.d. = £4.75; *requires manual dexterity to operate lever and slider to release each dose into the mouthpiece before breath-activation.*
Breath-actuated inhaler Easi-Breathe®, 50microgram, 100microgram/puff, 28 days @ 100microgram b.d. = £4.75.
Qvar® is approximately twice as potent as Clenil Modulite® and Soprobec®.

Budesonide (generic)
Dry powder inhaler 100microgram, 200microgram, 400microgram/inhalation, 28 days @ 200microgram b.d. = £5; *available as Budesonide Easyhaler®.*
Nebulizer solution (single-dose units), 250microgram/mL, 20 x 2mL (500microgram) = £26; 500microgram/mL, 20 x 2mL (1,000microgram) = £39.

Ciclesonide
Alvesco® (AstraZeneca)
Pressurized metered-dose inhaler 80microgram, 160microgram/puff, 28 days @ 160microgram once daily = £9.

Fluticasone
Flixotide® (GlaxoSmithKline)
Pressurized metered-dose inhaler Evohaler®, 50microgram, 125microgram, 250microgram/puff, 28 days @ 100microgram b.d. = £6.
Dry powder inhaler blisters for use with Accuhaler® device, 50microgram, 100microgram, 250microgram, 500microgram/blister, 28 days @ 100microgram b.d. = £7.50.
Nebulizer solution (single-dose units) Nebules®, 250microgram/mL, 10 x 2mL (500microgram) = £9.50; 1mg/mL, 10 x 2mL (2mg) = £37.50.

Mometasone
Asmanex® (Organon)
Dry powder inhaler Twisthaler®, 200microgram, 400microgram/inhalation, 28 days @ 400microgram once daily = £16; *restricted to second-line use only in Scotland on the advice of the Scottish Medicines Consortium.*

For combination products containing inhaled corticosteroids and LABAs, see Inhaled long-acting β_2 agonists (LABAs), p.132.

1 MHRA (2008) Inhaled products that contain corticosteroids. *Drug Safety Update*. **1**: www.gov.uk/drug-safety-update.
2 Tattersfield AE *et al.* (2004) Safety of inhaled corticosteroids. *Proceedings of the American Thoracic Society*. **1**: 171–175.
3 Simpson H *et al.* (2020) Guidance for the prevention and emergency management of adult patients with adrenal insufficiency. *Clinical Medicine*. **20**: 371–378.
4 DTB (2000) The use of inhaled corticosteroids in adults with asthma. *Drug and Therapeutics Bulletin*. **38**: 5–8.
5 BTS/SIGN (2019) British guideline on the management of asthma. A National Clinical Guideline. Revised edition July 2019. *British Thoracic Society and Scottish Intercollegiate Guidelines Network*. Available from: www.brit-thoracic.org.uk.
6 NICE (2018) Chronic obstructive pulmonary disease in over 16s: diagnosis and management. *Clinical Guideline*. NG115. Updated July 2019. www.nice.org.uk.
7 Nannini LJ *et al.* (2012) Combined corticosteroid and long-acting beta(2)-agonist in one inhaler versus long-acting beta(2)-agonists for chronic obstructive pulmonary disease. *Cochrane Database of Systematic Reviews*. **9**: CD006829. www.cochranelibrary.com.
8 NHLBI/WHO (2017) Global initiative for chronic obstructive lung disease. Global strategy for the diagnosis, management and prevention of chronic obstructive pulmonary disease. www.goldcopd.com.
9 Daley-Yates PT *et al.* (2001) Beclomethasone dipropionate: absolute bioavailability, pharmacokinetics and metabolism following intravenous, oral, intranasal and inhaled administration in man. *British Journal of Clinical Pharmacology*. **51**: 400–409.
10 Harrison LI *et al.* (2002) Pharmacokinetics of beclomethasone 17-monopropionate from a beclomethasone dipropionate extrafine aerosol in adults with asthma. *European Journal of Clinical Pharmacology*. **58**: 197–201.
11 Woodcock A *et al.* (2002) Modulite technology: pharmacodynamic and pharmacokinetic implications. *Respiratory Medicine*. **96 (Suppl D)**: S9–15.
12 Harrison TW and Tattersfield AE (2003) Plasma concentrations of fluticasone propionate and budesonide following inhalation from dry powder inhalers by healthy and asthmatic subjects. *Thorax*. **58**: 258–260.
13 CHM (2006) High dose inhaled steroids: new advice on supply of steroid treatment cards. *Current Problems in Pharmacovigilance*. **31 (May)**: 5.
14 MHRA (2010) Inhaled and intranasal corticosteroids: risk of psychological and behavioural side effects. *Drug Safety Update*. **4**. www.gov.uk/drug-safety-update.
15 Smeeth L *et al.* (2003) A population based case-control study of cataract and inhaled corticosteroids. *British Journal of Ophthalmology*. **87**: 1247–1251.
16 Carnahan M and Goldstein D (2000) Ocular complications of topical, peri-ocular, and systemic corticosteroids. *Current Opinion in Ophthalmology*. **11**: 478–483.
17 MHRA (2017) Corticosteroids: rare risk of central serous chorioretinopathy with local as well as systemic administration. *Drug Safety Update*. www.gov.uk/drug-safety-update.
18 Suissa S *et al.* (2010) Inhaled corticosteroids and the risks of diabetes onset and progression. *American Journal of Medicine*. **123**: 1001–1006.
19 Loke YK *et al.* (2011) Risk of fractures with inhaled corticosteroids in COPD: systematic review and meta-analysis of randomised controlled trials and observational studies. *Thorax*. **66**: 699–708.
20 Kew KM and Seniukovich A (2014) Inhaled steroids and risk of pneumonia for chronic obstructive pulmonary disease. *Cochrane Database of Systematic Reviews*. **3**: CD010115. www.cochranelibrary.com.
21 McKeever T *et al.* (2013) Inhaled corticosteroids and the risk of pneumonia in people with asthma: a case-control study. *Chest*. **144**: 1788–1794.

Updated (minor change) October 2021

OXYGEN

Oxygen is used to correct hypoxaemia. It should *not* be used to relieve breathlessness unless the patient is hypoxic and/or other treatment options are ineffective.[1,2] It should be prescribed only after careful consideration, particularly if for home use. Used inappropriately, oxygen can have serious effects or even be fatal (see Cautions and Box A).[3]

Indications: Acute and chronic hypoxaemia; breathlessness unrelieved by other measures in, e.g. severe COPD, pulmonary fibrosis, heart failure or cancer.

3

Pharmacology

Oxygen is prescribed for *hypoxaemic* patients to increase alveolar oxygen tension and decrease the work of breathing necessary to maintain a given arterial oxygen tension. The appropriate concentration varies with the underlying condition, and the dose is generally titrated to achieve normoxaemia/near normoxaemia, which is associated with better outcomes than hyperoxaemia.[4,5]

Medical emergencies involving critically ill patients, e.g. anaphylaxis, carbon monoxide poisoning, cardiopulmonary resuscitation, sepsis, are an exception when high-concentration oxygen should initially be used (15L/min via a reservoir mask). Nonetheless, as soon as reliable oximetry readings are available (and the patient has spontaneous circulation), the oxygen dose is reduced to maintain the appropriate target SpO_2 range (see below).[4]

Most of the available evidence does *not* support the use of oxygen to relieve breathlessness *at rest.*[2,4,6] One short-term study in cancer-related breathlessness suggests that oxygen is generally better than medical air in moderate–severe hypoxaemia (SpO_2 <90%).[7] However, studies involving patients with mild–moderate hypoxaemia have found no additional benefit from oxygen over that seen with medical air delivered by nasal prongs.[8-11] This suggests that a sensation of airflow is an important determinant of benefit.[12-16] Thus, these patients should be encouraged to test the benefit of a cool draught, e.g. open window or electric fan (table or hand-held).[17,18] Consequently, national guidelines recommend that home oxygen should *not* be prescribed for the relief of breathlessness unless the patient is hypoxaemic (SpO_2 <92%) and/or other treatment options (e.g. opioids, breathing control, hand-held fan) are ineffective.[1,2]

Generally, the use of ambulatory oxygen is limited to patients who fulfil the criteria for long-term oxygen therapy (see below). However, oxygen can improve breathlessness *on exertion* in patients with COPD or fibrotic lung disease who desaturate with exercise, even when they would not otherwise qualify for home oxygen.[19,20] Thus, national guidelines recommend the use of ambulatory oxygen in patients with exercise desaturation who objectively benefit from oxygen.[2,21]

Ideally, patients should undergo a formal evaluation, e.g. shuttle walk test, symptom scores/diaries, to examine the benefit of oxygen, e.g. on exercise capacity, breathlessness, quality of life.[6] The evaluation should be tailored to the circumstances of each patient. As a minimum, a pulse oximeter will help identify those patients who are hypoxaemic at rest for whom it appears reasonable to give sufficient oxygen to achieve an SpO_2 of 94–98% (or 88–92% for those at risk of hypercapnic respiratory failure). A trial of oxygen therapy can be given for 10–15min and the impact on any breathlessness evaluated.

When oxygen is being used in hypoxaemic patients for purely palliative purposes (i.e. to improve breathlessness rather than impact on long-term survival), the degree of symptom relief rather than the SpO_2 should be used to help guide the dose of oxygen given. If benefit is obtained, review again after a longer period of use, e.g. 2–3 days. If the patient has persisted in using the oxygen and has found it useful it can be continued, but if the patient has any doubts about its benefit it should be stopped.[11]

Other methods to correct hypoxaemia include non-invasive ventilation (NIV) and, increasingly, high-flow nasal oxygen (HFNO). Both are used when simpler delivery methods are inadequate. NIV has been compared with oxygen therapy (via Venturi or reservoir mask) in patients with cancer and acute respiratory failure caused by disease complications, e.g. bronchial obstruction, lymphangitis.[22] Compared with oxygen, NIV provided greater relief of breathlessness and reduced opioid requirements, particularly in patients with hypercapnia, although about 10% of patients were unable to tolerate it. In patients with advanced cancer with moderate breathlessness despite usual oxygen therapy, HFNO improved breathlessness to a similar degree to NIV and was better tolerated (fewer dropouts, better sleep).[23] The wider clinical relevance of these findings remains to be determined.[24]

When death is imminent, the findings of one study suggest that in the absence of respiratory distress, even with severe hypoxaemia, oxygen should *not* be routinely given.[25] Further, in 90% of those already receiving oxygen, it was possible to discontinue it without causing distress.[25]

Helium 79%–oxygen 21% mixture (Heliox®) is less dense and viscous than air.[26] Its use helps to reduce the respiratory work needed to overcome upper airway obstruction.[27-29] It can be used as a temporary measure in patients breathless at rest while more definitive treatment is arranged. A high-concentration non-rebreathing mask must be used for optimal benefit, and the patient's voice will be squeaky. Mixtures containing higher concentrations of oxygen are also available, e.g. **helium** 72%–oxygen 28%. This improves exercise capacity, oxygen saturation and breathlessness in patients with lung cancer.[30] However, this approach is expensive (each cylinder lasts only 2–3h) and limited by the practical difficulties of transporting a large cylinder. Nonetheless, there is interest in the use of **helium**–oxygen mixtures in various settings, e.g. severe asthma attacks or COPD, or to improve exercise capacity in patients with COPD.[31-34] However, in a study of patients with COPD undergoing pulmonary rehabilitation, there was no overall benefit from breathing **helium**–oxygen (or supplemental oxygen) during exercise training.[35]

Cautions

Patients with hypercapnic respiratory failure who are dependent upon hypoxia for their respiratory drive, e.g. some patients with COPD, cystic fibrosis, neuromuscular disease, kyphoscoliosis or morbid obesity. Patients with a prior episode of hypercapnic respiratory failure should have been issued with an oxygen alert card.

Fire risks

Patients and carers must be warned verbally and in writing of the fire risks of oxygen therapy:

- *no smoking near the cylinder*; this includes use of e-cigarettes and their chargers
- *no open flames*, including candles, matches and gas stoves
- *keep away from sources of heat*, e.g. radiators and direct sunlight
- *use only water-based skin products* on the face and hands; oil-based emollients and petroleum jelly support combustion in the presence of oxygen.

Patients who smoke should be offered help to stop. The risk of prescribing oxygen when the patient ± carers are smokers should be evaluated on an individual basis; oxygen can be declined on the grounds of safety.

Oxygen cylinders carried in cars should be made secure so as not to move during travel or in the event of an accident.

Patients should notify the fire brigade and their home insurer that they have oxygen at home, and their car insurer if oxygen is carried in the car.

Undesirable effects (Box A)

Box A Undesirable effects of oxygen therapy[6]

Hypercapnic respiratory failure

Psychological dependence:
- increased anxiety
- increased probability of excessive use
- excessive restriction of normal activities
- withdrawal difficult

Apparatus restricts activities

Oxygen mask may cause claustrophobia

Nasal prongs may cause dryness and soreness of the nasal mucosa

Humidification is noisy and not always effective

Impaired communication

Social stigma

Additional burden on carers

Cost

Patients who benefit from oxygen under the care of a home palliative care service report that the advantages outweigh the disadvantages.[36]

Equipment

Delivery devices

A high-concentration reservoir (non-rebreathe) mask is used in medical emergencies. Otherwise, either constant (e.g. Venturi) or variable performance masks are used.

Venturi masks provide an almost constant supply of oxygen over a wide range of oxygen flow rates. *Venturi masks should be used when an accurate delivery of oxygen is necessary, i.e. in patients at risk of hypercapnic respiratory failure.* The masks are colour-coded, with the oxygen concentration delivered (24%, 28%, 35%, 40% or 60%) and the minimum recommended flow rate written on each mask. For patients with a respiratory rate >30 breaths/min, the minimum recommended flow rate may be insufficient; flow rates generally 50–100% higher than the minimum should be used.

With variable performance masks, the concentration of oxygen supplied to the patient varies with the rate of flow of the oxygen (2L/min is recommended and provides 24% oxygen) and with the patient's breathing pattern.

Nasal cannulae permit talking, eating and drinking and are thus better suited to chronic use. However, they are the least accurate, with the concentration of oxygen delivered dependent on factors other than flow rate, e.g. breathing pattern. At 2L/min, oxygen concentrations can vary from 24–35%.[37] Although oxygen concentration continues to increase with flow rates >6L/min (the usual maximum), nasal discomfort and dryness limit tolerability, particularly with flow rates >4L/min.

High-flow nasal oxygen delivery devices that deliver humidified oxygen at 40–70L/min are now available and are increasingly used in hospitals outside of intensive care units.[38,39]

Containers

Oxygen can be provided via a cylinder (large for home and small for ambulatory use), oxygen concentrator or liquid oxygen system. It is more economical to use an oxygen concentrator for long-term oxygen therapy and other situations where use is likely to exceed 1.5h/day. Modern concentrators are compact, quiet and cheap to run (2p per hour, reimbursed to the patient).

Generally, concentrators deliver flow rates of up to 4L/min, although some high-flow models deliver 8L/min. However, performance tends to decline with increasing flow rates. If necessary, two concentrators can be linked by tubing and a Y-connector to deliver higher flow rates (e.g. 12L/min, using two high-flow models set at 6L/min); both concentrators must be set to the same flow rate. A backup oxygen cylinder is provided to all patients using a concentrator. Transportable and portable concentrators are also available.

Liquid oxygen systems make use of the fact that 1L of liquid oxygen produces 860L of gaseous oxygen. Relatively compact base units can provide home oxygen or be used to fill portable units to provide ambulatory oxygen; these are lighter and last longer than a portable cylinder, e.g. about 8h vs. 2h at 2L/min. Liquid oxygen systems are the most expensive, but they are quiet and need no electric power; the base unit is refilled as needed.

Oxygen-conserving devices significantly increase the duration of use of a cylinder or liquid oxygen system and should be considered for use out of the home. These permit gas flow during inspiration only, generally either as a fixed volume per breath (pulsed devices) or as a variable volume according to the length of inspiration (demand devices). However, they vary in their ability to maintain SaO_2 levels during exertion, and some patients have difficulty triggering them.

Home oxygen equipment for ambulatory use can be carried in backpacks, trolleys or wheeled carts.

Prescribing oxygen

Oxygen is generally poorly prescribed and monitored.[40] A specific oxygen prescription chart should be used that includes details of:[4,41,42]

- target SpO_2 range
- name of delivery device
- flow rate/oxygen concentration
- duration of use
- method for monitoring to avoid under- or over-dosing of oxygen.

For domiciliary use, the home oxygen order form (HOOF) requires the prescriber to specify:

- number of hours per day that oxygen will be used
- nasal cannulae or a mask
- flow rate
- oxygen concentration (if using a mask)
- need for humidification (only when oxygen given via a tracheostomy).

Completion of a home oxygen record form (HORF) is also recommended to document initial and ongoing evaluations. Generally, these will be needed unless home oxygen is provided on a palliative basis.

Emergency oxygen therapy

This is primarily used to treat hypoxaemia resulting from acute illness, e.g. severe anaemia, acute heart failure, pleural effusion, pneumonia, pneumothorax, pulmonary embolism, severe asthma attack. Specialty guidelines exist.[4]

In brief, for patients not at risk of hypercapnic respiratory failure, initial oxygen therapy is via:

- preferably nasal cannulae at 2–6L/min *or*
- simple face mask at 5–10L/min *or*
- when SpO_2 <85%, a high-concentration reservoir (non-rebreathe) mask at 15L/min.

Avoid flow rates <5L/min with a simple face mask because this may result in carbon dioxide rebreathing. Subsequently, the delivery device and flow rate are adjusted to maintain the SpO_2 within 94–98%. Wait at least 5min before evaluating the effect of a dose adjustment.

Greater caution is needed in patients at risk of hypercapnic respiratory failure (see Cautions); oxygen therapy should commence via:

- preferably a 24% Venturi mask (2–3L/min) *or*
- a 28% Venturi mask (4L/min) *or*
- nasal cannulae (1–2L/min).

Aim for a target SpO_2 of 88–92%, pending urgent blood gas results:

- if $PaCO_2$ normal or low (≤6kPa):
  - ▷ + no risk factor(s) for hypercapnia, adjust oxygen therapy to achieve SpO_2 target of 94–98%
  - ▷ + risk factor(s) for hypercapnia, maintain SpO_2 target of 88–92%
- if $PaCO_2$ raised (>6kPa) but pH ≥7.35 (or H^+ ≤45nmol/L), maintain SpO_2 target of 88–92%
- for all of the above, recheck blood gases after 30–60min
- if at any time $PaCO_2$ raised and pH <7.35 (or H^+ >45nmol/L), consider non-invasive ventilation (seek experienced help urgently).

A clinical evaluation is recommended if the SpO_2 falls ≥3% below the target range.

In the emergency setting, humidification is generally reserved for patients:

- with a tracheostomy or artificial airway
- with difficulty clearing viscous airway secretions (nebulized sodium chloride 0.9% is an alternative)
- needing high-flow oxygen >24h, with upper airway discomfort because of dryness.

Humidification requires the use of a large-volume oxygen humidifier device (essentially a large nebulizer); *bubble bottles should not be used, because they are ineffective and pose an infection risk.*

Oxygen can be progressively reduced once a patient is stable and the SpO_2 is either above or has been at the upper end of the target range for ≥4h; it can be discontinued when, with the patient breathing air, the SpO_2 is maintained above or within the target range or has returned to their usual baseline. A repeat SpO_2 is recommended after 1h to confirm that it is safe to discontinue oxygen therapy.

Long-term oxygen therapy

Long-term oxygen (≥15h/day) can be considered for use in patients with cancer or other life-threatening diseases who are hypoxaemic (SpO_2 ≤92%, or ≤94% when secondary complications are present).[1] More specifically, in patients with:

- COPD, cystic fibrosis, heart failure or interstitial lung disease with PaO_2 ≤7.3kPa, or ≤8kPa when peripheral oedema, polycythaemia (haematocrit ≥55%) or pulmonary hypertension present
- pulmonary hypertension, without parenchymal lung involvement and PaO_2 ≤8kPa
- obstructive sleep apnoea who remain hypoxic during sleep despite nasal continuous positive airway pressure (CPAP)
- neuromuscular or chest wall disorders causing inspiratory muscle weakness, when hypoxaemia is not corrected by non-invasive ventilation.

The oxygen is used overnight and for several hours during the day. Evidence of benefit from such use relates mainly to patients with COPD, where correction of severe hypoxaemia improves survival (particularly with use for 20h/day) and quality of life.[2,43] The precise mechanism for the improved survival is unknown, but possibilities include a reduction in pulmonary vascular resistance and the subsequent load on the right side of the heart.

When long-term oxygen is considered appropriate (if in doubt, obtain advice from a specialist respiratory physician), a referral should be made to a specialist home oxygen service for further evaluation, provision of long-term ± ambulatory oxygen and ongoing review. For example, in patients with COPD, arterial blood gas tensions should be measured before treatment when the patient's condition has been stable for at least 8 weeks, to ensure the criteria are met (see first bullet above). Supplemental oxygen is given for 20min to ensure a PaO_2 of >8kPa is achieved without an unacceptable rise in $PaCO_2$ (capillary blood gases are sufficient for titration purposes, unless hypercapnia present at baseline). Arterial blood gas tensions should be measured at the end of titration and ≥3 weeks later, to confirm the need for long-term therapy.[2] Generally, these measurements should be detailed on the home oxygen record form (see Prescribing oxygen).

A full evaluation is not always appropriate when home oxygen is purely palliative in end-of-life care.[1]

Nocturnal oxygen therapy

This is recommended when nocturnal hypoxaemia occurs in patients with:

- COPD, cystic fibrosis or interstitial lung disease *and* who meet the criteria for long-term oxygen therapy (see above)
- heart failure with evidence of sleep-disordered breathing and daytime symptoms, even when not meeting the criteria for long-term oxygen therapy, provided heart failure treatment has been optimized and other causes excluded, e.g. obstructive sleep apnoea.

When nocturnal hypoxaemia is caused by ventilatory failure, e.g. due to neuromuscular weakness, nocturnal oxygen therapy can be considered as part of non-invasive ventilation support.

Ambulatory oxygen

This can be prescribed for patients who fulfil the criteria for long-term oxygen therapy, are mobile, and wish to leave the home (see above).[2]

Some patients, e.g. with interstitial lung disease, who do not qualify for long-term oxygen therapy but desaturate on exercise (defined as a fall in SpO_2 ≥4% to <90%), can also be considered for ambulatory oxygen provided other treatments have been optimized.[2]

Ambulatory oxygen is also used to enhance participation in pulmonary rehabilitation or exercise programmes for patients who are not hypoxaemic at rest but desaturate on exertion, providing it improves exercise capacity >10% in a formal evaluation, e.g. shuttle walk test.[2]

In some patients, ambulatory oxygen fails to prevent significant desaturation on exertion. Failure varied with different delivery devices but was as high as 20% in COPD and 40% in interstitial lung disease.[44] This emphasizes the importance of individual evaluation.

A breath-activated conserver can be added into ambulatory oxygen circuits using nasal cannulae to extend the life of the cylinder. However, conservers are unsuitable for patients who mouth breathe.

Palliative oxygen therapy

Opioids are more effective than oxygen in reducing breathlessness at rest in patients with advanced disease with and without hypoxaemia (see p.412).[2,45]

Generally, patients with advanced cancer or end-stage cardiorespiratory disease with intractable breathlessness should *not* be given oxygen unless they meet the long-term oxygen therapy thresholds (see above).[1,2] However, palliative oxygen therapy may be considered when breathlessness is unresponsive to opioids and non-drug approaches, e.g. breathing control, hand-held fan. A formal evaluation of benefit and quality of life should be made.[2]

When death is imminent, if severe intractable breathlessness is present, oxygen may be used when hypoxaemia cannot be confirmed without discomfort to the patient (this should be rare, given the wide availability of pulse oximeters).[1] Conversely, oxygen can often be discontinued when death is imminent (see Pharmacology).

Short-burst oxygen therapy

This is not recommended in the absence of hypoxaemia. When the underlying cause is irreversible, patients should be evaluated for long-term oxygen therapy ± ambulatory oxygen as above.[1,2]

Short-term (intermittent) home oxygen therapy may be needed for patients rendered temporarily hypoxaemic, e.g. as a result of a chest infection or episode of heart failure. These patients should also undergo a specialist evaluation. For those likely to continue to experience recurrent episodes of hypoxaemia, an intermittent source of home oxygen, probably in the form of cylinders, may be appropriate.[1]

Previously, for exercise-induced breathlessness, some patients used oxygen before the exercise and others afterwards to aid recovery. However, in patients with COPD, most studies fail to show benefit from this strategy. Thus, it is no longer recommended.[2]

Travel by air

Patients with lung conditions and certain other co-morbidities who wish to travel by air should be given specific advice (Box B).

In-flight oxygen provision

- generally, airlines charge for providing in-flight oxygen (fees and services vary)
- passengers may carry their own small full oxygen cylinders with them as hand luggage for medical use, provided they have airline approval; a charge may be made for this service, in addition to a charge for in-flight oxygen
- certain types of lightweight battery-operated portable oxygen concentrators may be permitted with airline approval; sufficient batteries are needed to cover the flight and possible delays
- the airline must be informed at the time of the booking and at least 1 month before the flight
- the airline will issue a Medical Information Form (MEDIF) to be completed by the patient and GP/hospital specialist; the airline's medical officer then evaluates the patient's needs; regular flyers can obtain a frequent traveller's medical card from the airline, which avoids the need to complete multiple forms
- in-flight oxygen is generally prescribed at a rate of 2–4L/min through nasal cannulae and has to be used in accordance with the airline's instructions
- pulsed dose (breath-actuated) systems are increasingly used by airlines; if there is concern over the patient's suitability for such a system, e.g. the patient is frail or has an irregular or shallow breathing pattern, a trial should be undertaken and, if necessary, an alternative system arranged with the airline.

For guidance on specific diseases, patients oxygen-dependent at sea level, those needing ventilation, and infants and children, see the full guidance.[46]

General advice

- *medical insurance:* travel with a European Health Insurance Card (if visiting a European Economic Area country) and ensure fully covered for medical costs that may arise related to the lung disease, including the cost of an air ambulance
- *documentation:* have a medical letter on their person detailing condition and medication
- *medication:* take a full supply of all medication as hand luggage, e.g. well-filled reliever and preventer inhalers (also see Chapter 23, p.815)
- *equipment:* e.g. portable battery-operated nebulizers may be used at the discretion of the cabin crew, but the airline must be notified in advance (an inhaler + spacer is an alternative)
- *ground transportation:* airports can generally provide transport assistance
- *DVT prophylaxis:* see LMWH, p.106.

Free booklets/fact sheets are also available from various patient organisations, e.g.:

- 'Going on holiday with a lung condition', British Lung Foundation (tel: 0300 222 5800, www.blf.org.uk)
- 'Air travel for people affected by chest, heart or stroke illness' and 'Holiday information', Chest Heart & Stroke Scotland Advice Line (tel: 0808 801 0899, www.chss.org.uk).

Supply

Oxygen is classified as a General Sale List (GSL) product; some companies will sell or rent cylinders privately if needed, e.g. for travel outside the UK (see below) or as an emergency back-up supply in a care home.[47]

Box B Fitness to undertake air travel in adults[46]

Air travel exacerbates hypoxaemia in patients with lung disease and may cause compensatory hyperventilation and tachycardia.

Aircraft cabins are pressurized, generally to reflect an altitude of about 8,000ft. This is equivalent to breathing air containing 15% oxygen instead of 21% at sea level. Even in the healthy, blood oxygen levels (PaO_2) will fall to 8–10kPa (60–75mmHg; SpO_2 89–94%) or lower during exercise or sleep.

Contra-indications to commercial air travel

- need for >4L/min of oxygen (at sea level)
- infectious tuberculosis
- pneumothorax
- major haemoptysis.

Evaluation

Undertake a clinical history and examination, ± simple spirometry, to determine if the patient is low or high risk.

Low risk

Patients who can walk 50m on the level at a steady pace without oxygen, breathlessness or needing to stop are unlikely to experience problems with reduced cabin pressure.

High risk

Referral for a more detailed evaluation by a specialist respiratory physician is advised when any of the following are present:

- previous air travel intolerance with respiratory symptoms (breathlessness, chest pain, confusion or syncope)
- use of oxygen, continuous positive airway pressure or ventilator support
- severe COPD (FEV_1 <30% predicted) or asthma
- bullous lung disease
- severe (vital capacity <1L) restrictive disease (including chest wall and respiratory muscle disease), particularly with blood gas abnormalities
- cystic fibrosis
- co-morbidity worsened by hypoxaemia (cerebrovascular disease, cardiac disease, pulmonary hypertension)
- pulmonary tuberculosis
- <6 weeks since hospital discharge for acute respiratory illness
- recent pneumothorax (avoid flights for at least 7 days (spontaneous) or 14 days (traumatic) *after* full radiographic resolution)
- risk of VTE, or previous VTE (avoid flights for ≥4 weeks unless no residual symptoms and no hypoxaemia at rest or after exercise)
- other concerns regarding the patient's fitness to fly.

Further evaluation can include the hypoxic challenge test, where the patient breathes 15% oxygen at sea level for 20min to mimic air cabin conditions:

- if PaO_2 ≥6.6kPa (>50mmHg) or SpO_2 ≥85%, in-flight oxygen is not needed
- if PaO_2 <6.6kPa (<50mmHg) or SpO_2 <85%, in-flight oxygen is needed at 2L/min via nasal cannulae.

For guidance on specific diseases, patients oxygen-dependent at sea level, those needing ventilation and infants and children, see the full guidance.[46]

England and Wales[2,47-49]

Any registered health professional can order home oxygen from regional suppliers (see Table 1) using a home oxygen order form (HOOF). Patient consent, using the combined initial home oxygen risk mitigation (IHORM) consent form and home oxygen consent form (HOCF), *must* also be obtained to allow their details to be passed on to the supplier and relevant authorities, e.g. the fire service. The following types of oxygen therapy can be ordered:

- short-burst (intermittent) oxygen
- long-term oxygen; unless for palliative care, patients should be referred to the hospital home oxygen service for a full evaluation
- nocturnal oxygen
- ambulatory oxygen.

Standard delivery is generally within 3 days of receipt of order, during working hours. Other delivery services can also be specified but will incur a higher charge:

- urgent response (4-hour delivery)
- next day (clinical assessment services and hospital discharges only).

A breath-activated conserver can be added into ambulatory oxygen circuits using nasal cannulae to extend the life of the cylinder. However, conservers are unsuitable for patients who mouth breathe.

The supplier will ensure that the appropriate equipment is provided (cylinder or oxygen concentrator), contact the patient to arrange its delivery, installation and maintenance, organise payment of the patient's electricity costs in relation to use of equipment supplied, and train the patient in its use. The supplier will continue the service until a revised order is received or until notified that the patient no longer needs home oxygen. For more information, contact the relevant supplier (Table 1).

Table 1 Regional suppliers of home oxygen in England and Wales[48]

Supplier	*Region covered*	*Contact details*
Air Liquide (Homecare)	London East Midlands North West South West	Tel: 0808 1439991/1439992 (North West)/1439993 (East Midlands)/1439999 (South West) www.airliquidehealthcare.co.uk
Baywater Healthcare	Yorkshire & Humberside West Midlands Wales	Tel: 0800 373580 Fax: 0800 214709 www.baywater.co.uk
BOC Healthcare	East of England North East	Tel: 0800 136603 Fax: 0800 1699989 www.bochomeoxygen.co.uk
Dolby Vivisol	South East Coast South Central	Tel: 0800 9179840 Fax: 0800 7814610 www.dolbyvivisol.com

Scotland[50]

The Scottish home oxygen order form (SHOOF) should be completed and e-mailed to Health Facilities Scotland, which works in partnership with Dolby Vivisol to provide the equipment needed and arrange installation in the patient's home. The ordering/prescribing of oxygen via the NHS must be by a specialist, generally a respiratory or paediatric consultant, who is specified by the local health authority.

For palliative care patients, each health board should have a local solution developed, e.g. access by palliative care teams to portable concentrators or facilities placed in local cottage hospitals. For further details, including the national guidance document, see the Health Facilities Scotland website www.hfs.scot.nhs.uk. Alternatively, contact Health Facilities Scotland by: tel. 0131 275 6860; fax 0131 314 0724; e-mail nss.oxycon@nhs.net.

Northern Ireland[51]

Home oxygen is supplied via the home oxygen service contractor BOC using the Northern Ireland home oxygen order form (HOOF NI). The prescription form can only be signed by a qualified prescriber listed on the BOC register of authorized oxygen prescribers. In primary care, GPs can also use a HS21 prescription to obtain oxygen cylinders (portable and non-portable) from community pharmacy oxygen contractors. For further details, the HOOF and guidelines, see 'Home Oxygen Services' in the 'FPS Pharmaceutical Services' section of the Business Services Organisation website: http://www.hscbusiness.hscni.net/services/2359.htm.

Note. Community Pharmacy Palliative Care Network (CPPCN) pharmacies all provide oxygen cylinders.

Temporary supplies for when travelling[48]

Patients travelling to other parts of the UK, e.g. for holidays, can obtain a temporary supply at the alternative address through reciprocal arrangements between the various UK authorities and oxygen suppliers. This is organized as a holiday order on a HOOF; contact the usual regional supplier for information. Ideally, at least 2 weeks' notice should be given, but up to 4 weeks may be needed during peak holiday periods in popular tourist destinations or remote areas such as the Scottish Isles. Permission has to be obtained from the householder/hotel to allow oxygen onto the premises.

Patients travelling outside the UK (including the Isle of Man, the Channel Islands, and on cruises that start in the UK) need to arrange a private supply with their local oxygen supplier. Some specialist travel companies can help organize this. Their details can be obtained from the Chest Heart & Stroke Scotland 'Holiday Information' fact sheet (see above).

1 NHS (2011) Service specification: home oxygen service assessment and review. Gateway reference 17874 www.gov.uk (archived).
2 Hardinge M *et al.* (2015) British Thoracic Society guidelines for home oxygen use in adults. *Thorax.* **70 (Suppl 1)**: i1–43.
3 Lamont T *et al.* (2010) Improving the safety of oxygen therapy in hospitals: summary of a safety report from the National Patient Safety Agency. *British Medical Journal.* **340**: C187.
4 O'Driscoll BR *et al.* (2017) BTS guideline for oxygen use in adults in healthcare and emergency settings. *Thorax.* **72 (Suppl 1)**: ii1–90.
5 Chu DK *et al.* (2018) Mortality and morbidity in acutely ill adults treated with liberal versus conservative oxygen therapy (IOTA): a systematic review and meta-analysis. *Lancet.* **391**: 1693–1705.
6 Booth S *et al.* (2004) The use of oxygen in the palliation of breathlessness. A report of the expert working group of the scientific committee of the association of palliative medicine. *Respiratory Medicine.* **98**: 66–77.
7 Bruera E *et al.* (1993) Effects of oxygen on dyspnoea in hypoxaemic terminal cancer patients. *Lancet.* **342**: 13–14.
8 Uronis HE *et al.* (2008) Oxygen for relief of dyspnoea in mildly- or non-hypoxaemic patients with cancer: a systematic review and meta-analysis. *British Journal of Cancer.* **98**: 294–299.
9 Bruera E *et al.* (2003) A randomized controlled trial of supplemental oxygen versus air in cancer patients with dyspnea. *Palliative Medicine.* **17**: 659–663.
10 Philip J *et al.* (2006) A randomized, double-blind, crossover trial of the effect of oxygen on dyspnea in patients with advanced cancer. *Journal of Pain and Symptom Management.* **32**: 541–550.
11 Abernethy AP *et al.* (2010) Effect of palliative oxygen versus room air in relief of breathlessness in patients with refractory dyspnoea: a double-blind, randomised controlled trial. *Lancet.* **376**: 784–793.
12 Schwartzstein R *et al.* (1987) Cold facial stimulation reduces breathlessness induced in normal subjects. *American Review of Respiratory Disease.* **136**: 58–61.
13 Burgess K and Whitelaw W (1988) Effects of nasal cold receptors on pattern of breathing. *Journal of Applied Physiology.* **64**: 371–376.
14 Freedman S (1988) Cold facial stimulation reduces breathlessness induced in normal subjects. *American Review of Respiratory Diseases.* **137**: 492–493.
15 Kerr D (1989) A bedside fan for terminal dyspnea. *American Journal of Hospice Care.* **89**: 22.
16 Liss H and Grant B (1988) The effect of nasal flow on breathlessness in patients with chronic obstructive pulmonary disease. *American Review of Respiratory Disease.* **137**: 1285–1288.
17 Luckett T *et al.* (2017) Contributions of a hand-held fan to self-management of chronic breathlessness. *European Respiratory Journal.* **50**: 1700262.
18 Qian Y *et al.* (2019) Fan therapy for the treatment of dyspnea in adults: a systematic review. *Journal of Pain and Symptom Management.* **50**: [Epub ahead of print].
19 Ekstrom M *et al.* (2016) Oxygen for breathlessness in patients with chronic obstructive pulmonary disease who do not qualify for home oxygen therapy. *Cochrane Database of Systematic Reviews.* **11**: CD006429.
20 Visca D *et al.* (2018) Effect of ambulatory oxygen on quality of life for patients with fibrotic lung disease (AmbOx): a prospective, open-label, mixed-method, crossover randomised controlled trial. *Lancet Respiratory Medicine.* **6**: 759–770.
21 NICE (2018) Chronic obstructive pulmonary disease in over 16s: diagnosis and management. *Clinical Guideline.* NG115. Updated July 2019. www.nice.org.uk.
22 Nava S *et al.* (2013) Palliative use of non-invasive ventilation in end-of-life patients with solid tumours: a randomised feasibility trial. *Lancet Oncology.* **14**: 219–227.
23 Hui D *et al.* (2013) High-flow oxygen and bilevel positive airway pressure for persistent dyspnea in patients with advanced cancer: a phase II randomized trial. *Journal of Pain and Symptom Management.* **46**: 463–473.
24 Shah N *et al.* (2017) High-flow nasal cannula oxygen therapy in palliative care. *Journal of Palliative Medicine.* **20**: 679–680.
25 Campbell ML *et al.* (2013) Oxygen is nonbeneficial for most patients who are near death. *Journal of Pain and Symptom Management.* **45**: 517–523.
26 Boorstein J *et al.* (1989) Using helium-oxygen mixtures in the emergency management of acute upper airway obstruction. *Annals of Emergency Medicine.* **18**: 688–690.
27 Lu T-S *et al.* (1976) Helium-oxygen in treatment of upper airway obstruction. *Anesthesiology.* **45**: 678–680.
28 Rudow M *et al.* (1986) Helium-oxygen mixtures in airway obstruction due to thyroid carcinoma. *Canadian Anaesthesiology Society Journal.* **33**: 498–501.

29 Khanlou H and Eiger G (2001) Safety and efficacy of heliox as a treatment for upper airway obstruction due to radiation-induced laryngeal dysfunction. *Heart and Lung*. **30**: 146–147.
30 Ahmedzai SH *et al.* (2004) A double-blind, randomised, controlled Phase II trial of Heliox28 gas mixture in lung cancer patients with dyspnoea on exertion. *British Journal of Cancer*. **90**: 366–371.
31 Laude EA and Ahmedzai SH (2007) Oxygen and helium gas mixtures for dyspnoea. *Current Opinion in Supportive and Palliative Care*. **1**: 91–95.
32 Chiappa GR *et al.* (2009) Heliox improves oxygen delivery and utilization during dynamic exercise in patients with chronic obstructive pulmonary disease. *American Journal of Respiratory and Critical Care Medicine*. **179**: 1004–1010.
33 Eves ND *et al.* (2009) Helium-hyperoxia: a novel intervention to improve the benefits of pulmonary rehabilitation for patients with COPD. *Chest*. **135**: 609–618.
34 Hunt T *et al.* (2010) Heliox, dyspnoea and exercise in COPD. *European Respiratory Review*. **19**: 30–38.
35 Scorsone D *et al.* (2010) Does a low-density gas mixture or oxygen supplementation improve exercise training in COPD? *Chest*. **138**: 1133–1139.
36 Jaturapatporn D *et al.* (2010) Patients' experience of oxygen therapy and dyspnea: a qualitative study in home palliative care. *Supportive Care in Cancer*. **18**: 765–770.
37 Bazuaye E *et al.* (1992) Variability of inspired oxygen concentration with nasal cannulas. *Thorax*. **47**: 609–611.
38 Ward JJ (2013) High-flow oxygen administration by nasal cannula for adult and perinatal patients. *Respiratory Care*. **58**: 98–122.
39 Epstein AS *et al.* (2011) Humidified high-flow nasal oxygen utilization in patients with cancer at Memorial Sloan-Kettering Cancer Center. *Journal of Palliative Medicine*. **14**: 835–839.
40 O'Driscoll R (2012) Emergency oxygen use. *British Medical Journal*. **345**: e6856.
41 Bateman NT and Leach RM (1998) ABC of oxygen. Acute oxygen therapy. *British Medical Journal*. **317**: 798–801.
42 Dodd ME *et al.* (2000) Audit of oxygen prescribing before and after the introduction of a prescription chart. *British Medical Journal*. **321**: 864–865.
43 Eaton T *et al.* (2004) Long-term oxygen therapy improves health-related quality of life. *Respiratory Medicine*. **98**: 285–293.
44 Marti S *et al.* (2013) Are oxygen-conserving devices effective for correcting exercise hypoxemia? *Respiratory Care*. **58**: 1606–1613.
45 Clemens KE *et al.* (2009) Use of oxygen and opioids in the palliation of dyspnoea in hypoxic and non-hypoxic palliative care patients: a prospective study. *Supportive Care in Cancer*. **17**: 367–377.
46 BTS (2011) Air Travel Working Group. Managing passengers with stable respiratory disease planning air travel: British Thoracic Society recommends. Available from: http://www.brit-thoracic.org.uk.
47 UKMI (2015) Do oxygen cylinders need to be prescribed on an individual patient basis in residential nursing homes? *Medicines Q&A*. www.evidence.nhs.uk.
48 NHSBSA (2019) The November 2019 Electronic Drug Tariff. www.nhsbsa.nhs.uk/prescriptions.
49 NHS England (2017) Home oxygen risk management (letter). Gateway number 06381.
50 NHS Scotland Home Oxygen Service. www.hfs.scot.nhs.uk (accessed November 2019).
51 Business Services Organisation Home oxygen services. http://www.hscbusiness.hscni.net/2359.htm (accessed November 2019).

Updated November 2019

DRUGS FOR COUGH

General strategy

Coughing helps clear the central airways of foreign matter, secretions or pus, and should generally be encouraged.[1] It is pathological when:

- ineffective, e.g. dry or unproductive
- it adversely affects sleep, rest, eating, or social activities
- it causes other symptoms such as muscle strain, rib fracture, vomiting, syncope, headache or urinary incontinence.

Generally, the primary aim is to identify and treat the underlying cause(s) and remove any aggravating factors, e.g. smoking. However, when this is not possible, a symptomatic approach is appropriate in palliative care. Drugs for cough can be divided into two main categories (Box A):

- *protussives (expectorants):* make coughing more effective and less distressing
- *antitussives:* reduce the intensity and frequency of coughing.

The choice of drug depends largely on whether the cough is 'wet' or 'dry' (Figure 1).

The choice and use of antitussives (including demulcents) is discussed on p.158.

Nebulized sodium chloride 0.9% is generally the protussive of choice, but sometimes an irritant mucolytic (e.g. **guaifenesin**, available OTC) or a chemical mucolytic (e.g. **carbocisteine**, p.156) may be preferable. Nebulized sodium chloride 3–7% (hypertonic saline) is used in cystic fibrosis, and this is extending to other conditions, e.g. bronchiectasis (also see Nebulized drugs, p.904). Further specialist options are authorized for use in cystic fibrosis, e.g. **dornase alpha, mannitol**.

The evidence supporting the use of protussives or antitussives in acute or chronic cough is generally low level.[6-9] However, recent advances in the understanding of cough and the mechanism of mucin production may lead to more targeted treatments.[10] For example, receptors important

Box A Examples of drugs for cough (modified from[2,3])

Protussives (expectorants)

Topical mucolytics

Nebulized sodium chloride 0.9% (normal saline) or 3–7% (hypertonic saline)

Chemical inhalations
- benzoin tincture, compound, BP (Friars' balsam)
- menthol and eucalyptus BP

Irritant mucolytics[a]

Ambroxol (not UK)
Ammonium chloride
Bromhexine (not UK)
Capsicum
Guaifenesin[b]
Ipecacuanha[b]
Potassium iodide

Chemical mucolytics

Acetylcysteine
Carbocisteine
Erdosteine

Antitussives

Peripheral

Simple linctus BP (demulcent)
Benzonatate (not UK)
Levocloperastine (not UK)
Levodropizine (not UK)
Local anaesthetics (nebulized)
Sodium cromoglicate

Central

Anti-epileptics
- gabapentin
- pregabalin

Baclofen

Opioids/opioid derivatives
- codeine[b]
- dextromethorphan[b]
- diamorphine
- dihydrocodeine
- hydrocodone (not UK)
- hydromorphone
- morphine
- methadone
- pholcodine[b]

a. generally found as constituents in OTC cough products
b. restricted use in children;[4,5] also see mucolytics (p.156) and antitussives (p.158).

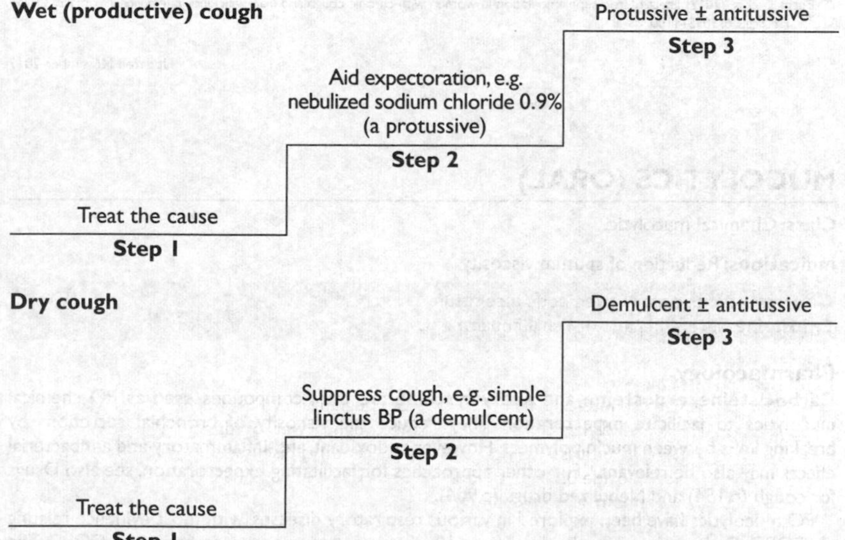

Figure 1 Treatment ladders for cough. Non-drug approaches, generally provided by physiotherapists ± speech and language therapists, should also be considered.

in cough generation have been identified (e.g. P2X purinoceptor), and specific antagonists are under development.[11] **Menthol**, long used in OTC cough remedies, is now known to be an agonist at the inhibitory TRP melastatin 8 receptor.[12]

Sensitization of the cough reflex, resulting in cough hypersensitivity, appears important in chronic cough of various causes.[3,13] Thus, there are parallels with neuropathic pain:

- paraesthesia ~ laryngeal paraesthesia, abnormal throat sensation or tickle
- hyperalgesia ~ hypertussia, increased cough sensitivity to known tussigens
- allodynia ~ allotussia, cough triggered by non-tussive stimuli, e.g. talking, cold air.

This probably explains the benefit from drugs that target such sensitization, either generally, e.g. **amitriptyline** (p.228), **baclofen** (p.658), **gabapentin** (p.297),[3,9,14,15] or more specifically, e.g. correction of iron deficiency.[16]

1 Twycross R and Wilcock A (2016) *Introducing Palliative Care* (5e). palliativedrugs.com, Nottingham, pp166–170.
2 Homsi J *et al.* (2001) Important drugs for cough in advanced cancer. *Supportive Care in Cancer*. **9**: 565–574.
3 Smith JA and Woodcock A (2016) Chronic Cough. *New England Journal of Medicine*. **375**: 1544–1551.
4 MHRA (2009) Over-the-counter cough and cold medicines for children. *Drug Safety Update*. www.gov.uk/drug-safety-update.
5 MHRA (2015) Codeine for cough and cold: restricted use in children. *Drug Safety Update*. www.gov.uk/drug-safety-update.
6 Wee B *et al.* (2012) Management of chronic cough in patients receiving palliative care: review of evidence and recommendations by a task group of the Association for Palliative Medicine of Great Britain and Ireland. *Palliative Medicine*. **26**: 780–787.
7 Smith SM *et al.* (2014) Over-the-counter (OTC) medications for acute cough in children and adults in community settings. *Cochrane Database of Systematic Reviews*. **11**: CD001831. www.cochranelibrary.com.
8 Molassiotis M *et al.* (2015) Interventions for cough in cancer. *Cochrane Database of Systematic Reviews*. **5**: CD007881. www.cochranelibrary.com.
9 Gibson P *et al.* (2016) Treatment of unexplained chronic cough: CHEST guideline and expert panel report. *Chest*. **149**: 27–44.
10 Nadel JA (2013) Mucous hypersecretion and relationship to cough. *Pulmonary Pharmacology and Therapeutics*. **26**: 510–513.
11 Smith JA and Badri H (2019) Cough: New Pharmacology. *Journal of Allergy and Clinical Immunology: In Practice*. **7**: 1731–1738.
12 Millqvist E *et al.* (2013) Inhalation of menthol reduces capsaicin cough sensitivity and influences inspiratory flows in chronic cough. *Respiratory Medicine*. **107**: 433–438.
13 Chung KF (2017) Advances in mechanisms and management of chronic cough: The Ninth London International Cough Symposium 2016. *Pulmonary Pharmacology and Therapeutics*. **47**: 2–8.
14 Wei W *et al.* (2016) The efficacy of specific neuromodulators on human refractory chronic cough: a systematic review and meta-analysis. *Journal of Thoracic Diseases*. **8**: 2942–2951.
15 Atreya S *et al.* (2016) Gabapentin for chronic refractory cancer cough. *Indian Journal of Palliative Care*. **22**: 94–96.
16 Bucca C *et al.* (2012) Effect of iron supplementation in women with chronic cough and iron deficiency. *International Journal of Clinical Practice*. **66**: 1095–1100.

Updated November 2019

MUCOLYTICS (ORAL)

Class: Chemical mucolytic.

Indications: Reduction of sputum viscosity.

Contra-indications: Active peptic ulceration.
Erdosteine: severe hepatic or renal impairment.

Pharmacology

Carbocisteine, **erdosteine** and **acetylcysteine** are thiol compounds used as PO chemical mucolytics to facilitate expectoration. They reduce the viscosity of bronchial secretions by breaking links between mucin polymers. However, antioxidant, anti-inflammatory and antibacterial effects may also be relevant.[1] For other approaches for facilitating expectoration, see also Drugs for cough (p.154) and Nebulized drugs (p.904).

PO mucolytics have been explored in various respiratory diseases, with most evidence relating to COPD. **Erdosteine** is authorized for ≤10 days use during an exacerbation of COPD. The long-term use of other mucolytics, at best, produces only a small reduction in the likelihood of an acute exacerbation (NNT = 8 (95% CI 7–10) for 1 less patient with an exacerbation over a mean of 9 months) and days of disability (<0.5 days/month); the impact of other effects is limited (lung function, quality of life), inconsistent (hospitalisations) or unclear (mortality).[2] UK guidelines recommend that mucolytics should only be considered for patients with a chronic productive cough, and continued only when there is symptomatic benefit.[3]

There is only low-level evidence to support the use of mucolytics in bronchiectasis, and other airway clearance approaches are preferred (e.g. positional drainage ± nebulized sterile water or sodium chloride 0.9%).[4,5] Nonetheless, guidelines note that **carbocisteine** appears widely used and consider a 6 month therapeutic trial reasonable in patients who struggle to expectorate sputum, continuing only when there is clinical benefit.

Mucolytics have no established role in interstitial lung disease, although there is interest in exploring a possible disease-modifying effect of **acetylcysteine.**[6,7]

Carbocisteine, **erdosteine** and **acetylcysteine** are all metabolized in the liver and excreted in the urine as unchanged drug or metabolites. A dose reduction is advised for **erdosteine** in mild–moderate hepatic impairment. For pharmacokinetic details, see Table 1.

Table 1 Pharmacokinetics of mucolytics

	Carbocisteine	*Erdosteine*	*Acetylcysteine*
Bio-availability	<10%	No data	<10%
Peak plasma concentration	1–3h	1h; 1.5h (active metabolite)	0.5–1h
Plasma halflife	1.5–2.5h	1.5h	6.5h; increased by ≤80% in severe hepatic impairment

Cautions

History of peptic ulcer disease (mucolytics can disrupt the gastric mucosal barrier).
Erdosteine: hepatic impairment (see below).

Undesirable effects

Occasional dyspepsia, rash.
Rare (<0.1%, ≥0.001%): GI haemorrhage.

Dose and use

Carbocisteine

- start with 750mg PO t.d.s.
- reduce to 750mg b.d. when there is a satisfactory decrease in cough and sputum production.

Erdosteine

- give 300mg PO b.d. for up to 10 days
- limit dose to 300mg/24h in mild–moderate hepatic impairment; avoid in severe hepatic impairment and renal impairment (CrCl <25mL/min), due to a lack of data.

Acetylcysteine

- give 600mg PO once daily; dissolve the effervescent tablet in half a glass of water.

Supply

Carbocisteine (generic)
Capsules 375mg, 750mg, 28 days @ 750mg t.d.s. = £3.25 or £27 respectively.
Oral solution 250mg/5mL, 750mg/5mL, 28 days @ 750mg t.d.s. = £26 or £40 respectively.
Oral solution sachets 750mg/10mL sachet, 28 days @ 1 sachet t.d.s. = £22.

Erdosteine
Erdotin® (Galen)
Capsules 300mg, 10 days @ 300mg b.d. = £5. *Not prescribable on NHS prescriptions in Scotland.*

Acetylcysteine (generic)
Effervescent tablets (sugar-free) 600mg, 28 days @ 600mg once daily = £5; *contains* Na^+ *5mmol/tablet.*

1 Cazzola M *et al.* (2019) Thiol-based drugs in pulmonary medicine: much more than mucolytics. *Trends in Pharmacological Sciences.* **40**: 452–463.
2 Poole P and Black P (2019) Mucolytic agents versus placebo for chronic bronchitis or chronic obstructive pulmonary disease. *Cochrane Database of Systematic Reviews.* **5**: CD001287. www.thecochranelibrary.com
3 NICE (2018) Chronic obstructive pulmonary disease in over 16s: diagnosis and management. *Clinical Guideline.* NG115. Updated July 2019. www.nice.org.uk.
4 Wilkinson M *et al.* (2014) Mucolytics for bronchiectasis. *Cochrane Database of Systematic Reviews.* **5**: CD001289. www.cochranelibrary.com.
5 Hill AT *et al.* (2019) British Thoracic Society Guideline for bronchiectasis in adults. *Thorax.* **74 (Suppl 1)**: 1–69.
6 Sun T *et al.* (2016) Efficacy of N-acetylcysteine in idiopathic pulmonary fibrosis: a systematic review and meta-analysis. *Medicine.* **95**: e3629.
7 Oldham JM *et al.* (2015) TOLLIP, MUC5B, and the response to N-Acetylcysteine among individuals with idiopathic pulmonary fibrosis. *American Journal of Respiratory and Critical Care Medicine.* **192**: 1475–1482.

Updated (minor change) December 2021

ANTITUSSIVES

Cough is a complicated vagally mediated reflex that includes peripheral and central nervous system components.[1] Although antitussives can be considered predominantly peripherally acting (e.g. local anaesthetics) or centrally acting (e.g. opioids), most have a complicated mechanism of action, including a strong placebo effect. Generally, the evidence supporting the use of antitussives in palliative care is low level.[2-5]

Opioid antitussives are given precedence in *PCF* because they are commonly needed for concurrent symptoms in patients with advanced disease receiving palliative care. Guidelines for cough due to lung cancer also favour the use of opioids.[4]

Increasingly, non-opioid neuromodulating drugs are being developed/used, particularly when hypersensitivity of the cough reflex is present/suspected, e.g. idiopathic chronic cough (cough hypersensitivity syndrome).[1,5,6]

Preliminary data suggest benefit from non-drug approaches encompassed in speech pathology therapy,[7] and several chronic cough guidelines recommend their use (idiopathic, interstitial lung disease, lung cancer).[4-6] In part, benefit may relate to improved voluntary suppression. Generally, these approaches are provided by speech and language therapists or physiotherapists.

Demulcents

Most OTC cough syrups contain soothing substances, e.g. syrup, **glycerol**. The high sugar content stimulates the production of saliva and soothes the oropharynx. The associated swallowing may also interfere with the cough reflex. The sweet taste itself may be antitussive by stimulating the release of endogenous opioids in the brain stem, and this may contribute to the large placebo effect seen in RCTs of demulcents.[8] Honey, a traditional remedy, presumably acts in the same way.[9]

However, the antitussive effect of demulcents is generally short-lived, often no better than placebo, and there is no evidence that combination products are better than **simple linctus BP** (5mL t.d.s.–q.d.s.). Thus, if **simple linctus BP** is ineffective, there is little point in trying OTC combination products.

Opioids and opioid derivatives

Opioids (e.g. **codeine, pholcodine, hydrocodone** (not UK), **morphine**) and their derivatives (e.g. **dextromethorphan**) are predominantly centrally acting antitussives. All are common ingredients in OTC combination antitussive products, but often in small and probably ineffective doses.[10] Thus, the benefit of OTC combination products may reside mainly in the sugar content (see Demulcents above).[8] The MHRA has advised against the use of OTC cough products containing **codeine** for those under 18 years old (contra-indicated in under 12 years old) and **dextromethorphan** and **pholcodine** for those under 6 years old.[11,12]

For analgesia in palliative care, strong opioids are increasingly preferred over weak opioids (p.376).[3] The same rationale can also be applied to cough, particularly because higher quality evidence supports **morphine** (but *not* **codeine**) as an effective antitussive, albeit in a non-cancer chronic cough setting.[13,14]

For opioid-naïve patients, the initial dose is generally **morphine** 10–20mg/24h (see Drug treatment below). For those already receiving strong opioids, there is no evidence to guide practice. A pragmatic approach is to evaluate the effect of a p.r.n. dose; if this relieves the cough, continue to use it in this way or increase the regular dose. However, if no benefit is obtained from a p.r.n. dose, this suggests there would be little point in further regular dose increments. Some patients with cough but no pain benefit from a bedtime dose of **morphine** to prevent cough disturbing sleep.

If a weak opioid is used, **codeine** is preferred to **pholcodine**, which has little analgesic effect. **Pholcodine** has been withdrawn in some countries because of concerns that it may cause IgE sensitization to neuromuscular blocking agents.[15] However, the EMA concluded that the evidence for this is weak and that the risk–benefit ratio for **pholcodine** remains favourable.[16] If **codeine** or **hydrocodone** (not UK)[17] is ineffective, **morphine** should be prescribed. *If a patient is already receiving a strong opioid for pain relief, it is a nonsense to prescribe* ***codeine*** *as well.*

Local anaesthetics

Nebulized local anaesthetics have been used as antitussives in patients with chronic cough and also cancer.[18-20] They probably act locally by inhibiting the sensory nerves in the airways involved in the cough reflex, but there could be a central effect as well. Their use has not been evaluated in an RCT, and they should be considered only when other measures have failed.

Typical doses are 5mL of either **lidocaine** 2% or **bupivacaine** 0.25% nebulized t.d.s.–q.d.s. In a case series of 100 patients with chronic cough given nebulized **lidocaine**, only about 20% considered their cough much improved and would definitely recommend it to other patients.[19] Undesirable effects include:

- unpleasant taste; irritation of the mouth or throat[19]
- oropharyngeal numbness → reduced gag/cough reflex; patients should be advised not to eat or drink for 1h after treatment to reduce risk of aspiration
- risk of bronchoconstriction; consider pretreatment with **salbutamol** in asthmatic patients[20]
- a short duration of action (10–30min).[10]

Even so, there are anecdotal reports of patients with chronic lung disease, sarcoidosis or cancer in whom a single treatment with nebulized **lidocaine** 400mg relieved cough for 1–8 weeks.[21-23] Also see Chapter 31, p.904.

Benzonatate (not UK) is chemically related to the **procaine** class of local anaesthetics. It acts peripherally by inhibiting the stretch receptors in the lower respiratory tract, lungs and pleura. It acts in 15–20min, and the effect lasts 3–8h. It is used PO at some centres in the USA when opioids fail or are poorly tolerated.[24]

Management strategy

Correct the correctable

If possible, the cause of the cough should be treated specifically, e.g. antibacterials for infection, and aggravating factors removed, e.g. smoking. However, when the cause of the cough is not amenable to specific treatment or is unknown, measures should be taken to suppress the cough (see Drugs for cough, Figure 1, p.155).

Non-drug treatment

Speech pathology therapy includes patient education, cough suppression techniques, breathing exercises and laryngeal hygiene.

Drug treatment

If a locally soothing demulcent (e.g. **simple linctus BP** 5mL t.d.s.–q.d.s.) is inadequate, consider a centrally acting opioid antitussive (see also Opioids above):

- **morphine**, starting with:
  - ▷ an *immediate-release* formulation 2.5–5mg PO q.d.s.–q4h *or*
  - ▷ a *modified-release* formulation 5–10mg PO b.d.
- if necessary, increase the dose until the cough is relieved or until undesirable effects prevent further escalation (see p.404).

If a patient is already receiving a strong opioid for pain relief, it is a nonsense to prescribe a second strong opioid (or **codeine**) for cough suppression.

If opioid antitussives are unsatisfactory, other possible treatments include:

- **sodium cromoglicate** 10mg inhaled q.d.s. improves cough in patients with lung cancer within 36–48h[25]
- **gabapentin** 300–600mg PO t.d.s. is more effective than placebo in idiopathic chronic cough (NNT = 3.6 for a meaningful reduction in Leicester Cough Questionnaire score);[26] case reports, including patients with cancer, have used smaller starting doses, e.g. 100–300mg PO once daily, titrated upwards every 3–4 days.[27,28] **Pregabalin** is also of benefit in idiopathic cough[29]
- **diazepam**, e.g. 5mg PO once daily/at bedtime, is reported to have an effect in intractable cough associated with lung metastases[30]
- **baclofen** 10mg PO t.d.s. or 20mg PO once daily has an antitussive effect in healthy volunteers and in patients with ACE inhibitor cough; maximum effect is seen after 2–4 weeks[31]
- **amitriptyline** 10mg PO at bedtime improves cough in post-viral vagal neuropathy.[13,32]

Amitriptyline (p.228), **baclofen** (p.658), **diazepam** (p.163) and **gabapentinoids** (p.297) all have neuro-inhibitory effects. They may act by interfering with the cough reflex and/or central sensitization which leads to cough hypersensitivity, present in most patients with chronic cough.[33] **Baclofen** also inhibits relaxation of the lower oesophageal sphincter, and this was considered a possible advantage in chronic cough associated with gastro-oesophageal reflux. However, in patients failing to benefit from a PPI and a prokinetic, **baclofen** and **gabapentin** are equally effective, with the latter better tolerated.[34]

Other (non-UK) options include:

- **levodropropizine** 75mg PO t.d.s. (not UK) is as effective as **dihydrocodeine** 10mg PO t.d.s. in patients with lung cancer and causes less drowsiness[35,36]
- **benzonatate** 100mg PO t.d.s. (not UK); if necessary, increase to 200mg t.d.s. It has a narrow safety margin. The capsules must not be chewed or opened, because of the risk of enhanced absorption producing toxic plasma levels.[37]

Supply

Simple linctus BP

Oral syrup 28 days @ 5mL q.d.s. = £3.
Available OTC.

Morphine sulfate

Oral solution 2mg/mL (10mg/5mL), 28 days @ 5mg q.d.s. = £6.
Also see **Morphine**, p.404, for other formulations.

Morphine solution is available in two strengths: 2mg/mL and a high-potency concentrate of 20mg/mL supplied with a calibrated syringe. *Deaths have occurred from accidental overdose with the concentrated solution*, mostly when doses prescribed in *mg* were administered as *mL*, resulting in *20 times* the prescribed dose being given.[38]

Sodium cromoglicate
Intal® (Sanofi)
Aerosol inhalation 5mg/dose, 28 days@ 2 puffs q.d.s. = £36.

Also see **gabapentin** and **pregabalin** (p.297), **amitriptyline** (p.228), benzodiazepines and Z-drugs (for **diazepam**, p.163) and **baclofen** monographs (p.658).

1 Smith JA and Badri H (2019) Cough: New Pharmacology. *Journal of Allergy and Clinical Immunology: In Practice*. **7**: 1731–1738.
2 Molassiotis M *et al.* (2015) Interventions for cough in cancer. *Cochrane Database of Systematic Reviews*. **5**: CD007881. www.thecochranelibrary.com.
3 Wee B *et al.* (2012) Management of chronic cough in patients receiving palliative care: review of evidence and recommendations by a task group of the Association for Palliative Medicine of Great Britain and Ireland. *Palliative Medicine*. **26**: 780–787.
4 Molassiotis A *et al.* (2017) Symptomatic treatment of cough among adult patients with lung cancer: CHEST guideline and expert panel report. *Chest*. **151**: 861–874.
5 Gibson P *et al.* (2016) Treatment of unexplained chronic cough: CHEST guideline and expert panel report. *Chest*. **149**: 27–44.
6 Birring SS *et al.* (2018) Treatment of interstitial lung disease associated cough: CHEST guideline and expert panel report. *Chest*. **154**: 904–917.
7 Slinger C *et al.* (2018) Speech and language therapy for management of chronic cough. *Cochrane Database of Systematic Reviews*. CD013067.

8 Eccles R (2006) Mechanisms of the placebo effect of sweet cough syrups. *Respiratory Physiology and Neurobiology*. **152**: 340–348.
9 Oduwole O *et al.* (2018) Honey for acute cough in children. *Cochrane Database of Systematic Reviews*. CD007094.
10 Fuller R and Jackson D (1990) Physiology and treatment of cough. *Thorax*. **45**: 425–430.
11 MHRA (2015) Codeine for cough and cold: restricted use in children. *Drug Safety Update*. www.gov.uk/drug-safety-update.
12 MHRA (2009) Over-the-counter cough and cold medicines for children. *Drug Safety Update*. www.gov.uk/drug-safety-update.
13 Ryan NM *et al.* (2018) An update and systematic review on drug therapies for the treatment of refractory chronic cough. *Expert Opinion on Pharmacotherapy*. **19**: 687–711.
14 Dicpinigaitis PV *et al.* (2014) Antitussive drugs – past, present, and future. *Pharmacology Review*. **66**: 468–512.
15 Florvaag E and Johansson SG (2012) The pholcodine case. Cough medicines, igE-sensitization, and anaphylaxis: a devious connection. *World Allergy Organ Journal*. **5**: 73–78.
16 EMA (2011) Questions and answers on the review of the marketing authorisations for medicines containing pholcodine. Available from: www.ema.europa.eu.
17 Homsi J *et al.* (2002) A phase II study of hydrocodone for cough in advanced cancer. *American Journal of Hospice and Palliative Care*. **19 (1)**: 49–56.
18 Truesdale K and Jurdi A (2013) Nebulized lidocaine in the treatment of intractable cough. *American Journal of Hospital Palliative Care*. **30**: 587–589.
19 Lim KG *et al.* (2013) Long-term safety of nebulized lidocaine for adults with difficult-to-control chronic cough: a case series. *Chest*. **143**: 1060–1065.
20 Slaton RM *et al.* (2013) Evidence for therapeutic uses of nebulized lidocaine in the treatment of intractable cough and asthma. *Annals of Pharmacotherpy*. **47**: 578–585.
21 Howard P *et al.* (1977) Lignocaine aerosol and persistent cough. *British Journal of Diseases of the Chest*. **71**: 19–24.
22 Stewart C and Coady T (1977) Suppression of intractable cough. *British Medical Journal*. **1**: 1660–1661.
23 Sanders RV and Kirkpatrick MB (1984) Prolonged suppression of cough after inhalation of lidocaine in a patient with sarcoid. *Journal of the American Medical Association*. **252**: 2456–2457.
24 Doona M and Walsh D (1998) Benzonatate for opioid-resistant cough in advanced cancer. *Palliative Medicine*. **12**: 55–58.
25 Moroni M *et al.* (1996) Inhaled sodium cromoglycate to treat cough in advanced lung cancer patients. *British Journal of Cancer*. **74**: 309–311.
26 Ryan NM *et al.* (2012) Gabapentin for refractory chronic cough: a randomised, double-blind, placebo-controlled trial. *Lancet*. **380**: 1583–1589.
27 Shi G *et al.* (2018) Efficacy and safety of gabapentin in the treatment of chronic cough: A systematic review. *Tuberculosis and Respiratory Diseases*. **81**: 167–174.
28 Razzak R *et al.* (2017) Gabapentin for cough in cancer. *Journal of Pain and Palliative Care Pharmacotherapy*. **31**: 195–197.
29 Vertigan AE *et al.* (2016) Pregabalin and speech pathology combination therapy for refractory chronic cough: A randomized controlled trial. *Chest*. **149**: 639–648.
30 Estfan B and Walsh D (2008) The cough from hell: diazepam for intractable cough in a patient with renal cell carcinoma. *Journal of Pain and Symptom Management*. **36**: 553–538.
31 Dicpinigaitis P *et al.* (1998) Inhibition of capsaicin-induced cough by the gamma-aminobutyric acid agonist baclofen. *Journal of Clinical Pharmacology*. **38**: 364–367.
32 Jeyakumar A *et al.* (2006) Effectiveness of amitriptyline versus cough suppressants in the treatment of chronic cough resulting from postviral vagal neuropathy. *Laryngoscope*. **116**: 2108–2112.
33 Smith JA and Woodcock A (2016) Chronic Cough. *New England Journal of Medicine*. **375**: 1544–1551.
34 Dong R *et al.* (2019) Randomised clinical trial: gabapentin vs baclofen in the treatment of suspected refractory gastro-oesophageal reflux-induced chronic cough. *Alimentary Pharmacology & Therapeutics*. **49**: 714–722.
35 Luporini G *et al.* (1998) Efficacy and safety of levodropropizine and dihydrocodeine on nonproductive cough in primary and metastatic lung cancer. *European Respiratory Journal*. **12**: 97–101.
36 Birring S *et al.* (2019) Antitussive therapy: A role for levodropropizine. *Pulmonary Pharmacology & Therapeutics*. **56**: 79–85.
37 Bishop-Freeman SC *et al.* (2017) Benzonatate Toxicity: Nothing to cough at. *Journal of Analytical Toxicology*. **41**: 461–463.
38 FDA (2011) Medwatch safety alert. Morphine sulfate oral solution 100mg per 5mL (20mg/mL): medication use error - reports of accidental overdose. Available from: www.fda.gov/Safety/MedWatch/SafetyInformation (archived).

Updated November 2019

4: CENTRAL NERVOUS SYSTEM

4

BENZODIAZEPINES AND Z-DRUGS

Class: GABAmimetics; hypnotics (Z-drugs and short-acting benzodiazepines); anxiolytics (long-acting benzodiazepines).

Indications: Authorized indications vary; see individual SPCs for details. Insomnia; anxiety and panic disorder; seizures; myoclonus; skeletal muscle spasm; alcohol withdrawal; sedation; †agitation in the imminently dying; †catatonia; †restless legs syndrome; †drug-induced movement disorders; †neuropathic pain; †spasticity; †nausea and vomiting; †intractable pruritus; †intractable hiccup.

Contra-indications: Unless in the imminently dying: acute severe pulmonary insufficiency, untreated sleep apnoea syndrome, severe hepatic impairment, myasthenia gravis. Also see individual SPCs.

Pharmacology

GABA is the major inhibitory neurotransmitter of the nervous system. Several drug classes enhance its action (GABAmimetics):[1-4]

- $GABA_A$ modulators: benzodiazepines, Z-drugs (e.g. **zopiclone**), ethanol, barbiturates, some general anaesthetics (e.g. **propofol**), valerian (herbal product)
- $GABA_B$ agonists: **baclofen**, **sodium oxybate**
- inhibitors of GABA transaminase (e.g. **vigabatrin**) or re-uptake (e.g. **tiagabine**).

The $GABA_A$ receptor is a chloride channel formed by five subunits comprising varying subtypes (Figure 1). $GABA_A$ modulators bind to sites distinct from GABA itself (allosteric modulation), increasing the receptor's affinity for GABA (benzodiazepines) or prolonging channel opening (barbiturates).[5] The α subunit of the $GABA_A$ receptor, of which there are six subtypes, is the predominant determinant of benzodiazepine affinity and function (Table 1).

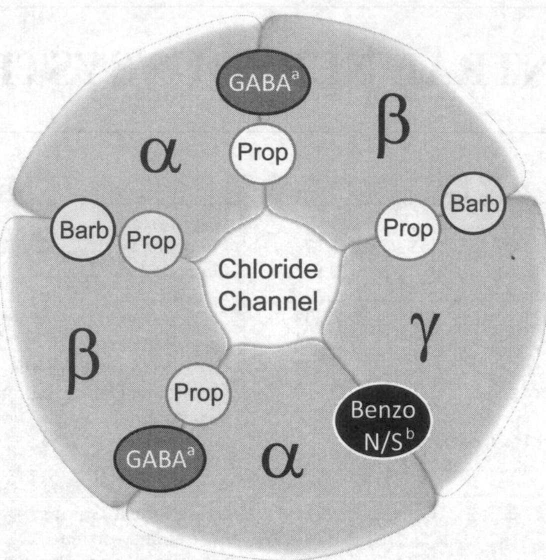

Figure 1 The $GABA_A$ receptor and selected drug binding sites.[5,6]

Abbreviations: Barb = barbiturates; Benzo = benzodiazepines; N/S = neurosteroids; Prop = propofol

a. the central chloride channel is opened by the concurrent binding of two GABA molecules

b. benzodiazepines bind to the same site as endogenous neurosteroids.

Synaptic channels (α1–3) detect intermittent (phasic) release of GABA within the synapse. GABA is then partly removed by a re-uptake transporter, with the remainder diffusing away from the synapse forming a diffuse tonic (i.e. relatively stable) background. The latter is detected by extra-synaptic (α4–6) channels.[7] Synaptic channels are more likely than extra-synaptic channels to become desensitized by repeated stimulation.[8] This partly explains why some actions (e.g. hypnotic and anti-epileptic effects) diminish over time more quickly than others (e.g. undesirable cognitive effects; also see Table 1).[9]

The sedative effects of benzodiazepines and Z-drugs result from α1-$GABA_A$ receptor-mediated inhibition of the wakefulness-promoting system (see Melatonin, Figure 2, p.181).[10] Their anxiolytic effects result from α2-$GABA_A$ receptor-mediated inhibition of 'fear circuits', which are co-ordinated by the amygdala (Figure 2). Further, benzodiazepines increase the synthesis of neurosteroids with anxiolytic effects.[5] The location and α-subunits involved in the anti-epileptic effects of benzodiazepines vary depending on seizure type.

Selective modulation of α-subunits might improve tolerability by separating desirable from undesirable effects. **Clobazam** and its active *N*-desmethyl metabolite bind relatively selectively to α2-subunits.[11,12] This may explain the lower incidence of sedation and cognitive impairment with **clobazam** compared with other benzodiazepines.[13] More selective α2-modulators are under investigation, e.g. as non-sedating anxiolytics and antihyperalgesics.[12,14] Z-drugs are more α1-selective, but the clinical relevance is questionable because many undesirable effects are direct consequences of sedation. Although indirect comparisons find fewer undesirable effects with Z-drugs compared with benzodiazepine hypnotics,[15] this may reflect their shorter halflives rather than subunit selectivity.

Most benzodiazepines and Z-drugs are well absorbed PO, widely distributed and hepatically metabolized before being eliminated. **Clobazam**, **diazepam** and **midazolam** all have active metabolites (Table 2). Their receptor profiles are similar (Table 1) but their halflives (Table 2) and potency (Table 3) differ. Their varied metabolic pathways affect their pharmacogenetic profiles and drug interactions (see below and individual SPCs).

Table 1 $GABA_A$ α-subunit subtypes and relative activity of selected GABAmimetics[1,7-9,11,12,14,16,17]

Location		*GABAergic synapses (phasic response to GABA release)*			*Extra-synaptic (tonic response to background GABA)*		
Alpha-subunit subtype		*1*	*2*	*3*	*4*[a]	*5*	*6*[a]
Function of agonists		*Addiction* *Amnesia* *Anti-epilepsis*[b] *Sleep*	*Anxiolysis* *Antihyperalgesia* *Muscle relaxation*	*Antihyperalgesia* *Muscle relaxation*		*Amnesia* *Cognitive impairment* *Benzodiazepine tolerance*	
Benzodiazepines	Clobazam[c]	+	++	+	–	++	+[c]
	Clonazepam	++	++	++	–	++	–
	Diazepam	++	++	++	–	++	–
	Flunitrazepam	++	++	++	–	++	–
	Midazolam	++		++	–	++	–
Z-drugs	Zolpidem[d]	++	+	+	–	–	–
	Zopiclone	++	++	–/+[d]	–	+	–
Other	Ethanol[e]	+	+	+	++	+	+
	Neurosteroids	+	+	+	++	++	++
	Pentobarbital	++	++	++	++	++	

Activity: ++ high, + low, – negligible or none; blank = no data

a. benzodiazepines do not bind to α4- and α6-subunits, or to receptors lacking α- and γ-subunits (benzodiazepine-insensitive $GABA_A$ receptors)

b. relative importance of subunits varies with different seizure models

c. clobazam and its active *N*-desmethyl metabolite are α2-selective. The clinical significance of clobazam binding to the (generally benzodiazepine-insensitive) α6 channel is unclear

d. subunit affinity varies with different β- and γ-subunit configurations. Before cloning, $GABA_A$ classifications encompassed more than one subunit configuration, which may account for earlier conflicting affinity data

e. tonic α4(δ)-mediated inhibition predominates at lower doses, whereas synaptic (α1, 2 and 3) effects are responsible for severe intoxication. Ethanol also enhances release of GABA and GABAmimetic neurosteroids.

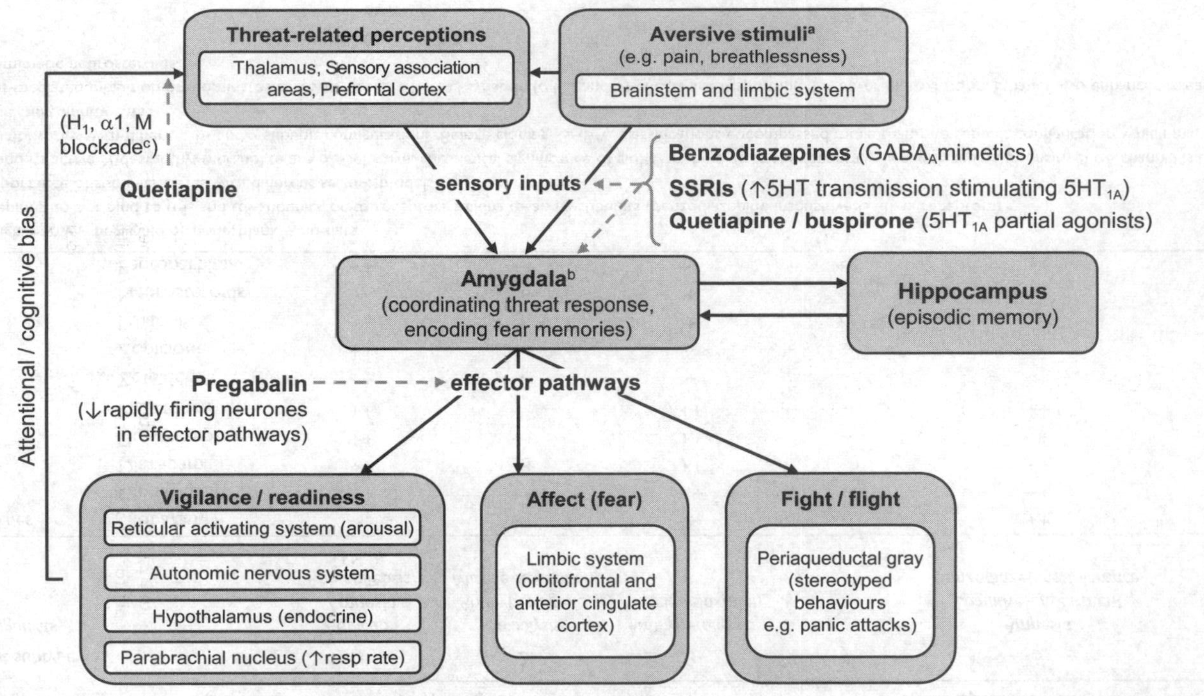

Figure 2 Putative sites of action of anxiolytics on fear circuits.[3,4,18-20]

Abbreviations: α_1 = alpha adrenergic type 1 receptor; $GABA_A$ = gamma-aminobutyric acid type A; H_1 = histamine type 1 receptor; 5HT = 5-hydroxytryptamine (serotonin); $5HT_{1A}$ = serotonin type 1A receptor; M = muscarinic acetylcholine receptor

a. aversive stimuli are conveyed to the amygdala both directly and after 'higher' processing, e.g. perceived context

b. $GABA_A$ and $5HT_{1A}$ receptors alter both sensory input and amygdala circuits. Not all antipsychotics are $5HT_{1A}$ agonists, and thus their anxiolytic properties vary (see Antipsychotics, Table 1, p.188)

c. quetiapine also affects monoamines involved in arousal and attention, but their relative importance to its anxiolytic effects are unclear.

Table 2 Pharmacokinetics of selected benzodiazepines and related drugs; PO unless stated otherwise[21-25]

Drug	*Bio-availability PO (%)*	T_{max} *(h)*	*Plasma halflife (h)*	*Metabolism*
Alprazolam	≥90[a]	1–2	12–15	CYP3A4
Clobazam	85	0.5–4	35; (80)[b]	CYP3A4[b]; metabolite inactivated by CYP2C19
Clonazepam	>80	1–4	20–60	Multiple non-P450 pathways[b]
Diazepam	>90 65–85 (PR)	0.5–1.5 ≤0.5 (PR) ≤0.25 (IV) 1–2 (IM)[c]	25–50; (≤200)[b]	Multiple P450 pathways[b]
Lorazepam	90	2.5 2.5 (SL)	10–20	Non-P450 glucuronidation
Midazolam	40 95 (SC) 85 (buccal)	0.5–1 0.5 (SC) ≤0.5 (buccal)	1–4[d]; (1)[b]	CYP3A4[b]
Oxazepam	≥90[a]	1–5	6–20	Non-P450 glucuronidation
Temazepam	≥90[a]	1	8–15	Non-P450 glucuronidation
Zolpidem	70	1.5	2	CYP3A4 and CYP1A2
Zopiclone	75	1.5	3.5	CYP3A4[b]

a. estimated
b. active metabolite(s)
c. 1–1.5h for oil-based formulation; 2h for emulsion formulation
d. up to 24h when given by CIVI in critical care.

Cautions

Chronic respiratory disease (risk of respiratory depression, particularly when given IV); history of substance abuse.

Renal or hepatic impairment

Benzodiazepines and Z-drugs differ in their potential to cause toxicity in renal and hepatic impairment (see Chapter 17, p.741 and Chapter 18, p.771 respectively). Lower starting doses and slower titration may be necessary (see individual SPCs), particularly for those drugs with a long halflife, e.g. **clonazepam**, **diazepam, lorazepam** or renally excreted active metabolites, e.g. **midazolam**.[26] Unless in the imminently dying, all are contra-indicated in severe hepatic impairment (see Chapter 18, Box D, p.779).

Suicide risk

It is not known if benzodiazepines are associated with suicidal thoughts and behaviour; the manufacturer of **clonazepam** advises similar caution to that for other anti-epileptics (see p.287).

Drug interactions

Concurrent treatment with ≥2 CNS depressants (e.g. benzodiazepines, gabapentinoids, opioids) increases the risk of respiratory depression, particularly in susceptible groups, e.g. the elderly and those with renal or hepatic impairment.[27]

Fatalities from oversedation or cardiorespiratory depression have occurred after concurrent use of **midazolam** with higher than approved doses of parenteral **olanzapine** (not UK) (see p.204).

The metabolism of Z-drugs and several benzodiazepines is mostly CYP3A4 dependent (Table 2), and plasma concentrations may be decreased or increased to a clinically relevant degree by moderate or potent CYP3A4 inducers (e.g. **carbamazepine**, **enzalutamide**, **phenytoin**, **rifampicin**) or inhibitors (e.g. antifungal azoles, **clarithromycin**, **diltiazem**, **erythromycin**, protease inhibitors, **verapamil**) respectively (see Chapter 19, Table 8, p.790). Adjust doses, increase monitoring and/or explain the need for increased caution (e.g. the likelihood of increased morning impairment with hypnotics). For example, the use of CYP3A4 inducers and inhibitors is clinically significant with **midazolam**, particularly with PO **midazolam** (not UK):

- overall exposure to **midazolam** can be reduced by ≤90% after the addition of a CYP3A4 inducer; use of a different benzodiazepine is recommended if a moderate or potent inducer is essential[28]
- plasma concentrations of **midazolam** can be eight times higher after the addition of a CYP3A4 inhibitor.[29] Thus ≥50% reduction in the midazolam dose may be needed when a moderate or potent inhibitor is used concurrently.

Diazepam clearance is reduced by ≤65% by **fluvoxamine** (a potent CYP2C19 inhibitor).[28]

Together, **phenytoin** and either **diazepam** or **clonazepam** have unpredictable effects on each other's plasma concentrations. Monitor the **phenytoin** plasma concentration.

Clinically significant pharmacokinetic interactions are less likely with **lorazepam**, **oxazepam** or **temazepam**, because of their non-P450 metabolism (Table 2).

Undesirable effects

Benzodiazepines with long halflives accumulate when given repeatedly, and undesirable effects may manifest only after several days or weeks. Appropriate monitoring is required, particularly for those at greater risk of drowsiness, falls and memory and cognitive impairment, e.g. the elderly or frail patients.

Dose-dependent drowsiness, impaired psychomotor skills (e.g. impaired driving ability), reduced independence, fatigue, cognitive impairment, hypotonia (manifesting as unsteadiness/ataxia) with an increased (almost double) risk of femoral fracture in the elderly.[30,31]

Paradoxical arousal, agitation and aggression can occur in <10%; risk factors include high-trait anxiety, borderline personality disorder and alcohol misuse.[32-34]

Less commonly, complex actions while apparently asleep (e.g. driving, eating, cooking, conversations) occur with both benzodiazepines and Z-drugs.[35]

Benzodiazepines and Z-drugs can cause physical and psychological dependence.

Clonazepam has been associated with salivary hypersecretion and drooling in children.

Diazepam may cause painful thrombophlebitis when given IV.

Toxicity from propylene glycol, an excipient in parenteral **lorazepam**, has been reported with prolonged high-dose IVI, resulting in confusion, drowsiness, seizures, cardiac arrhythmias and/or renal failure.[36] However, the doses necessary in palliative care are unlikely to approach the mean dose of **lorazepam** (270mg/24h) required to achieve toxic levels of propylene glycol.

Zopiclone commonly causes an unpleasant taste.

Risk of cancer, dementia and increased mortality

Observational studies have explored the association of benzodiazepine and Z-drug use with risk of dementia, cancer and overall mortality, with conflicting results. Interpretation is made difficult by multiple confounding factors (e.g. smoking, obesity, alcohol, higher use in those with more severe illness) and use of benzodiazepines and Z-drugs for the prodromal sleep disturbance and anxiety that commonly precede a diagnosis of dementia.[37-46] Thus, no definite causal link has been established.

In US veterans with chronic non-cancer pain, the concurrent use of a benzodiazepine with an opioid was associated with higher mortality and morbidity than with an opioid alone. However, the strongest association was with self-inflicted injury.[47] Notably, most pains were poorly opioid-responsive and patients under an oncologist or palliative care were excluded from the study. Thus, it is unclear how these findings relate to patients with opioid-responsive pains due to advanced life-limiting illness. However, in the last days–weeks of life, the use of a benzodiazepine ± an opioid is *not* associated with shortened survival.[48]

Dose and use of benzodiazepines and Z-drugs in palliative care

Consider alternatives if using for ≥4 weeks; dependence can occur.[49]

Benzodiazepines are generally safer in overdose than barbiturates and tricyclic antidepressants. However, fatal iatrogenic overdoses of IV **midazolam** have occurred during procedural sedation. Thus, regulators recommend that **flumazenil** is available for emergency use wherever **midazolam** is used clinically.[50]

Benzodiazepines are included in a law in England, Wales and Scotland relating to driving with certain drugs above specified plasma concentrations, see, p.809.

Insomnia

Initial treatment includes:

- correcting contributory factors if possible:[51-54]
  - ▷ pain
  - ▷ delirium
  - ▷ depression, anxiety or rumination
  - ▷ drugs, e.g. alcohol, corticosteroids (see p.556)
  - ▷ obstructive sleep apnoea
  - ▷ parasomnias, e.g. nightmares, sleep walking (Box A)
- non-drug measures, e.g. sleep hygiene, increased daytime lighting, psychological and complementary therapies.[55]

Where drug treatment is required, consider a hypnotic drug that may help the underlying cause (e.g. delirium → **quetiapine** (p.208); depression → **mirtazapine** (p.241)). Otherwise, use a Z-drug or a short-halflife benzodiazepine, ideally for <4 weeks:

- **zolpidem** (halflife 2h) 10mg PO at bedtime (5mg initially if elderly or frail) *or*
- **zopiclone** (halflife 3.5h) 7.5mg PO at bedtime (3.75mg initially if elderly or frail) *or*
- **midazolam** (halflife 1–4h) 2.5mg SC at bedtime,[56] e.g. when PO route unavailable.

Generic Z-drugs are cheaper than **temazepam** (halflife 8–15h). Although the latter is available as an oral solution, it is significantly more expensive. See Chapter 28 (p.853) for other options for patients with swallowing difficulties or an EFT.

Box A Parasomnias (nightmares, sleep walking and related phenomena)[59,61-63]

Classification

Parasomnias are behaviours or fear responses occurring during sleep. Nightmares and REM sleep behaviour disorder (RBD) occur during rapid eye movement (REM) sleep and are thus generally recalled once awake; conversely, sleep walking and night terrors occur during non-REM sleep and are not.

Causes

- Drug-related, including:
  - ▷ antidepressants (on starting/stopping)
  - ▷ β-blockers
  - ▷ cholinesterase inhibitors
  - ▷ hypnotics (particularly zolpidem)
  - ▷ levodopa
  - ▷ tramadol (other opioids are *not* implicated)
- Neurodegenerative disease (particularly RBD; may precede diagnosis by several years):
  - ▷ Parkinson's disease
  - ▷ multi-system atrophy.

Treatment

Nightmares due to post-traumatic stress disorder

Prazosin, an α-blocker, is effective:

- start prazosin 1mg PO at bedtime
- increase by 1mg every 2–3 days
- mean effective dose 6–10mg/24h.

Monitor blood pressure; postural hypotension and dizziness are common undesirable effects. Because other α-blockers cross the blood–brain barrier less readily, benefit for nightmares is unlikely to be a class effect.

Other parasomnias

Seek advice from a sleep specialist. Clonazepam and melatonin (p.180) are commonly used, but no symptomatic treatment has been consistently effective in RCTs.

A meta-analysis confirmed that, in people >60 years of age, benzodiazepines and Z-drugs had an NNT of 13 but an NNH of 6.[57] The undesirable effects were cognitive impairment, daytime drowsiness, ataxia and falls. Even low doses of short halflife benzodiazepines increase the risk of falls.[58] Alternatives include sedating antidepressants (e.g. **doxepin**, **mirtazapine**, **trazodone**; see p.222) and **melatonin** (p.180).[59]

For sleep disturbance in dementia, neither benzodiazepines nor Z-drugs have been examined in RCTs; **trazodone** may be beneficial, but **melatonin** is *ineffective*.[60]

Anxiety and panic disorder

The efficacy of cognitive behavioral therapy and of drug treatment are comparable.[64] Choice of drug is largely influenced by likely duration of use:

- benzodiazepine, if prognosis is days to weeks:
  - ▷ **diazepam** 2–10mg PO at bedtime and p.r.n. *or*
  - ▷ **lorazepam** 500microgram–1mg PO b.d. and p.r.n. *or*
  - ▷ **midazolam** 5–10mg/24h CSCI
- SSRI (± a benzodiazepine initially), if prognosis is months.

Pregabalin (p.297) and **quetiapine** (p.208) act within days but are less effective and less well tolerated, respectively, than SSRIs.[65,66] Thus, they are reserved for second-/third-line use or where there are concurrent indications, e.g. neuropathic pain, delirium.

If anxiety persists, anxiolytics with different sites of action (Figure 2) are combined, e.g. a monoamine re-uptake inhibitor with **pregabalin**.

Because of dependence and undesirable effects, long-term (>4 weeks) use of benzodiazepines is reserved for severe anxiety refractory to other treatments.[49] Tolerance to their anxiolytic effects may not occur.[9]

Seizures

Acute treatment

Benzodiazepines are first-line treatments for acute seizures (also see Anti-epileptics, p.290), including status epilepticus.[67] Although IV **lorazepam** is generally recommended for the control of status epilepticus, IM **midazolam** is as effective:

- **lorazepam** 4mg IV (diluted 1:1 with sodium chloride 0.9% or WFI) over 2min; repeat once after 10–20min if needed *or*
- **midazolam** 10mg buccal/SC/IM stat or IV over 2min; repeat once after 10min if needed.

The **midazolam** injection formulation can be given buccally in status epilepticus. **Midazolam** oromucosal solutions for buccal administration, authorized for children and adolescents, are available (see Buccal administration, below). In children, buccal **midazolam** is more effective than rectal **diazepam**.[68]

In the imminently dying

- manage acute seizures with **midazolam** 10mg buccal/SC/IM stat or IV over 2min; repeat once after 10min if needed
- for prophylaxis, commence **midazolam** 20–30mg/24h CSCI
- if seizures persist, consider switching to **phenobarbital** (p.315).

If it is desirable to avoid sedation, consider alternative SC/CSCI anti-epileptics, e.g. **lacosamide**,[69] **levetiracetam** (p.312), **valproate** (p.307).

Chronic treatment

Long-term use is limited by the development of tolerance; thus, benzodiazepines are reserved for epilepsy refractory to other measures:

- **clobazam**
  - ▷ start with 20–30mg PO at bedtime
  - ▷ if necessary, increase by 20–30mg every 5–7 days up to 60mg/24h
- **clonazepam**
  - ▷ start with 500microgram–1mg PO at bedtime
  - ▷ if necessary, increase by 500microgram every 3–5 days up to 2–4mg, occasionally more
  - ▷ doses above 2mg can be divided, e.g. 2mg at bedtime and 1mg each morning.

Myoclonus

Treat the underlying cause if possible:

- drug-related, e.g. opioids, **gabapentin**, **pregabalin**: consider dose reduction or switching to an alternative
- metabolic disturbance, e.g. hyponatraemia, uraemia.

Otherwise, consider a benzodiazepine, e.g.:

- **clonazepam** 500microgram PO at bedtime *or*
- **midazolam** 2.5mg SC stat and 10mg/24h CSCI in imminently dying patients.

If necessary, give p.r.n. doses and consider increasing the regular dose.

†Spasticity and skeletal muscle spasm

Benzodiazepines are reserved for spasticity where **baclofen**, **dantrolene** and **tizanidine** are ineffective or where short-term SC/CSCI administration is desirable (see Skeletal muscle relaxants, p.655).

Benzodiazepines are also alternatives to **baclofen** for pain due to skeletal muscle spasm, if the anticipated duration of use is ≤4 weeks or parenteral treatment is required:

- **diazepam** 2–5mg PO at bedtime and p.r.n. *or*
- **midazolam** 10mg/24h CSCI.

Alcohol withdrawal

Benzodiazepines reduce withdrawal symptoms, particularly seizures.[70] The choice is as for acute treatment of seizures (see above), with dose and route dependent on severity of withdrawal syndrome. **Gabapentin** (p.297) and barbiturates are alternatives if benzodiazepines are insufficient.[71,72]

†Agitation in the imminently dying

Because this is often a feature of hyperactive delirium, some centres use antipsychotics first-line to treat agitation in the imminently dying (Box B). When insufficient, the use of an antipsychotic and a benzodiazepine together is more effective than continuing with an antipsychotic alone.[73]

Benzodiazepines are an alternative first-line choice, particularly when anxiety is prominent. In various case series, the mean effective dose of **midazolam** was 15–60mg/24h (range 5–200mg/24h).[74-83]

†Catatonia

Because it is exacerbated by antipsychotics, it is important to differentiate catatonia from delirium (Box C).

†Sedation for massive haemorrhage

Readily available 'crisis' medication is often recommended (e.g. **midazolam**), but unless immediately available it is of no use in the event of a massive haemorrhage: the patient would be left alone during those final seconds of consciousness while **midazolam** was obtained and administered and/or die before the medication could take effect. Sitting with the patient and holding their hand is the only realistic comfort measure.[87] However, if the patient does not die immediately and is distressed, give:

- **midazolam** 5–10mg buccal/SC/IM/IV.

†Breathlessness

Benzodiazepines do not relieve breathlessness per se,[88] but anxiolytics do have a role when *anxiety* exacerbates breathlessness. Either a benzodiazepine or an SSRI is used, depending on prognosis (see above). In an RCT (n=432), **buspirone** 20mg/24h, a $5HT_{1A}$ partial agonist, was ineffective for breathlessness and anxiety in cancer.[89]

In the last days of life, for patients with distressing breathlessness at rest, the combined use of an opioid with a benzodiazepine is more effective than either alone (see Morphine, p.414).[90] Start with:

- **midazolam** 2.5mg SC q1h p.r.n. and 10mg/24h CSCI.

†Restless legs syndrome

Clonazepam is sometimes used when first-line options (e.g. **gabapentin**, **pregabalin**, **ropinirole**, **rotigotine**) are ineffective or inappropriate (see p.297):[91-93]

- **clonazepam** 500microgram PO at bedtime, increased if necessary to 1mg at bedtime.[92]

Box B Drugs for agitation in the imminently dying

First-line drugs

Haloperidol (particularly if delirium present or probable)

- start with 1.5–5mg SC stat and q1h p.r.n. (0.5–2.5mg in the elderly)
- maintain with 2.5–10mg/24h CSCI (see p.198).

When ≥5mg/24h is required, consider adding midazolam. If the patient fails to settle with 10mg/24h together with midazolam, consider switching haloperidol to levomepromazine.

Midazolam (particularly if anxiety is prominent)

- start with 2.5–5mg SC/IV stat and q1h p.r.n.
- if necessary, increase progressively to 10mg SC/IV q1h p.r.n.
- maintain with 10–60mg/24h CSCI/CIVI.

Although some centres titrate up to 200mg/24h,[29] it is probably better to add in an antipsychotic before increasing above 30mg/24h.

Second-line drugs

Levomepromazine

Note. Some centres use smaller doses first-line, e.g. 12.5mg SC stat and q1h p.r.n. (6.25mg in the elderly):

- start with 25mg SC stat and q1h p.r.n. (12.5mg in the elderly)
- if necessary, titrate dose according to response
- maintain with 50–200mg/24h CSCI. Alternatively, smaller doses can be given as an SC bolus at bedtime–b.d. and p.r.n. (see p.201).

Third-line drugs

Specialist use only. For patients who fail to respond to adequate titration and p.r.n. use of the above, e.g. midazolam together with levomepromazine.

Phenobarbital

Because of the irritant nature of the injection and the volume after dilution, stat doses are generally given IM/IV, followed by CSCI (see p.315).

Propofol

Necessitates the use of an IVI and a variable-rate syringe driver (see p.702).[30]

Other drugs

Successful use of sodium oxybate (parenteral preparation; not UK) or dexmedetomidine has been reported.[84]

†*Drug-induced movement disorders*

Benzodiazepines may have a possible role in the treatment of acute akathisia, dystonia and tardive dyskinesia, if other measures are ineffective or contra-indicated, see Chapter 21, p.805.

Acute movement disorders

Reduce or stop the causal drug if possible (see p.805). Otherwise, switch to an alternative with a lower risk of extrapyramidal reactions, e.g. **metoclopramide → domperidone, haloperidol → quetiapine**. If symptoms are causing distress, give an antimuscarinic, e.g. **procyclidine**; if the latter ineffective or contra-indicated, RCTs indicate a *possible* role for benzodiazepines in acute akathisia and dystonia:

- **clonazepam** 500microgram–1mg PO at bedtime, increased if necessary to 2.5mg at bedtime[94] *or*
- **diazepam** 5mg IV (about equipotent to **midazolam** 2.5mg SC).[95]

Tardive dyskinesia

Seek specialist advice. No symptomatic treatment has been found to be consistently effective. Small RCTs have found **clonazepam** (mean dose 5mg/24h) to be of modest benefit.[96]

Box C Catatonia[85,86]

Clinical features

Catatonia is characterized by abnormal:

- posture, e.g. passive induction of a posture that is held against gravity
- movements, e.g. stereotyped movements, grimacing
- mutism
- stupor
- mimicry of another person's movements or speech.

Severe (malignant) catatonia is also associated with fever, autonomic instability and 20% mortality; some consider this is a variant of acute dopamine depletion syndrome, see p.192).

Causes

- physical illness:
  - ▷ neurological, e.g. encephalitis, epilepsy, neurodegeneration, space occupying lesion, vascular injury
  - ▷ drug-related, e.g. alcohol/benzodiazepine withdrawal, antipsychotics, corticosteroids
  - ▷ metabolic/systemic, e.g. hyponatraemia, sepsis, uraemia
- psychiatric illness, e.g. bipolar disorder, depression, schizophrenia.

Treatment

If fever or autonomic instability occur, seek urgent advice from a psychiatrist or intensivist.

Benzodiazepines are the treatment of choice:

- lorazepam 1–2mg IV (diluted 1:1 with sodium chloride 0.9% or WFI) over 2min and q4–8h p.r.n. (0.5–1mg in the elderly) *or* midazolam 5–10mg SC stat and q4–8h p.r.n.
- second-line options include electroconvulsive therapy and dopaminergics, e.g. bromocriptine.

†Neuropathic pain

Clonazepam is reported to improve both cancer-related and non-cancer neuropathic pain.[97-100] Antihyperalgesic properties have been demonstrated in healthy volunteers.[101] Its anxiolytic and muscle-relaxant properties and the ability to administer it SC in some countries (not UK) has led to its use in selected palliative care patients, despite the absence of supporting RCTs.[102] Start with:

- **clonazepam** 500microgram PO stat and p.r.n.; usual range is 0.5–4mg/24h in divided doses.

†Nausea and vomiting

Benzodiazepines are effective for chemotherapy-related[103-107] and postoperative[108] nausea and vomiting:

- **lorazepam** 500microgram SL p.r.n. *or*
- **midazolam** 10mg/24h CSCI.

Although a specific role for benzodiazepines in *anticipatory* nausea has been proposed, there is limited evidence to support this over and above their general anti-emetic effect. Alternative approaches to anticipatory nausea include relaxation, hypnosis and other psychological interventions.[109,110]

†Pruritus

Benzodiazepines are not consistently effective for pruritus; their role, if any, is limited to patients refractory to other measures, see Chapter 26 (p.825).[111-113]

†Hiccup

Midazolam is reported to improve hiccup refractory to other approaches (see Prokinetics, Table 2, p.25), e.g. **baclofen**, **gabapentin**, **haloperidol**, **metoclopramide**, **simeticone**, alone or in combination.[114]

Buccal and sublingual administration

Midazolam oromucosal solutions in prefilled buccal syringes, authorized for children and adolescents, may be preferable when a rapid onset of action is required and parenteral injections are impractical, e.g. at home (see Chapter 15, p.721). However, they are significantly more expensive.

In some countries, specific SL **lorazepam** tablets are available, *but not in the UK*. Thus, in the UK, proprietary tablets that dissolve easily are often used SL, e.g. the generic tablets made by Genus (the manufacturer's name should be stipulated on the prescription). However, although one pharmacokinetic study suggested more rapid absorption SL than PO, others have found no difference.[115-118] Thus, it is probable that the amount of **lorazepam** absorbed SL is variable and formulation-dependent. Tablets will not dissolve SL in patients with a dry mouth; dissolve the tablet in a few drops of warm water, draw up in a 1mL oral syringe and put between the patient's cheek and gum (i.e. buccally).[119] Alternatively, the **lorazepam** *injection* solution can be placed in the buccal cavity.

†Subcutaneous administration

Clonazepam (not UK), **flunitrazepam** (not UK), **lorazepam** and **midazolam** can be given SC or by CSCI. The SC and IV routes are generally considered equipotent.[120,121] Because an IV dose acts more rapidly, the minimum interval between p.r.n. doses is typically 10min, compared with 1h if SC, allowing dose titration with smaller more frequent doses.

Generally, for **clonazepam** and **lorazepam**, the same dose can be used when converting from PO to SC/IV. However, when converting from PO **midazolam** (not UK) to SC/IV **midazolam**, the SC/IV dose should be 50% less than the PO dose, because of the low PO bio-availability (Table 2 and Table 3).

Diazepam is strongly irritant and *must not* be given SC or CSCI. Note. For IV administration, the emulsion formulation is preferred.

Clonazepam CSCI should be administered using non-PVC tubing (e.g. IVAC®); up to 50% of infused clonazepam is adsorbed onto PVC tubing.[122] However, because of the long halflife (20–60h), a bolus injection at bedtime can be given.

Lorazepam may also adsorb to PVC; it is also poorly soluble and can precipitate when diluted. The solubilizing agents polyethylene and propylene glycol and preservative benzyl alcohol may cause irritation by SC bolus injection. Accidental intra-arterial administration or extravasation close to an artery has been associated with thrombosis and gangrene. Thus, CSCI **lorazepam** is rarely used.

Midazolam can be diluted with WFI or sodium chloride 0.9% or glucose 5% for administration by CSCI.

CSCI compatibility with other drugs:

Midazolam

There are 2-drug compatibility data for midazolam in WFI with **alfentanil**, **diamorphine**, **glycopyrronium**, **haloperidol**, **hydromorphone**, **hyoscine *butylbromide***, **hyoscine *hydrobromide***, **ketamine**, **levomepromazine**, **metoclopramide**, **morphine sulfate**, **octreotide** and **oxycodone**.

Concentration-dependent *incompatibility* may occur with **cyclizine** or **ranitidine**. Midazolam is *incompatible* with **dexamethasone** and **ketorolac**.

Clonazepam

There are 2-drug compatibility data for clonazepam in WFI with **alfentanil**, **diamorphine**, **glycopyrronium**, **haloperidol**, **hyoscine *butylbromide***, **hyoscine *hydrobromide***, **morphine sulfate** and **oxycodone**.

Concentration-dependent *incompatibility* may occur with **cyclizine** or **dexamethasone**.

For more details and 3-drug compatibility data, see Appendix 3 (p.933). Compatibility charts for mixing **midazolam** or **clonazepam** (not UK) with other drugs in sodium chloride 0.9%, can be found in the extended Appendix 3 of the on-line *PCF*. Combinations including **flunitrazepam** (not UK) are included in the www.palliativedrugs.com Syringe Driver Survey Database (SDSD).

Switching between benzodiazepines

Dose conversion is not straightforward, and switching is best avoided when possible. However, when necessary, use the dose equivalence table (Table 3) to provide a starting point. Equivalent doses are always approximations, and appropriate caution and monitoring is required. Particularly when switching at a high dose, it is prudent to use, say, a 30–40% lower dose than predicted and to ensure that both **flumazenil** and additional benzodiazepine doses are available for p.r.n. use.

Table 3 Approximate equivalent anxiolytic-sedative doses[123-127]

Drug	*Dose (PO)*	*Dose (SC)*
Alprazolam	0.25–0.5mg	
Chlordiazepoxide	12.5–15mg	
Clobazam	10mg	
Clonazepam	250–500microgram	250–500microgram (not UK)
Diazepam	5mg	
Flurazepam	7.5–15mg	
Loprazolam	0.5–1mg	
Lorazepam	500microgram	500microgram
Lormetazepam	0.5–1mg	
Midazolam	5mg (not UK)	2.5mg
Nitrazepam	5mg	
Oxazepam	10–15mg	
Temazepam	10mg	
Zolpidem	10mg	
Zopiclone	7.5mg	

Stopping benzodiazepines and Z-drugs

Abrupt cessation of long-term treatment can precipitate withdrawal symptoms, e.g. anxiety and seizures, *even if not present before starting treatment.* Taper gradually, e.g. by 5–10% every 1–2 weeks. Peak–trough variability can be sufficient to cause withdrawal symptoms when tapering short-acting benzodiazepines; consider switching to an equivalent dose of **diazepam** first (Table 3).[49,127]

Supply

Clobazam

All products are Schedule 4 Part 1 **CD**.
Tablets 10mg, 28 days @ 20mg at bedtime = £7.
Oral suspension 5mg/5mL, 10mg/5mL, 28 days @ 20mg at bedtime = £190.

Clonazepam (generic)
All products are Schedule 4 Part 1 **CD**.
Tablets 500microgram, 2mg, 28 days @ 500microgram at bedtime = £8.
Oral solution 500microgram/5mL, 2mg/5mL, 28 days @ 500microgram at bedtime = £74 and £25 respectively; *may contain ethanol and not suitable for children; do not further dilute with water.*
Oral drops 2.5mg/mL, 10mL = £51 (unauthorized product, available as a special order; see Chapter 24, p.817). *Price based on Specials tariff in community.*
Injection (concentrate) 1mg/mL, 1mL amp and 1mL amp of solvent = £10 (not UK, obtainable via import; see Chapter 24, p.817).

Diazepam (generic)
All products are Schedule 4 Part 1 **CD**.
Tablets 2mg, 5mg, 10mg, 28 days @ 5mg at bedtime = £0.75.
Oral solution (sugar-free) 2mg/5mL, 28 days @ 5mg at bedtime = £143.
Oral suspension 2mg/5mL, 28 days @ 5mg at bedtime = £111.
Injection (oil-based solution) 5mg/mL, 2mL amp = £0.50; *excipients include ethanol and propylene glycol.*
Injection (emulsion) *Diazemuls®* 5mg/mL, 2mL amp = £1.
Rectal solution 2mg/mL, 2.5mg or 5mg = £1.25; 4mg/mL, 10mg = £1.50.

Lorazepam (generic)
All products are Schedule 4 Part I **CD**.
Tablets 1mg, 2.5mg, 28 days @ 1mg b.d. = £6; *tablets manufactured by Genus are scored.*
Oral solution 1mg/mL, 28 days @ 1mg b.d. = £39.

Ativan® (Pfizer)
Injection 4mg/mL, 1mL amp = £0.50; *excipients include benzyl alcohol and propylene glycol.*

Midazolam
All products are Schedule 3 **CD**.
Oromucosal products

Buccolam® (Shire Pharmaceuticals)
Oromucosal solution (prefilled oral syringe) 5mg/mL, 2.5mg, 5mg, 7.5mg and 10mg = £23.

Epistatus® (Veriton Pharma)
Oromucosal solution (prefilled oral syringe) 10mg/mL, 10mg = £46.

Note. Buccolam® oromucosal products are 5mg/mL. Do not confuse with Epistatus® and unauthorized special order products, which are 10mg/mL.[128]

Parenteral products

Midazolam (generic)
Injection 1mg/mL, 2mL amp, 5mL amp, 50mL vial = £0.50, £0.75 and £10 respectively.
High-strength injections 2mg/mL, 5mL amp, 50mL vial = £0.75 and £10 respectively; 5mg/mL, 2mL amp, 10mL amp = £0.75 and £2.50 respectively.

Many hospitals restrict the availability of high-strength midazolam injections (2mg/mL and 5mg/mL) after fatal dose errors.[129]

Zolpidem (generic)
All products are Schedule 4 Part I **CD**.
Tablets 5mg, 10mg, 28 days @ 10mg at bedtime = £1.

Zopiclone (generic)
All products are Schedule 4 Part I **CD**.
Tablets 3.75mg, 7.5mg, 28 days @ 7.5mg at bedtime = £0.75.
Oral solution 3.75mg/5mL, 7.5mg/5mL, 28 days @ 7.5mg at bedtime = £81 (unauthorized product, available as a special order; see Chapter 24, p.817). *Price based on Specials tariff in community.*
Oral suspension 3.75mg/5mL, 7.5mg/5mL, 28 days @ 7.5mg at bedtime = £47 (unauthorized product, available as a special order; see Chapter 24, p.817). *Price based on Specials tariff in community.*

1 Rudolph U and Knoflach F (2011) Beyond classical benzodiazepines: novel therapeutic potential of GABAA receptor subtypes. *Nature Reviews Drug Discovery*. **10**: 685-697.
2 Benke D *et al.* (2009) GABA A receptors as in vivo substrate for the anxiolytic action of valerenic acid, a major constituent of valerian root extracts. *Neuropharmacology*. **56**: 174-181.
3 Stahl SM (2013) Chapter 9: Anxiety disorders and anxiolytics. In: *Essential Psychopharmacology: Neuroscientific Basis and Practical Applications (4e)*. Cambridge University Press, USA. 388-419.
4 Yeh LF *et al.* (2018) Dysregulation of aversive signaling pathways: a novel circuit endophenotype for pain and anxiety disorders. *Curr Opin Neurobiol*. **48**: 37-44.
5 Poisbeau P *et al.* (2018) Anxiolytics targeting GABA A receptors: Insights on etifoxine. p. S36-S45.
6 Olsen RW (2018) GABAA receptor: Positive and negative allosteric modulators. *Neuropharmacology*. **136**: 10-22.
7 Carver CM and Reddy DS (2013) Neurosteroid interactions with synaptic and extrasynaptic GABA(A) receptors: regulation of subunit plasticity, phasic and tonic inhibition, and neuronal network excitability. *Psychopharmacology* **230**: 151-188.
8 Brickley SG and Mody I (2012) Extrasynaptic GABA(A) receptors: their function in the CNS and implications for disease. *Neuron*. **73**: 23-34.
9 Vinkers CH and Olivier B (2012) Mechanisms underlying tolerance after long-term benzodiazepine use: a future for subtype-selective GABA(A) receptor modulators? *Advances in Pharmacological Sciences*. **2012**: 416864.
10 Idzikowski C (2014) The pharmacology of human sleep, a work in progress? *Current Opinion in Pharmacology*. **14**: 90-96.
11 Jensen HS *et al.* (2014) Clobazam and its active metabolite N-desmethylclobazam display significantly greater affinities for alpha(2)- versus alpha(1)-GABA(A)-receptor complexes. *PLoS One*. **9**: e88456.

12 Ralvenius WT *et al.* (2016) The clobazam metabolite N-desmethyl clobazam is an alpha2 preferring benzodiazepine with an improved therapeutic window for antihyperalgesia. *Neuropharmacology.* **109**: 366-375.

13 Sankar R (2012) GABA(A) receptor physiology and its relationship to the mechanism of action of the 1,5-benzodiazepine clobazam. *CNS Drugs.* **26**: 229-244.

14 Mohler H (2011) The rise of a new GABA pharmacology. *Neuropharmacology.* **60**: 1042-1049.

15 Buscemi N *et al.* (2007) The efficacy and safety of drug treatments for chronic insomnia in adults: a meta-analysis of RCTs. *Journal of General Internal Medicine.* **22**: 1335-1350.

16 Hammer H *et al.* (2015) Functional characterization of the 1,5-benzodiazepine clobazam and its major active metabolite N-desmethylclobazam at human GABA(A) receptors expressed in Xenopus laevis oocytes. *PLoS One.* **10**: e0120239.

17 Olsen RW and Sieghart W (2008) International Union of Pharmacology. LXX. Subtypes of gamma-aminobutyric acid(A) receptors: classification on the basis of subunit composition, pharmacology, and function. Update. *Pharmacological Reviews.* **60**: 243-260.

18 Dias BG *et al.* (2013) Towards new approaches to disorders of fear and anxiety. *Current Opinion in Neurobiology.* **23**: 346-352.

19 Hill JL and Martinowich K (2016) Activity-dependent signaling: influence on plasticity in circuits controlling fear-related behavior. *Current Opinion in Neurobiology.* **36**: 59-65.

20 Grunfeld IS and Likhtik E (2018) Mixed selectivity encoding and action selection in the prefrontal cortex during threat assessment. *Curr Opin Neurobiol.* **49**: 108-115.

21 Riss J *et al.* (2008) Benzodiazepines in epilepsy: pharmacology and pharmacokinetics. *Acta Neurologica Scandinavica.* **118**: 69-86.

22 Drover DR (2004) Comparative pharmacokinetics and pharmacodynamics of short-acting hypnosedatives: zaleplon, zolpidem and zopiclone. *Clinical Pharmacokinetics.* **43**: 227-238.

23 Pecking M *et al.* (2002) Absolute bioavailability of midazolam after subcutaneous administration to healthy volunteers. *British Journal of Clinical Pharmacology.* **54**: 357-362.

24 Scott LJ *et al.* (2012) Oromucosal midazolam: a guide to its use in paediatric patients with prolonged acute convulsive seizures. *CNS Drugs.* **26**: 893-897.

25 Beigmohammadi MT *et al.* (2013) Pharmacokinetics alterations of midazolam infusion versus bolus administration in mechanically ventilated critically ill patients. *Iranian Journal of Pharmaceutical Research.* **12**: 483-488.

26 Franken LG *et al.* (2017) Hypoalbuminaemia and decreased midazolam clearance in terminally ill adult patients, an inflammatory effect? *Br J Clin Pharmacol.* **83**: 1701-1712.

27 MHRA (2020) Benzodiazepines and opioids: reminder of risk of potentially fatal respiratory depression. *Drug Safety Update.* www.gov.uk/drug-safety-update

28 Baxter K, and Preston, C.L. Stockley's Drug Interactions. *Pharmaceutical Press,* London. www.medicinescomplete.com (Accessed May 2019)

29 Kotlinska-Lemieszek A (2013) Should Midazolam Drug-Drug Interactions be of Concern to Palliative Care Physicians? *Drug Safety.* **36**: 789-790.

30 Grad R (1995) Benzodiazepines for insomnia in community-dwelling elderly: a review of benefit and risk. *Journal of Family Practice.* **41**: 473–481.

31 Petrov ME *et al.* (2014) Benzodiazepine (BZD) use in community-dwelling older adults: Longitudinal associations with mobility, functioning, and pain. *Archives of Gerontology and Geriatrics.* **59**: 331-337.

32 Mancuso CE *et al.* (2004) Paradoxical reactions to benzodiazepines: literature review and treatment options. *Pharmacotherapy.* **24**: 1177-1185.

33 Weinbroum AA *et al.* (2001) The midazolam-induced paradox phenomenon is reversible by flumazenil. Epidemiology, patient characteristics and review of the literature. *European Journal of Anaesthesiology.* **18**: 789-797.

34 Saias T and Gallarda T (2008) Paradoxical aggressive reactions to benzodiazepine use: a review. *Encephale.* **34**: 330-336.

35 Dolder CR and Nelson MH (2008) Hypnosedative-induced complex behaviours : incidence, mechanisms and management. *CNS Drugs.* **22**: 1021-1036.

36 Horinek EL *et al.* (2009) Propylene glycol accumulation in critically ill patients receiving continuous intravenous lorazepam infusions. *Annals of Pharmacotherpy.* **43**: 1964-1971.

37 Park TW *et al.* (2015) Benzodiazepine prescribing patterns and deaths from drug overdose among US veterans receiving opioid analgesics: case-cohort study. *British Medical Journal.* **350**: h2698.

38 Ekstrom MP *et al.* (2014) Safety of benzodiazepines and opioids in very severe respiratory disease: national prospective study. *British Medical Journal.* **348**: g445.

39 Patorno E *et al.* (2017) Benzodiazepines and risk of all cause mortality in adults: cohort study. *Bmj.* **358**: j2941.

40 Pariente A *et al.* (2016) The benzodiazepine-dementia disorders link: current state of knowledge. *CNS Drugs.* **30**: 1-7.

41 Gray SL *et al.* (2016) Benzodiazepine use and risk of incident dementia or cognitive decline: prospective population based study. *British Medical Journal.* **352**: i90.

42 Billioti de Gage S *et al.* (2014) Benzodiazepine use and risk of Alzheimer's disease: case-control study. *British Medical Journal.* **349**: g5205.

43 Pottegard A *et al.* (2013) Use of benzodiazepines or benzodiazepine related drugs and the risk of cancer: a population-based case-control study. *British Journal of Clinical Pharmacology.* **75**: 1356-1364.

44 Weich S *et al.* (2014) Effect of anxiolytic and hypnotic drug prescriptions on mortality hazards: retrospective cohort study. *British Medical Journal.* **348**: g1996.

45 Kao CH *et al.* (2012) Relationship of zolpidem and cancer risk: a Taiwanese population-based cohort study. *Mayo Clinic Proceedings.* **87**: 430-436.

46 Kao CH *et al.* (2012) Benzodiazepine use possibly increases cancer risk: a population-based retrospective cohort study in Taiwan. *Journal of Clinical Psychiatry.* **73**: e555-560.

47 Gressler LE *et al.* (2018) Relationship between concomitant benzodiazepine-opioid use and adverse outcomes among US veterans. *Pain.* **159**: 451-459.

48 Golcic M *et al.* (2018) The Impact of Combined Use of Opioids, Antipsychotics, and Anxiolytics on Survival in the Hospice Setting. *J Pain Symptom Manage.* **55**: 22-30.

49 Baldwin DS *et al.* (2013) Benzodiazepines: risks and benefits. A reconsideration. *Journal of Psychopharmacology.* **27**: 967-971.

50 National Patient Safety Agency (2008) Reducing risk of overdose with midazolam injection in adults. *Rapid Response Report.* NPSA/2008/RRR2011.

51 Mercadante S *et al.* (2015) Sleep disturbances in patients with advanced cancer in different palliative care settings. *Journal of Pain and Symptom Management.* **50**: 786-792.

52 Induru RR and Walsh D (2014) Cancer-related insomnia. *American Journal of Hospice and Palliative Care.* **31**: 777-785.

53 Renom-Guiteras A *et al.* (2014) Insomnia among patients with advanced disease during admission in a Palliative Care Unit: a prospective observational study on its frequency and association with psychological, physical and environmental factors. *BMC Palliative Care*. **13**: 40-52.
54 Mercadante S *et al.* (2017) Sleep disturbances in advanced cancer patients admitted to a supportive/palliative care unit. *Support Care Cancer*. **25**: 1301-1306.
55 Capezuti E *et al.* (2018) An Integrative Review of Nonpharmacological Interventions to Improve Sleep among Adults with Advanced Serious Illness. *J Palliat Med*. **21**: 700-717.
56 Kaneishi K *et al.* (2015) Single-dose subcutaneous benzodiazepines for insomnia in patients with advanced cancer. *Journal of Pain and Symptom Management*. **49**: e1-2.
57 Glass J *et al.* (2005) Sedative hypnotics in older people with insomnia: meta-analysis of risks and benefits. *British Medical Journal*. **331**: 1169.
58 Wang PS *et al.* (2001) Hazardous benzodiazepine regimens in the elderly: effects of half-life, dosage, and duration on risk of hip fracture. *American Journal of Psychiatry*. **158**: 892–898.
59 Wilson SJ *et al.* (2019) British Association for Psychopharmacology consensus statement on evidence-based treatment of insomnia, parasomnias and circadian rhythm disorders: an update. *Journal of Psychopharmacology*. **33**: 923–947.
60 McCleery J *et al.* (2016) Pharmacotherapies for sleep disturbances in dementia. *Cochrane Database of Systematic Reviews*. **11**: CD009178. www.thecochranelibrary.com.
61 Davies AN *et al.* (2017) Observational study of sleep disturbances in advanced cancer. *BMJ Supportive & Palliative Care*. **7**: 435.
62 Khachatryan D *et al.* (2016) Prazosin for treating sleep disturbances in adults with posttraumatic stress disorder: a systematic review and meta-analysis of randomized controlled trials. *Gen Hosp Psychiatry*. **39**: 46-52.
63 Proserpio P (2018) Drugs Used in Parasomnia. *Sleep Medicine Clinics*. **13**: 191-202.
64 Bandelow B *et al.* (2007) Meta-analysis of randomized controlled comparisons of psychopharmacological and psychological treatments for anxiety disorders. *World Journal of Biological Psychiatry*. **8**: 175-187.
65 Baldwin (2011) Efficacy of drug treatments for generalised anxiety disorder: systemic review and meta-analysis. *British Medical Journal*. **342**: 1199.
66 Baldwin DS *et al.* (2014) Evidence-based pharmacological treatment of anxiety disorders, post-traumatic stress disorder and obsessive-compulsive disorder: a revision of the 2005 guidelines from the British Association for Psychopharmacology. *Journal of Psychopharmacology*. **28**: 403–439.
67 NICE (2012) The epilepsies: the diagnosis and management of the epilepsies in adults and children in primary and secondary care. *Clinical Guideline*. CG137 www.nice.org.uk.
68 McKee HR and Abou-Khalil B (2015) Outpatient pharmacotherapy and modes of administration for acute repetitive and prolonged seizures. *CNS Drugs*. **29**: 55-70.
69 Remi C *et al.* (2016) Subcutaneous use of lacosamide. *Journal of Pain Symptom Management*. **51**: e2–e4.
70 Amato L *et al.* (2010) Benzodiazepines for alcohol withdrawal. *Cochrane Database of Systematic Reviews*. **3**: CD05063. www.thecochranelibrary.com.
71 Hammond CJ *et al.* (2015) Anticonvulsants for the treatment of alcohol withdrawal syndrome and alcohol use disorders. *CNS Drugs*. **29**: 293-311.
72 Martin K and Katz A (2016) The role of barbiturates for alcohol withdrawal syndrome. *Psychosomatics*. **57**: 341-347.
73 Hui D *et al.* (2017) Effect of Lorazepam With Haloperidol vs Haloperidol Alone on Agitated Delirium in Patients With Advanced Cancer Receiving Palliative Care: A Randomized Clinical Trial. *Jama*. **318**: 1047-1056.
74 Ensor B and Cohen D (2012) Benchmarking benzodiazepines and antipsychotics in the last 24 hours of life. *New Zealand Medical Journal*. **125**: 19-30.
75 Alonso-Babarro A *et al.* (2010) At-home palliative sedation for end-of-life cancer patients. *Palliative Medicine*. **24**: 486-492.
76 Mercadante S *et al.* (2014) Palliative sedation in patients with advanced cancer followed at home: a prospective study. *Journal of Pain Symptom Management*. **47**: 860-866.
77 Muller-Busch HC *et al.* (2003) Sedation in palliative care - a critical analysis of 7 years experience. *BMC Palliative Care*. **2**: 2.
78 Goncalves F *et al.* (2016) A protocol for the control of agitation in palliative care. *American Journal of Hospice and Palliative Care*. **33**: 948-951.
79 Chater S *et al.* (1998) Sedation for intractable distress in the dying - a survey of experts. *Palliative Medicine*. **12**: 255-269.
80 Cowan JD and Walsh D (2001) Terminal sedation in palliative medicine - definition and review of the literature. *Supportive Care in Cancer*. **9**: 403-407.
81 Mercadante S *et al.* (2012) Palliative sedation in advanced cancer patients followed at home: a retrospective analysis. *Journal of Pain Symptom Management*. **43**: 1126-1130.
82 Cherny NI and Radbruch L (2009) European Association for Palliative Care (EAPC) recommended framework for the use of sedation in palliative care. *Palliative Medicine*. **23**: 581-593.
83 Radha Krishna LK *et al.* (2012) The use of midazolam and haloperidol in cancer patients at the end of life. *Singapore Medical Journal*. **53**: 62-66.
84 Ciais JF *et al.* (2015) Using sodium oxybate (gamma hydroxybutyric acid) for deep sedation at the end o flife. *Journal of Palliative Medicine*. **18**: 822.
85 Oldham M (2018) The Probability That Catatonia in the Hospital has a Medical Cause and the Relative Proportions of Its Causes: A Systematic Review. *Psychosomatics*. **59**: 333-340.
86 Weinberg R *et al.* (2018) Catatonia #349. *Journal of Palliative Medicine*. **21**: 565-566.
87 Harris DG *et al.* (2011) The use of crisis medication in the management of terminal haemorrhage due to incurable cancer: a qualitative study. *Palliative Medicine*. **25**: 691-700.
88 Simon ST *et al.* (2016) Benzodiazepines for the relief of breathlessness in advanced malignant and non-malignant diseases in adults. *Cochrane Database of Systematic Reviews*. **10**: CD007354. www.theochranelibrary.com.
89 Peoples AR *et al.* (2016) Buspirone for management of dyspnea in cancer patients receiving chemotherapy: a randomized placebo-controlled URCC CCOP study. *Supportive Care in Cancer*. **24**: 1339–1347.
90 Navigante AH *et al.* (2006) Midazolam as adjunct therapy to morphine in the alleviation of severe dyspnea perception in patients with advanced cancer. *Journal of Pain and Symptom Management*. **31**: 38–47.
91 Mackie S and Winkelman JW (2015) Long-term treatment of restless legs syndrome (RLS): an approach to management of worsening symptoms, loss of efficacy, and augmentation. *CNS Drugs*. **29**: 351-357.
92 Aurora RN *et al.* (2012) The treatment of restless legs syndrome and periodic limb movement disorder in adults--an update for 2012: practice parameters with an evidence-based systematic review and meta-analyses: an American Academy of Sleep Medicine Clinical Practice Guideline. *Sleep*. **35**: 1039-1062.

93 Garcia-Borreguero D *et al.* (2012) European guidelines on management of restless legs syndrome: report of a joint task force by the European Federation of Neurological Societies, the European Neurological Society and the European Sleep Research Society. *European Journal of Neurology*. **19**: 1385-1396.
94 Lima AR *et al.* (2002) Benzodiazepines for neuroleptic-induced acute akathisia. *Cochrane Database of Systematic Reviews*. **1**: CD001950. www.thecochranelibrary.com.
95 Gagrat D *et al.* (1978) Intravenous diazepam in the treatment of neuroleptic-induced acute dystonia and akathisia. *American Journal of Psychiatry*. **135**: 1232–1233.
96 Bergman H *et al.* (2018) Benzodiazepines for antipsychotic-induced tardive dyskinesia. *Cochrane Database Syst Rev*. **1**: CD000205. www.thecochranelibrary.com
97 Swerdlow M and Cundill J (1981) Anticonvulsant drugs used in the treatment of lancinating pain: a comparison. *Anaesthesia*. **36**: 1129–1132.
98 Bouckoms AJ and Litman RE (1985) Clonazepam in the treatment of neuralgic pain syndrome. *Psychosomatics*. **26**: 933-936.
99 Hugel H *et al.* (2003) Clonazepam as an adjuvant analgesic in patients with cancer-related neuropathic pain. *Journal of Pain and Symptom Management*. **26**: 1073-1074.
100 Bartusch S *et al.* (1996) Clonazepam for the treatment of lancinating phantom limb pain. *Clinical Journal of Pain*. **12**: 59–62.
101 Vuilleumier PH *et al.* (2013) Evaluation of anti-hyperalgesic and analgesic effects of two benzodiazepines in human experimental pain: a randomized placebo-controlled study. *PLoS One*. **8**: e43896.
102 Corrigan R *et al.* (2012) Clonazepam for neuropathic pain and fibromyalgia in adults. *Cochrane Database of Systematic Reviews*. **5**: CD009486. www.thecochranelibrary.com.
103 Bishop J *et al.* (1984) Lorazepam: a randomized, double-blind, crossover study of a new antiemetic in patients receiving cytotoxic chemotherapy and prochlorperazine. *Journal of Clinical Oncology*. **2**: 691–695.
104 Tsavaris N *et al.* (1994) Comparison of ondansentron (GR 38032F) versus ondansentron plus alprazolam as antiemetic prophylaxis during cisplatin-containing chemotherapy. *American Journal of Clinical Oncology*. **17**: 516-521.
105 Bauduer F *et al.* (1999) Granisetron plus or minus alprazolam for emesis prevention in chemotherapy of lymphomas: a randomized multicenter trial. Granisetron Trialists Group. *Leukemia and Lymphoma*. **34**: 341-347.
106 Razavi D *et al.* (1993) Prevention of adjustment disorders and anticipatory nausea secondary to adjuvant chemotherapy: a double-blind, placebo-controlled study assessing the usefulness of alprazolam. *Journal of Clinical Oncology*. **11**: 1384-1390.
107 Malik IA *et al.* (1995) Clinical efficacy of lorazepam in prophylaxis of anticipatory, acute, and delayed nausea and vomiting induced by high doses of cisplatin. A prospective randomized trial. *American Journal of Clinical Oncology*. **18**: 170-175.
108 Di Florio T and Goucke CR (1999) The effect of midazolam on persistent postoperative nausea and vomiting. *Anaesthesia and Intensive Care*. **27**: 38–40.
109 Mandala M *et al.* (2005) Midazolam for acute emesis refractory to dexamethasone and granisetron after highly emetogenic chemotherapy: a phase II study. *Supportive Care in Cancer*. **13**: 375–380.
110 Aapro MS *et al.* (2005) Anticipatory nausea and vomiting. *Supportive Care in Cancer*. **13**: 117–121.
111 Hagermark O (1973) Influence of antihistamines, sedatives, and aspirin on experimental itch. *Acta Dermato-Venereologica*. **53**: 363–368.
112 Muston H *et al.* (1979) Differential effect of hypnotics and anxiolytics on itch and scratch. *Journal of Investigative Dermatology*. **72**: 283.
113 Ebata T *et al.* (1998) Effects of nitrazepam on nocturnal scratching in adults with atopic dermatitis: a double-blind placebo-controlled crossover study. *British Journal of Dermatology*. **138**: 631–634.
114 Calsina-Berna A *et al.* (2012) Treatment of chronic hiccups in cancer patients: a systematic review. *Journal of Palliative Medicine*. **15**: 1142-1150.
115 Caille G *et al.* (1983) Pharmacokinetics of two lorazepam formulations, oral and sublingual, after multiple doses. *Biopharmaceutics and Drug Disposition*. **4**: 31-42.
116 Greenblatt DJ *et al.* (1982) Pharmacokinetic comparison of sublingual lorazepam with intravenous, intramuscular, and oral lorazepam. *Journal of Pharmaceutical Sciences*. **71**: 248-252.
117 Spenard J *et al.* (1988) Placebo-controlled comparative study of the anxiolytic activity and of the pharmacokinetics of oral and sublingual lorazepam in generalized anxiety. *Biopharmaceutics and Drug Disposition*. **9**: 457–464.
118 Gram-Hansen P and Schultz A (1988) Plasma concentrations following oral and sublingual administration of lorazepam. *International Journal of Clinical Pharmacology Therapy and Toxicology*. **26**: 323-324.
119 Nicholson A (2007) Lorazepam. *Palliativedrugs.com Ltd.* www.palliativedrugs.com
120 Nelson KA *et al.* (1997) A prospective within-patient crossover study of continuous intravenous and subcutaneous morphine for chronic cancer pain. *Journal of Pain and Symptom Management*. **13**: 262–267.
121 Moulin D *et al.* (1991) Comparisons of continuous subcutaneous and intravenous hydromorphone infusion for management of cancer pain. *Lancet*. **337**: 465–468.
122 Schneider JJ *et al.* (2006) Effect of tubing on loss of clonazepam administered by continuous subcutaneous infusion. *Journal of Pain and Symptom Management*. **31**: 563–567.
123 Whitwam JG *et al.* (1983) Comparison of midazolam and diazepam in doses of comparable potency during gastroscopy. *British Journal of Anaesthesia*. **55**: 773-777.
124 Cole SG *et al.* (1983) Midazolam, a new more potent benzodiazepine, compared with diazepam: a randomized, double-blind study of preendoscopic sedatives. *Gastrointestinal Endoscopy*. **29**: 219-222.
125 UK Medicines Information (2014) *What are the equivalent doses of oral benzodiazepines? Q&A* 293.3. www.evidence.nhs.uk.
126 McEvoy GK *American Hospital Formulary Service*. Maryland, USA: American Society of Health-System Pharmacists www.medicinescomplete.com (accessed April 2017).
127 NICE (2018) Benzodiazepine and Z-drug withdrawal. *Clinical Knowledge Summaries*. www.nice.org.uk.
128 MHRA (2011) Buccal midazolam (Buccolam): new authroised medicine for paediatric use - care needed when transferring from unlicensed formulations. *Drug Safety Update*. **5**: www.mhra.gov.uk/safetyinformation.
129 Department of Health (2015) Never events list for 2015/2016. www.gov.uk.

Updated (minor change) January 2021

MELATONIN

Class: Melatonin receptor agonist.

Indications: Primary insomnia in adults ≥55 years old, jet-lag (short-term), †secondary insomnia, †sleep phase disorders, †migraine prophylaxis.

Pharmacology

Melatonin is a hormone released during darkness by the pineal gland. It is one of several mechanisms through which the central circadian clock synchronizes the day/night cycle with numerous physiological rhythms (Figure 1).[1–4] Melatonin also modifies the circadian clock sleep phase through a feedback loop.[5] These circadian rhythms separate mutually exclusive processes (e.g. catabolism from anabolism) and help to evenly distribute resources (e.g. maximizing immune activity at night when fewer other processes are active).[6]

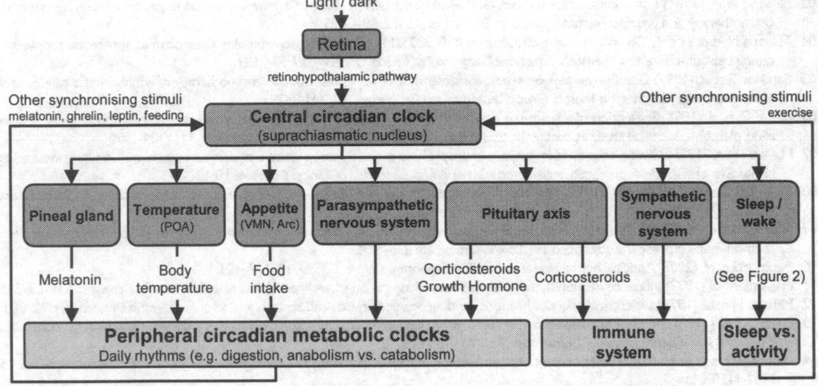

Figure 1 The circadian rhythm.[1–4,7]

Abbreviations: Arc = arcuate nucleus; POA = pre-optic area; VMN = ventromedial nucleus

Circadian desynchronization is implicated in sleep disorders, neuropsychiatric disorders (e.g. delirium, dementia, depression, psychosis)[8] and metabolic disorders (e.g. atherosclerosis, diabetes, hypertension, obesity).[1,2] The relative importance of melatonin to the above disorders is unclear.

Sleep disorders: Sleep is considered important for learning. New memories, temporarily held in the hippocampus, are reviewed during sleep when underlying patterns are identified, allowing these memories to be moved into long-term storage throughout the neocortex.

The drive to sleep arises from energy depletion, neuroplasticity (synaptic re-modelling) and immune activation. Sleep can be postponed by goal-directed and threat-related drives (Figure 2).[5,14] Melatonin's main action is to set the circadian clock sleep phase. Its direct soporific properties are modest.[15,16] Thus, while melatonin is effective for some sleep phase disorders, melatonin and **ramelteon** (a melatonin receptor agonist; not UK) are less effective for insomnia than Z-drugs, reducing sleep latency (the delay in getting to sleep) by 5–10min compared with 20min.[17–19] Head-to-head comparisons found no clinically significant differences between melatonin doses[20] or formulations (immediate-release vs. m/r).[21,22] Reduced melatonin production does not predict response.[23] The marketing authorization for primary insomnia (i.e. insomnia not due to a known physiological condition or drug), is restricted to adults ≥55 years old, reflecting its poorer efficacy in younger adults.[24]

Although melatonin is authorized for primary insomnia, greater reductions in sleep latency, along with improvements in sleep quality and fragmentation, are seen in specific groups, e.g. patients with autism (40min),[25–27] intellectual disabilities (35min),[28–30] and with short-term use in those on haemodialysis (30min).[31]

Modest reductions in sleep latency (≤10min) are seen in patients with Parkinson's disease,[32–34] and COPD.[35] A case series found melatonin improved self-reported sleep quality and reduced sleep fragmentation in 32 patients with advanced breast cancer.[36]

Melatonin and **ramelteon** are not consistently effective for sleep disturbance in dementia.[37]

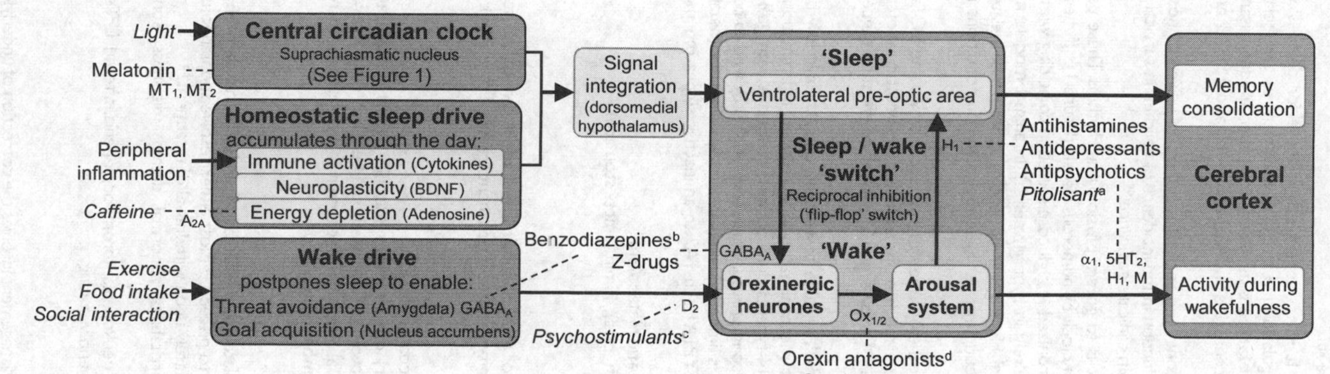

Figure 2 Putative targets of selected drugs and other influences on sleep and wakefulness.[3,6,7,9–13]

Key: Italics = wakefulness-promoting drugs and influences

Abbreviations: BDNF = brain-derived neurotrophic factor; the remainder refer to receptor types: A_{2A} = adenosine type 2_A; α_1 = α_1-adrenergic; D_2 = dopamine type 2; $GABA_A$ = gamma-aminobutyric acid type A; H_1 = histamine type 1; $5HT_2$ = 5-hydroxytriptamine (serotonin) type 2; M = muscarinic acetylcholine; MT_1, MT_2 = melatonin type 1, type 2; Ox_1, Ox_2 = orexin type 1, type 2

a. Pitolisant increases histaminergic transmission by antagonizing pre-synaptic (type 3) histamine autoreceptors
b. GABAmimetic hypnotics inhibit both orexinergic neurones and the amygdala. Thus, the latter is implicated in both their hypnotic and anxiolytic properties (also see Benzodiazepines and Z-drugs, p.163)
c. Psychostimulants increase dopamine release (see p.246), stimulating orexinergic neurones
d. Suvorexant (not UK), an orexin receptor antagonist, has recently been authorized for insomnia in the USA.

Neuropsychiatric disorders: Neuropsychiatric disorders are commonly associated with altered sleep/wake rhythms.[13] Variations in circadian clock genes predispose to such disorders, suggesting a possible *causal* role for circadian dysregulation.[38–40]

Melatonin reduces peri-operative anxiety.[41] It is not consistently effective for depression.[42] The association of depression with circadian dysregulation led to the development of the melatonergic antidepressant **agomelatine**. Although **agomelatine** is as effective as other antidepressants,[43] the significance, if any, of its affinity for melatonin receptors is unclear, because it is also a $5HT_{2C}$ antagonist (c.f. **mirtazapine**).

A meta-analysis examining *prophylactic* melatonin and **ramelteon** (not UK) given to hospitalized older patients found a statistically significant reduction in the incidence of delirium in surgical and ICU (but not medical) patients, but this is of uncertain clinical significance.[44]

Metabolic disturbance: Many organs use clocks to govern physiological rhythms. These peripheral clocks are synchronized to the central circadian clock by numerous signals (Figure 1).[1] If these signals conflict, peripheral clocks can become desynchronized (e.g. glucose secretion coinciding with daytime food intake rather than overnight fasting, resulting in hyperglycaemia). In animal models, metabolic syndrome can be caused by altering peripheral clock genes or feeding times. Thus, melatonin and peripheral clock genes are of potential therapeutic interest in several common conditions including diabetes, obesity and atherosclerosis.[1,2]

Cancer and immunity: When added to chemotherapy, melatonin was found by some RCTs to have a beneficial effect on cancer survival.[45] Possible mechanisms include immunomodulation, reduced angiogenesis and direct anti-proliferative effects.[46–48] However, RCTs found no effect on cancer-related fatigue, anorexia or weight loss.[49,50]

Pain: Melatonin reduced pain from fibromyalgia[51], irritable bowel syndrome, chronic low back pain, migraine and cluster headaches.[52,53] Potential mechanisms include reduced inflammation, altered descending pain modulation, and inhibition of N-type calcium channels (compare with **gabapentin** and **pregabalin** (p.297)).[52,54] However, sleep also improved, which could indirectly lead to benefit.

Oral bio-availability of exogenous melatonin is limited by extensive first-pass hepatic metabolism. It is 60% protein-bound and is metabolized by CYP1A1 and 1A2 to an inactive sulphatoxy metabolite, which is renally excreted.

Bio-availability 15% (because of first-pass hepatic metabolism).
Time to peak plasma concentration 3h (with food), 45min (empty stomach).
Plasma halflife 3.5–4h.

Cautions

Auto-immune disease (although there are no data in humans, melatonin can cause deleterious immunostimulation in animals with auto-immunity); hepatic impairment (reduced clearance).

Drug interactions

Melatonin may enhance the sedative effect of sedative drugs.

Fluvoxamine (a potent CYP1A2 inhibitor) can increase melatonin plasma concentrations 12-fold, and concurrent administration should be avoided. Caution should be taken with other CYP1A2 inhibitors (e.g. **ciprofloxacin**; see Chapter 19, Table 8, p.790). Melatonin can increase or decrease INR when taken with warfarin (consider increased monitoring).

Undesirable effects

No undesirable effects occurred in >1% for melatonin m/r (Circadin®). In RCTs and open-label follow-up, rates of undesirable effects are comparable to placebo.[23] Most either resolve spontaneously within a few days with no dose adjustment or immediately upon withdrawal of treatment.[55]

Uncommon (<1%, >0.1%): Restlessness, irritability, abnormal dreams, dizziness, somnolence, constipation, dry mouth, hyperbilirubinaemia.

Rare (<0.1%, >0.01%): Laboratory changes (leukopenia, thrombocytopenia, altered LFTs), rashes, mood alteration, vertigo, blurred vision, nausea and vomiting.

Dose and use

Sleep disturbance is common in palliative care. Management involves the correction of underlying causes (sleep-disturbing symptoms, fears, concurrent depression, delirium, opioid-related obstructive sleep apnoea), non-drug approaches (e.g. relaxation techniques), as well as sedative drugs.[56–58] The efficacy of both conventional hypnotics (see Benzodiazepines and Z-drugs, p.163) and melatonin is modest.

The place of melatonin for sleep problems in palliative care remains uncertain. Because melatonin lacks the undesirable motor and memory effects of conventional GABAmimetic hypnotics,[59] it could be considered as an alternative when tolerability is an issue:

- melatonin m/r 2mg PO 1–2h before bedtime.

Supply

Melatonin (generic)
Tablets 1mg, 2mg, 3mg, 28 days @ 2mg at night = £14.
Oral solution (sugar-free) 1mg/mL, 28 days @ 2mg at night = £49.

Modified-release products
Circadin® (Flynn)
Tablets m/r 2mg, 28 days @ 2mg at night = £14.

Note. Immediate-release tablets are authorized for the short-term treatment of jet-lag; m/r tablets are authorized for the short-term treatment of primary insomnia in adults ≥55 years old. Melatonin m/r tablets 1mg and 5mg are available and authorized for the treatment of insomnia in children 2–18 years old with autism spectrum disorder and/or Smith-Magenis syndrome. Several unauthorized oral suspensions are available as a special order.

1 Kanki M and Young MJ (2021) Corticosteroids and circadian rhythms in the cardiovascular system. *Current Opinion in Pharmacology*. **57**: 21–27.
2 Cardinali DP and Vigo DE (2017) Melatonin, mitochondria, and the metabolic syndrome. *Cellular and Molecular Life Sciences*. **74**: 3941–3954.
3 Astiz M *et al.* (2019) Mechanisms of communication in the mammalian circadian timing system. *International Journal of Molecular Sciences*. **20**: 343.
4 Patel A *et al.* (2021) Melatonin in neuroskeletal biology. *Current Opinion in Pharmacology*. **61**: 42–48.
5 Rihel J and Schier AF (2013) Sites of action of sleep and wake drugs: insights from model organisms. *Current Opinion in Neurobiology*. **23**: 831–840.
6 Borbély AA *et al.* (2016) The two-process model of sleep regulation: a reappraisal. *Journal of Sleep Research*. **25**: 131–143.
7 Irwin MR (2019) Sleep and inflammation: partners in sickness and in health. *Nature Reviews – Immunology*. **19**: 702–715.
8 Riemann D *et al.* (2020) Sleep, insomnia, and depression. *Neuropsychopharmacology*. **45**: 74–89.
9 Scammell TE *et al.* (2017) Neural circuitry of wakefulness and sleep. *Neuron*. **93**: 747–765.
10 Feld GB and Born J (2020) Neurochemical mechanisms for memory processing during sleep: basic findings in humans and neuropsychiatric implications. *Neuropsychopharmacology*. **45**: 31–44.
11 Jones BE (2020) Arousal and sleep circuits. *Neuropsychopharmacology*. **45**: 6–20.
12 Grippo RM and Güler AD (2019) Dopamine signaling in circadian photoentrainment: consequences of desynchrony. *Yale Journal of Biology and Medicine*. **92**: 271–281.
13 Krystal AD (2020) Sleep therapeutics and neuropsychiatric illness. *Neuropsychopharmacology*. **45**: 166–175.
14 Porkka-Heiskanen T (2013) Sleep homeostasis. *Current Opinion in Neurobiology*. **23**: 799–805.
15 Idzikowski C (2014) The pharmacology of human sleep, a work in progress? *Current Opinion in Pharmacology*. **14**: 90–96.
16 Lazarus M *et al.* (2013) Role of the basal ganglia in the control of sleep and wakefulness. *Current Opinion in Neurobiology*. **23**: 780–785.
17 Ferracioli-Oda E *et al.* (2013) Meta-analysis: melatonin for the treatment of primary sleep disorders. *PLoS One*. **8**: e63773.
18 Kuriyama A *et al.* (2014) Ramelteon for the treatment of insomnia in adults: a systematic review and meta-analysis. *Sleep Medicine*. **15**: 385–392.
19 Huedo-Medina TB *et al.* (2012) Effectiveness of non-benzodiazepine hypnotics in treatment of adult insomnia: meta-analysis of data submitted to the Food and Drug Administration. *British Medical Journal*. **345**: e8343.
20 Zhdanova IV *et al.* (2001) Melatonin treatment for age-related insomnia. *Journal of Clinical Endocrinology and Metabolism*. **86**: 4727–4730.
21 Haimov I *et al.* (1995) Melatonin replacement therapy of elderly insomniacs. *Sleep*. **18**: 598–603.
22 Hughes RJ *et al.* (1998) The role of melatonin and circadian phase in age-related sleep-maintenance insomnia: assessment in a clinical trial of melatonin replacement. *Sleep*. **21**: 52–68.
23 Wade AG *et al.* (2010) Nightly treatment of primary insomnia with prolonged release melatonin for 6 months: a randomized placebo controlled trial on age and endogenous melatonin as predictors of efficacy and safety. *BMC Medicine*. **8**: 51.
24 Wang L *et al.* (2021) A network meta-analysis of the long- and short-term efficacy of sleep medicines in adults and older adults. *Neuroscience and Biobehavioral Reviews*. **131**: 489–496.
25 Rossignol DA and Frye RE (2011) Melatonin in autism spectrum disorders: a systematic review and meta-analysis. *Developmental Medicine and Child Neurology*. **53**: 783–792.
26 Yan T and Goldman RD (2020) Melatonin for children with autism spectrum disorder. *Canadian Family Physician*. **66**: 183–185.
27 Lalanne S *et al.* (2021) Melatonin: from pharmacokinetics to clinical use in autism spectrum disorder. *International Journal of Molecular Sciences*. **22**: 1490.
28 Gringras P *et al.* (2012) Melatonin for sleep problems in children with neurodevelopmental disorders: randomised double masked placebo controlled trial. *British Medical Journal*. **345**: e6664.
29 Braam W *et al.* (2009) Exogenous melatonin for sleep problems in individuals with intellectual disability: a meta-analysis. *Developmental Medicine and Child Neurology*. **51**: 340–349.
30 Gringras P *et al.* (2017) Efficacy and safety of pediatric prolonged-release melatonin for insomnia in children with autism spectrum disorder. *Journal of the American Academy of Child and Adolescent Psychiatry*. **56**: 948–957.e4.

31 Koch BC *et al.* (2009) The effects of melatonin on sleep-wake rhythm of daytime haemodialysis patients: a randomized, placebo-controlled, cross-over study (EMSCAP study). *British Journal of Clinical Pharmacology.* **67**: 68–75.
32 Dowling GA *et al.* (2005) Melatonin for sleep disturbances in Parkinson's disease. *Sleep Medicine.* **6**: 459–466.
33 Medeiros CA *et al.* (2007) Effect of exogenous melatonin on sleep and motor dysfunction in Parkinson's disease. A randomized, double blind, placebo-controlled study. *Journal of Neurology.* **254**: 459–464.
34 Ahn JH *et al.* (2020) Prolonged-release melatonin in Parkinson's disease patients with a poor sleep quality: a randomized trial. *Parkinsonism and Related Disorders.* **75**: 50–54.
35 Nunes DM *et al.* (2008) Effect of melatonin administration on subjective sleep quality in chronic obstructive pulmonary disease. *Brazilian Journal of Medical and Biological Research.* **41**: 926–931.
36 Innominato PF *et al.* (2016) The effect of melatonin on sleep and quality of life in patients with advanced breast cancer. *Supportive Care in Cancer.* **24**: 1097–1105.
37 McCleery J and Sharpley AL (2020) Pharmacotherapies for sleep disturbances in dementia. *Cochrane Database of Systematic Reviews.* **11**: CD009178. www.cochranelibrary.com.
38 Mattis J and Sehgal A (2016) Circadian rhythms, sleep, and disorders of aging. *Trends in Endocrinology and Metabolism.* **27**: 192–203.
39 Jagannath A *et al.* (2013) Sleep and circadian rhythm disruption in neuropsychiatric illness. *Current Opinion in Neurobiology.* **23**: 888–894.
40 Comai S and Gobbi G (2014) Unveiling the role of melatonin MT2 receptors in sleep, anxiety and other neuropsychiatric diseases: a novel target in psychopharmacology. *Journal Psychiatry and Neuroscience.* **39**: 6–21.
41 Madsen BK *et al.* (2020) Melatonin for preoperative and postoperative anxiety in adults. *Cochrane Database of Systematic Reviews.* **12**: CD009861. www.cochranelibrary.com.
42 Hansen MV *et al.* (2014) The therapeutic or prophylactic effect of exogenous melatonin against depression and depressive symptoms: a systematic review and meta-analysis. *European Neuropsychopharmacology.* **24**: 1719–1728.
43 Guaiana G *et al.* (2013) Agomelatine versus other antidepressive agents for major depression. *Cochrane Database of Systematic Reviews.* **12**: CD008851. www.cochranelibrary.com.
44 Khaing K and Nair BR (2021) Melatonin for delirium prevention in hospitalized patients: a systematic review and meta-analysis. *Journal of Psychiatric Research.* **133**: 181–190.
45 Ginzac A *et al.* (2020) Quality of life for older patients with cancer: a review of the evidence supporting melatonin use. *Aging Clinical and Experimental Research.* **32**: 2459–2468.
46 Westermann J *et al.* (2015) System consolidation during sleep – a common principle underlying psychological and immunological memory formation. *Trends in Neurosciences.* **38**: 585–597.
47 Lin GJ *et al.* (2013) Modulation by melatonin of the pathogenesis of inflammatory autoimmune diseases. *International Journal of Molecular Sciences.* **14**: 11742–11766.
48 Di Bella G *et al.* (2013) Melatonin anticancer effects: review. *International Journal of Molecular Sciences.* **14**: 2410–2430.
49 Lund Rasmussen C *et al.* (2015) Effects of melatonin on physical fatigue and other symptoms in patients with advanced cancer receiving palliative care: A double-blind placebo-controlled crossover trial. *Cancer.* **121**: 3727–3736.
50 Del Fabbro E *et al.* (2013) Effects of melatonin on appetite and other symptoms in patients with advanced cancer and cachexia: a double-blind placebo-controlled trial. *Journal of Clinical Oncology.* **31**: 1271–1276.
51 de Zanette SA *et al.* (2014) Melatonin analgesia is associated with improvement of the descending endogenous pain-modulating system in fibromyalgia: a phase II, randomized, double-dummy, controlled trial. *BMC Pharmacology and Toxicology.* **15**: 40.
52 Danilov A and Kurganova J (2016) Melatonin in chronic pain syndromes. *Pain and Therapy.* **5**: 1–17.
53 Liampas I *et al.* (2020) Endogenous melatonin levels and therapeutic use of exogenous melatonin in migraine: systematic review and meta-analysis. *Headache.* **60**: 1273–1299.
54 Chen WW *et al.* (2016) Pain control by melatonin: Physiological and pharmacological effects. *Experimental and Therapeutics Medicine.* **12**: 1963–1968.
55 Besag FM *et al.* (2019) Adverse events associated with melatonin for the treatment of primary or secondary sleep disorders: a systematic review. *CNS Drugs.* **33**: 1167–1186.
56 Mercadante S *et al.* (2017) Sleep disturbances in advanced cancer patients admitted to a supportive/palliative care unit. *Support Care Cancer.* **25**: 1301–1306.
57 Nzwalo I *et al.* (2020) Systematic review of the prevalence, predictors, and treatment of insomnia in palliative care. *American Journal of Hospice and Palliative Care.* **37**: 957–969.
58 Jehangir W *et al.* (2020) Opioid-related sleep-disordered breathing: an update for clinicians. *American Journal of Hospice and Palliative Care.* **37**: 970–973.
59 Wilson S *et al.* (2019) British Association for Psychopharmacology consensus statement on evidence-based treatment of insomnia, parasomnias and circadian rhythm disorders: an update. *Journal of Psychopharmacology.* **33**: 923–947.

Updated February 2022

ANTIPSYCHOTICS

Indications: Authorized indications vary among products; consult SPC for details. Psychosis, mania and bipolar disorders, intractable hiccup, nausea and vomiting, delirium, †treatment-resistant anxiety and/or depression, †agitation in the imminently dying.

Pharmacology

Antipsychotics act predominantly through D_2-receptor antagonism, countering the symptoms of dopamine excess in delirium (Figure 1), psychosis (Figure 2), nausea (stimulation of the area postrema) and aggression (stimulation of the nucleus accumbens).[1] However, *unopposed* D_2 antagonism causes *dopamine depletion* symptoms in other pathways (e.g. the extrapyramidal system) and may worsen 'negative' psychotic symptoms (e.g. apathy, anhedonia).[2,3] Thus, the development of antipsychotics has been driven, with partial success, by attempts to reduce extrapyramidal symptoms and improve efficacy for 'negative' psychotic symptoms.

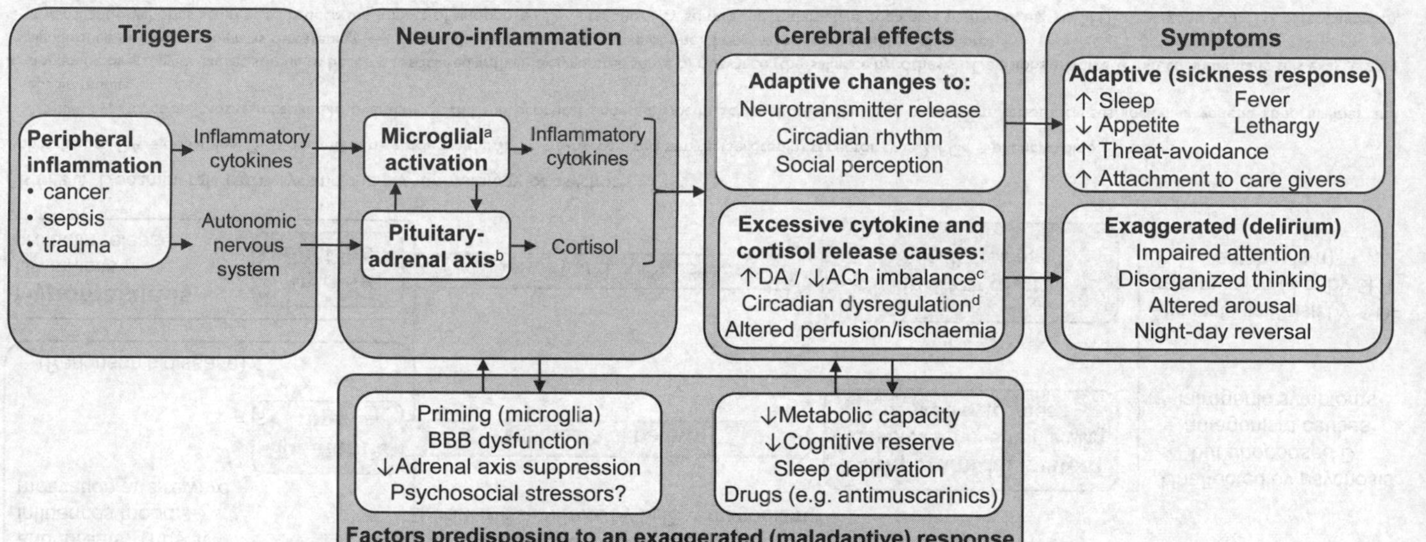

Figure 1 Delirium results from a breakdown in neuronal network connectivity arising from a maladaptive exaggeration of the neuro-inflammatory symptoms that aid recovery from acute illness.[4-6]

Abbreviations: ACh = acetylcholine; BBB = blood-brain barrier; DA = dopamine

a. microglia are CNS-resident macrophages. On detecting inflammatory cytokines, they release similar cytokines, promoting adaptive responses to sickness. When excessive, the response becomes maladaptive, i.e. delirium. Further, once activated, they respond more strongly to ongoing stimuli, thereby lowering the delirium threshold. They are implicated in other neurodegenerative diseases, e.g. dementia, which may partly explain why delirium and dementia predispose to each other

b. the pituitary–adrenal axis, via cortisol, protects against excessive peripheral inflammation. Conversely, in the CNS, cortisol increases microglial activation, synaptic dysfunction and cerebral hypoperfusion. Thus, impaired negative feedback of the pituitary–adrenal axis, which is common in older age, lowers the delirium threshold

c. in addition to cytokines and cortisol, synaptic function is also changed by hypoperfusion/hypoxia, which results in ↑DA and ↓ACh; these further exacerbate neuroinflammation and thereby delirium. This may explain why antipsychotics reduce, and antimuscarinics predispose to, delirium

d. ↓melatonin disinhibits dopaminergic neurones.

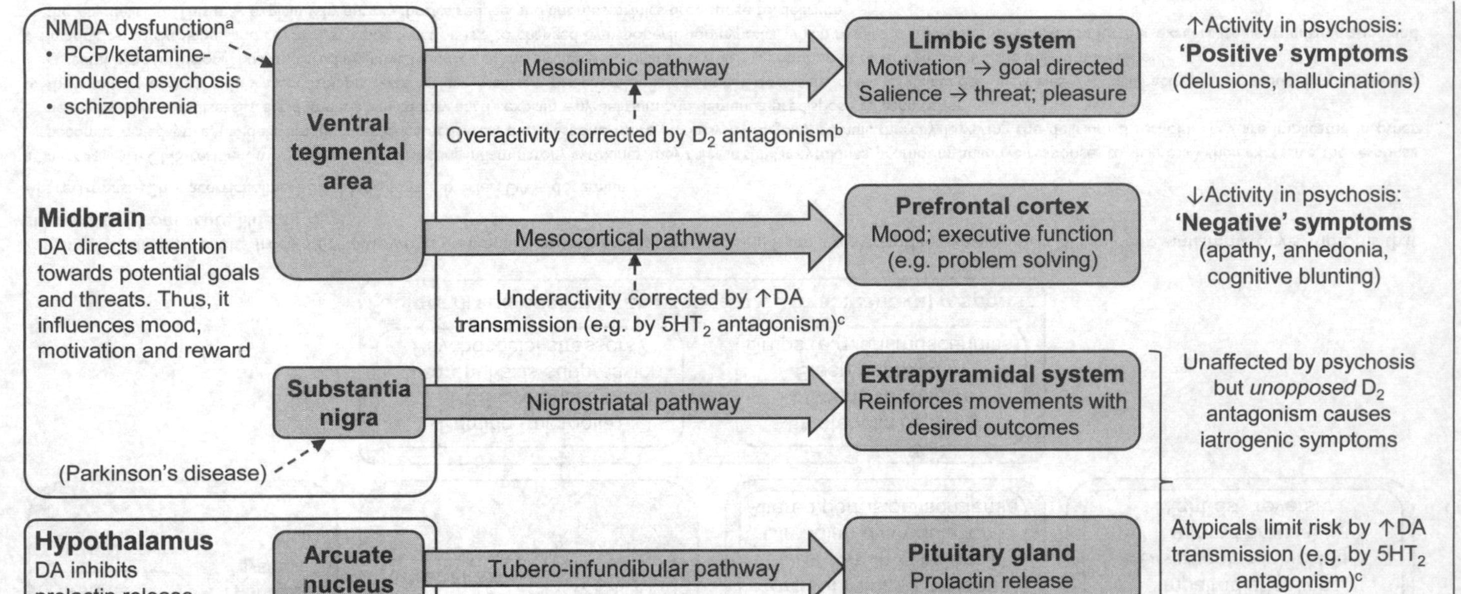

Figure 2 Dopaminergic pathways and the pathophysiology of psychosis.[2,3,7-10]

Abbreviations: DA = dopamine; D_2 = dopamine receptor type 2; $5HT_2$ = 5-hydroxytryptamine (serotonin) receptor type 2; PCP = phencyclidine

a. NMDA hypofunction causes mesolimbic overactivity and mesocortical underactivity. In schizophrenia, this may arise from various causes, including genetic abnormalities and autoimmunity

b. dopamine overactivity causes stimuli to become associated with an exaggerated sense of relevance (the 'salience hypothesis'). Delusions are an attempt to understand this exaggerated significance by interpreting it as threatening (e.g. paranoid delusions) or indicative of one's importance (e.g. grandiose delusions)

c. *atypical* antipsychotics attempt to reduce the impact of unopposed D_2 antagonism by stimulating underactive dopamine pathways, e.g. via $5HT_{2A}$ antagonism, $5HT_{1A}$ partial agonism, D_2 partial agonism (see text).

Serotonin receptors and D_2 partial agonists

$5HT_{2A}$ receptors *inhibit*, and $5HT_{1A}$ receptors *stimulate*, dopaminergic neurones. Thus, both $5HT_{2A}$ antagonists and $5HT_{1A}$ partial agonists increase activity in underactive dopaminergic pathways, countering the extrapyramidal impact of D_2 antagonism and improving 'negative' symptoms.[3]

Other antipsychotics (e.g. **aripiprazole**) use D_2 *partial agonism* to reduce the problem of unopposed D_2 antagonism. Such drugs displace dopamine from, but only partially activate, the D_2-receptor. Thus, they reduce overall transmission in overactive pathways. However, in *underactive* pathways, the partial D_2-receptor activation is sufficient to *increase* overall transmission. Thus, a D_2 partial agonist antipsychotic can potentially improve both 'positive' (e.g. hallucinations, delusions) and 'negative' symptoms and limit undesirable extrapyramidal effects.[3,11]

Other actions

Some antipsychotics have additional actions that alleviate non-dopaminergic symptoms (e.g. depression, anxiety; Table 1).[3,12] The beneficial effect of **olanzapine** on cancer-related anorexia may relate to $5HT_{2C}$ and H_1 antagonism.[13] Muscarinic antagonism reduces the risk of acute extrapyramidal symptoms, because cholinergic neurones affect dopamine release in the nigrostriatal pathway.[8] Differences in receptor profile result in varying anti-emetic properties (see Anti-emetics, p.258). Some antipsychotics antagonise sigma receptors (implicated in the pathophysiology of neuropathic and opioid poorly responsive pain).[14,15] Dopamine also modulates pain pathways.[16]

Classification

Antipsychotic classification reflects the varying propensity to cause extrapyramidal symptoms and treat 'negative' psychotic symptoms (in descending order):[3]

- typical ('first generation'):
  - ▷ less sedating (butyrophenones; highest extrapyramidal risk), e.g. **haloperidol**
  - ▷ more sedating (phenothiazines), e.g. **levomepromazine**, **chlorpromazine**, **prochlorperazine**, **perphenazine**
- atypical ('second generation'):
  - ▷ less sedating, e.g. **risperidone**
  - ▷ more sedating (lowest extrapyramidal risk), e.g. **olanzapine**, **quetiapine**.

Although atypical antipsychotics reduce dopamine depletion symptoms, none completely avoid them.[17] Further, non-dopaminergic actions themselves cause undesirable effects (Table 3). Thus, although both desirable and undesirable effects vary, the overall tolerability of antipsychotics is comparable.[17,18] In an RCT, although extrapyramidal effects accounted for more discontinuations of **perphenazine** than of several atypicals (8% vs. 2–4%), overall discontinuation rates for undesirable effects or lack of efficacy were comparable.[17] Further, all treatment groups experienced some degree of involuntary movement (13–17%), akathisia (5–9%) or extrapyramidal signs (4–8%).

Pharmacokinetics and pharmacogenetics

Pharmacokinetic details of selected antipsychotics are summarized in Table 2.

Numerous alleles are associated with efficacy or tolerability. Many relate to monoamine receptors, transporters, synthesis and degradation (e.g. extrapyramidal effects, hyperprolactinaemia). Others influence glutamate transmission (efficacy in psychosis), immunoregulation (**clozapine**-induced agranulocytosis) or energy metabolism (weight gain).[19]

Table 1 Beneficial actions and receptor affinities for selected antipsychotics[3,12,14,20-24]

Action[a]	*Reduced 'positive' symptoms*	*Reduced extrapyramidal and 'negative' symptoms*		*Antidepressant effect*[b]			*Anxiolytic effect*[c]			*Analgesic effect*[d]
Receptor	D_2	$5HT_{1A}$	$5HT_{2A}$	$5HT_{2C}$	$5HT_3$	α_2	α_1	H_1	*M*	*Sigma*
Amisulpride[e]	++	–	–	–	–	–	–	–	–	–
Aripiprazole	+++PA	++PA	++	++	–	++	++	++	–	–
Chlorpromazine	++	–	+++	++	–	+	+++	+++	++	–
Clozapine	+	++PA	+++	++	+	+	+++	+++	+++	–
Flupentixol	+++	–	+	+	+AM	–		+++		
Haloperidol	+++	–	+	–	+AM	–	+++	–	–	+++
Levomepromazine	++		+++		+AM	+	+++	+++	++	
Olanzapine	++	–	+++	++	+	+	++	+++	++	–
Perphenazine	+++	+	+++	+		+	+++	+++	–	++
Prochlorperazine	++	–	++	+	–	–	++	++	+	
Quetiapine	+	+PA	+	+	–	++	+++	+++	–	+
Risperidone	+++	+	+++	++	–	+++	+++	++	–	–

Affinity: +++ high, ++ moderate, + low, – negligible or none, blank = no data

Abbreviations: AM = allosteric modulator; PA = partial agonist; D = dopamine receptor; 5HT = serotonin receptor; α = alpha-adrenergic receptor; H = histamine receptor; M = muscarinic acetylcholine receptor

a. anti-emetic actions are associated with several receptors, including D_2, $5HT_2$, $5HT_3$, H_1 and M (also see Anti-emetics, p.258)
b. other actions implicated in an antidepressant effect include $5HT_{1A}$ and D_2 partial agonism, $5HT_7$ antagonism (amisulpride, quetiapine), and monoamine re-uptake inhibition (norquetiapine, an active metabolite of quetiapine)
c. $5HT_{1A}$ partial agonism is also implicated in the anxiolytic effect of some antipsychotics
d. clinical significance unknown
e. amisulpride preferentially binds to presynaptic D_2- and D_3-receptors in the limbic system.

Table 2 Pharmacokinetic details for selected antipsychotics[23,25,26]

	Oral bio-availability (%)	*Time to peak plasma concentration*	*Halflife (h)*	*Metabolism (predominant P450 isoenzyme)*
Amisulpride	50	1h	12	Mostly excreted unchanged
Aripiprazole	85–90	3–5h (PO)	75–145[a]	CYP2D6, CYP3A4
Chlorpromazine	10–25	2–4h (PO)	30	CYP2D6
Clozapine	50–60	2h	12	CYP1A2, CYP3A4
Haloperidol	40–85	2–6h (PO) 20–30min (IM)	12–38	CYP2D6, CYP3A4
Levomepromazine	20–50	2–3h (PO) 30–90min (SC)	15–30	CYP3A4[b]
Olanzapine	60	5–8h	34[c] (52[d])	CYP1A2, CYP2D6
Prochlorperazine	6 14 (buccal)	4h (PO) 8h (buccal; 4h with multiple doses)	14–21	Multiple
Quetiapine	≥75	1.5h	7[e] (10–14[d]) (12[b])	CYP3A4
Risperidone	70	1–2h	24[f,g]	CYP2D6, CYP3A4[h]

a. 75h in ultra-rapid metabolizers; 145h in slow metabolizers
b. active metabolite(s)
c. unaffected by hepatic or renal impairment
d. in the elderly
e. clearance reduced by both renal and hepatic impairment
f. for risperidone + active 9-hydroxy metabolite
g. clearance reduced by renal impairment
h. activity of 9-hydroxyrisperidone, the predominant CYP2D6 metabolite, is comparable to risperidone; thus, overall clinical effect is not altered by CYP2D6 polymorphisms or inhibitors.

Cautions

Stroke risk and mortality

Meta-analysis of RCTs in the elderly with dementia indicates that the risk of stroke and death with antipsychotics is ≤2 and ≤1.6 times higher respectively, compared with placebo.[27] The mechanism of this association is not known. The risk is greatest within the first month of starting treatment and with higher doses. It is a class effect.[27-29] An association with myocardial infarction is also reported; this may be due to confounding lifestyle factors and co-morbidities, rather than a causal association.[30]

Seizure risk

Most antipsychotics are reported to cause seizures, particularly in those with epilepsy or dementia. **Clozapine** carries the highest risk and **haloperidol** probably the lowest risk;[31] other antipsychotics fall between these two, with no clear separation in relative risk.[32-34] When an antipsychotic is necessary in patients at risk of seizure, use the lowest effective dose and avoid depot formulations, because they cannot be withdrawn quickly if problems occur.

Parkinsonism and Parkinson's disease

All antipsychotics, through D_2 antagonism, can cause or exacerbate parkinsonism. The risk is lowest with **clozapine** and **quetiapine**. In patients with parkinsonism, alternatives to antipsychotics should be used where possible; e.g. for agitation, consider **trazodone** (p.244) or a benzodiazepine (p.163); for nausea and vomiting, consider:

- domperidone (p.271)
- ondansetron (p.277). Note. Concurrent use with apomorphine contra-indicated
- hyoscine *hydrobromide* (p.18) but may exacerbate delirium
- cyclizine (p.273).

Although there are reports of a worsening of Parkinson's symptoms with all, the risk is less than with antipsychotics or **metoclopramide** (p.268).

Where delirium or psychotic symptoms occur in the context of Parkinson's disease or Lewy body dementia, look for potentially reversible causes of delirium, e.g. urinary retention, faecal impaction, sepsis. If symptoms persist, seek specialist advice. Options include:[35-37]

- trial reduction of antiparkinsonian medication
- **quetiapine** 12.5–25mg/24h PO (generally no deterioration in motor symptoms, but not consistently effective in RCTs)
- **clozapine** (effective in RCTs, but specialist monitoring needed)
- in the last days of life, if the PO route is unavailable and **midazolam** is insufficient alone, small doses of **levomepromazine** (p.201).

Also see End-stage idiopathic Parkinson's disease, p.717.

Cardiovascular disease

All antipsychotics have the potential to predispose to arrhythmias through muscarinic antagonism and QT interval prolongation. For those typically used in palliative care, a known link between prolonged QT interval and *torsade de pointes* exists for **haloperidol** and **levomepromazine** (for implications for practice, see Chapter 20, p.800); for others, the relationship is either possible or is conditional on the presence of other factors, e.g. high doses, drug interactions, hypokalaemia, hypomagnesaemia (see Chapter 20, p.797).

Renal and hepatic impairment

Antipsychotics differ in their potential to cause toxicity when renal or hepatic function is impaired. See Chapter 17, p.741 and Chapter 18, p.771 for general information on the choice of antipsychotic and use in ESRF and hepatic impairment respectively.

Drug interactions

Several pharmacodynamic interactions (additive sedation, hypotension, reduced effect of antiparkinsonian drugs) can be predicted from the receptor profile of antipsychotics (Table 1).

Antipsychotics are one of several classes of drugs that can prolong the QT interval and at least theoretically increase the risk of cardiac tachyarrhythmias, including potentially fatal *torsade de pointes*. Generally, concurrent prescribing of two drugs that can significantly prolong the QT interval should be avoided (see Chapter 20, p.797).

Potentially serious interactions may result from the concurrent use of antipsychotics with potent inhibitors or inducers of the relevant CYP450 enzyme, resulting in undesirable effects or failure of treatment. See the individual drug monographs and Chapter 19, Table 8, p.790 for more details.

Severe neurotoxic or extrapyramidal undesirable effects have been reported with **lithium** and several antipsychotics including **haloperidol**, **levomepromazine**, **prochlorperazine** or **quetiapine**, but appear to be uncommon and the mechanism unexplained.

Undesirable effects

These are summarized in Table 3.

Clozapine may be associated with a small increased risk of leukaemia. Animal studies suggest other antipsychotics may also have carcinogenic properties. However, human trials and observational studies have found either no difference or a small *protective* effect on the risk of cancer.[38]

Severe bone pain has been reported with **aripiprazole**.[39]

Table 3 Relative frequency and putative mechanisms of undesirable effects[3,28,29,31,40-43]

Undesirable effect		*Mechanism*	*Relative frequency with selected antipsychotics*							
			Aripiprazole	*Clozapine*	*Haloperidol*	*Levomepromazine*	*Olanzapine*	*Prochlorperazine*	*Quetiapine*	*Risperidone*
Extrapyramidal		D_2 antagonism	+/++	+	++++	+++	+/++	+++	+	++
Cardiovascular	Postural hypotension	α_1 antagonism	++	+++	++	+++	++	+++	+++	++
	QT prolongation (see text)	K-channel blockade								
	Stroke, mortality[a]	Unknown	++	++	++[a]	++[a]	++	++	++[a]	++
	Venous thrombo-embolism	Unknown	++	+++	++	+++	+++	+++	++	++
Metabolic	Hyperprolactinaemia (amenorrhoea, gynaecomastia, sexual dysfunction)	D_2 antagonism	+	+	++++	+++	++	+++	+	+++
	Weight gain, dyslipidaemia, type 2 diabetes mellitus	H_1, $5HT_{2C}$ and M_3 antagonism[b]	++	++++	+	++	++++	++	+++	++
Miscellaneous	Agranulocytosis	Immune-mediated	+	++++	+	+	+	+	+	+
	Dry mouth, constipation	M_1 and M_3 antagonism	+	+++	+	++++	++	+++	++	+
	Lowered seizure threshold	Unknown	++	+++	+	++	++	++	++	++
	Sedation	M_1, H_1 and α_1 antagonism	++	++++	+	++++	+++	+++	++++	+

Relative frequency: + = lowest risk; ++++ = highest risk

Abbreviations: α_1 = alpha adrenergic receptor type 1; D_2 = dopamine receptor type 2; K = potassium; H_1 = histamine receptor type 1; $M_{1/3}$ = muscarinic acetylcholine receptor type 1 or 3; $5HT_{2C}$ = serotonin receptor type 2C

a. confounding may explain the higher and lower risk seen with typical antipsychotics and quetiapine in observational studies[28,29]

b. H_1 and $5HT_{2C}$ antagonism increase appetite and weight; M_3 antagonism reduces insulin secretion (thus diabetes can occur rapidly and in the absence of weight gain).

Acute dopamine depletion syndrome (antipsychotic/neuroleptic malignant syndrome)

Acute dopamine depletion syndrome (Box A) is a potentially life-threatening idiosyncratic reaction to:

- starting, or increasing the dose of, dopamine antagonists, e.g. antipsychotics, **metoclopramide** *or*
- abruptly stopping antiparkinsonian dopamimetics, e.g. **levodopa**, dopamine agonists.

The incidence among those starting antipsychotics is 0.01%. The higher incidence (<3%) in older studies may reflect higher doses, higher risk with 'typical' antipsychotics, and/or changes in diagnostic criteria.[44,45] The incidence with dopamimetic withdrawal is unknown.

Box A Acute dopamine depletion syndrome[44,45]

Diagnosis

Requires 4 features unexplained by other diagnoses or frailty:

- recent dopaminergic medication change (most cases <2 weeks) *and*
- severe muscle rigidity *and*
- pyrexia *and*
- ≥2 additional features:
  - ▷ altered consciousness
  - ▷ dysphagia
  - ▷ incontinence
  - ▷ mutism
  - ▷ sweating
  - ▷ tremor
  - ▷ tachycardia
  - ▷ labile blood pressure
  - ▷ leukocytosis
  - ▷ muscle injury, e.g.
    - myoglobinuria
    - raised creatine phosphokinase.

Treatment

- discontinuation (or re-instatement) of the causal drug
- supportive care, e.g. hydration
- muscle relaxants[a], e.g. benzodiazepine and/or dantrolene (causes hepatotoxicity, thus reserved for severe symptoms and withdrawn when symptoms resolve)
- dopamimetics[a] (if caused by dopamine antagonists), e.g. bromocriptine; generally continued for 10 days (longer if caused by *depot* antipsychotics).

Prognosis

- resolves in 1–2 weeks (longer if caused by a depot antipsychotic)
- residual extrapyramidal symptoms can occur, particularly if treatment was delayed
- 10% mortality
- 30–50% risk of recurrence if antipsychotic-associated and an alternative is tried.

a. although benefit has not been confirmed in RCTs, mortality is lower in case reports employing such measures (10% vs. 20–30%).

Use of antipsychotics in palliative care

When long-term use of **olanzapine**, **quetiapine** or phenothiazines is anticipated, consider monitoring weight, glucose and lipids at baseline and 3-monthly thereafter.

Doses are described in individual monographs: **haloperidol** (p.198), **levomepromazine** (p.201), **olanzapine** (p.203), **risperidone** (p.206), **quetiapine** (p.208). For buccal use of **prochlorperazine**, see below. For agitation in the imminently dying, also see p.171.

Acute mania

Haloperidol, **olanzapine**, **quetiapine** or **risperidone** are used first-line because they act more quickly than 'mood stabilizers'.[46] The latter (e.g. **valproate**, p.307) are added if antipsychotics are insufficient.[47] **Lithium** is *not* generally used for mania caused by drugs or cerebral disease; it requires specific experience and monitoring, and may be less effective than for 'classical' bipolar mania.

Intractable hiccup

Chlorpromazine and **haloperidol** are authorized for hiccup, but their reported benefits remain unconfirmed by RCTs. Thus, they are used when more specific treatment, e.g. **metoclopramide** (p.268) ± **simeticone** (an antifoaming agent; see p.1) for gastric distension, or **baclofen**, is ineffective. Also see Prokinetics, Table 2, p.25. Antipsychotics occasionally *cause* hiccup.[48]

Nausea and vomiting

Haloperidol is used where specific D_2 antagonism is needed in the area postrema (chemoreceptor trigger zone; see Anti-emetics, p.258), e.g. for most chemical causes of nausea. RCTs find benefit in postoperative and chemotherapy-related nausea and vomiting and in patients referred to specialist gastro-enterology clinics with multifactorial nausea. Open-label series also suggest benefit from **haloperidol** in palliative care patients (see p.198).

Many antipsychotics bind to other receptors involved in the transduction of emetic signals and are used second-line as broad-spectrum anti-emetics (p.258). **Levomepromazine** (p.201) is widely used because it can be administered SC/CSCI. However, it has not been compared with placebo in an RCT; used first-line in unselected patients, its efficacy is comparable to **haloperidol**.[49] The buccal formulation of **prochlorperazine** is a convenient alternative for patients at home (see below). **Olanzapine** (p.203) is effective for chemotherapy-related nausea and vomiting (15 RCTs; n=1,552), and case series report benefit for nausea and vomiting in advanced cancer. However, in the UK, the parenteral preparation is available only as a special order and is expensive.

Recently, IV **amisulpride** (not UK) has been found effective in postoperative and chemotherapy-related nausea and vomiting.[50-54]

Buccal administration

Prochlorperazine can be administered buccally, although it is expensive (see Supply). Like **levomepromazine**, it is a broad-spectrum anti-emetic (Table 1). Because buccal administration avoids first-pass hepatic metabolism, buccal bio-availability is about 2.5 times higher than PO.[26] The manufacturer advises that it is contra-indicated in bone marrow depression, epilepsy, hepatic impairment (see Chapter 18, p.767), narrow-angle glaucoma and prostatism. Avoid direct contact with the skin, because irritant. Because of the risk of photosensitivity, advise patients to use a high-factor (25–30) sunscreen cream and a wide brimmed hat in sunny weather:

- **prochlorperazine** 3–6mg buccally b.d.

Delirium

Delirium is common, distressing and associated with poorer outcomes (including higher symptom burden and mortality).[55-58] Delirium may be hyperactive (e.g. patient obviously agitated), hypo-active (e.g. patient withdrawn) or a mixture of both. Because it is less immediately obvious and often erroneously put down to, e.g. fatigue or depression, a diagnosis of hypo-active delirium is often delayed, with consequently poorer outcomes. Despite differences in their 'appearance', both hyperactive and hypo-active delirium are equally distressing to patients. Note. Because treatment differs, it is important to distinguish hypo-active delirium from catatonia (see p.173).

Management of delirium includes addressing the underlying cause(s) when possible and appropriate, as well as non-drug approaches, e.g. ensure adequate vision and hearing, presence of a carer to reassure and re-orientate. Drug treatment is generally reserved for when there is severe distress or behavioural disturbance, non-drug approaches are inadequate, or when there are safety concerns.

Until recently, there has been a clear consensus that antipsychotics are the drug treatment of choice based on three RCTs, numerous open-label series and extensive clinical experience in psychiatry, critical care and palliative medicine.[55,59-63] They improve symptoms in 75% of patients, *irrespective of delirium type*.[59] The efficacy and tolerability of **haloperidol**, **olanzapine**, **quetiapine** and **risperidone** appear comparable.[59,64-68] **Aripiprazole**, the only parenteral 'atypical' antipsychotic available in a formulation for acute use in the UK, also appears effective in open-label series (n=78) at a mean IM dose of 20mg/24h (range 5–30mg/24h).[69]

A recent RCT in palliative care inpatients cast doubt on this consensus.[70] Patients with delirium with an expected survival of >1 week were randomized to receive either b.d. PO placebo, **haloperidol** or **risperidone** (both titrated to a maximum of 2–4mg/day, depending on age).

After 72h, there was improvement in delirium symptom scores in all groups; the improvement was significantly greater in those receiving placebo, although probably not to a clinically relevant degree. For those receiving an antipsychotic, extrapyramidal symptom scores were higher (probably not to a clinically relevant degree), median survival was shorter (16 vs. 26 days) and the probability of death 1.5 times greater (hazard ratio 1.47; 95% CI 0.2–2.0; p=0.01).[71] This has led to the suggestion that antipsychotics should no longer be used for delirium.[72] However, the study population and methodology used raise questions about its generalizability. Half of the patients had mild delirium (Memorial Delirium Assessment Scale ≤15; rated only 'a bit worse' by a relative) and in all groups only 1–2 doses of 'rescue' midazolam 2.5mg SC were needed over 72h. This suggests the study included patients who may not have received an antipsychotic in usual clinical practice. Further, interpretation of the differences among the groups is difficult because of the use of a non-validated primary outcome measure, a lack of data on the potential cause(s) of the delirium, and uncertainty as to whether reversible and irreversible causes of delirium were distributed evenly among treatment groups. Thus, although this RCT suggests that antipsychotics add little to corrective and non-drug approaches in mild–moderate delirium, it does not definitively exclude potential for benefit from antipsychotics in delirium, particularly when severe and/or occurring in the last days of life.

Thus, antipsychotics continue to be considered for use in selected patients with distressing symptoms.[63,70,73,74] However, antipsychotics do *not* improve survival or outcome from the underlying acute illness.[75]

When antipsychotics alone are insufficient, the concurrent use of a benzodiazepine provides additional benefit and is a common clinical practice in delirium during the last days of life (see Benzodiazepines and Z-drugs, Box B, p.172).[76,77] Benefit from the addition of **trazodone** (see p.244) or **valproate** (p.307) to an antipsychotic is also reported.

Although benzodiazepines can paradoxically worsen agitation, they are preferred for delirium related to alcohol withdrawal, acute dopamine depletion (antipsychotic/neuroleptic malignant) syndrome or Parkinson's disease.

Cholinesterase inhibitors, e.g. **rivastigmine**, are not consistently effective.[78]

Used *prophylactically*, antipsychotics do not prevent delirium in high-risk patients.[79-81] Results of RCTs examining prophylactic **melatonin** (p.180) are conflicting.

Agitation in the imminently dying

Because agitation in the imminently dying is often a feature of hyperactive delirium, some centres use antipsychotics (e.g. **haloperidol**, **levomepromazine**) first-line to treat this. Benzodiazepines (e.g. **midazolam**) are an alternative first-line choice, particularly when anxiety is prominent. An antipsychotic and a benzodiazepine are commonly combined when either alone is insufficient (see Benzodiazepines, Box B, p.172).

Challenging behaviours in dementia

Patients with dementia may become agitated for many reasons, including an *appropriate* response to a distressing situation. Possible precipitants should be treated or modified:

- intercurrent infections
- pain and/or other distressing symptoms
- environmental factors.

If carers or the care setting changes, seek information about the patient's daily routine. Consider the use of 'This is me' or a similar tool.[82]

If no cause is found, consider an empirical trial of **paracetamol**. Pain can be difficult to identify.[83] In an RCT, an empirical stepwise trial of analgesia (**paracetamol** → opioid → **pregabalin**) reduced agitation in unselected patients (i.e. without any specific indicator of pain).[84]

Psychotropic medication should be used only where other measures have failed. Training in non-drug management of behavioural disturbance reduces the use of psychotropic medication.[85] The efficacy of antipsychotics for challenging behaviour is marginal and generally outweighed by their undesirable effects (including increased risk of stroke, seizures and overall mortality).[86] Antidepressants, benzodiazepines and anti-epileptics are not consistently effective. Where drug treatment is needed, consider seeking specialist advice. Options include:[87,88]

- antipsychotics, e.g. **risperidone**
- cholinesterase inhibitors (benefit is marginal, but they may be better tolerated)
- **trazodone** 50mg PO at bedtime (where sleep disturbance predominates).

Whichever drug is selected, use the lowest effective dose for the shortest possible time; attempt dose reduction ≤4 months; many patients do not deteriorate when medication is withdrawn.[87,89]

Treatment-resistant depression

Certain antipsychotics have been used as adjuncts for depression refractory to conventional antidepressants, particularly when switching antidepressants has been unsuccessful. Generally, **aripiprazole** or **quetiapine** is added to an SSRI or **venlafaxine** (see Antidepressants, p.220). Alternatives include **risperidone** or **olanzapine**.[90]

Treatment-resistant anxiety

Prochlorperazine is authorized for short-term adjunctive treatment. However, most RCTs in treatment-resistant anxiety examined **quetiapine**, which is generally reserved for anxiety refractory to antidepressants ± benzodiazepines ± **pregabalin**.[91]

Anorexia

In open studies, **olanzapine** (p.203) improved cancer-related anorexia.

Pain

Antipsychotics are no longer used as analgesics. RCTs in acute, arthritic, neuropathic and fibromyalgic pain yield conflicting results,[92,93] and alternatives are better tolerated (see Adjuvant analgesics, p.325).

Switching antipsychotics

Equivalent PO doses of typical antipsychotics have been estimated, predominantly from surveys of psychiatric practice, and provide a starting point if switching PO from one to another (Table 4). Equivalent SC doses can be estimated from their bio-availability. However, doses of atypical antipsychotics are less variable and starting doses are generally unaffected by the dose of a previous antipsychotic.

Table 4 Equivalent PO doses of typical antipsychotics used for psychosis[94]

Drug	*PO dose*
Chlorpromazine	100mg
Flupentixol	2mg
Haloperidol	2–3mg
Levomepromazine	50–100mg
Promazine	100mg
Perphenazine	5–10mg
Sulpiride	150–300mg
Trifluoperazine	3–6mg

Supply

Prochlorperazine (generic)

Buccal tablets (as maleate) 3mg, 28 days @ 3mg b.d. = £36.

1 Aleyasin H *et al.* (2018) Neurocircuitry of aggression and aggression seeking behavior: nose poking into brain circuitry controlling aggression. *Current Opinion in Neurobiology*. **49**: 184–191.

2 Stahl SM (2013) Chapter 4: Psychosis and schizophrenia. In: *Essential Psychopharmacology: Neuroscientific Basis and Practical Applications* (4e), Cambridge University Press. pp. 79–128.

3 Stahl SM (2013) Chapter 5: Antipsychotic agents. In: *Essential Psychopharmacology: Neuroscientific Basis and Practical Applications* (4e), Cambridge University Press. pp. 129–236.

4 Maldonado JR (2018) Delirium pathophysiology: an updated hypothesis of the etiology of acute brain failure. *International Journal of Geriatric Psychiatry*. **33**: 1428–1457.

5 Eisenberger NI *et al.* (2017) In sickness and in health: the co-regulation of inflammation and social behavior. *Neuropsychopharmacology Reviews*. **42**: 242–253.

6 Hennessy E *et al.* (2017) Systemic TNF-alpha produces acute cognitive dysfunction and exaggerated sickness behavior when superimposed upon progressive neurodegeneration. *Brain, Behavior, and Immunity*. **59**: 233–244.
7 Laruelle M (2014) Schizophrenia: from dopaminergic to glutamatergic interventions. *Current Opinion in Pharmacology*. **14**: 97–102.
8 Surmeier DJ *et al.* (2014) Dopaminergic modulation of striatal networks in health and Parkinson's disease. *Current Opinion in Neurobiology*. **29**: 109–117.
9 Masdeu JC (2017) Detecting synaptic autoantibodies in psychoses: need for more sensitive methods. *Current Opinion in Neurology*. **30**: 317–326.
10 Supekar K *et al.* (2019) Dysregulated brain dynamics in a triple-network saliency model of schizophrenia and its relation to psychosis. *Biological Psychiatry*. **85**: 60–69.
11 Tadori Y *et al.* (2011) In vitro pharmacology of aripiprazole, its metabolite and experimental dopamine partial agonists at human dopamine D2 and D3 receptors. *European Journal of Pharmacology*. **668**: 355–365.
12 Stahl SM *et al.* (2013) Serotonergic drugs for depression and beyond. *Current Drug Targets*. **14**: 578–585.
13 Heisler LK and Lam DD (2017) An appetite for life: brain regulation of hunger and satiety. *Current Opinion in Pharmacology*. **37**: 100–106.
14 Cobos EJ and Baeyens JM (2015) Use of very-low-dose methadone and haloperidol for pain control in palliative care patients: are the sigma-1 receptors involved? *Journal of Palliative Medicine*. **18**: 660.
15 Davis MP (2015) Sigma-1 receptors and animal studies centered on pain and analgesia. *Expert Opinion on Drug Discovery*. **10**: 885–900.
16 Abdallah K *et al.* (2015) GABAAergic inhibition or dopamine denervation of the A11 hypothalamic nucleus induces trigeminal analgesia. *Pain*. **156**: 644–655.
17 Lieberman JA *et al.* (2005) Effectiveness of antipsychotic drugs in patients with chronic schizophrenia. *New England Journal of Medicine*. **353**: 1209–1223.
18 Jones PB *et al.* (2006) Randomized controlled trial of the effect on quality of life of second- vs first-generation antipsychotic drugs in schizophrenia: cost utility of the latest antipsychotic drugs in schizophrenia study (CUtLASS 1). *Archives of General Psychiatry*. **63**: 1079–1087.
19 Zai CC *et al.* (2018) New findings in pharmacogenetics of schizophrenia. *Current Opinion in Psychiatry*. **31**: 200–212.
20 Lal S *et al.* (1993) Levomepromazine receptor binding profile in human brain--implications for treatment-resistant schizophrenia. *Acta Psychiatrica Scandinavica*. **87**: 380–383.
21 Binding Database (2015) Skaggs School of Pharmacy and Pharmaceutical Sciences. http://bindingdb.org/as/search.html
22 Rammes G *et al.* (2004) Antipsychotic drugs antagonize human serotonin type 3 receptor currents in a noncompetitive manner. *Molecular Psychiatry*. **9**: 846–858.
23 McKeage K and Plosker GL (2004) Amisulpride: a review of its use in the management of schizophrenia. *CNS Drugs*. **18**: 933–956.
24 Sykes DA *et al.* (2017) Extrapyramidal side effects of antipsychotics are linked to their association kinetics at dopamine D2 receptors. *Nature Communications*. **8**: 763.
25 Eiermann B *et al.* (1997) The involvement of CYP1A2 and CYP3A4 in the metabolism of clozapine. *British Journal of Clinical Pharmacology*. **44**: 439–446.
26 Finn A *et al.* (2005) Bioavailability and metabolism of prochlorperazine administered via the buccal and oral delivery route. *Journal of Clinical Pharmacology*. **45**: 1383–1390.
27 Mittal V *et al.* (2011) Risk of cerebrovascular adverse events and death in elderly patients with dementia when treated with antipsychotic medications: a literature review of evidence. *American Journal of Alzheimer's Disease and Other Dementias*. **26**: 10–28.
28 Huybrechts KF *et al.* (2012) Differential risk of death in older residents in nursing homes prescribed specific antipsychotic drugs: population based cohort study. *British Medical Journal*. **344**: e977.
29 Murray-Thomas T *et al.* (2013) Risk of mortality (including sudden cardiac death) and major cardiovascular events in atypical and typical antipsychotic users: a study with the general practice research database. *Cardiovascular Psychiatry Neurology*. **2013**: 247486.
30 Brauer R *et al.* (2011) The association between antipsychotic agents and the risk of myocardial infarction: a systematic review. *British Journal of Clinical Pharmacology*. **72**: 871–878.
31 Druschky K *et al.* (2018) Seizure rates under treatment with antipsychotic drugs: data from the AMSP project. *The World Journal of Biological Psychiatry*. **20**: 732–741.
32 Khoury R and Ghossoub E (2019) Antipsychotics and seizures: what are the risks? *Current Psychiatry*. **18**: 21–33.
33 Maguire M *et al.* (2018) Epilepsy and psychosis: a practical approach. *Practical Neurology*. **18**: 106–114.
34 Mula M (2016) The pharmacological management of psychiatric comorbidities in patients with epilepsy. *Pharmacological Research*. **107**: 147–153.
35 NICE (2017) Parkinson's disease in adults: diagnosis and management. *NICE Guideline*. NG71. www.nice.org.uk.
36 Desmarais P *et al.* (2016) Quetiapine for psychosis in Parkinson disease and neurodegenerative parkinsonian disorders: a systematic review. *Journal of Geriatric Psychiatry and Neurology*. **29**: 227–236.
37 Samudra N *et al.* (2016) Psychosis in Parkinson Disease: A Review of Etiology, Phenomenology, and Management. *Drugs & Aging*. **33**: 855–863.
38 Fond G *et al.* (2012) Antipsychotic drugs: pro-cancer or anti-cancer? A systematic review. *Medical Hypotheses*. **79**: 38-42.
39 Wilson MS, 2nd (2005) Aripiprazole and bone pain. *Psychosomatics*. **46**: 187.
40 Peuskens J *et al.* (2014) The effects of novel and newly approved antipsychotics on serum prolactin levels: a comprehensive review. *CNS Drugs*. **28**: 421–453.
41 Rummel-Kluge C *et al.* (2012) Second-generation antipsychotic drugs and extrapyramidal side effects: a systematic review and meta-analysis of head-to-head comparisons. *Schizophrenia Bulletin*. **38**: 167–177.
42 Rummel-Kluge C *et al.* (2010) Head-to-head comparisons of metabolic side effects of second generation antipsychotics in the treatment of schizophrenia: a systematic review and meta-analysis. *Schizophrenia Research*. **123**: 225–233.
43 Weston-Green K *et al.* (2013) Second generation antipsychotic-induced type 2 diabetes: a role for the muscarinic M3 receptor. *CNS Drugs*. **27**: 1069–1080.
44 Perry PJ and Wilborn CA (2012) Serotonin syndrome vs neuroleptic malignant syndrome: a contrast of causes, diagnoses, and management. *Annals of Clinical Psychiatry*. **24**: 155–162.
45 Berman BD (2011) Neuroleptic malignant syndrome: a review for neurohospitalists. *Neurohospitalist*. **1**: 41–47.
46 NICE (2014) Bipolar disorder: assessment and management. *Clinical Guideline*. CG185. www.nice.org.uk.
47 Grande I and Vieta E (2015) Pharmacotherapy of acute mania: monotherapy or combination therapy with mood stabilizers and antipsychotics? *CNS Drugs*. **29**: 221–227.
48 Silverman MA *et al.* (2014) Aripiprazole-associated hiccups: a case and closer look at the association between hiccups and antipsychotics. *Journal of Pharmacy Practice*. **27**: 587–590.
49 Hardy JR *et al.* (2019) Methotrimeprazine versus haloperidol in palliative care patients with cancer-related nausea: a randomised, double-blind controlled trial. *BMJ Open*. **9**: e029942.

50 Gan TJ *et al.* (2017) Intravenous amisulpride for the prevention of postoperative nausea and vomiting: two concurrent, randomized, double-blind, placebo-controlled trials. *Anesthesiology*. **126**: 268–275.
51 Kranke P *et al.* (2018) Amisulpride prevents postoperative nausea and vomiting in patients at high risk: a randomized, double-blind, placebo-controlled trial. *Anesthesiology*. **128**: 1099–1106.
52 Kranke P *et al.* (2013) I.V. APD421 (amisulpride) prevents postoperative nausea and vomiting: a randomized, double-blind, placebo-controlled, multicentre trial. *British Journal of Anaesthesia*. **111**: 938–945.
53 Herrstedt J *et al.* (2018) Amisulpride in the prevention of nausea and vomiting induced by cisplatin-based chemotherapy: a dose-escalation study. *Supportive Care in Cancer*. **26**: 139–145.
54 Candiotti KA *et al.* (2019) Randomized, double-blind, placebo-controlled study of intravenous amisulpride as treatment of established postoperative nausea and vomiting in patients who have had no prior prophylaxis. *Anesthesia & Analgesia*. **128**: 1098–1105.
55 Bush SH *et al.* (2014) Treating an established episode of delirium in palliative care: expert opinion and review of the current evidence base with recommendations for future development. *Journal of Pain Symptom and Management*. **48**: 231–248.
56 Rainsford S et *al.* (2014) Delirium in advanced cancer: screening for the incidence on admission to an inpatient hospice unit. *Journal of Palliative Medicine*. **17**: 1045–1048.
57 Hosie A *et al.* (2013) Delirium prevalence, incidence, and implications for screening in specialist palliative care inpatient settings: a systematic review. *Palliative Medicine*. **27**: 486–498.
58 de la Cruz M *et al.* (2017) Increased symptom expression among patients with delirium admitted to an acute palliative care unit. *Journal of Palliative Medicine*. **20**: 638–641.
59 Meagher DJ *et al.* (2013) What do we really know about the treatment of delirium with antipsychotics? Ten key issues for delirium pharmacotherapy. *American Journal of Geriatric Psychiatry*. **21**: 1223–1238.
60 Morandi A et *al.* (2013) Consensus and variations in opinions on delirium care: a survey of European delirium specialists. *International Psychogeriatrics*. **25**: 2067–2075.
61 Kishi T *et al.* (2016) Antipsychotic medications for the treatment of delirium: a systematic review and meta-analysis of randomised controlled trials. *Journal of Neurology Neurosurgery and Psychiatry*. **87**: 767–774.
62 Grassi L et *al.* (2015) Management of delirium in palliative care: a review. *Current Psychiatry Reports*. **17**: 550.
63 NICE (2019) Delirium. *Clinical Guideline*. CG103 www.nice.org.uk.
64 Grover S *et al.* (2011) Comparative efficacy study of haloperidol, olanzapine and risperidone in delirium. *Journal of Psychosomatic Research*. **71**: 277–281.
65 Yoon HJ *et al.* (2013) Efficacy and safety of haloperidol versus atypical antipsychotic medications in the treatment of delirium. *BMC Psychiatry*. **13**: 240.
66 Maneeton B *et al.* (2013) Quetiapine versus haloperidol in the treatment of delirium: a double-blind, randomized, controlled trial. *Drug design, development and therapy*. **7**: 657–667.
67 van der vorst M *et al.* (2017) Efficacy and side effect profile of olanzapine versus haloperidol for symptoms of delirium in hospitalized patients with advanced cancer: A multicenter, investigator-blinded, randomized, controlled trial (RCT). *Journal of Clinical Oncology*. **35 (31)**: 231.
68 Jain R *et al.* (2017) Comparison of efficacy of haloperidol and olanzapine in the treatment of delirium. *Indian Journal of Psychiatry*. **59**: 451–456.
69 Kirino E (2015) Use of aripiprazole for delirium in the elderly: a short review. *Psychogeriatrics*. **15**: 75–84.
70 Meagher D *et al.* (2018) Debate article: Antipsychotic medications are clinically useful for the treatment of delirium. *International Journal of Geriatric Psychiatry*. **33**: 1420–1427.
71 Agar MR *et al.* (2017) Efficacy of oral risperidone, haloperidol, or placebo for symptoms of delirium among patients in palliative care: a randomized clinical trial. *JAMA Internal Medicine*. **177**: 34–42.
72 Maust DT and Kales HC (2017) Medicating Distress. *JAMA Internal Medicine*. **177**: 42–43.
73 Bush SH *et al.* (2018) Delirium in adult cancer patients: ESMO Clinical Practice Guidelines. *Annals of Oncology*. **29**: 1–23: doi:10.1093/annonc/mdy1147.
74 Marcantonio ER (2017) Delirium in hospitalized older adults. *New England Journal of Medicine*. **377**: 1456–1466.
75 Girard TD *et al.* (2018) Haloperidol and ziprasidone for treatment of delirium in critical illness. *New England Journal of Medicine*. **379**: 2506–2516.
76 Hui D *et al.* (2017) Effect of lorazepam with haloperidol vs haloperidol alone on agitated delirium in patients with advanced cancer receiving palliative care: a randomized clinical trial. *JAMA*. **318**: 1047–1056.
77 Wu YC *et al.* (2019) Association of delirium response and safety of pharmacological interventions for the management and prevention of delirium: a network meta-analysis. *JAMA Psychiatry*. **76**: 526–535.
78 Yu A *et al.* (2018) Cholinesterase inhibitors for the treatment of delirium in non-ICU settings. *Cochrane Database of Systematic Reviews*. **6**: CD012494. www.cochranelibrary.com.
79 Page VJ *et al.* (2013) Effect of intravenous haloperidol on the duration of delirium and coma in critically ill patients (Hope-ICU): a randomised, double-blind, placebo-controlled trial. *Lancet Respiratory Medicine*. **1**: 515–523.
80 Schrijver EJM *et al.* (2018) Haloperidol versus placebo for delirium prevention in acutely hospitalised older at risk patients: a multi-centre double-blind randomised controlled clinical trial. *Age and Ageing*. **47**: 48–55.
81 van den Boogaard M *et al.* (2018) Effect of haloperidol on survival among critically ill adults with a high risk of delirium: the REDUCE randomized clinical trial. *JAMA*. **319**: 680–690.
82 Royal College of Nursing and Alzheimer's Society This is me tool. Available from: www.alzheimers.org.uk.
83 Achterberg WP *et al.* (2013) Pain management in patients with dementia. *Clinical Interventions in Aging*. **8**: 1471–1482.
84 Husebo BS *et al.* (2011) Efficacy of treating pain to reduce behavioural disturbances in residents of nursing homes with dementia: cluster randomised clinical trial. *British Medical Journal*. **343**: d4065.
85 Fossey J *et al.* (2006) Effect of enhanced psychosocial care on antipsychotic use in nursing home residents with severe dementia: cluster randomised trial. *British Medical Journal*. **332**: 756–761.
86 Bloechliger M *et al.* (2015) Antipsychotic drug use and the risk of seizures: follow-up study with a nested case-control analysis. *CNS Drugs*. **29**: 591–603.
87 APA (2016) The American Psychiatric Association Practice Guideline on the Use of Antipsychotics to Treat Agitation or Psychosis in Patients With Dementia. https://doi.org/10.1176/appi.books.9780890426807.
88 McCleery J *et al.* (2016) Pharmacotherapies for sleep disturbances in dementia. *Cochrane Database of Systematic Reviews*. **11**: CD009178. www.cochranelibrary.com.
89 Van Leeuwen E *et al.* (2018) Withdrawal versus continuation of long-term antipsychotic drug use for behavioural and psychological symptoms in older people with dementia. *Cochrane Database of Systematic Reviews*. CD007726. www.cochranelibrary.com.

90 Cleare A *et al.* (2015) Evidence-based guidelines for treating depressive disorders with antidepressants: a revision of the 2008 British Association for Psychopharmacology guidelines. *Journal of Psychopharmacology*. **29**: 459–525.
91 Baldwin DS *et al.* (2014) Evidence-based pharmacological treatment of anxiety disorders, post-traumatic stress disorder and obsessive-compulsive disorder: a revision of the 2005 guidelines from the British Association for Psychopharmacology. *Journal of Psychopharmacology*. **28**: 403–439.
92 Seidel (2013) Antipsychotics for acute and chronic pain in adults. *Cochrane Database of Systematic Reviews*. **8**: CD004844. www.cochranelibrary.com
93 Walitt B *et al.* (2016) Antipsychotics for fibromyalgia in adults. *Cochrane Database of Systematic Reviews*. **6**: CD011804. www.cochranelibrary.com.
94 Cunningham Owens D (2012) Meet the relatives: a reintroduction to the clinical pharmacology of 'typical' antipsychotics (Part 1). *Advances in Psychiatric Treatment*. **18**: 323–336.

Updated (minor change) March 2022

HALOPERIDOL

Class: Butyrophenone antipsychotic.

Indications: Authorized indications vary among products; consult SPC for details. Psychosis, nausea and vomiting, intractable hiccup, delirium, †agitation in the imminently dying.

Contra-indications: Parkinson's disease (but also see Antipsychotics, p.189); Lewy body dementia; significant cardiac disorders, including QTc interval prolongation, recent myocardial infarction, uncompensated heart failure, but see Cautions below; concurrent use of other QT prolonging drugs (but also see Antipsychotics, p.190).

Pharmacology

Haloperidol is a D_2, α_1-adrenergic and sigma receptor antagonist. Compared with other antipsychotics, haloperidol causes less drowsiness, fewer antimuscarinic and metabolic effects, but more extrapyramidal symptoms (see Antipsychotics, p.184).[1] Haloperidol is widely used in palliative care for delirium and as an anti-emetic.

For delirium, it is as effective as **risperidone**, **olanzapine** and **quetiapine** (but see Antipsychotics, p.193).

For nausea and vomiting, RCTs find benefit in postoperative and chemotherapy-related nausea and vomiting and in patients referred to specialist gastro-enterology clinics with nausea due to various causes. Open-label series also suggest benefit in palliative care patients.[2-4] As a D_2 antagonist, haloperidol might have a gastric prokinetic effect (comparable with **domperidone** and **metoclopramide**); this remains unconfirmed. The benefit reported for hiccup has not been confirmed in RCTs. Also see Prokinetics, Table 2, p.25.

Data from a large cohort of palliative care patients (n=494), mostly with advanced cancer, suggest haloperidol (median dose 1.5mg/24h) is relatively well tolerated, with sedation (≤6%) the most common undesirable effect. Few (<1%) extrapyramidal reactions were reported; none were severe.[5]

Haloperidol has variable PO bio-availability, in part due to enterohepatic recycling during first-pass metabolism. It is metabolized in the liver, principally by CYP3A4 and possibly CYP2D6; some metabolites are biologically active.[1]

Bio-availability 40–85% (mean 60%) PO.
Onset of action 10–15min SC; >1h PO.
Time to peak plasma concentration 2–6h PO; 20–30min IM.[1]
Plasma halflife 12–38h.
Duration of action up to 24h, sometimes longer.

Cautions

Dementia (increased mortality and stroke risk, see Antipsychotics, p.189; also see use for challenging behaviours in dementia, p.194); epilepsy (lowered seizure threshold, although the risk is probably smaller than for more sedating antipsychotics; see p.189); renal and hepatic impairment (see Chapter 17, p.737 and Chapter 18, p.771 respectively); hyperthyroidism (uncorrected); cardiac disease (may prolong QT interval, particularly IV or in those with risk factors (see Chapter 20,

Box C, p.800).[6] Although the manufacturer advises against use in 'significant' cardiac disorders, one series reporting low doses of haloperidol for peri-operative delirium found no effect on QT interval; for implications for practice see Chapter 20, p.800).[7]

Drug interactions

See Antipsychotics (p.190) for class-wide interactions.

Use caution with drugs that inhibit or induce CYP3A4 or CYP2D6 (see Chapter 19, Table 8). In particular, close monitoring ± dosage adjustment are needed for:

- **carbamazepine**, **phenobarbital**, **phenytoin** and **rifampicin** (potent CYP3A4 inducers); can decrease haloperidol concentrations ≤50% (≤70% for rifampicin)
- **itraconazole** (potent CYP3A4 inhibitor); can increase haloperidol plasma concentrations and neurological undesirable effects
- **fluoxetine** (potent CYP2D6 inhibitor); can increase haloperidol plasma concentrations.

Other drugs known to significantly increase haloperidol plasma concentrations (mechanism of action is unknown) include **fluvoxamine** and **venlafaxine**.

Undesirable effects

Very common (>10%): extrapyramidal effects (see Chapter 21, p.805).
Common (<10%, >1%): altered LFTs, dizziness, sedation, depression, visual disturbance, hypotension.
Uncommon (<1%, >0.1%): blood disorders, endocrine effects, hyperthermia.
Rare (<0.1%) or not known: acute dopamine depletion (neuroleptic/antipsychotic malignant) syndrome (see p.192), prolongation of the QT interval, and *torsade de pointes* (see Chapter 20, p.797).

Dose and use

The PO bio-availability of haloperidol suggests that when converting from PO to SC, a dose reduction of ≤50% may be needed. This is unlikely to be problematic when titrating to effect and a 1:1 ratio is convenient. However, monitor for undesirable effects when switching route at higher doses; some patients will need a dose reduction.

Anti-emetic

For chemical/toxic causes of nausea and vomiting:

- start with 500microgram–1.5mg/24h CSCI or PO/SC at bedtime and q2h p.r.n.
- if necessary, titrate dose according to response
- maintain with 500microgram–10mg/24h
- if 5–10mg/24h ineffective, review the cause; consider switching to **levomepromazine** (p.201).

Also see QCG: Nausea and vomiting, p.264 and QCG: Inoperable bowel obstruction, p.266.

Intractable hiccup

Haloperidol is generally used when more specific treatment, e.g. **metoclopramide** (p.268) ± an antifoaming agent (see **simeticone**, p.1) or **baclofen** (p.658) are ineffective (see Prokinetics, Table 2, p.25):

- give haloperidol 1.5–3mg PO b.d.–t.d.s. (≤5mg t.d.s. if severe)
- maintenance dose 500microgram–1mg t.d.s. (≤3mg t.d.s. if severe).

Delirium

Also see Antipsychotics, p.193.

- start with 500microgram/24h CSCI or PO/SC at bedtime and q2h p.r.n.
- if necessary, increase in 0.5–1mg increments
- median effective dose 2.5mg/24h; range 250microgram–10mg/24h[8-10]
- consider a higher starting dose (1.5–3mg PO/SC) when a patient's distress is severe and/or there is immediate danger to self or others.

If insufficient, consider switching to an alternative antipsychotic (e.g. **olanzapine**, p.203 or **quetiapine**, p.208) *or* concurrent use of a benzodiazepine (p.163) *or* **trazodone** (p.244).

†Agitation in the imminently dying

- start with 1.5–5mg SC stat and q1h p.r.n. (500microgram–2.5mg in the elderly)
- median effective dose 2.5–10mg/24h CSCI; range 500microgram–25mg/24h.[11-17]

If the patient fails to settle with 10mg/24h together with **midazolam**, consider switching haloperidol to **levomepromazine** (see Benzodiazepines, Box B, p.172).

CSCI compatibility with other drugs: there are 2-drug compatibility data for haloperidol in WFI with **alfentanil, clonazepam, cyclizine, glycopyrronium, hyoscine *butylbromide*, hyoscine *hydrobromide*, metoclopramide, midazolam** and **oxycodone**.

Haloperidol is *incompatible* with **ketorolac**. Concentration-dependent *incompatibility* occurs with **dexamethasone, diamorphine, hydromorphone** and **morphine sulfate**. For more details and 3-drug compatibility data, see Appendix 3 charts and tables (p.933).

Compatibility charts for mixing drugs in sodium chloride 0.9% can be found in the extended appendix section of the on-line *PCF* on *www.medicinescomplete.com*. Note. High concentrations of haloperidol (>1mg/mL after mixing) are incompatible with sodium chloride 0.9% (see Chapter 29, p.889).

Supply

Do not confuse haloperidol injection 5mg/mL with haloperidol decanoate depot injection 50mg/mL and 100mg/mL.

Haloperidol (generic)
Tablets 500microgram, 1.5mg, 5mg, 10mg, 28 days @ 1.5mg at bedtime = £10.00.
Oral solution 200microgram/mL, 1mg/mL, 2mg/mL, 28 days @ 1.5mg at bedtime = £3.
Injection 5mg/mL, 1mL amp = £3.50.

Serenace® (Teva)
Capsules 500microgram, 28 days @ 1.5mg at bedtime = £3.50.

1 Prommer E (2012) Role of haloperidol in palliative medicine: an update. *American Journal of Hospice and Palliative Care*. **29**: 295–301.
2 McLean SL *et al.* (2013) Using haloperidol as an antiemetic in palliative care: informing practice through evidence from cancer treatment and postoperative contexts. *Journal of Pain and Palliative Care Pharmacotherapy*. **27**: 132–135.
3 Buttner M *et al.* (2004) Is low-dose haloperidol a useful antiemetic?: A meta-analysis of published and unpublished randomized trials. *Anesthesiology*. **101**: 1454–1463.
4 Digges M *et al.* (2018) Pharmacovigilance in hospice/palliative care: net effect of haloperidol for nausea or vomiting. *Journal of Palliative Medicine*. **21**: 37–43.
5 Matsuoka H *et al.* (2019) Harms from haloperidol for symptom management in palliative care-a post hoc pooled analysis of three randomized controlled studies and two consecutive cohort studies. *Journal of Pain and Symptom Management*. (published online ahead of print).
6 MHRA (2021) Haloperidol (Haldol): reminder of risks when used in elderly patients for the acute treatment of delirium. *Drug Safety Update*. www.gov.uk/drug-safety-update.
7 Blom MT *et al.* (2015) In-hospital haloperidol use and perioperative changes in QTc-duration. *Journal of Nutrition of Health and Aging*. **19**: 583–589.
8 Kang JH *et al.* (2013) Comprehensive approaches to managing delirium in patients with advanced cancer. *Cancer Treatment Reviews*. **39**: 105–112.
9 Bush SH *et al.* (2014) Treating an established episode of delirium in palliative care: expert opinion and review of the current evidence base with recommendations for future development. *Journal of Pain Symptom and Management*. **48**: 231–248.
10 Meagher DJ *et al.* (2013) What do we really know about the treatment of delirium with antipsychotics? Ten key issues for delirium pharmacotherapy. *American Journal of Geriatric Psychiatry*. **21**: 1223–1238.
11 Ensor B and Cohen D (2012) Benchmarking benzodiazepines and antipsychotics in the last 24 hours of life. *New Zealand Medical Journal*. **125**: 19–30.
12 Radha Krishna LK *et al.* (2012) The use of midazolam and haloperidol in cancer patients at the end of life. *Singapore Medical Journal*. **53**: 62–66.
13 Mercadante S *et al.* (2014) Palliative sedation in patients with advanced cancer followed at home: a prospective study. *Journal of Pain Symptom Management*. **47**: 860–866.
14 Goncalves F *et al.* (2016) A protocol for the control of agitation in palliative care. *American Journal of Hospice and Palliative Care*. **33**: 948–951.
15 Chater S *et al.* (1998) Sedation for intractable distress in the dying - a survey of experts. *Palliative Medicine*. **12**: 255–269.
16 Cowan JD and Walsh D (2001) Terminal sedation in palliative medicine - definition and review of the literature. *Supportive Care in Cancer*. **9**: 403–407.
17 Mercadante S *et al.* (2012) Palliative sedation in advanced cancer patients followed at home: a retrospective analysis. *Journal of Pain Symptom Management*. **43**: 1126–1130.

Updated (minor change) March 2022

LEVOMEPROMAZINE

Class: Phenothiazine antipsychotic.

Indications: Authorized indications vary among products: consult SPC for details. Psychosis. Pain and agitation in the imminently dying, nausea and vomiting.

Pharmacology

Levomepromazine is a D_2, $5HT_{2A}$, α_1- and α_2-adrenergic, H_1 and muscarinic antagonist.[1] It binds to an allosteric site in the $5HT_3$ receptor, reducing its responsiveness (negative allosteric modulation).[2] It is structurally and functionally similar to **chlorpromazine**, but is more widely used in palliative care, in part because it can be administered SC/CSCI.

Despite the absence of placebo-controlled RCT evidence,[3,4] levomepromazine is widely used in palliative care in the UK for agitation in the imminently dying and as a second-line anti-emetic (see p.258).[3,5] Doses ≥25mg/24h tend to cause drowsiness and postural hypotension. **Olanzapine** (p.203) is an alternative broad-spectrum anti-emetic, although in the UK the lack of a parenteral formulation is a disadvantage.

Although authorized for pain and accompanying distress in the terminally ill, RCTs for pain are small, results conflicting, and undesirable effects (particularly sedation and extrapyramidal effects) common.[6] Thus for pain, other adjuvant analgesics, which have more supporting evidence and are better tolerated, should generally be used in preference.

Levomepromazine is largely metabolized by CYP3A4 to desmethyl- and sulfoxide metabolites.[7] It accumulates within brain tissue, particularly the basal ganglia, where its elimination halflife is 1 week.[8]

Bio-availability 20–50% PO.[9,10]

Onset of action 30min.

Time to peak plasma concentration 2–3h PO; 30–90min SC.

Plasma halflife 15–30h, sometimes longer.[11]

Duration of action 12–24h.

Cautions

Dementia (increased mortality and stroke risk (see Antipsychotics, p.189); also see use for challenging behaviours in dementia (p.194)); cardiac disease (QT interval prolongation, particularly IV or in those with risk factors; see Chapter 20, Box B, p.799; other antipsychotics are less commonly affected, see p.190); parkinsonism (exacerbation); postural hypotension; epilepsy (lowered seizure threshold p.189); renal and hepatic impairment (see Chapter 17, p.737 and Chapter 18, p.771, respectively), diabetes mellitus.

Drug interactions

See Antipsychotics, p.190 for class-wide interactions.

Levomepromazine is largely metabolized by CYP3A4; it inhibits CYP2D6 and, to a lesser extent, CYP1A2 and CYP3A4.[12] There are no clinically significant reports of interactions with CYP3A4 inhibitors or inducers, nor levomepromazine affecting other drugs via this mechanism. Caution is advised with the concurrent use of drugs metabolized by CYP2D6 (see Chapter 19, Table 8, p.790) e.g. TCAs, some beta-blockers, as theoretically levomepromazine may cause plasma concentrations to increase, or reduce conversion of pro-drugs to the active metabolite, e.g. **codeine → morphine**.

Undesirable effects

Very common (>10%): dry mouth, sedation.

Common (<10%, >1%): hyperthermia, hypotension, QT alterations.

Uncommon (<1%, >0.1%): extrapyramidal effects (see Chapter 21, p.805), blood disorders.

Not known: seizures (see p.189), *torsade de pointes* (see p.190), endocrine effects, photosensitivity. Painful glossitis has been reported.[13]

Dose and use

When long term use is anticipated, consider monitoring weight, glucose and lipids at baseline and 3-monthly thereafter.

Although the PO bio-availability of levomepromazine suggests that when converting from PO to SC a dose reduction may be required, most centres use the same dose regardless of route.[5]

Anti-emetic

- start with 6–6.25mg PO/SC at bedtime and q2h p.r.n.
- if necessary, progressively increase every 4–5 days to ≤25mg/24h.

To obtain 6.25mg and 12.5mg doses, a 25mg tablet can be quartered or halved; a tablet cutter can be requested on the prescription to facilitate this. A 6mg tablet is an authorized alternative to the 6.25mg dose but is expensive, as are the unauthorized oral solutions available via special order (see Supply).

Some centres report benefit with lower starting doses, e.g. 2.5–5mg PO/SC. If drowsiness limits dose titration, switch to **olanzapine** (p.203) or reduce the dose and combine with an anti-emetic of a different profile of action (e.g. **ondansetron**; see Anti-emetics, Table 1, p.260).[5] Also see QCG: Nausea and vomiting, p.264 and QCG: Inoperable bowel obstruction, p.266.

Agitation in the imminently dying

Generally, levomepromazine is a second-line treatment (see Benzodiazepines and Z-drugs, Box B, p.172), given only if it is intended to reduce a patient's level of consciousness:

- start with 25mg SC stat and q1h p.r.n. (12.5mg in the elderly)
- if necessary, titrate dose according to response
- maintain with 50–200mg/24h CSCI. Alternatively, smaller doses can be given as an SC bolus at bedtime–b.d. and p.r.n.

Some centres use smaller doses first-line, e.g. 12.5mg SC stat and q1h p.r.n. (6.25mg in the elderly).[3]

Analgesic

Seek advice from specialist palliative care or pain teams before such use (see Pharmacology). RCTs started with 12.5–25mg PO/SC and titrated according to response. Reported maximum doses vary widely; typically 75mg/24h.[6]

Subcutaneous administration

To reduce the likelihood of inflammatory reactions at the skin infusion site, dilute CSCI to the largest practical volume and consider the use of sodium chloride 0.9% as the diluent (see Chapter 29, p.889). Syringes and lines must be protected from light to prevent degradation of the drug and must be discarded if a yellow/pink/purple colour occurs, see Chapter 29, Box B, p.891.

Alternatively, given its halflife, levomepromazine can be given as an SC bolus at bedtime–b.d. (see Chapter 29, Table 1, p.888).

CSCI compatibility with other drugs: there are 2-drug compatibility data for levomepromazine in WFI with **alfentanil, diamorphine, glycopyrronium, hydromorphone, hyoscine *butylbromide*, hyoscine *hydrobromide*, midazolam, morphine sulfate** and **oxycodone**.

Levomepromazine is *incompatible* with **ketorolac**. Concentration-dependent *incompatibility* occurs with **dexamethasone, ranitidine** and **octreotide**.

For more details and 3-drug compatibility data, see Appendix 3 charts and tables (p.933).

Compatibility charts for mixing drugs in sodium chloride 0.9% can be found in the extended appendix section of the on-line *PCF* on *www.medicinescomplete.com*.

Supply

The approximate cost of a 6mg tablet is £9; the equivalent cost of one quarter of a 25mg tablet is £0.06.

Levomepromazine (generic)
Tablets *(scored)* 6mg, 28 days @ 6mg at bedtime = £240.
Tablets *(scored)* 25mg, 28 days @ 6.25mg at bedtime = £7.
Injection 25mg/mL, 1mL amp = £2.

For patients who have swallowing difficulties, whole, halved or quartered tablets may be dispersed in water see Chapter 28, p.856 and p.863.

Unauthorized oral products

Oral suspension 2.5mg/5mL, 28 days @ 6.25mg at bedtime = £48 (unauthorized product, available as a special order; see Chapter 24, p.817). *Price based on specials tariff in community.*

Oral suspension 6mg/5mL, 28 days @ 6mg at bedtime = £259 (unauthorized product, available as a special order; see Chapter 24, p.817). *Price based on specials tariff in community.*

1 Lal S *et al.* (1993) Levomepromazine receptor binding profile in human brain--implications for treatment-resistant schizophrenia. *Acta Psychiatrica Scandinavica.* **87**: 380–383.

2 Rammes G *et al.* (2004) Antipsychotic drugs antagonize human serotonin type 3 receptor currents in a noncompetitive manner. *Molecular Psychiatry.* **9**: 846–858.

3 Dietz I *et al.* (2013) Evidence for the use of Levomepromazine for symptom control in the palliative care setting: a systematic review. *BMC Palliative Care.* **12**: 2.

4 Cox L *et al.* (2015) Levomepromazine for nausea and vomiting in palliative care. *Cochrane Database of Systematic Reviews.* **11**: CD009420. www.cochranelibrary.com

5 Palliativedrugs.com (2016) Levomepromazine for anti-emesis – how do you use it? *Latest additions: Survey results (June).* www.palliativedrugs.com

6 Seidel (2013) Antipsychotics for acute and chronic pain in adults. *Cochrane Database of Systematic Reviews.* **8**: CD004844. www.cochranelibrary.com

7 Wojcikowski J *et al.* (2014) The cytochrome P450-catalyzed metabolism of levomepromazine: a phenothiazine neuroleptic with a wide spectrum of clinical application. *Biochemical Pharmacology.* **90**: 188–195.

8 Kornhuber J *et al.* (2006) Region specific distribution of levomepromazine in the human brain. *Journal of Neural Transmission.* **113**: 387–397.

9 Bagli M *et al.* (1995) Bioequivalence and absolute bioavailability of oblong and coated levomepromazine tablets in CYP2D6 phenotyped subjects. *International Journal of Clinical Pharmacology and Therapeutics.* **33**: 646–652.

10 Dahl SG (1975) Pharmacokinetics of methotrimeprazine after single and multiple doses. *Clinical Pharmacology and Therapeutics.* **19**: 435–442.

11 Dahl SG *et al.* (1977) Pharmacokinetics and relative bioavailability of levomepromazine after repeated administration of tablets and syrup. *European Journal of Clinical Pharmacology.* **11**: 305–310.

12 Basinska-Ziobron A *et al.* (2015) Inhibition of human cytochrome P450 isoenzymes by a phenothiazine neuroleptic levomepromazine: an in vitro study. *Pharmacological reports.* **67**: 1178–1182.

13 Murray-Brown FL (2012) A case of possible glossitis in a patient with non small cell carcinoma of the lung secondary to levomepromazine. *Palliative Medicine.* **26**: 860–861.

Updated (minor change) February 2021

OLANZAPINE

Class: Atypical antipsychotic.

Indications: Psychosis, mania and bipolar disorders, †nausea and vomiting, †delirium, †treatment-resistant depression, †serotonin toxicity (IM; not UK).

Contra-indications: Narrow angle glaucoma.

Pharmacology

Olanzapine is a potent D_1, D_2, D_3, D_4, $5HT_{2A}$, $5HT_{2C}$, $5HT_3$, $5HT_6$ and $5HT_7$ antagonist. It also binds to other receptors, including α_1- and α_2-adrenergic, H_1 and muscarinic receptors.[1]

For delirium, olanzapine is as effective as **haloperidol**, **quetiapine** and **risperidone** (but see Antipsychotics, p.193).

For nausea and vomiting, most RCT evidence comes from its use alongside chemotherapy in addition to standard anti-emetics (e.g. $5HT_3$ antagonists and **dexamethasone**), where olanzapine increases the likelihood of complete control by 30–100%.[2,3] For other causes of nausea and vomiting in patients with advanced cancer, three case series (n=76) report benefit from olanzapine, even when one or more other anti-emetic had failed.[4-6] However, generally, **levomepromazine** (p.201) had *not* been used. Given the actions of **levomepromazine** and olanzapine are similar, choice will be influenced by the local availability of the parenteral formulation (see Supply).

Benefit is also reported in paraneoplastic sweating[7] and serotonin toxicity (see Antidepressants, Box A, p.217).

Olanzapine, **quetiapine** and **clozapine** cause fewer drug-induced movement disorders than other antipsychotics.[8] However, other undesirable effects are more common, e.g. drowsiness, weight gain. Thus, overall, tolerability is comparable.[9,10]

Because of the frequent increase in appetite and weight, a potential role for olanzapine in cancer-related anorexia is being explored. Benefit is reported with olanzapine either alone (in doses as low as 1.5mg/24h) or in combination with **megestrol**,[11,12] but has *not* been confirmed in an RCT.

Olanzapine is metabolized in the liver by glucuronidation and, to a lesser extent, by oxidation via the cytochrome P450 system, primarily via CYP1A2 with a minor contribution via CYP2D6 (see Antipsychotics, Table 2). The major metabolite is the 10-N-glucuronide, which does not pass the blood-brain barrier. Elimination of metabolites is both renal (60%) and faecal (30%).[13]

Bio-availability 60%, sometimes >80% PO.

Onset of action hours–days in delirium; days–weeks in psychoses.

Time to peak plasma concentration 5–8h PO, unaffected by food; 15–45min IM.

Plasma halflife 34h; 52h in the elderly; shorter in smokers; unchanged in hepatic and renal impairment.

Duration of action 12–48h, situation dependent.

Cautions

Injections (not UK): fatalities from oversedation or cardiorespiratory depression have occurred after higher than approved doses or *concurrent use with benzodiazepines*. Monitor blood pressure, heart rate, respiratory rate and level of consciousness for ≥4h after IM olanzapine, and do not give parenteral benzodiazepines within 1h of IM olanzapine.

Dementia (increased mortality and stroke risk (see Antipsychotics, p.189); also see use for challenging behaviours in dementia (p.194)); elderly patients; renal and hepatic impairment (see Dose and use); Parkinson's disease (exacerbation); epilepsy (lowers seizure threshold; consider an alternative, e.g. **haloperidol**; also see p.189);[14] history of bulimia (recurrence reported when used for nausea in advanced cancer).[15] May cause or adversely affect diabetes mellitus; rare reports of keto-acidosis.

Drug interactions

See Antipsychotics, p.190 for class-wide interactions.

Carbamazepine and tobacco exposure induce CYP1A2 and decrease the plasma concentration of olanzapine; in contrast, **fluvoxamine**, a potent inhibitor of CYP1A2, increases the plasma concentration ≤80%, and a lower dose of olanzapine should be considered if concurrent administration cannot be avoided. Caution should be taken with other CYP1A2 inhibitors (e.g. **ciprofloxacin**; see Chapter 19, Table 8, p.790).

Undesirable effects

Very common (>10%): drowsiness, weight gain, orthostatic hypotension.

Common (<10%, >1%): extrapyramidal symptoms (see Chapter 21, p.805), neutropenia.

Uncommon (<1%, >0.1%): dry mouth, constipation, agitation, nervousness, dizziness, peripheral oedema.

Common (<10%, >1%): neutropenia, oedema.

The incidence and severity of extrapyramidal symptoms are less than with **haloperidol**, but greater than with **quetiapine**.[16]

Dose and use

When long-term use is anticipated, consider monitoring weight, glucose and lipids at baseline and every 3 months thereafter.

Psychosis or mania

- Generally, start with 10mg PO at bedtime, 15mg for acute severe mania
- if necessary, increase to 20mg at bedtime.

†Delirium

Also see Antipsychotics, p.193:

- start with 2.5mg PO at bedtime and p.r.n.
- titrate if necessary; mean effective dose 5mg/24h (range 1.25–20mg/24h).[17]

†Anti-emetic

- start with 2.5–5mg PO at bedtime
- typical effective dose 2.5–5mg/24h, occasionally 10mg/24h.[4-6,18]

Most chemotherapy RCTs added olanzapine 5–10mg at bedtime to the standard anti-emetic regimen for 4–5 nights. Although generally started on the day of chemotherapy, some gave 5mg on the preceding 1–2 nights.[2,3,5]

†Treatment-resistant depression

As adjunct therapy to an SSRI or SNRI (also see Antidepressants, p.220):

- start with 5mg PO at bedtime, 2.5mg if frail
- typical effective dose 10mg/24h
- maximum dose 20mg at bedtime.[19]

†Subcutaneous administration

Although available in some countries, the injection formulation was withdrawn from the UK in 2012 for commercial reasons. It can be obtained as a special order product, but the cost is prohibitive (see Supply).

SC use is reported without evidence of site reactions.[20] CSCI use is also reported, but, because of the long halflife, this is generally unnecessary.

When converting small doses (≤5mg) of olanzapine from PO to SC, a PO:SC conversion ratio of 1:1 is probably reasonable. However, because the PO bio-availability of olanzapine varies between 60–80%, with larger doses or frail patients consider reducing the SC dose by about one third.

Renal or hepatic impairment

A maximum starting dose of 5mg PO at bedtime is recommended in patients with renal impairment or moderate hepatic impairment, or frail patients (see SPC). For use in severe renal or hepatic impairment, see Chapter 17, p.741 and Chapter 18, p.771.

Supply

Olanzapine (generic)

Tablets 2.5mg, 5mg, 7.5mg, 10mg, 15mg, 20mg, 28 days @ 5mg at bedtime = £1.50.

Tablets orodispersible (sugar-free) 5mg, 10mg, 15mg, 20mg, 28 days @ 5mg at bedtime = £6.50; *may be placed on the tongue and allowed to dissolve and then swallowed, or dispersed in water, orange juice, apple juice, milk or coffee immediately before administration.*

Zyprexa® (Lilly)

Injection (powder for reconstitution) 10mg single-use vial for IM injection = £42 (unauthorized product, available as a special order; see Chapter 24, p.817). The vial contains a calculated overage; reconstitute with 2.1mL water for injection to give a final concentration of 5mg/mL.

Note. Do not confuse this product with olanzapine embonate 210mg, 300mg or 405mg depot injection (Zypadhera®), which is available in the UK for the long-term treatment of schizophrenia.

1 Stahl SM (2013) Chapter 5: Antipsychotic agents. In: *Essential Psychopharmacology: Neuroscientific Basis and Practical Applications* (4e). Cambridge University Press, USA. 129–236.

2 Sutherland A *et al.* (2018) Olanzapine for the prevention and treatment of cancer-related nausea and vomiting in adults. *Cochrane Database of Systematic Reviews*. Cd012555. www.cochranelibrary.com

3 Yoodee J *et al.* (2017) Efficacy and safety of olanzapine for the prevention of chemotherapy-induced nausea and vomiting: a systematic review and meta-analysis. *Critical Reviews in Oncology/Hematology*. **112**: 113–125.

4 Harder S *et al.* (2019) Antiemetic use of olanzapine in patients with advanced cancer: results from an open-label multicenter study. *Supportive Care in Cancer*. **27**: 2849–2856.

5 MacKintosh D (2016) Olanzapine in the management of difficult to control nausea and vomiting in a palliative care population: a case series. *Journal of Palliative Medicine*. **19**: 87–90.

6 Kaneishi K *et al.* (2012) Olanzapine for the relief of nausea in patients with advanced cancer and incomplete bowel obstruction. *Journal of Pain and Symptom Management.* **44**: 604–607.
7 Zylicz Z and Krajnik M (2003) Flushing and sweating in an advanced breast cancer patient relieved by olanzapine. *Journal of Pain and Symptom Management.* **25**: 494–495.
8 Rummel-Kluge C *et al.* (2012) Second-generation antipsychotic drugs and extrapyramidal side effects: a systematic review and meta-analysis of head-to-head comparisons. *Schizophrenia Bulletin.* **38**: 167–177.
9 Lieberman JA *et al.* (2005) Effectiveness of antipsychotic drugs in patients with chronic schizophrenia. *New England Journal of Medicine.* **353**: 1209–1223.
10 Jones PB *et al.* (2006) Randomized controlled trial of the effect on quality of life of second- vs first-generation antipsychotic drugs in schizophrenia: cost utility of the latest antipsychotic drugs in schizophrenia study (CUtLASS 1). *Archives of General Psychiatry.* **63**: 1079–1087.
11 Navari RM and Brenner MC (2010) Treatment of cancer-related anorexia with olanzapine and megestrol acetate: a randomized trial. *Supportive Care in Cancer.* **18**: 951–956.
12 Okamoto H *et al.* (2019) Low-dose of olanzapine has ameliorating effects on cancer-related anorexia. *Cancer Management and Research.* **11**: 2233–2239.
13 Prommer E (2013) Olanzapine: palliative medicine update. *American Journal Hospice and Palliative Care.* **30**: 75–82.
14 Adachi N *et al.* (2013) Basic treatment principles for psychotic disorders in patients with epilepsy. *Epilepsia.* **54 (Suppl 1)**: 19–33.
15 Wu KL *et al.* (2019) Resurgence of eating disorders with olanzapine. *Journal of Palliative Medicine.* **22**: 231–233.
16 Rummel-Kluge C *et al.* (2010) Head-to-head comparisons of metabolic side effects of second generation antipsychotics in the treatment of schizophrenia: a systematic review and meta-analysis. *Schizophrenia Research.* **123**: 225–233.
17 Meagher DJ *et al.* (2013) What do we really know about the treatment of delirium with antipsychotics? Ten key issues for delirium pharmacotherapy. *American Journal of Geriatric Psychiatry.* **21**: 1223–1238.
18 Kaneishi K *et al.* (2016) Use of olanzapine for the relief of nausea and vomiting in patients with advanced cancer: a multicenter survey in Japan. *Supportive Care in Cancer.* **24**: 2393–2395.
19 Kato M and Chang CM (2013) Augmentation treatments with second-generation antipsychotics to antidepressants in treatment-resistant depression. *CNS Drugs.* **27 Suppl 1**: S11–19.
20 Elsayem (2010) Subcutaneous olanzapine for hyperactive or mixed delirium in patients with advanced cancer: a preliminary study. *Journal of Pain and Symptom Management.* **40**: 774–782.

Updated November 2019

RISPERIDONE

Class: Atypical antipsychotic.

Indications: Psychosis, mania and bipolar disorders, †delirium.

Pharmacology

Risperidone is a potent D_2 and $5HT_{2A}$ antagonist. It also binds to $5HT_{2C}$, H_1, α_1- and α_2-adrenergic, but *not* muscarinic, receptors.[1]

Risperidone is as effective as **haloperidol**, **olanzapine** and **quetiapine** in treating delirium (but see Antipsychotics, p.193). The benefit reported for refractory opioid-induced nausea and vomiting[2] has not been confirmed in RCTs.

The incidence of drug-induced movement disorders is less than with **haloperidol** and phenothiazines, but greater than with more sedating atypical antipsychotics (e.g. **olanzapine**, **quetiapine**; see p.184).[3] Weight gain and appetite stimulation is generally less than with other atypical antipsychotics.[4]

Risperidone is metabolized by CYP2D6 to 9-OH-risperidone (**paliperidone**, which is also commercially available). Both are active; risperidone is less readily removed from the brain by active transport, but has a higher affinity for $5HT_2$ receptors (believed to reduce undesirable extrapyramidal effects; see p.184).[5] Their overall activity is similar. Thus, although risperidone's halflife varies (17h, 5h and 3h in poor, extensive and ultra-rapid metabolizers, respectively),[6] the effect of CYP2D6 metabolizer status on dose requirements is small.[7] 9-OH-risperidone is renally excreted unchanged (75%) or further metabolized (25%; multiple pathways including CYP3A4).
Bio-availability 70%.
Time to peak plasma concentration 1–2h, not affected by food.
Onset of action hours–days in delirium; days–weeks in psychoses.
Plasma halflife 24h (for risperidone + 9-OH-risperidone; see text).
Duration of action 12–48h, situation dependent.

Cautions

Dementia (increased mortality and stroke risk (see Antipsychotics, p.189); also see use for challenging behaviours in dementia (p.194)); elderly patients; renal and hepatic impairment (see Chapter 17, p.741 and Chapter 18, p.771, respectively);[8] Parkinson's disease (exacerbation); epilepsy (lowers seizure threshold, although the risk is possibly lower than with more sedating atypical antipsychotics; see p.189).

Drug interactions

See Antipsychotics, p.190 for class-wide interactions.

Use caution with drugs that inhibit or induce CYP3A4 and possibly CYP2D6 (see Chapter 19, Table 8). In particular, close monitoring ± dosage adjustment may be required for:

- **carbamazepine** and **rifampicin** (potent CYP3A4 inducers); can decrease risperidone plasma concentrations (≤50% for rifampicin)
- **verapamil** (potent CYP3A4 inhibitor); can increase risperidone plasma concentrations.

Some CYP3A4 or CYP2D6 inhibitors, e.g. **itraconazole**, **paroxetine**, may increase the risperidone plasma concentration, but not the overall combined active antipsychotic effect of risperidone and its metabolite, unless high doses are used.

Undesirable effects

Very common (>10%): parkinsonism.

Common (<10%, >1%): akathisia, dystonia, dyskinesia (see Dose and use); insomnia, agitation, anxiety, headache, drowsiness, weight gain.

Uncommon (<1%, >0.1%): drowsiness, fatigue, dizziness, impaired concentration, seizures, blurred vision, syncope, dyspepsia, nausea and vomiting, constipation, sexual dysfunction (including priapism and erectile dysfunction), urinary incontinence, rhinitis.

Dose and use

Despite being commonly given b.d., there is no advantage in dividing the total daily dose, which can conveniently be given at bedtime.[9] Doses above 10mg/24h generally do not provide added benefit and may increase the risk of drug-induced movement disorders.

Psychosis and mania

- start with 2mg PO at bedtime
- if necessary, increase to 4mg and 6mg at bedtime on successive days
- in elderly patients and those with severe renal or hepatic impairment, the starting dose should be halved to 1mg at bedtime and titration extended over 6 days (see Chapter 17, p.741 and Chapter 18, p.771).

†Delirium

Also see p.193:

- start with 0.5–1mg PO at bedtime and p.r.n.
- if necessary, increase by 0.5–1mg after 2 days
- mean effective dose 1.5mg/24h (range 0.5–3mg).[10]

Supply

Risperidone (generic)

Tablets 500microgram, 1mg, 2mg, 3mg, 4mg, 6mg, 28 days @ 1mg at bedtime = £6.

Tablets orodispersible 500microgram, 1mg, 2mg, 3mg, 4mg, 28 days @ 1mg at bedtime = £21; *tablets should be placed on the tongue, allowed to dissolve, then swallowed.*

Oral solution 1mg/mL, 28 days @ 1mg at bedtime = £1.25; *may be diluted with any non-alcoholic drink except tea.*

1 Stahl SM (2013) Chapter 5: Antipsychotic agents. In: Essential Psychopharmacology: Neuroscientific Basis and Practical Applications (4e). Cambridge University Press, USA. 129-236.

2 Okamoto Y *et al.* (2007) A retrospective chart review of the antiemetic effectiveness of risperidone in refractory opioid-induced nausea and vomiting in advanced cancer patients. *Journal of Pain and Symptom Management.* **34**: 217-222.

3 Rummel-Kluge C *et al.* (2012) Second-generation antipsychotic drugs and extrapyramidal side effects: a systematic review and meta-analysis of head-to-head comparisons. *Schizophrenia Bulletin*. **38**: 167–177.
4 Rummel-Kluge C *et al.* (2010) Head-to-head comparisons of metabolic side effects of second generation antipsychotics in the treatment of schizophrenia: a systematic review and meta-analysis. *Schizophrenia Research*. **123**: 225–233.
5 de Leon J *et al.* (2010) The pharmacokinetics of paliperidone versus risperidone. *Psychosomatics*. **51**: 80-88.
6 Xiang Q *et al.* (2010) Effect of CYP2D6, CYP3A5, and MDR1 genetic polymorphisms on the pharmacokinetics of risperidone and its active moiety. *Journal of Clinical Pharmacology*. **50**: 659-666.
7 Mas S *et al.* (2012) Intuitive pharmacogenetics: spontaneous risperidone dosage is related to CYP2D6, CYP3A5 and ABCB1 genotypes. *Pharmacogenomics Journal*. **12**: 255-259.
8 Snoecke E *et al.* (1995) Influence of age, renal and liver impairment on the pharmacokinetics of risperidone in man. *Psychopharmacology (Berl)*. **122**: 223–229.
9 Nair N (1998) Therapeutic equivalence of risperidone given once daily and twice daily in patients with schizophrenia. The Risperidone Study. *Journal of Clinical Psychopharmacology*. **18**: 10–110.
10 Meagher DJ *et al.* (2013) What do we really know about the treatment of delirium with antipsychotics? Ten key issues for delirium pharmacotherapy. *American Journal of Geriatric Psychiatry*. **21**: 1223–1238.

Updated November 2019

QUETIAPINE

Class: Atypical antipsychotic.

Indications: Psychosis, mania and bipolar disorders, †delirium, †treatment-resistant depression and/or anxiety.

Pharmacology

Quetiapine is an α_1-adrenergic, D_2, D_3, H_1, $5HT_{2A}$ and muscarinic antagonist and a $5HT_{1A}$ partial agonist. Like **mirtazapine** (an antidepressant; p.241), it is an α_2 and $5HT_{2C}$ antagonist,[1,2] and an active metabolite (norquetiapine) is a noradrenaline re-uptake inhibitor; all may contribute to quetiapine's antidepressant effect.[3]

For delirium, quetiapine is as effective as **haloperidol**, **olanzapine** and **risperidone** (but see Antipsychotics, p.193). For anxiety, it is generally reserved for symptoms refractory to antidepressants ± benzodiazepines ± **pregabalin**.[4] For depression, it is added when the response to a monoamine re-uptake inhibitor is insufficient (see Antidepressants, p.220).

Quetiapine and **clozapine** have the lowest risk of extrapyramidal effects of all antipsychotics (see Chapter 21, p.805).[5] The Movement Disorder Society recommends **clozapine** for Parkinson's-related psychosis, but quetiapine is used more commonly because the former requires specialist haematological monitoring. When directly compared in two small RCTs (n=72), the efficacy and tolerability (including worsening of motor symptoms) of quetiapine and **clozapine** were comparable (also see Antipsychotics, p.189).[6-8]

Quetiapine shares the undesirable metabolic effects, and the increased mortality in patients with dementia, of the other atypical antipyschotics.[9,10] Compared with **olanzapine** and **risperidone**, it causes more antimuscarinic effects. Like **olanzapine**, it is more sedating than **risperidone**.

It is rapidly absorbed after oral administration. Although not known precisely, bio-availability is at least 75% (the proportion of radio-labelled quetiapine excreted in urine).[11] Metabolism is predominantly by CYP3A4. Elimination is both renal (75%) and faecal (25%); <1% of quetiapine is excreted unchanged.[11]
Bio-availability ≥75%.[11]
Onset of action hours–days in delirium; 1–2 weeks in psychoses.
Time to peak plasma concentration 1.5h.
Plasma halflife 7h (10–14h in the elderly).
Duration of action 12h (although serotoninergic activity may persist for much longer).[11]

Cautions

Dementia (increased mortality and stroke risk (see Antipsychotics, p.189); also see use for challenging behaviours in dementia (p.194)); elderly patients; renal and hepatic impairment (see Chapter 17, p.741 and Chapter 18, p.771, respectively); Parkinson's disease (exacerbation, but lower risk than for other antipsychotics (see p.189)); epilepsy (lowers seizure threshold; consider an alternative, e.g. **haloperidol**; also see p.189).[12] May cause or adversely affect diabetes mellitus. Possibly an increased risk of neutropenia.

Drug interactions

See Antipsychotics, p.190 for class-wide interactions.

Plasma quetiapine concentrations can be significantly increased by CYP3A4 inhibitors (e.g. azole antifungals, macrolide antibiotics; see Chapter 19, Table 8, p.790) and concurrent use is contra-indicated by the manufacturer. Quetiapine plasma concentrations can be significantly reduced by enzyme inducers (e.g. **carbamazepine, phenytoin**), and concurrent administration should be avoided where possible.

Undesirable effects

Very common (>10%): drowsiness, dizziness, extrapyramidal symptoms (but see Pharmacology above and Chapter 21, p.805).
Common (<10%, >1%): dry mouth, constipation, leukopenia, tachycardia, orthostatic hypotension, peripheral oedema; altered liver transaminases, thyroid hormone and glucose levels.
Uncommon (<1%, >0.1%): neutropenia, thrombocytopenia, QT prolongation (see p.184).
Frequency unknown: aphasia.[13]

Dose and use

When long-term use is anticipated, consider monitoring weight, glucose and lipids at baseline and 3-monthly thereafter.

Reduce starting dose and rate of titration in the elderly and those with renal or hepatic impairment or Parkinson's disease (also see Chapter 17, p.741 and Chapter 18, p.771, respectively). Doses can be split asymmetrically (e.g. 12.5mg in the morning, 25mg at bedtime) if daytime drowsiness and/or insomnia are present.

†Delirium

Also see p.193:
- start with 12.5mg PO b.d. (halve a 25mg immediate-release tablet)
- if necessary, increase in 12.5–25mg increments
- mean effective dose 75mg/24h (range 25–300mg/24h).[14]

†Anxiety, †depression and psychosis

- start with 12.5–25mg PO b.d.
- if necessary, increase in 12.5–25mg increments
- can be titrated rapidly over 3–4 days for severe symptoms, e.g. → 50mg b.d. → 100mg b.d. → 150mg b.d.
- typical effective dose:
  - ▷ anxiety 50–150mg/24h; occasionally titrated ≤400mg/24h[15]
  - ▷ depression 150–300mg/24h; occasionally titrated ≤600mg/24h[16]
  - ▷ psychosis 300–450mg/24h.

Bipolar mania

As monotherapy or as adjunct therapy to mood stabilizers:
- start with 50mg PO b.d.
- increase to 100mg b.d. (day 2) → 150mg b.d. (day 3) → 200mg b.d. (day 4)
- typical effective dose 400–800mg/24h.

Supply

Immediate-release
Quetiapine (generic)
Tablets 25mg, 100mg, 150mg, 200mg, 300mg, 28 days @ 100mg b.d.= £6.
Oral solution 20mg/mL 28 days @ 100mg b.d.= £185.
Note. Once daily modified-release tablets are available but generally more expensive (see *BNF*).

1 NIMH (National Institute of Mental Health) (2015) Psychoactive Drug Screening Program. *University of North Carolina*. Available from: https://pdspdb.unc.edu/pdspWeb (accessed August 2017).
2 Stahl SM (2013) Chapter 5: Antipsychotic agents. In: *Essential Psychopharmacology: Neuroscientific Basis and Practical Applications* (4e). Cambridge University Press, USA. 129–236.

3 Stahl SM *et al.* (2013) Serotonergic drugs for depression and beyond. *Current Drug Targets.* **14**: 578–585.
4 Baldwin DS *et al.* (2014) Evidence-based pharmacological treatment of anxiety disorders, post-traumatic stress disorder and obsessive-compulsive disorder: a revision of the 2005 guidelines from the British Association for Psychopharmacology. *Journal of Psychopharmacology.* **28**: 403–439.
5 Rummel-Kluge C *et al.* (2012) Second-generation antipsychotic drugs and extrapyramidal side effects: a systematic review and meta-analysis of head-to-head comparisons. *Schizophrenia Bulletin.* **38**: 167–177.
6 Seppi K *et al.* (2011) The Movement Disorder Society evidence-based medicine review update: treatments for the non-motor symptoms of Parkinson's disease. *Movement Disorders.* **26 (Suppl 3)**: S42–80.
7 Weintraub D *et al.* (2011) Patterns and trends in antipsychotic prescribing for Parkinson disease psychosis. *Archives of Neurology.* **68**: 899–904.
8 Starkstein SE *et al.* (2012) Psychiatric syndromes in Parkinson's disease. *Current Opinion in Psychiatry.* **25**: 468–472.
9 Rummel-Kluge C *et al.* (2010) Head-to-head comparisons of metabolic side effects of second generation antipsychotics in the treatment of schizophrenia: a systematic review and meta-analysis. *Schizophrenia Research.* **123**: 225–233.
10 Mittal V *et al.* (2011) Risk of cerebrovascular adverse events and death in elderly patients with dementia when treated with antipsychotic medications: a literature review of evidence. *American Journal of Alzheimer's Disease and Other Dementias.* **26**: 10–28.
11 DeVane CL and Nemeroff CB (2001) Clinical pharmacokinetics of quetiapine: an atypical antipsychotic. *Clinical Pharmacokinetics.* **40**: 509–522.
12 Adachi N *et al.* (2013) Basic treatment principles for psychotic disorders in patients with epilepsy. *Epilepsia.* **54 (Suppl 1)**: 19–33.
13 Chien C-F *et al.* (2017) Reversible global aphasia as a side effect of quetiapine: a case report and literature review. *Neuropsychiatric disease and treatment.* **13**: 2257–2260.
14 Meagher DJ *et al.* (2013) What do we really know about the treatment of delirium with antipsychotics? Ten key issues for delirium pharmacotherapy. *American Journal of Geriatric Psychiatry.* **21**: 1223–1238.
15 Hershenberg R *et al.* (2014) Role of atypical antipsychotics in the treatment of generalized anxiety disorder. *CNS Drugs.* **28**: 519–533.
16 Kato M and Chang CM (2013) Augmentation treatments with second-generation antipsychotics to antidepressants in treatment-resistant depression. *CNS Drugs.* **27 Suppl 1**: S11–19.

Updated November 2019

ANTIDEPRESSANTS

Indications: Authorized indications vary; see individual SPCs for details. Depression, anxiety, panic and post-traumatic stress disorders, neuropathic pain, stress incontinence and urgency, †bladder spasm, †hyperactive delirium, †insomnia, †pathological laughing and crying, †drooling, †refractory cough, †sweating, †hot flushes, †pruritus.

Pharmacology

Conventional antidepressants enhance monoamine transmission. Because monoamines regulate activity in numerous circuits, antidepressants are of benefit in many symptoms:

- pre-frontal cortex: depression (see Figure 1)[1]
- fear circuits: anxiety (see Benzodiazepines, Figure 2, p.166)
- descending pain modulation pathways: neuropathic pain (see Adjuvant analgesics, Figure 1, p.326)
- descending bladder control pathways: urinary incontinence.

Enhanced monoamine transmission is also believed to underlie the action of antidepressants in cough, hot flushes, pruritus (see p.825) and pathological laughing and crying, although their site of action is less well characterized.[2-5]

Some have additional actions of relevance to both beneficial and undesirable effects (Table 1), e.g.:

- histamine type 1 receptor antagonism: insomnia
- muscarinic receptor antagonism: bladder spasm, drooling
- sodium channel blockade (tricyclic antidepressants): neuropathic pain (but in overdose: coma, arrhythmias, seizures).

Classification

Antidepressants are classified according to their mechanism(s) of action (Table 1). However, many have multiple actions, and some labels are applied inconsistently. For example, 'SNRI' (serotonin and noradrenaline (norepinephrine) re-uptake inhibitor) can refer to all SNRIs or be reserved for those without additional receptor-binding affinities (e.g. **venlafaxine** and **duloxetine**).

SRIs (serotonin re-uptake inhibitors) with relatively minor additional actions ('selective' SRIs; SSRIs) are generally considered separately from those with more significant additional actions (e.g. **clomipramine, trazodone, vortioxetine**). However, all SSRIs except **escitalopram** have additional actions and, thus, their differences form a spectrum.

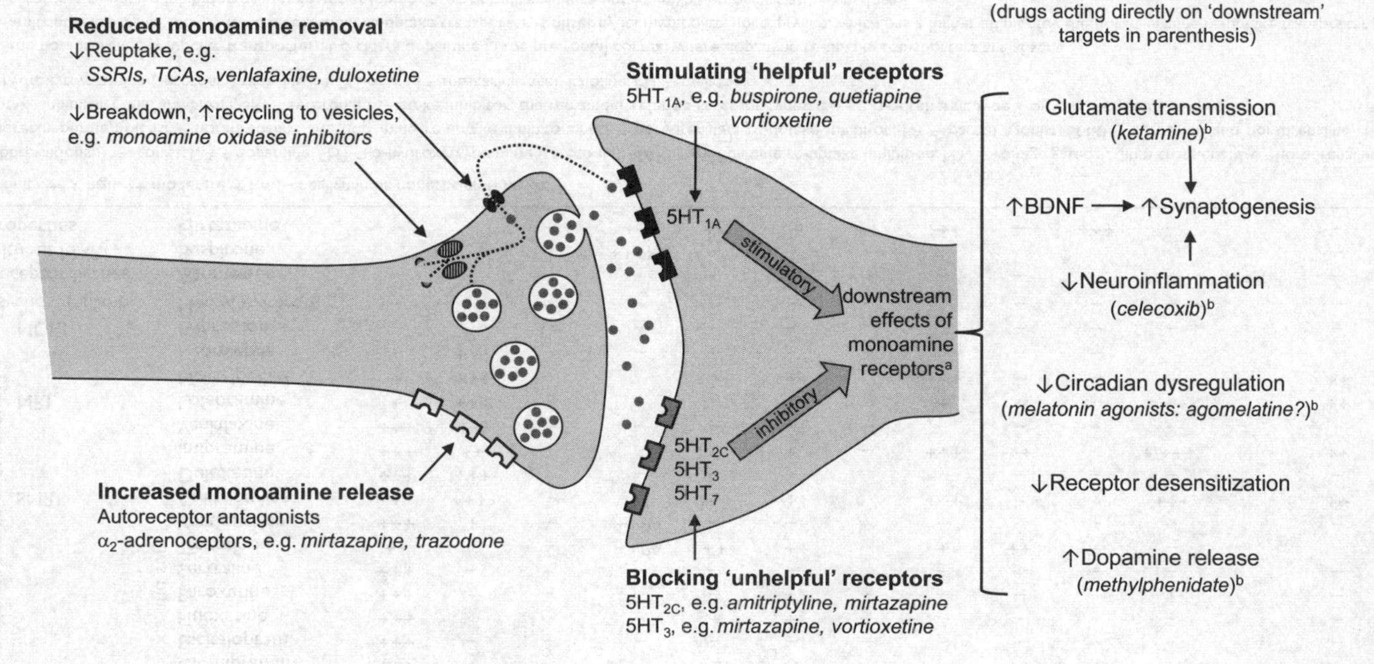

Figure 1 Mechanism of action of antidepressants and related drugs[1,6,7]

a. monoamines are not directly mood elevating; they act on depression through a variety of downstream effects (see text); this partly explains the delayed improvement in depression despite antidepressants increasing monoamine transmission within hours of commencing

b. drugs acting directly on these downstream effects might act faster (e.g. ketamine, methylphenidate) or improve residual symptoms (e.g. celecoxib).

Table 1 Classification and action of selected antidepressants[8-15]

Classification		Drug	Re-uptake transporters			Receptors									Ion channels
			5HT	NA[a]	DA	$5HT_{1A}$	$5HT_{2A}$	$5HT_{2C}$	$5HT_3$	H_1	α_1	α_2	M	MT	Na_v
Monoamine re-uptake inhibitors	SRI	Citalopram	+++	–	–	–	–	–	–	+	–	–	–		–
		Clomipramine	+++	+	–	–	+++	++	++	++	++	+	+++		++
		Escitalopram	+++	–	–	–	–	–	–	–	–	–	–		–
		Fluoxetine	+++	–	–	–	+	+	–	–	–	–	–		–
		Paroxetine	+++	+	–	–	–	–	–	–	–	–	+		–
		Sertraline	+++	–	+	–	–	–	–	–	+	–	–		–
		Trazodone	++	–	–	++PA	++	+	–	+	++	+	–		–
		Vortioxetine	+++	+	–	++PA	–	–	++	–	–	–	–		–
	SNRI	Amitriptyline	+++	+++[b]	–	+[d]	+++	+++		+++	+++	+	+++		++
		Duloxetine	+++	+++	+	–	–	–		–	–	–	–		–
		Imipramine	+++	++	–	–	+	+	–	+++	++	–	+/+++[e]		++
		Venlafaxine	+++	++[c]	–	–	–	–	–	–	–	–	–		–
	NRI	Lofepramine	+	+++	–	–	–			+	+	–	–/++[e]		++
		Nortriptyline	+	+++	–		+++	+++		+++	++	–	++		++
		Reboxetine	–	+++	–	–	–	–	–		–	–			–
	NDRI	Bupropion	–	+	++	–	–	–			–	–	–		–
Psychostimulants		Methylphenidate	–	–	+++	–	–	–	–		–	–	–		–
Receptor ligands without MARI properties		Agomelatine					–	+	–	–	–		–	++A	–
		Buspirone				+++PA	–	–	–						–
		Mirtazapine	–	–	–	++[d]	++	++	++	+++	–	+++	–		–

Affinity: +++ high, ++ moderate, + low, – negligible or none; blank = no data

Abbreviations: A = agonist; DA = dopamine; 5HT = 5-hydroxytryptamine (serotonin); MARI = monoamine re-uptake inhibition; Na_V = voltage gated sodium channels; NA = noradrenaline (norepinephrine); NDRI = noradrenaline and dopamine re-uptake inhibitor; NRI = noradrenaline re-uptake inhibitor; PA = partial agonist; SNRI = serotonin and noradrenaline re-uptake inhibitor ('dual' inhibitor); SRI = serotonin re-uptake inhibitor; the remainder refer to receptor types: $\alpha_{1/2}$ = α-adrenergic type 1 or 2; H_1 = histamine type 1; $5HT_{1A/2A/2C/3}$ = 5-hydroxytryptamine (serotonin) type 1A, 2A, 2C or 3; M = muscarinic acetylcholine; MT = melatonin.

a. the noradrenaline re-uptake transporter also clears dopamine in the prefrontal cortex, where dopamine re-uptake transporters are absent
b. amitriptyline's higher affinity for the serotonin re-uptake transporter is offset by its metabolite, nortriptyline, which has a higher affinity for the noradrenaline re-uptake transporter
c. serotonin re-uptake inhibition predominates at lower doses; noradrenaline re-uptake inhibition occurs at higher doses
d. assay measured *affinity* for $5HT_{1A}$ receptor but not whether the drug bound as an agonist, partial agonist or antagonist
e. varies with different M receptor subtypes.

The tricyclic antidepressants (TCAs) are structurally related but functionally variable, encompassing SRIs (e.g. **clomipramine**), SNRIs (e.g. **amitriptyline**) and NRIs (e.g. **lofepramine**, **nortriptyline**). They all inhibit voltage-gated sodium channels, making TCAs more dangerous in overdose than other antidepressants.

Psychostimulants are generally considered separately. They *reverse*, rather than inhibit, re-uptake transporters (i.e. actively pump neurotransmitters, particularly dopamine, out of the neurone; see p.246).

Only the monoamine oxidase inhibitors (MAOIs) form a clear discrete subclass, but their use requires specialist oversight. MAO type A breaks down serotonin, noradrenaline (norepinephrine) and dopamine. Type B breaks down dopamine. Antidepressant MAOIs are either non-selective or type A selective. Antiparkinsonian MAOIs (e.g. **selegiline**) are type B selective.

Depression

Conventional antidepressants increase the synaptic concentration of monoamines within hours. This triggers a cascade of events within the post-synaptic neurone that alter secondary messengers and genes controlling synaptogenesis (e.g. brain-derived neurotrophic factor), circadian rhythm (clock genes), inflammation and receptor sensitivity (see Figure 1).[1,6,7,16] Thus, an improvement in symptoms is slower to manifest. Drugs acting directly on these downstream events act faster (e.g. **ketamine**, **methylphenidate**) and/or improve symptoms refractory to conventional treatment (e.g. **celecoxib**).[12,17,18]

Various monoamines contribute to different depressive symptoms, e.g. reduced serotonin to low mood and reduced dopamine to anhedonia, demotivation and inattention.[1] Thus, for depression refractory to a single monoamine antidepressant (e.g. SRI, NRI), a first-line strategy is to switch to a broader acting antidepressant (e.g. an SNRI). Attempts to further refine drug selection using symptom profiles are ongoing.[19]

Not all monoamine receptors are helpful in depression. Some have regulatory roles that *reduce* the release of monoamines within the synapse (e.g. type 2 α-adrenergic autoreceptors) or elsewhere (e.g. post-synaptic $5HT_{2C}$ and $5HT_7$ receptors, which inhibit the downstream release of dopamine and serotonin, respectively). Thus, monoamine re-uptake inhibitors increase transmission at both helpful and unhelpful receptors. A second-line strategy for refractory depression is to block one or more unhelpful monoamine receptor (e.g. adding **mirtazapine** to an existing SNRI).

Some monoamine receptors mediate opposing effects, depending on their location. For example, *post-synaptic* $5HT_{1A}$ receptors mediate many helpful effects, whereas *pre-synaptic* $5HT_{1A}$ receptors inhibit serotonin release (i.e. are unhelpful autoreceptors). Some antidepressants and antipsychotics use $5HT_{1A}$ *partial* agonism to enable them to stimulate underactive post-synaptic receptors while reducing transmission at overstimulated autoreceptors.[15]

St John's wort (hypericum extract) is superior to placebo for mild depression.[20] However, NICE discourages its use because of:
- uncertainty about appropriate doses
- variation in the nature of products
- potential serious interactions with other drugs (including oral contraceptives, anticoagulants and anti-epileptics).[21]

Anxiety and panic disorder

Antidepressants and benzodiazepines inhibit the amygdala's 'fear circuits' through $5HT_{1A}$ and $GABA_A$ receptors, respectively (see Benzodiazepines, Figure 1, p.164).[22,23] The amygdala is a threat sensor which integrates sensory information with contextual information (e.g. interpretations, memories). If a fear response is required, the amygdala's effector pathway activates the relevant circuits (respiratory and cardiovascular centres, pituitary–adrenal axis, sympathetic autonomic nervous system, and fear-related areas of the cerebral cortex).

Breathlessness

Serotonergic neurones have a regulatory role in brainstem respiratory control. Thus, in addition to reducing coexistent anxiety, antidepressants might influence refractory breathlessness directly.[24] However, this is unconfirmed in RCTs.

Pain

The analgesic effect of antidepressants is predominantly due to enhanced noradrenaline transmission in descending pain modulation pathways, acting upon spinal α_2-adrenoceptors.[25] Noradrenaline also influences pain transmission in the brain (e.g. the limbic system) and reduces neuroinflammation in the spinal cord and peripheral nervous system.[25,26] The α_2-adrenoceptor agonists **clonidine** and **dexmedetomidine** are likely to act at the same sites (see p.82).

The effect of serotonin transmission is more variable; it can induce either analgesia or hyperalgesia depending on the location and subtype of serotonin receptor, and this probably explains the inconsistent analgesic effect of SSRIs.[27]

Duloxetine and, to a lesser extent, **amitriptyline**, inhibit P2X4 receptors. These purine-gated calcium channels are upregulated on spinal microglia in neuropathic pain.[28]

Sodium-channel blockade may also contribute to the analgesic efficacy of some antidepressants, including the modest effect of topical TCAs.[29,30]

Urological symptoms

Antidepressants act through parasympatholytic and sympathomimetic mechanisms. Antimuscarinic antidepressants (e.g. **amitriptyline**) inhibit detrusor stimulation and thus overactive bladder symptoms. Monoamine re-uptake inhibitors (e.g. **duloxetine**, and probably **amitriptyline**) enhance monoamine transmission in descending bladder control pathways, thus stimulating the sympathetic fibres that control sphincter tone. This explains their modest effect on urinary incontinence.[31]

Pharmacokinetics and pharmacogenetics

The pharmacokinetics of antidepressants are summarized in Table 2. The clearance of many antidepressants is significantly affected by CYP2D6 metabolizer phenotype, and to a lesser extent by CYP2C19. Further, serotonin re-uptake and drug transporter polymorphisms influence SSRI and TCA efficacy, respectively.[32,33] However, clinical benefit from genotyping has yet to be demonstrated.[34]

Cautions

In patients with a history of mania, antidepressants may precipitate a recurrent episode, particularly if administered without a mood stabilizer.

Suicide risk

The risk of antidepressant-related suicidal ideation needs to be balanced against the greater risk of non-fatal self-harm and completed suicide from untreated depression.[44]

In those aged ≤25 years, antidepressants are associated with suicidal ideation and non-fatal self-harm (NNH=143). Some studies found a greater risk with SSRIs than TCAs.[45] In adults ≥25 years, there is a smaller increase in risk (NNH around 700) and no association with the type of antidepressant.[45,46] *The risk is present even when an antidepressant is used for non-depressive indications.*[47]

There *is* a clear association between type of antidepressant and the risk of dying from an overdose: TCAs and MAO inhibitors (highest risk); **mirtazapine** and **venlafaxine** (intermediate); SSRIs (lowest risk).[45]

Suicidal ideation should be evaluated when treating depression in all age groups. Consider the safety in overdose of both the antidepressant and concurrent medicines. In both Europe and the USA, regulators have emphasized the need for close monitoring of adherence to treatment, treatment response, and emergence of thoughts of self-harm, particularly during the first month after starting or stopping an antidepressant, and to encourage patients to report to their doctor any deterioration in mood or behaviour.[46,48,49]

Cardiovascular disease and QT prolongation

Citalopram, **escitalopram**, **venlafaxine** and TCAs exhibit dose-related QT prolongation.[50] **Citalopram** and **escitalopram** have a known risk of *torsade de pointes* (see Chapter 20, p.797), even when taken as recommended, and specific restrictions are listed in the individual SPCs. **Fluoxetine**, **paroxetine** and **sertraline** are less affected, and the risk of *torsade de pointes* is

Table 2 Pharmacokinetic details for selected antidepressants[35-43]

	Bio-availability PO (%)	T_{max} *(h)*	*Plasma halflife (h)*	*Metabolism*
Agomelatine	<5	1–2	1–2	CYP1A2
Amitriptyline	45–55	4–6	9–25	Multiple pathways[a] (nortriptyline[a])
Bupropion	>87	1.5	21	CYP2B6[a]
Citalopram	80[b]	3	36	Multiple pathways[a]
Clomipramine	50[c]	1–5	12–36	Multiple pathways[a]
Doxepin	27[c]	2–4	8–24	Multiple pathways[a]
Duloxetine	90	6	8–17	CYP1A2, CYP2D6
Escitalopram	80	4	30	Multiple pathways[a]
Fluoxetine	90	4–8	1–4 days 7–15 days[a]	Multiple pathways[a]
Imipramine	45	3	21 12–24[a]	Multiple pathways[a] (desipramine[a])
Lofepramine	≤10[c]	1–2 4[a]	1.6 12–24[a]	Multiple pathways[a] (desipramine[a])
Methylphenidate	30	1–3	2	Non-CYP hepatic carboxylesterase
Mirtazapine	50	2	20–40	CYP1A2, CYP2D6, CYP3A4[a]
Nortriptyline	60	7–8.5	15–39	CYP2D6[a]
Paroxetine	50[d]	5	15–20	Multiple pathways
Reboxetine	95	2–4	12	CYP3A4
Sertraline	>44	6–8	26	CYP3A4
Trazodone	65	1	5–13	CYP2D6, CYP3A4[a]
Venlafaxine	40–45[c]	2.5 5.5[e]	5 11[a]	CYP2D6, CYP3A4[a]
Vortioxetine	75	7–11	66	CYP2D6

Blank = no data

a. active metabolite(s); listed in table if can be administered separately
b. for tablets; bio-availability of drops is nearly 100%
c. reflects significant first-pass metabolism limiting amount of parent drug reaching systemic circulation; however, more is absorbed, reaching the systemic circulation as active metabolite(s)
d. increases with multiple dosing
e. m/r product.

associated with other risk factors, e.g. excessive dose, hypokalaemia, interacting drugs. The risk is lowest with **paroxetine**, but drug interactions and withdrawal reactions are more common.[51]

Compared with other antidepressants, **citalopram** and **mirtazapine** are associated with a small increase in overall mortality in people aged >65 years,[52] but not in those aged 24–65 years.[53]

Consider alternatives (e.g. **sertraline**) in those with cardiovascular disease and/or risk factors for QT prolongation (see Chapter 20, p.797). If **citalopram** or **escitalopram** is required, note the specific precautions and dose limits recommended by regulatory authorities (see Selective serotonin re-uptake inhibitors, p.232).

Epilepsy

Although all antidepressants cause seizures in *overdose* (and perhaps also in slow metabolizers), only **amoxapine** (not UK), **bupropion**, **clomipramine** and **maprotiline** (not UK) are confirmed to reduce seizure threshold at therapeutic levels.[54] Antidepressants also cause seizures through hyponatraemia or by altering anti-epileptic drug concentrations as a result of a drug–drug interaction.[55]

Citalopram and **escitalopram** are widely favoured for use in patients with epilepsy, because of the lack of significant interactions with anti-epileptic drugs.[54] **Sertraline** is an alternative.[56]

Low-dose TCAs for neuropathic pain have not been studied in patients with previous seizures, but the risk is dose-related and animal studies even suggest a possible *anti*-epileptic action at low doses.[57]

Epilepsy is associated with both mood disorders and psychosis. Symptoms may occur in between (inter-ictal), during (ictal) or in the days or weeks after (post-ictal) seizures. Optimization of anti-epileptic medication should be considered alongside antidepressant treatment, particularly for ictal and post-ictal mood-related symptoms.[58] Further, anti-epileptic drugs can *cause* (and treat) mood disorders; seek specialist advice if negative mood changes occur after anti-epileptics are started.

Parkinson's disease

SSRIs can worsen extrapyramidal symptoms, because serotonin reduces nigrostriatal dopamine release via inhibitory $5HT_2$ receptors. However, the risk appears small; few RCTs report any worsening.[59] SSRIs are thus still often used in preference to TCAs, which can worsen autonomic dysfunction (α blockade) and cognitive impairment (M blockade).

$5HT_2$ antagonist antidepressants might be expected to avoid serotonin-mediated exacerbations. In small pilot RCTs, parkinsonian symptoms improved with **nefazodone**[60] but not **mirtazapine**.[61]

Antiparkinsonian D_2 agonists can themselves improve mood. In RCTs evaluating **pramipexole** for motor symptoms, mood and motivation also improved.[62] Further, in an RCT, **pramipexole** was more effective than **sertraline** for depression in patients with Parkinson's disease.[63]

Monoamine oxidase inhibitors (MAOIs)

Included for general information. MAOIs are *not recommended* in palliative care. They can cause serious undesirable effects when prescribed concurrently with various other drugs.

Seek advice from a psychiatrist if caring for a patient already receiving an MAOI; their previous mental illness is likely to have been difficult to treat, and switching or adding other psychotropics is difficult and risky.

MAOIs are potentially dangerous because of the risk of serious dietary and drug interactions. Hypertensive crises are mainly associated with the consumption of tyramine-containing foods (high levels present in aged or fermented foods, e.g. red wine, beer, old cheese, some beans, pickled foods, aged meat, yeast extracts). Typically, the patient experiences severe headache, and may suffer an intracranial haemorrhage.

Drug interactions occur with sympathomimetics (e.g. **ephedrine**, **pseudoephedrine**, **methylphenidate**, **modafinil**, **nefopam**), **levodopa** and serotoninergics (Box A). Serotonin toxicity has been reported with serotoninergic opioids (e.g. **fentanyl**, **pethidine**, **tramadol**; see Box A). Although companies marketing **morphine** and **oxycodone** also advise against concurrent use with MAOIs, their affinity for the serotonin re-uptake transporter is negligible,[64] and toxicity has not been reported.[65] Insisting on a 2-week washout before treating pain is unnecessary.

Renal and hepatic impairment

Antidepressants differ in their potential to cause toxicity when renal or hepatic function is impaired; see Chapter 17, p.737 and Chapter 18, p.763 for general information on the choice of antidepressant and use in ESRF or severe hepatic impairment respectively.

Drug interactions

MAOIs have numerous clinically significant drug interactions, which may result in hypertensive crises (see Cautions) and serotonin toxicity (Box A).

Because of the multiple actions of individual antidepressants, there is a risk of additive toxicity with the concurrent prescription of other drugs with the same pharmacodynamic effects, e.g. serotonin toxicity, bleeding risk, hyponatraemia, antimuscarinic effects, QT prolongation.

In addition, potentially serious interactions may result from induction or inhibition of hepatic metabolism. Some antidepressants inhibit cytochrome P450 enzymes:
- CYP1A2 inhibition by **fluvoxamine**, e.g. **tizanidine** levels increased ≤33 times
- CYP2C19 inhibition by **fluvoxamine**, e.g. **diazepam** clearance reduced by ≤65%
- CYP2D6 inhibition by **duloxetine**, **fluoxetine** and **paroxetine**, e.g. TCA levels increased ≤10 times; may reduce the efficacy of **tamoxifen** (a pro-drug).[66,67]

The metabolism of some antidepressants is affected by other potent P450 inhibitors and inducers:
- **duloxetine**, **mirtazapine**, by CYP1A2 inducers and/or inhibitors
- most TCAs, **duloxetine**, by CYP2D6 inhibitors
- **mirtazapine**, **trazodone**, **venlafaxine**, by CYP3A4 inducers and/or inhibitors.

See Chapter 19, Table 8, p.790, and individual monographs for more detail.

Box A Serotonin toxicity[68-73]

Cause

Ingestion of drug(s) which in combination and/or high doses (e.g. overdose) increase synaptic levels of serotonin in the CNS, mostly via:
- decreased metabolism, e.g. MAOIs
- decreased re-uptake, e.g. SSRIs
- increased release, e.g. MDMA, 'ecstasy'.

Severe life-threatening serotonin toxicity is generally associated with combinations of two or more serotonergic drugs that act via different mechanisms, e.g. MAOI + SSRI. An overdose of a single serotonergic drug or combinations of drugs that share the same mechanism is more likely to be associated with mild–moderate serotonin toxicity. Associations between some drugs and serotonin toxicity are debated. Those implicated in *severe* toxicity are:

Antidepressants
Monoamine oxidase inhibitors
Serotonin re-uptake inhibitors
Dual re-uptake inhibitors
TCAs (particularly clomipramine, imipramine)

Opioids
Dextromethorphan
Fentanyl
Methadone
Pentazocine
Pethidine
Tapentadol
Tramadol
(for other opioids, see below)

Other psychotropic drugs
Psychostimulants (amfetamines, cocaine, MDMA/'ecstasy')
Sibutramine (anorectic)
Ziprasidone (not UK)

Miscellaneous
Chlorphenamine, brompheniramine (but not reported with other H_1 antihistamines)
Linezolid
Lithium
Metaxalone (not UK)
Methylene blue

The above opioids are weak serotonin re-uptake inhibitors and/or $5HT_{2A}$ receptor agonists; the latter is probably the most relevant receptor in serotonin toxicity, given the benefit from $5HT_{2A}$ receptor *antagonists* (see Treatment below). Fatalities have been seen with dextromethorphan, pethidine, tramadol and possibly fentanyl.

Although serotonin toxicity is also reported with oxycodone, it lacks serotonergic properties and other serotonergic drugs were generally also administered. Nonetheless, some authors suggest using alternative opioids (e.g. alfentanil, buprenorphine or morphine) in those receiving multiple or high-dose serotonergic drugs.[64]

SPCs of various other drugs warn of the potential for serotonin toxicity, e.g. bupropion, granisetron, linezolid, metoclopramide, ondansetron, selegiline, triptans. However, interpretation of case reports is often hampered by ingestion of multiple drugs or alternative potential explanations (e.g. acute dopamine depletion syndrome, p.192). Thus, their association, if any, with serotonin toxicity is uncertain.

continued

Box A Continued

Clinical features

Diagnosis is based on a triad of neuro-excitatory features in the presence of serotonergic drugs and the absence of alternative explanations (e.g. sepsis). Symptoms can develop rapidly (e.g. after 1 or 2 doses) or gradually (e.g. mild symptoms for weeks before the development of severe toxicity):

- *autonomic hyperactivity:* sweating, fever, mydriasis, tachycardia, hypertension, tachypnoea, sialorrhoea, diarrhoea
- *neuromuscular hyperactivity:* tremor, hyperreflexia, hypertonia, myoclonus, clonus
- *altered mental status:* agitation, altered consciousness, hypomania, delirium.

Treatment

In severe cases (e.g. rigidity, rhabdomyolysis, haemodynamic instability, temperature >38.5°C, deteriorating blood gases), seek urgent advice from a critical care specialist; ventilation and paralysis ± inotropic support may be required.

Discontinue all serotinergic medication (toxicity generally resolves within 24h).
Provide supportive care, e.g. IV fluids, oxygen.
Symptomatic measures in mild–moderate cases:

- benzodiazepines for agitation, myoclonus and seizures, e.g. midazolam 5–10mg SC p.r.n.
- beta-blocker for hypertension and tachycardia[64]
- $5HT_{2A}$ antagonist[a], either:
  - ▷ cyproheptadine 8–12mg PO stat followed by 8mg q6h until symptoms resolve; tablets can be dispersed (or crushed if necessary) and given by enteral feeding tube (see Chapter 28, p.853) *or*
  - ▷ chlorpromazine 50–100mg IM stat[b].

a. benefit from $5HT_{2A}$ antagonists is reported but has *not* been confirmed in an RCT[68,73]
b. in most case reports, only a single dose was given.

Undesirable effects

A synopsis is contained in Table 3. Overall, discontinuation rates are marginally lower with SSRIs than with TCAs.[74]

GI bleeding and platelet function

SSRIs and SNRIs decrease serotonin uptake from the blood by platelets. Because platelets do not synthesize serotonin, the amount of serotonin in platelets is reduced.[77] This reduces platelet aggregation.[78] After confounding factors have been controlled for, SRIs increase the risk of GI bleeding, and possibly also intracranial haemorrhage, particularly when used in combination with an NSAID.[79-81] If an antidepressant is indicated in high-risk patients, safer alternatives would include an NRI (e.g. **nortriptyline**) or **mirtazapine**.[82]

Fracture risk

Although observational studies report an increased fracture risk with SSRIs, SNRIs and TCAs,[83,84] a subsequent study noted that an increased falls risk was present *before* the antidepressant was started, suggesting a confounded (non-causal) association.[85]

Sweating

In an RCT, the α_1-adrenoceptor antagonist **terazosin** alleviated SSRI-related sweating within 14 days of starting 1mg PO at bedtime.[86]

Use of antidepressants in palliative care

See individual monographs for doses and titration. For advice relating to driving, see Chapter 22, p.809.

Table 3 Relative frequency and putative mechanisms of undesirable effects of antidepressants[45,75,76]

Undesirable effect	*Mechanism*	*Relative frequency*													
		SNRI				*NRI*			*SRI*					*RA*	
		Amitriptyline	*Duloxetine*	*Imipramine*	*Venlafaxine*	*Desipramine*	*Lofepramine*	*Nortriptyline*	*Citalopram*	*Clomipramine*	*Fluoxetine*	*Paroxetine*	*Sertraline*	*Mirtazapine*	*Trazodone*
GI (nausea, diarrhoea)	↑ Serotonin (acting on $5HT_3$)	–	++	–	++	–	–	–	++	+	++	++	++	–	–
CNS (agitation, restlessness, anxiety, insomnia)	↑ Serotonin (acting on $5HT_2$)	–	+	+	+	+	+	+	+	+	+	+	+	–	–
Weight gain	$5HT_2$ and H_1 antagonism	++	–	+	–	–	–	–	–	+	–	–	–	++	+
Sedation	H_1, M and α_1-adrenergic antagonism	++	–	+	–	+	–	+	–	++	–	–	–	++	++
Postural hypotension	α_1-adrenergic antagonism	++	–	++	–	+	+	+	–	++	–	–	–	–	++
QT prolongation	Cardiac potassium channel blockade	+	+	+	+	+	+	+	++	+	+	–	+	–	+
Sexual dysfunction	↑ Serotonin (acting on $5HT_2$)	+	++	+	++	+	+	+	++	++	++	++	++	–	–
Dry mouth, constipation	M antagonism	++	–	++	–	+	+	+	–	++	–	–	–	–	–
Hyponatraemia (SIADH)	↑ Serotonin (acting on $5HT_2$); ↑ noradrenaline (norepinephrine) (acting on α_1)	+	+	+	+	+	+	+	++	+	++	++	++	+	+

Relative frequency: ++ = relatively common or strong, + = may occur or moderately strong, – = absent or rare/weak

Abbreviations: NRI = noradrenaline (norepinephrine) re-uptake inhibitor; RA = receptor antagonist; SNRI = serotonin and noradrenaline re-uptake inhibitor; SRI = serotonin re-uptake inhibitor; SIADH = syndrome of inappropriate anti-diuretic hormone secretion; the remainder refer to receptor types: $\alpha_{1/2}$ = α-adrenergic type 1 or 2; H_1 = histamine type 1; $5HT_{2/3}$ = 5-hydroxytryptamine (serotonin) type 2 or 3; M = muscarinic acetylcholine.

4

Depression

Treatment is tailored to the severity of symptoms, their functional impact and patient preference (Figure 2). The efficacy of cognitive behavioural and drug therapy is comparable.[87] First-line drug treatment is generally with **sertraline** or **citalopram**. They have fewer drug interactions, lower risk in overdose, and are marginally better tolerated than alternatives.[21,88] Efficacy has been confirmed in palliative populations.[89] An exception is dementia, where antidepressants appear less effective.[90] **Mirtazapine** may be preferred if there is concurrent nausea, insomnia or reduced appetite. An SNRI (e.g. **duloxetine**) may be considered if depression and neuropathic pain co-exist. Frequent re-evaluation of response, adherence, and alternative and concurrent sources of distress is required throughout.

Both **methylphenidate** (p.246) and **ketamine** (p.691) act within days and are sometimes used where prognosis is thought to be ≤4 weeks. However, trials are of short duration; conventional antidepressants should be used if the patient has a sufficient prognosis for a response to manifest.

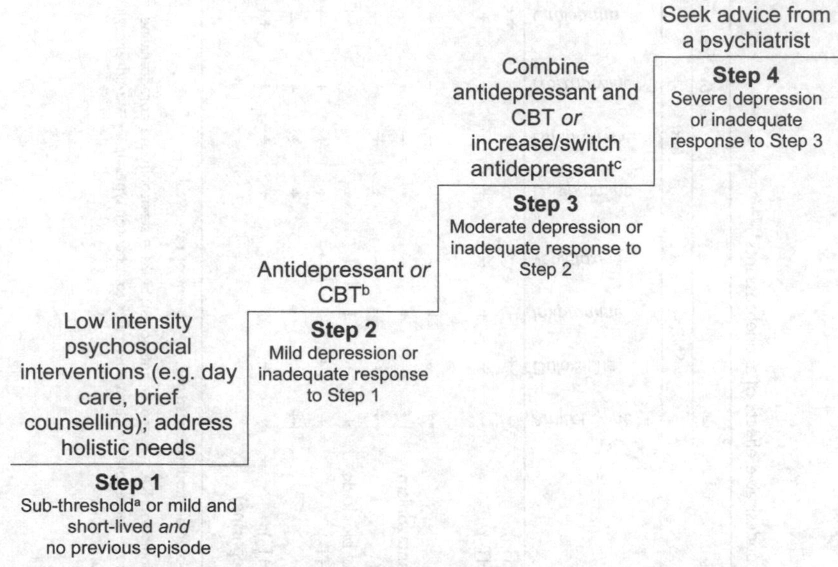

Figure 2 Overview of the management of depression.[21,89,91]

a. sub-threshold symptoms = patients with <5 DSM IV symptoms required for a diagnosis of depression
b. CBT = cognitive behavioural therapy
c. see Next-step treatments, below.

Next-step treatments: titrating, switching and combining antidepressants

If there is *no* response after 2–4 weeks or only a partial response after 6–8 weeks:

- increase the dose, particularly if there has been a partial response and minimal undesirable effects *or*
- switch antidepressants, particularly if there has been minimal improvement or bothersome undesirable effects *or*
- combine with a second antidepressant or adjuvant psychotropic drug, particularly if a previous switch was unhelpful.[21,45,92]

Dose titration is straightforward but, for SSRIs and **duloxetine**, of uncertain value. A systematic review found dose titration in patients not responding to SSRIs taken for 3–6 weeks no more effective than continuing the dose unaltered.[93] Nonetheless, many guidelines highlight individual variation in effective doses and therefore recommend dose titration if the existing drug is well tolerated.[21,45] A dose–response effect is more clearly established with some TCAs and **venlafaxine**.

Switching to a second-line antidepressant with a different mode of action (e.g. from SSRI to **mirtazapine** or **venlafaxine**) appears more effective than switching within a class (also see Switching antidepressants).[19,45] The effect of **mirtazapine** on additional monoamines is theoretically advantageous, and its onset may be faster. **Venlafaxine** has a marginally higher response rate compared with switching to a second SSRI, but is less well tolerated.[45]

A partial response to an antidepressant can be increased ('augmented') by adding a second psychotropic drug to an SSRI or SNRI. This avoids potential loss of the initial improvement, but is generally less well tolerated than monotherapy.[21] Options include:[19,45,94]

- antipsychotics (e.g. **quetiapine**)
- **mirtazapine** (particularly if concurrent anxiety)[95]
- a range of options used only by psychiatrists (e.g. **lithium**, **tri-iodothyronine**).

NICE suggests primary care clinicians seek advice before adding a second drug.[21] Palliative care specialists using some of the above drugs for other indications should be aware of their potential benefit when concurrent depression has only partially responded to an antidepressant.

Duration of treatment

Consider stopping treatment 6 months after full remission in those without risk factors for relapse. Risk factors include previous episodes of depression, severity, duration and degree of treatment resistance of current episode, presence of residual symptoms, and possibly older age. Treatment is tapered slowly (see Stopping antidepressants). Treat those with risk factors for longer:

- 1 year if full remission but 1 risk factor
- ≥2 years if ≥2 risk factors.[21,45]

In palliative care, the latter is likely to mean lifelong/indefinitely.

Anxiety and panic disorders

The efficacy of cognitive behavioural and drug therapy is comparable.[96] Choice of drug is largely influenced by likely duration of use:

- benzodiazepine, if prognosis is days to weeks
- SSRI (± a benzodiazepine initially), if prognosis is months.

Supporting evidence (and market authorization) for SSRIs varies for different anxiety disorders.[96] **Citalopram** and **sertraline** are authorized for panic disorder, well tolerated, have fewer drug interactions, and are generally more familiar to prescribers. All SSRIs can initially exacerbate anxiety; start low and consider a concurrent benzodiazepine for the first few weeks. If response is inadequate, consider:

- combining with cognitive behavioural therapy
- switching to **venlafaxine** or **duloxetine** (see Switching antidepressants)
- combining with or switching to **pregabalin** or a benzodiazepine (see Stopping antidepressants).

In general psychiatry, switching is not advocated within 3 months, because benefit from SSRIs can take longer to manifest than in depression.[96,97] However, in patients with a short prognosis, adding **pregabalin** or a benzodiazepine may bring more rapid benefit. **Quetiapine** also acts quickly but is less well tolerated and so is generally reserved for anxiety refractory to antidepressants ± benzodiazepines ± **pregabalin**.[96]

Post-traumatic stress disorder

Evidence-based treatments include psychological therapies and SSRIs, but benefit from the latter takes several weeks to manifest.[98] In the last weeks of life, antipsychotics and benzodiazepines may act more quickly.[99] **Prazosin** (p.169) reduces the frequency and severity of nightmares.

Neuropathic pain

Amitriptyline, **imipramine**, **nortriptyline** and **duloxetine** are commonly used for neuropathic pain.[100] In both direct comparisons and network analyses, their efficacy and tolerability appear to be similar to each other and to **gabapentin/pregabalin**.[101-115] Most trials examined chronic pain, particularly painful diabetic neuropathy and post herpetic neuralgia. In smaller trials in cancer-related and chemotherapy-related neuropathic pain, efficacy appears comparable.[106,111,114,116-118] Inhibition of noradrenaline re-uptake is important to their analgesic action. This may explain why SSRIs are not consistently effective and why **venlafaxine** appears less effective at lower doses (see p.236).[100] The benefit reported with **mirtazapine**[119] has *not* been confirmed in RCTs.

If the first-choice treatment is poorly tolerated, consider switching to an alternative antidepressant (e.g. from **amitriptyline** to **duloxetine**; see Switching antidepressants). However, switching is unlikely to improve efficacy unless undesirable effects have prevented dose titration; all predominantly act on noradrenaline transmission; the clinical relevance of their dissimilar actions is unclear (e.g. **amitriptyline** upon sodium channels, **duloxetine** upon P2X4 receptors; see Pharmacology).[28]

If the first-choice treatment fails, switch to or combine with an anti-epileptic (see p.289; see Stopping antidepressants below). The combination of **amitriptyline**, **imipramine** or **nortriptyline** with **gabapentin**, **pregabalin** or **morphine** is more effective and/or better tolerated than any treatment alone.[120-124]

Other pain syndromes

Antidepressants are of benefit for various pain syndromes, including migraine and tension headache (TCAs),[125] †fibromyalgia (**amitriptyline, duloxetine, milnacipran** (not UK),[126,127] and †post-operative pain (**duloxetine**).[128]

Stress incontinence, urgency and †bladder spasm

Antimuscarinic antidepressants (e.g. **amitriptyline**) reduce detrusor contractions associated with urgency, although authorized alternatives have additional direct effects on the detrusor muscle.[129] **Duloxetine** has a limited role in stress incontinence.[130]

†Hyperactive delirium

The benefit reported with **trazodone** (p.244) remains unconfirmed in clinical trials. Treatment of underlying causes, non-drug management (e.g. orientation strategies, correction of sensory deprivation) and prevention of complications are central to delirium management. Antipsychotics are generally used first-line when medication is needed (see p.193).

†Impulsivity and aggression

Serotonin is implicated in the regulation of impulsivity and aggression.[131] Antipsychotics, SSRIs and mood stabilisers (e.g. **valproate**) reduce these symptoms in personality disorders and traumatic brain injury.[131-133] Their role in similar symptoms due to brain tumours has not been studied.

†Agitation and challenging behaviours in dementia

Evidence for antidepressants is insufficient to justify routine use. Although **citalopram** was more effective than placebo, a subgroup of patients appeared to deteriorate more rapidly compared with controls.[134] A small RCT (n=30) found **trazodone** improved sleep disturbance.[135]

†Insomnia

When insomnia co-exists with other indications, sedating antidepressants are often selected (e.g. TCAs, **mirtazapine, trazodone**). Limited evidence suggests that **doxepin** and **trazodone** may be effective for primary insomnia.[136] However, **doxepin** is significantly more expensive than other TCAs and the dose used in trials (3–6mg PO at bedtime) is lower than that available in the UK (25mg).

†Pathological laughing and crying

Frequent brief uncontrollable laughter and/or crying incongruent with external events can complicate numerous neurological disorders, including strokes, Parkinson's disease, cerebral tumours, multiple sclerosis, MND/ALS and dementia. It can be socially disabling. Functional imaging suggests dysregulation of serotoninergic and glutaminergic pathways.[2] The differential diagnosis includes:

- seizures: generally complex partial seizures and thus an alteration of consciousness during/after episodes
- depression or other mood disorders; mood alteration is persistent, whereas the emotion that may accompany pathological laughing and crying is short-lived.

Validated assessment tools are available to aid diagnosis.[137] First-line treatment is with **citalopram** or **sertraline**; doses can be lower than those required for depression. Benefit is often seen within days. Second-line options include **amitriptyline, nortriptyline, mirtazapine** and **memantine**.[2] A **quinidine–dextromethorphan** combination (not UK) is also effective,[138] but is expensive and has not been compared with established treatments.[2]

†*Refractory cough*
Amitriptyline is more effective than **codeine** for cough that persists despite resolution of the initial cause.[139] **Gabapentin** (p.297) is an alternative. Benefit probably relates to reducing cough reflex hypersensitivity, which is generally present in this group of patients (see Drugs for cough, p.154).[4]

†*Breathlessness*
In addition to their use for secondary anxiety, a potential role for antidepressants has been suggested in refractory breathlessness *per se*. However, to date, RCTs have found no benefit with **buspirone**[140] or **sertraline** (p.232); an RCT of **mirtazapine** (p.241) is ongoing.

†*Sweating*
Like other antimuscarinics, **amitriptyline** is used for paraneoplastic sweating unresponsive to NSAIDs.[141] However, like all monoamine re-uptake inhibitors, it can also *cause* sweating.[142]

†*Hot flushes*
Trials in patients with breast cancer have found benefit from SSRIs (p.232), **venlafaxine** (p.236), **gabapentin** (p.297) and **duloxetine** (p.239).[143] **Venlafaxine** works faster than **clonidine** (p.82), and participants prefer **venlafaxine** over **gabapentin**.[143] **Venlafaxine** and SSRIs are also reported to improve hot flushes resulting from medical or surgical castration in men.[144-146]

†*Pruritus*
Sertraline (p.232) is a first-line choice for cholestatic pruritus and a second-line choice for uraemic pruritus refractory to **gabapentin** (see Drugs for pruritus, p.825). Benefit is reported for pruritus in advanced cancer (**paroxetine**, **mirtazapine**), neuropathic pruritus (**amitriptyline**, p.228) and idiopathic pruritus (**mirtazapine**); see Drugs for pruritus, p.825.

†*Drooling*
Like other antimuscarinics (p.4), **amitriptyline** reduces salivation.

Switching antidepressants
Usual doses of most PO SSRIs can be switched to PO **duloxetine, mirtazapine** or **venlafaxine** in a single step; only **fluoxetine** needs a washout gap due to its longer halflife, i.e. from:[45,147]
- **sertraline** ≤50mg/24h, **citalopram** ≤20mg/24h, **escitalopram** ≤10mg/24h or **paroxetine** ≤20mg/24h: stop the SSRI and start the second-line antidepressant the following day
- **fluoxetine** 20mg/24h: stop, wait 4–7 days, then start the second-line antidepressant.

Higher doses of SSRIs require cross-tapering, e.g. reducing in weekly steps to the above level and then switching. If the symptoms being treated are severe, consider adding the second-line antidepressant sooner provided adequate monitoring for serotonin toxicity is possible.[94,147]

Switching from TCAs requires additional care because of the potential for pharmacokinetic drug interactions and withdrawal reactions (e.g. rebound insomnia). Switching to **duloxetine** in a single step might be possible with low doses (e.g. **amitriptyline** PO ≤25mg/24h) taken for ≤6 weeks; otherwise, cross-taper. Careful monitoring for both withdrawal reactions and serotonin toxicity is required for either approach.[94,147]

Switching to or from MAOIs requires specialist advice.

Stopping antidepressants
Abrupt cessation of antidepressant therapy (particularly **paroxetine**, **venlafaxine,** TCAs or an MAOI) after regular administration for >8 weeks may result in a discontinuation reaction (withdrawal syndrome; Box B).[148] Discontinuation reactions depend on the class of antidepressant, and are more common with drugs with shorter halflives. Thus, with SSRIs, discontinuation reactions are most common with **paroxetine** and least common with **fluoxetine**.

Discontinuation reactions differ from a depressive relapse or a panic disorder. They generally start abruptly within a few days of stopping the antidepressant (*or reducing its dose*). In contrast, a depressive relapse is uncommon in the first week after stopping an antidepressant, and symptoms tend to build up gradually and persist. Discontinuation reactions generally resolve within 24h of re-instating antidepressant therapy, whereas the response is slower with a depressive relapse.

Ideally, antidepressants taken for >8 weeks should be progressively reduced over 4 weeks. If a mild discontinuation reaction is suspected, re-assurance alone may be adequate. If distressing, restart the antidepressant and reduce more gradually.

Some patients experience discontinuation symptoms even during tapering. When this happens, increase the dose and, before continuing with tapering, consider:

- using a liquid formulation and reducing the dose in smaller steps *or*
- switching from **venlafaxine** or a short-halflife SSRI to **fluoxetine**.[148]

Box B Antidepressant discontinuation reactions[148]

SSRIs and venlafaxine: *'FINISH'*[149]

Flu-like symptoms (fatigue, lethargy, myalgia, chills)
Insomnia (including vivid dreams)
Nausea
Imbalance (ataxia, vertigo, dizziness)
Sensory disturbances (paraesthesia, sensations of electric shock)
Hyperarousal (restlessness, anxiety, agitation)

TCAs

Flu-like symptoms (fatigue, lethargy, myalgia, chills)
Insomnia (including vivid dreams)
GI disorders (nausea, diarrhoea)
Mood disorders (depression or mania)
Movement disorders (rare: akathisia, parkinsonism)

Trazodone

Flu-like symptoms (fatigue, lethargy, myalgia, chills)
GI disorders (nausea, diarrhoea)
Restlessness
Tremor
Headache

Mirtazapine

Nausea
Dizziness
Hyperarousal (anxiety, agitation)
Headache

MAOIs

Insomnia
Movement disorders (ataxia, athetosis, catatonia, myoclonus)
Mood disorders (lability, depression, agitation, aggression)
Paranoia
Hallucinations
Seizures
Altered speech (pressured, slow)

1 Stahl SM (2021) Chapter 6: Mood disorders. In: *Essential Psychopharmacology: Neuroscientific Basis and Practical Applications* (5e). Cambridge University Press, USA. pp. 244–282.
2 Finegan E *et al.* (2019) Pathological crying and laughing in motor neuron disease: pathobiology, screening, intervention. *Frontiers in Neurology*. **10**: 260.
3 Grajales-Reyes JG and Samineni VK (2019) Untangling a canopy of spinal itch circuits. *Pain*. **5**: 987–988.
4 Turner RD and Birring SS (2019) Chronic cough: ATP, afferent pathways and hypersensitivity. *European Respiratory Journal*. **54**: 1900889.
5 O'Neill S and Eden J (2017) The pathophysiology of menopausal symptoms. *Obstetrics, Gynaecology and Reproductive Medicine*. **27**: 303–310.
6 Yang T *et al.* (2020) The role of BDNF on neural pasticity in depression. *Frontiers in Cellular Neuroscience*. **14**: 82.
7 Troubat R *et al.* (2021) Neuroinflammation and depression: a review. *European Journal of Neuroscience*. **53**: 151–171.

8 Stahl SM *et al.* (2004) A review of the neuropharmacology of bupropion, a dual norepinephrine and dopamine reuptake inhibitor. *Primary Care Companion Journal of Clinical Psychiatry*. **6**: 159–166.

9 Beique JC *et al.* (1998) Affinities of venlafaxine and various reuptake inhibitors for the serotonin and norepinephrine transporters. *European Journal of Pharmacology*. **349**: 129–132.

10 Hamon M and Bourgoin S (2006) Pharmacological profile of antidepressants: a likely basis for their efficacy and side effects? *European Neuropsychopharmacology*. **16 (Suppl 5)**: S625–632.

11 Garnock-Jones KP (2014) Vortioxetine: a review of its use in major depressive disorder. *CNS Drugs*. **28**: 855–874.

12 Stahl SM (2021) Chapter 7: Treatments for mood disorders. In: *Essential Psychopharmacology: Neuroscientific Basis and Practical Applications* (5e). Cambridge University Press, USA. pp. 283–358.

13 Gillman PK (2007) Tricyclic antidepressant pharmacology and therapeutic drug interactions updated. *British Journal of Pharmacology*. **151**: 737–748.

14 Binding Database (2015) Skaggs School of Pharmacy and Pharmaceutical Sciences. http://bindingdb.org/as/search.html (accessed June 2015).

15 Stahl SM *et al.* (2013) Serotonergic drugs for depression and beyond. *Current Drug Targets*. **14**: 578–585.

16 Planchez B *et al.* (2020) Adult hippocampal neurogenesis and antidepressants effects. *Current Opinion in Pharmacology*. **50**: 88–95.

17 Williams NR and Schatzberg AF (2016) NMDA antagonist treatment of depression. *Current Opinion in Neurobiology*. **36**: 112–117.

18 Kohler-Forsberg O *et al.* (2019) Efficacy of anti-inflammatory treatment on major depressive disorder or depressive symptoms: meta-analysis of clinical trials. *Acta Psychiatrica Scandinavica*. **139**: 404–419.

19 Haddad PM and Nutt DJ (2020) Chapter 7: Drugs to treat depression. In: *Seminars in Clinical Psychopharmacology* (3e). Cambridge University Press, UK. pp. 227–267.

20 Apaydin EA (2016) A systematic review of St. John's wort for major depressive disorder. *Systematic Reviews*. **5**: 148.

21 NICE (2009) Depression. *Clinical Guidelines*. CG90 and CG91. www.nice.org.uk.

22 Capogna M (2014) GABAergic cell type diversity in the basolateral amygdala. *Current Opinion in Neurobiology*. **26**: 110–116.

23 Stahl SM (2021) Chapter 8: Anxiety, trauma and treatment. In: *Essential Psychopharmacology: Neuroscientific Basis and Practical Applications* (5e). Cambridge University Press, USA. pp. 359–378.

24 Lovell N *et al.* (2018) Mirtazapine for chronic breathlessness? A review of mechanistic insights and therapeutic potential. *Expert Review of Respiratory Medicine*. **13**: 173–180.

25 Kremer M *et al.* (2018) A dual noradrenergic mechanism for the relief of neuropathic allodynia by the antidepressant drugs duloxetine and amitriptyline. *Journal of Neuroscience*. **38**: 9934–9954.

26 Caraci F *et al.* (2019) Rescue of noradrenergic system as a novel pharmacological strategy in the treatment of chronic pain: focus on microglia activation. *Frontiers in Pharmacology*. **10**: 1024.

27 Liu QQ *et al.* (2020) Role of 5-HT receptors in neuropathic pain: potential therapeutic implications. *Pharmacological Research*. **159**: 104949.

28 Yamashita T *et al.* (2016) Duloxetine inhibits microglial P2X4 receptor function and alleviates neuropathic pain after peripheral nerve injury. *PLoS One*. **11**: e0165189.

29 Genevois A-L *et al.* (2020) Analgesic effects of topical amitriptyline in patients with chemotherapy-induced peripheral neuropathy: mechanistic insights from studies in mice. *The Journal of Pain*. **22**: 440–453.

30 Casale R *et al.* (2017) Topical treatments for localized neuropathic pain. *Current Pain and Headache Reports*. **21**: 15.

31 Deepak P and Kumar TN (2011) Duloexetine – pharmacological aspects. *International Journal of Biological and Medical Research*. **2**: 589–592.

32 Porcelli S *et al.* (2012) Meta-analysis of serotonin transporter gene promoter polymorphism (5-HTTLPR) association with antidepressant efficacy. *European Neuropsychopharmacology*. **22**: 239–258.

33 Benavides R *et al.* (2020) A functional polymorphism in the ATP-Binding Cassette B1 transporter predicts pharmacologic response to combination of nortriptyline and morphine in neuropathic pain patients. *Pain*. **161**: 619–629.

34 Kirchheiner J and Rodriguez-Antona C (2009) Cytochrome P450 2D6 genotyping: potential role in improving treatment outcomes in psychiatric disorders. *CNS Drugs*. **23**: 181–191.

35 Wen B *et al.* (2008) Detection of novel reactive metabolites of trazodone: evidence for CYP2D6-mediated bioactivation of m-chlorophenylpiperazine. *Drug Metabolism and Disposition*. **36**: 841–850.

36 Jefferson JW *et al.* (2005) Bupropion for major depressive disorder: pharmacokinetic and formulation considerations. *Clinical Therapeutics*. **27**: 1685–1695.

37 Hiemke C and Härtter S (2000) Pharmacokinetics of selective serotonin reuptake inhibitors. *Pharmacology and Therapeutics*. **85**: 11–28.

38 Fleishaker JC (2000) Clinical pharmacokinetics of reboxetine, a selective norepinephrine reuptake inhibitor for the treatment of patients with depression. *Clinical Pharmacokinetics*. **39**: 413–427.

39 Venkatakrishnan K *et al.* (1998) Five distinct human cytochromes mediate amitriptyline N-demethylation in vitro: dominance of CYP 2C19 and 3A4. *Journal of Clinical Pharmacology*. **38**: 112–121.

40 Richelson E (1997) Pharmacokinetic drug interactions of new antidepressants: a review of the effects on the metabolism of other drugs. *Mayo Clinic Proceedings*. **72**: 835–847.

41 Kaye CM *et al.* (1989) A review of the metabolism and pharmacokinetics of paroxetine in man. *Acta Psychiatrica Scandinavica Supplementum*. **350**: 60–75.

42 Schulz P *et al.* (1985) Discrepancies between pharmacokinetic studies of amitriptyline. *Clinical Pharmacokinetics*. **10**: 257–268.

43 Abernethyl DR *et al.* (1984) Absolute bioavailability of imipramine: influence of food. *Psychopharmacology*. **83**: 104–106.

44 Lu CY *et al.* (2014) Changes in antidepressant use by young people and suicidal behavior after FDA warnings and media coverage: quasi-experimental study. *British Medical Journal*. **348**: G3596.

45 Cleare A *et al.* (2015) Evidence-based guidelines for treating depressive disorders with antidepressants: a revision of the 2008 British Association for Psychopharmacology guidelines. *Journal of Psychopharmacology*. **29**: 459–525.

46 Coupland C *et al.* (2015) Antidepressant use and risk of suicide and attempted suicide or self harm in people aged 20 to 64: cohort study using a primary care database. *British Medical Journal*. **350**: H517.

47 Pereira A *et al.* (2014) Suicidal ideation and behavior associated with antidepressant medications: implications for the treatment of chronic pain. *Pain*. **155**: 2471–2475.

48 MHRA (2008) Antidepressants: suicidal thoughts and behaviour. *Drug Safety Update*. www.gov.uk/drug-safety-update.

49 Sinyor M and Cheung AH (2015) Antidepressants and risk of suicide. *British Medical Journal*. **350**: H783.

50 Jasiak NM and Bostwick JR (2014) Risk of QT/QTc prolongation among newer non-SSRI antidepressants. *Annals of Pharmacotherpy*. **48**: 1620–1628.

51 Funk KA and Bostwick JR (2013) A comparison of the risk of QT prolongation among SSRIs. *Annals of Pharmacotherapy*. **47**: 1330–1341.

52 Danielsson B *et al.* (2016) Antidepressants and antipsychotics classified with torsades de pointes arrhythmia risk and mortality in older adults – a Swedish nationwide study. *British Journal of Clinical Pharmacology.* **81**: 773–783.
53 Coupland C *et al.* (2016) Antidepressant use and risk of cardiovascular outcomes in people aged 20 to 64: cohort study using primary care database. *British Medical Journal.* **352**: i1350.
54 Kanner AM (2013) The treatment of depressive disorders in epilepsy: what all neurologists should know. *Epilepsia.* **54 (Suppl 1)**: 3–12.
55 Kerr MP *et al.* (2011) International consensus clinical practice statements for the treatment of neuropsychiatric conditions associated with epilepsy. *Epilepsia.* **52**: 2133–2138.
56 Specialist Pharmacy Service (2021) Using antidepressants for depression in people with epilepsy. www.sps.nhs.uk (accessed December 2021).
57 Dailey JW and Naritoku DK (1996) Antidepressants and seizures: clinical anecdotes overshadow neuroscience. *Biochemical Pharmacology.* **52**: 1323–1329.
58 Blumer D *et al.* (2004) The interictal dysphoric disorder: recognition, pathogenesis, and treatment of the major psychiatric disorder of epilepsy. *Epilepsy and Behaviour.* **5**: 826–840.
59 Skapinakis P *et al.* (2010) Efficacy and acceptability of selective serotonin reuptake inhibitors for the treatment of depression in Parkinson's disease: a systematic review and meta-analysis of randomized controlled trials. *BMC Neurology.* **10**: 49.
60 Avila A *et al.* (2003) Does nefazodone improve both depression and Parkinson disease? A pilot randomized trial. *Journal of Clinical Psychopharmacology.* **23**: 509-513.
61 Zhang LS *et al.* (2006) Mirtazapine vs fluoxetine in treating Parkinson's disease with depression and anxiety. *Medical Journal of Chinese People's Health.*
62 Leentjens AF *et al.* (2009) The effect of pramipexole on mood and motivational symptoms in Parkinson's disease: a meta-analysis of placebo-controlled studies. *Clinical Therapeutics.* **31**: 89–98.
63 Barone P *et al.* (2006) Pramipexole versus sertraline in the treatment of depression in Parkinson's disease: a national multicenter parallel-group randomized study. *Journal of Neurology.* **253**: 601–607.
64 Baldo BA and Rose MA (2020) The anaesthetist, opioid analgesic drugs, and serotonin toxicity: a mechanistic and clinical review. *British Journal of Anaesthesia.* **124**: 44–62.
65 Preston CL. Stockley's Drug Interactions. London: Pharmaceutical Press www.medicinescomplete.com (accessed December 2021).
66 Kelly CM *et al.* (2010) Selective serotonin reuptake inhibitors and breast cancer mortality in women receiving tamoxifen: a population based cohort study. *British Medical Journal.* **340**: C693.
67 Specialist Pharmacy Service (2018) Tamoxifen and SSRI or SNRI antidepressants – is there an interaction? www.sps.nhs.uk (accessed December 2021).
68 Nguyen H *et al.* (2018) An 11-year retrospective review of cyproheptadine use in serotonin syndrome cases reported to the California Poison Control System. *Journal of Clinical Pharmacology and Therapeutics.* **44**: 327–334.
69 Werneke U *et al.* (2016) Conundrums in neurology: diagnosing serotonin syndrome – a meta-analysis of cases. *Boston Medical Center Neurology.* **16**: 97.
70 Moss MJ *et al.* (2019) Serotonin toxicity: Associated agents and clinical characeteristics. *Journal of Clinical Psychopharmacology.* **39**: 628–633.
71 Chow R *et al.* (2020) Serotonin syndrome in palliative care #403. *Journal of Palliative Medicine.* **23**: 1678–1680.
72 Baldo BA and Rose MA (2020) The anaesthetist, opioid analgesic drugs, and serotonin toxicity: a mechanistic and clinical review. *British Journal of Anaesthesia.* **124**: 44–62.
73 Gillman PK (1999) The serotonin syndrome and its treatment. *Journal of Psychopharmacology.* **13**: 100–109.
74 Anderson IM (2000) Selective serotonin reuptake inhibitors versus tricyclic antidepressants: a meta-analysis of efficacy and tolerability. *Journal of Affective Disorders.* **58**: 19–36.
75 Bhuvaneswar CG *et al.* (2009) Adverse endocrine and metabolic effects of psychotropic drugs: selective clinical review. *CNS Drugs.* **23**: 1003–1021.
76 Jacob S and Spinler SA (2006) Hyponatremia associated with selective serotonin-reuptake inhibitors in older adults. *Annals of Pharmacotherapy.* **40**: 1618–1622.
77 Ross S *et al.* (1980) Inhibition of 5-hydroxytryptamine uptake in human platelets by antidepressant agents in vivo. *Psychopharmacology.* **67**: 1–7.
78 Li N *et al.* (1997) Effects of serotonin on platelet activation in whole blood. *Blood Coagulation Fibrinolysis.* **8**: 517–523.
79 van Walraven C *et al.* (2001) Inhibition of serotonin reuptake by antidepressants and upper gastrointestinal bleeding in elderly patients: retrospective cohort study. *British Medical Journal.* **323**: 655–657.
80 Paton C and Ferrier IN (2005) SSRIs and gastrointestinal bleeding. *British Medical Journal.* **331**: 529–530.
81 Shin JY *et al.* (2015) Risk of intracranial haemorrhage in antidepressant users with concurrent use of non-steroidal anti-inflammatory drugs: nationwide propensity score matched study. *British Medical Journal.* **351**: H3517.
82 de Abajo FJ and Garcia-Rodriguez LA (2008) Risk of upper gastrointestinal tract bleeding associated with selective serotonin reuptake inhibitors and venlafaxine therapy: interaction with nonsteroidal anti-inflammatory drugs and effect of acid-suppressing agents. *Archives of General Psychiatry.* **65**: 795–803.
83 European Medicines Agency (2010) Pharmacovigilance Working Party March 2010 plenary meeting report. www.ema.europa.eu.
84 Lanteigne A *et al.* (2015) Serotonin-norepinephrine reuptake inhibitor and selective serotonin reuptake inhibitor use and risk of fractures: a new-user cohort study among US adults aged 50 years and older. *CNS Drugs.* **29**: 245–252.
85 Brännström J *et al.* (2019) Association between antidepressant drug use and hip fracture in older people before and after treatment initiation. *JAMA Psychiatry.* **76**: 172–179.
86 Ghaleiha A *et al.* (2013) Effect of terazosin on sweating in patients with major depressive disorder receiving sertraline: a randomized controlled trial. *International Journal of Psychiatry in Clinical Practice.* **17**: 44–47.
87 Amick HR *et al.* (2015) Comparative benefits and harms of second generation antidepressants and cognitive behavioral therapies in initial treatment of major depressive disorder: systematic review and meta-analysis. *British Medical Journal.* **351**: h6019.
88 Cipriani A *et al.* (2018) Comparative efficacy and acceptability of 21 antidepressant drugs for the acute treatment of adults with major depressive disorder: a systematic review and network meta-analysis. *The Lancet.* **391**: 1357–1366.
89 Perusinghe M *et al.* (2021) Evidence-based management of depression in palliative care: a systematic review. *Journal of Palliative Medicine.* **24**: 767–781.
90 Dudas R *et al.* (2018) Antidepressants for treating depression in dementia. *Cochrane Database of Systematic Reviews.* **8**: CD003944. www.thecochranelibrary.com.
91 Pitman A *et al.* (2018) Depression and anxiety in patients with cancer. *British Medical Journal.* **361**: k1415.
92 Kudlow PA *et al.* (2014) Early switching strategies in antidepressant non-responders: current evidence and future research directions. *CNS Drugs.* **28**: 601–609.

93 Adli M *et al.* (2005) Is dose escalation of antidepressants a rational strategy after a medium-dose treatment has failed? A systematic review. *European Archives of Psychiatry and Clinical Neuroscience*. **255**: 387–400.
94 Taylor DM *et al.* (2021) *The Maudsley Prescribing Guidelines in Psychiatry* (14e). Informa Healthcare, London.
95 Rifkin-Zybutz R *et al.* (2020) Does anxiety moderate the effectiveness of mirtazapine in patients with treatmentresistant depression? A secondary analysis of the MIR trial. *Journal of Psychopharmacology*. **34**: 1342–1349.
96 Baldwin DS *et al.* (2014) Evidence-based pharmacological treatment of anxiety disorders, post-traumatic stress disorder and obsessive-compulsive disorder: a revision of the 2005 guidelines from the British Association for Psychopharmacology. *Journal of Psychopharmacology*. **28**: 403–439.
97 NICE (2011) Generalised anxiety disorder and panic disorder (with or without agoraphobia) in adults: management in primary, secondary and community care. *Clinical Guideline*. CG113 (updated 2020). www.nice.org.uk.
98 Sable-Smith A *et al.* (2020) Assessment and treatment of post-traumatic stress disorder at the end of life #398. *Journal of Palliative Medicine*. **23**: 1270–1272.
99 Glick DM *et al.* (2018) Assessment and treatment considerations for post traumatic stress disorder at end of life. *American Journal of Hospice and Palliative Medicine*. **35**: 1133–1139.
100 Finnerup NB *et al.* (2016) Pharmacotherapy for neuropathic pain in adults: a systematic review and meta-analysis. *Lancet Neurology*. **14**: 162–173.
101 Watson CP *et al.* (1998) Nortriptyline versus amitriptyline in postherpetic neuralgia: a randomized trial. *Neurology*. **51**: 1166–1171.
102 Boyle J *et al.* (2012) Randomized, placebo-controlled comparison of amitriptyline, duloxetine, and pregabalin in patients with chronic diabetic peripheral neuropathic pain: impact on pain, polysomnographic sleep, daytime functioning, and quality of life. *Diabetes Care*. **35**: 2451–2458.
103 Bansal D *et al.* (2009) Amitriptyline vs. pregabalin in painful diabetic neuropathy: a randomized double blind clinical trial. *Diabetic Medicine*. **26**: 1019–1026.
104 Morello C *et al.* (1999) Randomized double-blind study comparing the efficacy of gabapentin with amitriptyline on diabetic peripheral neuropathy pain. *Archives of Internal Medicine*. **159**: 1931–1937.
105 Chandra K *et al.* (2006) Gabapentin versus nortriptyline in post-herpetic neuralgia patients: a randomized, double-blind clinical trial--the GONIP Trial. *International Journal of Clinical Pharmacology and Therapeutics*. **44**: 358–363.
106 Mishra S *et al.* (2012) A comparative efficacy of amitriptyline, gabapentin, and pregabalin in neuropathic cancer pain: a prospective randomized double-blind placebo-controlled study. *American Journal of Hospice and Palliative Care*. **29**: 177–182.
107 Kaur H *et al.* (2011) A comparative evaluation of amitriptyline and duloxetine in painful diabetic neuropathy: a randomized, double-blind, cross-over clinical trial. *Diabetes Care*. **34**: 818–822.
108 Sindrup SH *et al.* (2003) Venlafaxine versus imipramine in painful polyneuropathy: a randomized, controlled trial. *Neurology*. **60**: 1284–1289.
109 Watson CP *et al.* (2011) Nontricyclic antidepressant analgesics and pain: are serotonin norepinephrine reuptake inhibitors (SNRIs) any better? *Pain*. **152**: 2206–2210.
110 Griebeler ML *et al.* (2014) Pharmacologic interventions for painful diabetic neuropathy: an umbrella systematic review and comparative effectiveness network meta-analysis. *Annals of Internal Medicine*. **161**: 639–649.
111 Banerjee M *et al.* (2013) A comparative study of efficacy and safety of gabapentin versus amitriptyline as coanalgesics in patients receiving opioid analgesics for neuropathic pain in malignancy. *Indian Journal of Pharmacology*. **45**: 334–338.
112 NICE (2013) Neuropathic pain – pharmacological management (appendix G). *Clinical Guideline*. CG173. www.nice.org.uk.
113 Bayani MM *et al.* (2021) Analgesic effect of duloxetine compared to nortriptyline in patients with painful neuropathy: a randomized double–blind placebo–controlled trial. *Caspian Journal of Internal Medicine*. **12**: 29–34.
114 Gül ŞK *et al.* (2020) Duloxetine and pregabalin in neuropathic pain of lung cancer patients. *Brain and Behaviour*. **10**: e01527.
115 Barohn RJ *et al.* (2021) Patient assisted intervention for neuropathy: comparison of treatment in real life situations (PAIN-CONTRoLS). Bayesian Adaptive Comparative Effectiveness Randomised Trial. *JAMA Neurology*. **78**: 68–76.
116 Matsuoka H *et al.* (2019) Additive duloxetine for cancer-related neuropathic pain nonresponsive or intolerant to opioid-pregabalin therapy: a randomized controlled trial (JORTC-PAL08). *Journal of Pain and Symptom Management*. **58**: 645–653.
117 Smith EML *et al.* (2013) Effect of duloxetine on pain, function, and quality of life among patients with chemotherapy-induced painful peripheral neuropathy: a randomized clinical trial. *Journal of the American Medical Association*. **309**: 1359–1367.
118 Farshchian N *et al.* (2018) Comparative study of the effects of venlafaxine and duloxetine on chemotherapy-induced peripheral neuropathy. *Cancer Chemotherapy and Pharmacology*. **82**: 787–793.
119 Christodoulou C *et al.* (2010) Effectiveness of mirtazapine in the treatment of postherpetic neuralgia. *Journal of Pain and Symptom Management*. **39**: e3–e6.
120 Gilron I *et al.* (2009) Nortriptyline and gabapentin, alone and in combination for neuropathic pain: a double-blind, randomised controlled crossover trial. *The Lancet*. **374**: 1252–1261.
121 Holbech JV *et al.* (2015) Imipramine and pregabalin combination for painful polyneuropathy: a randomized controlled trial. *Pain*. **156**: 958–966.
122 Gilron I *et al.* (2015) Combination of morphine with nortriptyline for neuropathic pain. *Pain*. **156**: 1440–1448.
123 Tesfaye S *et al.* (2013) Duloxetine and pregabalin: high-dose monotherapy or their combination? The "COMBO-DN study" a multinational, randomized, double-blind, parallel-group study in patients with diabetic peripheral neuropathic pain. *Pain*. **154**: 2616–2625.
124 Chakrabarty S *et al.* (2019) Pregabalin and amitriptyline as monotherapy or as low-dose combination in patients with neuropathic pain: a randomized, controlled trial to evaluate efficacy and safety in an eastern India teaching hospital. *Annals of Indian Academy of Neurology*. **22**: 437–441.
125 Jackson JL *et al.* (2010) Tricyclic antidepressants and headaches: systematic review and meta-analysis. *British Medical Journal*. **341**: C5222.
126 Hauser W *et al.* (2012) The role of antidepressants in the management of fibromyalgia syndrome: a systematic review and meta-analysis. *CNS Drugs*. **26**: 297–307.
127 Lunn MP *et al.* (2014) Duloxetine for treating painful neuropathy, chronic pain or fibromyalgia. *Cochrane Database of Systematic Reviews*. **1**: CD007115. www.thecochranelibrary.com.
128 Schnabel A *et al.* (2021) Efficacy and adverse events of selective serotonin noradrenaline reuptake inhibitors in the management of postoperative pain: a systematic review and meta-analysis. *Journal of Clinical Anaesthesia*. **75**: 110451.
129 Twycross R *et al.* (eds) (2021) *Introducing Palliative Care* (6e). Pharmaceutical Press, London. pp. 179–186.
130 NICE (2006) Urinary incontinence: the management of urinary incontinence in women. *Clinical Guideline*. CG40. www.nice.org.uk.
131 da Cunha-Bang S and Knudsen GM (2021) The modulatory role of serotonin on human impulsive aggression. *Biological Psychiatry*. **90**: 447–457.

132 Mungo A *et al.* (2020) Impulsivity and its therapeutic management in borderline personality disorder: a systematic review. *Psychiatric Quarterly*. **91**: 1333–1362.

133 Nicholl J and LaFrance WC Jr. (2009) Neuropsychiatric sequelae of traumatic brain injury. *Seminars in Neurology*. **29**: 247–255.

134 Forlenza OV *et al.* (2017) Recent advances in the management of neuropsychiatric symptoms in dementia. *Current Opinion in Psychiatry*. **30**: 151–158.

135 McCleery J *et al.* (2014) Pharmacotherapies for sleep disturbances in Alzheimer's disease. *Cochrane Database of Systematic Reviews*. **3**: CD009178. www.thecochranelibrary.com.

136 Everitt H *et al.* (2018) Antidepressants for insomnia in adults. *Cochrane Database of Systematic Reviews*. **5**: CD010753. www.thecochranelibrary.com.

137 Chang YD *et al.* (2016) Pseudobulbar affect or depression in dementia? *Journal of Pain and Symptom Management*. **51**: 954–958.

138 Pioro EP *et al.* (2010) Dextromethorphan plus ultra low-dose quinidine reduces pseudobulbar affect. *Annals of Neurology*. **68**: 693–702.

139 Gibson PG and Vertigan AE (2015) Management of chronic refractory cough. *British Medical Journal*. **351**: H5590.

140 Peoples AR *et al.* (2016) Buspirone for management of dyspnea in cancer patients receiving chemotherapy: a randomized placebo-controlled URCC CCOP study. *Supportive Care in Cancer*. **24**: 1339–1347.

141 Twycross R *et al.* (eds) (2021) *Introducing Palliative Care* (6e). Pharmaceutical Press, London. p. 345.

142 Marcy TR and Britton ML (2005) Antidepressant-induced sweating. *Annals of Pharmacotherapy*. **39**: 748–752.

143 Johns C *et al.* (2016) Informing hot flash treatment decisions for breast cancer survivors: a systematic review of randomized trials comparing active interventions. *Breast Cancer Research and Treatment*. **156**: 415–426.

144 Quella S *et al.* (1999) Pilot evaluation of venlafaxine for the treatment of hot flashes in men undergoing androgen ablation therapy for prostate cancer. *Journal of Urology*. **162**: 98–102.

145 Loprinzi CL *et al.* (2011) Nonestrogenic management of hot flashes. *Journal of Clinical Oncology*. **29**: 3842–3846.

146 Roth AJ and Scher HI (1998) Sertraline relieves hot flashes secondary to medical castration as treatment of advanced prostate cancer. *Psychooncology*. **7**: 129–132.

147 Specialist Pharmacy Service (2019) How do you switch between tricyclic, SSRI and related antidepressants? www.sps.nhs.uk (accessed December 2021).

148 Haddad PM (2001) Antidepressant discontinuation syndromes: clinical relevance, prevention and management. *Drug Safety*. **24**: 183–197.

149 Berber MJ (1998) FINISH: remembering the discontinuation syndrome. Flu-like symptoms, insomnia, nausea, imbalance, sensory disturbances, and hyperarousal (anxiety/agitation). *Journal of Clinical Psychiatry*. **59**: 255.

Updated December 2021

TRICYCLIC ANTIDEPRESSANTS

Class: Antidepressant.

Indications: Authorized indications vary; see individual SPCs for details. Depression, anxiety and panic disorders, neuropathic pain, nocturnal enuresis, †urgency and urge incontinence, †bladder spasm, †pathological laughing and crying, †drooling, †refractory cough, †sweating, †neuropathic pruritus.

Contra-indications: Concurrent use with an MAOI or within 2 weeks of its cessation (see Antidepressants, Box A, p.217), coronary artery insufficiency, recent myocardial infarction, arrhythmias (particularly any degree of heart block), mania, severe hepatic impairment.

Pharmacology

Tricyclic antidepressants (TCAs) are monoamine re-uptake inhibitors, sodium-channel blockers, and muscarinic, $5HT_{2A}$, $5HT_{2C}$, H_1, and α_1-adrenergic receptor antagonists.[1] They differ in their relative effects on serotonin and noradrenaline re-uptake, risk in overdose, antimuscarinic effects and cost (Table 1).

For depression, **amitriptyline** is marginally more effective than other antidepressants. However, because it is less well tolerated and more dangerous in overdose, it is generally reserved for severe unresponsive depression.[3]

For neuropathic pain, the efficacy and tolerability of **amitriptyline** and **nortriptyline** are comparable with alternatives (see Antidepressants, p.221). Onset of action is generally <1 week. Noradrenaline re-uptake inhibition is the predominant action. Sodium-channel blockade and NMDA–glutamate-receptor antagonism may also contribute.[4] Generally, a dose–response effect is evident, with patients benefiting from higher doses. However, for some patients benefit is *lost* at higher doses.[5] One potential explanation is that at higher doses, pro-nociceptive effects (e.g. serotonin re-uptake inhibition, α_2 antagonism) predominate over anti-nociceptive effects.

For pathological laughing and crying, **nortriptyline** is more effective than placebo;[6] benefit is also reported with **amitriptyline**.[7,8]

Table 1 Differences between selected TCAs[1,2]

	Re-uptake inhibition		*Antimuscarinic effects*	*Risk in overdose*[a]	*Cost*[b]
	5HT	*NA*			
Amitriptyline[c]	+++	+++	+++	++	+
Clomipramine	+++	+	+++	++	+
Desipramine (not UK)	+	+++	+	++	
Dosulepin (dothiepin)[d]	+++	+++	++	+++	+
Doxepin[d]	++	+++	+++	++	+++
Imipramine	+++	++	++	++	+
Lofepramine	+	+++	+	+	++
Nortriptyline	+	+++	+	++	+

Key: +++ high, ++ moderate, + low, blank = no data
Abbreviations: 5HT = 5-hydroxytryptamine (serotonin); NA = noradrenaline (norepinephrine)

a. all TCAs are more dangerous in overdose than SSRIs, venlafaxine, duloxetine and mirtazapine
b. typical monthly cost of UK tablet/capsule formulation: + (<£10), ++ (£10–80), +++ (>£80)
c. amitriptyline's higher affinity for the serotonin re-uptake transporter is offset by its metabolite, nortriptyline, which has a higher affinity for the noradrenaline re-uptake transporter
d. use is discouraged in the UK because of higher risk in overdose (dosulepin) or higher cost (doxepin).

For cough which persists despite resolution of the initial cause, **amitriptyline** is more effective than **codeine**;[9] benefit is also reported with **nortriptyline**.[10,11] Both TCAs probably reduce cough reflex hypersensitivity, which is generally present in this group of patients (see Drugs for cough, p.154).

For neuropathic pruritus, benefit is reported with **amitriptyline**.[12] For uraemic pruritus, although PO **doxepin** is more effective than placebo, it is expensive and less effective than **gabapentin** or **pregabalin** (see Drugs for pruritus, p.825).

For pharmacokinetic details, see Table 2.

Table 2 Pharmacokinetic details for selected TCAs[13]

	Bio-availability PO (%)	T_{max} *(h)*	*Plasma halflife (h)*	*Metabolism*
Amitriptyline	45–55	4–6	9–25	Multiple pathways (nortriptyline)[a]
Clomipramine	50[b]	1–5	12–36	Multiple pathways[a]
Doxepin	27[b]	2–4	8–24	Multiple pathways[a]
Imipramine	45	3	21 12–24[a]	Multiple pathways (desipramine)[a]
Lofepramine	≤10[b]	1–2 4[a]	1.6 12–24[a]	Multiple pathways (desipramine)[a]
Nortriptyline	60	7–8.5	15–39	CYP2D6[a]

a. active metabolite(s); listed in table if can be administered separately
b. reflects significant first-pass metabolism limiting amount of parent drug reaching systemic circulation; however, more is absorbed, reaching the systemic circulation as active metabolite(s).

Cautions

Suicide risk: the possibility of a suicide attempt is inherent in major depression and persists until remission. Antidepressants may themselves cause suicidal ideation, particularly in those aged ≤25 years (see p.214). If there is concern about suicide, consider alternatives that are safer in overdose (e.g. an SSRI). If a TCA cannot be avoided, the lowest risk is with **lofepramine.**

Bipolar disorder (can transform into manic phase); epilepsy (may lower seizure threshold); cardiac disease (risk of arrhythmia); renal or hepatic impairment (see Chapter 17, p.737 and Chapter 18, p.763); urinary hesitancy and narrow-angle glaucoma (antimuscarinic).

Drug interactions

Additive pharmacodynamic interactions with other drugs (see Antidepressants, p.216), notably QT prolongation, hyponatraemia and serotonin toxicity (see Antidepressants, Box A, p.217). Concurrent administration with an MAOI or within 2 weeks of its cessation is contra-indicated (see above).

Amitriptyline is metabolized mainly by CYP2D6 (as is **nortriptyline**) and to a lesser degree by CYP1A2 and possibly other hepatic enzymes. Caution should be taken with concurrent use of drugs which inhibit or induce these enzymes, particularly in those who are poor CYP2D6 metabolizers (see Chapter 19, p.783).

Specific significant interactions[14]

- TCAs and SSRIs: **fluoxetine**, **paroxetine** (strong CYP2D6 inhibitors) and **fluvoxamine** (strong CYP1A2 inhibitor) have the greatest effect, *increasing* plasma concentrations of TCAs by *≤10 times*. In addition, the plasma concentration of the SSRI may also *increase*. If an SSRI and a TCA are prescribed concurrently, use an alternative SSRI (e.g. **citalopram** or **sertraline**) or reduce the dose of the TCA to 25–33% of the previous dose (and possibly prescribe a relatively low SSRI dose)
- other drugs shown to *increase* the plasma concentrations of **amitriptyline** and **nortriptyline** are **cimetidine**, **fluconazole**, **quinidine** (strong CYP2D6 inhibitor) and **terbinafine**
- concurrent prescription of **carbamazepine** *decreases* the plasma concentrations of **amitriptyline** and **nortriptyline** by ≤60%.

Undesirable effects

Frequencies based on **amitriptyline**.

Very common (>10%): aggression, somnolence, dizziness, speech disorders, tremor, headache, postural hypotension, tachycardia, palpitations, dry mouth, accommodation disorder, nausea, constipation, weight gain, sweating.

Common (<10%, >1%): agitation, confusion, fatigue, paraesthesia, QT prolongation, AV or bundle branch block, hyponatraemia, mydriasis, urinary disorders, sexual dysfunction.

Uncommon (<1%, >0.1%): anxiety, mania, seizures, tinnitus, vomiting, hepatic impairment.

Rare (<0.01%) or unknown incidence: delirium, hallucinations, acute glaucoma, movement disorders (e.g. akathisia), *torsade de pointes*, arrythmias, agranulocytosis, jaundice, hepatitis, paralytic ileus, decreased appetite.

Nortriptyline and **lofepramine** cause less dry mouth than **amitriptyline** and **dosulepin**.[15,16]

Dose and use

Because of the potential for undesirable effects, low doses should be used initially, particularly in the frail elderly. **Amitriptyline** has the most potent antimuscarinic effects, making it the TCA of choice in sweating, drooling and urinary symptoms. For other indications, consider a TCA with fewer antimuscarinic effects (e.g. **nortriptyline**).

TCAs can be given as a single dose at bedtime for all indications. For patients that take a long time to settle at night, give 2h before bedtime.

Avoid abrupt withdrawal after prolonged use (see Stopping antidepressants, p.223).

A small number of patients are stimulated by TCAs and experience insomnia, unpleasant vivid dreams, myoclonus and physical restlessness. In these patients, administer in the morning or switch to an alternative antidepressant, see p.220.

Neuropathic pain

For **amitriptyline** or **nortriptyline**:

- start with 10mg PO at bedtime
- if tolerated, increase to 25mg after 3–7 days
- if necessary, increase by 25mg every 1–2 weeks

- usual effective dose is 25–75mg at bedtime. If successive increases are well tolerated *and bring additional benefit*, continue to titrate up to a maximum of 150mg/24h (seldom required) in divided doses
- if a TCA is helpful but poorly tolerated, consider switching to **duloxetine** (p.239), for information on switching, see p.223
- if no response, switch to an anti-epileptic (p.280); see Stopping antidepressants, p.223.

If switching from **amitriptyline** to **nortriptyline**, some centres use a direct switch with a 1:1 dose ratio; consider using a lower dose if undesirable effects are moderate–severe, or if switching doses ≥75mg/24h.

Depression, anxiety and panic disorders

TCAs are *not* first-line treatments for depression, panic or anxiety disorders, but **amitriptyline** might retain a place for depression refractory to other treatments. Seek advice from a psychiatrist before use. For depression with co-existent neuropathic pain, **duloxetine** is generally preferred.

Amitriptyline is titrated as for neuropathic pain; 75–100mg/24h PO is generally as effective as higher doses and better tolerated.[17] Maximum authorized dose is 150mg/24h in two divided doses.

†Pathological laughing and crying

SSRIs (p.232) are first-line treatments. **Nortriptyline** or **amitriptyline** are second-line alternatives:

- start with 10mg PO at bedtime
- effective dose 25–100mg/24h.[6–8]

†Refractory cough

For **amitriptyline** or **nortriptyline**:

- start with 10mg PO at bedtime
- mean effective dose 25mg/24h (range 10–50mg/24h).[10,11]

†Urgency and urge incontinence, bladder spasm

TCAs are *not* first-line treatments for urinary symptoms (see p.611). Use **amitriptyline**; dose as for neuropathic pain. If antimuscarinic CNS effects occur, consider switching to a peripherally acting antimuscarinic (e.g. **propantheline**, p.21).

†Sweating, drooling

Use **amitriptyline**; dose as for neuropathic pain. If antimuscarinic CNS effects occur, consider switching to a peripherally acting antimuscarinic (e.g. **propantheline**, p.21).

†Neuropathic pruritus

Use **amitriptyline**; dose as for neuropathic pain.[12] For other causes of pruritus, see Drugs for pruritus, p.825.

Supply

Amitriptyline (generic)

Tablets 10mg, 25mg, 50mg, 28 days @ 50mg at bedtime = £0.50.

Oral solution (sugar-free) 10mg/5mL, 25mg/5mL, 50mg/5mL, 28 days @ 50mg at bedtime = £16.

Nortriptyline (generic)

Tablets 10mg, 25mg, 50mg, 28 days @ 50mg at bedtime = £0.50.

Oral solution (sugar-free) 10mg/5mL, 25mg/5mL, 28 days @ 50mg at bedtime = £363.

1 Binding Database Skaggs School of Pharmacy and Pharmaceutical Sciences. Available from: http://bindingdb.org/as/search.html (accessed June 2015).

2 Gillman PK (2007) Tricyclic antidepressant pharmacology and therapeutic drug interactions updated. *British Journal of Pharmacology*. **151**: 737–748.

3 Leucht C *et al.* (2012) Amitriptyline versus placebo for major depressive disorder. *Cochrane Database of Systematic Reviews*. **12**: CD009138. www.thecochranelibrary.com

4 Kremer M *et al.* (2016) Antidepressants and gabapentinoids in neuropathic pain: mechanistic insights. *Neuroscience*. **338**: 183–206.

5 Watson CP (1984) Therapeutic window for amitriptyline analgesia. *Canadian Medical Association Journal*. **130**: 105–106.
6 Robinson RG *et al.* (1993) Pathological laughing and crying following stroke: validation of a measurement scale and a double-blind treatment study. *American Journal of Psychiatry*. **150**: 286–293.
7 Szczudlik A *et al.* (1995) The effect of amitriptyline on the pathological crying and other pseudobulbar signs. *Neurologia i Neurochirurgia Polska*. **29**: 663–674.
8 Tateno A *et al.* (2004) Pathological laughing and crying following traumatic brain injury. *The Journal of Neuropsychiatry and Clinical Neurosciences*. **16**: 426–434.
9 Gibson PG and Vertigan AE (2015) Management of chronic refractory cough. *British Medical Journal*. **351**: h5590.
10 Bowen AJ *et al.* (2018) Tachyphylaxis and dependence in pharmacotherapy for unexplained chronic cough. *Otolaryngology–Head and Neck Surgery*. **159**: 705–711.
11 Song SA *et al.* (2020) The effectiveness of nortriptyline and tolerability of side effects in neurogenic cough patients. *Annals of Otology, Rhinology and Laryngology*. **130**: 781–787.
12 Kaur R and Sinha VR (2018) Antidepressants as antipruritic agents: a review. *European Neuropsychopharmacology*. **28**: 341–352.
13 Schulz P *et al.* (1985) Discrepancies between pharmacokinetic studies of amitriptyline. *Clinical Pharmacokinetics*. **10**: 257–268.
14 Preston CL (2011) *Stockley's Drug Interactions*. London: Pharmaceutical Press. www.medicinescomplete.com (accessed December 2021).
15 Fairbairn AF *et al.* (1989) Lofepramine versus dothiepin in the treatment of depression in elderly patients. *British Journal of Clinical Practice*. **43**: 55–60.
16 Watson CP *et al.* (1998) Nortriptyline versus amitriptyline in postherpetic neuralgia: a randomized trial. *Neurology*. **51**: 1166–1171.
17 Furukawa T *et al.* (2003) Low dosage tricyclic antidepressants for depression. *Cochrane Database of Systematic Reviews*. CD003197. www.thecochranelibrary.com

Updated December 2021

SELECTIVE SEROTONIN RE-UPTAKE INHIBITORS

Class: Antidepressant.

Indications: Authorized indications vary; see individual SPCs for details. Depression, anxiety, panic and post-traumatic stress disorders, †pathological laughing and crying, †hot flushes, †pruritus.

Contra-indications: Concurrent use with an MAOI or within 2 weeks of its cessation (see Antidepressants, Box A, p.217); known prolonged QT interval or concurrent use with other drugs that prolong the QT interval (**citalopram, escitalopram**); concurrent use with **pimozide**; mania.

Pharmacology

SSRIs inhibit the serotonin re-uptake transporter. They differ in their propensity for causing pharmacokinetic drug interactions and discontinuation reactions. They also have varying additional actions, which may partly explain why some individuals respond when switched to an alternative SSRI (Table 1).

In palliative care, **citalopram** or **sertraline** are generally the SSRIs of choice; they combine a low risk of both drug interactions and discontinuation reactions. They are first-line treatments for depression (see p.220), anxiety and panic disorders (see p.221), and pathological laughter and crying (see p.222). **Sertraline** is preferred in patients with risk factors for QT interval prolongation (see below).

For anxiety secondary to breathlessness, trials are small but SSRIs appear effective.[7,8] A potential role for antidepressants for refractory breathlessness *per se* has been suggested. However, **sertraline** was no better than placebo in patients with advanced respiratory disease.[9]

SSRIs are not consistently effective for neuropathic pain; an SNRI (e.g. **amitriptyline, duloxetine**) or an anti-epileptic is preferable (see p.221).

For the role of SSRIs in pruritus, particularly due to cholestasis, see Dose and use and also Drugs for pruritus, p.825. The benefit reported for dry cough in cancer has not been confirmed in an RCT.[10,11]

Escitalopram is the S-enantiomer of **citalopram**. *R*-citalopram does not inhibit the serotonin re-uptake transporter but may hinder the binding of S-citalopram. Some fixed-dose comparisons do find a marginally higher response rate with **escitalopram** 10mg vs. **citalopram** 20mg,[12] but titrating **citalopram** might be expected to achieve the same result.

For pharmacokinetic details, see Table 2.

Table 1 Differences between SSRIs[1–6]

Drug	*Additional actions*	*Hepatic enzyme inhibitor*					*Discontinuation reaction risk*[a]
		CYP1A2	*CYP2C9*	*CYP2C19*	*CYP2D6*	*CYP3A4*	
Citalopram	H_1 antagonist (*R*-enantiomer)				+		Low
Escitalopram	None				+		Low
Fluoxetine	$5HT_{2C}$ antagonist[b]		++	++	+++	+	Minimal
Fluvoxamine	Sigma-1 agonist[c]	+++		+++		++	Moderate
Paroxetine	Noradrenaline (norepinephrine) re-uptake inhibitor[b], P2X4 receptor inhibitor[d]				+++		High
Sertraline	Dopamine re-uptake inhibitor[b]				+		Low

Key: + = weak inhibitor; ++ = moderate inhibitor; +++ = strong inhibitor (also see Chapter 19, p.781)

a. approximates to halflife (see Antidepressants, Table 2, p.215)

b. these actions theoretically contribute to the antidepressant effects of the drugs (see Antidepressants, p.210), but the affinity, and overall contribution of these additional actions is much less than the predominant serotonin re-uptake inhibition

c. the action of sigma-1 receptors is poorly defined, but sigma-1 receptor agonists may have antidepressant, pro-seizure, euphoric and/or dysphoric effects

d. P2X4 receptors are expressed by microglia and implicated in neuro-inflammation and neuropathic pain (see Antidepressants, p.214).

Table 2 Pharmacokinetic details for selected SSRIs[12–14]

Drug	*Bio-availability PO (%)*	T_{max} *(h)*	*Plasma halflife*	*Metabolism*
Citalopram	80[a]	3	36h	Multiple pathways[b]
Escitalopram	80[c]	4	30h	Multiple pathways[b]
Fluoxetine	90	4–8	1–4 days; 1–2 *weeks*[b]	Multiple pathways[b]
Paroxetine	50[d]	5	15–20h	Multiple pathways
Sertraline	>44	6–8	26h	CYP3A4

a. for tablets; bio-availability of drops is nearly 100%

b. active metabolite(s)

c. the bio-availability of tablets and oral solution is comparable

d. increases with multiple dosing.

Cautions

Suicide risk: the possibility of a suicide attempt is inherent in major depression and persists until remission. Antidepressants may themselves cause suicidal ideation, particularly in those aged ≤25 years (see p.214).

Bipolar disorder (can transform into manic phase); epilepsy (may lower seizure threshold, but less than other antidepressants; ***citalopram*** *or* ***escitalopram*** *are generally preferred because they lack significant interactions with anti-epileptics,* see p.215); QT prolongation risk factors (particularly **citalopram** and **escitalopram**; see below and Chapter 20, p.797); renal impairment (see Chapter 17, p.737) hepatic impairment (see Chapter 18, p.763); diabetes mellitus (reduced hypoglycaemic awareness); peptic ulceration or bleeding disorders (SSRIs increase the risk of GI bleeding,[15] particularly in those aged >80 years);[16] narrow angle glaucoma.

Drug interactions

Fluoxetine, fluvoxamine and **paroxetine** are potent hepatic enzyme inhibitors (see Chapter 19, Table 8, p.790), and potentially serious interactions can result when used with other drugs that are metabolized by these enzymes (see p.216).[17]

Citalopram, escitalopram and **sertraline** are only weak hepatic enzyme inhibitors and are less likely to affect the metabolism of other drugs.[4,5]

Additive pharmacodynamic interactions with other drugs (see Antidepressants, p.216), notably bleeding risk, QT prolongation (**citalopram** and **escitalopram**), hyponatraemia and serotonin toxicity (see Antidepressants, Box A, p.217). Concurrent administration with an MAOI or within 2 weeks of its cessation is contra-indicated (see above).

Sertraline is metabolized mainly by CYP3A4, and to a minor degree by CYP2D6. Caution should be taken with concurrent use of drugs that inhibit or induce these enzymes, particularly in those who are poor CYP2D6 metabolizers (see Chapter 19, p.783). However, generally **sertraline** rarely requires dose reduction with other enzyme inhibitors; consider only if symptoms of toxicity occur.

Citalopram and **escitalopram** are metabolized by CYP2C19, CYP2D6 and CYP3A4. Although the FDA recommends a reduced dose of **citalopram** when used with **cimetidine, omeprazole** or other drugs that inhibit CYP2C19, the effect on plasma citalopram levels is likely to be small.[18]

Undesirable effects

Frequencies based on **sertraline** and **citalopram**.

Very common (>10%): somnolence, insomnia, dizziness, headache, dry mouth, nausea, diarrhoea, sweating.

Common (<10%, >1%): agitation, anxiety, nervousness, confusion, tremor, tinnitus, yawning, fatigue, dizziness, paraesthesia, bruxism (teeth grinding), palpitations, altered taste, decreased appetite, vomiting, sexual dysfunction, myalgia, arthralgia, pruritus.

Uncommon (<1%, >0.1%): aggression, depersonalization, hallucinations, mania.

Rare (<0.01%) or unknown incidence: psychosis, hyponatraemia, seizures, movement disorders (e.g. dyskinesia), hepatitis, haemorrhage, fracture risk (see p.218).

Myocardial infarction

The manufacturer reports myocardial infarction as a rare consequence of taking **sertraline**. However, this would be expected, because depression is an independent risk factor for myocardial infarction. Further, case control studies suggest that SSRIs confer a protective effect,[19] possibly because they impact negatively on platelet aggregation (see p.218). **Sertraline** has been used safely in patients with unstable angina and after myocardial infarction.[20]

QT prolongation

Citalopram and **escitalopram** exhibit dose-related QT prolongation. Regulators recommend correction of hypokalaemia and hypomagnesaemia, and advise ECG monitoring in those with cardiac disease, and contra-indication in patients receiving other QT prolonging drugs (see Chapter 20, Box B, p.799).[21] **Sertraline** and other SSRIs appear safer in this respect.[19] Also see Chapter 20, p.797.

Dose and use

Treatment should not be discontinued abruptly (see Stopping antidepressants, p.223).

Depression, anxiety and panic

For **sertraline**:

- if anxiety/panic symptoms are prominent, start with 25mg PO each morning and increase to 50mg each morning after 1 week
- otherwise, start with 50mg each morning; if necessary, increase the dose to 100mg after 2–4 weeks
- if no response after 4 weeks, or only a partial response after 6–8 weeks, consider further increases to a maximum of 200mg each morning or an alternative (see p.220)

- if effective, continue until the patient has been symptom-free for ≥6 months (see p.221); after this, discontinue over 2–4 weeks.

For **citalopram**:
Because of concerns regarding QT prolongation, do not exceed the maximum dose (also see comments above).[21]

- start with 10mg PO each morning and increase to 20mg each morning after 1 week
- if no response after 4 weeks, or only a partial response after 6–8 weeks, consider further increases to a maximum of 40mg each morning or switch to an alternative (see p.220)
- restrict maximum dose to 20mg each morning in those >60 years and in hepatic impairment, and consider with patients also taking **cimetidine, omeprazole** or other inhibitors of CYP2C19[18,21]
- if effective, continue until the patient has been symptom-free for ≥6 months (see p.221); after this, discontinue over 2–4 weeks.

†*Cholestatic pruritus* (also see Drugs for pruritus, p.825)

For **sertraline**:

- start with 25mg PO each morning; if necessary, increase in 25mg increments
- doses above 100mg each morning rarely give additional relief.[22]

†*Pathological laughter and crying*

Often responds to lower doses than required for depression.[23]
For **sertraline**:

- start with 12.5mg PO each morning; if necessary, increase in 12.5–25mg increments to a maximum of 200mg each morning.

For **citalopram**:

- start with 5mg PO each morning; if necessary, increase in 5–10mg increments to a maximum of 40mg each morning (20mg in those with risk factors; see above).

†*Hot flushes*

For **citalopram**:

- start with 10mg PO each morning; if necessary, increase in 10mg increments to a maximum of 30mg each morning (20mg in those with risk factors; see above).[24]

Supply

Citalopram (generic)
Tablets (as *hydrobromide*) 10mg, 20mg, 40mg, 28 days @ 20mg each morning = £0.50.
Oral liquid drops (as *hydrochloride*) 40mg/mL, 28 days @ 16mg (8 drops) each morning = £7; *16mg as oral liquid (8 drops) is equivalent to 20mg as tablets. Mix with water, orange juice or apple juice before taking. May contain alcohol.*

Sertraline (generic)
Tablets 25mg, 50mg, 100mg, 28 days @ 50mg each morning = £0.50.
Oral suspension (sugar-free) 25mg/mL, 50mg/5mL, 100mg/5mL, 28 days @ 50mg each morning = £16 (unauthorized product, available as a special order; see Chapter 24, p.817). *Price based on Specials tariff in community.*

1 Hashimoto K (2009) Sigma-1 receptors and selective serotonin reuptake inhibitors: clinical implications of their relationship. *Central Nervous System Agents in Medicinal Chemistry*. **9**: 197–204.

2 Carrasco JL and Sandner C (2005) Clinical effects of pharmacological variations in selective serotonin reuptake inhibitors: an overview. *International Journal of Clinical Practice*. **59**: 1428–1434.

3 Haddad PM (2001) Antidepressant discontinuation syndromes: clinical relevance, prevention and management. *Drug Safety*. **24**: 183–197.

4 Preskorn SH (1997) Clinically relevant pharmacology of selective serotonin reuptake inhibitors. An overview with emphasis on pharmacokinetics and effects on oxidative drug metabolism. *Clinical Pharmacokinetics*. **32 (Suppl 1)**: 1–21.

5 Rao N (2007) The clinical pharmacokinetics of escitalopram. *Clinical Pharmacokinetics*. **46**: 281–290.

6 Yamashita T *et al.* (2016) Duloxetine inhibits microglial P2X4 receptor function and alleviates neuropathic pain after peripheral nerve injury. *PLoS One*. **11**: e0165189.

7 Usmani ZA *et al.* (2018) A randomized placebo-controlled trial of paroxetine for the management of anxiety in chronic obstructive pulmonary disease (PAC Study). *Journal of Multidisciplinary Healthcare*. **11**: 287–293.

8 Eiser N *et al.* (2005) Effect of treating depression on quality-of-life and exercise tolerance in severe COPD. COPD: *Journal of Chronic Obstructive Pulmonary Disease*. **2**: 233–241.
9 Currow DC *et al.* (2019) Sertraline in symptomatic chronic breathlessness: a double blind, randomised trial. *European Respiratory Journal.* **53**: 1801270.
10 Thakerar A *et al.* (2020) Paroxetine for the treatment of intractable and persistent cough in patients diagnosed with cancer. *Journal of Oncology Pharmacy Practice.* **26**: 803–808.
11 Zylicz Z and Krajnik M (2004) What has dry cough in common with pruritus? Treatment of dry cough with paroxetine. *Journal of Pain and Symptom Management.* **27**: 180–184.
12 Garnock-Jones KP and McCormack PL (2010) Escitalopram: a review of its use in the management of major depressive disorder in adults. *CNS Drugs*. **24**: 769–796.
13 Hiemke (2000) Pharmacokinetics of selective serotonin reuptake inhibitors. *Pharmacology and Therapeutics*. **85**: 11–28.
14 Kaye CM *et al.* (1989) A review of the metabolism and pharmacokinetics of paroxetine in man. *Acta Psychiatrica Scandinavica Supplementum*. **350**: 60–75.
15 Paton C and Ferrier IN (2005) SSRIs and gastrointestinal bleeding. *British Medical Journal*. **331**: 529–530.
16 van Walraven C *et al.* (2001) Inhibition of serotonin reuptake by antidepressants and upper gastrointestinal bleeding in elderly patients: retrospective cohort study. *British Medical Journal*. **323**: 655–657.
17 Preston CL *Stockley's Drug Interactions*. London: Pharmaceutical Press. www.medicinescomplete.com (accessed December 2021).
18 FDA (2012) Celexa (citalopram hydrobromide) Revised recommendations, potential risk of abnormal heart rhythms. *Drug Safety Communication*. www.fda.gov/Safety/MedWatch..
19 Edinoff AN *et al.* (2021) Selective serotnonin reuptake inhibitors and adverse effects: a narrative review. *Neurology International* **13**: 387–401.
20 Glassman AH *et al.* (2002) Sertraline treatment of major depression in patients with acute MI or unstable angina. *Journal of the American Medical Association*. **288**: 701–709.
21 Medicines and Healthcare products Regulatory Agency (2011) Citalopram and escitalopram: QT interval prolongation – new maximum daily dose restrictions (including in elderly patients), contraindications, and warnings. *Drug Safety Update*. **5**. www.gov.uk/drug-safety-update.
22 Mayo MJ *et al.* (2007) Sertraline as a first-line treatment for cholestatic pruritus. *Hepatology*. **45**: 666–674.
23 Wortzel HS *et al.* (2008) Pathological laughing and crying: epidemiology, pathophysiology and treatment. *CNS Drugs*. **22**: 531–545.
24 Johns C *et al.* (2016) Informing hot flash treatment decisions for breast cancer survivors: a systematic review of randomized trials comparing active interventions. *Breast Cancer Research and Treatment*. **156**: 415–426.

Updated December 2021

*VENLAFAXINE

Class: Antidepressant; serotonin and noradrenaline (norepinephrine) re-uptake inhibitor (SNRI).

Indications: Depression, anxiety and panic disorders, †neuropathic pain, †hot flushes.

Contra-indications: Concurrent use with an MAOI or within 2 weeks of its cessation (see Antidepressants, Box A, p.217); uncontrolled hypertension.

Pharmacology

Like **duloxetine**, venlafaxine inhibits serotonin and noradrenaline (norepinephrine) re-uptake transporters, but lacks the sodium-channel blockade and muscarinic, α-adrenergic and H_1-receptor antagonism of **amitriptyline** and other tricyclic SNRIs.[1,2] Inhibition of noradrenaline re-uptake transporters increases with higher doses.[3] Because these also clear dopamine in the prefrontal cortex, which lacks separate dopamine re-uptake transporters, venlafaxine enhances dopamine transmission here too.

For depression, venlafaxine is generally reserved for second-line use, where it is marginally more effective than switching to an alternative SSRI, but less well tolerated (see Antidepressants, p.220).[4,5]

For neuropathic pain, benefit from venlafaxine ≥150mg/24h appears similar to that of **duloxetine**. Lower doses (≤75mg/24h) are not consistently effective.[6-8] In a comparative trial, venlafaxine 225mg/24h was as effective as **imipramine** 150mg/24h.[9] Dry mouth was more common with **imipramine**, and tiredness more common with venlafaxine.

For hot flushes, trials in patients with breast cancer have found benefit from venlafaxine, SSRIs (p.232), **gabapentin** (p.297) and **duloxetine** (p.239).[10] Venlafaxine works faster than **clonidine** (p.82), and participants prefer venlafaxine to **gabapentin**.[10] Venlafaxine and SSRIs are also reported to improve hot flushes resulting from medical or surgical castration in men.[11,12]

Venlafaxine is metabolized by CYP2D6 to a pharmacologically active metabolite, O-desmethylvenlafaxine (ODV), which has a similar pharmacodynamic profile, and by CYP3A4 to a minor, less active metabolite. Venlafaxine and its metabolites are primarily renally excreted.
Bio-availability 40–45%.
Onset of action >2 weeks for depression.
Time to peak plasma concentration about 2.5h; 5.5h m/r.
Plasma halflife 5h; 11h for ODV.
Duration of effect 12–24h, situation-dependent.

Cautions

Suicide risk: the possibility of a suicide attempt is inherent in major depression and persists until remission. Antidepressants may themselves cause suicidal ideation, particularly in those aged ≤25 years (see p.214). If there is concern about suicide, the MHRA advises that supply should be limited to 2 weeks.[13] The risk in overdose is greater than with SSRIs, similar to **mirtazapine** and less than with TCAs.[5]

Bipolar disorder (can transform into manic phase); epilepsy (lowers seizure threshold); cardiac disease (risk of hypertension and arrhythmia); renal impairment (see Dose and use, and Chapter 17, p.737); mild–moderate hepatic impairment (see Dose and use, and Chapter 18, p.763); narrow-angle glaucoma (mydriasis reported).

Drug interactions

Additive pharmacodynamic interactions with other drugs (see Antidepressants, p.216), notably bleeding risk, QT prolongation and serotonin toxicity (see Antidepressants, Box A, p.217). Concurrent administration with an MAOI or within 2 weeks of its cessation is contra-indicated (see above).

Venlafaxine is metabolized by CYP2D6 and CYP3A4. Concurrent use with drugs that inhibit these enzymes may result in higher plasma concentrations (see Chapter 19, Table 8, p.790), and should generally be avoided in order to prevent clinically important interactions in poor metabolizers.[13]

Venlafaxine may increase concurrent **haloperidol** plasma concentrations (≤70% increase in AUC).[14] The mechanism is unknown and the dose of haloperidol may need to be reduced. The dose of **warfarin** may need to be reduced when used concurrently with venlafaxine (reports of increased prothrombin times; unknown mechanism).[14]

Undesirable effects

Very common (>10%): drowsiness, dizziness, insomnia, nervousness, dry mouth, nausea, constipation, sexual dysfunction, asthenia, headache, sweating.
Common (<10%, >1%): abnormal dreams, agitation, confusion, abnormal vision/accommodation, mydriasis, tinnitus, tremor, hypertonia, paraesthesia, dyspnoea, hypertension, palpitations, postural hypotension, vasodilation, anorexia, diarrhoea, dyspepsia, vomiting, abdominal pain, urinary frequency, decreased libido, impotence, menstrual disorders, arthralgia, myalgia, weight gain/loss, chills, pyrexia, pruritus, rash, ecchymosis.
Uncommon (<1%): hallucinations, urinary retention, muscle spasm, hyponatraemia, increased liver enzymes, angioedema, maculopapular eruptions, urticaria.

Dose and use

Remains of m/r tablets may appear in the patient's faeces ('ghost tablets'). These are inert residues and do not affect the efficacy of the products.

May be taken with or after food to improve tolerability (see Chapter 14, p.707). If severe renal or mild–moderate hepatic impairment, reduce the dose by 50% and give once daily; avoid in ESRF and severe hepatic impairment (see Chapter 17, p.737 and Chapter 18, p.763).

Check blood pressure before and after starting and after dose increases; consider dose reduction or discontinuation in those who show a sustained increase.

Withdraw gradually over 2-4 weeks after prolonged use (see Stopping antidepressants, p.223); in some patients, discontinuation could take several months.

Depression

Because of concerns about its tolerability and safety in overdose, venlafaxine is reserved for depression refractory to other antidepressants (see p.220).

- generally, start with 75mg m/r PO once daily
- in frail or elderly patients, start with 37.5mg m/r once daily for 4–7 days
- if necessary, increase by 75mg m/r once daily every 2 weeks
- maximum recommended dose 375mg/24h. Specialist supervision required if a dose of ≥300mg is necessary in severely depressed or hospitalized patients
- if effective, continue until the patient has been symptom-free for ≥6 months (see p.220); after this, discontinue over 2–4 weeks or longer if withdrawal symptoms occur.

Anxiety and panic

Venlafaxine is reserved for anxiety or panic disorders refractory to other antidepressants (see p.221).

- use as for depression
- maximum recommended dose 225mg/24h.

†Neuropathic pain

Venlafaxine is not a first-line treatment for neuropathic pain (see p.221).[15]

- use as for depression
- maximum recommended dose 150–225mg/24h.[8]

†Hot flushes

- start with 37.5mg m/r PO once daily
- if necessary, increase to 75mg m/r once daily; generally, higher doses offer no additional benefit but more undesirable effects.[10]

Supply

Venlafaxine (generic)

Tablets 37.5mg, 75mg, 28 days @ 75mg b.d. = £3; *authorized for depression only.*

Capsules m/r 37.5mg, 75mg, 150mg, 225mg, 28 days @ 150mg once daily = £4.

Tablets m/r 37.5mg, 75mg, 150mg, 225mg, 300mg, 28 days @ 150mg once daily = £4.

Oral solution (sugar free) 37.5mg/5mL, 75mg/5mL, 28 days @ 150mg once daily = £387.

1 Bymaster FP *et al.* (2001) Comparative affinity of duloxetine and venlafaxine for serotonin and norepinephrine transporters in vitro and in vivo, human serotonin receptor subtypes, and other neuronal receptors. *Neuropsychopharmacology.* **25**: 871–880.

2 Beique JC *et al.* (1998) Affinities of venlafaxine and various reuptake inhibitors for the serotonin and norepinephrine transporters. *European Journal of Pharmacology.* **349**: 129–132.

3 Arakawa R (2019) Venlafaxine ER blocks the norepinephrine transporter in the brain of patients with major depressive disorder: a PET study using [18F]FMeNER-D2. *International Journal of Neuropsychopharmacology.* **22**: 278–285.

4 NICE (2009) Depression. *Clinical Guidelines.* CG90 and CG91. www.nice.org.uk.

5 Cleare A *et al.* (2015) Evidence-based guidelines for treating depressive disorders with antidepressants: a revision of the 2008 British Association for Psychopharmacology guidelines. *Journal of Psychopharmacology.* **29**: 459–525.

6 Finnerup NB *et al.* (2015) Pharmacotherapy for neuropathic pain in adults: a systematic review and meta-analysis. *Lancet Neurology.* **14**: 162–173.

7 Farshchian N *et al.* (2018) Comparative study of the effects of venlafaxine and duloxetine on chemotherapy-induced peripheral neuropathy. *Cancer Chemotherapy and Pharmacology.* **82**: 787–793.

8 Aiyer R *et al.* (2017) Treatment of neuropathic pain with venlafaxine: a systematic review. *Pain Medicine.* **18**: 1999–2012.

9 Sindrup SH *et al.* (2003) Venlafaxine versus imipramine in painful polyneuropathy: a randomized, controlled trial. *Neurology.* **60**: 1284–1289.

10 Johns C *et al.* (2016) Informing hot flash treatment decisions for breast cancer survivors: a systematic review of randomized trials comparing active interventions. *Breast Cancer Research and Treatment.* **156**: 415–426.

11 Quella S *et al.* (1999) Pilot evaluation of venlafaxine for the treatment of hot flashes in men undergoing androgen ablation therapy for prostate cancer. *Journal of Urology.* **162**: 98–102.

12 Loprinzi CL *et al.* (2011) Nonestrogenic management of hot flashes. *Journal of Clinical Oncology.* **29**: 3842–3846.

13 MHRA (2006) Updated prescribing advice for venlafaxine (Efexor/Effexor XL). Letter from the chairman of the Commission on Human Medicines, 31 May 2006. Available from: http://www.mhra.gov.uk/Safetyinformation/.

14 Preston CL. *Stockley's Drug Interactions.* London: Pharmaceutical Press. www.medicinescomplete.com (accessed December 2021).

15 Gallagher HC *et al.* (2015) Venlafaxine for neuropathic pain in adults. *Cochrane Database of Systematic Reviews.* **8**: CD011091. www.cochranelibrary.com.

Updated December 2021

DULOXETINE

Class: Antidepressant, serotonin and noradrenaline (norepinephrine) re-uptake inhibitor (SNRI).

Indications: Depression, generalized anxiety disorder, diabetic neuropathic pain, †other neuropathic pain, moderate–severe stress incontinence in women, †hot flushes.

4

Contra-indications: Concurrent use with an MAOI or within 2 weeks of its cessation (see Antidepressants, Box A, p.217); concurrent use with strong CYP1A2 inhibitors, e.g. **fluvoxamine, ciprofloxacin**;[1] uncontrolled hypertension; hepatic impairment; creatinine clearance <30mL/min.

Pharmacology

Like **venlafaxine**, duloxetine inhibits serotonin and noradrenaline (norepinephrine) re-uptake transporters, but lacks the sodium-channel blockade and muscarinic, α-adrenergic and H_1-receptor antagonism of **amitriptyline** and other tricyclic SNRIs.[2] Duloxetine also inhibits P2X4 receptors, a subset of purine-gated calcium channels upregulated on microglia in neuropathic pain.[3]

For depression, duloxetine is less well tolerated than **venlafaxine** and SSRIs.[4] For neuropathic pain, the NNT for a 50% reduction in pain score is 5. Although most trials examined painful diabetic neuropathy,[5] benefit has also been seen in chemotherapy- and cancer-related neuropathic pain.[6-9] In one study, the presence of tingling pain increased the likelihood of response.[10] A dose–response effect up to 120mg/24h has been seen in diabetic neuropathy.[11] In two RCTs, efficacy was comparable to **amitriptyline**, and undesirable effects were similar, although in one of the RCTs, dry mouth occurred less with duloxetine, and constipation more.[12,13] Duloxetine is also of benefit in fibromyalgia (authorized in the USA).[5] An RCT for pain related to Parkinson's Disease found duloxetine was no better than placebo, but duloxetine was not titrated above 40mg daily.[14]

For stress incontinence, duloxetine has a limited role;[15] serotonin and noradrenaline increase urethral sphincter tone (see Antidepressants, p.210). For hot flushes in patients with breast cancer, the efficacy and tolerability of duloxetine is similar to **escitalopram**.[16] For pathological laughter and crying, benefit is reported.[17]

Duloxetine is extensively metabolized in the liver to inactive metabolites that are principally excreted in the urine.

Bio-availability 90%.

Onset of action 2 weeks in depression.[18]

Time to peak plasma concentration 6h.

Plasma halflife 8–17h.

Duration of action >24h, situation-dependent.

Cautions

Suicide risk: the possibility of a suicide attempt is inherent in major depression and persists until remission. Antidepressants themselves may cause suicidal ideation, particularly in those aged ≤25 years (see p.214).

Bipolar disorder (can transform into manic phase); epilepsy (lowers seizure threshold); cardiac disease (risk of hypertension and arrhythmia); renal impairment (see Dose and use, and Chapter 17, p.737); hepatic impairment (see Dose and use, and Chapter 18, p.763); urinary hesitancy and narrow-angle glaucoma (may exacerbate).

Drug interactions

Additive pharmacodynamic interactions with other drugs (see Antidepressants, p.216), notably serotonin toxicity (see Antidepressants, Box A, p.217). Concurrent administration with an MAOI or within 2 weeks of its cessation is contra-indicated.

Duloxetine is metabolized by CYP1A2 and CYP2D6. Caution should be taken with concurrent use of drugs that inhibit or induce these enzymes, particularly in those who are poor CYP2D6 metabolizers (see Chapter 19, Table 8, p.790).

Duloxetine is a moderate *inhibitor* of CYP2D6 and can increase plasma levels of TCAs, and may *reduce* the efficacy of a pro-drug, e.g. **tamoxifen**.[19]

Specific significant interactions[1]

- **fluvoxamine** (strong CYP1A2 inhibitor) *significantly increases* duloxetine plasma concentrations, and **ciprofloxacin** probably does the same; concurrent use of these drugs with duloxetine is contra-indicated
- **fluoxetine**, **paroxetine** and **quinidine** (strong CYP2D6 inhibitors) can increase duloxetine plasma concentrations
- smoking (CYP1A2 inducer) can *decrease* duloxetine plasma concentration by ≤50%; however, a routine dose increase in smokers is not recommended.

Undesirable effects

Very common (>10%): drowsiness, headache, dry mouth, nausea.
Common (<10%, >1%): dizziness, tremor, paraesthesia, blurred vision, tinnitus, sleep disturbance, agitation, palpitations, hypertension, diarrhoea, constipation, anorexia, rash, sweating, dysuria, sexual dysfunction.
Uncommon (<1%, >0.1%): altered taste, extrapyramidal symptoms, postural hypotension, arrhythmias, urinary hesitancy and retention.
Rare (<0.1%): hypertensive crises, Stevens-Johnson syndrome.

Like SSRIs and **venlafaxine**, duloxetine increases the risk of bleeding.[20]

Dose and use

The timing of once daily doses is immaterial, although it should be constant. Monitor blood pressure; consider dose reduction or discontinuation if there is a sustained increase.

No dose reduction is required in mild–moderate renal impairment; use is contra-indicated in patients with creatinine clearance <30mL/min and in hepatic impairment (see Chapter 17, p.737 and Chapter 18, p.763).

Avoid abrupt withdrawal after prolonged use (see Stopping antidepressants, p.223).

Neuropathic pain

Although authorized for painful *diabetic* neuropathy, duloxetine is commonly advocated as a first-line choice for neuropathic pain of any cause:[21]

- start at 30mg PO once daily and increase to 60mg after 1–2 weeks
- if necessary, increase to 60mg b.d.

Depression

Duloxetine is less effective and less well tolerated than alternatives (see above). It may have a role in depression with concurrent neuropathic pain:

- start at 30mg PO once daily and increase to 60mg after 1–2 weeks.

Although there is no direct evidence of benefit, increasing the dose to 60mg b.d. is one of several options if the response to the starting dose is inadequate (see p.220).[18]

†Hot flushes

- start at 30mg PO once daily and increase to 60mg after 1–2 weeks.[16]

Stress incontinence in women

In physically fit women, management is primarily non-drug, e.g. pelvic floor muscle training (sometimes followed by surgery).[15] If prescribing duloxetine, the manufacturer recommends twice daily dosing:

- start with 20mg PO b.d.
- if necessary, increase to 40mg b.d. after 2 weeks.

However, this has not been directly compared to once daily dosing, which may be more convenient.

Supply

Duloxetine (generic)
Capsules enclosing e/c pellets 20mg, 30mg, 40mg, 60mg, 28 days @ 60mg once daily = £2.

1 Preston CL. *Stockley's Drug Interactions*. London: Pharmaceutical Press. www.medicinescomplete.com (accessed December 2021).
2 Bymaster FP *et al.* (2001) Comparative affinity of duloxetine and venlafaxine for serotonin and norepinephrine transporters in vitro and in vivo, human serotonin receptor subtypes, and other neuronal receptors. *Neuropsychopharmacology*. **25**: 871–880.
3 Yamashita T *et al.* (2016) Duloxetine inhibits microglial P2X4 receptor function and alleviates neuropathic pain after peripheral nerve injury. *PLoS One*. **11**: e0165189.
4 Cipriani A *et al.* (2012) Duloxetine versus other anti-depressive agents for depression. *Cochrane Database of Systematic Reviews*. **10**: CD006533. www.cochranelibrary.com.
5 Lunn MP *et al.* (2014) Duloxetine for treating painful neuropathy, chronic pain or fibromyalgia. *Cochrane Database of Systematic Reviews*. **1**: CD007115. www.cochranelibrary.com.
6 Farshchian N *et al.* (2018) Comparative study of the effects of venlafaxine and duloxetine on chemotherapy-induced peripheral neuropathy. *Cancer Chemotherapy and Pharmacology*. **82**: 787–793.
7 Gül ŞK *et al.* (2020) Duloxetine and pregabalin in neuropathic pain of lung cancer patients. *Brain and Behaviour*. **10**: e01527.
8 Matsuoka H *et al.* (2019) Additive duloxetine for cancer-related neuropathic pain nonresponsive or intolerant to opioid-pregabalin therapy: a randomised controlled trial (JORTC-PAL08). *Journal of Pain and Symptom Management*. **58**: 645–653.
9 Smith EM *et al.* (2013) Effect of duloxetine on pain, function, and quality of life among patients with chemotherapy-induced painful peripheral neuropathy: a randomized clinical trial. *Journal of the American Medical Association*. **309**: 1359–1367.
10 Matsuoka H *et al.* (2020) Predictors of duloxetine response in patients with neuropathic cancer pain: a secondary analysis of a randomised controlled trial – JORTC-PAL08 (DIRECT) study. *Supportive Care in Cancer*. **28**: 2931–2939.
11 Goldstein DJ *et al.* (2005) Duloxetine vs. placebo in patients with painful diabetic neuropathy. *Pain*. **116**: 109–118.
12 Kaur H *et al.* (2011) A comparative evaluation of amitriptyline and duloxetine in painful diabetic neuropathy: a randomized, double-blind, cross-over clinical trial. *Diabetes Care*. **34**: 818–822.
13 Boyle J *et al.* (2012) Randomized, placebo-controlled comparison of amitriptyline, duloxetine, and pregabalin in patients with chronic diabetic peripheral neuropathic pain: impact on pain, polysomnographic sleep, daytime functioning, and quality of life. *Diabetes Care*. **35**: 2451–2458.
14 Iwaki H *et al.* (2020) A double-blind randomized controlled trial of duloxetine for pain in Parkinson's disease. *Journal of the Neurological Sciences*. **414**: 116833.
15 NICE (2019) Urinary incontinence and pelvic organ prolapse in women: management. *NICE guideline* NG123. www.nice.org.uk.
16 Biglia N *et al.* (2018) Duloxetine and escitalopram for hot flushes: efficacy and compliance in breast cancer survivors. *European Journal for Cancer Care*. **27**: e12484.
17 Shin S *et al.* (2019) Treatment of poststroke pathologic laughing with duloxetine: a case series. *Clinical Neuropharmacology*. **42**: 60–63.
18 Cleare A *et al.* (2015) Evidence-based guidelines for treating depressive disorders with antidepressants: a revision of the 2008 British Association for Psychopharmacology guidelines. *Journal of Psychopharmacology*. **29**: 459–525.
19 UKMI (2018) Tamoxifen and SSRI or SNRI antidepressants – is there an interaction Medicines Q&A. www.sps.nhs.uk (accessed December 2021).
20 Perahia DG *et al.* (2013) The risk of bleeding with duloxetine treatment in patients who use nonsteroidal anti-inflammatory drugs (NSAIDs): analysis of placebo-controlled trials and post-marketing adverse event reports. *Drug Healthcare and Patient Safety*. **5**: 211–219.
21 Finnerup NB *et al.* (2016) Pharmacotherapy for neuropathic pain in adults: a systematic review and meta-analysis. *Lancet Neurology*. **14**: 162–173.

Updated December 2021

MIRTAZAPINE

Class: α_2 Adrenergic and $5HT_{2A/2C}$ antagonist antidepressant.

Indications: Depression, †anxiety and panic disorders, †gastroparesis, †pruritus.

Contra-indications: Concurrent use with an MAOI or within 2 weeks of its cessation (see Drug interactions).

Pharmacology

Mirtazapine antagonizes receptors that inhibit monoamine release:[1]

- pre-synaptic α_2-adrenergic antagonism disinhibits serotonin and noradrenaline (norepinephrine) release
- post-synaptic $5HT_{2A}$, $5HT_{2C}$ and $5HT_3$ antagonism disinhibits noradrenaline and dopamine release.

In addition, H_1 antagonistic activity is responsible for its sedative properties. At lower doses, the sedative antihistaminic effect of mirtazapine predominates. With higher doses, sedation is reduced as noradrenergic and dopaminergic neural transmission increases. At therapeutic doses, it has no significant antimuscarinic activity and is not associated with cardiovascular toxicity or sexual dysfunction,[2] but arrhythmias are reported with overdoses.

The antidepressant effects of mirtazapine manifest faster than with SSRIs.[3] There are also fewer relapses compared with **amitriptyline**.[2] For refractory depression, mirtazapine is sometimes combined with an SSRI or **venlafaxine**, particularly if a previous switch of antidepressant monotherapy was unhelpful. (see Antidepressants, p.220). For anxiety disorders, mirtazapine is *not* consistently effective.[4]

Mirtazapine has anti-emetic properties that may be due to H_1, $5HT_2$ and/or $5HT_3$ antagonism.[5,6] In RCTs of patients with functional dyspepsia (± depression), mirtazapine 15–30mg/day improved dyspepsia symptoms (particularly early satiety and nutrient volume tolerance) and produced a mean weight gain of about 4kg/8 weeks.[7,8] An improvement in gastric accommodation is considered one mechanism of benefit in functional dyspepsia. In other settings, mirtazapine improves gastric emptying;[9] this may contribute to the rapid and sometimes dramatic improvement reported with mirtazapine in patients with gastroparesis of various causes who had failed to respond to usual prokinetic treatments.[10-13] Mirtazapine does not appear to be a prokinetic *per se*,[14] and improved gastric emptying may be secondary to, e.g. reduced levels of nausea, anxiety, changes in GI hormone levels.

Appetite stimulation and weight gain are common as a result of blockade of $5HT_2$ and H_1 receptors and changes in levels of hormones regulating energy intake.[7] Although there are reports of mirtazapine improving appetite in patients with cancer-related anorexia,[15] an RCT found the improvement in appetite to be no better than placebo.[16]

Mirtazapine is of benefit in uraemic pruritus, and anecdotally pruritus related to cancer or lymphoma (see Drugs for pruritus, p.825).

The benefit reported for cancer-related bone and neuropathic pain has not been confirmed in RCTs.[5,17] There are reports of benefit in refractory breathlessness,[18,19] with a phase III RCT currently underway.

Mirtazapine displays linear pharmacokinetics at usual doses. Food does not affect absorption, binding to plasma proteins is about 85%, and steady-state is reached after 5 days. Mirtazapine is extensively metabolized in the liver and eliminated primarily via the urine. It is a racemic mixture of two active enantiomers: the *R*-enantiomer is metabolized by CYP3A4 to the active metabolite, demethylmirtazapine, whereas the *S*-enantiomer is metabolized by CYP2D6 and CYP1A2.[2] Clearance in the elderly may be reduced by ≤40%.

Bio-availability 50% PO.

Onset of action hours–days (off-label indications); 1–2 weeks (antidepressant).

Time to peak plasma concentration 2h.

Plasma halflife 20–40h; often shorter in men (26h) than women (37h), but can extend up to 65h.

Duration of action variable; up to several days.

Cautions

Suicide risk: the possibility of a suicide attempt is inherent in major depression and persists until remission. Antidepressants may themselves cause suicidal ideation, particularly in those aged ≤25 years (see p.214).

Bipolar disorder (can transform into manic phase); epilepsy (seizures occur rarely; risk relative to other antidepressants is uncertain); cardiac disease (manufacturer advises increased monitoring with ischaemic heart disease or risk of arrhythmia); renal impairment (see Dose and use); hepatic impairment (see Dose and use); diabetes mellitus (may alter glycaemic control); narrow-angle glaucoma (mydriasis reported).

Drug interactions

Additive pharmacodynamic interactions with other drugs (see Antidepressants, p.216). The concurrent administration with an MAOI or within 2 weeks of its cessation is contra-indicated by the manufacturer because of the theoretical risk of serotonin toxicity (no serious cases have been reported).[20] There are isolated reports of serotonin toxicity with **venlafaxine** and possibly some SSRIs, leading to warnings of caution with the concurrent use of mirtazapine and other serotinergic drugs (see Antidepressants, Box A, p.217).[20] However, generally, the risk of serotonin toxicity appears to be low. Conversely, mirtazapine has been suggested as a treatment for serotonin toxicity.[17]

Mirtazapine is metabolized by CYP1A2, CYP2D6 and CYP3A4. Caution should be taken with concurrent use of drugs that inhibit or induce these enzymes, particularly in those who are poor CYP2D6 metabolizers (see Chapter 19, Table 8, p.790).

Specific significant interactions[20]

- **ketoconazole** (strong CYP3A4 inhibitor) can *increase* the plasma concentrations of mirtazapine by ≤40%; other strong CYP3A4 inhibitors (e.g. azole antifungals, HIV protease inhibitors, and macrolides) will probably have a similar effect; a dose reduction of mirtazapine may be necessary
- **fluvoxamine** (strong CYP1A2 inhibitor) can *increase* the plasma concentrations of mirtazapine up to four times and **cimetidine** by 50%
- **carbamazepine** and **phenytoin** (hepatic enzyme inducers) *decrease* mirtazapine plasma concentrations by up to 40%; other enzyme-inducing drugs (e.g. other anti-epileptic drugs and **rifampicin**) probably have a similar effect.

Undesirable effects

Very common (>10%): increase in appetite and weight gain;[21] drowsiness during the first few weeks of treatment. *Dose reduction reduces the likelihood of an antidepressant effect and does not necessarily alleviate drowsiness.*
Uncommon (<1%, >0.1%): hepatic impairment.
Very rare (<0.01%): agranulocytosis.

Dose and use

In elderly or frail patients and those with hepatic impairment or renal impairment with creatinine clearance <40mL/min, titrate slowly to a maximum dose of 30mg PO at bedtime. In ESRF, clearance is halved and mirtazapine should be avoided (see Chapter 17, p.737 and Chapter 18, p.763).

Avoid abrupt withdrawal after prolonged use (see Stopping antidepressants, p.223).

Depression[2]

- start with 15mg PO at bedtime
- if necessary, increase the dose by 15mg every 2 weeks up to 45mg at bedtime
- if no response after 2-4 weeks on 45mg, switch to an alternative antidepressant (see p.220)
- if effective, continue until the patient has been symptom-free for ≥6 months (see p.220); then discontinue over 2–4 weeks.

†Gastroparesis

Consider when a lack of benefit from usual prokinetic treatments (see Pharmacology, and also Prokinetics, p.22). Generally, onset of benefit is within 1–2 days:

- start with 15mg PO at bedtime (although some use the orodispersible formulation SL, all absorption occurs after swallowing)
- if necessary, increase the dose by 15mg every 5 days up to 45mg at bedtime
- usual effective dose 15–30mg/24h.

†Intractable pruritus

As for depression, see Chapter 26, Table 1, p.829.

†Panic and anxiety disorders

As for depression, although mirtazapine is *not* a first-line treatment (see Antidepressants, p.221).[4]

Supply

Mirtazapine (generic)
Tablets 15mg, 30mg, 45mg, 28 days @ 30mg at bedtime = £1.50.
Tablets orodispersible 15mg, 30mg, 45mg, 28 days @ 30mg at bedtime = £1.25; *tablets should be placed on the tongue, allowed to disperse, then swallowed.*
Oral solution (sugar-free) 15mg/mL, 28 days @ 30mg at bedtime = £68.

1 Stahl SM (2021) Chapter 7: Treatments for mood disorders. In: *Essential Psychopharmacology: Neuroscientific Basis and Practical Applications* (5e). Cambridge University Press, USA. pp. 283-358.
2 Croom KF *et al.* (2009) Mirtazapine: a review of its use in major depression and other psychiatric disorders. *CNS Drugs.* **23**: 427–452.
3 Watanabe N *et al.* (2011) Mirtazapine versus other antidepressive agents for depression. *Cochrane Database of Systematic Reviews.* **12**: CD006528. www.cochranelibrary.com

4 Baldwin DS *et al.* (2014) Evidence-based pharmacological treatment of anxiety disorders, post-traumatic stress disorder and obsessive-compulsive disorder: a revision of the 2005 guidelines from the british association for psychopharmacology. *Journal of Psychopharmacology*. **28**: 403–439.
5 Economos *et al.* (2020) What is the evidence for mirtazapine in treating cancer-related symptomatology? A systematic review. *Supportive Care in Cancer.* **28**: 1597–1606.
6 Chen CC *et al.* (2008) Premedication with mirtazapine reduces preoperative anxiety and postoperative nausea and vomiting. *Anesthesia and Analgesia*. **106**: 109–113.
7 Jiang SM *et al.* (2016) Beneficial effects of antidepressant mirtazapine in functional dyspepsia patients with weight loss. *World Journal of Gastroenterology*. **22**: 5260–5266.
8 Tack J *et al.* (2016) Efficacy of mirtazapine in patients with functional dyspepsia and weight loss. *Clinical Gastroenterology and Hepatology*. **14**: 385–392.e4.
9 Kumar N *et al.* (2017) Effect of mirtazapine on gastric emptying in patients with cancer-associated anorexia. *Indian Journal of Palliative Care*. **23**: 335–337.
10 Malamood M *et al.* (2017) Mirtazapine for symptom control in refractory gastroparesis. *Drug Design, Development and Therapy*. **11**: 1035–1041.
11 Kundu S *et al.* (2014) Rapid improvement in post-infectious gastroparesis symptoms with mirtazapine. *World Journal of Gastroenterology*. **20**: 6671–6674.
12 Song J *et al.* (2014) Successful treatment of gastroparesis with the antidepressant mirtazapine: a case report. *Journal of Nippon Medical School*. **81**: 392–394.
13 Kim SW *et al.* (2006) Mirtazapine for severe gastroparesis unresponsive to conventional prokinetic treatment. *Psychosomatics*. **47**: 440–442.
14 Carbone F *et al.* (2017) The effect of mirtazapine on gastric accommodation, gastric sensitivity to distension and nutrient tolerance in healthy subjects. *Neurogastroenterology and Motility*. **29**: e13146.
15 Riechelmann RP *et al.* (2010) Phase II trial of mirtazapine for cancer-related cachexia and anorexia. *American Journal of Hospice and Palliative Medicine*. **27**: 106–110.
16 Hunter CM *et al.* (2021) Mirtazapine in cancer-associated anorexia and cachexia: a double-blind placebo-controlled randomized trial. *Journal of Pain and Symptom Management*. **62**: 1207–1215.
17 Hoes MJ and Zeijpveld JH (1996) Mirtazapine as treatment for serotonin syndrome. *Pharmacopsychiatry*. **29**: 81.
18 Lovell N *et al.* (2018) Use of mirtazapine in patients with chronic breathlessness: a case series. *Palliative Medicine* **32**: 1518–1521
19 Higginson IJ *et al.* (2020) Randomised double blind multicentre mixed methods dose escalation feasibility trial of mirtazapine for better treatment of severe breathlessness in advanced lung disease (BETTER-B feasibility). *Thorax* **75**: 176–179
20 Preston CL. *Stockley's drug interactions*. London: Pharmaceutical Press. www.medicinescomplete.com (accessed December 2021).
21 Abed R and Cooper M (1999) Mirtazapine causing hyperphagia. *British Journal of Psychiatry*. **174**: 181–182.

Updated December 2021

TRAZODONE

Class: α-Adrenergic and $5HT_{2A/2C}$ antagonist antidepressant; serotonin re-uptake inhibitor.

Indications: Depression, †anxiety and panic disorders, †hyperactive delirium, †insomnia.

Contra-indications: Concurrent use with an MAOI or within 2 weeks of its cessation (see Antidepressants, Box A, p.217). Avoid use in the initial recovery period after an acute myocardial infarction.

Pharmacology

Trazodone is an α_1-adenergic, α_2-adrenergic, H_1, $5HT_{2A}$ and $5HT_{2C}$ receptor antagonist, a $5HT_{1A}$ partial agonist, and, at higher doses, a serotonin re-uptake inhibitor.[1] It is devoid of antimuscarinic activity. Trazodone has an active metabolite, m-chlorophenylpiperazine. Excretion is almost entirely as free or conjugated metabolites.

Trazodone Is *not* a first-line treatment for depression (p.220) or anxiety (p.221). However, adjunctive use of doses lower than those authorized may have a place in selected patients. The benefit reported for insomnia and delirium is unconfirmed in RCTs.[2-5] In dementia, trazodone is *not* effective for challenging behaviours,[6] but *may* improve sleep disturbance.[7] Trazodone is *not* effective for neuropathic pain.[8,9]

Bio-availability 65%.
Onset of action 30–60min for insomnia or agitation; 1–4 weeks as an antidepressant.
Time to peak plasma concentration 1h if taken fasting; 2h if taken after food.
Plasma halflife 5–13h.
Duration of action variable, situation-dependent.

Cautions

Suicide risk: the possibility of a suicide attempt is inherent in major depression and persists until remission. Antidepressants may themselves cause suicidal ideation, particularly in those aged ≤25 years (see p.214).

Bipolar disorder (can transform into manic phase); epilepsy (lowers seizure threshold); risk factors for QT prolongation (see Chapter 20, p.797) and cardiac disease (risk of arrhythmia); renal impairment (see Chapter 17, p.737); severe hepatic impairment (increased drowsiness; see Chapter 18, p.763).

Drug interactions

Additive pharmacodynamic interactions with other drugs (see Antidepressants, p.216) notably QT prolongation (see p.799) and serotonin toxicity (see Antidepressants, Box A, p.217). Concurrent administration with an MAOI or within 2 weeks of its cessation is contra-indicated (see above).

Trazodone is metabolized by CYP3A4 and possibly CYP2D6. Caution should be taken with concurrent use of drugs that inhibit or induce these enzymes, particularly in those who are poor CYP2D6 metabolizers (see Chapter 19, Table 8, p.790).

Specific significant interactions[10]

- **clarithromycin** and **ritonavir** (strong CYP3A4 inhibitors) can *increase* plasma concentrations of trazodone by one third and double the elimination halflife; thus, strong CYP3A4 inhibitors should be avoided where possible or a lower dose of trazodone used
- **carbamazepine** can *decrease* plasma concentrations of trazodone by ≤75%.

If trazodone is prescribed concurrently, the dose of **warfarin** may need to be *increased*[11] and, because of reports of toxicity, the dose of **digoxin** and **phenytoin** *decreased*; the mechanism for these interactions is unknown.

Undesirable effects

Common: drowsiness, headaches, dizziness, dry mouth.[2]

Other: include agitation, restlessness, myoclonus, altered taste, nausea, vomiting, sweating, diarrhoea, constipation, hyponatraemia, postural hypotension, rash.

Rare: include hepatic impairment (may be severe), increased libido, priapism, arrhythmias, blood dyscrasias.

Dose and use

Trazodone is not a first-line treatment for any indication. Undesirable effects are minimized by a low starting dose. An oral solution is available, but it is expensive:

- start with 50mg PO at bedtime
- usual effective dose:
  - ▷ †insomnia 50mg at bedtime (occasionally ≤150mg/24h)[2,3,7,12]
  - ▷ depression or †anxiety ≤300mg/24h in divided doses
  - ▷ †delirium 25–50mg at bedtime (occasionally ≤200mg/24h).[4,5]

Avoid abrupt withdrawal after prolonged use (see Stopping antidepressants, p.223).

Supply

Trazodone (generic)

Capsules 50mg, 100mg, 28 days @ 100mg at bedtime = £1.75.

Tablets (scored) 50mg, 100mg, 150mg, 28 days @ 150mg at bedtime = £2.

Oral solution (sugar-free) 50mg/5mL, 100mg/5mL, 28 days @ 100mg at bedtime = £37 and £181 respectively.

1 Settimo L and Taylor D (2018) Evaluating the dose-dependent mechanism of action of trazodone by estimation of occupancies for different brain neurotransmitter targets. *Journal of Psychopharmacology*. **32**: 96–104.

2 Fagiolini A *et al.* (2012) Rediscovering trazodone for the treatment of major depressive disorder. *CNS Drugs*. **26**: 1033–1049.

3 Tanimukai H *et al.* (2013) An observational study of insomnia and nightmare treated with trazodone in patients with advanced cancer. *American Journal of Hospice and Palliative Care*. **30**: 359–362.
4 Okamoto Y *et al.* (1999) Trazodone in the treatment of delirium. *Journal of Clinical Psychopharmacology*. **19**: 280–282.
5 Maeda I *et al.* (2021) Low-dose trazodone for delirium in patients with cancer who received specialist palliative care: a multicenter prospective study. *Journal of Palliative Medicine* **24**: 914–918.
6 Seitz D *et al.* (2011) Antidepressants for agitation and psychosis in dementia. *Cochrane Database of Systematic Reviews*. **2**: CD008191. www.cochranelibrary.com
7 McCleery J *et al.* (2020) Pharmacotherapies for sleep disturbances in dementia. *Cochrane Database of Systematic Reviews*. **11**: CD009178. www.cochranelibrary.com
8 Davidoff G *et al.* (1987) Trazodone hydrochloride in the treatment of dysesthetic pain in traumatic myelopathy: a radomized double-blind, placebo controlled study. *Pain*. **29**: 151–161.
9 Lipone P (2020) Efficacy and safety of low doses of trazodone in patients affected by painful diabetic neuropathy and treated with gabapentin: a randomised controlled pilot study. *CNS Drugs* **34**: 1177–1189
10 Preston CL. *Stockley's Drug Interactions*. London: Pharmaceutical Press www.medicinescomplete.com (accessed December 2021).
11 Small NL and Giamonna KA (2000) Interaction between warfarin and trazodone. *Annals of Pharmacotherapy*. **34**: 734–736.
12 Everitt H *et al.* (2018) Antidepressants for insomnia in adults. *Cochrane Database of Systematic Reviews*. **5**: CD010753. www.cochranelibrary.com

Updated December 2021

*PSYCHOSTIMULANTS

Indications: Attention deficit hyperactivity disorder in children (**methylphenidate**), daytime drowsiness due to narcolepsy (**modafinil**), †obstructive sleep apnoea or chronic shift work-related sleep disorder (discouraged by regulators),[1] †depression when prognosis limited (i.e. ≤4 weeks), †fatigue refractory to correction of underlying contributory factors, †opioid-related drowsiness, †apathy in Alzheimer's disease.

Contra-indications: Severe cardiovascular disease (e.g. uncontrolled hypertension or angina, arrhythmias; also see Cautions); use within the last 2 weeks of a monoamine oxidase inhibitor (MAOI), including **procarbazine** (an antineoplastic drug and a weak MAOI, see p.216).

Manufacturers of **methylphenidate** also recommend avoiding in cerebrovascular disorders, glaucoma, phaeochromocytoma, thyrotoxicosis and history of severe psychiatric illness.

Pharmacology

The psychostimulants **dexamfetamine**, **methylphenidate** and **modafinil** inhibit or reverse dopamine re-uptake transporters, thereby increasing synaptic dopamine.[2,3] Dopamine has a central role in attention, arousal and motivation. It is released in response to stimuli and thoughts perceived as relevant, particularly with regard to 'threat' or 'reward'.[4,5] Thus, psychostimulants can improve alertness, motivation and mood.

Dopaminergic dysfunction in the mesolimbic and mesocortical systems is implicated in several disorders. In attention deficit hyperactivity disorder, psychostimulants may improve attention by correcting a deficit in dopamine release in response to relevant stimuli.[6] Conversely, in psychoses, dopamine excess increases the importance attached to thoughts and perceptions, e.g. the actions of others gain an enhanced relevance and are interpreted as evidence of threat (paranoid delusions) or importance (grandiose delusions). This explains the beneficial effects of D_2 antagonists in patients experiencing hallucinations and delusions (see Antipsychotics, p.184).[4,7]

Methylphenidate and **modafinil** have the best evidence base to support use in palliative care,[8] with **methylphenidate** probably the most widely used.[9,10] Although **methylphenidate** is available in m/r formulations, these may increase the risk of insomnia further, particularly if taken later in the day.

Modafinil is sometimes suggested as an alternative where **methylphenidate** is poorly tolerated. However, its undesirable cardiovascular and psychotropic effects appear similar. Further, regulators have withdrawn marketing authorizations for all indications except narcolepsy, because of concerns about undesirable skin and neuropsychiatric effects, and its abuse potential.[1]

The milder psychostimulant **caffeine** also acts indirectly via dopamine. Adenosine receptors are co-localized with and inhibit D_1 and D_2 receptors, and, as adenosine accumulates during the daytime, dopamine-mediated arousal is reduced; **caffeine**, which acts as an adenosine receptor antagonist, helps prevent this. Present in some OTC combination analgesics, **caffeine** appears beneficial for headache.[11] Although IV **caffeine** is better than placebo in cancer pain, the degree of benefit is unlikely to be clinically relevant.[12]

Table 1 contains selected pharmacokinetic data.

Table 1 Pharmacokinetic details for selected psychostimulants[13–16]

	Oral bio-availability (%)	*Time to peak plasma concentration (h)*	*Halflife (h)*	*Metabolism*
Dexamfetamine	No data	2–4	6–12	Multiple routes; ≤50% renally excreted unchanged
Methylphenidate	30[a]	1–3	2	Non-CYP carboxylesterase[b]
Modafinil	40–65[c]	1.5–4	15[d]	CYP3A4; non-CYP esterase[b]

a. almost completely absorbed but undergoes extensive first-pass hepatic metabolism
b. metabolites are inactive
c. estimated from urinary recovery of radio-labelled doses; absolute bio-availability unknown because of the lack of an IV preparation
d. modafinil is a racemic compound; enantiomers are equipotent.

Cautions

Psychostimulants may exacerbate cardiovascular disease (e.g. severe hypertension, angina, arrhythmia; manufacturers recommend specialist cardiac evaluation; also see Contra-indications). Psychostimulants may also exacerbate psychiatric illness (e.g. anxiety, agitation, psychosis, addiction disorders), epilepsy (possible lowering of seizure threshold), hyperthyroidism and closed-angle glaucoma (*not* **modafinil**).

Severe hepatic impairment (**modafinil**; see Dose and use).

Modafinil may be teratogenic; ensure adequate contraception (also see Drug interactions).[17]

Although rare in adults, serious skin reactions occur with **modafinil** in 1% of children; consider alternatives where possible (e.g. **methylphenidate**).

Drug interactions

Pharmacodynamic interactions include those with sympathomimetics (e.g. MAOIs; see Contra-indications) and antipsychotics (reduced stimulant effect).

Methylphenidate and **modafinil** may increase plasma concentrations of TCAs, **phenytoin** and **warfarin** (check INR at least weekly until stabilized). **Modafinil** may also increase the plasma concentrations of **diazepam**.

Modafinil is considered a weak–moderate inducer of CYP3A4/5 enzymes, potentially resulting in reduced efficacy of **ciclosporin**, HIV protease inhibitors, **midazolam**, L-type calcium-channel blockers, statins and hormonal contraception (use alternative methods of contraception because of teratogenic risk; see Cautions). **Modafinil** also inhibits CYP2C19 and thus may decrease the plasma concentrations of the active metabolites of **clopidogrel**.

Undesirable effects

Undesirable effects have been reported in ≤30% of patients.

Neuropsychiatric: insomnia, agitation and anorexia (generally settle after 2–3 weeks if the drug is continued, or resolve after 2–3 days if the drug is discontinued), psychosis, movement disorders.

Cardiovascular: tachyarrhythmias, hypertension, angina (rare).

Other: headache (common and responds to slower dose titration); nausea; reduced seizure threshold (**methylphenidate**); *very rarely cerebral arteritis occurs with* ***methylphenidate***. Mild rashes are common with **modafinil**; serious skin reactions occur in 1% of children.

Use of psychostimulants in palliative care

†*Depression*

Psychostimulants are used where prognosis is thought to be ≤4 weeks. Trials generally show psychostimulants to be well tolerated in the short term, but methodological limitations preclude firm conclusions about their efficacy as antidepressants.[8,18,19] Thus, conventional antidepressants should be used if the patient has a prognosis sufficient for a response to manifest.[8,18]

Methylphenidate is the most commonly used psychostimulant for depression in palliative care. Although undesirable effects are similar for all psychostimulants, some patients may benefit by switching to an alternative (e.g. **modafinil**) if the first choice is ineffective or poorly tolerated. Concurrent use of **methylphenidate** with **mirtazapine** may hasten the response compared with the latter alone.[20] This effect has not been demonstrated in conjunction with SSRIs.[21]

Ketamine (p.691) is an alternative rapid-onset antidepressant.

†*Fatigue*

Psychological and exercise-based interventions are first-line options for cancer-related fatigue (n=11,525).[22] However, the use of psychostimulants is controversial. Two meta-analyses (n=146, n=498) found **methylphenidate** may be moderately more effective for cancer-related fatigue than placebo,[23,24] although several subsequent RCTs showed no benefit.[25–27] **Modafinil** (two RCTs; n=197) and **armodafinil** (n=50) were also ineffective.[28–30] An RCT (n=28) of **methylphenidate** p.r.n. found benefit of uncertain clinical significance.[31] Psychostimulants are not consistently effective for fatigue related to chemotherapy,[32–36] cranial radiotherapy,[37] or cancer-associated cognitive impairment.[38]

In Parkinson's disease, NICE suggests that **modafinil** can be considered for excessive daytime sleepiness,[39] although results of RCTs (n=76) are conflicting.[40–42] In multiple sclerosis, one RCT (n=21)[43] found **modafinil** improved fatigue, but two larger RCTs (n=256) found no such benefit with either **modafinil** or **methylphenidate**.[44,45] **Modafinil** may be beneficial for fatigue related to MND/ALS (n=32)[46] and HIV (n=115).[47]

Many trials found large placebo responses. Psychostimulants were generally well tolerated, and some 'negative' RCTs noted clinically meaningful responses in subgroups (e.g. those with more severe fatigue).[26,33]

Given this uncertainty, psychostimulants should be reserved for fatigue refractory to other measures such as:

- correction of underlying causal factors, e.g. anaemia, depression, electrolyte disturbance, medication
- modification of daily routine, e.g. exercise, energy conservation, practical help to aid adjustment to changing circumstances.[48–52]

†*Opioid-related drowsiness*

Drowsiness is common when opioids are commenced or the dose is increased; it is generally transient, lasting about 1 week. Persistent drowsiness may indicate opioid toxicity; a trial dose reduction should be made and other drug and non-drug approaches considered to provide adequate analgesia (see Adjuvant analgesics, p.325). However, some patients experience persistent drowsiness despite adjusting the opioid dose. In this circumstance, switching to an alternative opioid may be of benefit (see Appendix 2, p.925).

Psychostimulants are occasionally used for opioid-related drowsiness refractory to these measures. They may improve psychomotor performance and allow opioid dose escalation to a higher level than would otherwise be possible, including in some instances of difficult to manage break-through pain.[53] However, these reports pre-date the availability of other potential options, e.g. transmucosal **fentanyl** (p.450).

†*Apathy in Alzheimer's disease*

A meta-analysis of three RCTs (n=145) found **methylphenidate** may improve apathy, cognition and functional performance in patients with Alzheimer's disease.[54] Insomnia, agitation and delusions were reported, but overall adverse events were comparable to placebo. Nevertheless, caution is advised in prescribing for this population, particularly patients with cardiovascular disease and epilepsy. Improvement in excessive daytime sleepiness has also been reported.[55]

Dose

SPCs recommend that heart rate, BP and an ECG (**modafanil**) are assessed at baseline and after each dose increase. If used long-term, heart rate and BP should be monitored at regular intervals (e.g. every 6 months).

Methylphenidate

- start with 2.5–5mg PO b.d. (on waking/breakfast time and noon/lunchtime)
- if necessary, increase by *daily* increments of 2.5–5mg b.d. (every third day for apathy in Alzheimer's disease)
- usual maximum:
  - ▷ fatigue: 20–40mg/24h
  - ▷ apathy in Alzheimer's disease: 20mg/24h
  - ▷ depression: ≤60mg/24h has been used.[18]

Modafinil

Dose titration is slower:

- start with 100mg PO each morning
- if necessary after *1 week*, increase to 200mg each morning
- maximum dose 400mg/24h (200mg/24h in severe hepatic impairment).

The manufacturer recommends either a single morning dose or divided doses in the morning and at noon. However, given the relatively long halflife of **modafinil**, the latter may increase the risk of sleep disturbance.

Supply

Methylphenidate

All products are **CDs**.

Methylphenidate hydrochloride (generic)

Tablets *(scored)* 5mg, 10mg, 20mg, 28 days @ 10mg b.d. = £8.

Oral suspension 5mg/5mL, 28 days @ 10mg b.d. = £27 (unauthorized product, available as a special order; see Chapter 24, p.817). *Price based on the Specials tariff in the community.*

Note. M/r products are available but are not appropriate as daytime stimulants in palliative care.

Modafinil

Modafinil (generic)

Tablets 100mg, 200mg, 28 days @ 200mg each morning = £7.

1 MHRA (2010) European Medicines Agency recommends restricting the use of modafinil. *Drug Safety Update*. **4**: www.gov.uk/drug-safety-update.

2 Heal DJ *et al.* (2014) Dopamine reuptake transporter (DAT) "inverse agonism"–a novel hypothesis to explain the enigmatic pharmacology of cocaine. *Neuropharmacology*. **87**: 19–40.

3 Schmitt KC *et al.* (2013) Nonclassical pharmacology of the dopamine transporter: atypical inhibitors, allosteric modulators, and partial substrates. *Journal of Pharmacology and Experimental Therapeutics*. **346**: 2–10.

4 Stahl SM (2013) Chapter 4: Psychosis and schizophrenia. In: *Essential Psychopharmacology: Neuroscientific Basis and Practical Applications* (4e). Cambridge University Press, pp. 79–128.

5 Phillips JM *et al.* (2016) A subcortical pathway for rapid, goal-driven, attentional filtering. *Trends Neurosciences*. **39**: 49–51.

6 del Campo N *et al.* (2013) A positron emission tomography study of nigro-striatal dopaminergic mechanisms underlying attention: implications for ADHD and its treatment. *Brain*. **136**: 3252–3270.

7 Stahl SM (2013) Chapter 5: Antipsychotic agents. In: *Essential Psychopharmacology: Neuroscientific Basis and Practical Applications* (4e). Cambridge University Press, pp. 129–236.

8 Candy *et al.* (2008) Psychostimulants for depression. *Cochrane Database of Systematic Reviews*. **2**: CD006722. www.cochranelibrary.com.

9 Dein S and George R (2002) A place for psychostimulants in palliative care? *Journal of Palliative Care*. **18**: 196–199.

10 Masand PS and Tesar GE (1996) Use of stimulants in the medically ill. *Psychiatric Clinics of North America*. **19**: 515–547.

11 Sawynok J (2011) Caffeine and pain. *Pain*. **152**: 726–729.

12 Suh SY *et al.* (2013) Caffeine as an adjuvant therapy to opioids in cancer pain: a randomized, double-blind, placebo-controlled trial. *Journal of Pain and Symptom Management*. **46**: 474–482.

13 Challman TD and Lipsky JJ (2000) Methylphenidate: its pharmacology and uses. *Mayo Clinic Proceedings*. **75**: 711–721.

14 de la Torre R *et al.* (2004) Clinical pharmacokinetics of amfetamine and related substances: monitoring in conventional and non-conventional matrices. *Clinical Pharmacokinetics*. **43**: 157–185.

15 Connor DF and Steingard RJ (2004) New formulations of stimulants for attention-deficit hyperactivity disorder: therapeutic potential. *CNS Drugs*. **18**: 1011–1030.

16 Robertson P, Jr. and Hellriegel ET (2003) Clinical pharmacokinetic profile of modafinil. *Clinical Pharmacokinetics*. **42**: 123–137.

17 MHRA (2020) Modafinil (Provigil): increased risk of congenital malformations if used during pregnancy. *Drug Safety Update*. www.gov.uk/drug-safety-update.

18 Orr K and Taylor D (2007) Psychostimulants in the treatment of depression: a review of the evidence. *CNS Drugs.* **21**: 239–257.
19 Centeno C *et al.* (2012) Multi-centre, double-blind, randomised placebo-controlled clinical trial on the efficacy of methylphenidate on depressive symptoms in advanced cancer patients. *BMJ Supportive and Palliative Care.* **2**: 328–333.
20 Ng C *et al.* (2014) Rapid response to methylphenidate as an add-on therapy to mirtazapine in the treatment of major depressive disorder in terminally ill cancer patients: a four-week, randomized, double-blinded, placebo-controlled study. *European Neuropsychopharmacology.* **24**: 491–498.
21 Sullivan D *et al.* (2017) Randomized, double-blind, placebo-controlled study of methylphenidate for the treatment of depression in SSRI-treated cancer patients receiving palliative care. *Psychooncology.* **26**: 1763–1769.
22 Mustian K *et al.* (2017) Comparison of pharmaceutical, psychological, and exercise treatments for cancer-related fatigue: a meta-analysis. *JAMA Oncology.* **3**: 961–968.
23 Mücke M *et al.* (2015) Pharmacological treatments for fatigue associated with palliative care. *Cochrane Database of Systematic Reviews.* **5**: CD006788. www.cochranelibrary.com.
24 Gong S *et al.* (2014) Effect of methylphenidate in patients with cancer-related fatigue: a systematic review and meta-analysis. *PLoS One.* **9**: e84391.
25 Bruera E *et al.* (2013) Methylphenidate and/or a nursing telephone intervention for fatigue in patients with advanced cancer: a randomized, placebo-controlled, phase II trial. *Journal of Clinical Oncology.* **31**: 2421–2427.
26 Mitchell GK *et al.* (2015) The effect of methylphenidate on fatigue in advanced cancer: an aggregated N-of-1 trial. *Journal of Pain and Symptom Management.* **50**: 289–296.
27 Centeno C *et al.* (2020) Improved cancer-related fatigue in a randomised clinical trial: methylphenidate no better than placebo. *BMJ Supportive & Palliative Care.*
28 Spathis A *et al.* (2014) Modafinil for the treatment of fatigue in lung cancer: results of a placebo-controlled, double-blind, randomized trial. *Journal of Clinical Oncology.* **32**: 1882–1888.
29 Boele FW *et al.* (2013) The effect of modafinil on fatigue, cognitive functioning, and mood in primary brain tumor patients: a multicenter randomized controlled trial. *Neuro-Oncology.* **15**: 1420–1428.
30 Berenson JR *et al.* (2015) A phase 3 trial of armodafinil for the treatment of cancer-related fatigue for patients with multiple myeloma. *Supportive Care in Cancer.* **23**: 1503–1512.
31 Pedersen L *et al.* (2020) Methylphenidate as needed for fatigue in patients with advanced cancer. A prospective, double-blind, and placebo-controlled study. *Journal of Pain and Symptom Management.* **60**: 992–1002.
32 Lower EE *et al.* (2009) Efficacy of dexmethylphenidate for the treatment of fatigue after cancer chemotherapy: a randomized clinical trial. *Journal of Pain and Symptom Management.* **38**: 650–662.
33 Jean-Pierre P *et al.* (2010) A phase 3 randomized, placebo-controlled, double-blind, clinical trial of the effect of modafinil on cancer-related fatigue among 631 patients receiving chemotherapy: a University of Rochester Cancer Center Community Clinical Oncology Program Research base study. *Cancer.* **116**: 3513–3520.
34 Mar Fan HG *et al.* (2008) A randomised, placebo-controlled, double-blind trial of the effects of d-methylphenidate on fatigue and cognitive dysfunction in women undergoing adjuvant chemotherapy for breast cancer. *Supportive Care in Cancer.* **16**: 577–583.
35 Hovey E *et al.* (2014) Phase III, randomized, double-blind, placebo-controlled study of modafinil for fatigue in patients treated with docetaxel-based chemotherapy. *Supportive Care in Cancer.* **22**: 1233–1242.
36 Heckler CE *et al.* (2016) Cognitive behavioral therapy for insomnia, but not armodafinil, improves fatigue in cancer survivors with insomnia: a randomized placebo-controlled trial. *Supportive Care in Cancer.* **24**: 2059-2066.
37 Butler JM, Jr. *et al.* (2007) A phase III, double-blind, placebo-controlled prospective randomized clinical trial of d-threo-methylphenidate HCl in brain tumor patients receiving radiation therapy. *International Journal of Radiation Oncology, Biology, Physics.* **69**: 1496–1501.
38 Miladi N *et al.* (2019) Psychostimulants for cancer-related cognitive impairment in adult cancer survivors: a systematic review and meta-analysis. *Supportive Care in Cancer.* **27**: 3717–3727.
39 NICE (2017) Parkinson's disease in adults. *NICE Guideline* NG71. www.nice.org.uk.
40 Adler C *et al.* (2003) Randomized trial of modafinil for treating subjective daytime sleepiness in patients with Parkinson's disease. *Movement Disorders.* **18**: 287–293.
41 Högl B *et al.* (2002) Modafinil for the treatment of daytime sleepiness in Parkinson's disease: a double-blind, randomized, crossover, placebo-controlled polygraphic trial. *Sleep.* **25**: 905–909.
42 Ondo W *et al.* (2005) Modafinil for daytime somnolence in Parkinson's disease: double blind, placebo controlled parallel trial. *Journal of Neurology, Neurosurgery and Psychiatry.* **76**: 1636–1639.
43 Lange R *et al.* (2009) Modafinil effects in multiple sclerosis patients with fatigue. *Journal of Neurology.* **256**: 645–650.
44 Stankoff B *et al.* (2005) Modafinil for fatigue in MS: a randomized placebo-controlled double-blind study. *Neurology.* **64**: 1139–1143.
45 Nourbakhsh B *et al.* (2021) Safety and efficacy of amantadine, modafinil, and methylphenidate for fatigue in multiple sclerosis: a randomised, placebo-controlled, crossover, double-blind trial. *Lancet Neurology.* **20**: 38–48.
46 Rabkin JG *et al.* (2009) Modafinil treatment of fatigue in patients with ALS: a placebo-controlled study. *Muscle and Nerve.* **39**: 297–303.
47 Rabkin JG *et al.* (2010) Modafinil treatment for fatigue in HIV/AIDS: a randomized placebo-controlled study. *Journal of Clinical Psychiatry.* **71**: 707-715.
48 National Comprehensive Care Network (2014) Cancer related fatigue. In: *Clinical practice guidelines in oncology.* www.nccn.org.
49 Radbruch L *et al.* (2008) Fatigue in palliative care patients -- an EAPC approach. *Palliative Medicine.* **22**: 13–32.
50 Minton O *et al.* (2008) A systematic review and meta-analysis of the pharmacological treatment of cancer-related fatigue. *Journal of the National Cancer Institute.* **100**: 1155–1166.
51 Cramp F and Byron-Daniel J (2012) Exercise for the management of cancer-related fatigue in adults. *Cochrane Database of Systematic Reviews.* **11**: CD006145. www.cochranelibrary.com.
52 ESMO (2020) Cancer-related fatigue: ESMO Clinical Practice Guidelines for diagnosis and treatment. *Annals of oncology.* 713–723.
53 Stone P and Minton O (2011) European Palliative Care Research collaborative pain guidelines. Central side-effects management: what is the evidence to support best practice in the management of sedation, cognitive impairment and myoclonus? *Palliative Medicine.* **25**: 431–441.
54 Ruthirakuhan M *et al.* (2018) Pharmacological interventions for apathy in Alzheimer's disease. *Cochrane Database of Systematic Reviews.* **5**: CD012197. www.cochranelibrary.com.
55 Bidzan L and Bidzan M (2020) Use of methylphenidate in excessive daytime sleepiness in Alzheimer's patients treated with donepezil: case series. *Neuropsychiatric Disease and Treatment.* **16**: 2677–2680.

Updated June 2021

*CANNABINOIDS

Indications: Refractory chemotherapy-induced nausea and vomiting (**nabilone, dronabinol** (not UK)); refractory spasticity in multiple sclerosis (**Δ^9-THC** with **cannabidiol**; Sativex®); †pain unresponsive to standard treatments; Lennox–Gastaut or Dravet syndrome (**cannabidiol**); AIDS-related anorexia (**dronabinol**; not UK).

Contra-indications: History (including family history) of psychosis.

Pharmacology

Endocannabinoids have important regulatory roles throughout the nervous system, immune system and elsewhere, making them potential therapeutic targets for a wide range of disorders, including pain, spasticity, nausea, itch, epilepsy, obesity and cancer.[1-6]

Cannabinoids containing the psychoactive constituent of *Cannabis sativa*, Δ^9-tetrahydrocannabinol (**Δ^9-THC**), or a synthetic analogue, are currently used for pain, spasticity and nausea. However, they are only modestly effective, generally less well tolerated than alternative drugs, and relatively expensive. **Cannabidiol** (CBD) is authorized for two rare childhood epilepsy syndromes, Lennox–Gastaut and Dravet syndrome, in conjunction with **clobazam**, but its place, if any, in adult-onset epilepsy is unknown (also see below).[7]

Although an improved understanding of the endocannabinoid system in pain has led to RCTs of more selective cannabinoids (CB_2-selective agonists) and inhibitors of endocannabinoid breakdown (fatty acid amide hydrolase inhibitors), they are no better than placebo.[8,9] In part, this may be due to endocannabinoids having both antinociceptive and pronociceptive properties. Further, cannabinoids acting at the *same* receptor can trigger *different* secondary messenger systems (biased agonism); this may be why the promising preclinical effects of CB_2 agonists were not seen in human trials.[9] Potential future avenues include exploiting:[1,9-12]

- *Cannabis sativa*'s many non-psychoactive compounds
- cannabinoids that affect multiple parts of the endocannabinoid system, e.g. dual fatty acid amide hydrolase (FAAH) and monoacylglycerol lipase (MAGL) inhibitors (see below)
- cannabinoids that also affect other lipid signalling systems, e.g. cyclooxygenase (see NSAIDs, p.341), transient receptor potential channels (see below)
- allosteric modulators of cannabinoid transmission
- cannabinoid-biased agonists.

Endocannabinoid system

The endocannabinoid system comprises:[9,10]

- two known receptors:
  - ▷ CB_1, expressed mainly by central and peripheral neurones
  - ▷ CB_2, expressed mainly by immune cells
- endogenous cannabinoids (endocannabinoids), mainly fatty acids derived from arachidonic acid, produced *de novo* as required and then rapidly removed by hydrolysis. Several have been identified, notably:
  - ▷ 2-arachidonyl glycerin (2-AG)
  - ▷ anandamide (arachidonylethanolamide, AEA)
- enzymes and re-uptake systems involved in endocannabinoid metabolism, including MAGL and fatty acid amide hydrolase-1 (FAAH-1).

CB_1 (an inhibitory receptor) reduces neuronal excitability and neurotransmitter release by opening potassium channels and blocking N/P/Q-type calcium channels respectively. It is part of a negative-feedback loop which regulates neurotransmitter release (Figure 1). CB_1 is also present on adjacent astrocytes, where it stimulates the release of gliotransmitters that influence nearby synapses.[1,13]

CB_2 is implicated in immune regulation. Located on antigen-presenting cells, it inhibits the production of pro-inflammatory cytokines.[11] Its expression on microglia is upregulated in the dorsal root ganglia and spinal cord following sciatic nerve injury. It is also expressed on neurones, but its role is uncertain.[12]

Endocannabinoids also act at receptors shared with other transmitter systems, including the capsaicin TRPV1 receptor involved in pain signalling (see Capsaicin, p.651) and the lipid GPR18, GPR55 and GPR119 receptors involved in the regulation of appetite, inflammation and metabolism.[1,14]

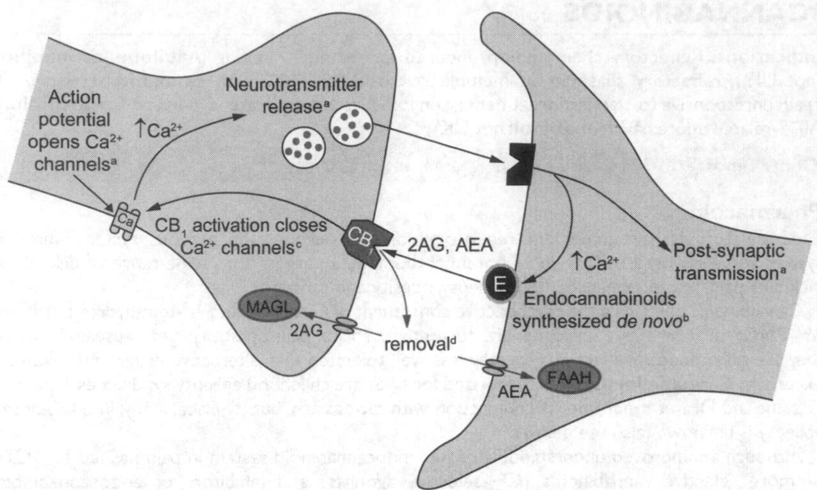

Figure 1 Cannabinoids and neurotransmission. Endocannabinoids are retrograde neurotransmitters, travelling from the postsynaptic to the presynaptic neurone as part of a negative-feedback loop that regulates neurotransmitter release.[1,13]

a. arriving action potential opens voltage-gated calcium channels; increasing *presynaptic* intracellular calcium triggers the release of stored neurotransmitter. Postsynaptic events depend on the neurotransmitter but include an increase in intracellular calcium

b. increasing *postsynaptic* intracellular calcium triggers the *de novo* synthesis of the endocannabinoids anandamide (AEA) and 2-acylglycerol (2AG), which cross back across the synapse

c. activation of CB_1 closes *presynaptic* calcium channels, preventing further calcium influx and thereby terminating neurotransmitter release. These channels are also targeted by other drugs of analgesic relevance, e.g. gabapentin, pregabalin, ziconotide

d. removal of endocannabinoids is by re-uptake pumps and degradation by the enzymes fatty acid amide hydrolase-1 (FAAH-1) and monoacylglycerol lipase (MAGL).

Pain

Pro-inflammatory signalling between neurones and surrounding glial cells is central to the pathophysiology of neuropathic pain (also see Adjuvant analgesics, p.325).[12] Although endocannabinoids can reduce such neurone–glial signalling, they also have pronociceptive effects. This, along with other undesirable effects, limits the efficacy of currently available cannabinoid analgesics.[9]

The antinociceptive effects of cannabinoids are mediated by both CB_1 and CB_2 activation at multiple sites including:[1,9,12]

- peripheral nerves (CB_1) and inflamed tissue (antigen-presenting cell CB_2)
- spinal cord microglia (CB_2) within the dorsal columns
- brainstem; CB_1 agonists, like μ-opioid agonists (see Strong opioids, p.389), disinhibit antinociceptive neurones of a descending pain-modulatory pathway (CB_1 on the pathway's GABAergic 'brake')
- thalamus; CB_1 inhibition of ascending nociceptive pathways
- limbic system and cerebral cortex; CB_1 altering affective and cognitive processing.

Cannabinoids have pronociceptive actions at other sites (e.g. CB_1 on antinociceptive neurones) and receptors (e.g. pronociceptive and pro-inflammatory actions at TRPV1 and GPR55, respectively).[9]

Nausea and vomiting

In the laboratory, cannabinoids acting on CB_1 receptors in the interoceptive insular cortex reduce both acute and anticipatory nausea.[2,15] However, current cannabinoid anti-emetics are less well tolerated and more expensive than alternatives.[16]

Appetite and energy metabolism

The endocannabinoid system modulates appetite and energy metabolism. Activation of hypothalamic and limbic CB_1 receptors increases appetite. Activation of CB_1 and CB_2 receptors on adipocytes, skeletal muscle cells and hepatocytes promotes fat deposition and insulin resistance.[3,17]

Rimonabant, a CB_1 inverse agonist (i.e. results in a *reduction* in basal activity of the receptor), was approved for appetite suppression in obesity. However, it also caused depression, anxiety and aggression, and has been withdrawn. CB_1 antagonists that do not cross the blood–brain barrier are being developed.[18]

Dronabinol (not UK) is authorized in some countries for AIDS-related anorexia. However, its effect, if any, on performance status is unclear.[19] In cancer-related anorexia, cannabinoids are inferior to **megestrol acetate** (see Progestogens, p.599) and no more effective than placebo.[20-22] Although a small RCT in advanced cancer (n=46) suggested improvement in taste disturbance with **dronabinol**, there were serious methodological limitations.[23]

Cardiorespiratory regulation

Animal studies suggest that central and peripheral CB_1 receptors impact on the cardiorespiratory system. In the brainstem, CB_1 stimulation elicits respiratory depression, bradycardia and hypertension.[24] In the lung and peripheral vasculature, effects are variable.[25,26]

Currently available exogenous cannabinoids

Δ^9-THC analogues

Δ^9-**THC** is a CB_1 and CB_2 partial agonist. Its effects include muscle relaxation, analgesia and anti-emesis, but it can also cause sedation, anxiety and psychosis. **Dronabinol** (not UK) is a synthetic preparation of its (-)-*trans* isomer, the best studied of several isomers present in *Cannabis sativa*; **nabilone** is a synthetic analogue.

Cannabidiol (CBD)

Cannabidiol is a negative allosteric CB_1 modulator[27] and a FAAH inhibitor (the enzyme that degrades anandamide; see Figure 1).[28] It is also a $5HT_{1A}$ partial agonist (see Antidepressants, p.210), an adenosine re-uptake inhibitor (see Psychostimulants, p.246) and a PPARγ agonist (a nuclear receptor with anti-inflammatory effects).[28]

A **cannabidiol** medicinal product (Epidyolex®) is authorized for two rare childhood epilepsy syndromes (Lennox–Gestault and Dravet), although the RCTs used to obtain these marketing authorizations have been strongly criticized (see Drug interactions, below). It is important to note that their mechanism and response to treatment differ significantly from other forms of epilepsy. Beyond these specific syndromes, cannabinoids do not have an established role in epilepsy.

Despite claims in the wider media, benefit for anxiety, depression, post-traumatic stress disorder and cancer cell growth has *not* been confirmed in RCTs.[4,19,29] Trials examining cannabinoids for *symptom relief* generally use Δ^9-**THC** or a synthetic analogue, ± **cannabidiol**, and *not* **cannabidiol** *alone*. Further, a national registry of cannabinoid use found patient self-reported improvements in pain, insomnia and depressive symptoms were associated with the use of preparations containing higher ratios of Δ^9-THC:CBD.[30]

Products containing **cannabidiol** are legally sold in the UK as food supplements provided there are no health claims (which would then automatically classify them as medicinal products).[31] They are available as oils or as food products containing **cannabidiol**, e.g. chocolate, coffee syrups. Topical products, e.g. oils, sprays and creams, are also available. These products are unregulated, thus there is no standard for quality, safety or the amount of **cannabidiol** that they contain. Such unregulated products may also unknowingly retain traces of Δ^9-**THC**, subjecting them to Schedule 1 controlled drug legislation, which does not permit prescribing, supply or administration.[32]

Δ^9-THC–cannabidiol combinations

The effects of Δ^9-**THC** are modified by other cannabinoids present in *Cannabis sativa*. For example, **cannabidiol** reduces Δ^9-**THC**-induced anxiety in healthy volunteers. In an attempt to improve the efficacy/tolerability profile of Δ^9-**THC**, a combined formulation of Δ^9-**THC** with **cannabidiol** (Sativex®, also known as **nabiximols**) has been developed; each oromucosal spray contains Δ^9-**THC** 2.7mg and **cannabidiol** 2.5mg. It is authorized for refractory spasticity in multiple sclerosis and, in some countries, for pain (e.g. Canada, but not UK). However, results of RCTs in patients with pain comparing Δ^9-**THC** and **cannabidiol**, in combination, with Δ^9-**THC** alone have been mixed: two RCTs found modest improvements in tolerability and patient preference,[33,34] one found modest improvements in efficacy but not tolerability,[35] and one found no difference.[36]

Other cannabis-based medicinal products

Currently the only other cannabis-based medicinal products are unauthorized. They are classified as Schedule 2 controlled drugs, are subject to additional prescribing restrictions and require special manufacture or importation (see Chapter 24, p.817).[7] There is no clear justification for using such products in palliative care in preference to the *authorized* cannabis-based medicinal products, **Sativex®**, **nabilone** and **cannabidiol**.

The pharmacokinetic profiles of selected cannabinoids are summarized in Table 1. Food increases the absorption of **cannabidiol** and Sativex®, suggesting a proportion of the latter is swallowed before absorption. There is a high degree of variability in the pharmacokinetics of Sativex® within and between patients following single and repeat doses.

Table 1 Pharmacokinetic profiles of selected cannabinoids[37,38]

	Oral bio-availability (%)	*Time to peak plasma concentration (h)*	*Halflife (h)*	*Metabolism*
Cannabidiol (CBD)	Not known	1–5	55–60	Multiple pathways[a, b]
Nabilone	85	1–4	2 5–10[a]	Multiple pathways[a, b]
Tetrahydrocannabinol (Δ^9-THC)	≥50	1–4	2–5	CYP2C9[c]

a. has active metabolite(s)

b. eliminated by both biliary and renal pathways

c. affected by combined use: cannabidiol reduces Δ^9-THC-induced anxiety in healthy volunteers, perhaps by inhibiting the metabolism of Δ^9-THC to a more psychoactive metabolite, 11-hydroxyTHC.

Cautions

Psychiatric history (mood, cognitive and behavioural changes can occur); severe ischaemic heart disease, heart failure or arrhythmias (risk of postural hypotension or reflex tachycardia); renal or hepatic impairment (no data, but active hepatic metabolites undergo biliary and renal clearance; also see Chapter 17, p.731 and Chapter 18, p.753); epilepsy (cannabinoids can either lower or raise seizure threshold).

Cannabidiol: elevated transaminase and bilirubin levels (>3 and 2 times the upper limit of normal respectively); see SPC for details. Dose adjustment is needed for **cannabidiol** in moderate–severe hepatic impairment.

Drug interactions

Additive CNS-depressant effects with other psychotropics.

The metabolism of Sativex® is marginally inhibited by CYP3A4 inhibitors (e.g. **clarithromycin**, **ritonavir**) and may be induced by CYP3A4 inducers (e.g. **carbamazepine**, **rifampicin**).

Cannabinoids inhibit numerous CYP450 enzymes, although generally not at typical therapeutic concentrations. Caution is advised when substrates for CYP2C19, 2D6 (e.g. **amitriptyline**) and 3A4 (e.g. **alfentanil**, **fentanyl**, **sufentanil**) are used concurrently with Sativex®.

The fivefold increase in levels of the active metabolites of **clobazam** resulting from inhibition of CYP2C19 and 3A4 by **cannabidiol** has been suggested as an alternative explanation for the apparent anti-epileptic effect of the latter; ≤2/3 of participants in the RCTs used to obtain the marketing authorization for **cannabidiol** were also taking **clobazam**.[39]

4

Undesirable effects

Box A Undesirable effects of cannabinoids[a]

Psychological[b]
Common (<10%, >1%): depression, euphoria, disorientation, dissociation
Uncommon (<1%, >0.1%): hallucinations, paranoia, delusions, suicidal ideation

Neurological[c]
Very common (>10%): dizziness (Sativex®, particularly during titration)
Common: ataxia, amnesia, drowsiness, blurred vision

Gastro-intestinal
Common: appetite (↑ or ↓), nausea
Uncommon: abdominal pain, hyperemesis (see text below)
Variable frequency: altered LFTs (see text below)

Cardiovascular
Uncommon: palpitations, tachycardia, syncope, hyper/hypotension

Buccal irritation[d] (Sativex® only)
Common: ulceration, pain
Uncommon: discolouration

a. frequencies relate to Sativex®. Other cannabinoids have similar undesirable effects, although frequencies will differ; see individual SPCs
b. illicit use is a risk factor for schizophrenia[40]
c. tolerance to CNS-depressant effects generally develops after a few days
d. Sativex® contains 50% v/v ethanol and propylene glycol. Two reports of suspected leukoplakia occurred in RCTs.

Cannabinoid hyperemesis

Delayed-onset nausea and vomiting are described with illicit use of *Cannabis sativa*. Symptoms are generally worst in the morning (70%), associated with abdominal colic (85%), often relieved by hot baths, and resolve when the cannabinoid is discontinued. Although most patients have used cannabis weekly for at least 2 years before symptom onset, a third have symptoms within 1 year.[41] In a patient using cannabinoids for spasticity, hyperemesis resolved within 3 weeks of reducing the dose.[42]

Cannabidiol and altered LFTs

In RCTs examining **cannabidiol** for Lennox–Gastaut and Dravet syndrome, 30% of participants had dose-related elevations of ALT and/or AST. The median age was 15 years. Most (90%) were taking **valproate** concomitantly (see SPC). In RCTs examining Sativex® for cancer pain, deranged LFTs were uncommon (1–3% compared with 0–2% with placebo),[35,43] or too infrequent to be reported.[44,45]

Use of cannabinoids in palliative care

Food increases the absorption of Sativex®, resulting in both an increased C_{max} (2–3 times) and AUC (3–5 times). Consistent timing of administration with regard to mealtimes may be important in some patients.

The spray should only be directed beneath the tongue or inside the cheeks. The site of application should be varied and the buccal mucosa inspected regularly for signs of irritation caused by the excipients (ethanol (50% v/v), propylene glycol). Additional information for health professionals is available from the palliativedrugs.com Document library.

Δ^9-**THC** is included in the law in England and Wales relating to driving with certain drugs above specified plasma concentrations (see Chapter 22, p.809).

Chemotherapy-induced nausea and vomiting (nabilone)

Although cannabinoids are moderately beneficial for chemotherapy-related nausea and vomiting,[19] $5HT_3$ antagonists are more effective and better tolerated and should generally be used instead.[16] NICE recommends that **nabilone** is reserved for chemotherapy-induced nausea and vomiting refractory to usual measures.[7] The manufacturer advises against the use of **nabilone** for non-chemotherapy related nausea.

Nabilone should be given the night before, during and for 2 days after each chemotherapy treatment (see SPC):

- start with 1mg PO b.d.
- if necessary, increase to 2mg b.d.
- maximum recommended dose 2mg t.d.s.

Dronabinol (not UK) is authorized in the USA for this indication for patients who have failed to respond to conventional anti-emetics.

Refractory spasticity in multiple sclerosis (Sativex®)

The place, if any, of cannabinoids is uncertain. A meta-analysis found statistically significant benefit of uncertain clinical significance.[19] NICE recommends that it is reserved for spasticity refractory to usual measures.[7]

- start with 1 oromucosal spray at bedtime
- increase over 2 weeks to a maximum of 12 sprays/24h given in divided doses, e.g. 1–2 sprays b.d.–3 sprays q.d.s.
- treatment should be stopped if benefit is not seen after 4 weeks.

†Refractory pain (Sativex®, nabilone)

For chronic non-cancer pain, systematic reviews and meta-analyses reveal statistically significant benefit of uncertain clinical significance.[19,46-48] Most trials were short (<6 weeks), but open-label extension studies found that analgesia was maintained without dose escalation for up to 1.5 years.[49-51] NICE recommends that cannabinoids should *not* be used for chronic non-cancer pain.[7]

For cancer pain, five RCTs examining Sativex® found mixed results. In three RCTs, Sativex® was titrated to optimal effect over 2 weeks. One found it was more effective than placebo or **Δ⁹-THC** alone (NNT 4.5 for 30% pain reduction).[35] The other two found no difference in pain reduction, although participants' global impression of change was greater with Sativex® (NNT 16 for much or very much improved).[44,45,52] Withdrawal due to undesirable effects was higher with Sativex® than placebo (15–20% vs. 5–18%).[35,44,45] A fourth study randomized participants to three fixed dose ranges; although low (1–4 sprays/day) and moderate (6–10 sprays/day) doses of Sativex® were more effective than placebo, high doses (11–16 sprays/day) were not.[43] A meta-analysis of the above four RCTs found no clinically meaningful reduction in overall pain or need for break-through analgesia.[52] An enriched enrolment study found no difference between Sativex® and placebo.[45] NICE concluded that the place, if any, of cannabinoids for intractable cancer pain was uncertain.[7]

For chemotherapy-related neuropathic pain, a small cross-over study found Sativex® no better than placebo.[53]

Sativex® (adapted from the Canadian Product Monograph):

- start with 1 oromucosal spray b.d.
- titrate up on a daily basis (but more slowly if dizziness occurs)
- most patients require ≤12 sprays/24h (median dose = 5–8 sprays/24h).

Nabilone:

- start with 250–500microgram PO b.d.
- titrate in 500microgram increments on a weekly basis
- maximum dose 1mg b.d.[54]

Supply

Nabilone (generic) is a Schedule 2 **CD**.

Capsules 250microgram, 20 = £150.

Capsules 1mg, 20 = £196.

Δ⁹-THC–cannabidiol combination

Sativex® (Bayer) is a Schedule 4 (part 1) **CD**.

Oromucosal spray *Cannabis sativa* extract (**dronabinol**) 27mg and **cannabidiol** 25mg/mL each spray = 0.1mL, pack of 3 x 10mL (approx. 90 sprays/bottle) = £375; *the unopened pack should be stored in a refrigerator. Once opened, store at room temperature and use within 6 weeks.*

Cannabidiol
Epidyolex® (GW Pharma)
Oral solution Cannabidiol 100mg/mL; price unavailable at time of print. *Contains ethanol 8%.*

4

Records must be kept for 2 years for cannabis-based medicines (1961 UN Convention on Narcotic Drugs); this includes the quantities possessed or destroyed by those authorized to do so (patients and their representatives are exempt). The Home Office strongly recommends using a standard **CD** register for this.

1 Huang WJ *et al.* (2016) Endocannabinoid system: role in depression, reward and pain control (Review). *Molecular Medicine Reports*. **14**: 2899–2903.
2 Sticht MA *et al.* (2016) Endocannabinoid regulation of nausea is mediated by 2-arachidonoylglycerol (2-AG) in the rat visceral insular cortex. *Neuropharmacology*. **102**: 92–102.
3 Lau BK *et al.* (2017) Endocannabinoid modulation of homeostatic and non-homeostatic feeding circuits. *Neuropharmacology*. **124**: 38–51.
4 Fowler CJ (2015) Delta(9) -tetrahydrocannabinol and cannabidiol as potential curative agents for cancer: a critical examination of the preclinical literature. *Clinical Pharmacology & Therapeutics*. **97**: 587–596.
5 Mounessa JS *et al.* (2017) The role of cannabinoids in dermatology. *Journal of the American Academy of Dermatology*. **77**: 188–190.
6 Devinsky O *et al.* (2014) Cannabidiol: pharmacology and potential therapeutic role in epilepsy and other neuropsychiatric disorders. *Epilepsia*. **55**: 791–802.
7 NICE (2019) Cannabis-based medicinal products. *Clinical Guideline*. CG144. www.nice.org.uk.
8 Huggins JP *et al.* (2012) An efficient randomised, placebo-controlled clinical trial with the irreversible fatty acid amide hydrolase-1 inhibitor PF-04457845, which modulates endocannabinoids but fails to induce effective analgesia in patients with pain due to osteoarthritis of the knee. *Pain*. **153**: 1837–1846.
9 Woodhams SG *et al.* (2017) The cannabinoid system and pain. *Neuropharmacology*. **124**: 105–120.
10 Malek N and Starowicz K (2016) Dual-acting compounds targeting endocannabinoid and endovanilloid systems-a novel treatment option for chronic pain management. *Frontiers in Pharmacology*. **7**: 257.
11 Zhou J *et al.* (2016) CB2 and GPR55 receptors as therapeutic targets for systemic immune dysregulation. *Frontiers in Pharmacology*. **7**: 264.
12 Maldonado R *et al.* (2016) The endocannabinoid system and neuropathic pain. *Pain*. **157 (Suppl 1)**: S23–32.
13 Araque A *et al.* (2017) Synaptic functions of endocannabinoid signaling in health and disease. *Neuropharmacology*. **124**: 13–24.
14 Guerrero-Alba R *et al.* (2018) Some prospective alternatives for treating pain: The endocannabinoid system and its putative receptors GPR18 and GPR55. *Frontiers in Pharmacology*. **9**: 1496.
15 Parker LA *et al.* (2015) Cannabinoids suppress acute and anticipatory nausea in preclinical rat models of conditioned gaping. *Clinical Pharmacology & Therapeutics*. **97**: 559–561.
16 Tafelski S *et al.* (2016) Efficacy, tolerability, and safety of cannabinoids for chemotherapy-induced nausea and vomiting--a systematic review of systematic reviews. *Schmerz*. **30**: 14–24.
17 Rossi F *et al.* (2016) Cannabinoid receptor 2 as antiobesity target: Inflammation, fat storage, and browning modulation. *Journal of Clinical Endocrinology and Metabolism*. **101**: 3469–3478.
18 Tam J *et al.* (2018) The therapeutic potential of targeting the peripheral endocannabinoid/CB1 receptor system. *European Journal of Internal Medicine*. **49**: 23–29.
19 Whiting PF *et al.* (2015) Cannabinoids for medical use: A systematic review and meta-analysis. *JAMA*. **313**: 2456–2473.
20 Strasser F *et al.* (2006) Comparison of orally administered cannabis extract and delta-9-tetrahydrocannabinol in treating patients with cancer-related anorexia-cachexia syndrome: a multicenter, phase III, randomized, double-blind, placebo-controlled clinical trial from the Cannabis-In-Cachexia-Study-Group. *Journal of Clinical Oncology*. **24**: 3394–3400.
21 Jatoi A *et al.* (2002) Dronabinol versus megestrol acetate versus combination therapy for cancer-associated anorexia: a North Central Cancer Treatment Group study. *Journal of Clinical Oncology*. **20**: 567–573.
22 Mucke M *et al.* (2018) Systematic review and meta-analysis of cannabinoids in palliative medicine. *Journal of Cachexia, Sarcopenia and Muscle*. **9**: 220–234.
23 Brisbois TD *et al.* (2011) Delta-9-tetrahydrocannabinol may palliate altered chemosensory perception in cancer patients: results of a randomized, double-blind, placebo-controlled pilot trial. *Annals of Oncology*. **22**: 2086–2093.
24 Pfitzer T *et al.* (2004) Central effects of the cannabinoid receptor agonist WIN55212-2 on respiratory and cardiovascular regulation in anaesthetised rats. *British Journal of Pharmacology*. **142**: 943–952.
25 Calignano A *et al.* (2000) Bidirectional control of airway responsiveness by endogenous cannabinoids. *Nature*. **408**: 96–101.
26 Stanley C and O'Sullivan SE (2014) Vascular targets for cannabinoids: animal and human studies. *British Journal of Pharmacology*. **171**: 1361–1378.
27 Khurana L *et al.* (2017) Modulation of CB1 cannabinoid receptor by allosteric ligands: Pharmacology and therapeutic opportunities. *Neuropharmacology*. **124**: 3–12.
28 Campos AC *et al.* (2016) Cannabidiol, neuroprotection and neuropsychiatric disorders. *Pharmacological Research*. **112**: 119–127.
29 White CM (2019) A review of human studies assessing cannabidiol's (CBD) therapeutic actions and potential. *Journal of Clinical Pharmacology*. **59**: 923–934.
30 Casarett DJ *et al.* (2019) Benefit of tetrahydrocannabinol versus cannabidiol for common palliative care symptoms. *Journal of Palliative Medicine*. **22**: 1180–1184.
31 MHRA (2016) MHRA statement on products containing Cannabidiol (CBD). www.gov.uk

32 Home Office (2018) Drug Licensing Fact Sheet : Cannabis, CBD and other cannabinoids. www.gov.uk.
33 Wade DT *et al.* (2003) A preliminary controlled study to determine whether whole-plant cannabis extracts can improve intractable neurogenic symptoms. *Clinical Rehabilitation*. **17**: 21–29.
34 Notcutt W *et al.* (2004) Initial experiences with medicinal extracts of cannabis for chronic pain: results from 34 'N of 1' studies. *Anaesthesia*. **59**: 440–452.
35 Johnson JR *et al.* (2010) Multicenter, double-blind, randomized, placebo-controlled, parallel-group study of the efficacy, safety, and tolerability of THC:CBD extract and THC extract in patients with intractable cancer-related pain. *Journal of Pain and Symptom Management*. **39**: 167–179.
36 Berman JS *et al.* (2004) Efficacy of two cannabis based medicinal extracts for relief of central neuropathic pain from brachial plexus avulsion: results of a randomised controlled trial. *Pain*. **112**: 299–306.
37 Barnes MP (2006) Sativex: clinical efficacy and tolerability in the treatment of symptoms of multiple sclerosis and neuropathic pain. *Expert Opinion on Pharmacotherpy*. **7**: 607–615.
38 Grotenhermen F (2003) Pharmacokinetics and pharmacodynamics of cannabinoids. *Clinical Pharmacokinetics*. **42**: 327–360.
39 Groeneveld (2019) Parasitic pharmacology: a plausible mechanism of action for cannabidiol. *British journal of clinical pharmacology*. 1–3.
40 Crocker CE and Tibbo PG (2015) Cannabis and the maturing brain: role in psychosis development. *Clinical Pharmacology & Therapeutics*. **97**: 545–547.
41 Simonetto DA *et al.* (2012) Cannabinoid hyperemesis: a case series of 98 patients. *Mayo Clinic Proceedings*. **87**: 114–119.
42 Howard I (2019) Cannabis hyperemesis syndrome in palliative care: a case study and narrative review. *Journal of Palliative Medicine*. **22**: 1227–1231.
43 Portenoy RK *et al.* (2012) Nabiximols for opioid-treated cancer patients with poorly-controlled chronic pain: a randomized, placebo-controlled, graded-dose trial. *Journal of Pain*. **13**: 438–449.
44 Lichtman AH *et al.* (2018) Results of a double-blind, randomized, placebo-controlled study of nabiximols oromucosal spray as an adjunctive therapy in advanced cancer patients with chronic uncontrolled pain. *Journal of Pain and Symptom Management*. **55**: 179–188.
45 Fallon MT *et al.* (2017) Sativex oromucosal spray as adjunctive therapy in advanced cancer patients with chronic pain unalleviated by optimized opioid therapy: two double-blind, randomized, placebo-controlled phase 3 studies. *British Journal of Pain*. **11**: 119–133.
46 Aviram J and Samuelly-Leichtag G (2017) Efficacy of cannabis-based medicines for pain management: a systematic review and meta-analysis of randomized controlled trials. *Pain Physician*. **20**: E755–796.
47 Hauser W *et al.* (2017) Cannabinoids in pain management and palliative medicine. *Deutsches Arzteblatt International*. **114**: 627–634.
48 Stockings E *et al.* (2018) Cannabis and cannabinoids for the treatment of people with chronic noncancer pain conditions: a systematic review and meta-analysis of controlled and observational studies. *Pain*. **159**: 1932–1954.
49 Wade DT *et al.* (2006) Long-term use of a cannabis-based medicine in the treatment of spasticity and other symptoms in multiple sclerosis. *Multiple Sclerosis*. **12**: 639–645.
50 Nurmikko TJ *et al.* (2007) Sativex successfully treats neuropathic pain characterised by allodynia: a randomised, double-blind, placebo-controlled clinical trial. *Pain*. **133**: 210–220.
51 Johnson JR *et al.* (2013) An open-label extension study to investigate the long-term safety and tolerability of THC/CBD Oromucosal spray and Oromucosal THC spray in patients with terminal cancer-related pain refractory to strong opioid analgesics. *Journal of Pain and Symptom Management*. **46**: 207–218.
52 Hauser W *et al.* (2019) Efficacy, tolerability and safety of cannabis-based medicines for cancer pain : a systematic review with meta-analysis of randomised controlled trials. *Schmerz*. **33**: 424–436.
53 Lynch ME *et al.* (2014) A double-blind, placebo-controlled, crossover pilot trial with extension using an oral mucosal cannabinoid extract for treatment of chemotherapy-induced neuropathic pain. *Journal of Pain and Symptom Management*. **47**: 166–173.
54 CADTH (2011) Nabilone for chronic pain management: a review of clinical efectiveness, safety and guidelines. www.cadth.ca

Updated January 2020

ANTI-EMETICS

Indications: Authorized indications vary among products; consult SPC for details. Nausea and vomiting, †delayed gastric emptying, †hiccup, †pruritus, †diarrhoea associated with carcinoid syndrome.

Pharmacology

Anti-emetics are a functionally diverse group of drugs acting on one or more sites implicated in nausea and/or vomiting (Figure 1). Because there is little direct RCT evidence to guide drug selection in palliative care,[1-3] choice of anti-emetic is guided by the probable mechanism by which the drug acts (Table 1). This 'mechanistic approach' brings more rapid relief compared with an unselected approach[4] and is successful in most patients.[5,6] Other factors to consider include the response to anti-emetics already given and the undesirable effects, cost and available routes of alternatives (see individual monographs).

The model underlying this approach is extrapolated from experimental data, RCTs in postoperative and chemotherapy-related nausea and vomiting, and neuroimaging.[7-12] For example, while **droperidol** (a dopamine antagonist) reduces *nausea* more successfully than vomiting, $5HT_3$ antagonists are more effective for *vomiting*; thus, they might be expected to act in the effector pathways responsible for these respective symptoms (Figure 1).[7] Neuroimaging confirms that D_2 and $5HT_3$ receptors respectively, *are* present in these locations.

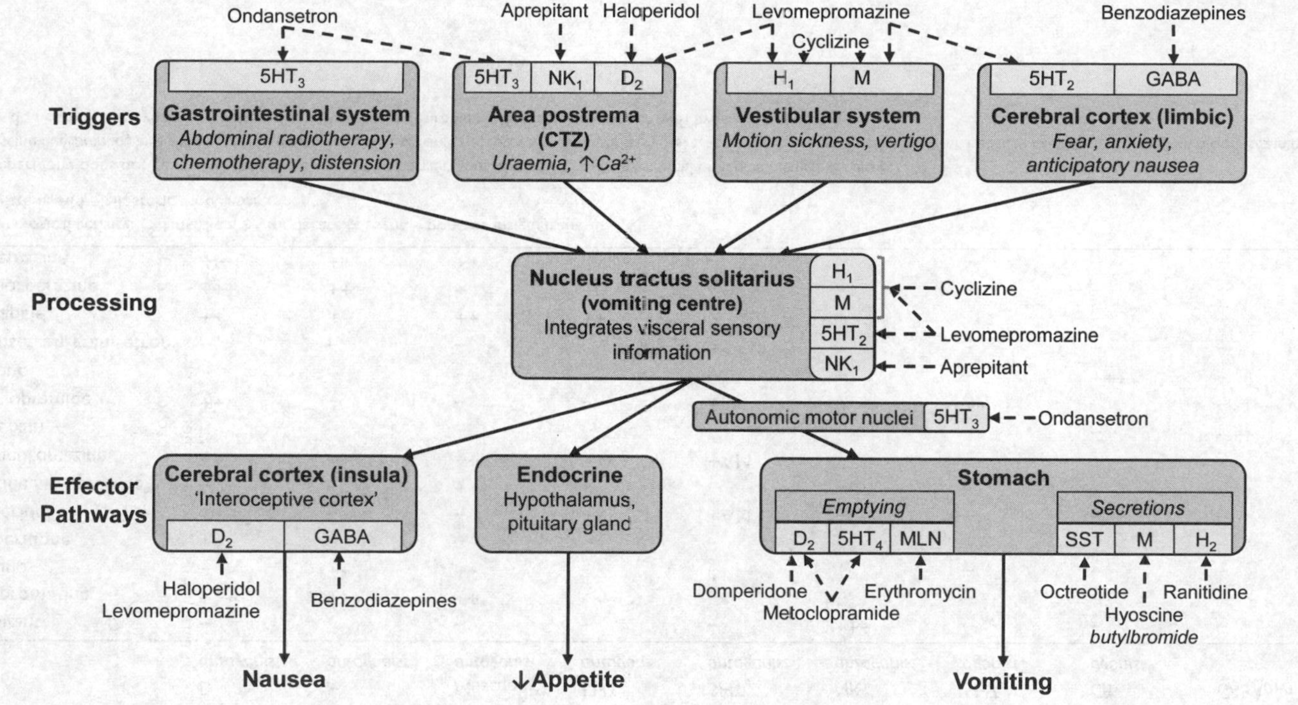

Figure 1 Putative peripheral and central sites of action of selected anti-emetics. Also see individual drug monographs.[7-12]

Abbreviations: Ca^{2+} = calcium, CTZ = chemoreceptor trigger zone. Other abbreviations refer to receptor types: D_2 = dopamine type 2; $5HT_2$, $5HT_3$ = 5-hydroxytriptamine (serotonin) type 2, type 3; H_1, H_2 = histamine type 1, type 2; M = muscarinic cholinergic; NK_1 = neurokinin 1. Note. Anti-emetics act as *antagonists* at these receptors, whereas the effects on $5HT_4$ (5-hydroxytriptamine type 4), MLN (motilin), SST (somatostatin) and GABA (gamma-aminobutyric acid) are *agonistic*.

Table 1 Receptor site affinities of selected anti-emetics[13-18]

	D_2 *antagonist*	H_1 *antagonist*	*Muscarinic antagonist*	$5HT_2$ *antagonist*	$5HT_3$ *antagonist*	NK_1 *antagonist*	$5HT_4$ *agonist*	CB_1 *agonist*	*GABAmimetic*
Aprepitant	–	–	–	–	–	+++	–	–	–
Chlorpromazine	+++	+++	++	++	–	–	–	–	–
Cyclizine	–	++	++	–	–	–	–	–	–
Domperidone	++[a]	–	–	–	–	–	–	–	–
Haloperidol	+++	–	–	–	+AM	–	–	–	–
Hyoscine *hydrobromide*[b]	–	–	+++	–	–	–	–	–	–
Levomepromazine	++	+++	++	+++	+AM	–	–	–	–
Lorazepam	–	–	–	–	–	–	–	–	+++
Metoclopramide	++	–	–	–	+	–	++	–	–
Nabilone	–	–	–	–	–	–	–	+++	–
Ondansetron, granisetron	–	–	–	–	+++	–	–	–	–
Olanzapine	++	+	++	++	+	–	–	–	–
Prochlorperazine	+++	++	+	+/++	–	–	–	–	–
Promethazine	+/++	++	++	–	–	–	–	–	–

Pharmacological activity: +++ marked, ++ moderate, + slight, – none or insignificant

Abbreviation: AM = allosteric modulator

a. domperidone does not generally cross the blood–brain barrier; thus, the risk of extrapyramidal effects is negligible (see p.271)

b. hyoscine *butylbromide* and glycopyrronium also act on muscarinic receptors in the periphery (GI tract antisecretory effect). However, because they do not cross the blood–brain barrier, they do not act in the vestibular system (or cause the undesirable CNS effects associated with hyoscine *hydrobromide*).

The model is also based on clinical experience. Thus, H_1 receptors were hypothesized to exist in the vestibular system, because H_1 antagonists appear effective for nausea related to vestibular irritation. Although neuroimaging is starting to corroborate these locations, there are knowledge gaps in the 'mechanistic approach'.

Cautions

For information on the use of anti-emetics in renal and hepatic impairment, see Chapter 17, p.737 and Chapter 18, p.767.

Use in palliative care

Nausea and vomiting

Also see QCG: Nausea and vomiting (p.264) and QCG: Inoperable bowel obstruction (p.266).

First-line anti-emetics

Generally, in palliative care, the initial choice depends upon the cause:

- for vestibular irritation or raised intracranial pressure use an anti-emetic acting principally in the vestibular system and vomiting centre, e.g. **cyclizine** (p.273)
- for most chemical causes of vomiting, e.g. **morphine**, hypercalcaemia, renal impairment use an anti-emetic acting principally in chemoreceptor trigger zone, e.g. **haloperidol** (p.198)
- for gastritis, gastric stasis or functional bowel obstruction (peristaltic failure) use a prokinetic, e.g. **domperidone** (p.271), **metoclopramide** (p.268).

Drug-induced nausea and vomiting can be caused by several different mechanisms (Table 2), each of which requires a distinct therapeutic response.

Table 2 Causes of drug-induced nausea and vomiting

Mechanism	*Drugs*
Gastric irritation	Antibacterials Corticosteroids Iron supplements Misoprostol NSAIDs Spironolactone Tranexamic acid
Gastric stasis	Antimuscarinics (e.g. TCAs) Opioids
Area postrema stimulation (chemoreceptor trigger zone)	Antibacterials Cytotoxics Digoxin Imidazoles Opioids
$5HT_3$-receptor stimulation	Antibacterials Cytotoxics SSRIs

Second-line anti-emetics

If symptoms persist, consider an alternative first-line anti-emetic or switch to a broader spectrum drug, e.g. **levomepromazine** (p.201), **olanzapine** (p.203); these have affinity at many receptors and may be as effective as, and easier for patients to handle than, two or more different anti-emetics simultaneously.

Third-line anti-emetics

If **levomepromazine** or **olanzapine** alone fail to relieve nausea and vomiting, they can be *combined* with an anti-emetic with different receptor affinities, typically a $5HT_3$ antagonist (p.277).

Alternatives include **dexamethasone** (see Systemic corticosteroids, p.556) and benzodiazepines (p.163). Although a specific role for benzodiazepines in *anticipatory* nausea has been proposed, there is limited evidence to support this over and above their general anti-emetic effect (see p.173).

Although **aprepitant**, a neurokinin 1 (NK_1) antagonist, and **nabilone** (p.251), a cannabinoid, also act at distinct sites, their place, if any, in the palliative care setting is unclear. Both are expensive. Further, **aprepitant** is a CYP3A4 inhibitor (see Chapter 19, Table 8, p.790). A parenteral pro-drug, **fosaprepitant**, is available for IV use.

†Hiccup and delayed gastric emptying

In palliative care, prokinetics (p.22) are used for hiccup, early satiety and other symptoms of delayed gastric emptying. First-line options include **domperidone** (p.271) and **metoclopramide** (p.268). Alternatives include **clonidine** (p.82) and **erythromycin** (p.22). All are unauthorized and have important safety considerations (see individual monographs).

†Carcinoid-related diarrhoea

Ondansetron is reported to be beneficial for diarrhoea refractory to **octreotide** (see p.277).

†Pruritus

Ondansetron relieves pruritus related to spinal **morphine**, but not cholestatic or uraemic pruritus (see $5HT_3$ antagonists, p.277; also see Chapter 26, p.825).

Aprepitant is reported to improve pruritus due to mycosis fungoides,[19] chemotherapy (mainly **cetuximab** or **erlotinib**)[20] and immunotherapy-related Stevens–Johnson syndrome,[21] and chronic pruritus of mixed cause (including uraemic, diabetic and idiopathic pruritus).[22] Most reports used 80mg once daily and benefit was often seen in ≤2 days. Although **aprepitant** is also reported to be of benefit in Sezary syndrome,[23] an RCT (n=5) found pruritus *increased*.[24] **Aprepitant** is expensive and a CYP3A4 inhibitor.

Pain

In an RCT of postoperative nausea and vomiting, a reduction in analgesic requirements was noted in those receiving **aprepitant**.[25] **Fosaprepitant** is reported to improve painful paraneoplastic dermatomyositis.[26] A potential analgesic effect of $5HT_3$ antagonists has also been investigated, with conflicting results (see p.277). Thus, the place, if any, of NK_1 and $5HT_3$ antagonists in analgesia is uncertain.

1 Davis MP *et al.* (2010) A systematic review of the treatment of nausea and/or vomiting in cancer unrelated to chemotherapy or radiation. *Journal of Pain and Symptom Management.* **39**: 756–767.

2 Glare P *et al.* (2011) Treating nausea and vomiting in palliative care: a review. *Clinical Interventions in Aging.* **6**: 243–259.

3 Glare P *et al.* (2004) Systematic review of the efficacy of antiemetics in the treatment of nausea in patients with far-advanced cancer. *Supportive Care in Cancer.* **12**: 432–440.

4 Hardy J *et al.* (2018) A randomized open-label study of guideline-driven antiemetic therapy versus single agent antiemetic therapy in patients with advanced cancer and nausea not related to anticancer treatment. *BMC Cancer.* **18**: 510.

5 Bentley A and Boyd K (2001) Use of clinical pictures in the management of nausea and vomiting: a prospective audit. *Palliative Medicine.* **15**: 247–253.

6 Stephenson J and Davies A (2006) An assessment of aetiology-based guidelines for the management of nausea and vomiting in patients with advanced cancer. *Supportive Care in Cancer.* **14**: 348–353.

7 Stern RM (2011) Section II: Physiology of Nausea. In: *Nausea mechanisms and management.* Oxford University Press, USA, 39–167.

8 Santana TA *et al.* (2015) Meta-analysis of adjunctive non-NK1 receptor antagonist medications for the control of acute and delayed chemotherapy-induced nausea and vomiting. *Supportive Care in Cancer.* **23**: 213–222.

9 Saulin A *et al.* (2012) Serotonin and molecular neuroimaging in humans using PET. *Amino Acids.* **42**: 2039–2057.

10 Farmer AD *et al.* (2015) Visually induced nausea causes characteristic changes in cerebral, autonomic and endocrine function in humans. *Journal of Physiology.* **593**: 1183–1196.

11 Napadow V *et al.* (2013) The brain circuitry underlying the temporal evolution of nausea in humans. *Cerebral Cortex.* **23**: 806–813.

12 Becker DE (2010) Nausea, vomiting, and hiccups: a review of mechanisms and treatment. *Anesthesia Progress.* **57**: 150–156.

13 Peroutka SJ and Snyder SH (1982) Antiemetics: neurotransmitter receptor binding predicts therapeutic actions. *Lancet.* **1**: 658–659.

14 Fleming M and Hawkins C (2005) Use of atypical antipsychotic olanzapine as an anti-emetic. *European Journal of Palliative Care.* **12**: 144–146.

15 Saito R *et al.* (2003) Roles of substance P and NK(1) receptor in the brainstem in the development of emesis. *Journal of Pharmacology Science.* **91**: 87–94.

16 Aapro MS *et al.* (2005) Anticipatory nausea and vomiting. *Supportive Care in Cancer.* **13**: 117–121.

17 Davis M *et al.* (2007) The emerging role of cannabinoid neuromodulators in symptom management. *Supportive Care in Cancer.* **15**: 63–71.

18 Rammes G *et al.* (2004) Antipsychotic drugs antagonize human serotonin type 3 receptor currents in a noncompetitive manner. *Molecular Psychiatry.* **9**: 846–858.

19 Jimenez Gallo D *et al.* (2014) Treatment of pruritus in early-stage hypopigmented mycosis fungoides with aprepitant. *Dermatologic Therapy*. **27**: 178–182.
20 Santini D *et al.* (2012) Aprepitant for management of severe pruritus related to biological cancer treatments: a pilot study. *Lancet Oncology*. **13**: 1020–1024.
21 Ito J *et al.* (2017) Aprepitant for refractory nivolumab-induced pruritus. *Lung Cancer*. **109**: 58–61.
22 Pojawa-Golab M *et al.* (2019) NK-1 receptor antagonists and pruritus: review of current literature. *Dermatology and Therapy*. **9**: 391–405.
23 Torres T *et al.* (2012) Aprepitant: evidence of its effectiveness in patients with refractory pruritus continues. *Journal of the American Academy of Dermatology*. **66**: e14–15.
24 Zic JA *et al.* (2018) Aprepitant for the treatment of pruritus in Sézary syndrome: a randomized crossover clinical trial. *JAMA Dermatology*. **154**: 1221–1222.
25 Kakuta N *et al.* (2011) Neurokinin-1 receptor antagonism, aprepitant, effectively diminishes post-operative nausea and vomiting while increasing analgesic tolerance in laparoscopic gynecological procedures. *Journal of Medical Investigation*. **58**: 246–251.
26 Dulin JD *et al.* (2017) Fosaprepitant for the management of refractory pain in a patient with cancer-related dermatomyositis. *Journal of Palliative Medicine*. **20**: 1415–1419.

Updated November 2019

Quick Clinical Guide: Nausea and vomiting

1 From the patient's history and physical examination, decide what is the most likely cause (or causes) of the nausea and vomiting. Take a blood sample if biochemical derangement is suspected. For bowel obstruction, see QCG: Inoperable bowel obstruction (p.266).

2 Correct correctable causes/exacerbating factors, e.g. drugs, severe pain, cough, infection, hypercalcaemia. *(Remember: antibacterial treatment and correction of hypercalcaemia are not always appropriate in a dying patient.)*

3 Prescribe the most appropriate anti-emetic regularly and p.r.n.

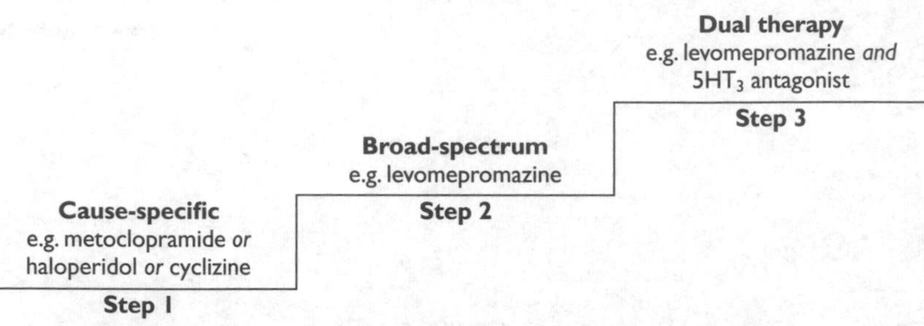

Commonly used Step 1 (cause-specific) anti-emetics

For gastritis, gastric stasis, functional bowel obstruction (peristaltic failure)

Prokinetic anti-emetic:

- metoclopramide
  - ▷ PO: 10mg t.d.s.–q.d.s. and 10mg q2h p.r.n.
  - ▷ CSCI: 30–40mg/24h and 10mg SC q2h p.r.n.
  - ▷ PO/CSCI: usual maximum 100mg/24h
- domperidone
  - ▷ PO: 10mg b.d.–t.d.s.

For most chemical causes of vomiting, e.g. morphine, hypercalcaemia, renal failure

Anti-emetic acting principally in chemoreceptor trigger zone:

- haloperidol
  - ▷ PO/SC: 500microgram–1.5mg at bedtime and q2h p.r.n.
  - ▷ CSCI: 500microgram–1.5mg/24h and 1mg SC q2h p.r.n.
  - ▷ PO/SC/CSCI: usual maximum 10mg/24h.

Metoclopramide also has a central action.

For raised intracranial pressure (in conjunction with dexamethasone) and/or vestibular symptoms

Anti-emetic acting principally in the vestibular system and vomiting centre:

- cyclizine
  - ▷ PO: 50mg b.d.–t.d.s. and 50mg p.r.n.
  - ▷ CSCI: 75–150mg/24h and 25–50mg SC p.r.n.
  - ▷ PO/CSCI: usual maximum 200mg/24h.

If a dominant cause is not apparent, metoclopramide or haloperidol are reasonable Step 1 treatment options.

4 Give by SC injection or CSCI if continuous nausea or frequent vomiting.

5 Start with a stat p.r.n. dose to cover the period before the first regular dose or the delay in reaching therapeutic levels by CSCI.

6 Initially, review anti-emetic dose each day; take note of p.r.n. use and adjust the regular dose accordingly.

7 If little benefit despite upward titration of the dose, reconsider the likely cause(s) and review the choice of anti-emetic and route of administration. Sometimes it is necessary to convert to a broad-spectrum anti-emetic, and occasionally dual therapy will be needed.

Commonly used Step 2 and 3 anti-emetics
Step 2: Broad-spectrum • levomepromazine ▷ PO/SC: 6–6.25mg at bedtime and q2h p.r.n. ▷ usual maximum 25mg/24h ▷ at home, consider CSCI if a bedtime SC injection is impractical. **Step 3: Dual-therapy (combining anti-emetics with different mechanisms)** • levomepromazine + a $5HT_3$ antagonist, e.g. granisetron 1–2mg SC once daily or CSCI, or ondansetron 16mg/24h CSCI • levomepromazine + a benzodiazepine, e.g. lorazepam 0.5–1mg SL b.d. or midazolam 10mg/24h CSCI, *particularly when anxiety or anticipatory nausea* • levomepromazine + dexamethasone 6.6mg SC or 8mg PO stat and thereafter once or twice daily *when all else fails*; stop dexamethasone if no benefit after 1 week; otherwise taper weekly by 1.65–3.3mg SC or 2–4mg PO to the minimum effective dose.

8 Prokinetics act through a cholinergic system which is competitively antagonized by antimuscarinics; concurrent use is best avoided.

9 Seizures occasionally present as nausea (e.g. with meningeal carcinomatosis); this responds to anti-epileptic drugs or benzodiazepines.

10 Continue the anti-emetic(s) unless the cause is self-limiting. Except in mechanical bowel obstruction (see QCG: Inoperable bowel obstruction, p.266), consider changing to PO after 3 days of good control with CSCI.

11 With successful dual therapy, it may be possible to simplify the regimen after 1–2 weeks by tapering the dose of one of the two anti-emetics.

Updated (minor change) February 2021

Quick Clinical Guide: Inoperable bowel obstruction

Initial management

1 Resting the GI tract for several days may allow an obstruction to settle spontaneously:
- restrict PO intake to sips of fluid to keep the mouth comfortable, and hydrate IV/SC, e.g. 10–20mL/kg/24h
- a nasogastric (NG) tube can be reserved for patients experiencing large-volume vomits more than 2–3 times/24h
- correct electrolyte imbalances that may contribute to peristaltic failure, e.g. low potassium, low magnesium
- a combination of analgesics (opioids and antispasmodics), anti-emetics and antisecretory drugs should be used to manage abdominal pain, colic, and nausea and vomiting (see below)
- some centres add dexamethasone, e.g. 6.6mg SC once daily for 5–7 days (evidence suggests only a trend towards benefit) with antacid cover (e.g. omeprazole 40mg by IV/SC infusion once daily).

Ongoing management (≥1 week)

2 If the obstruction does not settle with the above measures, the aim (*although not always achieved*) is to:
- control pain and nausea *and*
- minimize vomiting so as to avoid the need for an NG tube *and*
- permit sufficient oral fluids to maintain hydration.

Symptom management

3 For constant background cancer pain, morphine should be given regularly by the clock and p.r.n. For those with colic, an antispasmodic antisecretory anti-emetic should be given (see below).

4 Drugs for inoperable bowel obstruction are best given by CSCI (for more information on anti-emetic doses, see QCG: Nausea and vomiting), but some, e.g. dexamethasone, levomepromazine, can be given as a single SC daily dose.

5 The ladder shows a general approach; dose titration over several days may be necessary before optimum relief is achieved:
- start on Step 1 if *no* colic: probable functional obstruction (i.e. peristaltic failure):
  - ▷ metoclopramide 30–40mg/24h CSCI and 10mg SC q2h p.r.n.
  - ▷ if beneficial, optimize the dose up to 100mg/24h
- start on Step 2 if colic: probable mechanical obstruction:
  - ▷ hyoscine *butylbromide* 60–120mg/24h CSCI and 20mg SC q1h p.r.n.
  - ▷ maximum reported dose 300mg/24h.

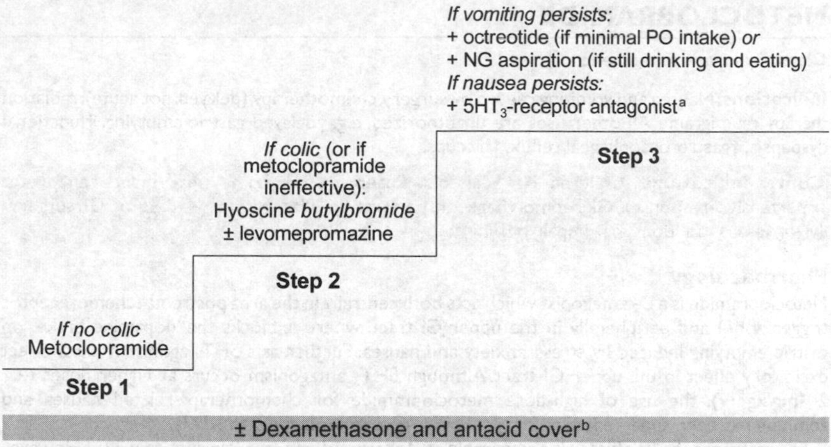

If vomiting persists:
+ octreotide (if minimal PO intake) *or*
+ NG aspiration (if still drinking and eating)
If nausea persists:
+ $5HT_3$-receptor antagonist[a]

Step 3

If colic (or if metoclopramide ineffective):
Hyoscine *butylbromide*
± levomepromazine

Step 2

If no colic
Metoclopramide

Step 1

± Dexamethasone and antacid cover[b]

a. e.g. granisetron 1–2mg SC once daily, ondansetron 16mg/24h CSCI
b. see point 1 above.

6 Instead of levomepromazine 6.25–25mg/24h CSCI, some centres use:
- cyclizine 75–150mg/24h CSCI and 25–50mg SC p.r.n. (maximum 200mg/24h) *or*
- haloperidol 500micrograms–1.5mg/24h CSCI and 1mg SC q2h p.r.n. (maximum 10mg/24h) *or*
- cyclizine *and* haloperidol, if levomepromazine is too sedative.

Note. Cyclizine mixed with hyoscine *butylbromide* may be incompatible.

7 If heartburn/acid reflux occurs, start/continue a PPI (see point 1).

8 If hyoscine *butylbromide* is inadequate to control vomiting, or to obtain more rapid relief, consider octreotide (a somatostatin analogue and antisecretory agent):
- if colic, add to hyoscine *butylbromide*
- if no colic, substitute or use instead of hyoscine *butylbromide:*
  - ▷ octreotide 100microgram SC stat
  - ▷ CSCI 500microgram/24h
  - ▷ usual maximum 750microgram/24h, occasionally higher.

9 If vomiting persists, review the patient's oral intake. Antisecretory drugs cannot fully alleviate the vomiting of ingested fluid and food; consider NG tube or venting gastrostomy.

10 In partial obstruction, there may be passage of flatus and faeces. When a laxative is required, use a stool softener that does not distend the bowel, e.g. docusate sodium 100–200mg PO b.d.

Nutrition

11 Some patients and carers are concerned about a restricted oral caloric intake and need sensitive counselling. Note:
- with a distal obstruction, a patient may still manage and absorb small amounts of oral fibre-free nutritional supplements and/or readily digestible food
- sometimes a patient chooses a long-term NG tube or considers a venting gastrostomy to permit unrestricted oral intake
- parenteral nutrition generally has no role in patients with limited options for anticancer treatment or poor performance status.

Updated (minor change) February 2022

METOCLOPRAMIDE

Class: Prokinetic anti-emetic.

Indications: Nausea and vomiting caused by surgery, chemotherapy (delayed, not acute), radiation therapy or migraine. All other uses are unauthorized, e.g. †delayed gastric emptying, †functional dyspepsia, †gastro-oesophageal reflux, †hiccups.

Contra-indications: Children <1 year old. Phaeochromocytoma (may induce an acute hypertensive response). GI haemorrhage or perforation. Use within <4 days of GI surgery (vigorous contractions may impair healing).

Pharmacology

Metoclopramide is a D_2 antagonist which acts both centrally in the area postrema (chemoreceptor trigger zone) and peripherally in the upper GI tract, where it blocks the 'dopamine brake' on gastric emptying induced by stress, anxiety and nausea. Further, as a $5HT_4$ agonist, it has a direct excitatory effect in the upper GI tract. Although $5HT_3$ antagonism occurs at higher doses (e.g. 2–4mg/kg IV), the use of high-dose metoclopramide for chemotherapy-related nausea and vomiting has been superseded by specific $5HT_3$-receptor antagonists (p.277).

For gastroparesis, its efficacy is comparable to **domperidone** (see Prokinetics, p.22).[1] However, it causes more frequent and more severe undesirable effects, including drowsiness, loss of mental acuity, and extrapyramidal symptoms.[2]

Metoclopramide is metabolized in the liver, with CYP2D6 the main CYP450 enzyme involved. It is eliminated mainly via the kidney, either as conjugated metabolites or unchanged (20–30%). Both hepatic and renal impairment reduce the clearance of metoclopramide, resulting in higher plasma levels and a prolonged halflife, and the SPC advises a reduced dose. Thus, in patients with moderate–severe renal impairment or ESRF or severe cirrhosis, reduce the usual starting dose and monitor carefully (also see Chapter 17, p.737 and Chapter 18, p.767).[3]

Metoclopramide is a commonly used anti-emetic in palliative care. In RCTs, cancer-related nausea and vomiting resolved in about ≤33% and ≤50%, respectively.[4,5] Although metoclopramide often has immediate effect, benefit may increase throughout the first week of use.[6–8]

Bio-availability 50–80% PO.
Onset of action 10–15min IM, 15–60min PO.
Time to peak plasma concentration 1–2.5h PO.
Plasma halflife 2.5–5h.
Duration of action 1–2h (data for single dose and relating to gastric emptying).

Cautions

Cardiac disease, enhanced effects of catecholamines in patients with essential hypertension[9,10] (also see Undesirable effects), epilepsy (lowers seizure threshold), Parkinson's disease, mechanical GI obstruction (but is commonly used in palliative care to restore peristalsis in functional GI obstruction),[11,12] moderate–severe renal impairment or ESRF, severe hepatic impairment (see Pharmacology and Chapter 17, p.737 and Chapter 18, p.767).

Drug interactions

Serious drug interaction: a combination of IV metoclopramide and IV **ondansetron** occasionally causes cardiac arrhythmias.[13] $5HT_3$-receptors influence various aspects of cardiac function, including inotropy, chronotropy and coronary arterial tone,[14] effects which are mediated by both the parasympathetic and the sympathetic nervous systems. Thus, in any given patient, blockade of $5HT_3$-receptors will produce effects dependent on the pre-existing serotoninergic activity in both arms of the autonomic nervous system.

Risk of serotonin toxicity when used in combination with other serotoninergic drugs, e.g. SSRIs (see Antidepressants, Box A, p.217).

Because antimuscarinics competitively block the final common (cholinergic) pathway through which prokinetics act, concurrent prescription with metoclopramide should be avoided if possible. Opioids may also impede this action.

Metoclopramide may increase the rate of absorption of **morphine** via increased gastric emptying.

Undesirable effects

Because of concerns about tardive dyskinesia, the EMA has reduced the authorized indications for metoclopramide and limited the maximum daily dose and duration of use to 30mg (0.5mg/kg) for 5 days. High-dose formulations have been withdrawn.[15] The FDA has issued similar restrictions.[16] Use of metoclopramide has subsequently declined.[17] However, the EMA recognizes that the risk:benefit ratio may be different in populations where off-label use is accepted practice, e.g. palliative care.[18]

Also see Drug-induced movement disorders, p.805. The risk of extrapyramidal effects is dose-related and increased by the co-administration of other drugs known to cause extrapyramidal effects, e.g. antipsychotics, $5HT_3$ antagonists, antidepressants. Other risk factors include female sex, age (<20 and >80 years), past psychiatric history, Parkinson's disease, diabetes mellitus and renal or hepatic failure.[19]

Acute dystonic reactions occur in <5% of patients receiving metoclopramide, and are more common in the young, particularly girls and young women. They generally occur ≤5 days of starting treatment and subside within 24h of stopping the drug. When possible, use alternatives in patients 1–20 years old.

Acute akathisia occurs in 10–15% of patients receiving a single dose of metoclopramide 20mg IV, and is severe enough to require treatment in 1–3%.[20] In a small series of palliative care patients, 10% exhibited acute akathisia after 2 weeks of metoclopramide, median dose 30mg/24h (range 10–60mg).[21] Acute akathisia is easily missed; patients may not spontaneously volunteer the symptoms, or clinicians misinterpret them as anxiety-related or another psychiatric condition.[22] Paradoxically, this can result in the use of neuroleptic drugs which, via their dopamine antagonist effects, exacerbates the situation.

Drug-induced parkinsonism generally develops <3 months after starting metoclopramide. The exact incidence is unknown. In one series, 30% of patients had signs of parkinsonism after ≥3 months of use.[19] In another series, tremor was present in 5% after 2 weeks of use.[21]

The overall incidence of tardive dyskinesia is probably <1%.[23] The risk increases with duration of treatment and total cumulative dose. Onset is generally after months of use; in one series, after a median of 14 months (range 4–44 months).[24] However, about 20% of palliative care clinicians report seeing tardive dyskinesia in their patients, sometimes after only 2 weeks of use.[25] Further, it has occurred in a 16 year old male after only 2 days of 30mg/24h PO.[26] A possible mechanism is a direct neurotoxic effect of metoclopramide.[27] The likelihood of recovery is inversely related to age, probably reflecting capacity for CNS repair.

Patients experiencing extrapyramidal effects should be counselled against future use and the reaction clearly documented in their medical records.

Other undesirable effects include neuroleptic (antipsychotic) malignant syndrome (see Antipsychotics, p.184), drowsiness, depression, diarrhoea. Very rarely: hypotension, cardiac arrhythmia and cardiac arrest; mainly with IV use in at risk patients.

Dose and use

Avoid metoclopramide in patients in whom it has previously caused extrapyramidal effects.

If a long-term prokinetic is necessary, consider **domperidone** (p.271) instead. When this is not possible (e.g. because of contra-indications or the need for parenteral administration), review the use of metoclopramide frequently (e.g. at least every week) and discontinue if an optimal dose fails to provide benefit.

With long-term use, continue to monitor the patient regularly, particularly when higher than usual doses are being used, and discontinue metoclopramide if extrapyramidal signs or symptoms develop.

Nausea and vomiting, †delayed gastric emptying, †peristaltic failure

Also see QCG: Nausea and vomiting, p.264 and QCG: Inoperable bowel obstruction, p.266.

- start 10mg PO t.d.s. or 30mg/24h CSCI, and 10mg PO/SC q2h p.r.n.
- titrate if necessary to a maximum dose of 20mg PO q.d.s. or 100mg/24h CSCI.

†*Hiccup*

If caused by delayed gastric emptying, gastric distension or acid reflux:

- as above ± an antifoaming agent (see Prokinetics, Table 2, p.25)
- if no response to PO treatment, consider stat dose of 10–20mg IV; give over ≥3min.[15]

Note. Increasing IV administration time to 15min reduced the incidence of acute akathisia in one study but not another.[20,28]

For CSCI, dilute with WFI or sodium chloride 0.9%.

CSCI compatibility with other drugs: there are 2-drug compatibility data for metoclopramide in WFI with **alfentanil**, **diamorphine**, **glycopyrronium**, **haloperidol**, **hydromorphone**, **ketamine**, **midazolam**, **morphine sulfate**, **octreotide** and **oxycodone**. For more details and 3-drug compatibility charts, see Appendix 3 (p.933).

Compatibility charts for mixing drugs in sodium chloride 0.9% can be found in the extended Appendix section of the on-line *PCF* on *www.medicinescomplete.com*.

Supply

Metoclopramide (generic)

Tablets 10mg, 28 days @ 10mg q.d.s. = £2.50.

Oral solution 5mg/5mL, 28 days @ 10mg q.d.s. = £116.

Injection 5mg/mL, 2mL and 20mL amp = £0.25 and £2.75 respectively.

1 Barone J (1999) Domperidone: a peripherally acting dopamine$_2$-receptor antagonist. *Annals of Pharmacotherapy*. **33**: 429–440.
2 Patterson D *et al.* (1999) A double-blind multicenter comparison of domperidone and metoclopramide in the treatment of diabetic patients with symptoms of gastroparesis. *American Journal of Gastroenterology*. **94**: 1230–1234.
3 Magueur E *et al.* (1991) Pharmacokinetics of metoclopramide in patients with liver cirrhosis. *British Journal of Clinical Pharmacology*. **31**: 185–187.
4 Davis MP *et al.* (2010) A systematic review of the treatment of nausea and/or vomiting in cancer unrelated to chemotherapy or radiation. *Journal of Pain and Symptom Management*. **39**: 756–767.
5 Glare P *et al.* (2004) Systematic review of the efficacy of antiemetics in the treatment of nausea in patients with far-advanced cancer. *Support Care Cancer*. **12**: 432–440.
6 Bruera E *et al.* (2004) Dexamethasone in addition to metoclopramide for chronic nausea in patients with advanced cancer: a randomized controlled trial. *Journal of Pain and Symptom Management*. **28**: 381–388.
7 Bruera E *et al.* (1996) Chronic nausea in advanced cancer patients: a retrospective assessment of a metoclopramide-based antiemetic regimen. *Journal of Pain and Symptom Management*. **11**: 147–153.
8 Bruera E *et al.* (2000) A double-blind, crossover study of controlled-release metoclopramide and placebo for the chronic nausea and dyspepsia of advanced cancer. *Journal of Pain and Symptom Management*. **19**: 427–435.
9 Kuchel O *et al.* (1985) Effect of metoclopramide on plasma catecholamine release in essential hypertension. *Clinical Pharmacology and Therapeutics*. **37**: 372–375.
10 Agabiti-Rosei E (1995) Hypertensive crises in patients with phaeochromocytoma given metoclopramide. *Annals of Pharmacology*. **29**: 381–383.
11 Twycross RG and Back I (1998) Nausea and vomiting in advanced cancer. *European Journal of Palliative Care*. **5**: 39–45.
12 Ripamonti C *et al.* (2001) Clinical-practice recommendations for the management of bowel obstruction in patients with end-stage cancer. *Supportive Care in Cancer*. **9**: 223–233.
13 Baguley W *et al.* (1997) Cardiac dysrhythmias associated with the intravenous administration of ondansetron and metoclopramide. *Anesthesia and Analgesia*. **84**: 1380–1381.
14 Saxena P and Villalon C (1991) 5-Hydroxytryptamine: a chameleon in the heart. *Trends in Pharmacological Sciences*. **12**: 223–227.
15 MHRA (2013) Metoclopramide: risk of neurological adverse effects - restricted dose and duration of use. *Drug Safety Update*. **7**: www.mhra.gov.uk/safetyinformation
16 FDA (2009) Summary of warnings for metoclopramide containing products. *Medwatch*. www.fda.gov/Safety/MedWatch/SafetyInformation
17 Ehrenpreis ED *et al.* (2013) The metoclopramide black box warning for tardive dyskinesia: effect on clinical practice, adverse event reporting, and prescription drug lawsuits. *American Journal of Gastroenterology*. **108**: 866–872.
18 EMA (2013) Personal communication.
19 Ganzini L *et al.* (1993) The prevalence of metoclopramide-induced tardive dyskinesia and acute extrapyramidal movement disorders. *Archives of Internal Medicine*. **153**: 1469–1475.
20 Egerton-Warburton D and Povey K (2013) Administration of metoclopramide by infusion or bolus does not affect the incidence of drug-induced akathisia. *Emergency Medicine Australasia*. **25**: 207–212.
21 Currow DC *et al.* (2012) Pharmacovigilance in hospice/palliative care: rapid report of net clinical effect of metoclopramide. *Journal of Palliative Medicine*. **15**: 1071–1075.
22 Akagi H and Kumar TM (2002) Lesson of the week: Akathisia: overlooked at a cost. *British Medical Journal*. **324**: 1506–1507.
23 Rao A and Camilleri M (2009) Review article: metoclopramide and tardive dyskinesia. *Alimentary Pharmacology and Therapeutics*. **31**: 11–19.
24 Wiholm BE *et al.* (1984) Tardive dyskinesia associated with metoclopramide. *British Medical Journal*. **288**: 545–547.
25 Palliativedrugs.com (2014) Metoclopramide – What is your experience? Survey November-December 2013. www.palliativedrugs.com

26 Karimi Khaledi M *et al.* (2012) Tardive dyskinesia after short-term treatment with oral metoclopramide in an adolescent. *International Journal of Clinical Pharmacy*. **34**: 822–824.
27 Lai TK *et al.* (2012) Cell membrane lytic action of metoclopramide and its relation to tardive dyskinesia. *Synapse*. **66**: 273–276.
28 Tura P *et al.* (2012) Slow infusion metoclopramide does not affect the improvement rate of nausea while reducing akathisia and sedation incidence. *Emergency Medical Journal*. **29**: 108–112.

Updated November 2019

4

DOMPERIDONE

Class: Prokinetic anti-emetic.

Indications: Nausea and vomiting. All other uses are unauthorized, e.g. †delayed gastric emptying, †functional dyspepsia, †gastro-oesophageal reflux, †hiccups.

Contra-indications: Prolactinoma; conditions where cardiac conduction is, or could be, impaired, e.g. prolonged QT interval (congenital or acquired); underlying cardiac disease, e.g. CHF; concurrent use with potent CYP3A4 inhibitors or other drugs known to prolong QT interval (see Drug interactions); GI haemorrhage or perforation, mechanical GI obstruction; moderate–severe hepatic impairment.

Pharmacology

Like **metoclopramide**, domperidone antagonizes D_2-receptors in:

- the chemoreceptor trigger zone (CTZ) in the area postrema
- the gastro-oesophageal and gastroduodenal junctions, counteracting the gastric 'dopamine brake' associated with nausea from any cause.[1]

Unlike **metoclopramide**, domperidone's blood–brain barrier penetration is negligible; thus, domperidone causes less frequent and less severe undesirable effects, including drowsiness, loss of mental acuity,[2] and extrapyramidal symptoms. It is the anti-emetic of choice for nausea related to antiparkinsonian dopamimetics.[3]

However, the usefulness of domperidone is limited by the absence of a parenteral formulation and concern about QT prolongation. Epidemiological studies found domperidone was associated with an increased risk of serious ventricular arrhythmia/sudden cardiac death of ≤60%.[4] The risk was higher in those >60 years old, receiving doses >30mg/24h, and/or receiving a CYP3A4 inhibitor or drug known to cause QT prolongation.[4-6] Although some consider that the risk has been overstated,[7,8] regulators have restricted its marketing authorization to nausea and vomiting for ≤1 week and added new contra-indications (see above).[9] Further, the maximum authorized dose is now 30mg/24h, and many studies found benefit only with 40–80mg/24h.[10]

For gastroparesis, the efficacy of domperidone and **metoclopramide** are similar, despite the latter's additional prokinetic $5HT_4$ agonist action (see Prokinetics, Table 1, p.23).[11] Domperidone may be effective even when there is no response to **metoclopramide**.[12,13] In diabetic patients, the prokinetic effect for solids attenuates after 1–2 months, although the effect on liquid emptying persists.[14,15]

Although domperidone is almost completely absorbed from the GI tract, bio-availability is relatively poor because of extensive first-pass metabolism in the wall of the GI tract and the liver. Bio-availability in healthy volunteers is nearly doubled if taken *after* a meal.[16] Maximal absorption requires an acid environment; H_2 antagonists, PPIs and antacids all reduce absorption. PO and PR bio-availability are almost the same, but suppositories are not available in the UK.

Domperidone is metabolized in the liver to inactive compounds, principally via CYP3A4. Because of safety concerns regarding high plasma levels of domperidone (see Undesirable effects), the manufacturer suggests moderate–severe hepatic impairment is a contra-indication to its use. However, domperidone has previously been used in this setting and is the anti-emetic of choice in many liver centres; thus, if domperidone is considered necessary, a reduction in dose and careful monitoring is recommended (see Chapter 18, p.767).

Renal clearance is a minor route of elimination (<1% unchanged). In renal failure, although the plasma halflife is increased by ≤3 times, plasma concentration does not increase (possibly because of an altered volume of distribution).[17] However, most sources recommend limiting the maximum daily dose in severe renal impairment/ESRF (see Chapter 17, p.737).

Bio-availability 12–18% PO (fasting), 24% PO (after food).
Onset of action 30min.
Time to peak plasma concentration 0.5–2h PO.
Plasma halflife 7–16h; increasing up to 21h in severe renal impairment.[12]
Duration of action 12–24h (estimate based on halflife).

Cautions

Underlying cardiac disease and other risk factors for prolonged QT, e.g. electrolyte disturbances (also see Chapter 20, p.797); severe renal impairment or ESRF, hepatic impairment (see Pharmacology, and Chapter 17, p.737 and Chapter 18, p.767).

In patients with Parkinson's disease, the use of domperidone is associated with an increased risk of death from all causes.[18] However, the need for symptom-relieving drugs often reflects worsening disease or an intercurrent illness, and the difficulty of controlling for these confounding factors limits meaningful conclusions being drawn from such studies.

Drug interactions

Avoid concurrent use with drugs known to:
- increase the QT interval (see Chapter 20, p.797)
- inhibit the metabolism of domperidone, i.e. CYP3A4 inhibitors. These may increase the domperidone plasma concentration, increasing the risk of QT prolongation and thus *torsade de pointes*.

Examples of strong CYP3A4 inhibitors include **aprepitant**, azoles (**fluconazole**, **itraconazole**), grapefruit juice, macrolide antibiotics (**clarithromycin**, **erythromycin**), protease inhibitors (**ritonavir**), SSRIs (**fluvoxamine, fluoxetine**). Also see Chapter 19, Table 8, p.790.

Because antimuscarinics competitively block the final common (cholinergic) pathway through which prokinetics act, concurrent prescription with domperidone should be avoided if possible. Opioids may also impede this action.

H_2 antagonists, PPIs and antacids reduce absorption and bio-availability.

Undesirable effects

Very rare (<0.01%): transient colic, gynaecomastia, galactorrhoea, amenorrhoea (secondary to increased prolactin secretion), reduced libido, cramp, pruritus, rash;[12] headache; extrapyramidal effects (acute dystonias).[19] In two women with polycystic ovaries, hyperoestrogenism may have been a predisposing factor.[12]

Paradoxical vomiting has been reported in children with severe brain injury requiring tube feeding. Inhibition of pyloric relaxation was considered the likely cause, due to the D_2 antagonist effect of domperidone in the presence of a severe reduction in vagal tone.[20]
Unknown frequency: QT prolongation (p.797).

Dose and use

In 2014, because of a small increased risk of serious ventricular arrhythmia, particularly in those >60 years old receiving >30mg/24h and/or receiving a CYP3A4 inhibitor or drug known to cause QT prolongation, regulators concluded that the risk:benefit ratio was only acceptable for nausea and vomiting, and recommended restricting dose and duration of use to 10mg t.d.s. and ≤1 week, respectively. Further, they added new contra-indications related to cardiovascular disease and drug interactions (see above).

However, the risk:benefit balance should be determined on an individual patient basis, taking circumstances and other options into account. For example, if a patient with end-stage CHF requires a long-term anti-emetic, domperidone may be preferable to **cyclizine** (also pro-arrhythmic) or **metoclopramide** (risk of extrapyramidal effects).

Advise patients to seek prompt medical attention should symptoms such as syncope or cardiac arrhythmias occur.

The manufacturer recommends giving domperidone t.d.s. (previously up to q.d.s. 15–30min before meals in patients with upper GI dysmotility). However, given its halflife, b.d. may suffice, and its bio-availability is higher if taken after food:

- start with 10mg PO b.d.
- increase to 10mg t.d.s., the *authorized* maximum dose
- If symptoms persist, consider increasing to 20mg b.d. → 20mg t.d.s. → 20mg q.d.s. (the *previous* authorized maximum dose, used in many trials).[10]

Alternative options to higher-dose domperidone are **metoclopramide** (p.268) and **erythromycin** (see Prokinetics, Box B, p.24).

Also see QCG: Nausea and vomiting, p.264.

Supply

Domperidone (generic)

Tablets 10mg, 28 days @ 10mg q.d.s. = £2.50.

Oral suspension 5mg/5mL, 28 days @ 10mg q.d.s. = £75.

1 Barone J (1999) Domperidone: a peripherally acting dopamine$_2$-receptor antagonist. *Annals of Pharmacotherapy*. **33**: 429–440.
2 Patterson D *et al.* (1999) A double-blind multicenter comparison of domperidone and metoclopramide in the treatment of diabetic patients with symptoms of gastroparesis. *American Journal of Gastroenterology*. **94**: 1230–1234.
3 Langdon N *et al.* (1986) Comparison of levodopa with carbidopa, and levodopa with domperidone in Parkinson's disease. *Clinical Neuropharmacology*. **9**: 440–447.
4 Johannes CB *et al.* (2010) Risk of serious ventricular arrhythmia and sudden cardiac death in a cohort of users of domperidone: a nested case-control study. *Pharmacoepidemiology and Drug Safety*. **19**: 881–888.
5 van Noord C *et al.* (2010) Domperidone and ventricular arrhythmia or sudden cardiac death: a population-based case-control study in the Netherlands. *Drug Safety*. **33**: 1003–1014.
6 Leelakanok N *et al.* (2016) Domperidone and risk of ventricular arrhythmia and cardiac death: a systematic review and meta-analysis. *Clinical Drug Investigation*. **36**: 97–107.
7 Buffery PJ and Strother RM (2015) Domperidone safety: a mini-review of the science of QT prolongation and clinical implications of recent global regulatory recommendations. *New Zealand Medical Journal*. **128**: 66–74.
8 Ortiz A *et al.* (2015) Cardiovascular safety profile and clinical experience with high-dose domperidone therapy for nausea and vomiting. *American Journal of the Medical Sciences*. **349**: 421–424.
9 MHRA (2014) Domperidone: risk of cardiac side effects - indication restricted to nausea and vomiting, new contraindications, and reduced dose and duration of use. *Drug Safety Update*. **7**: www.mhra.gov.uk/safetyinformation.
10 Reddymasu SC *et al.* (2007) Domperidone: review of pharmacology and clinical applications in gastroenterology. *American Journal of Gastroenterology*. **102**: 2036–2045.
11 Sturm A *et al.* (1999) Prokinetics in patients with gastroparesis: a systematic analysis. *Digestion*. **60**: 422–427.
12 Prakash A and Wagstaff AJ (1998) Domperidone. A review of its use in diabetic gastropathy. *Drugs*. **56**: 429–445.
13 Dumitrascu D and Weinbeck M (2000) Domperidone versus metoclopramide in the treatment of diabetic gastroparesis. *American Journal of Gastroenterology*. **95**: 316–317.
14 Horowitz M *et al.* (1985) Acute and chronic effects of domperidone on gastric emptying in diabetic autonomic neuropathy. *Digestive Diseases and Sciences*. **30**: 1–9.
15 Koch KL *et al.* (1989) Gastric emptying and gastric myoelectrical activity in patients with diabetic gastroparesis: effect of long-term domperidone treatment. *American Journal of Gastroenterology*. **84**: 1069–1075.
16 Heykants J *et al.* (1981) On the pharmacokinetics of domperidone in animals and man. IV. The pharmacokinetics of intravenous domperidone and its bioavailability in man following intramuscular, oral and rectal administration. *European Journal of Drug Metabolism and Pharmacokinetics*. **6**: 61–70.
17 Brogden RN *et al.* (1982) Domperidone. A review of its pharmacological activity, pharmacokinetics and therapeutic efficacy in the symptomatic treatment of chronic dyspepsia and as an antiemetic. *Drugs*. **24**: 360–400.
18 Simeonova M *et al.* (2018) Increased risk of all-cause mortality associated with domperidone use in Parkinson's patients: a population-based cohort study in the UK. *British journal of clinical pharmacology*. **84**: 2551–2561.
19 Casteels-Van Daele M *et al.* (1984) Refusal of further cancer chemotherapy due to antiemetic drug. *Lancet*. **1**: 57.
20 Pozzi M *et al.* (2013) Case series: paradoxical action of domperidone leads to increased vomiting. *European Journal of Clinical Pharmacology*. **69**: 289–290.

Updated November 2019

CYCLIZINE

Class: Antihistaminic antimuscarinic anti-emetic.

For alternative antihistaminic antimuscarinic anti-emetics used in countries where cyclizine is unavailable, see Table 1.

Indications: Nausea and vomiting, motion sickness, vertigo and labyrinthine disorders.

Pharmacology

Cyclizine is an H_1 and muscarinic antagonist. It is thought to act on the vestibular system and the nucleus tractus solitarius (vomiting centre; see Anti-emetics, Figure 1, p.259).

Because of its sedative and antimuscarinic properties, cyclizine is generally reserved for nausea related to vestibular system irritation or raised intracranial pressure, or when dopaminergic anti-emetics are contra-indicated (e.g. Parkinson's disease).[1-4]

Cyclizine is extensively hepatically metabolized to inactive metabolites that are predominantly renally excreted.[5,6] The long halflife means that with the t.d.s. dosing interval recommended in the SPC, accumulation is probable, and/or undesirable effects may arise only after several days–weeks of regular use.

Bio-availability 50% PO.[6]

Onset of action 30–60min.

Time to peak plasma concentration 2h PO.

Plasma halflife 20h.

Duration of action 4–6h (may be longer).

Cautions

See Antimuscarinics, p.6. Renal and hepatic impairment see Chapter 17, p.737 and Chapter 18, p.767, respectively.

Drug interactions

Concurrent treatment with ≥2 antimuscarinic drugs (including antihistamines, phenothiazines and TCAs; see Antimuscarinics, Box B, p.4) will increase the probability of undesirable effects and (when centrally acting) of central toxicity, e.g. restlessness, agitation, delirium (see Antimuscarinics, Box C, p.5). Children, the elderly, and patients with renal or hepatic impairment are more susceptible to the central effects of antimuscarinics.

See Antimuscarinics (p.7).

Undesirable effects

Central and peripheral antimuscarinic effects (see Antimuscarinics, Box C, p.5). Rarely, movement disorders, e.g. tremor, dyskinesia, dystonia;[4,7] potential for misuse/abuse of the injection;[4,8,9] paralysis (case reports after IV use in neuromuscular disorders).

Dose and use

Review the need to continue other antihistaminic or antimuscarinic drugs, because cyclizine may render them unnecessary.

Cyclizine can accumulate with repeated use, and undesirable effects may arise only after several days–weeks. Particular caution is needed in the elderly and in renal and hepatic impairment (see Cautions), when a reduced frequency of dosing, e.g. b.d., may suffice.

- give 50mg PO b.d.–t.d.s. and 50mg p.r.n.
- usual maximum dose 200mg/24h.

Also see QCG: Nausea and vomiting (p.264), QCG: Inoperable bowel obstruction (p.266) and QCG: Vertigo (p.276).

†Subcutaneous administration

Because PO bio-availability of cyclizine is 50%, the PO:SC dose conversion ratio is 2:1.

- start with 75mg/24h CSCI and 25mg SC p.r.n.; if necessary, increase to 150mg/24h CSCI and 50mg SC p.r.n.
- usual maximum dose 200mg/24h.

For CSCI, dilute cyclizine with WFI or glucose 5%; cyclizine is *incompatible* with sodium chloride 0.9% and will precipitate; see Chapter 29, p.889.

CSCI compatibility with other drugs: there are 2-drug compatibility data for cyclizine in WFI with **haloperidol**, **hyoscine *hydrobromide***, **morphine sulfate** and **morphine tartrate** (not UK).

Concentration-dependent *incompatibility* occurs with **alfentanil**, **dexamethasone**, **diamorphine** and **oxycodone**. *Incompatibility* has also been reported with **clonazepam**, **hydromorphone**, **hyoscine *butylbromide***, **ketorolac**, **midazolam** and **octreotide**.

See Appendix 3, p.933 for more details and 3-drug compatibility data.

Alternative antihistaminic antimuscarinic anti-emetics

Table 1 Examples of anti-emetics used in countries without access to cyclizine[a]

	Nausea	*Vomiting*	*Vertigo*
Dimenhydrinate	50–100mg PO q4–6h p.r.n.; maximum 400mg/24h	50–100mg IM/IV q4–6h p.r.n.; maximum 400mg/24h	
Diphenhydramine	25–50mg PO q4–6h p.r.n.; maximum 300mg/24h	10–50mg IM/IV q6h p.r.n.	
Hydroxyzine		25–100mg IM q4–6h p.r.n.	
Meclizine	25–50mg PO once daily		25–100mg/24h PO in divided doses

a. based on doses generally used for nausea, vomiting or vertigo; authorized indications and doses vary between countries; check product information for details.

Supply

Oral products

Cyclizine *hydrochloride* (generic)

Tablets 50mg, 28 days @ 50mg t.d.s. = £5.50.

Oral suspension 50mg/5mL, 28 days @ 50mg t.d.s. = £69 (unauthorized product, available as a special order; see Chapter 24, p.817). *Price based on Specials tariff in community.*

Parenteral products

Cyclizine *lactate* (generic)

Injection 50mg/mL, 1mL amp = £1.75.

1 Brandt T (2005) *Vertigo and Dizziness: Common Complaints*. Second Edition. London: Springer.

2 Bisdorff A *et al.* (2013) The epidemiology of vertigo, dizziness, and unsteadiness and its links to co-morbidities. *Frontiers in Neurology*. **4**: 29.

3 Karatas M (2008) Central vertigo and dizziness: epidemiology, differential diagnosis, and common causes. *Neurologist*. **14**: 355–364.

4 Palliativedrugs.com (2018) Cyclizine – What is your experience? *Latest additions: Survey results (April 2018)*. www.palliativedrugs.com

5 Vella-Brincat JW *et al.* (2012) The pharmacokinetics and pharmacogenetics of the antiemetic cyclizine in palliative care patients. *Journal of Pain and Symptom Management*. **43**: 540–548.

6 Walker RB (1995) HPLC analysis and pharmacokinetics of cyclizine. Rhodes University PhD thesis. School of Pharmaceutical Sciences, Rhodes University, Grahamstown, South Africa.

7 Lee P (2013) Locked-in syndrome as a result of cyclizine administration. *Journal of Pain and Symptom Management*. **45**: e5–7.

8 Bailey F and Davies A (2008) The misuse/abuse of antihistamine antiemetic medication (cyclizine) by cancer patients. *Palliative Medicine*. **22**: 869–871.

9 Thursby-Pelham FW *et al.* (2009) Cyclizine dependence in patients with complex nutritional requirements. *Proceedings of the Nutrition Society*. **68**: E21.

Updated (minor change) September 2021

Quick Clinical Guide: Vertigo

Vertigo is an unpleasant spinning sensation generally related to dysfunction of the vestibular system, and is often associated with nausea and vomiting, and difficulties with standing or walking. It is distinct from dizziness, which (in Europe) is widely regarded as a synonym for non-rotational light-headedness. Vertigo can be continuous or paroxysmal, with episodes ranging from seconds/minutes–days/weeks.

In the general population, the main causes are excessive alcohol, benign paroxysmal positional vertigo, Ménière's disease, vestibular neuritis, and labyrinthitis. Vertigo may also be caused by brain tumours (primary or secondary), stroke, and neurodegenerative disorders, e.g. Parkinson's disease, multiple sclerosis.

Clinical evaluation

Vertigo needs to be differentiated from non-rotational light-headedness:

'Does everything spin like a top?', 'Is it like being on a merry-go-round?'

'Or is it more a feeling of light-headedness?'

Precipitating factors

- after drugs/alcohol?
- when moving (e.g. walking, turning the head) or when resting/lying down?
- when stressed?

Associated symptoms

- nausea, vomiting?
- difficulties with standing or walking?
- aural symptoms, e.g. tinnitus, impaired hearing?
- headache?
- visual disturbances, e.g. oscillopsia, diplopia?
- anxiety?

Differential diagnosis

The main differential diagnosis is light-headedness, most cases of which are associated with orthostatic (postural) hypotension (Box A). However, some are psychosomatic, e.g. hyperventilation syndrome, panic attack, phobic postural vertigo, agoraphobia.

Box A Common somatic causes of light-headedness

Cardiogenic

- orthostatic hypotension
- presyncope (near-faint)
- vasovagal syncope
- cardiac arrhythmia

Hypoglycaemia

Exogenous substances

- alcohol
- drugs (Box B)

Box B Drugs and orthostatic hypotension[a]

Cardiac

ACE inhibitors
α-blockers (e.g. prazosin, tamsulosin)
β-blockers (e.g. carvedilol, labetalol)
Clonidine
Diuretics (e.g. furosemide)
Nitrates (e.g. glyceryl trinitrate)

Central nervous system

Antidepressants (e.g. TCAs, trazodone)
Antiparkinsonian drugs (e.g. bromocriptine, levodopa)
Antipsychotics (e.g. chlorpromazine, clozapine)
Opioids
Skeletal muscle relaxants (e.g. baclofen, tizanidine)

Urological

Phosphodiesterase type-5 inhibitors (e.g. sildenafil)
Urinary antimuscarinics (e.g. oxybutynin)

a. there may be additive effects with polypharmacy (the norm in palliative care).

Management

Correct the correctable

The cause of the vertigo should be determined and specific treatment considered; *seek specialist advice if necessary.*

When drug-induced orthostatic hypotension is the cause, discontinue or reduce the dose of potential causal drugs.

Non-drug treatment

Particularly in benign paroxysmal positional vertigo, certain manoeuvres can reduce the impact of the vertigo but need to be used appropriately and taught correctly; obtain advice from an otologist.

Drug treatment

Specific: e.g. Ménière's disease, betahistine initially 16mg t.d.s.

Symptomatic relief of acute episodes:

- if vertigo related to a brain tumour (primary or secondary), give a benzodiazepine, e.g. lorazepam 1mg PO or midazolam 2.5mg SC/IV, and repeat 30–60min p.r.n.; combine with an anti-emetic if necessary (see below)
- for vestibular causes:
  - ▷ first-line anti-emetic: antihistaminic antimuscarinic, e.g. cyclizine 50mg PO or 25–50mg SC/IV p.r.n.; maximum dose 200mg/24h
  - ▷ alternative anti-emetic: prokinetic, metoclopramide 10mg PO/SC/IV.

Antimuscarinic drugs should be avoided long term because they may inhibit compensatory mechanisms; for the management of prolonged continuous vertigo, seek advice from an otologist.

Updated November 2019

5HT$_3$ ANTAGONISTS

Indications: Nausea and vomiting after surgery, chemotherapy and radiotherapy, †intractable vomiting due to chemical, abdominal and cerebral causes when usual approaches have failed, †diarrhoea associated with carcinoid syndrome,[1] †opioid-induced pruritus.

Contra-indications: Congenital long QT syndrome (**ondansetron**).

Pharmacology

5HT$_3$ antagonists were developed specifically to control emesis associated with highly emetogenic chemotherapy, e.g. **cisplatin**. They block the effect of excess 5HT on vagal nerve fibres, and are thus of particular value in situations when excessive amounts of 5HT are released from the body's stores, i.e. from enterochromaffin cells after chemotherapy or radiation-induced damage of the GI mucosa, or because of intestinal distension, or from leaky platelets when there is severe renal impairment.

In an open RCT, **tropisetron** (not UK) was shown to be of benefit in patients with far-advanced cancer and nausea and vomiting of indeterminate cause when given either as a sole agent or with a second anti-emetic, particularly **dexamethasone**.[2] 5HT$_3$ antagonists also relieve nausea and vomiting associated with head injury, brain stem radiotherapy[3,4] or gastro-enteritis,[5] and in multiple sclerosis with brain stem disease.[6]

A TD **granisetron** patch is authorized for the *prevention* of nausea and vomiting associated with moderately or highly emetogenic chemotherapy. It has a slow onset of action and must be applied 24–48h before chemotherapy. It can be worn for ≤7 days if required and is removed ≥24h after completion of chemotherapy. Because TD **granisetron** is no more effective than PO, its use is limited to situations where the PO route is not available.[7]

Ondansetron relieves pruritus related to spinal **morphine**, but not cholestatic or uraemic pruritus (also see Chapter 26, p.825).[8-10]

In carcinoid syndrome, benefit is reported for diarrhoea refractory to **octreotide**. In a case series (n=6), **ondansetron** 8mg b.d. provided satisfactory control within 2–3 days. Subsequently, the dose was reduced to the minimum effective maintenance dose (4–8mg daily).[1]

5HT$_3$ receptors are involved in the transmission of pain, both centrally and peripherally, and the potential analgesic effect of 5HT$_3$ antagonists has been explored. However, in RCTs, 5HT$_3$ antagonists given systemically were of inconsistent benefit.[11-13] An RCT of weekly injections of **granisetron** into muscle trigger points improved chronic temporomandibular pain;[14] locally injected **tropisetron** (not UK) is also reported to relieve chronic back pain and myofascial pain.[15,16]

For pharmacokinetic details, see Table 1.

Table 1 Pharmacokinetic details of 5HT$_3$ antagonists

		Ondansetron	*Granisetron*	*Palonosetron*
Bio-availability	PO	56–71% (60% PR)[a]	60%	n/a
Onset of action	PO	<30min	<30min	n/a
	IV	<5min	<15min	
Plasma halflife		3–5h (6h PR)[a]	10–11h	40h
Time to peak plasma concentration	PO	1.5h	No data	n/a
	IM	10min		n/a
	PR[a]	6h		n/a
Duration of action		12h	24h	>24h[17]

a. suppositories not UK.

Cautions

Risk factors for QT prolongation (particularly **ondansetron**; see Chapter 20, p.797); moderate–severe hepatic impairment (**ondansetron**; see Dose and use and Chapter 18, p.767); reduced colonic motility (can cause or worsen constipation).

Drug interactions

Serious drug interaction: a combination of IV **metoclopramide** and IV **ondansetron** occasionally causes cardiac arrhythmias (see p.268).

Additive effects with other drugs that cause QT interval prolongation (see p.797) and serotonin toxicity (e.g. SSRIs; see Antidepressants, Box A, p.217).

There are mixed reports of the analgesic effect of **tramadol** (p.383) and **paracetamol** (p.331) being reduced by 5HT$_3$ antagonists, possibly by blocking the action of serotonin at presynaptic 5HT$_3$-receptors on primary afferent nociceptive neurones in the spinal dorsal horn.

Undesirable effects

Very common (>10%): headache.[18]
Common (<10%, >1%): light-headedness, dizziness, nervousness, tremor, ataxia, asthenia, drowsiness, fever, sensation of warmth or flushing (particularly when given IV), thirst, constipation or diarrhoea.
Uncommon (<1%, >0.1%): **ondansetron**: dystonic reactions, arrhythmia, hypotension, raised LFTs.
Rare (<0.1%, >0.01%): hiccup.
Very rare (<0.01%): **ondansetron**: transient blindness during IV administration (sight generally returns within 20min).

Dose and use

Although commonly used first-line in chemotherapy-related and post-operative nausea and vomiting, first-line use is rarely appropriate in palliative care. 5HT$_3$ antagonists are typically *added* to an antipsychotic with affinity for multiple receptors (e.g. **levomepromazine**, **olanzapine**) if the latter is ineffective alone (see Anti-emetics, p.258).

Granisetron can be given once daily, whereas **ondansetron** is given b.d.–t.d.s. $5HT_3$ antagonists are equally effective PO, by injection or TD.[7,19-21]

Regimens include:

- **granisetron** 1–2mg PO/SC once daily for 3 days *or*
- **ondansetron** 4–8mg PO/SC b.d.–t.d.s. (or 16–24mg/24h CSCI) for 3 days
- if clearly of benefit, continue indefinitely unless the cause is self-limiting
- some patients benefit from higher doses, occasionally as high as **granisetron** 9mg daily[22]
- in patients with moderate–severe hepatic impairment, the dose of **ondansetron** should be limited to 8mg daily, whereas no dose reduction is necessary for **granisetron** (in renal impairment, no dose reduction is necessary with either drug).

Also see QCG: Nausea and vomiting, p.264 and QCG: Inoperable bowel obstruction, p.266. For use in pruritus associated with spinally administered **morphine** or for diarrhoea in carcinoid syndrome, see Pharmacology.

For CSCI dilute with WFI, sodium chloride 0.9% or glucose 5%.

CSCI compatibility with other drugs: there are 2-drug compatibility data for **ondansetron** in WFI with **alfentanil**, **diamorphine**, and **octreotide**. For more details and 3-drug compatibility data, see Appendix 3 (p.933).

Compatibility charts for mixing drugs in sodium chloride 0.9% can be found in the extended appendix of the on-line *PCF* on *www.medicinescomplete.com*.

To control nausea and vomiting caused by severely emetogenic chemotherapy, **granisetron** (or other $5HT_3$ antagonist) is used with other anti-emetics, typically **dexamethasone** and **metoclopramide**.[23]

For IV **ondansetron** in chemotherapy-induced nausea and vomiting only, the MHRA provides specific dose and administration advice for patients >65 years, based on the risk of dose-dependent QT interval prolongation.[24]

Supply

Granisetron (generic)

Tablets 1mg, 2mg, 28 days @ 1mg once daily = £115.

Injection 1mg/mL, for dilution and use as an injection or infusion, 1mL amp = £2, 3mL amp = £6.

Sancuso® (Kyowa Kirin)

Transdermal patches (for up to 7 days) 3.1mg/24h, 1 = £56. *Similar considerations apply as for other medical transdermal products, e.g. skin hair should be clipped rather than shaved, fold patches in half and dispose of safely, remove before MRI scans (see Chapter 30, p.901).*

Ondansetron (generic)

Tablets 4mg, 8mg, 28 days @ 8mg b.d. = £8.

Orodispersible tablet 4mg, 8mg, 28 days @ 8mg b.d. = £403.

Oral solution (sugar-free) 4mg/5mL, 28 days @ 8mg b.d. = £202.

Injection 2mg/mL, 2mL amp = £1, 4mL amp = £1.75.

Setofilm (Norgine)

Orodispersible film 4mg, 8mg, 28 days @ 8mg b.d. = £319.

1 Kiesewetter B and Raderer M (2013) Ondansetron for diarrhea associated with neuroendocrine tumors. *New England Journal of Medicine*. **368**: 1947-1948.

2 Mystakidou K *et al.* (1998) Comparison of the efficacy and safety of tropisetron, metoclopramide, and chlorpromazine in the treatment of emesis associated with far advanced cancer. *Cancer*. **83**: 1214–1223.

3 Kleinerman K *et al.* (1993) Use of ondansetron for control of projectile vomiting in patients with neurosurgical trauma: two case reports. *Annals of Pharmacotherapy*. **27**: 566–568.

4 Bodis S *et al.* (1994) The prevention of radiosurgery-induced nausea and vomiting by ondansetron: evidence of a direct effect on the central nervous system chemoreceptor trigger zone. *Surgery and Neurology*. **42**: 249–252.

5 Cubeddu L *et al.* (1997) Antiemetic activity of ondansetron in acute gastroenteritis. *Alimentary Pharmacology and Therapeutics*. **11**: 185–191.

6 Rice G and Ebers G (1995) Ondansetron for intractable vertigo complicating acute brainstem disorders. *Lancet*. **345**: 1182–1183.

7 Boccia RV *et al.* (2011) Efficacy and tolerability of transdermal granisetron for the control of chemotherapy-induced nausea and vomiting associated with moderately and highly emetogenic multi-day chemotherapy: a randomized, double-blind, phase III study. *Supportive Care in Cancer.* **19**: 1609-1617.
8 To TH *et al.* (2012) The role of ondansetron in the management of cholestatic or uremic pruritus--a systematic review. *Journal of Pain and Symptom Management.* **44**: 725–730.
9 Wang W *et al.* (2017) Ondansetron for neuraxial morphine-induced pruritus: A meta-analysis of randomized controlled trials. *Journal of Clinical Pharmacy and Therapeutics.* **42**: 383–393.
10 Rashid S *et al.* (2018) Is there a role for 5-HT3 receptor antagonists in the treatment of pioid-induced pruritus? *American Journal of Hospice and Palliative Medicine.* **35**: 740–744.
11 Farber L *et al.* (2001) Short-term treatment of primary fibromyalgia with the 5-HT3-receptor antagonist tropisetron. Results of a randomized, double-blind, placebo-controlled multicenter trial in 418 patients. *International Journal of Pharmacology Research.* **21**: 1–13.
12 Bhosale UA *et al.* (2015) Randomized, double-blind, placebo-controlled study to investigate the pharmacodynamic interaction of 5-HT3 antagonist ondansetron and paracetamol in postoperative patients operated in an ENT department under local anesthesia. *Journal of Basic and Clinical Physiology and Pharmacology.* **26**: 217–222.
13 Neziri AY *et al.* (2012) Effect of intravenous tropisetron on modulation of pain and central hypersensitivity in chronic low back pain patients. *Pain.* **153**: 311–318.
14 Christidis N *et al.* (2015) Repeated tender point injections of granisetron alleviate chronic myofascial pain--a randomized, controlled, double-blinded trial. *Journal of Headache and Pain.* **16**: 104.
15 Stratz T and Muller W (2004) Treatment of chronic low back pain with tropisetron. *Scandinavian Journal of Rheumatology.* **119**: 76–78.
16 Muller W and Stratz T (2004) Local treatment of tendinopathies and myofascial pain syndromes with the 5-HT3 receptor antagonist tropisetron. *Scandinavian Journal of Rheumatology.* **119**: 44–48.
17 Saito M *et al.* (2009) Palonosetron plus dexamethasone versus granisetron plus dexamethasone for prevention of nausea and vomiting during chemotherapy: a double-blind, double-dummy, randomised, comparative phase III trial. *Lancet Oncology.* **10**: 115-124.
18 Goodin S and Cunningham R (2002) 5-HT3-receptor antagonists for the treatment of nausea and vomiting: a reappraisal of their side-effect profile. *The Oncologist.* **7**: 424–436.
19 Perez EA *et al.* (1997) Efficacy and safety of different doses of granisetron for the prophylaxis of cisplatin-induced emesis. *Support Care Cancer.* **5**: 31–37.
20 Perez E *et al.* (1997) Efficacy and safety of oral granisetron versus IV ondansetron in prevention of moderately emetogenic chemotherapy-induced nausea and vomiting. *Proceedings of the American Society of Clinical Oncology.* **16**: 149.
21 Gralla R *et al.* (1997) Can an oral antiemetic regimen be as effective as intravenous treatment against cisplatin: results of a 1054 patient randomized study of oral granisetron versus IV ondansetron. *Proceedings of the American Society of Clinical Oncology.* **16**: 178.
22 Minami M (2003) Granisetron: is there a dose-response effect on nausea and vomiting? *Cancer Chemotherapy and Pharmacology.* **52**: 89–98.
23 Kris MG *et al.* (2006) American Society of Clinical Oncology guideline for antiemetics in oncology: update 2006. *Journal of Clinical Oncology.* **24**: 2932-2947.
24 MHRA (2013) Ondansetron for intravenous use: dose dependent QT interval prolongation – new posology. *Drug Safety Update.* **6**: www.mhra.gov.uk/safetyinformation

Updated (minor change) November 2021

ANTI-EPILEPTICS

Indications: (Authorized indications vary between products; consult SPC for details.) Neuropathic pain, epilepsy, status epilepticus, mania, anxiety, †hyperactive delirium, †agitation and anxiety in dementia, †refractory agitation in the imminently dying, †sweats and hot flushes, †refractory hiccup, †restless legs syndrome, †spasticity, †refractory cough, †nausea and vomiting, †pruritus, †alcohol withdrawal.

Pharmacology

Anti-epileptic drugs inhibit rapidly firing neurones and can thereby impact on symptoms arising from excessive neuronal activity in any part of the nervous system. They are structurally and functionally diverse. Some reduce action potential generation or excitatory neurotransmission. Others increase the GABA-mediated inhibition of rapidly firing neurones (Table 1 and Figure 1).

The relationship between clinical activity and mode of action is not fully understood. Further, clinically relevant differences exist between anti-epileptics acting in similar ways, and additional actions contribute to the beneficial and/or undesirable effects of some. Thus, the choice of drug remains partly empirical.[1]

Table 1 Mechanisms of action of selected anti-epileptics[1–10]

	Membrane stabilizers		*↓Neurotransmitter release*			*↓Excitatory transmission*	*↑Inhibitory transmission (GABAmimetics)*	*Altered excitability/ neuroplasticity*	
	Na-channel blocker	*K-channel opener*	*Ca-channel blocker*		*↓Vesicle release (SV2A)*	*AMPA antagonist*	*↑GABA$_A$-receptor activation*	*↓NMDA receptor*	*Ca-channel blocker (T type)*
			(N, P/Q type)	*(R type)*					
Benzodiazepines							++		
Carbamazepine	++								
Ethosuximide									++
Gabapentin		+	++					+	
Lacosamide	++					+			
Lamotrigine	++		++	++					
Levetiracetam/ brivaracetam					++				
Oxcarbazepine/ eslicarbazepine *acetate*[a]	++	+							
Phenobarbital							++		
Phenytoin	++								
Pregabalin			++					+	
Topiramate	++			++			++		
Valproate	+[c]	+					+[b,c]	+[c]	+[c]

++ predominant action, + putative or non-predominant action.

a. eslicarbazepine *acetate* and oxcarbazepine are pro-drugs of the same active metabolite, (es)licarbazepine (also see p.304)

b. valproate affects both synthesis and re-uptake/breakdown of GABA in selected brain regions

c. although many anti-epileptics have more than one mode of action, valproate in particular is thought to have no predominant mode of action, helping to explain its broad spectrum of activity (see p.307).

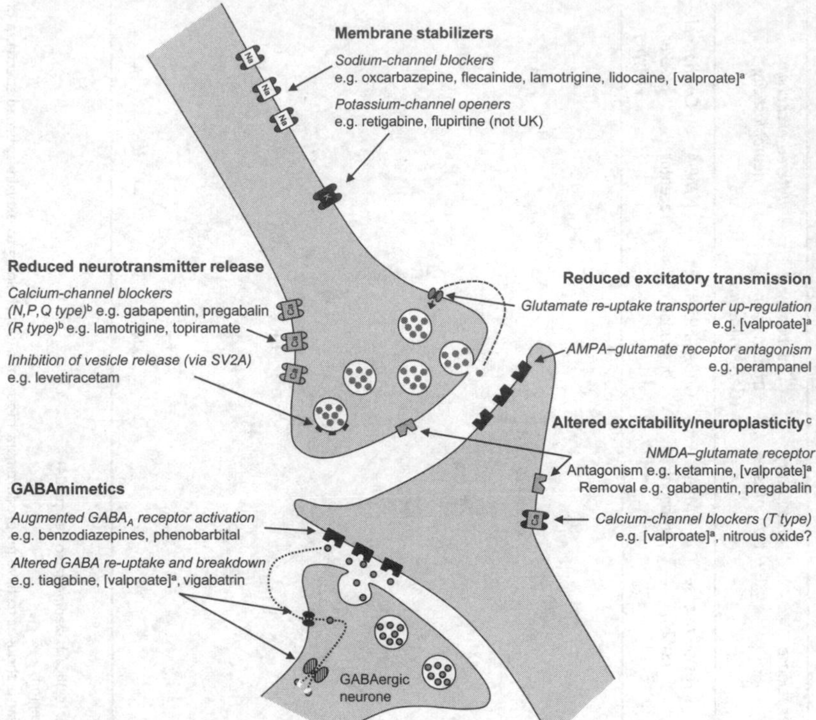

Figure 1 Mechanisms of action of anti-epileptics and related drugs.[1–8,11,12] Square brackets indicate a contributory, but not predominant, action of the anti-epileptic.

a. although many anti-epileptics have more than one mode of action, valproate in particular is thought to have no single predominant action (see p.307)
b. arriving action potentials open pre-synaptic N-, P-, Q- and R-type calcium channels. The resulting calcium influx triggers neurotransmitter release (see p.297)
c. both NMDA–glutamate receptors and T-type calcium channels affect neuronal excitability, threshold setting and neuroplasticity. T-type calcium channels also affect neuronal firing patterns, e.g. tonic or burst firing, in nociceptive neurones and the thalamus (burst firing in the latter is implicated in absence seizures).

Membrane stabilizers: sodium-channel blockers and potassium-channel openers

Sodium channels initiate and propagate action potentials (nerve 'firing') by transiently opening to allow sodium to enter the nerve, reversing the voltage across its membrane (depolarisation). Potassium channels open more slowly, allowing potassium to leave the nerve and return the voltage to normal (repolarisation). The transport of sodium channels is disrupted by nerve injury, leading to their accumulation, creating foci of ectopic action potential generation.[13]

Sodium-channel blockers have two distinct effects, depending on their concentration. *High* concentrations, seen with local administration, block action potential propagation, resulting in local anaesthesia. *Low* concentrations, seen with systemic administration, are insufficient to affect action potential propagation but can selectively accumulate on rapidly firing neurones ('use-dependent block'). Thus, they inhibit the ectopic foci seen on damaged neurones ('membrane stabilization'), thereby relieving neuropathic pain.[14] Several classes of drug act in this way:

- some anti-epileptics, e.g. **oxcarbazepine** (p.304), **carbamazepine**, **lamotrigine**, **lacosamide**, **phenytoin**
- local anaesthetics, e.g. **lidocaine** (p.77)
- class I anti-arrhythmics, e.g. **flecainide** (p.80).

However, the duration of blockade before the drug dissociates from the channel, and the relative impact of the drug on different rates of channel inactivation (slow vs. fast), varies.[15] Further, some drugs act on targets other than sodium channels. This creates important clinical differences between such drugs.

Subtype-selective blockers are of interest because some sodium-channel subtypes have distinct functions; e.g. inherited abnormalities of one subtype ($Na_v1.7$) cause congenital insensitivity to pain while leaving other senses unaffected.[16] However, results of RCTs have been disappointing.[17,18]

The analgesic **flupirtine** (not UK) and the anti-epileptic **retigabine** exert a membrane-stabilizing effect by prolonging the duration of potassium channel opening, thus hyperpolarizing the cell membrane.[12]

Reduced neurotransmitter release: $\alpha 2\delta$ and SV2A ligands

Gabapentin and **pregabalin** bind to the $\alpha 2\delta$ subunit responsible for channel trafficking. Thus, they remove pre-synaptic NMDA-receptor and voltage-gated calcium channels (N-, P/Q-type) from the cell surface, reducing excitability and the calcium influx responsible for triggering neurotransmitter release (see p.297). Spinal calcium channels are also targeted by **lamotrigine**, **topiramate** and **ziconotide** (an analgesic given IT).

Levetiracetam and **brivaracetam** bind SV2A, a synaptic vesicle protein involved in neurotransmitter release from the vesicle (see p.312).

GABAmimetics

Barbiturates and benzodiazepines affect $GABA_A$-receptors, binding at sites distinct from GABA itself (allosteric modulation). Benzodiazepines increase the receptors' affinity for GABA; barbiturates prolong channel opening (see p.163, p.315 and Table 1).[9]

Tiagabine and **vigabatrin** inhibit GABA re-uptake transporters and GABA transaminase, the enzyme responsible for GABA breakdown, respectively. **Valproate** probably also affects GABA metabolism.

Miscellaneous modes of action

The broad spectrum of efficacy of **valproate** is explained by its multiple actions, including blockade of sodium channels and T-type calcium channels. The latter are involved in the regulation of pain excitation thresholds in a 'T-rich' subset of peripheral nociceptors and have been implicated in neuropathic pain.[19,20] However, an RCT of the T-type calcium channel blocker **ethosuximide** for neuropathic pain was stopped early because of poor tolerability.[21]

The endocannabinoid system is another important inhibitory neurotransmitter system. However, cannabinoids have a generally disappointing analgesic effect (see p.251). Although **cannabidiol** is authorized for two rare childhood epilepsy syndromes, their response to treatment differs significantly from that of other forms of epilepsy. Further, the RCTs used to obtain the marketing authorizations for these syndromes have been strongly criticized. Thus, beyond these specific syndromes, cannabinoids do not have an established role in epilepsy.

Pharmacogenetics and pharmacokinetics

The genes responsible for some inherited epilepsies (genes encoding sodium and potassium channels, NMDA and GABA receptors) have been identified, leading to improved classification and drug selection; e.g. a polymorphism in the gene (SCN1A) encoding the sodium-channel α-subunit has been linked to **carbamazepine**-resistant epilepsy.[22]

Genetic factors also affect pharmacokinetics and the risk of undesirable effects. Two poor metabolizer CYP2C9 alleles (which occur in 10–20% of Caucasians, 10% of Japanese, and 1–5% of Asians and Africans) reduce the mean effective daily **phenytoin** dose by 20–40%.[23] Human leukocyte antigen (HLA) genotype is associated with the risk of serious skin reactions, e.g. Stevens–Johnson syndrome, toxic epidermal necrolysis (TEN) and drug rash with eosinophilia (DRESS) in patients taking **carbamazepine**, **eslicarbazepine** ***acetate***, **oxcarbazepine**, **phenytoin** or **lamotrigine**.[24,25] The UK MHRA recommends testing HLA B*1502 status before **carbamazepine** is started in people of Han Chinese, Hong Kong Chinese or Thai origin.[26] Similarly, the manufacturers of **oxcarbazepine** and **eslicarbazepine** ***acetate*** recommend HLA B*1502 testing where possible.

Table 2 Pharmacokinetic details of selected anti-epileptics[27–37]

Drug	*Bio-availability PO (%)*	*T_{max} (h)*	*Plasma protein binding (%)*	*Plasma halflife (h)*	*Fate*
Brivaracetam	≥95	1	≤20	9	CYP2C19; hepatic and non-hepatic hydrolysis
Carbamazepine	80	4–8	75	8–24	CYP3A4, CYP2C8[a]
Clonazepam	≥80	1–4	80–90	30–40	CYP3A
Diazepam	≥80	1–3	95–98	24–48, 48–120[b]	CYP2C19, CYP3A4[a]
Eslicarbazepine *acetate*[c]	>90	2–3	<40	<2 10-20h[a]	Hepatic hydrolysis to eslicarbazepine[c], which then undergoes glucuronidation
Gabapentin	30–75[d]	2–3	0	5–9	Excreted unchanged
Lacosamide	≥95	0.5–4	<30	13	CYP2C19 (40% excreted unchanged)
Lamotrigine	98	1–4	55	15–35, 8–20[e], 30–90[f]	Glucuronidation
Levetiracetam	≥95	1–2	<10	6–8	Non-hepatic hydrolysis (70% excreted unchanged)
Oxcarbazepine[c]	≥95	1–6	65, 40[a]	1–5, 7–20[a]	Cytosolic keto-reduction to licarbazepine[c], which then undergoes glucuronidation[a]
Perampanel	≥95	0.25–2	95	66–90	CYP3A4, then glucuronidation
Phenobarbital	≥90	2–12	50	72–144	CYP2C9 (25% excreted unchanged)
Phenytoin	90–95	4–8	90	10–70[d]	CYP2C9
Pregabalin	>90	1–2	0	5–9[g]	Excreted unchanged
Topiramate	≥80	1–4	13	20–30, 8–15[e]	Multiple pathways (>60% excreted unchanged)
Valproate	95	1–2[h]	90	9–18, 5–12[e]	Multiple pathways[a]
Zonisamide	≥50	1–4	50	50–70, 25–35[e]	CYP3A4 (15–30% excreted unchanged)

a. biologically active metabolites
b. nordiazepam, active metabolite
c. eslicarbazepine *acetate* and oxcarbazepine are pro-drugs of the same active metabolite, (es)licarbazepine (also see p.304)
d. dose or plasma-concentration dependent
e. with concurrent enzyme inducers
f. with concurrent valproate
g. >2 days in severe renal impairment and haemodialysis patients

The pharmacokinetics of anti-epileptics are summarized in Table 2. Whereas absorption is generally unaffected by increasing age, the volume of distribution may change (reduced albumin, total body water and lean:fat mass ratio) and elimination rates slow (altered metabolism, renal function and volume of distribution).[26,27]

Cautions

Safety concerns with **vigabatrin** (visual field deficits) and **felbamate** (not UK; aplastic anaemia and hepatic failure) limit their use to refractory epilepsy under specialist supervision when all other measures have failed.

Driving

In the UK, patients with epilepsy must notify the DVLA. Generally, a seizure-free period of 1 year is required before driving can resume (longer for heavy goods vehicles), although this varies (e.g. where a seizure was due to a transient illness). The DVLA must also be notified of any subsequent change of anti-epileptic medication, when a further 6-month seizure-free period may be required.[38]

Skin rashes and cross-reactive hypersensitivity

In relation to skin rashes:[24]

- cross-reactive hypersensitivity between **carbamazepine**, **eslicarbazepine *acetate***, **oxcarbazepine**, **phenobarbital**, **phenytoin** and TCAs: use alternative if possible
- **zonisamide**: avoid if hypersensitive to sulfonamides
- **lamotrigine**: increased risk of rash if rapidly titrated, with concurrent **valproate** or if a rash occurred with a previous anti-epileptic.

Hepatic impairment

With the exception of **gabapentin**, **pregabalin** and **vigabatrin**, the manufacturers advise caution with all the anti-epileptics listed in Table 2 (i.e. lower initial doses, slower titration and careful monitoring). Additional advice is given in the individual monographs and summarized in Chapter 18, p.769. Previous or concurrent hepatic disease increases the risk of **valproate**- and **carbamazepine**-related hepatic failure. However, no specific information is available about the risks with hepatic metastases, which do not generally affect the hepatic metabolism of drugs unless there is severe hepatic impairment/cirrhosis.[39,40]

Renal impairment

Caution should be taken with all the anti-epileptics listed in Table 2 (i.e. lower initial doses, slower titration and careful monitoring); anti-epileptics differ in their potential to cause toxicity when renal function is impaired (see Chapter 17, p.738). Specific advice on dose adjustment in all stages of renal impairment is available in the individual monographs for **gabapentin** (see p.300), **levetiracetam** (see p.313) and **pregabalin** (see p.301). Further, there are occasional reports of renal failure possibly caused by **gabapentin** and **pregabalin**.

Females of childbearing age

Consider teratogenicity when choosing an anti-epileptic; for **valproate**, specific additional precautions apply (see p.308).[41] Enquire about existing oral contraceptive use if starting an enzyme-inducing anti-epileptic (see Drug interactions).

Additional cautions with specific anti-epileptics

- atrioventricular block: **carbamazepine** and **oxcarbazepine** may cause complete block
- previous bone marrow suppression: **carbamazepine**; possible increased risk
- heart failure: **oxcarbazepine** and **pregabalin**; fluid retention can exacerbate; monitor weight and plasma sodium
- patients at high risk of drug abuse: **gabapentin** and **pregabalin**.[42–44]

Drug interactions

Interactions are described in individual drug monographs:

- **gabapentin** (p.297), **levetiracetam** (p.312) and **pregabalin** (p.297) have no clinically significant pharmacokinetic interactions
- **oxcarbazepine** (p.304) can induce some hepatic enzymes, but not often to a clinically significant extent (an exception is hormonal oral contraceptives)
- **valproate** (p.307) has a few important drug interactions via different mechanisms
- **carbamazepine** (Table 3), **phenobarbital** (p.315) and **phenytoin** (Table 3) are potent hepatic enzyme inducers (see Chapter 19, p.785) resulting in numerous clinically important interactions
- **carbamazepine** and **phenytoin** are metabolized by various CYP450 enzymes (Table 2) and are thus affected by CYP450 enzyme inhibitors and inducers:
  - ▷ **diltiazem, fluconazole, fluoxetine, fluvoxamine, miconazole, verapamil** can cause **carbamazepine** and **phenytoin** toxicity
  - ▷ **clarithromycin, erythromycin** can cause **carbamazepine** toxicity
  - ▷ **cimetidine, ticlopidine, voriconazole** can cause **phenytoin** toxicity
  - ▷ **rifampicin** *reduces* **phenytoin** plasma concentrations
- interactions between two or more anti-epileptics can be complex and unpredictable; plasma concentrations of each drug may be increased, decreased or unchanged.[45]

For full details see the SPCs for the individual anti-epileptic drugs.

Undesirable effects

Despite their diverse actions and structures, anti-epileptics share many undesirable effects. Their relative incidence is often similar.[46,47]

All anti-epileptics cause psychotropic and CNS-depressant effects, including drowsiness, ataxia, cognitive impairment, agitation, diplopia and dizziness. Psychiatric effects (e.g. depression, psychosis, irritability, lability) are commonest with **levetiracetam, perampanel, phenobarbital, tiagabine, topiramate, vigabatrin** and **zonisamide.**[48,49] Cognitive impairment is worst with **phenobarbital** and least with newer anti-epileptics and **valproate.**[31,50] Ataxia is commonest with **phenytoin** and **carbamazepine.**[51]

Most anti-epileptics cause haematological derangements. These are often asymptomatic and may not require stopping the drug (see SPCs for advice). Severe derangement (e.g. aplastic anaemia, agranulocytosis) is reported particularly with **felbamate** (not UK; limiting use) and **carbamazepine** (monitor blood counts). Folate deficiency occurs with enzyme inducers, e.g. **phenytoin**.

Biochemical derangements (particularly of LFTs) are also common but are generally asymptomatic. Albeit rarely, hepatic failure is seen with many anti-epileptics, again particularly with **felbamate** (also limiting its use) and **carbamazepine** (where symptoms of hepatic disease and LFTs should be monitored), as well as with newer anti-epileptics. The incidence of hepatic failure for other anti-epileptics compared with that for **carbamazepine** is unknown. Pancreatitis affects 1 in 3,000 users of **valproate.**[52] It also occurs with many newer anti-epileptics, but the incidence of pancreatitis for newer anti-epileptics compared with that for **valproate** is unknown. Hyponatraemia is commonest with **carbamazepine** and **oxcarbazepine.**[53] Transient rashes are particularly associated with **lamotrigine**, **carbamazepine** and **oxcarbazepine**. Risk factors include rashes with previous anti-epileptics, higher starting doses and rapid titration (and, with **lamotrigine**, childhood and concurrent **valproate**).

Undesirable effects seen with particular anti-epileptics include: urolithiasis (**topiramate** and **zonisamide**); vitamin deficiencies (hepatic enzyme inducers);[53] hyperammonaemic encephalopathy (**valproate**); coarse facies, acne, hirsutism and gingival hypertrophy (**phenytoin**); complex regional pain syndrome (**phenobarbital**). **Phenytoin** also exhibits distinct undesirable effects at supratherapeutic levels (Box A) or after rapid high-dose IV infusion (purple glove syndrome, a painful discolouration seen distal to the infusion site in <6% of patients).[54] Although severe rashes, e.g. Stevens–Johnson syndrome, are reported with all anti-epileptics, they are commonest with **carbamazepine**, **clorazepate**, **lamotrigine**, **phenytoin**, **rufinamide** and **zonisamide.**[55] Specific HLA types are known to predispose specific groups to **carbamazepine**-, **eslicarbazepine** ***acetate***-, **oxcarbazepine**- and **phenytoin**-related serious skin reactions (see Pharmacogenetics and pharmacokinetics, p.283).

Table 3 Clinically important drug interactions with the potent enzyme-inducing drugs carbamazepine and phenytoin resulting in *decreased* plasma concentrations and possible lack of effect[a,45]

Drug class	*Drug plasma concentration decreased by carbamazepine or phenytoin*
Anti-arrhythmics	Amiodarone[b,c], disopyramide, mexiletine[b]
Antibacterials	Doxycycline
Anticoagulants	Apixaban, dabigatran, edoxaban, rivaroxaban, warfarin (and other coumarins)
Antidepressants	Citalopram[d], mianserin, mirtazapine, paroxetine, sertraline, TCAs (all)[d]
Anti-epileptics[e]	Carbamazepine, ethosuximide, lamotrigine, perampanel, phenytoin, primidone, tiagabine, topiramate, valproate, zonisamide
Antifungals	Itraconazole[c], posaconazole[c], voriconazole[c]
Antipsychotics	Clozapine, haloperidol[c], olanzapine[d], quetiapine, risperidone
Antiretrovirals/antivirals	Seek specialist advice
Benzodiazepines[c] and z-drugs	Alprazolam, diazepam, midazolam, zolpidem[d]
Bronchodilators	Theophylline
Calcium-channel blockers	All[c]
Corticosteroids	All
Cytotoxics and immunomodulators	Seek specialist advice
Hormone antagonists	Toremifene
Hormonal contraceptives and hormone replacement therapy	All
Neurokinin-1 antagonists	Aprepitant, fosaprepitant
Non-opioid analgesics	Paracetamol[f]
Opioid analgesics	Alfentanil, buprenorphine, fentanyl, methadone, oxycodone, tramadol
Opioid antagonists	Naldemedine, naloxegol
Miscellaneous	Digoxin[b], levothyroxine, tolvaptan

a. limited to classes of drugs with the best evidence for clinically significant interactions in palliative care. However, this is not an exhaustive list, and interactions can occur unpredictably; seek advice, particularly if unexpected undesirable effects or loss of benefit occur

b. interaction only reported for phenytoin

c. increased carbamazepine or phenytoin plasma concentrations can also occur

d. interaction only reported for carbamazepine

e. interactions between anti-epileptic drugs are complex and unpredictable; plasma concentrations of either drug may be increased, decreased or unchanged

f. hepatotoxic metabolites may be increased (see p.334).

Suicide

Overall, anti-epileptic drugs are associated with suicidal thoughts or behaviour in 1 in 500 patients from the start of treatment onwards. Although a higher risk with **pregabalin** has been suggested compared with **gabapentin**, the findings were confounded by indication: psychiatric illness was twice as common among users of **pregabalin**.[56] Suicide risk is considered a class effect; all patients should be monitored for suicidal ideation and advised to report any mood disturbance or suicidal thoughts to a health professional.[48,57–59]

Box A Phenytoin toxicity[60]

Clinical features

Phenytoin toxicity generally manifests as a syndrome of cerebellar, vestibular and ocular effects, including some or all of the following:

- nystagmus:
  - ▷ on lateral gaze only (early sign)
  - ▷ spontaneous (more severe toxicity)
- blurred vision/diplopia
- slurred speech
- ataxia.

These may be accompanied by lethargy and/or delirium. Some patients experience break-through seizures (or an increase in the frequency of seizures) when the free phenytoin plasma concentration increases to toxic levels.

Evaluation

If phenytoin toxicity is suspected, check the plasma phenytoin concentration (and plasma albumin) just before the next dose is due. The normal therapeutic range is 40–80micromol/L (10–20microgram/mL). Because phenytoin is highly protein-bound, it is important to correct the observed concentration in patients with a low albumin:

$$\text{Corrected total phenytoin concentration (normal renal function)} = \frac{\text{observed concentration}}{(0.02 \times \text{albumin [g/L]}) + 0.1}$$

$$\text{Corrected total phenytoin concentration (in end-stage renal failure)} = \frac{\text{observed concentration}}{(0.01 \times \text{albumin [g/L]}) + 0.1}$$

Note: the units for albumin must be g/L; however, the formulae can be used for whatever units the phenytoin concentration is reported in.

Phenytoin toxicity can be present despite being within the therapeutic range; if necessary, make the diagnosis on clinical features alone and act accordingly.

Management

There is no specific antidote to phenytoin. If the patient has clinical features suggestive of toxicity, omit one or more doses, depending on severity of symptoms, and reduce subsequent doses to a previous non-toxic level. Generally, symptoms resolve when the plasma phenytoin concentration falls, although permanent cerebellar ataxia and peripheral neuropathy have been recorded.[61]

Treat break-through seizures with benzodiazepines (see p.290) because other anti-epileptic drugs may exacerbate toxicity. If the frequency of seizures increases as the phenytoin toxicity drops, obtain advice from a neurologist.

Use of anti-epileptics in palliative care

Particularly when prescribing more than one anti-epileptic, it is important to consider:

- pharmacokinetic drug–drug interactions
- seizure type (particularly in long-standing epilepsy; generalized seizures may be precipitated by **carbamazepine**, **oxcarbazepine**, **gabapentin**, **tiagabine** and **vigabatrin**)
- additive cognitive impairment.

Switching between formulations

The MHRA recommends *not* switching between brands of anti-epileptics *when used for epilepsy*, except for **brivaracetam**, **ethosuximide**, **gabapentin**, **lacosamide**, **levetiracetam**, **pregabalin**, **tiagabine** and **vigabatrin**.[62]

Switching between different manufacturers' products or brands should be avoided if possible, because bio-availability and duration of action may differ. Both loss of effect and new undesirable effects have been reported after switching.[62] However, if there is a delay in obtaining the patient's usual brand, *it is better to give a different brand than to miss a dose*.

Phenytoin 300mg as capsules is equivalent to 270mg as oral solution.

Neuropathic pain

Pregabalin and **gabapentin** are commonly used first-line choices.[63] They are authorized for peripheral neuropathic pain, have few drug interactions and have been studied in a range of settings, including cancer-related pain (see p.297).[64–75] Despite limited evidence of efficacy, the marketing authorization for **pregabalin** also includes central neuropathic pain.[74]

Carbamazepine is an authorized first-line treatment for trigeminal neuralgia. It has long been used off-label for other neuropathic pains. However, RCTs are small, short (mostly <4 weeks) and use outcome measures of uncertain clinical significance.[76] Further, it requires slow titration and particular care with regard to drug interactions. Although results of RCTs of **oxcarbazepine** in diabetic neuropathy show inconsistent benefit *overall*, clinical examination may identify subgroups who *are* likely to benefit (see p.304). Of other membrane stabilizers, **lamotrigine** appears ineffective[77] and RCTs of **phenytoin** are small, short (≤5 weeks) and give conflicting results.[78] **Lacosamide** is reported to improve oxaliplatin-related neuropathic pain[79] and can be given CSCI,[80] but in RCTs of other peripheral neuropathic pains, it is generally less effective than gabapentinoids (NNT 10–12 vs. 6).[81,82]

Valproate is used in some centres, particularly when the parenteral route is required (it can be given CSCI). Benefit is reported for cancer-related neuropathic pain,[83,84] but the results of RCTs in non-cancer pain are conflicting (see p.307)[85] and international guidelines do not recommend its use.[63,86] It appears to be well tolerated with lower rates of discontinuation because of undesirable effects (<5%)[85] compared with **gabapentin** (10%)[75] and **pregabalin** (20–30%)[74] in similar populations.

Clonazepam is reported to improve both cancer-related and non-cancer neuropathic pain (see p.173). It has anxiolytic and muscle-relaxant properties and can be given SC (not UK), leading to its use in selected palliative care patients despite the absence of supporting RCTs.[87]

Topiramate is as effective as **carbamazepine** for trigeminal neuralgia.[88] It is also reported to improve cancer-related neuropathic pain; most patients had already tried **gabapentin**, a tricyclic antidepressant and **methadone.**[89] In a cross-over RCT in multiple sclerosis, more patients preferred **topiramate** than placebo (12 vs. 2; n=32).[90] However, results of RCTs in non-cancer neuropathic pain (diabetic neuropathy, lumbar radicular pain) do not show consistent benefit.[91] Slow titration and adequate hydration are required to minimize undesirable CNS effects and the risk of urolithiasis, respectively. Studies often gave **topiramate** in divided doses, but because the halflife is 20–30h, this is unlikely to be necessary:

- start with **topiramate** 25mg PO at bedtime
- if necessary, increase in 25mg increments every 1–2 weeks
- typical effective dose ≤200mg/24h.[88–90]

Ethosuximide, **levetiracetam** (p.312) and **zonisamide** are ineffective for neuropathic pain.[21,92,93]

Few studies have compared gabapentinoids with anti-epileptics with different mechanisms of action. In painful diabetic neuropathy, although an RCT found **pregabalin** to be superior to **carbamazepine** and **venlafaxine**, doses were fixed, not titrated;[94] in a single-blind RCT, the efficacy of **pregabalin** and **oxcarbazepine** was similar, but neither was titrated to the maximum tolerated dose (see p.304).

Switching vs. combining anti-epileptics for neuropathic pain

If the first-choice treatment fails, switch to a drug with a different mechanism of action (e.g. an antidepressant; see p.210). For example, **duloxetine** is more effective than **pregabalin** for pain unresponsive to **gabapentin.**[95]

Drugs with different mechanisms of action are often used in combination (see Adjuvant analgesics, p.325), particularly if the first-choice treatment is partially successful. The combination of **gabapentin** or **pregabalin** with **morphine**, **imipramine** or **nortriptyline** is superior to any treatment alone.[96–100] An open-label trial in cancer pain with a neuropathic component also found combined treatment with **gabapentin** to be superior to **morphine** alone.[101]

Combinations of ≥2 anti-epileptics are used less commonly. Undesirable effects may be increased, and alternative options are often more appropriate (e.g. antidepressants, opioids, **ketamine**, interventional anaesthesia; also see Adjuvant analgesics, p.325). Where a second anti-epileptic drug is added, the first is generally withdrawn, although examples of combined use are reported. Improvements in efficacy and tolerability have been described in 11 patients with multiple sclerosis whose trigeminal neuralgia had been unsatisfactorily controlled by

carbamazepine or **lamotrigine**. The addition of **gabapentin** brought relief in 10 patients. The initial drug was reduced to the minimal effective dose, with improved overall tolerability, but could not be withdrawn completely in any patient, suggesting that both **carbamazepine/lamotrigine** and **gabapentin** were contributing to overall relief.[102]

Doses are described in individual monographs: **gabapentin** and **pregabalin** (p.297), **oxcarbazepine** (p.304) and **valproate** (p.307).

Epilepsy

Overtreatment with anti-epileptic drugs is common. Seek specialist advice where the diagnosis of seizures or the dose or choice of anti-epileptic drug is in doubt.

When to start treatment

Generally, anti-epileptic drugs are started after a first seizure when an irreversible underlying focal lesion makes further seizures likely, e.g. cerebral tumour, multiple sclerosis. In the absence of a focal lesion, the risk is lower and an anti-epileptic is generally withheld unless a second seizure occurs.[103]

Anti-epileptics should *not* be used *prophylactically* in the absence of a history of seizures; in RCTs, they do not reduce the risk.[104] Peri-neurosurgical use is a possible exception, but results are conflicting.[105–107]

Choice of drug

Seizures caused by focal brain lesions are, by definition, focal onset, even if this is obscured by rapid secondary generalization. Thus, generally in palliative care, factors other than seizure classification influence the choice of anti-epileptic, e.g. the potential for drug interactions, co-morbidities, route, and the time taken to reach a therapeutic dose.[108]

Levetiracetam is a first-line choice for seizures in palliative care. An observational study suggests it is more effective than **valproate** for seizures due to gliomas.[109] **Oxcarbazepine** and **valproate** are used second-line or in selected patients, e.g. those with co-existent neuropathic pain (Box B). Other anti-epileptic options for focal seizures are less preferable because of the need for gradual titration over several weeks (**carbamazepine, lamotrigine**),[110] greater cost (**lacosamide**),[111,112] poorer tolerability (**carbamazepine, gabapentin**)[113] and numerous drug interactions (**carbamazepine, phenobarbital, phenytoin**).[114]

Because of the risk of teratogenicity with some anti-epileptics, particularly **valproate**, obtain specialist advice when treating women of childbearing age (see Cautions and p.307).

Titrating, switching or combining for persistent seizures

A response, if it occurs, is generally seen with relatively low doses, e.g.:[122–126]

- **carbamazepine** 400–600mg/24h
- **lamotrigine** 150–200mg/24h
- **levetiracetam** 1,000–1,500mg/24h
- **oxcarbazepine** 600–900mg/24h
- **valproate** 750–1,000mg/24h.

If seizures persist, consider:[9,123,125,127,128]

- further titration, particularly if there has been a partial response and minimal undesirable effects
- switching to an alternative anti-epileptic drug, particularly if the initial choice is poorly tolerated
- adding a second anti-epileptic drug with a different mechanism of action (see Box B and Table 1), particularly if there has been an inadequate response to two trials of monotherapy.

Do not combine three or more anti-epileptics except on specialist advice; additional benefit is rare.[129]

For doses, see the individual monographs for **gabapentin** and **pregabalin** (p.297), **levetiracetam** (p.312), **oxcarbazepine** (p.304), **valproate** (p.307), or the manufacturer's SPC.

Convulsive status epilepticus

Figure 2 is modified from NICE guidance.[110] **Midazolam, levetiracetam** and **phenobarbital** have been given preference over **lorazepam** and **phenytoin** because they are more likely to be immediately available in many palliative care units and/or a maintenance dose can be given SC/CSCI.

Box B Anti-epileptics for seizures in palliative care[108,109,114–120]

First-line

***Levetiracetam*[a]**

Can be titrated rapidly, IV or SC if necessary (see p.312); no clinically significant drug interactions.

Second-line

***Oxcarbazepine*[a]**

Fewer drug interactions than with carbamazepine and phenytoin; effective doses achieved more quickly than with lamotrigine and carbamazepine; may have a role in neuropathic pain (see p.304).

***Valproate*[a,b]**

Can be titrated rapidly, IV or SC if necessary; may have a role in agitation and neuropathic pain (see p.307).

Last days of life

Midazolam

Generally first-line because of familiarity, availability, benefit in concurrent symptoms and compatibility with other drugs CSCI (see p.170).

Phenobarbital

Generally second-line where seizures are unresponsive to midazolam (see p.315).

a. although other anti-epileptic options for focal seizures exist, they are less preferable (see Choice of drug)

b. despite abnormal *in vitro* haemostasis, valproate has not been shown to increase neurosurgical bleeding complications.[121] Nonetheless, if surgery is planned, before starting valproate, discuss with the neurosurgical team.

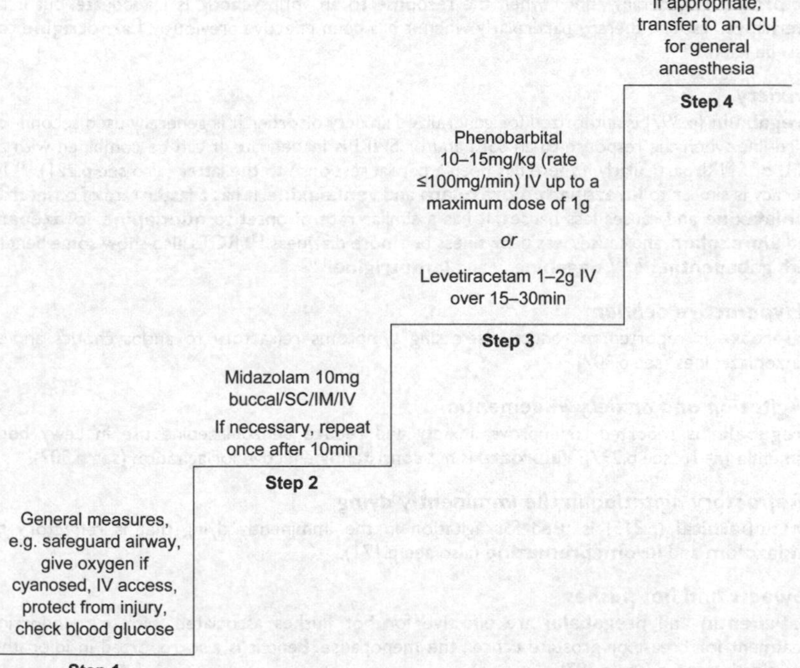
If appropriate, transfer to an ICU for general anaesthesia
Step 4
Phenobarbital 10–15mg/kg (rate ≤100mg/min) IV up to a maximum dose of 1g
or
Levetiracetam 1–2g IV over 15–30min
Step 3
Midazolam 10mg buccal/SC/IM/IV
If necessary, repeat once after 10min
Step 2
General measures, e.g. safeguard airway, give oxygen if cyanosed, IV access, protect from injury, check blood glucose
Step 1

Figure 2 Management of status epilepticus in adults. See text for more detail.

Hypoglycaemia should be excluded in all patients. If alcoholism or severely impaired nutrition is suspected, give **thiamine** 250mg IV (as one pair of Pabrinex IV high potency ampoules).

Although IV **lorazepam** is generally recommended for the control of status epilepticus, IM **midazolam** is as effective (see p.170). **Midazolam** 10mg †buccally/SC or **diazepam** 10–20mg PR are alternatives (see p.170).

Phenobarbital injection is diluted 1 in 10 with sodium chloride 0.9% for IV administration. It can also be given IM undiluted. Some centres administer an initial 10–15mg/kg loading dose up to a maximum of 600mg in 100mL of sodium chloride 0.9% by SC infusion over 30min, with the subsequent maintenance dose given CSCI or by SC injection once daily (see p.317).

Levetiracetam is diluted in 100mL sodium chloride 0.9% or glucose 5% and infused IV over 15–30min. Its efficacy is comparable to **phenytoin**.[130] It can also be given by SC infusion over 30min (≤1g), with the subsequent maintenance dose given CSCI (see p.313).

Fosphenytoin, **phenytoin** and **valproate** are alternatives. **Fosphenytoin** can be given IV more rapidly than **phenytoin**. Both have narrow therapeutic ranges and require careful monitoring and safeguards to avoid toxicity;[131] see SPCs for details. **Valproate** is diluted in 50mL sodium chloride 0.9% and infused IV over 15–20min, with the subsequent maintenance dose given CIVI or CSCI (see p.309); its efficacy is comparable to that of **levetiracetam** and **phenytoin**.[130]

Non-convulsive seizures

Non-convulsive status epilepticus (NCSE) is characterized by seizure activity on an EEG but without associated tonic-clonic activity. The commonest presentations are confusion, blank staring and automatisms. Others include agitation, aggression, altered speech, hallucinations and myoclonus.[132] In one report, NCSE was diagnosed in 5% of patients admitted to a palliative care unit; of these, half responded to treatment with anti-epileptics.[133] If an EEG is not possible, consider a trial of treatment.[132]

Non-convulsive seizures are also common in dementia, and may present with recurrent episodes of transient symptoms, e.g. loss of speech, staring, déjà vu, metallic taste, epigastric discomfort.[120]

Mania

Valproate is generally added when the response to an antipsychotic is inadequate, but is an alternative first-line therapy particularly when it has been effective previously. **Lamotrigine** can also be used.[134]

Anxiety

Pregabalin (p.297) is authorized for generalized anxiety disorder. It is generally used second- or third-line when the response to an SSRI and/or SNRI is inadequate. It can be combined with an SSRI or SNRI, particularly if there has been a partial response to the latter (also see p.221).[135] Its efficacy is similar to **lorazepam**, **alprazolam** and **venlafaxine**. It has a faster rate of onset than **venlafaxine** and causes less nausea. It has a similar rate of onset to **quetiapine**, **lorazepam** and **alprazolam**, and causes less drowsiness but more dizziness.[136] RCTs also show some benefit with **gabapentin**,[137–139] **tiagabine**[140] and **lamotrigine**.[141]

†Hyperactive delirium

Valproate is reported to reduce distressing symptoms refractory to antipsychotics and/or benzodiazepines (see p.307).

†Agitation and anxiety in dementia

Pregabalin is reported to improve anxiety and reduce benzodiazepine use in Lewy body dementia (n=16; see p.297). **Valproate** is *not* consistently effective for agitation (see p.307).

†Refractory agitation in the imminently dying

Phenobarbital (p.315) is used for agitation in the imminently dying that is refractory to **midazolam** and **levomepromazine** (also see p.171).

†Sweats and hot flushes

Gabapentin and **pregabalin** are effective for hot flushes associated with, e.g. endocrine treatment for breast or prostate cancer, the menopause. Benefit is also reported in idiopathic sweating in cancer (see p.297).

†Refractory hiccup

Gabapentin and **pregabalin** are reported to be effective for hiccup (see p.297).

†Restless legs syndrome

Correct the correctable: treat iron deficiency; if taking antipsychotics or **metoclopramide**, reduce or switch to alternatives (see akathisia, p.805); consider regular exercise.[142,143] For symptomatic treatment, guidelines recommend:

- **gabapentin** or **pregabalin** first-line
- dopamimetics (e.g. **rotigotine**, **ropinirole**) second-line
- **opioids** third-line.[144]

Dopamimetics are not recommended first-line because they can exacerbate symptoms in the longer term (≥months). However, in palliative care, choice will be modified by prognosis and concurrent indications (e.g. pain).

†Spasticity

Gabapentin (p.297) and **levetiracetam** (p.312) are reported to improve spasticity in multiple sclerosis and hypoxic ischaemic encephalopathy, respectively.

†Refractory cough

Gabapentin and **pregabalin** improve cough that persists despite resolution of the initial cause.[145] Benefit probably relates to reducing cough reflex hypersensitivity, which is generally present in this group of patients (see p.154).

†Nausea and vomiting

Nausea and vomiting in those with CNS lesions (e.g. meningeal carcinomatosis)[146,147] or focal seizures[148] is reported to respond to **carbamazepine**, **valproate** or **levetiracetam**.

Given prophylactically, **gabapentin** reduces both postoperative and chemotherapy-induced nausea and vomiting (CINV).[149,150] Although a second RCT found no benefit, this may reflect good control of CINV in both the placebo and **gabapentin** groups; most received a long-acting $5HT_3$ antagonist.[151]

†Pruritus

Gabapentin and **pregabalin** (p.297) are used for uraemic, neuropathic and burns-related pruritus (also see p.825).

†Alcohol withdrawal

Benzodiazepines (p.171) reduce withdrawal symptoms, particularly seizures. **Gabapentin** (p.297) and **phenobarbital** (p.315) are alternatives if benzodiazepines are insufficient.[152,153]

Subcutaneous administration of anti-epileptics

The following anti-epileptics can be given SC/CSCI (see monographs for full details):

- **clonazepam** (not UK), **lorazepam** and **midazolam** (see Benzodiazepines, p.163)
- **lacosamide** (see below)
- **levetiracetam** (p.312)
- **phenobarbital** (p.315)
- **valproate** (p.307).

Lacosamide 200mg/20mL was administered undiluted SC over 10min. It was well tolerated and serum levels suggested a PO:SC dose ratio of 1:1.[80]

Stopping anti-epileptics

Abrupt cessation of long-term anti-epileptic therapy should be avoided because rebound seizures may be precipitated, even if use is for indications other than epilepsy.

The optimal rate of withdrawal is unknown, but a slow reduction (i.e. over many months) is believed to be particularly important for barbiturates and benzodiazepines.[154] Even with slow withdrawal, seizures recur in ≤60%.[155] Thus, specialist advice should be sought, particularly when seizure recurrence would be dangerous (e.g. for those driving, swimming).

For patients who lose the ability to swallow anti-epileptic medication, consider substituting PO medication with an SC alternative (see Subcutaneous administration of anti-epileptics). In the last days of life, generally **midazolam** is used (Box B). However, some anti-epileptics have a long halflife (Table 2) and, in a moribund patient, might continue to be effective for 2–3 days after the last PO dose. When patients are not imminently dying, a less-sedative alternative to **midazolam** is more appropriate, e.g. **levetiracetam, valproate** (Box B).

1 Perucca E (2011) The pharmacology of new antiepileptic drugs: does a novel mechanism of action really matter? *CNS Drugs*. **25**: 907–912.

2 Kay HY *et al.* (2015) M-current preservation contributes to anticonvulsant effects of valproic acid. *Journal of Clinical Investigation*. **125**: 3904–3914.

3 Loscher W (2002) Basic pharmacology of valproate: a review after 35 years of clinical use for the treatment of epilepsy. *CNS Drugs*. **16**: 669–694.

4 Holtkamp D *et al.* (2017) Activity of the anticonvulsant lacosamide in experimental and human epilepsy via selective effects on slow Na+ channel inactivation. *Epilepsia*. **58**: 27–41.

5 Klitgaard H *et al.* (2016) Brivaracetam: rationale for discovery and preclinical profile of a selective SV2A ligand for epilepsy treatment. *Epilepsia*. **57**: 538–548.

6 Kremer M *et al.* (2016) Antidepressants and gabapentinoids in neuropathic pain: Mechanistic insights. *Neuroscience*. **338**: 183–206.

7 Bourinet E *et al.* (2016) T-type calcium channels in neuropathic pain. *Pain*. **157 Suppl 1**: S15–S22.

8 Wormuth C *et al.* (2016) Review: Cav2.3 R-type voltage-gated Ca2+ channels - functional implications in convulsive and non-convulsive seizure activity. *Open Neurology Journal*. **10**: 99–126.

9 Brodie MJ (2016) Pharmacological treatment of drug-resistant epilepsy in adults: a practical guide. *Current Neurology and Neuroscience Reports*. **16**: 82.

10 Deng M *et al.* (2019) Presynaptic NMDA receptors control nociceptive transmission at the spinal cord level in neuropathic pain. *Cellular and Molecular Life Sciences*. **76**: 1889–1899.

11 Hobo S (2012) Valproate upregulates glutamate transporters in rat spinal cord after peripheral nerve injury. *Journal of Pain*. **13 (Suppl 1)**: S62.

12 Abd-Elsayed A *et al.* (2019) Neuropathic pain and Kv7 voltage-gated potassium channels: The potential role of Kv7 activators in the treatment of neuropathic pain. *Molecular Pain*. **15**: DOI 1744806919864256.

13 Bennett D *et al.* (2019) The role of voltage-gated sodium channels in pain signaling. *Physiological Reviews*. **99**: 1079–1151.

14 Devor M (2006) Sodium channels and mechanisms of neuropathic pain. *Journal of Pain*. **7**: S3–S12.

15 Hebeisen S *et al.* (2015) Eslicarbazepine and the enhancement of slow inactivation of voltage-gated sodium channels: a comparison with carbamazepine, oxcarbazepine and lacosamide. *Neuropharmacology*. **89**: 122–135.

16 Dib-Hajj S *et al.* (2017) Sodium channels in pain disorders: pathophysiology and prospects for treatment. *Pain*. **158 Suppl 1**: S97–S107.

17 McDonnell A *et al.* (2018) Efficacy of the Nav1.7 blocker PF-05089771 in a randomised, placebo-controlled, double-blind clinical study in subjects with painful diabetic peripheral neuropathy. *Pain*. **159**: 1465–1476.

18 Jensen T (2017) Selective sodium channel blockers in trigeminal neuralgia. *Lancet Neurology*. **16**: 255–256.

19 Takahashi T *et al.* (2010) Upregulation of Ca(v)3.2 T-type calcium channels targeted by endogenous hydrogen sulfide contributes to maintenance of neuropathic pain. *Pain*. **150**: 183–191.

20 Francois A *et al.* (2013) State-dependent properties of a new T-type calcium channel blocker enhance Ca(V)3.2 selectivity and support analgesic effects. *Pain*. **154**: 283–293.

21 Kerckhove N *et al.* (2018) Efficacy and safety of a T–type calcium channel blocker in patients with neuropathic pain: A proof-of-concept, randomized, double–blind and controlled trial. *European Journal of Pain*. **22**: 1321–1330.

22 Symonds J *et al.* (2017) Advances in epilepsy gene discovery and implications for epilepsy diagnosis and treatment. *Current Opinion in Neurology*. **30**: 193–199.

23 Su S-C *et al.* (2019) HLA alleles and CYP2C9*3 as predictors of phenytoin hypersensitivity in East Asians. *Clinical Pharmacology & Therapeutics*. **105**: 476–485.

24 Mullan K *et al.* (2019) HLA-associated antiepileptic drug-induced cutaneous adverse reactions. *HLA* **93**: 417–435.

25 MHRA (2012) Carbamazepine, oxcarbazepine and eslicarbazepine: potential risk of serious skin reactions. *Drug Safety Update*. www.gov.uk/drug-safety-update.

26 MHRA (2008) Carbamazepine: genetic testing in some Asian populations. *Drug Safety Update*. www.gov.uk/drug-safety-update.

27 Perucca E (2006) Clinical pharmacokinetics of new-generation antiepileptic drugs at the extremes of age. *Clinical Pharmacokinetics*. **45**: 351–363.

28 Perucca E (1999) The clinical pharmacokinetics of the new antiepileptic drugs. *Epilepsia*. **40 (Suppl 9)**: S7–S13.

29 Garnett WR (2000) Clinical pharmacology of topiramate: a review. *Epilepsia*. **41 (Suppl 1)**: S61–S65.

30 Anderson *et al.* (2002) *Handbook of clinical drug data*. (10e). McGraw Hill.

31 Perucca E (2002) Pharmacological and therapeutic properties of valproate: a summary after 35 years of clinical experience. *CNS Drugs*. **16**: 695–714.

32 May TW *et al.* (2003) Clinical pharmacokinetics of oxcarbazepine. *Clinical Pharmacokinetics*. **42**: 1023–1042.

33 Bang LM and Goa KL (2004) Spotlight on oxcarbazepine in epilepsy. *CNS Drugs*. **18**: 57–61.

34 Kwan P and Brodie MJ (2004) Phenobarbital for the treatment of epilepsy in the 21st century: a critical review. *Epilepsia*. **45**: 1141–1149.

35 Patsalos PN (2004) Clinical pharmacokinetics of levetiracetam. *Clinical Pharmacokinetics*. **43**: 707–724.

36 Rogawski MA and Hanada T (2013) Preclinical pharmacology of perampanel, a selective non-competitive AMPA receptor antagonist. *Acta Neurologica Scandinavica Supplementum*. **197**: 19–24.

37 Patsalos P (2013) Drug interactions with the newer antiepileptic drugs (AEDs)--part 1: pharmacokinetic and pharmacodynamic interactions between AEDs. *Clinical Pharmacokinetics*. **52**: 927–966.

38 DVLA (2021) Assessing fitness to drive – a guide for medical professionals. *UK Government*. www.gov.uk

39 Morgan DJ and McLean AJ (1995) Clinical pharmacokinetic and pharmacodynamic considerations in patients with liver disease. An update. *Clinical Pharmacokinetics*. **29**: 370–391.

40 Ford-Dunn S (2005) Managing patients with cancer and advanced liver disease. *Palliative Medicine*. **19**: 563–565.
41 MHRA (2021) Antiepileptic drugs in pregnancy: updated advice following comprehensive safety review. *Drug Safety Update*. www.gov.uk/drug-safety-update.
42 PHE (2014) Advice for prescribers on the risk of the misuse of pregabalin and gabapentin. *Letter from Public Health England and NHS England*. www.gov.uk.
43 Chiappini S and Schifano F (2016) A decade of gabapentinoid misuse: an analysis of the european medicines agency's 'Suspected Adverse Drug Reactions' database. *CNS Drugs*. **30**: 647–654.
44 Schjerning O *et al.* (2016) Abuse potential of pregabalin: a systematic review. *CNS Drugs*. **30**: 9–25.
45 Preston CL. *Stockley's Drug Interactions*. London: Pharmaceutical Press www.medicinescomplete.com (accessed April 2021).
46 Marson AG *et al.* (2007) The SANAD study of effectiveness of valproate, lamotrigine, or topiramate for generalised and unclassifiable epilepsy: an unblinded randomised controlled trial. *Lancet*. **369**: 1016–1026.
47 Marson AG *et al.* (2007) The SANAD study of effectiveness of carbamazepine, gabapentin, lamotrigine, oxcarbazepine, or topiramate for treatment of partial epilepsy: an unblinded randomised controlled trial. *Lancet*. **369**: 1000–1015.
48 Mula M *et al.* (2013) Antiepileptic drugs and suicidality: an expert consensus statement from the Task Force on Therapeutic Strategies of the ILAE Commission on Neuropsychobiology. *Epilepsia*. **54**: 199–203.
49 Ettinger AB *et al.* (2015) Psychiatric and behavioral adverse events in randomized clinical studies of the noncompetitive AMPA receptor antagonist perampanel. *Epilepsia*. **56**: 1252–1263.
50 Kwan P and Brodie MJ (2001) Neuropsychological effects of epilepsy and antiepileptic drugs. *Lancet*. **357**: 216–222.
5 1van Gaalen J *et al.* (2014) Drug-induced cerebellar ataxia: a systematic review. *CNS Drugs*. **28**: 1139–1153.
52 French JA (2007) First-choice drug for newly diagnosed epilepsy. *Lancet*. **369**: 970–971.
53 Gaitatzis A and Sander JW (2013) The long-term safety of antiepileptic drugs. *CNS Drugs*. **27**: 435–455.
54 Lalla R *et al.* (2012) Purple glove syndrome: a dreadful complication of intravenous phenytoin administration. *BMJ Case Reports*. **2012**.
55 Borrelli E *et al.* (2018) Stevens–Johnson syndrome and toxic epidermal necrolysis with antiepileptic drugs: An analysis of the US Food and Drug Administration Adverse Event Reporting System. *Epilepsia*. **59**: 2318–2324.
56 Molero Y *et al.* (2019) Associations between gabapentinoids and suicidal behaviour, unintentional overdoses, injuries, road traffic incidents, and violent crime: population based cohort study in Sweden. *British Medical Journal*. **365**: l2147.
57 FDA (2008) Safety information. Antiepileptic drugs. www.fda.gov/Safety/MedWatch (archived)
58 Pereira A *et al.* (2013) Suicidality associated with antiepileptic drugs: implications for the treatment of neuropathic pain and fibromyalgia. *Pain*. **154**: 345-349.
59 MHRA (2008) Antiepileptics: risk of suicidal thoughts and behavior. *Drug Safety Update*. **2**. www.gov.uk/drug-safety-update.
60 Wu MF and Lim WH (2013) Phenytoin: a guide to therapeutic drug monitoring. *Proceedings of Singapore Healthcare*. **22**: 198-203.
61 Perkin G. Ch. 24:5.1 Epilepsy in later childhood and adults. In: Firth J (ed.). *Oxford Textbook of Medicine (6e)*. Oxford University Press, Oxford.
62 MHRA (2017) Antiepileptic drugs: updated advice on switching between different manufacturers' products. *Drug Safety Update*. www.gov.uk/drug-safety-update.
63 Finnerup NB *et al.* (2016) Pharmacotherapy for neuropathic pain in adults: a systematic review and meta-analysis. *Lancet Neurology*. **14**: 162–173.
64 Bansal D *et al.* (2009) Amitriptyline vs. pregabalin in painful diabetic neuropathy: a randomized double blind clinical trial. *Diabetic Medicine*. **26**: 1019–1026.
65 Boyle J *et al.* (2012) Randomized, placebo-controlled comparison of amitriptyline, duloxetine, and pregabalin in patients with chronic diabetic peripheral neuropathic pain: impact on pain, polysomnographic sleep, daytime functioning, and quality of life. *Diabetes Care*. **35**: 2451–2458.
66 Morello C *et al.* (1999) Randomized double-blind study comparing the efficacy of gabapentin with amitriptyline on diabetic peripheral neuropathy pain. *Archives of Internal Medicine*. **159**: 1931–1937.
67 Chandra K *et al.* (2006) Gabapentin versus nortriptyline in post-herpetic neuralgia patients: a randomized, double-blind clinical trial--the GONIP Trial. *International Journal of Clinical Pharmacology and Therapeutics*. **44**: 358–363.
68 Mishra S *et al.* (2012) A comparative efficacy of amitriptyline, gabapentin, and pregabalin in neuropathic cancer pain: a prospective randomized double-blind placebo-controlled study. *American Journal of Hospice and Palliative Care*. **29**: 177–182.
69 Banerjee M *et al.* (2013) A comparative study of efficacy and safety of gabapentin versus amitriptyline as coanalgesics in patients receiving opioid analgesics for neuropathic pain in malignancy. *Indian Journal of Pharmacology*. **45**: 334–338.
70 Griebeler ML *et al.* (2014) Pharmacologic interventions for painful diabetic neuropathy: an umbrella systematic review and comparative effectiveness network meta-analysis. *Annals of Internal Medicine*. **161**: 639–649.
71 Kaydok E and Levendoglu F (2014) Comparison of the efficacy of gabapentin and pregabalin for neuropathic pain in patients with spinal cord injury: a crossover study. *Acta Medica Mediterranea*. **30**: 1343–1348.
72 Kelle B (2012) The efficacy of gabapentin and pregabalin in the treatment of neuropathic pain due to nerve injury. *Journal of Musculoskeletal Pain*. **20**: 300–305.
73 NICE (2013) Neuropathic pain. *Clinical Guideline*. CG173 (appendix G). www.nice.org.uk.
74 Derry S *et al.* (2019) Pregabalin for neuropathic pain in adults. *Cochrane Database Systematic Reviews*. **1**: CD007076. www.cochranelibrary.com.
75 Wiffen P *et al.* (2017) Gabapentin for chronic neuropathic pain in adults. *Cochrane Database Systematic Reviews*. **6**: CD007938. www.cochranelibrary.com.
76 Wiffen PJ *et al.* (2014) Carbamazepine for chronic neuropathic pain and fibromyalgia in adults. *Cochrane Database of Systematic Reviews*. **4**: CD005451. www.cochranelibrary.com.
77 Wiffen PJ *et al.* (2013) Lamotrigine for chronic neuropathic pain and fibromyalgia in adults. *Cochrane Database of Systematic Reviews*. **12**: CD006044. www.cochranelibrary.com.
78 Birse F *et al.* (2012) Phenytoin for neuropathic pain and fibromyalgia in adults. *Cochrane Database of Systematic Reviews*. **5**: CD009485. www.cochranelibrary.com.
79 Argyriou A *et al.* (2020) Real world, open label experience with lacosamide against acute painful oxaliplatin-induced peripheral neurotoxicity. *Journal of the Peripheral Nervous System*. **25**: 178–183.
80 Remi C *et al.* (2016) Subcutaneous use of lacosamide. *Journal of Pain Symptom Management*. **51**: e2–e4.
81 Hearn L *et al.* (2012) Lacosamide for neuropathic pain and fibromyalgia in adults. *Cochrane Database of Systematic Reviews*. **2**: CD009318. www.cochranelibrary.com.
82 de Greef B *et al.* (2019) Lacosamide in patients with Nav1.7 mutations-related small fibre neuropathy: a randomized controlled trial. *Brain*. **142**: 263–275.

83 Hardy J *et al.* (2001) A phase II study to establish the efficacy and toxicity of sodium valproate in patients with cancer-related neuropathic pain. *Journal of Pain and Symptom Management.* **21**: 204–209.
84 Snare AJ (1993) Sodium Valproate. Retrospective analysis of neuropathic pain control in patients with advanced cancer. *Journal of Pharmacy Technology.* **9**: 114–117.
85 Gill D *et al.* (2011) Valproic acid and sodium valproate for neuropathic pain and fibromyalgia in adults. *Cochrane Database of Systematic Reviews.* **10**: CD009183. www.cochranelibrary.com.
86 Attal N *et al.* (2010) EFNS guidelines on the pharmacological treatment of neuropathic pain: 2010 revision. *European Journal of Neurology.* **17**: 1113–e1188.
87 Corrigan R *et al.* (2012) Clonazepam for neuropathic pain and fibromyalgia in adults. *Cochrane Database of Systematic Reviews.* **5**: CD009486. www.cochranelibrary.com.
88 Wang QP and Bai M (2011) Topiramate versus carbamazepine for the treatment of classical trigeminal neuralgia: a meta-analysis. *CNS Drugs.* **25**: 847–857.
89 Bendaly EA *et al.* (2007) Topiramate in the treatment of neuropathic pain in patients with cancer. *Supportive Cancer Therapy.* **4**: 241–246.
90 Rog (2003) Double blind, randomised placebo controlled, crossover trial of topiramate in central neuropathic pain due to multiple sclerosis. *Journal of Neurology Neurosurgery and Psychiatry.* **74**: 1457.
91 Wiffen PJ *et al.* (2013) Topiramate for neuropathic pain and fibromyalgia in adults. *Cochrane Database of Systematic Reviews.* **8**: CD008314. www.cochranelibrary.com.
92 Moore RA *et al.* (2015) Zonisamide for neuropathic pain in adults. *Cochrane Database of Systematic Reviews.* **1**: CD011241. www.cochranelibrary.com.
93 Wiffen PJ *et al.* (2014) Levetiracetam for neuropathic pain in adults. *Cochrane Database of Systematic Reviews.* **7**: CD010943. www.cochranelibrary.com.
94 Razazian N *et al.* (2014) Evaluation of the efficacy and safety of pregabalin, venlafaxine, and carbamazepine in patients with painful diabetic peripheral neuropathy. A randomized, double-blind trial. *Neurosciences (Riyadh).* **19**: 192–198.
95 Tanenberg RJ *et al.* (2014) Duloxetine compared with pregabalin for diabetic peripheral neuropathic pain management in patients with suboptimal pain response to gabapentin and treated with or without antidepressants: a post hoc analysis. *Pain Practice.* **14**: 640–648.
96 Gilron I *et al.* (2015) Combination of morphine with nortriptyline for neuropathic pain. *Pain.* **156**: 1440–1448.
97 Tesfaye S *et al.* (2013) Duloxetine and pregabalin: high-dose monotherapy or their combination? The "COMBO-DN study"--a multinational, randomized, double-blind, parallel-group study in patients with diabetic peripheral neuropathic pain. *Pain.* **154**: 2616–2625.
98 Gilron I *et al.* (2009) Nortriptyline and gabapentin, alone and in combination for neuropathic pain: a double-blind, randomised controlled crossover trial. *Lancet.* **374**: 1252–1261.
99 Gilron I *et al.* (2005) Morphine, gabapentin, or their combination for neuropathic pain. *New England Journal of Medicine.* **352**: 1324–1334.
100 Holbech JV *et al.* (2015) Imipramine and pregabalin combination for painful polyneuropathy: a randomized controlled trial. *Pain.* **156**: 958–966.
101 Keskinbora K *et al.* (2007) Gabapentin and an opioid combination versus opioid alone for the management of neuropathic cancer pain: a randomized open trial. *Journal of Pain and Symptom Management.* **34**: 183–189.
102 Solaro C *et al.* (2000) Low-dose gabapentin combined with either lamotrigine or carbamazepine can be useful therapies for trigeminal neuralgia in multiple sclerosis. *European Neurology.* **44**: 45–48.
103 Angus-Leppan H (2014) First seizures in adults. *British Medical Journal.* **348**: g2470.
104 Chen C *et al.* (2019) Congress of neurological surgeons systematic review and evidence-based guidelines on the role of prophylactic anticonvulsants in the treatment of adults with metastatic brain tumors. *Neurosurgery.* **84**: E195–E197.
105 Greenhalgh J *et al.* (2020) Antiepileptic drugs as prophylaxis for postcraniotomy seizures. *Cochrane Database of Systematic Reviews.* **4**: CD007286. www.cochranelibrary.com.
106 Islim A *et al.* (2017) The role of prophylactic antiepileptic drugs for seizure prophylaxis in meningioma surgery: A systematic review. *Journal of Clinical Neuroscience.* **43**: 47–53.
107 Stocksdale B *et al.* (2020) Neuro-oncology practice clinical debate: long-term antiepileptics drug prophylaxis in patients with glioma. *Neuro-Oncology Practice.* **7**: 583–588.
108 Guerrini R *et al.* (2013) The medical and surgical treatment of tumoral seizures: current and future perspectives. *Epilepsia.* **54 (Suppl 9)**: 84–90.
109 van der Meer P *et al.* (2021) First-line antiepileptic drug treatment in glioma patients with epilepsy: Levetiracetam vs valproic acid. *Epilepsia.* **62**: 1119–1129.
110 NICE (2012) The epilepsies: the diagnosis and management of the epilepsies in adults and children in primary and secondary care. *Clinical Guideline.* CG137 www.nice.org.uk.
111 Toledo M *et al.* (2018) Outcome of cancer-related seizures in patients treated with lacosamide. *Acta Neurologica Scandinavica.* **137**: 67–75.
112 Rudà R *et al.* (2020) Effectiveness and tolerability of lacosamide as add-on therapy in patients with brain tumor–related epilepsy: Results from a prospective, noninterventional study in European clinical practice (VIBES). *Epilepsia.* **61**: 647–656.
113 Lattanzi S *et al.* (2019) Antiepileptic drug monotherapy for epilepsy in the elderly: A systematic review and network meta-analysis. *Epilepsia.* **60**: 2245–2254.
114 Perucca E (2013) Optimizing antiepileptic drug treatment in tumoral epilepsy. *Epilepsia.* **54 (Suppl 9)**: 97–104.
115 Lim DA *et al.* (2009) Safety and feasibility of switching from phenytoin to levetiracetam monotherapy for glioma-related seizure control following craniotomy: a randomized phase II pilot study. *Journal of Neuro-oncology.* **93**: 349–354.
116 Rossetti AO *et al.* (2014) Levetiracetam and pregabalin for antiepileptic monotherapy in patients with primary brain tumors. A phase II randomized study. *Neuro-oncology.* **16**: 584–588.
117 Koekkoek JAF (2014) Epilepsy in the end of life phase of brain tumor patients: a systematic review. *Neuro-Oncology Practice.* **1**: 134–140.
118 Kerrigan S and Grant R (2011) Antiepileptic drugs for treating seizures in adults with brain tumours. *Cochrane Database of Systematic Reviews.* **8**: CD008586. www.cochranelibrary.com.
119 Ruiz M *et al.* (2019) Guidelines for seizure management in palliative care: Proposal for an updated clinical practice model based on a systematic literature review. *Neurologia.* **34**: 165–197.
120 Vossel KA *et al.* (2017) Epileptic activity in Alzheimer's disease: causes and clinical relevance. *Lancet Neurology.* **16**: 311–322.
121 Zighetti ML *et al.* (2015) Effects of chronic administration of valproic acid to epileptic patients on coagulation tests and primary hemostasis. *Epilepsia.* **56**: e49–e52.
122 Kwan P and Brodie MJ (2001) Effectiveness of first antiepileptic drug. *Epilepsia.* **42**: 1255-1260.

123 Brodie M *et al.* (2013) Effect of dosage failed of first antiepileptic drug on subsequent outcome. *Epilepsia.* **54:**194–198.
124 Brodie MJ *et al.* (2007) Comparison of levetiracetam and controlled-release carbamazepine in newly diagnosed epilepsy. *Neurology.* **68**: 402–408.
125 Chi X *et al.* (2018) Response to treatment schedules after the first antiepileptic drug failed. *Epilepsia.* **59**: 2118–2124.
126 Zou X-M *et al.* (2015) Efficacy of low to moderate doses of oxcarbazepine in adult patients with newly diagnosed partial epilepsy. *Seizure.* **29**: 81–85.
127 Margolis J *et al.* (2014) Effectiveness of antiepileptic drug combination therapy for partial-onset seizures based on mechanisms of action. *JAMA Neurology.* **71**: 985–993.
128 Abou-Khalil B (2017) Selecting rational drug combinations in epilepsy. *CNS Drugs.* **31**: 835–844.
129 Perucca E and Kwan P (2005) Overtreatment in epilepsy: how it occurs and how it can be avoided. *CNS Drugs.* **19**: 897–908.
130 Chu S-S *et al.* (2020) Therapeutic effect of intravenous levetiracetam in status epilepticus: a meta-anlysis and systematic review. *Seizure: European Journal of Epilepsy.* **74**: 49–55.
131 NHS Improvement (2016) Risk of death and severe harm from error with injectable phenytoin. *Patient Safety Alert.* NHS/PSA/W/2016/2010. www.england.nhs.uk.
132 Kinney M *et al.* (2017) Hidden in plain sight: non-convulsive status epilepticus-recognition and management. *Acta Neurologica Scandinavica.* **136**: 280–292.
133 Lorenzl S *et al.* (2010) Nonconvulsive status epilepticus in palliative care patients. *Journal of Pain and Symptom Management.* **40**: 460–465.
134 NICE (2014) Bipolar disorder: assessment and management. *Clinical Guideline.* CG185. www.nice.org.uk.
135 Baldwin DS *et al.* (2014) Evidence-based pharmacological treatment of anxiety disorders, post-traumatic stress disorder and obsessive-compulsive disorder: a revision of the 2005 guidelines from the British Association for Psychopharmacology. *Journal of Psychopharmacology.* **28**: 403–439.
136 Frampton JE (2014) Pregabalin: a review of its use in adults with generalized anxiety disorder. *CNS Drugs.* **28**: 835-854.
137 Pande AC *et al.* (1999) Treatment of social phobia with gabapentin: a placebo-controlled study. *Journal of Clinical Psychopharmacology.* **19**: 341–348.
138 Pande AC *et al.* (2000) Placebo-controlled study of gabapentin treatment of panic disorder. *Journal of Clinical Psychopharmacology.* **20**: 467–471.
139 Lavigne JE *et al.* (2012) A randomized, controlled, double-blinded clinical trial of gabapentin 300 versus 900 mg versus placebo for anxiety symptoms in breast cancer survivors. *Breast Cancer Research and Treatment.* **136**: 479–486.
140 Pollack MH *et al.* (2005) The selective GABA reuptake inhibitor tiagabine for the treatment of generalized anxiety disorder: results of a placebo-controlled study. *Journal of Clinical Psychiatry.* **66**: 1401–1408.
141 Hertzberg MA *et al.* (1999) A preliminary study of lamotrigine for the treatment of posttraumatic stress disorder. *Biological Psychiatry.* **45**: 1226–1229.
142 Garcia-Borreguero D and Cano-Pumarega I (2017) New concepts in the management of restless legs syndrome. *British Medical Journal.* **356**: j104.
143 Song Y-Y *et al.* (2018) Effects of exercise training on Restless Legs Syndrome, depression, sleep quality, and fatigue among hemodialysis patients: a systematic review and meta-analysis. *Journal of Pain and Symptom Management.* **55**: 1184–1195.
144 Garcia-Borreguero D *et al.* (2016) Guidelines for the first-line treatment of restless legs syndrome/Willis-Ekbom disease, prevention and treatment of dopaminergic augmentation: a combined task force of the IRLSSG, EURLSSG, and the RLS-foundation. *Sleep Medicine.* **21**: 1–11.
145 Gibson PG and Vertigan AE (2015) Management of chronic refractory cough. *British Medical Journal.* **351**: H5590.
146 Strohscheer I and Borasio GD (2006) Carbamazepine-responsive paroxysmal nausea and vomiting in a patient with meningeal carcinomatosis. *Palliative Medicine.* **20**: 549–550.
147 Lee JW *et al.* (2008) Emesis responsive to levetiracetam. *Journal of Neurology, Neurosurgery and Psychiatry.* **79**: 847–849.
148 Yukselen V *et al.* (2003) Partial seizure: an unusual cause of recurrent vomiting. *Internartional Journal of Clinical Practice.* **57**: 742–743.
149 Pandey CK *et al.* (2006) Prophylactic gabapentin for prevention of postoperative nausea and vomiting in patients undergoing laparoscopic cholecystectomy: a randomized, double-blind, placebo-controlled study. *Journal of Postgraduate Medicine.* **52**: 97–100.
150 Cruz FM *et al.* (2012) Gabapentin for the prevention of chemotherapy-induced nausea and vomiting: a pilot study. *Supportive Care in Cancer.* **20**: 601–606.
151 Barton DL *et al.* (2014) Phase III double-blind, placebo-controlled study of gabapentin for the prevention of delayed chemotherapy-induced nausea and vomiting in patients receiving highly emetogenic chemotherapy, NCCTG N08C3 (Alliance). *Cancer.* **120**: 3575–3583.
152 Hammond CJ *et al.* (2015) Anticonvulsants for the treatment of alcohol withdrawal syndrome and alcohol use disorders. *CNS Drugs.* **29**: 293–311.
153 Martin K and Katz A (2016) The role of barbiturates for alcohol withdrawal syndrome. *Psychosomatics.* **57**: 341–347.
154 Hixson J (2010) Stopping antiepileptic drugs: when and why? *Current Treatment Options in Neurology.* **12**: 434–442.
155 Specchio L and Beghi E (2004) Should antiepileptic drugs be withdrawn in seizure-free patients. *CNS Drugs.* **18**: 201–212.

Updated June 2021

GABAPENTIN AND PREGABALIN

Class: Anti-epileptic (gabapentinoid).

Indications: Focal seizures, neuropathic pain, anxiety (**pregabalin**), †pruritus, †hot flushes, †sweating, †refractory hiccup, †restless legs syndrome, †spasticity, †refractory cough, †alcohol withdrawal.

Pharmacology

Gabapentin and pregabalin bind to the $\alpha 2\delta$ subunit responsible for trafficking N-, P/Q-type voltage-gated calcium channels and NMDA-receptors to the cell surface, thereby impeding their up-regulation and contribution to central sensitization in neuropathic pain. Thus, gabapentin and pregabalin reduce neuronal excitability, calcium influx and transmitter release in:[1,2]

- spinal dorsal horn (reducing pain transmission)
- brainstem locus coeruleus (restoring descending pain-inhibitory pathways; see p.325)
- anterior cingulate cortex (correcting altered limbic pain processing).

Gabapentin may also inhibit microglia (neuro-inflammatory cells), either directly or via the above actions. Despite being GABA analogues, neither gabapentin nor pregabalin is GABAmimetic. They are unrelated to L-type calcium-channel blockers, e.g. **diltiazem** (Table 1).

For pharmacokinetic details, see Table 2.

Table 1 Classification of calcium channel[3-5]

Type	*Location (function)*	*Blocked by*
L-type (Ca_v1.1–1.4)	Cardiovascular and GI tissues (smooth muscle tone, conductivity); neurones (function unknown)	Diltiazem, nifedipine (p.92), verapamil
N-, P/Q-type (Ca_v2.1–2.2)	Pre-synaptic neurones (calcium influx triggers neurotransmitter release; over-expressed in neuropathic pain)	Gabapentin and pregabalin (N- and P/Q-type), ziconotide (N-type)
R-type (Ca_v2.3)	Pre-synaptic neurones (calcium influx triggers neurotransmitter release)	Lamotrigine, topiramate
T-type (Ca_v3.1–3.3)	Nociceptive neurones (excitability/threshold setting, pacemaker activity/firing pattern); thalamic neurones (dysregulation responsible for absence seizures)	Ethosuximide, valproate (p.307), zonisamide

Table 2 Pharmacokinetic details

Drug	*Gabapentin*	*Pregabalin*
Bio-availability PO (%)	Dose-dependent[a]	≥90%[a]
T_{max} (h)	2–3	1
Protein-bound	No	No
Plasma halflife (h)	5–7	5–9
Elimination	Renally excreted unchanged	Renally excreted unchanged

a. both gabapentin and pregabalin are absorbed through amino acid transporters. At higher doses, gabapentin saturates the available transporters causing a dose-dependent reduction in bio-availability, e.g.: 100mg (74%), 300mg (60%), 600mg (49%), 1,200mg (33%). The absorption of pregabalin is unaffected by dose.

Gabapentin and pregabalin are first-line choices for neuropathic pain.[6,7] Both are authorized for peripheral neuropathic pain but only pregabalin for central neuropathic pain, although the strength of the supporting evidence for the latter has been questioned.[6] In network analyses,[8,9] and small direct comparisons, the efficacy and tolerability of gabapentin and pregabalin are similar to each other and to antidepressants across a range of different neuropathic pains, e.g. peripheral nerve injury,[10] spinal cord injury[11] and cancer-related.[12,13]

Gabapentin and/or pregabalin are of benefit in other pains with suspected neuropathic and/or central sensitization mechanisms, including burns,[14] fibromyalgia,[15] and chronic masticatory myalgia.[16] The 'routine' use of gabapentin or pregabalin in *unselected* cancer pain is no better than opioids alone.[17] Despite case reports of benefit in cancer-related bone pain,[18] results of RCTs are mixed,[19] with the most methodologically robust being negative.[20] In cancer treatment-related pain, an RCT found pregabalin to benefit neuropathic pain that had persisted years after radical radiotherapy treatment for head and neck cancer,[21] whereas two small RCTs found mixed benefit from gabapentin in painful radiation-induced mucositis.[22,23] An RCT found *prophylactic* pregabalin failed to prevent oxaliplatin-induced neuropathic pain,[24] although there is a case report of analgesic benefit from pregabalin in docetaxel-related hand-foot syndrome.[25]

If the first-line treatment fails, add or switch to a drug with a different mechanism of action, e.g. an antidepressant (p.210). For example, **duloxetine** is more effective than pregabalin for pain unresponsive to gabapentin.[26] Switching to pregabalin has been reported to improve pain unresponsive to gabapentin.[27] Although benefit has *not* been confirmed in an RCT, a difference in response is possible because of their varied absorption at higher doses and varied binding affinity.

Pregabalin is authorized for generalized anxiety disorder. It is as effective as **lorazepam**, **alprazolam** and **venlafaxine**. Compared with **venlafaxine**, pregabalin has a faster rate of onset and causes less nausea; it has a similar rate of onset to **quetiapine**, **lorazepam** and **alprazolam** and causes less drowsiness but more dizziness.[28-31] Gabapentin is also effective.[32-34] Pregabalin is also reported to improve anxiety and reduce benzodiazepine use in Lewy body dementia (n = 16).[35]

4

Neuronal dysregulation (e.g. central sensitization as in neuropathic pain) is implicated in several other symptoms. This may partly explain the benefit of gabapentin and/or pregabalin in a wide range of settings, including: chronic refractory cough due to cough reflex hyperexcitability (see p.158); neuropathic, idiopathic, uraemic and burns-related pruritus (see p.825); idiopathic sweating in cancer;[36] hot flushes associated with the menopause or endocrine treatment of breast or prostate cancer;[37-40] chemotherapy-related nausea and vomiting;[41] and refractory hiccup (see p.25).

Gabapentin and pregabalin have also been used in spasticity.[42-44] Gabapentin and pregabalin are first-line options for restless legs syndrome, and gabapentin is used for this indication in ESRF (see p.293 and p.738).[45,46]

Gabapentin and **phenobarbital** (p.315) are options for alcohol withdrawal when benzodiazepines are ineffective. Regimens vary, but typically gabapentin is started at 1,200mg/24h and tapered over a week. Lower doses are described for milder symptoms in the outpatient setting.[47]

Cautions

Absence seizures (may worsen), psychotic illness (may precipitate or exacerbate psychotic episodes), patients at high risk of drug abuse (evidence of misuse, mostly in high doses to augment the effect of opioids),[48-51] renal impairment (see Dose and use and Chapter 17, p.738; renal failure reported with pregabalin, which resolved on discontinuation), CHF (exacerbation reported).

Gabapentin is reported to cause false positive readings for urinary protein with Ames N-Multistix SG®.

Drug interactions

Concurrent treatment with ≥2 CNS depressants (e.g. benzodiazepines, gabapentinoids, opioids) increases the risk of respiratory depression, particularly in susceptible groups, e.g. the elderly and those with renal or hepatic impairment.[52,53] Further, the addition of an adjuvant analgesic such as gabapentin can have an opioid dose-sparing effect, necessitating a reduction in the dose of the previously well-tolerated opioid. Generally, this is indicated by a patient reporting improved analgesia but increasing drowsiness.

Clinically significant pharmacokinetic interactions are unlikely.

Antacids containing **aluminium** or **magnesium** reduce gabapentin's bio-availability by ≤24%; separate administration by ≥2h. **Cetirizine** can also reduce the systemic exposure to gabapentin.[54] **Morphine** and **naproxen** may increase gabapentin levels. High doses of gabapentin may decrease **hydrocodone** (not UK) levels; mechanism unknown.

Undesirable effects

Undesirable effects are generally similar:

Very common (>10%): drowsiness, dizziness, ataxia.

Common (<10%, >1%): amnesia, confusion, visual disturbance, dysarthria, tremor, arthralgia, myalgia, peripheral oedema, dry mouth, vomiting, constipation.

Uncommon (<1%, >0.1%): suicidal ideation 0.2% (1 in 500; advise patients to report mood or thought disturbance; also see p.287), impotence, gynaecomastia, myoclonus (may also indicate need to reduce dose of concurrent opioid).

Rare (<0.1%): respiratory depression (see below), rhabdomyolysis, pancreatitis, acute renal failure, Stevens–Johnson syndrome.

Drowsiness is generally treated by reducing the dose of gabapentin/pregabalin and subsequently titrating upwards more slowly. However, consider reducing the dose of a concurrent opioid when drowsiness is accompanied by significant pain relief. **Melatonin** and **donepezil** are reported to reduce gabapentin-related drowsiness.[55,56]

The frequencies of some symptoms differ between SPCs. It is uncertain if this reflects a difference in incidence or detection. For example, leukopenia and arthralgia occur commonly with gabapentin but not pregabalin.[57] Similarly, pregabalin is associated with cardiac conduction disturbance, QT prolongation and exacerbation of CHF, but gabapentin less so.[58,59]

Respiratory depression

The MHRA has highlighted the rare (0.001%) risk of respiratory depression with gabapentin and pregabalin.[52,53] The risk appears low with gabapentin or pregabalin *alone*, and even when gabapentin is misused in high doses.[52,60,61] Nonetheless, some patients may be at greater risk, e.g. the elderly and those with hepatic, neurological, renal or respiratory impairment, or those using other CNS depressants concurrently.[52,53,60]

However, in population studies, the concurrent use of gabapentin *and an opioid* trebles the prevalence of respiratory depression compared with either used alone (0.5% → 1.7%; 3.2% when both misused in higher doses) and increases the risk of an opioid-related death by 50%.[61-63] With postoperative analgesia involving opioids, when pre-existing gabapentinoids are continued, there is a six-times increase in the risk of respiratory depression requiring **naloxone**.[64]

Possible explanations include additive sedative effects and pharmacokinetic interactions; e.g. **morphine**, by slowing GI transit, increases absorption and overall exposure to gabapentin.[65] Further, gabapentinoids may reverse opioid tolerance; e.g. in opioid-tolerant mice, an additional dose of **morphine** had no effect on respiration, as expected. However, when the **morphine** was combined with pregabalin, respiratory depression occurred.[51,66]

Dose and use

Gabapentin

- start with 300mg PO at night
- if necessary, increase by 300mg/24h every 2–3 days, e.g.:
  - ▷ *day 3* give 300mg b.d.
  - ▷ *day 5* give 300mg t.d.s.
  - ▷ *day 8* give 300mg, 300mg, 600mg
  - ▷ *day 11* give 600mg, 300mg, 600mg
  - ▷ *day 14* give 600mg t.d.s.
- in frail patients, slower titration is advisable, e.g. 100mg at night, increased if necessary by 100mg/24h every 2–3 days
- typical effective doses
  - ▷ neuropathic pain: 600mg t.d.s.[67]
  - ▷ †hiccup: 100–300mg t.d.s., occasionally more (see Box A)
  - ▷ †hot flushes: 300mg t.d.s.[39]
  - ▷ †uraemic itch: 100–400mg after haemodialysis, see Chapter 26, Table 1, p.829
- maximum recommended dose 1,200mg t.d.s.

The starting and maximum doses of gabapentin should be reduced in adults with renal impairment (Table 3) and those on haemodialysis (HD) (see below and Chapter 17, p.738).

Table 3 Gabapentin dose adjustments in renal impairment, modified from SPC

Creatinine clearance (mL/min)	*Starting dose*[a,b]	*Maximum dose*
50–79	300mg at bedtime	600mg t.d.s.
30–49	300mg at bedtime	300mg t.d.s.
15–29	100mg at bedtime	300mg b.d.[b]
<15 (non-dialysis or peritoneal dialysis only)	100mg on alternate nights	300mg at bedtime[b]

a. starting doses are lower than those recommended by the SPC; a further reduction is advisable in elderly patients and those receiving other CNS depressants

b. the SPC recommends the daily dose be administered in three divided doses, but the prolonged halflife in renal impairment permits b.d. or once daily dosing as indicated.

For HD patients with a urine output >100mL/24h:

- start with 100mg PO at bedtime; consider either a supplementary dose after each HD session or timing the daily dose post-HD.

For anuric HD patients:

- start with 100mg PO stat and 100mg after every HD session; a regular maintenance dose is generally not required.

Pregabalin

- start with 75mg PO b.d.
  - ▷ if necessary, at intervals of 3–7 days, increase to 150mg b.d. → 225mg b.d. → 300mg b.d. (maximum recommended dose)
- in frail patients
  - ▷ start with 25–50mg b.d.
  - ▷ if necessary, increase the dose correspondingly cautiously
- typical effective doses:
  - ▷ neuropathic pain: 150–300mg b.d.[68]
  - ▷ †hiccup: 25–75mg b.d. (see Box A)
  - ▷ †hot flushes: 75–150mg b.d.[40]
  - ▷ †uraemic itch: 25–75mg after haemodialysis, see Chapter 26, Table 1, p.829
  - ▷ †spasticity: 150–300mg b.d.[44]
- maximum recommended dose 300mg b.d.

Dose reduction is necessary in renal impairment (Table 4). For patients on HD, the regular dose should be adjusted according to the creatinine clearance and a supplementary single dose given after each dialysis (Table 5); alternatively, some centres time the daily dose post-HD (see Chapter 17, p.738).

Table 4 Pregabalin dose adjustments in renal impairment; modified from SPC

Creatinine clearance (mL/min)	*Starting dose*	*Maximum dose*
>60	75mg b.d.	300mg b.d.
31–60	25mg t.d.s.[a]	150mg b.d.
15–30	25–50mg once daily	150mg once daily
<15	25mg once daily	75mg once daily

a. 37.5mg capsules not available, necessitating t.d.s. regimen.

Table 5 Post-haemodialysis supplementary doses of pregabalin

Daily dose	*Supplementary single dose after every 4h of haemodialysis*
25mg	25–50mg
50mg	50–75mg
75mg	100mg

Switching from gabapentin to pregabalin

A direct overnight switch is generally well tolerated for neuropathic pain but some patients may require dose increases or decreases for worsening pain or drowsiness respectively. The last dose of gabapentin is given at bedtime and the first dose of pregabalin the following morning, using a gabapentin to pregabalin 6:1 conversion ratio, e.g. gabapentin 900mg/24h → pregabalin 150mg/24h.[74,75]

Stopping gabapentin and pregabalin

To avoid precipitating pain or seizures, withdraw gradually over several weeks.

Box A †Gabapentin and pregabalin for hiccup

Generally reserved for persistent or refractory hiccup unresponsive to other measures, see Prokinetics, Table 2, p.25.

Regimens vary. Initially, trial short-term use over several days, stopping the gabapentin/ pregabalin if successful. If hiccup recurs, consider treating long-term, dose-titrating as for neuropathic pain.

Gabapentin[69,70]

- in relatively robust patients start with 300–400mg PO t.d.s. for 3 days and review
- in elderly, frail patients use a lower dose, e.g. 100mg t.d.s. and, if necessary, titrate upwards by 100mg every 2–3 days
- further dose reduction may be needed in renal impairment, see Table 3.

Pregabalin[71-73]

- in relatively robust patients start with 75mg PO b.d. for 3 days and review
- in elderly, frail patients use a lower dose, e.g. 25mg b.d. and, if necessary, titrate upwards by 25mg every 2–3 days
- further dose reduction may be needed in renal impairment, see Table 4.

Supply

All products are Schedule 3 **CD**.

Gabapentin (generic)

Capsules 100mg, 300mg, 400mg, 28 days @ 300mg t.d.s. = £3.
Tablets 600mg, 800mg, 28 days @ 600mg t.d.s. = £6.
Oral solution 50mg/mL, 28 days @ 300mg t.d.s. = £222. *Note. Contains propylene glycol which, in high doses, may exceed WHO daily intake limits; see SPC.*

For patients who have swallowing difficulties, gabapentin capsules may be opened and the contents dispersed in water, see Chapter 28, p.856 and p.863, or mixed with fruit juice or apple sauce.[76]

Pregabalin (generic)

Capsules 25mg, 50mg, 75mg, 100mg, 150mg, 200mg, 225mg, 300mg, 28 days @ 225mg b.d. = £3.50.
Oral solution 20mg/mL, 28 days @ 225mg b.d. = £95.

For patients who have swallowing difficulties, pregabalin capsules may be opened and the contents dispersed in water, see Chapter 28, p.856 and p.863.

1 Deng M *et al.* (2019) Presynaptic NMDA receptors control nociceptive transmission at the spinal cord level in neuropathic pain. *Cellular and Molecular Life Sciences*. **76**: 1889–1899.

2 Bannister K *et al.* (2017) Multiple sites and actions of gabapentin-induced relief of ongoing experimental neuropathic pain. *Pain*. **158**: 2386–2395.

3 Gong N *et al.* (2018) Injury-induced maladaptation and dysregulation of calcium channel $\alpha 2\delta$ subunit proteins and its contribution to neuropathic pain development. *British Journal of Pharmacology*. **175**: 2231–2243.

4 Wormuth C *et al.* (2016) Review: Cav2.3 R-type voltage-gated Ca2+ channels — functional implications in convulsive and non-convulsive seizure activity. *Open Neurology Journal*. **10**: 99–126.

5 Sekiguchi F *et al.* (2018) Involvement of voltage-gated calcium channels in inflammation and inflammatory pain. *Biological and Pharmaceutical Bulletin*. **41**: 1127–1134.

6 Derry S *et al.* (2019) Pregabalin for neuropathic pain in adults. *Cochrane Database Syst Rev*. **1**: CD007076. www.cochranelibrary.com.

7 Wiffen P *et al.* (2017) Gabapentin for chronic neuropathic pain in adults. *Cochrane Database Syst Rev*. **6**: CD007938. www.cochranelibrary.com.

8 Griebeler ML *et al.* (2014) Pharmacologic interventions for painful diabetic neuropathy: an umbrella systematic review and comparative effectiveness network meta-analysis. *Annals of Internal Medicine*. **161**: 639–649.

9 NICE (2013) Neuropathic pain — pharmacological management (appendix G). *Clinical Guideline*. CG173. www.nice.org.uk.

10 Kelle B (2012) The efficacy of gabapentin and pregabalin in the treatment of neuropathic pain due to nerve injury. *Journal of Musculoskeletal Pain*. **20**: 300–305.

11 Kaydok E and Levendoglu F (2014) Comparison of the efficacy of gabapentin and pregabalin for neuropathic pain in patients with spinal cord injury: a crossover study. *Acta Medica Mediterranea*. **30**: 1343–1348.

12 Mishra S *et al.* (2012) A comparative efficacy of amitriptyline, gabapentin, and pregabalin in neuropathic cancer pain: a prospective randomized double-blind placebo-controlled study. *American Journal of Hospice and Palliative Care*. **29**: 177–182.

13 Gül Ş *et al.* (2020) Duloxetine and pregabalin in neuropathic pain of lung cancer patients. *Brain and Behavior*. **10**: e01527.

14 Gray P *et al.* (2011) Pregabalin in severe burn injury pain: a double-blind, randomised placebo-controlled trial. *Pain*. **152**: 1279–1288.

15 Hauser W *et al.* (2009) Treatment of fibromyalgia syndrome with gabapentin and pregabalin – a meta-analysis of randomized controlled trials. *Pain*. **145**: 69–81.

16 Kimos P *et al.* (2007) Analgesic action of gabapentin on chronic pain in the masticatory muscles: a randomized controlled trial. *Pain*. **127**: 151–160.

17 Mercadante S *et al.* (2013) The effects of low doses of pregabalin on morphine analgesia in advanced cancer patients. *Clinical Journal of Pain*. **29**: 15–19.

18 Caraceni A *et al.* (2008) Gabapentin for breakthrough pain due to bone metastases. *Palliative Medicine*. **22**: 392–393.

19 Miller S (2017) P-126 Effectiveness of gabapentin and pregabalin for cancer-induced bone pain: a systematic review. *BMJ Supportive & Palliative Care*. **7**: A46.

20 Fallon M *et al.* (2016) Randomized double-blind trial of pregabalin versus placebo in conjunction with palliative radiotherapy for cancer-induced bone pain. *Journal of Clinical Oncology*. **34**: 550–556.

21 Jiang J *et al.* (2019) Effect of pregabalin on radiotherapy-related neuropathic pain in patient with head and neck cancer: a randomised controlled trial. *Journal of Clinical Oncology*. **37**: 135–143.

22 Starmer HM *et al.* (2014) Effect of gabapentin on swallowing during and after chemoradiation for oropharyngeal squamous cell cancer. *Dysphagia*. **29**: 396–402.

23 Kataoka T *et al.* (2016) Randomized trial of standard pain control with or without gabapentin for pain related to radiation-induced mucositis in head and neck cancer. *Auris Nasus Larynx*. **43**: 677–684.

24 de Andrade D *et al.* (2017) Pregabalin for the prevention of oxaliplatin-induced painful neuropathy: a randomized, double-blind trial. *Oncologist*. **22**: 1154–e105.

25 Orare K *et al.* (2019) Pregabalin for treatment of docetaxel-related Hand-Foot Syndrome. *Journal of Pain and Symptom Management*. **58**: e1–e2.

26 Tanenberg RJ *et al.* (2014) Duloxetine compared with pregabalin for diabetic peripheral neuropathic pain management in patients with suboptimal pain response to gabapentin and treated with or without antidepressants: a post hoc analysis. *Pain Practice*. **14**: 640–648.

27 Saldana MT *et al.* (2012) Pain alleviation and patient-reported health outcomes following switching to pregabalin in individuals with gabapentin-refractory neuropathic pain in routine medical practice. *Clinical Drug Investigation*. **32**: 401–412.

28 Feltner DE *et al.* (2003) A randomized, double-blind, placebo-controlled, fixed-dose, multicenter study of pregabalin in patients with generalized anxiety disorder. *Journal of Clinical Psychopharmacology*. **23**: 240–249.

29 Pande AC *et al.* (2003) Pregabalin in generalized anxiety disorder: a placebo-controlled trial. *American Journal of Psychiatry*. **160**: 533–540.

30 Rickels K *et al.* (2005) Pregabalin for treatment of generalized anxiety disorder: a 4-week, multicenter, double-blind, placebo-controlled trial of pregabalin and alprazolam. *Archives of General Psychiatry*. **62**: 1022–1030.

31 Montgomery SA *et al.* (2006) Efficacy and safety of pregabalin in the treatment of generalized anxiety disorder: a 6-week, multicenter, randomized, double-blind, placebo-controlled comparison of pregabalin and venlafaxine. *Journal of Clinical Psychiatry*. **67**: 771–782.

32 Lavigne JE *et al.* (2012) A randomized, controlled, double-blinded clinical trial of gabapentin 300 versus 900 mg versus placebo for anxiety symptoms in breast cancer survivors. *Breast Cancer Research and Treatment*. **136**: 479–486.

33 Pande AC *et al.* (1999) Treatment of social phobia with gabapentin: a placebo-controlled study. *Journal of Clinical Psychopharmacology*. **19**: 341–348.

34 Pande AC *et al.* (2000) Placebo-controlled study of gabapentin treatment of panic disorder. *Journal of Clinical Psychopharmacology*. **20**: 467–471.

35 Segers K *et al.* (2020) Pregabalin as a treatment for anxiety in patients with dementia with Lewy Bodies. A case series. *Journal of Clinical Psychopharmacology*. **40**: 297–299.

36 Porzio G *et al.* (2006) Gabapentin in the treatment of severe sweating experienced by advanced cancer patients. *Supportive Care in Cancer*. **14**: 389–391.

37 Loprinzi CL *et al.* (2009) A phase III randomized, double-blind, placebo-controlled trial of gabapentin in the management of hot flashes in men (N00CB). *Annals of Oncology*. **20**: 542–549.

38 Nelson HD *et al.* (2006) Nonhormonal therapies for menopausal hot flashes: systematic review and meta-analysis. *Journal of the American Medical Association*. **295**: 2057–2071.

39 Pandya KJ *et al.* (2005) Gabapentin for hot flashes in 420 women with breast cancer: a randomised double-blind placebo-controlled trial. *Lancet*. **366**: 818–824.

40 Loprinzi C *et al.* (2010) Phase III, randomized, double-blind, placebo-controlled evaluation of pregabalin for alleviating hot flashes, N07C1. *Journal of Clinical Oncology*. **28**: 641–647.

41 Cruz FM *et al.* (2012) Gabapentin for the prevention of chemotherapy-induced nausea and vomiting: a pilot study. *Supportive Care in Cancer*. **20**: 601–606.

42 Paisley S *et al.* (2002) Clinical effectiveness of oral treatments for spasticity in multiple sclerosis: a systematic review. *Multiple Sclerosis*. **8**: 319–329.

43 Cutter NC *et al.* (2000) Gabapentin effect on spasticity in multiple sclerosis: a placebo-controlled, randomized trial. *Archives of Physical Medicine and Rehabilitation*. **81**: 164–169.

44 Bradley L and Kirker S (2008) Pregabalin in the treatment of spasticity: A retrospective case series. *Disability and Rehabilitation*. **30**: 1230–1232.

45 Mackie S and Winkelman JW (2015) Long-term treatment of restless legs syndrome (RLS): an approach to management of worsening symptoms, loss of efficacy, and augmentation. *CNS Drugs*. **29**: 351–357.

46 Garcia-Borreguero D *et al.* (2012) European guidelines on management of restless legs syndrome: report of a joint task force by the European Federation of Neurological Societies, the European Neurological Society and the European Sleep Research Society. *European Journal of Neurology*. **19**: 1385–1396.

47 Hammond CJ *et al.* (2015) Anticonvulsants for the treatment of alcohol withdrawal syndrome and alcohol use disorders. *CNS Drugs*. **29**: 293–311.

48 PHE (2014) Advice for prescribers on the risk of the misuse of pregabalin and gabapentin. Letter from Public Health England and NHS England. www.gov.uk.

49 Chiappini S and Schifano F (2016) A decade of gabapentinoid misuse: an analysis of the european medicines agency's 'Suspected Adverse Drug Reactions' database. *CNS Drugs*. **30**: 647–654.

50 Schjerning O *et al.* (2016) Abuse potential of pregabalin: a systematic review. *CNS Drugs*. **30**: 9–25.
51 Lyndon A *et al.* (2017) Risk to heroin users of polydrug use of pregabalin or gabapentin. *Addiction*. **112**: 1580–1589.
52 MHRA (2017) Gabapentin (Neurontin): risk of severe respiratory depression. *Drug Safety Update*. **11**: 2. www.gov.uk/drug-safety-update.
53 MHRA (2021) Pregabalin (Lyrica): reports of severe respiratory depression. *Drug Safety Update*. **14**: www.gov.uk/drug-safety-update.
54 Costa A *et al.* (2020) Cetirizine reduces gabapentin plasma concentrations and effect: role of renal drug transporters for organic cations. *Journal of Clinical Pharmacology*. **60**: 1076–1086.
55 Kogure T *et al.* (2017) Donepezil, an acetylcholinesterase inhibitor, can attenuate gabapentinoid-induced somnolence in patients with neuropathic pain: a retrospective chart review. *Journal of Pain and Palliative Care Pharmacotherapy*. **31**: 4–9.
56 Altiparmak B *et al.* (2019) [Effect of melatonin on the daytime sleepiness side-effect of gabapentin in adults patients with neuropathic pain]. *Rev Bras Anestesiol*. **69**: 137–143.
57 Zaccara G *et al.* (2011) The adverse event profile of pregabalin: a systematic review and meta-analysis of randomized controlled trials. *Epilepsia*. **52**: 826–836.
58 Feldman AE and Gidal BE (2013) QTc prolongation by antiepileptic drugs and the risk of torsade de pointes in patients with epilepsy. *Epilepsy and Behavior*. **26**: 421–426.
59 MHRA Yellow card reports for gabapentin and pregabalin. *Drug Analysis Prints*. www.mhra.gov.uk/Safetyinformation (accessed March 2021).
60 Palliativedrugs.com Gabapentin, pregabalin and respiratory depression —What is your experience? *Latest additions: Survey results (July-September 2018)*. www.palliativedrugs.com.
61 Peckham AM *et al.* (2018) All-Cause and Drug-Related Medical Events Associated with Overuse of Gabapentin and/or Opioid Medications: A Retrospective Cohort Analysis of a Commercially Insured US Population. *Drug Safety*. **41**: 213–228.
62 Gomes T *et al.* (2017) Gabapentin, opioids, and the risk of opioid-related death: A population-based nested case-control study. *PLoS Med*. **14**: e1002396.
63 Gomes T *et al.* (2018) Pregabalin and the risk for opioid-related death: a nested case-control study. *Annals of Internal Medicine*. **169**: 732–734.
64 Deljou A *et al.* (2018) Pattern of perioperative gabapentinoid use and risk for postoperative naloxone administration. *British Journal of Anaesthesia*. **120**: 798–806.
65 Eckhardt K *et al.* (2000) Gabapentin enhances the analgesic effect of morphine in healthy volunteers. *Anesthesia & Analgesia*. **91**: 185–191.
66 Hill R *et al.* (2018) Oxycodone-induced tolerance to respiratory depression: reversal by ethanol, pregabalin and protein kinase C inhibition. *British Journal of Pharmacology*. **175**: 2492–2503.
67 Tremont-Lukats IW *et al.* (2000) Anticonvulsants for neuropathic pain syndromes: mechanisms of action and place in therapy. *Drugs*. **60**: 1029–1052.
68 Freynhagen R *et al.* (2005) Efficacy of pregabalin in neuropathic pain evaluated in a 12-week, randomised, double-blind, multicentre, placebo-controlled trial of flexible- and fixed-dose regimens. *Pain*. **115**: 254–263.
69 Moretti R *et al.* (2004) Gabapentin as a drug therapy of intractable hiccup because of vascular lesion: a three-year follow up. *Neurologist*. **10**: 102–106.
70 Thompson DF and Brooks KG (2013) Gabapentin therapy of hiccups. *Annals of Pharmacotherapy*. **47**: 897–903.
71 Nicoletti F *et al.* (2009) Lyrica cures the Tenor. *Clinical Neuropharmacology*. **32**: 119.
72 Fong Y-I *et al.* (2020) Pregabalin is effective in treating prolonged hiccups both with and without brainstem lesion: A report of 2 cases. *Journal of the Neurological Sciences*. 408: 116517.
73 Vandemergel X *et al.* (2006) Intractable hiccups successfully treated with pregabalin. *European Journal of Internal Medicine*. **17**: 522.
74 Toth C (2010) Substitution of gabapentin therapy with pregabalin therapy in neuropathic pain due to peripheral neuropathy. *Pain Medicine*. **11**: 456–465.
75 Ifuku M *et al.* (2011) Replacement of gabapentin with pregabalin in postherpetic neuralgia therapy. *Pain Medicine*. **12**: 1112–1116.
76 Gidal B *et al.* (1998) Gabapentin absorption: effect of mixing with foods of varying macronutrient composition. *Annals of Pharmacotherapy*. **32**: 405–409.

Updated April 2021

OXCARBAZEPINE

Class: Anti-epileptic (sodium-channel blocker).

Indications: Focal seizures, †neuropathic pain.

Pharmacology

Oxcarbazepine is structurally related to **carbamazepine**. Both act through sodium-channel blockade but differ in tolerability and propensity for drug interactions. Additional actions of uncertain significance include potassium-channel activation, N-, P- and R-type calcium-channel blockade, and antagonism of the NMDA-receptor–channel complex.[1] In neuropathic pain, it mostly acts upon peripheral neurones.[2]

Oxcarbazepine is a pro-drug which is activated by metabolism to licarbazepine (the monohydroxy derivative; often known as MHD). Licarbazepine is primarily responsible for the pharmacological effect. This is inactivated by glucuronidation and oxidation, and the metabolites are renally excreted.[3] In severe renal impairment, the elimination halflife of licarbazepine is prolonged (≤19h) and the starting dose of oxcarbazepine should be reduced (see Dose and use). Oxcarbazepine has fewer drug interactions than **carbamazepine**, because it is a weaker inducer of hepatic enzymes.

In RCTs for epilepsy, oxcarbazepine caused less drowsiness and fewer skin reactions, but more nausea than **carbamazepine**; overall, efficacy and rates of withdrawal due to undesirable effects were similar (see p.290).[4,5]

4

In RCTs for neuropathic pain (predominantly diabetic), two found benefit (NNT=7 for 50% reduction in pain severity; n=229), one was equivocal (NNT=12 for global assessment of improvement; n=247), and one found no benefit (n=141).[6] Certain clinical findings (i.e. allodynia, hyperalgesia, normal temperature sensation) may predict a greater response (NNT 4 vs. 13).[7] Although most RCTs titrated oxcarbazepine to 1,800–2,400mg/24h, a single-blind RCT comparing oxcarbazepine 600mg/24h to **pregabalin** 150mg/24h for painful diabetic neuropathy found similar efficacy. Doses were not optimized; titration was fixed. Oxcarbazepine caused less dizziness, oedema and drowsiness, but more nausea and vomiting, than **pregabalin**.[8]

Oxcarbazepine is reported to improve trigeminal neuralgia unresponsive to **carbamazepine**, post-herpetic neuralgia unresponsive to **carbamazepine** + **gabapentin**, and painful cryoglobulinaemic neuropathy unresponsive to **gabapentin** + **pregabalin**.[9-11]

Eslicarbazepine *acetate* and **lacosamide** are alternative sodium-channel blockers. Like oxcarbazepine, they have fewer drug interactions than **carbamazepine**. Although both are more expensive than oxcarbazepine, their efficacy and rates of withdrawal due to undesirable effects are similar.[12,13] **Eslicarbazepine *acetate*** is a pro-drug of the same active metabolite as oxcarbazepine, i.e. licarbazepine, but yields a higher ratio of the *S*-enantiomer. **Lacosamide** has been used successfully †CSCI.[14]

Bio-availability ≥95%.

Onset of action pain improved ≤1 week, maximum response ≤4 weeks.

Time to peak plasma concentration 1–3h.

Plasma halflife 1–5h; 7–20h licarbazepine.[3]

Duration of action no specific data.

Cautions

Hepatic impairment (potentially reduced bio-transformation to the active metabolite, with a reduced/unpredictable effect; see Chapter 18, p.769); renal impairment (see Dose and use, and also Chapter 17, p.738); HLA predisposition or previous hypersensitivity to **carbamazepine** (25–30% cross-reactivity); predisposition to hyponatraemia, cardiac insufficiency (fluid retention), abnormal cardiac conduction (arrhythmias and AV block occur rarely).

Drug interactions

Oxcarbazepine (and licarbazepine) can induce CYP3A4 and inhibit CYP2C19, but not often to a clinically significant extent. Oral hormonal contraception may become ineffective. **Lamotrigine** and **phenytoin** may require dose adjustment.

Undesirable effects

Very common (>10%): drowsiness, dizziness, fatigue, headache, diplopia, nausea and vomiting.

Common (<10%, >1%): confusion, agitation, amnesia, altered mood, vertigo, ataxia, tremor, nystagmus, reduced attention, diarrhoea, constipation, abdominal pain, rash, alopecia, acne, asymptomatic hyponatraemia.

Uncommon (<1%, >0.1%): include suicidal ideation 0.2% (1 in 500; advise patients to report mood or thought disturbance).

Rare (<0.1%): AV block, arrhythmia, pancreatitis, hepatitis, multi-organ hypersensitivity, systemic lupus erythematosus, angioedema, Stevens–Johnson syndrome, toxic epidermal necrolysis, bone marrow depression.

Dose and use

The MHRA advises that oxcarbazepine products available in the UK may differ in bio-availability, and, *when used for epilepsy*, it is best to avoid switching between different products.[15] However, if there is a delay in obtaining the patient's usual brand, *it is better to give a different brand than to miss a dose*.

Because of the association of oxcarbazepine with severe skin reactions, the SPC recommends testing those of Han Chinese and Thai descent for HLA-B*1502 before commencing treatment where possible.

Many palliative care patients have risk factors for hyponatraemia; monitor sodium at baseline, after 2 weeks, then monthly for 3 months. Doses lower than recommended by the manufacturer have been proposed:[3]

- start with 150mg PO b.d. (start with 75mg b.d. in elderly, frail or in severe renal impairment (creatinine clearance ≤30mL/min))
- increase the dose in 75–150mg increments weekly
- typical effective dose for epilepsy 600–900mg/24h (see p.290)
- maximum dose 1,200mg b.d.

Switching from carbamazepine

Carbamazepine has been switched to oxcarbazepine in a single step without cross-tapering, using a dose ratio of 2:3.[16] For example, **carbamazepine** 400mg PO b.d. was replaced with oxcarbazepine 600mg PO b.d.

Supply

Oxcarbazepine (generic)
Tablets 150mg, 300mg, 600mg, 28 days @ 300mg b.d. = £6.

Trileptal® (Novartis)
Tablets *(scored)* 150mg, 300mg, 600mg, 28 days @ 300mg b.d. = £27.
Oral suspension (sugar-free) 300mg/5mL, 28 days @ 300mg b.d. = £55; *may contain propylene glycol.*

1 Schmidt D and Elger CE (2004) What is the evidence that oxcarbazepine and carbamazepine are distinctly different antiepileptic drugs? *Epilepsy and Behaviour*. **5**: 627–635.
2 Patel R *et al.* (2018) Neuropathy following spinal nerve injury shares features with the irritable nociceptor phenotype: a back translational study of oxcarbazepine. *European Journal of Pain*. [published online ahead of print].
3 May TW *et al.* (2003) Clinical pharmacokinetics of oxcarbazepine. *Clinical Pharmacokinetics*. **42**: 1023–1042.
4 Marson AG *et al.* (2007) The SANAD study of effectiveness of carbamazepine, gabapentin, lamotrigine, oxcarbazepine, or topiramate for treatment of partial epilepsy: an unblinded randomised controlled trial. *Lancet*. **369**: 1000–1015.
5 Koch MW and Polman SK (2009) Oxcarbazepine versus carbamazepine monotherapy for partial onset seizures. *Cochrane Database of Systematic Reviews*. **4**: CD006453. www.thecochranelibrary.com.
6 Zhou M *et al.* (2017) Oxcarbazepine for neuropathic pain. *Cochrane Database of Systematic Reviews*. www.thecochranelibrary.com.
7 Demant DT *et al.* (2014) The effect of oxcarbazepine in peripheral neuropathic pain depends on pain phenotype: a randomised, double-blind, placebo-controlled phenotype-stratified study. *Pain*. **155**: 2263–2273.
8 Amir S *et al.* (2018) Pregabalin versus oxcarbazepine in painful diabetic neuropathy in elderly population: Efficacy and safety in terms of pain relief, cognitive function, and overall quality of life. *Indian J Pain*. **32**: 40–45.
9 Gomez-Arguelles JM *et al.* (2008) Oxcarbazepine monotherapy in carbamazepine-unresponsive trigeminal neuralgia. *Journal of Clinical Neuroscience*. **15**: 516–519.
10 Criscuolo S *et al.* (2005) Oxcarbazepine monotherapy in postherpetic neuralgia unresponsive to carbamazepine and gabapentin. *Acta Neurologica Scandinavica*. **111**: 229–232.
11 Moretti R *et al.* (2018) Hepatitis C-related cryoglobulinemic neuropathy: potential role of oxcarbazepine for pain control. *BMC Gastroenterology*. **18**: 19.
12 Trinka E (2018) Efficacy and safety of eslicarbazepine acetate versus controlled-release carbamazepine monotherapy in newly diagnosed epilepsy: A phase III double-blind, randomized, parallel-group, multicenter study. *Epilepsia*. **59**: 479–491.
13 Baulac M (2017) Efficacy, safety, and tolerability of lacosamide monotherapy versus controlled-release carbamazepine in patients with newly diagnosed epilepsy: a phase 3, randomised, double-blind, non-inferiority trial. *Lancet Neurology*. **16**: 43–54.
14 Remi C *et al.* (2016) Subcutaneous use of lacosamide. *Journal of Pain Symptom Management*. **51**: e2–e4.
15 MHRA (2017) Antiepileptic drugs: updated advice on switching between different manufacturers' products. *Drug Safety Update*. www.gov.uk/drug-safety-update.
16 Albani F *et al.* (2004) Immediate (overnight) switching from carbamazepine to oxcarbazepine monotherapy is equivalent to a progressive switch. *Seizure*. **13**: 254–263.

Updated (minor change) January 2021

VALPROATE

Class: Anti-epileptic (multimodal action).

Indications: Epilepsy (see SPC for details), mania associated with bipolar disorder, †status epilepticus, †neuropathic pain, †migraine prophylaxis, †hyperactive delirium, †intractable hiccup (see p.25).

Contra-indications: Females of child-bearing age, unless participating in a pregnancy prevention programme (see Dose and use). Manufacturer advises against use in active hepatic disease or past or family history of severe hepatic impairment (particularly drug-related). See Chapter 18, p.755.

Pharmacology

Valproate is a sodium-channel blocker, an NMDA-receptor–channel blocker, it increases potassium conductance and the secondary messenger PIP_3, and alters glutamate, GABA, dopamine and serotonin transmission.[1-3] The relative significance of these actions in epilepsy is unclear. Actions of possible relevance in pain also include correcting the down-regulation of glutamate re-uptake transporters[4,5] and blockade of T-type calcium channels;[6] the latter lower nociceptor excitation thresholds and are upregulated in nerve injury and peripheral sensitisation.[7-10]

Valproate is well absorbed orally. It is ≥90% plasma protein-bound and crosses the blood–brain barrier and neuronal membranes via active transporters. It is metabolized by direct microsomal UDP-mediated glucuronidation (50%), mitochondrial β-oxidation (40%) and CYP450-mediated oxidation (10%: CYP2A6, 2B6, 2C9 and 2C19). Some metabolites are active, but their cerebral concentrations are too low to contribute to valproate's overall effect. Metabolites may be responsible for idiosyncratic hepatic toxicity. CYP450 enzyme inducers, inhibitors and polymorphisms affect the proportion of CYP450 metabolites, perhaps altering this risk.[11,12]

Compared with immediate-release and enteric-coated preparations, m/r preparations halve the initial peak plasma level without reducing overall bio-availability. Further, plasma levels at 24h are 50% higher and thus peak to trough variability is significantly decreased.[13,14]

Valproate remains a first-line treatment for generalized seizures, its efficacy and tolerability comparing favourably to those of newer anti-epileptics.[15,16] It is effective for status epilepticus[17,18] and focal onset seizures in palliative care (see p.290).

Benefit has been reported for cancer-related neuropathic pain.[19,20] However, because results of RCTs in non-cancer pain are mixed, international guidelines do not recommend its use.[21-23] Valproate was well tolerated in all six studies, with fewer patients (≤5%) discontinuing because of undesirable effects compared with **gabapentin** (10%) and **pregabalin** (20–30%) in similar populations (see p.289). Valproate is used in some centres if **gabapentin** or **pregabalin** are insufficient. It can be given by CSCI (see below).

Case series have reported benefit with valproate for hyperactive delirium refractory to antipsychotics and/or benzodiazepines.[24-26] It is *not* consistently effective for agitation related to dementia.[27] Valproate has no effect on cancer survival.[28]

Bio-availability 95% PO/PR.[29]

Onset of action often within 24h (for neuropathic pain).[19]

Time to peak plasma concentration 1–2h (3–5h for e/c, 5–10h for m/r).

Plasma halflife 9–18h (5–12h with concurrent enzyme inducers).

Duration of action 12–24h.[12]

Cautions

Liver disease (Table 1 and see Chapter 18, p.769);[30,31] renal impairment (dose reduction may be required; see Chapter 17, p.738); diabetes (harmless ketone metabolites, detected by bedside urinalysis, may cause diagnostic confusion).

Drug interactions

The clearance of valproate is increased by hepatic enzyme inducers such as **carbamazepine**, **phenytoin**, **phenobarbital** and **rifampicin**.[12] Its clearance is inhibited by **isoniazid**.

Oestrogen-containing products (e.g. hormonal contraceptives) may also result in decreased valproate efficacy by inducing glucuronidation.

Valproate inhibits the metabolism of **carbamazepine**'s active epoxide metabolite (increasing undesirable effects), **ethosuximide**, **phenytoin**, **phenobarbital**, **lamotrigine** and some antiretrovirals.

The concurrent use of some drugs, e.g. **acetazolamide**, antipsychotics, **topiramate** or enzyme inducers can increase the risk of valproate-induced hyperammonaemic encephalopathy (Table 1).

Concurrent administration with carbapenem antibacterials (e.g. **ertapenem**, **imipenem**, **meropenem**) can decrease the plasma concentration of valproate dramatically by 85–90% through the combined impact on intestinal absorption, distribution and metabolism, with consequential loss of therapeutic effect.[32] Because increasing the dose may not overcome this drug–drug interaction, alternative antibacterials should be considered for patients taking valproate.

Undesirable effects

Common problems include gastric intolerance (particularly nausea; reduced by e/c formulations or taking with food), hair loss (transient, dose-related), drowsiness and postural tremor (a rarer flapping tremor is seen with hyperammonaemia), although the incidence varies markedly between individual studies.

Hyperammonaemic encephalopathy and hepatic failure (Table 1), teratogenicity and pancreatitis are the most important idiosyncratic effects.[12,33] Other rare effects include severe skin reactions (e.g. Stevens–Johnson syndrome), reversible parkinsonism, and dementia. Whether serious idiosyncratic reactions are any less common with newer anti-epileptics is unknown. As with all anti-epileptics there is a risk of suicidal ideation 0.2% (1 in 500; advise patients to report mood or thought disturbance; also see p.286).

Table 1 Valproate-induced encephalopathy[30,31,34-37]

	Hyperammonaemic encephalopathy	*Hepatic failure ± encephalopathy*
Prevalence	≤1%	≤1 in 3,000
Clinical features	Nausea and vomiting Drowsiness → coma Flapping tremor Fatigue Ataxia	Nausea and vomiting Drowsiness → coma Flapping tremor Fatigue Jaundice
Risk factors	Concurrent hepatic enzyme inducers, acetazolamide, topiramate or antipsychotics	Pre-existing liver disease and/or deranged LFTs Young age
Investigation findings	↑Blood ammonia	Deranged LFTs, coagulopathy
Management	*Asymptomatic mild hyperammonaemia:* common; does not require discontinuation but monitor closely *Mild symptoms*: reduce dose and monitor closely *Severe or worsening symptoms*: stop valproate and seek specialist advice	*Asymptomatic mildly deranged LFTs with normal coagulation:* does not require discontinuation but monitor closely *Coagulopathy, severely deranged LFTs and/or symptoms:* in the absence of an alternative explanation, stop valproate and seek specialist advice

Dose and use

Because it is teratogenic, valproate should not be used in females of child-bearing age unless alternatives have been exhausted *and* they are participating in the pregnancy prevention programme. The initiating specialist should:[38-40]

- explain the teratogenic and neurodevelopmental risks (≤10% and ≤40% of births, respectively)
- arrange with the patient's GP for 'highly effective' contraception before the first prescription is issued
- obtain signed acknowledgment of the discussions from the patient using the dedicated annual risk acknowledgment form (ARAF)

- send a copy of the ARAF to the GP
- if long-term use is envisaged, arrange to review annually the appropriateness of ongoing use and to re-complete the ARAF.

The GP should ensure that the patient: has received the patient guide, has an up-to-date signed ARAF, and is using 'highly effective' contraception.[41]

The MHRA advise that, at *every* dispensing, the pharmacist should: provide a patient warning card and PIL, ensure the patient has a patient guide, discuss the teratogenic risks and the need for highly effective contraception.[39]

For full details, see the health professional guide[40] and pan-college guidance document.[42]

The manufacturer recommends that LFTs, prothrombin time (PT) and FBC be checked before and during the first 6 months of treatment, although this may not improve the early detection of hepatotoxicity.

Generally, for PO use, m/r preparations are preferred (see Pharmacology). Note. Remains of m/r tablets may appear in the patient's faeces ('ghost tablets'), but these are inert residues and do not affect the efficacy of the products.

For patients with swallowing difficulties, m/r oral granules or the contents of m/r capsules can be sprinkled on cold, soft food or a cold drink and immediately swallowed without chewing (see SPCs). If necessary, immediate-release chewable tablets or oral solutions are available (see Supply, and also Chapter 28, Table 2, p.863). The oral solution can be given PR; prior dilution with water may help to avoid rapid expulsion. Valproate can also be given IV or by CSCI (see below).

Epilepsy

The MHRA advises that the products available in the UK may differ in bio-availability, and, *when used for epilepsy*, it is best to avoid switching between different manufacturers' products; however, if there is a delay in obtaining the patient's usual brand, *it is better to give a different brand than to miss a dose* (see p.288).

Valproate is a commonly used first- or second-line treatment in palliative care. In the last days of life, **midazolam** is generally preferred (see Anti-epileptics, Box B, p.291).

- start with valproate 150–200mg m/r PO b.d.
- if necessary, increase by 150–200mg every 3 days.

Although the maximum dose is 2.5g/24h, most respond to lower doses, i.e. 750–1,000mg/24h (see p.290).

When the PO route cannot be used, valproate can be given IV or †CSCI (also see below):

- if already on PO treatment, give the same daily dose by continuous or intermittent (over 3–5min) infusions
- if starting *de novo*, give 400–800mg IV (maximum 10mg/kg) over 3–5min, followed by continuous or intermittent infusions of ≤2.5g/24h.

†Status epilepticus

Higher doses used for status epilepticus are reported to be well tolerated:[17]

- give valproate 15–30mg/kg IV, diluted in 50mL sodium chloride 0.9%, over 15–20min, with the subsequent maintenance dose of 1–3mg/kg/h given CIVI.

Alternatives include **levetiracetam** (p.312) and **phenobarbital** (p.315).

Mania

Not all marketed products are authorized for mania, but they appear to be clinically equivalent:

- start with valproate 300mg m/r PO b.d.
- increase as rapidly as possible to achieve the optimal response, to a maximum of 60mg/kg/24h
- most patients respond to doses <2g/24h.[43,44]

†Neuropathic pain

Valproate is *not* a first-line choice (see Pharmacology):

- start with valproate 150–200mg m/r PO at bedtime
- if necessary, increase by 150–200mg/24h every 2–3 days; give as a b.d. dose
- maximum used in 'positive' RCTs was ≤1.2g/24h;[22] higher doses are reported in case series (<2g/24h).[19,20]

†*Hyperactive delirium*

Valproate is *not* a first-line choice (see Antipsychotics, p.193). Dose as for mania. In case series, the median effective dose was 1,000–1,800mg/24h (range 375–4,000mg/24h).[24-26]

†*Continuous subcutaneous administration*

Valproate has been used successfully CSCI.[45,46] The PO:SC/IV dose ratio is 1:1. A total of ten patients (nine with seizures, one with neuropathic pain) received a median dose of 1,000mg/24h CSCI (range 400–1,800mg/24h). Duration of use ranged from 2 to 39 days, with only one patient experiencing mild erythema at the infusion site. In one report, the valproate was diluted with 30mL of WFI.

Alternative SC/CSCI anti-epileptics include **lacosamide**,[47] **levetiracetam** (p.312), **midazolam** (p.174) and **phenobarbital** (p.315).

CSCI compatibility with other drugs: because there are no reports of combined use, valproate should be administered via a separate syringe driver (see Chapter 29, p.892).

Supply

Valproate is the UK generic term for valproic acid and its salts and esters, including sodium valproate. The pharmacokinetics, efficacy and tolerability of valproic acid and sodium valproate are similar; sodium valproate 579mg is equivalent to valproic acid 500mg,[48] and the manufacturer of valproic acid (Convulex®) advises that doses are regarded as the same for both sodium valproate and valproic acid. Note. Also see MHRA advice in Dose and use when using for epilepsy.

Immediate-release oral products (*m/r products are generally preferred;* see Pharmacology)
Sodium valproate (generic)
Tablets e/c 200mg, 500mg, 28 days @ 200mg b.d. = £5.50.
Oral solution 200mg/5mL, 28 days @ 200mg b.d. = £9.

Epilim® (Sanofi)
Tablets crushable (scored) sodium valproate 100mg, 28 days @ 200mg b.d. = £6.50.
Tablets e/c sodium valproate 200mg, 500mg, 28 days @ 200mg b.d. = £4.75.
Oral solution (sugar-free) sodium valproate 200mg/5mL, 28 days @ 200mg b.d. = £7.50.
Oral syrup sodium valproate 200mg/5mL, 28 days @ 200mg b.d. = £9.

Modified-release oral products
Epilim Chrono® (Sanofi)
Tablets m/r (*sodium valproate and valproic acid*) equivalent to sodium valproate 200mg, 300mg, 500mg, 28 days @ 200mg b.d. = £6.50.
Oral granules m/r Epilim Chronosphere® (*sodium valproate and valproic acid*) equivalent to sodium valproate 50mg, 100mg, 250mg, 500mg, 750mg, 1g/sachet, 28 days @ 500mg at bedtime = £28.

Episenta® (Desitin)
Capsules enclosing m/r granules sodium valproate 150mg, 300mg, 28 days @ 150mg b.d. = £4.
Oral granules m/r sodium valproate 500mg, 1g/sachet, 28 days @ 500mg at bedtime = £6.

Parenteral products
Sodium valproate (generic)
Injection 100mg/mL, 3mL amp = £7, 4mL amp = £11.50.
Injection (powder for reconstitution) 400mg vial = £13; supplied with a 4mL amp of WFI for reconstitution. *Significant displacement occurs (see SPC).*

Not an exhaustive list; other brands are available. For full details and valproic acid products, see the BNF.

1 Loscher W (2002) Basic pharmacology of valproate: a review after 35 years of clinical use for the treatment of epilepsy. *CNS Drugs.* **16**: 669-694.

2 Chang P *et al.* (2014) Seizure-induced reduction in PIP3 levels contributes to seizure-activity and is rescued by valproic acid. *Neurobiology of Disease.* **62**: 296-306.

3 Kay HY *et al.* (2015) M-current preservation contributes to anticonvulsant effects of valproic acid. *Journal of Clinical Investigation.* **125**: 3904-3914.

4 Hobo (2012) Valproate upregulates glutamate transporters in rat spinal cord after peripheral nerve injury. *Journal of Pain*. **13 (Suppl 1)**: s62.
5 Inquimbert P *et al.* (2012) Peripheral nerve injury produces a sustained shift in the balance between glutamate release and uptake in the dorsal horn of the spinal cord. *Pain*. **153**: 2422-2431.
6 Takahashi T *et al.* (2010) Upregulation of Ca(v)3.2 T-type calcium channels targeted by endogenous hydrogen sulfide contributes to maintenance of neuropathic pain. *Pain*. **150**: 183-191.
7 Jevtovic-Todorovic V *et al.* (2006) The role of peripheral T-type calcium channels in pain transmission. *Cell Calcium*. **40**: 197-203.
8 Francois A *et al.* (2013) State-dependent properties of a new T-type calcium channel blocker enhance Ca(V)3.2 selectivity and support analgesic effects. *Pain*. **154**: 283-293.
9 Sekiguchi F *et al.* (2018) Involvement of voltage-gated calcium channels in inflammation and inflammatory pain. *Biological Pharmaceutical Bulletin*. **41**: 1127—1134.
10 Li Y *et al.* (2017) Dorsal root ganglion neurons become hyperexcitable and increase expression of voltage-gated T-type calcium channels (Cav3.2) in paclitaxel-induced peripheral neuropathy. *Pain*. **158**: 417—429.
11 Mann MW and Pons G (2007) Various pharmacogenetic aspects of antiepileptic drug therapy: a review. *CNS Drugs*. **21**: 143-164.
12 Perucca E (2002) Pharmacological and therapeutic properties of valproate: a summary after 35 years of clinical experience. *CNS Drugs*. **16**: 695-714.
13 Wangemann M *et al.* (1999) Pharmacokinetic characteristics of a new multiple unit sustained release formulation of sodium valproate. *International Journal of Clinical Pharmacology and Therapeutics*. **37**: 100-108.
14 Genton P (2005) Progress in pharmaceutical development presentation with improved pharmacokinetics: a new formulation for valproate. *Acta Neurologica Scandinavica Supplementum*. **182**: 26-32.
15 Marson AG *et al.* (2007) The SANAD study of effectiveness of valproate, lamotrigine, or topiramate for generalised and unclassifiable epilepsy: an unblinded randomised controlled trial. *Lancet*. **369**: 1016–1026.
16 Karceski S *et al.* (2005) Treatment of epilepsy in adults: expert opinion. *Epilepsy and Behavior*. **7 (Suppl 1)**: S1-64.
17 Trinka E *et al.* (2014) Efficacy and safety of intravenous valproate for status epilepticus: a systematic review. *CNS Drugs*. **28**: 623-639.
18 Yasiry Z and Shorvon SD (2014) The relative effectiveness of five antiepileptic drugs in treatment of benzodiazepine-resistant convulsive status epilepticus: a meta-analysis of published studies. *Seizure*. **23**: 167-174.
19 Snare AJ (1993) Sodium Valproate. Retrospective analysis of neuropathic pain control in patients with advanced cancer. *Journal of Pharmacy Technology*. **9**: 114-117.
20 Hardy J *et al.* (2001) A phase II study to establish the efficacy and toxicity of sodium valproate in patients with cancer-related neuropathic pain. *Journal of Pain and Symptom Management*. **21**: 204–209.
21 Attal N *et al.* (2010) EFNS guidelines on the pharmacological treatment of neuropathic pain: 2010 revision. *European Journal of Neurology*. **17**: 1113-e1188.
22 Finnerup NB *et al.* (2016) Pharmacotherapy for neuropathic pain in adults: a systematic review and meta-analysis. *Lancet Neurology*. **14**: 162–173.
23 Gill D *et al.* (2011) Valproic acid and sodium valproate for neuropathic pain and fibromyalgia in adults. *Cochrane Database of Systematic Reviews*. **10**: CD009183. www.thecochranelibrary.com.
24 Bourgeois JA *et al.* (2005) Adjunctive valproic acid for delirium and/or agitation on a consultation-liaison service: a report of six cases. *Journal of Neuropsychiatry and Clinical Neurosciences*. **17**: 232-238.
25 Gagnon DJ *et al.* (2017) Valproate for agitation in critically ill patients: a retrospective study. *Journal of Critical Care*. **37**: 119-125.
26 Crowley K *et al.* (2020) Valproic acid for the management of agitation and delirium in the intensive care setting: a retrospective analysis. *Clin Ther*. **42**: e65—e73.
27 Baillon S *et al.* (2018) Valproate preparations for agitation in dementia. *Cochrane Database of Systematic Reviews*. **10**: CD003945. www.thecochranelibrary.com.
28 Happold C *et al.* (2016) Does valproic acid or levetiracetam improve survival in glioblastoma? A pooled analysis of prospective clinical trials in newly diagnosed glioblastoma. *Journal of Clinical Oncology*. **34**: 731—739.
29 Leppik IE and Patel SI (2015) Intramuscular and rectal therapies of acute seizures. *Epilepsy and Behavior*. **49**: 307-312.
30 Konig SA *et al.* (1994) Severe hepatotoxicity during valproate therapy: an update and report of eight new fatalities. *Epilepsia*. **35**: 1005-1015.
31 Koenig SA *et al.* (2006) Valproic acid-induced hepatopathy: nine new fatalities in Germany from 1994 to 2003. *Epilepsia*. **47**: 2027-2031.
32 Mancl EE and Gidal BE (2009) The effect of carbapenem antibiotics on plasma concentrations of valproic acid. *Annals of Pharmacotherapy*. **43**: 2082-2087.
33 French JA (2007) First-choice drug for newly diagnosed epilepsy. *Lancet*. **369**: 970-971.
34 Chopra A *et al.* (2012) Valproate-induced hyperammonemic encephalopathy: an update on risk factors, clinical correlates and management. *General Hospital Psychiatry*. **34**: 290-298.
35 Yamamoto Y *et al.* (2012) Risk factors for hyperammonemia associated with valproic acid therapy in adult epilepsy patients. *Epilepsy Research*. **101**: 202-209.
36 Tseng YL *et al.* (2014) Risk factors of hyperammonemia in patients with epilepsy under valproic acid therapy. *Medicine*. **93**: e66.
37 Kipervasser S *et al.* (2017) Gait instability in valproate-treated patients: Call to measure ammonia levels. *Acta Neurologica Scandinavica*. **136**: 401—406.
38 MHRA (2018) Valproate medicines (Epilim, Depakote): contraindicated in women and girls of childbearing potential unless conditions of Pregnancy Prevention Programme are met. *Drug Safety Update*. www.gov.uk/drug-safety-update.
39 MHRA (2018) Valproate medicines: are you acting in compliance with the pregnancy prevention measures? *Drug Safety Update*. www.gov.uk/drug-safety-update.
40 MHRA (2020) Information on the risks of Valproate use in girls (of any age) and women of childbearing potential (Epilim, Depakote, Convulex, Episenta, Epival, Kentlim, Orlept, Sodium valproate, Syonell, Valpal, Belvo & Dyzantil). *Guidance for healthcare professionals*. www.gov.uk
41 UK Government Department of Health and Social Care (2018) Valproate use by women and girls: Information about the risks of taking valproate medicines during pregnancy. *Guidance*. www.gov.uk.
42 Shakespeare J and Sisodiva S (2019) Guidance document on valproate use in women and girls of childbearing years. *Royal College of General Practitioners and Association of British Neurologists and Royal College of Physicians*. www.rcgp.org.uk
43 Keck PE, Jr. *et al.* (1993) Valproate oral loading in the treatment of acute mania. *Journal of Clinical Psychiatry*. **54**: 305-308.
44 Macritchie K *et al.* (2003) Valproate for acute mood episodes in bipolar disorder. *Cochrane Database of Systematic Reviews*. **1**: CD004052. www.thecochranelibrary.com.

45 O'Connor MN (2014) The use of sodium valproate in a continuous infusion (CSCI) as an anticonvulsant at the end of life - a case series. *Palliative Medicine*. **28**: 740-741.
46 McKenna M (2013) Personal communication.
47 Remi C *et al.* (2016) Subcutaneous use of lacosamide. *Journal of Pain Symptom Management*. **51**: e2–e4.
48 Fisher (2003) Sodium valproate or valproate semisodium: is there a difference in the treatment of bipolar disorder? *Psychiatric Bulletin*. **27**: 446-448.

Updated (minor change) October 2021

LEVETIRACETAM

Class: Anti-epileptic (SV2A ligand).

Indications: Focal seizures, adjunctive therapy of generalized myoclonic and tonic-clonic seizures, †status epilepticus.

Pharmacology

Levetiracetam binds to synaptic vesicle protein SV2A, interfering with the release of the neurotransmitter stored within the vesicle. It gains access after neurotransmitter release as the vesicles are recycled. Thus, it selectively accumulates in, and inhibits, rapidly firing neurons.[1] Levetiracetam also inhibits potassium and N-type calcium channels, and AMPA-glutamate receptors.[2]

Levetiracetam is a commonly used first-line choice for seizures in palliative care (see p.290). Such seizures are generally caused by focal brain lesions and are, thus, focal onset, even if this is obscured by rapid secondary generalization. Efficacy and tolerability compare favourably to other anti-epileptics used in focal seizures, both non-cancer and cancer-related.[3-10] It has few drug interactions, can be given IV or SC, and can be used when other anti-epileptics are contra-indicated because of hepatic or cardiac co-morbidities.[11] PR use is also reported; suppositories compounded from levetiracetam tablets produced therapeutic plasma levels.[12] Anti-epileptics should not be used *prophylactically* in the absence of a history of seizures; in RCTs, they do not reduce the risk (see p.290).

Although unauthorized, levetiracetam is also used for status epilepticus refractory to benzodiazepines, generally in a dose of 20–30mg/kg given as a single IV bolus over 15–30min (see Dose and use). Efficacy appears comparable to **phenytoin** and **valproate**.[13]

Levetiracetam is effective for migraine prophylaxis,[14] but *not* neuropathic pain[15] or social anxiety disorder.[16] Benefit for bipolar disorder, spasticity due to hypoxic brain injury, and hot flushes is reported,[4,17-19] but none have been confirmed in RCTs.

Compared to levetiracetam, **brivaracetam** has a higher affinity for SV2A.[2] However, it appears to be no more effective or better tolerated;[20] it costs more and may have a greater propensity for drug interactions.

Food affects the rate but not the extent of PO absorption of levetiracetam. It is well absorbed SC.[21,22] It does not bind to plasma proteins. It readily crosses the blood–brain barrier and its CSF halflife is 3 times longer than that for plasma. One-third is metabolized predominantly by non-hepatic hydrolysis to an inactive metabolite; the remainder is excreted by the kidneys unchanged.[2]

Bio-availability ≥95% PO.
Onset of action <3 days PO.
Time to peak plasma concentration 1–2h PO.
Plasma halflife 6–8h.
Duration of action 24h.

Cautions

Renal impairment (dose adjustment required, see Dose and use, and also p.738) or severe hepatic impairment (see Dose and use, and also p.769).

Drug interactions

Clinically significant interactions are unlikely; however, caution is advised with concurrent administration of **carbamazepine**, **methotrexate** or **phenytoin**, because of isolated reports of toxicity.[23]

Undesirable effects

Very common (>10%): fatigue, drowsiness, headache.
Common (<10%, >1%): ataxia, hyperkinesis, tremor, dizziness, diplopia, blurred vision, amnesia, abnormal thinking, attention disturbance, behavioural disturbances (emotional lability, irritability, agitation, hostility/aggression, personality disorders), depression, insomnia, anorexia, abdominal pain, diarrhoea, dyspepsia, nausea, vomiting, myalgia, rash, pruritus, thrombocytopenia.

Behavioural disturbances occur in 3–4% of patients with epilepsy, but only 0.5% of those being treated for other conditions. Risk factors include a history of aggression or psychiatric disturbance.[24,25] Onset after several months use of an otherwise tolerated dose has been reported.[26]
Uncommon (<1%, >0.1%): suicidal ideation 0.2% (1 in 500; advise patients to report mood or thought disturbance; also see p.287).
Rare (<0.1%): psychosis, worsening of seizures, pancreatitis, QT interval prolongation, hepatic failure, acute kidney injury, bone marrow suppression, hyponatraemia, extra-pyramidal symptoms, rhabdomyolysis, severe skin reactions.

4

Dose and use

Focal seizures

- start with 250–500mg PO/IV b.d.
- if starting with 250mg b.d., increase automatically after 2 weeks to 500mg b.d. (the minimum effective dose in most people)
- if necessary, increase by 250–500mg b.d. every 2 weeks.

Although the maximum dose is 1.5g b.d., most respond to lower doses. In one RCT, about 90% of those responding did so with levetiracetam 500mg b.d.[27]

In some countries (not UK) a once daily PO m/r product is available. An oral solution or oral granules are available for administration by enteral feeding tubes; see specific SPCs for full details and p.863.

†Status epilepticus refractory to benzodiazepines[13]

- give a loading dose of 1–2g IV (or 20–30mg/kg up to a maximum of 3g) diluted in 100mL sodium chloride 0.9% or glucose 5% and infused over 15–30min.

Parenteral administration

The dose is the same PO/IV/SC.

For IV use, dilute the dose in ≥100mL sodium chloride 0.9% or glucose 5% and infuse over 15–30min.

†Subcutaneous administration

Levetiracetam (≤1g) can be given SC b.d. diluted in 100mL sodium chloride 0.9% and infused over 30min.[21]

Levetiracetam can also be given by CSCI diluted with either WFI or sodium chloride 0.9% when necessary.[28-32]

CSCI compatibility with other drugs: limited clinical experience suggests that levetiracetam is compatible with **diamorphine**, **glycopyrronium**, **haloperidol**, **hyoscine *butylbromide***, **levomepromazine**, **metamizole (dipyrone**; not UK or USA), **methadone**, **metoclopramide**, **midazolam**, **morphine sulfate**, **oxycodone** and **ranitidine**. Generally, sodium chloride 0.9% is used as diluent and local skin reactions occur in about 5% of patients.[29,33-35] Also see Chapter 29, p.892 and the www.palliativedrugs.com Syringe Driver Survey Database.

Alternative SC/CSCI anti-epileptics include **lacosamide**, **midazolam** (p.174), **phenobarbital** (p.315) and **valproate** (p.310).[36,37]

Renal impairment

Because levetiracetam is largely excreted unchanged by the kidneys, the dose should be reduced in patients with renal impairment (Table 1).

Table 1 Dose adjustment for levetiracetam in renal impairment[a]

Creatinine clearance (mL/min/1.73m²)[b]	*Usual maintenance dose*[c] *(mg)*
≥80	500–1,500 b.d.
50–79	500–1,000 b.d.
30–49	250–750 b.d.
<30	250–500 b.d.

a. for patients weighing <50kg, the SPC recommends dosing on a mg/kg basis
b. based on the Cockcroft–Gault formula adjusted for body surface area (see Chapter 17, p.734)
c. in some countries (not UK) a PO m/r product is available, permitting the total maintenance dose to be given once daily.

If on peritoneal dialysis or haemodialysis:

- give 750mg PO/IV on the first day of treatment and 500–1,000mg *once daily* thereafter
- consider giving a 250–500mg supplementary dose immediately after each haemodialysis session or timing the daily dose after the dialysis session.

Hepatic impairment

Because metabolism is non-hepatic and the drug is not protein-bound, there is no need to reduce the dose in hepatic impairment unless there is associated renal impairment (see Table 1).

Stopping levetiracetam

Reduce by a maximum of 500mg b.d. every 2–4 weeks to avoid rebound seizures.

Supply

Levetiracetam (generic)
Tablets 250mg, 500mg, 750mg, 1g, 28 days @ 750mg b.d. = £5.50.
Oral solution (sugar-free) 100mg/mL, 28 days @ 750mg b.d. = £10.
Injection (concentrate for dilution and use as an intravenous infusion) 100mg/mL, 5mL vial = £13.

Desitrend® (Desitin Pharma)
Granules 250mg, 500mg and 1g sachet, 28 days @ 750mg b.d. = £57.

1 Klitgaard H *et al.* (2016) Brivaracetam: Rationale for discovery and preclinical profile of a selective SV2A ligand for epilepsy treatment. *Epilepsia*. **57**: 538–548.
2 Steinhoff BJ and Staack AM (2019) Levetiracetam and brivarecetam: a review of evidence from clinical trials and clincial experience. *Therapeutic Advances in Neurological Disorders*. **12**: 1–23.
3 Nevitt SJ *et al.* (2017) Antiepileptic drug monotherapy for epilepsy: a network meta-analysis of individual participant data. *Cochrane Database of Systematic Reviews*. **12**: CD011412. www.cochranelibrary.com.
4 Zaccara G *et al.* (2006) Comparison of the efficacy and tolerability of new antiepileptic drugs: what can we learn from long-term studies? *Acta Neurologica Scandinavica*. **114**: 157–168.
5 Lim DA *et al.* (2009) Safety and feasibility of switching from phenytoin to levetiracetam monotherapy for glioma-related seizure control following craniotomy: a randomized phase II pilot study. *Journal of Neuro-oncology*. **93**: 349–354.
6 Rossetti AO *et al.* (2014) Levetiracetam and pregabalin for antiepileptic monotherapy in patients with primary brain tumors. A phase II randomized study. *Neuro-oncology*. **16**: 584–588.
7 Werhahn KJ *et al.* (2015) A randomized, double-blind comparison of antiepileptic drug treatment in the elderly with new-onset focal epilepsy. *Epilepsia*. **56**: 450–459.
8 Glauser T *et al.* (2013) Updated ILAE evidence review of antiepileptic drug efficacy and effectiveness as initial monotherapy for epileptic seizures and syndromes. *Epilepsia*. **54**: 551–563.
9 Vossel KA *et al.* (2017) Epileptic activity in Alzheimer's disease: causes and clinical relevance. *Lancet Neurology*. **16**: 311–322.
10 Cardona AF *et al.* (2018) Efficacy and safety of levetiracetam vs. other antiepileptic drugs in hispanic patients with glioblastoma. *Journal of Neuro-oncology*. **136**: 363–371.
11 Karceski S *et al.* (2005) Treatment of epilepsy in adults: expert opinion. *Epilepsy and Behavior*. **7 (Suppl 1)**: S1–S64.
12 Remi C (2018) Personal communication.
13 Chu S-S *et al.* (2020) Therapeutic effect of intravenous levetiracetam in status epilepticus: a meta-anlysis and systematic review. *Seizure: European Journal of Epilepsy*. **74**: 49–55.
14 Watkins AK *et al.* (2018) Efficacy and safety of levetiracetam for migraine prophylaxis: a systematic review. *Journal of Clinical Pharmacy and Therapeutics*. **43**: 467–475.
15 Wiffen PJ *et al.* (2014) Levetiracetam for neuropathic pain in adults. *Cochrane Database of Systematic Reviews*. **7**: CD010943. www.cochranelibrary.com.
16 Stein MB *et al.* (2010) Levetiracetam in generalized social anxiety disorder: a double-blind, randomized controlled trial. *Journal of Clinical Psychiatry*. **71**: 627–631.

17 Dunteman ED (2005) Levetiracetam as an adjunctive analgesic in neoplastic plexopathies: case series and commentary. *Journal of Pain and Palliative Care Pharmacotherapy*. **19**: 35–43.
18 Thompson S *et al.* (2008) Levetiracetam for the treatment of hot flashes: a phase II study. *Supportive Care in Cancer*. **16**: 75–82.
19 Pingue V *et al.* (2020) Levetiracetam improves upper limb spasticity in a patient with unresponsive wakefulness syndrome: a case report. *Frontiers in Neuroscience*. **14**: 70.
20 Zhang L *et al.* (2016) Levetiracetam vs. brivaracetam for adults with refractory focal seizures: a meta-analysis and indirect comparison. *Seizure*. **39**: 28–33.
21 Lopez-Saca JM *et al.* (2013) Repeated use of subcutaneous levetiracetam in a palliative care patient. *Journal of Pain and Symptom Management*. **45**: e7–e8.
22 Papa P *et al.* (2021) Pharmacokinetics of subcutaneous levetiracetam in palliative care patients. *Journal of Palliative Medicine*. **24**: 248–251.
23 Preston CL *Stockley's Drug Interactions*. London: Pharmaceutical Press www.medicinescomplete.com (accessed March 2021).
24 Dinkelacker V *et al.* (2003) Aggressive behavior of epilepsy patients in the course of levetiracetam add-on therapy: report of 33 mild to severe cases. *Epilepsy Behaviour*. **4**: 537–547.
25 Cramer JA *et al.* (2003) A systematic review of the behavioral effects of levetiracetam in adults with epilepsy, cognitive disorders, or an anxiety disorder during clinical trials. *Epilepsy Behaviour*. **4**: 124–132.
26 Mohamudally A and Clark K (2020) Levetiracetam at the end of life: A case report and discussion. *Journal of Palliative Medicine*. **23**: 995–997.
27 Brodie MJ *et al.* (2007) Comparison of levetiracetam and controlled-release carbamazepine in newly diagnosed epilepsy. *Neurology*. **68**: 402–408.
28 Sutherland AE *et al.* (2018) Subcutaneous levetiracetam for the management of seizures at the end of life. *BMJ Supportive and Palliative Care*. **8**: 129–135.
29 Remi C *et al.* (2014) Continuous subcutaneous use of levetiracetam: a retrospective review of tolerability and clinical effects. *Journal of Pain and Palliative Care Pharmacotherpy*. **28**: 371–377.
30 Ryan S *et al.* (2016) The use of additional antiepileptic drugs with subcutaneous levetiracetam for the management of seizures at the end of life: a case series. *Palliative Medicine*. 30: NP262.
31 Wells GH *et al.* (2016) Continuous subcutaneous levetiracetam in the management of seizures at the end of life: a case report. *Age and Ageing*. **45**: 321–322.
32 Furtado I *et al.* (2018) Continuous subcutaneous levetiracetam in end-of-life care. *BMJ Case Reports*.
33 Murray-Brown FL and Stewart A (2016) Remember Keppra: seizure control with subcutaneous levetiracetam infusion. *BMJ Supportive and Palliative Care*. **6**: 12–13.
34 Munich University Hospital (2017) Syringe driver compatability database. *Palliative medicine department*. Available from: www.pall-iv.de.
35 Palliativedrugs.com Ltd. *Syringe Driver Survey Database*. www.palliativedrugs.com (accessed March 2021).
36 Remi C *et al.* (2016) Subcutaneous use of lacosamide. *Journal of Pain and Symptom Management*. **51**: e2–e4.
37 O'Connor N *et al.* (2017) Sodium Valproate as a continuous subcutaneous infusion: a case series. *Journal of Pain and Symptom Management*. **54**: e1–e2.

Updated April 2021

*PHENOBARBITAL

Class: Anti-epileptic (barbiturate GABAmimetic).

Indications: Epilepsy (except absence seizures), status epilepticus, †refractory agitation in the imminently dying, †alcohol withdrawal.

Contra-indications: Unless in the imminently dying: severe renal or severe hepatic impairment (see Chapter 17, p.738 and Chapter 18, p.769).

Pharmacology

Phenobarbital enhances the post-synaptic inhibitory action of GABA by prolonging the opening of the chloride channel in the GABA-receptor–channel complex (see Anti-epileptics, Figure 1, p.282).[1] Phenobarbital is also an AMPA-glutamate receptor antagonist. These actions depress CNS activity, and high doses result in general anaesthesia.

There is considerable interindividual variation in the pharmacokinetics of phenobarbital. Peak CNS concentrations occur 15–20min after peak plasma concentrations. Because phenobarbital has a long plasma halflife, 3–4 weeks of therapy may be required to achieve steady-state plasma concentrations unless a loading dose is given.[2] Clearance has been shown to be reduced by one third in patients in the last weeks of life.[3] About 25% is excreted unchanged by the kidney; the rest is converted in the liver, mainly to inactive oxidative metabolites via CYP450 enzymes. Phenobarbital is a potent inducer of CYP3A and may induce other enzymatic processes, e.g. glucuronidation, thus reducing plasma concentrations of many concurrently administered drugs (see Drug interactions) and inducing its own metabolism.[4]

Phenobarbital's efficacy in epilepsy is comparable to that of alternatives, but concerns about its cognitive and behavioural effects have led to a decline in its use other than for status epilepticus (see p.290).

Phenobarbital is used at some centres for refractory agitation in the imminently dying that fails to respond to the combined use of **midazolam** and an antipsychotic (see p.172).
Bio-availability >90% PO and PR.[5]
Onset of action 5min IV, maximum effect achieved within 30min; onset after SC or IM administration is slower.[2]
Time to peak plasma concentration 2–4h IM;[6] 2h PO (some authorities report ≤12h);[2,6-8] 2–4h PR (using oral tablets dissolved in water).[5,9]
Plasma halflife 2–6 *days*; 1–3 *days* in children.
Duration of action situation dependent; chronic administration >24h.

Cautions

Elderly, children, debilitated, respiratory depression, renal impairment (also see Chapter 17, p.738), hepatic impairment (also see Chapter 18, p.769). Avoid sudden withdrawal (see below).

Drug interactions

Phenobarbital is regarded as a potent inducer of CYP3A4 and thus reduces plasma concentrations of many drugs.[4] Table 1 lists selected drugs that have this clinically important interaction.

Conversely, some drugs can affect phenobarbital plasma concentrations, e.g.:
- **stiripentol** can significantly *increase* phenobarbital plasma concentrations
- **folic acid** and **St John's wort** can significantly *decrease* phenobarbital plasma concentrations.

Table 1 Clinically important CYP450 drug interactions for phenobarbital affecting other drugs[a,4]

Drug class	*Drug plasma concentration decreased by phenobarbital*
Anti-arrhythmics	Disopyramide
Antibacterials	Doxycycline, metronidazole, rifampicin
Anticoagulants	Apixaban, edoxaban, rivaroxaban, warfarin (and other coumarins)
Antidepressants	Mianserin, TCAs (all)
Anti-epileptics[b]	Carbamazepine, ethosuximide, lamotrigine, phenytoin, tiagabine, valproate, zonisamide
Antifungals	Griseofulvin, itraconazole, posaconazole, voriconazole
Antipsychotics	Chlorpromazine[c], haloperidol
Antiretrovirals/antivirals	Seek specialist advice
Benzodiazepines	Clonazepam
β-blockers	Metoprolol, timolol
Bronchodilators	Theophylline
Calcium-channel blockers	Felodipine, nifedipine, nimodipine, verapamil
Corticosteroids	Dexamethasone, methylprednisolone, prednisolone
Cytotoxics and immunomodulators	Seek specialist advice
Hormone antagonists	Toremifene
Hormonal contraceptives & hormone replacement therapy	All
Neurokinin-1 antagonists	Aprepitant, fosaprepitant
Non-opioid analgesics	Paracetamol[d]
Opioid analgesics	Fentanyl (IV; significance not known for TD), methadone

a. not an exhaustive list; limited to drugs most likely to be encountered in palliative care
b. interactions between anti-epileptic drugs are complex and unpredictable; plasma concentrations of either drug may be increased, decreased or unchanged
c. chlorpromazine also decreases phenobarbital plasma concentrations
d. hepatotoxic metabolites may be increased (see p.334).

Undesirable effects

Respiratory depression (high doses), drowsiness, lethargy, ataxia, skin reactions (<3%). Paradoxical excitement, irritability, restlessness/hyperactivity and delirium, particularly in the elderly and children.

Long-term treatment is occasionally complicated by folate-responsive megaloblastic anaemia, osteomalacia or complex regional pain syndrome.[10]

As with all anti-epileptics, there is a risk of suicidal ideation of 0.2% (1 in 500; advise patients to report mood or thought disturbance; also see p.287).

Toxicity from propylene glycol, an excipient in the injection, has been reported with prolonged high dose IVI, resulting in confusion, drowsiness, seizures, cardiac arrhythmias or renal failure.[11] However, the dose of phenobarbital required to achieve toxic levels of propylene glycol (~14g/24h) is unlikely to be necessary in palliative care (~3,000mg/24h, using 200mg/mL UK injection).

Dose and use

Route of administration

IV infusion: the injection is very alkaline (pH >9.2) and has a high osmolality. Consequently, it is recommended to dilute it with 10 times its own volume of sodium chloride 0.9% to reduce the risk of venous pain and phlebitis.[12]

IM injection: phenobarbital can be given undiluted.

CSCI: although a 1 in 10 dilution has been advocated,[13] this is probably unnecessary; many centres administer phenobarbital ≤1600mg/24h diluted to 17mL with WFI or sodium chloride 0.9% when using a 20mL syringe and a T34 syringe driver.[14]

SC bolus infusion: some centres infuse ≤600mg loading doses SC diluted in 100mL sodium chloride 0.9% over approximately 30min under gravity.

SC bolus injection *of the undiluted product is avoided in the UK* because there are reports of tissue necrosis. Although the North American preparation appears well tolerated by SC bolus,[15] it is unclear whether the formulations differ or tissue necrosis is a rare effect.

PR: phenobarbital tablets have been dissolved in 6mL tap water and given PR.[9] Successful use of compounded suppositories is also described.[16]

PO: rarely used in palliative care patients unless already taking under specialist neurological treatment.

CSCI compatibility with other drugs: phenobarbital should be administered via a separate syringe driver. Due to its alkaline pH, it is likely to be *incompatible* with most palliative care drugs (see Chapter 29, p.892).

Alternative SC/CSCI anti-epileptics include **lacosamide**,[17] **levetiracetam** (p.313), **midazolam** (p.174) and **valproate** (p.310).

Epilepsy

The MHRA advises that the oral products available in the UK may differ in bio-availability, and that to avoid changes in effectiveness or increased risk of undesirable effects, it is best to avoid switching between formulations (see also p.288).

Status epilepticus

Phenobarbital is used for the emergency treatment of seizures refractory to benzodiazepines ± **levetiracetam** (see Anti-epileptics, Figure 2, p.291):

- give a stat dose of 10–15mg/kg (up to a maximum dose of 1g):[18]
  - ▷ IV (each 1mL ampoule diluted with 10mL sodium chloride 0.9%; rate 100mg/min) *or*
  - ▷ IM *undiluted* (if the IV route is not available). Larger doses may be split between ≥2 sites. IM absorption is significantly slower than IV
- if seizures persist:
  - ▷ if ICU is appropriate, transfer for general anaesthesia
  - ▷ if imminently dying, give further p.r.n. doses and commence a CSCI (dose as for refractory agitation below).

Some centres administer an initial 10–15mg/kg loading dose, up to a maximum of 600mg, in 100mL of sodium chloride 0.9% by SC infusion over 30min, with the subsequent maintenance dose given CSCI or by SC injection once daily.

Maintenance anti-epileptic in patients unable to swallow

Phenobarbital is a second-line alternative to **midazolam, valproate** or **levetiracetam** (see p.291):

- give a stat dose of 100mg (0.5mL of a 200mg/mL ampoule) IM (*undiluted*) or IV (diluted with 5mL sodium chloride 0.9%, over 2min)
- then 100mg/24h CSCI
- if seizures occur, give a second stat dose of 100mg IM/IV and titrate the maintenance dose (maximum of 400mg/24h CSCI)
- if seizures persist, treat as for status epilepticus (see above, taking account of the phenobarbital already given) or, in the imminently dying, as for refractory agitation (see below).

†Refractory agitation in the imminently dying

Phenobarbital is generally used third-line for patients who fail to respond to the combined use of **midazolam** and an antipsychotic (see p.172):

- give a stat dose of 200mg (1mL of a 200mg/mL ampoule) IM (*undiluted*) or IV (diluted with sodium chloride 0.9%, over 2min)
- if the patient remains unsettled, give 1 or 2 further doses p.r.n. of 200mg IM/IV 30min apart (the median loading dose reported in case series is 600mg)
- if still unsettled or agitation recurs, give further doses of 200mg IM/IV q1h p.r.n.
- maintain with 800mg/24h CSCI, or more if total initial 'settling' dose was ≥600mg
- if necessary, increase the dose progressively, e.g. 800 → 1,200 → 1,600mg/24h
- a typical dose is 800–1,200mg/24h but can range 200–3,800mg/24h.[19-23]

Some centres infuse ≤600mg loading doses SC over 30min (see Routes of administration). Some centres use **propofol** (see p.702), **sodium oxybate** (not UK) or **dexmedetomidine** instead.[24-27]

†Alcohol withdrawal

Phenobarbital is reserved for symptoms refractory to benzodiazepines. Regimens vary widely, but typically start with 200mg IV stat, repeated p.r.n. (sometimes at a lower dose) until symptoms settle. It was used in settings equipped to manage airways and respiratory depression.[28] **Gabapentin** (p.297) is an alternative.

Stopping phenobarbital

Abrupt cessation of long-term PO anti-epileptic therapy, particularly barbiturates and benzodiazepines, should be avoided because rebound seizures may be precipitated (see p.293).

Supply

All products are Schedule 3 **CD**.

Phenobarbital sodium (generic)
Tablets 15mg, 30mg, 60mg, 28 days @ 60mg at night = £7.50.
Oral solution 15mg/5mL; 28 days @ 60mg at night = £93; *may contain significant amounts of ethanol.*
Injection 30mg/mL, 60mg/mL and 200mg/mL, 1mL amp = £12; *vehicle contains propylene glycol 90%. Must be diluted with 10 times its volume before IV use.*

1 Brodie MJ (2016) Pharmacological treatment of drug-resistant epilepsy in adults: a practical guide. *Current Neurology and Neuroscience Reports*. **16**: 82.
2 Miller J (ed.) *American Hospital Formulary Service*. Maryland, USA: American Society of Health-System Pharmacists www.medicinescomplete.com (accessed April 2021).
3 Nakayama H *et al.* (2018) Reduced clearance of phenobarbital in advanced cancer patients near the end of life. *European Journal of Drug Metabolism and Pharmacokinetics*. **44**: 77–82.
4 Preston C (ed.) *Stockley's Drug Interactions*. London: Pharmaceutical Press www.medicinescomplete.com (accessed April 2021).
5 Leppik IE and Patel SI (2015) Intramuscular and rectal therapies of acute seizures. *Epilepsy and Behavior*. **49**: 307–312.

6 Buckingham R (ed.) *Martindale: The Complete Drug Reference*. London: Pharmaceutical Press www.medicinescomplete.com (accessed April 2021).
7 Stirling LC *et al.* (1999) The use of phenobarbitone in the management of agitation and seizures at the end of life. *Journal of Pain and Symptom Management*. **17**: 363–368.
8 Holford N (ed.) (1998) *Clinical Pharmacokinetics: Drug Data Handbook* (3e). Auckland, New Zealand: Adis International.
9 Lam YW *et al.* (2016) Pharmacokinetics of phenobarbital in microenema via macy catheter versus suppository. *Journal of Pain and Symptom Management*. **51**: 994–1001.
10 Jha S *et al.* (2020) Phenobarbital rheumatism – a fresh look at an old malady: case report and systematic review of literature. *International Journal of Rheumatic Diseases*. **23**: 589–594.
11 Pillai U *et al.* (2014) Severe propylene glycol toxicity secondary to use of anti-epileptics. *American Journal of Therapeutics*. **21**: e106–e109.
12 Medusa. Phenobarbital monograph (version 8). *NHS Injectable Medicines Guide*. https://medusa.wales.nhs.uk (accessed April 2021).
13 Dickman A and Schneider J (2016) *The Syringe Driver: Continuous Subcutaneous Infusions in Palliative Care* (4e). Oxford, UK: Oxford University Press.
14 Palliativedrugs.com Ltd Phenobarbital CSCI – how do you dilute it? *Latest additions: Survey results (September 2015)*. www.palliativedrugs.com.
15 Hosgood JR *et al.* (2016) Evaluation of subcutaneous phenobarbital administration in hospice patients. *American Journal of Hospice and Palliative Care*. **33**: 209–213.
16 Setla J and Pasniciuc S (2019) Home palliative sedation using phenobarbital suppositories: time to death, patient characteristics, and administration protocol. *American Journal of Hospice and Palliative Medicine*. **36**: 871–876.
17 Remi C *et al.* (2016) Subcutaneous use of lacosamide. *Journal of Pain Symptom Management*. **51**: e2–e4.
18 NICE (2012) The epilepsies: the diagnosis and management of the epilepsies in adults and children in primary and secondary care. *Clinical Guideline* CG137 www.nice.org.uk.
19 de Graeff A and Dean M (2007) Palliative sedation therapy in the last weeks of life: a literature review and recommendations for standards. *Journal of Palliative Medicine*. **10**: 67–85.
20 Gillon S *et al.* (2010) Review of phenobarbitone use for deep terminal sedation in a UK hospice. *Palliative Medicine*. **24**: 100–101.
21 Chater S *et al.* (1998) Sedation for intractable distress in the dying – a survey of experts. *Palliative Medicine*. **12**: 255–269.
22 Cowan J and Walsh D (2001) Terminal sedation in palliative medicine – definition and review of the literature. *Supportive Care in Cancer*. **9**: 403–407.
23 Won Y-W *et al.* (2019) Clinical patterns of continuous and intermittent palliative sedation in patients with terminal cancer: a descriptive, observational study. *Journal of Pain and Symptom Management*. **58**: 65–71.
24 Gertler R *et al.* (2001) Dexmedetomidine: a novel sedative-analgesic agent. *Proceedings (Baylor University Medical Center)*. **14**: 13–21.
25 Soares L *et al.* (2002) Dexmedetomidine: a new option for intractable distress in the dying. *Journal of Pain and Symptom Management*. **24**: 6–8.
26 Jackson KC 3rd *et al.* (2006) Dexmedetomidine: a novel analgesic with palliative medicine potential. *Journal of Pain and Palliative Care Pharmacotherapy*. **20**: 23–27.
27 Ciais J *et al.* (2015) Using sodium oxybate (gamma hydroxybutyric acid) for deep sedation at the end of life. *Journal of Palliative Medicine*. **18**: 822.
28 Martin K and Katz A (2016) The role of barbiturates for alcohol withdrawal syndrome. *Psychosomatics*. **57**: 341–347.

Updated May 2021

5: ANALGESICS

PRINCIPLES OF USE OF ANALGESICS

Analgesics can be divided into three classes:
- non-opioid
- opioid
- adjuvant (Figure 1).

Drugs from different classes are used alone or in combination according to the type of pain and response to treatment in conjunction with non-drug measures.

Because cancer pain typically has an inflammatory component, it is generally appropriate to optimize treatment with an NSAID and an opioid before introducing adjuvant analgesics. However, with treatment-related pains (e.g. chemotherapy-induced neuropathic pain, chronic postoperative scar pain) and pains unrelated to cancer (e.g. post-herpetic neuralgia, muscle spasm pain), an adjuvant may be an appropriate first-line treatment,[1] e.g. an antidepressant or an anti-epileptic for neuropathic pain, or a benzodiazepine or **baclofen** for muscle spasm (also see Adjuvant analgesics, p.325).

The main broad principles governing analgesic use for persistent cancer pain can be summarized as:
- administer at regular intervals ('by the clock'); back up with doses for break-through pain
- when feasible, use PO route ('by the mouth')
- use the analgesic ladder (Figure 2); after optimising the dose, if a drug fails to relieve, move up the ladder ('by the ladder')
- evaluate the pain, select an appropriate analgesic and titrate the dose against individual need ('by the individual')
- monitor benefit and treat undesirable effects ('attention to detail').[2]

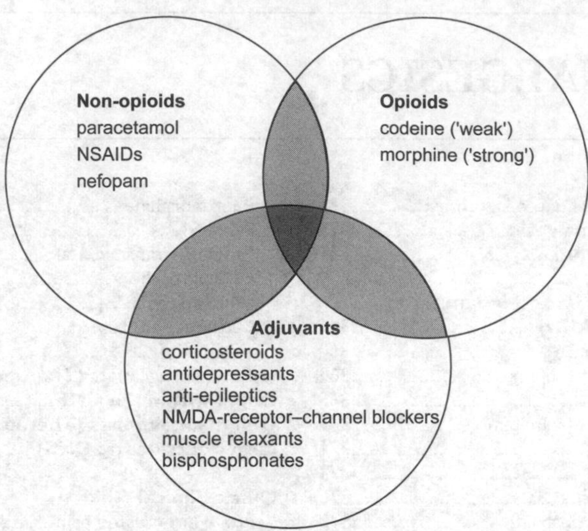

Figure 1 Broad-spectrum analgesia; drugs from different categories are used alone or in combination according to the type of pain and response to treatment.

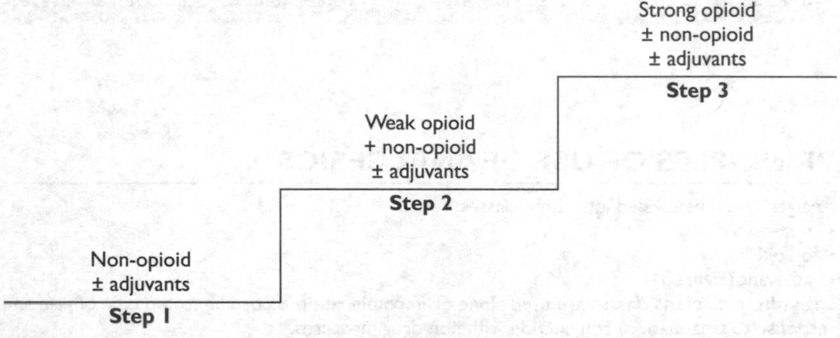

Figure 2 The World Health Organization 3-step analgesic ladder.[2] Step 2 is omitted in children and is unnecessary in countries where morphine is readily available (see text).

The WHO 3-step analgesic ladder for cancer pain in adults, created some 40 years ago, is still a useful educational tool (Figure 2).[2] However, there is no pharmacological need for Step 2.[3] Indeed, compared to a weak opioid, benefit from *low-dose* **morphine** (20–30mg/24h PO) is greater and more rapid.[4] Step 2 exists because in many countries accessing strong opioids is difficult (e.g. available only for inpatients, and then sparingly by injection) and sometimes impossible. Thus, in countries where **morphine** is readily available, by-passing a weak opioid is likely to become standard practice in adults with moderate–severe cancer pain.

Analgesic use in children is comparable to adults. However, because weak opioids (p.376) are generally contra-indicated in children, moving directly from a non-opioid to a strong opioid ± non-opioid is the norm (see Chapter 16, p.728).

Break-through pain

Several definitions of break-through pain exist.[5,6] Episodic pain, previously synonymous with break-through pain, has also been proposed as a broader overarching concept that encompasses all significant transient pain exacerbations, including those occurring in patients without background pain or requiring regular analgesia.[7] The focus in *PCF* is on break-through pain as defined below.

Break-through pain is a term used to describe a transient exacerbation of pain which occurs either spontaneously or in relation to a specific trigger despite relatively stable and adequately controlled background pain. It may or may not be at the same location as the background (controlled) pain.[8]

Patients with poorly relieved background pain are excluded because this suggests overall poor pain relief which requires an increase in regular analgesia. Similarly, pain recurring shortly before the next dose of a regular analgesic is due ('end-of-dose-interval pain') is not true break-through pain.

There are two main types of break-through pain:

- *predictable (incident) pain,* an exacerbation of pain caused by weight-bearing and/or activity (including swallowing, defaecation, coughing, nursing/medical procedures)
- *unpredictable (spontaneous) pain*, unrelated to movement or activity, e.g. colic, stabbing pain associated with nerve injury.

Break-through pain is common in cancer patients receiving opioid medication for persistent pain (≤80%).[5] In a large survey, the median number of episodes per day was 3 (range 0–24). These were generally moderate–severe in intensity and interfered with aspects of daily living, in particular, incident pain with walking and normal work, and spontaneous pain with sleep and mood.[9]

Break-through pain is often a resurgence of the background pain and may be either functional (e.g. tension headache) or pathological, and either nociceptive (associated with tissue distortion or injury) or neuropathic (associated with nerve compression or injury). Patients may experience more than one break-through pain, and these may have different causes. Various strategies reduce the impact of break-through pain (Figure 3).[10] Commonly used non-drug measures include rest, change of position and local heat.[9]

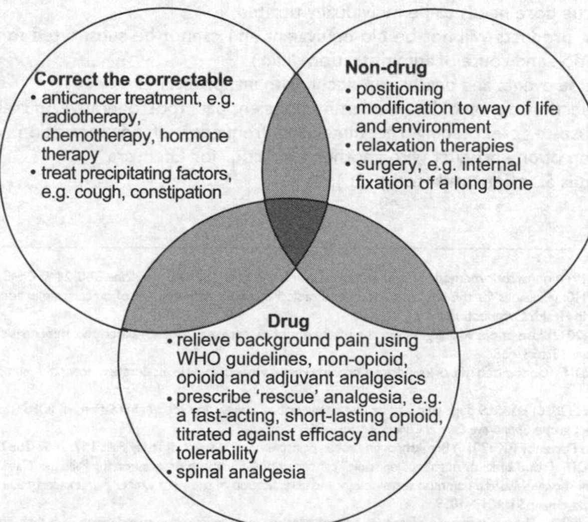

Figure 3 A multimodal approach to managing break-through pain.

Break-through cancer pain is commonly treated by giving an extra dose of the regular analgesic, e.g. a p.r.n. dose of immediate-release **morphine** for patients taking **morphine** regularly round-the-clock.[2,9] A traditional practice, dating from before m/r opioid products were available, was to give an extra dose of the regular q4h dose of oral **morphine** (i.e. one sixth of the total daily dose). However, many break-through pains are short-lived, and this approach effectively doubles the patient's opioid intake for the next 4h.

Accordingly, many centres now recommend that the patient initially takes, as an immediate-release formulation, 10% of the total daily regular dose as the p.r.n. dose.[11,12] However, a standard fixed dose is unlikely to suit all patients and all pains, particularly because the intensity and the impact of break-through pain vary considerably. Thus, when patients are encouraged to optimize their rescue dose, it varies from 5–20% of the total daily dose.[13,14] When prescribing a p.r.n. dose, it is recommended that:

- a maximum daily amount or frequency is stated
- an individual entry is used for each route, e.g. PO, SC
- patients/carers are taught how to use the formulation correctly
- the amount used is reviewed regularly and, where necessary, the background analgesia increased.[15]

Break-through cancer pain generally has a relatively rapid onset (median 5–10min) and short duration (45–60min), but ranging from <1min to 4–6h.[9] By comparison, oral **morphine**, on average, takes about 15–30min (solution quicker than tablet, see p.453) to achieve meaningful pain relief and has a longer duration of effect (3–6h).[16] This helps to explain why many patients choose *not* to take a rescue dose of PO opioid with every episode of break-through pain, particularly when predictable, mild in intensity, and of relatively short duration.[9]

Strategies to circumvent the mismatch between break-through pain duration and drug effect latency include:

- timing a predictable painful activity or procedure to coincide with the peak plasma concentration after a regular or rescue PO dose of **morphine** (1–2h) or another strong opioid
- using routes of administration, e.g. buccal, intranasal, SL, which permit more rapid absorption of some (lipophilic) opioids, e.g. **fentanyl**.[17,18]

Transmucosal **fentanyl** products (p.450) cost substantially more than short-acting PO opioids and generally their use is reserved for when the latter are unsatisfactory. Experience with them indicates:[19]

- there is little or no correlation between the dose of the regularly administered strong opioid and the satisfactory rescue dose
- that the rescue dose needs to be individually titrated
- that different products will not be bio-equivalent and cannot be substituted for one another (the formulation and route of administration differ)
- serious adverse events and deaths can occur with inappropriate:
  - ▷ patient selection, e.g. opioid non-tolerant, transient pain (postoperative, migraine)
  - ▷ product use, e.g.: exceeding recommended frequency of administration; dose-for-dose substitution of one product with another, e.g. Actiq® for Effentora®.

Another option is SL **alfentanil** (see p.420).

---

1 Finnerup NB (2019) Nonnarcotic methods of pain management. *New England Journal of Medicine*. **380**: 2440–2448.

2 WHO (2019) WHO guidelines for the pharmacological and radiotherapeutic management of cancer pain in adults and adolescents. Geneva: World Health Organization.

3 Caraceni A *et al.* (2012) Use of opioid analgesics in the treatment of cancer pain: evidence-based recommendations from the EAPC. *Lancet Oncology*. **13**: e58–e68.

4 Bandieri E *et al.* (2016) Randomized trial of low-dose morphine versus weak opioids in moderate cancer pain. *Journal of Clinical Oncology*. **34**: 436–442.

5 Mercadante S *et al.* (2016) Breakthrough pain and its treatment: critical review and recommendations of IOPS (Italian Oncologic Pain Survey) expert group. *Supportive Care in Cancer*. **24**: 961–968.

6 Mercadante S and Portenoy RK (2016) Breakthrough cancer pain: twenty-five years of study. *Pain*. **157**: 2657-2663.

7 Lohre ET *et al.* (2016) From "breakthrough" to "episodic" cancer pain? A European Association for Palliative Care Research Network Expert Delphi survey toward a common terminology and classification of transient cancer pain exacerbations. *Journal of Pain and Symptom Management*. **51**: 1013–1019.

8 Davies AN *et al.* (2009) The management of cancer-related breakthrough pain: recommendations of a task group of the Science Committee of the Association for Palliative Medicine of Great Britain and Ireland. *European Journal of Pain*. **13**: 331–338.

9 Davies A *et al.* (2013) Breakthrough cancer pain: an observational study of 1000 European oncology patients. *Journal of Pain and Symptom Management*. **46**: 619–628.

10 Zeppetella G and Ribeiro MD (2002) Episodic pain in patients with advanced cancer. *American Journal of Hospice and Palliative Care*. **19**: 267–276.

11 Davis MP *et al.* (2005) Controversies in pharmacotherapy of pain management. *Lancet Oncology.* **6:** 696–704.
12 Davis MP (2003) Guidelines for breakthrough pain dosing. *American Journal of Hospice and Palliative Care.* **20**: 334.
13 Portenoy K and Hagen N (1990) Breakthrough pain: definition, prevalence and characteristics. *Pain.* **41**: 273–281.
14 Mercadante S *et al.* (2002) Episodic (breakthrough) pain: consensus conference of an expert working group of the EAPC. *Cancer.* **94**: 832–839.
15 NICE (2016) Controlled drugs: safe use and management. *Clinical Guideline* NG46. www.nice.org.uk.
16 Zeppetella G (2008) Opioids for cancer breakthrough pain: a pilot study reporting patient assessment of time to meaningful pain relief. *Journal of Pain and Symptom Management.* **35**: 563–567.
17 Davies A *et al.* (2011) Multi-centre European study of breakthrough cancer pain: Pain characteristics and patient perceptions of current and potential management strategies. *European Journal of Pain.* **15**: 756–763.
18 Zeppetella G and Ribeiro MD (2006) Opioids for the management of breakthrough (episodic) pain in cancer patients. *Cochrane Database of Systematic Reviews.* CD004311. www.cochranelibrary.com.
19 Christie J *et al.* (1998) Dose-titration, multicenter study of oral transmucosal fentanyl citrate for the treatment of breakthrough pain in cancer patients using transdermal fentanyl for persistent pain. *Journal of Clinical Oncology.* **16**: 3238–3248.

Updated (minor change) December 2021

ADJUVANT ANALGESICS

Adjuvant analgesics are drugs with an effect on pain that is *circumstance specific*. Some reduce the painful stimulus directly:

- cancer-related bone pain (bisphosphonates)
- skeletal muscle spasm (skeletal muscle relaxants)
- smooth muscle spasm (smooth muscle relaxants)
- cancer-related oedema (corticosteroids).

Others correct changes in pain transmission caused by persistent severe pain and/or damage to the nervous system:

- peripheral sensitization (NSAIDs, corticosteroids)
- ectopic foci caused by nerve damage (e.g. some anti-epileptics)
- central sensitization of the spine and higher centres (e.g. NMDA-receptor–channel blockers, some anti-epileptics)
- altered descending pain modulation (some antidepressants).

Many act in more than one way (Figure 1). Most are marketed for indications other than pain. Unsurprisingly, adjuvant analgesics are *not* effective for *unselected* cancer-related pain.[1]

Some adjuvant analgesics take longer to act than standard analgesics, and complete pain relief is not always possible. Undesirable effects are often a limiting factor, particularly in frail patients.[2] As with any analgesic, it is important to discuss with the patient desired outcomes, potential problems and the probable timing of benefits.

Low-dose combined treatment may be preferable if a single drug (appropriately titrated) does not provide adequate relief. For example, when used together for neuropathic pain, **nortriptyline** with either **gabapentin** or **morphine** was more effective than each drug alone.[3,4]

Use relative to other measures

Because cancer pain typically has an inflammatory component, it is generally appropriate to optimize treatment with an NSAID and an opioid before introducing adjuvant analgesics. Subsequently, adjuvant analgesics are added to:

- relieve those pains that fail to respond, e.g. neuropathic, bone pain *and/or*
- reduce undesirable effects, e.g. by reducing the dose of opioid needed.

However, with treatment-related pains (e.g. chemotherapy-induced neuropathic pain, chronic postoperative scar pain) and pains unrelated to cancer (e.g. post-herpetic neuralgia, muscle spasm pain), an adjuvant may be an appropriate first-line treatment.

Neuropathic pain

Neuropathic pain is caused by multiple mechanisms including:

- overexpression of sodium channels at the site of peripheral nerve injury (see Anti-epileptics, p.280)
- overexpression of N-type calcium channels in the spine and brain (see **Gabapentin** and **pregabalin**, p.297)
- altered postsynaptic excitability (see **Ketamine**, p.691)
- neuro-inflammation in the spine and brain.[14]

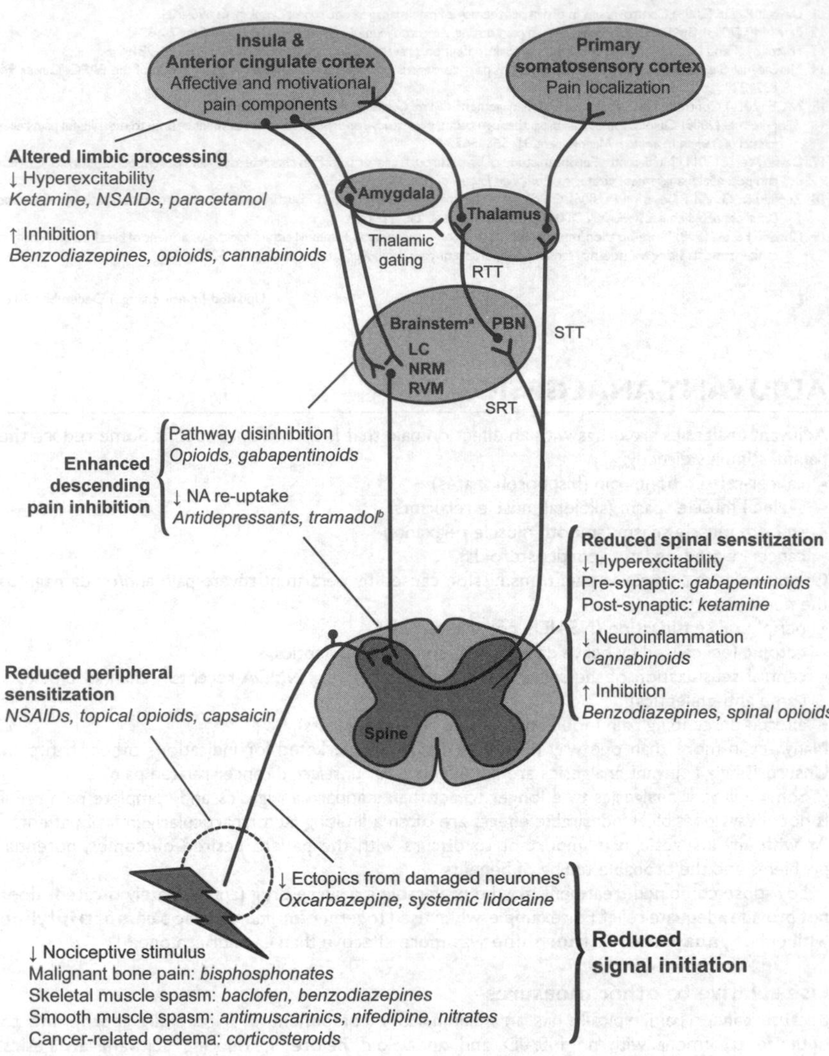

Figure 1 Putative sites of action of selected analgesics. See individual monographs for more detailed explanation and references.[5-13]

Abbreviations: NA = noradrenaline (norepinephrine), PBN = parabrachial nucleus, RTT = reticulothalamic tract, SRT = spinoreticulotract, STT = spinothalamic tract

a. important relay centres and neurotransmitters include the locus coeruleus (LC; noradrenaline; see Antidepressants, p.210), the nucleus raphe magnus (NRM; serotonin) and rostral ventral medulla (RVM; opioids)
b. also acts as a μ-opioid receptor agonist
c. reduces ectopic nerve signal transmission by damaged neurones (see Anti-epileptics, p.280); the higher concentrations of lidocaine used in local/regional anaesthesia completely inhibit nerve signal transmission.

First-line adjuvant choices for cancer-related neuropathic pain include **amitriptyline** (p.228), **duloxetine** (p.239), and **gabapentin** or **pregabalin** (p.297). These are also first-line choices for non-cancer neuropathic pain.[13] Because their efficacy and tolerability are comparable,[15-24] choice is influenced by cost and individual patient circumstances (Table 1). There is increasing interest in relating certain patterns of sensory findings (sensory phenotypic profiling) to the probability of response to particular classes of drug (e.g. **oxcarbazepine**, p.304).[25]

Drugs that act via different mechanisms can be combined if patients do not respond to a single drug (Figure 2).[3,4] In RCTs, opioids at least partly relieved neuropathic pain.[26,27]

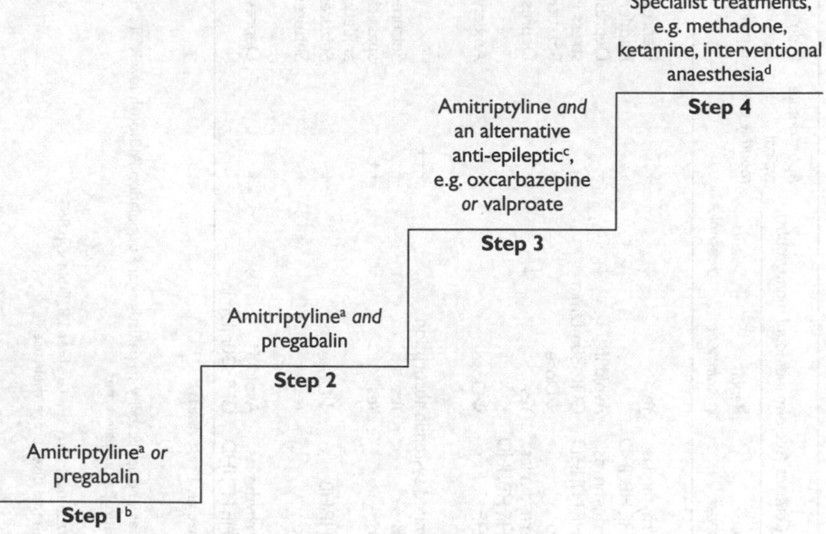

Figure 2 Suggested adjuvant analgesics for neuropathic pain.

a. consider duloxetine if amitriptyline is poorly tolerated but *not* if it is ineffective, because their mechanism of action is similar (see Antidepressants, p.221)
b. systemic corticosteroids are an alternative for *cancer-related* neuropathic pain, particularly if pain is associated with limb weakness or awaiting benefit from another treatment, e.g. radiotherapy
c. generally, the pregabalin is withdrawn once the new anti-epileptic has been titrated to an effective dose (see Anti-epileptics, p.289)
d. e.g. spinal analgesia, nerve block.

Systemic corticosteroids, by reducing oedema, are of benefit in some cancer-related neuropathic pains, e.g. nerve root or spinal cord compression (also see Systemic corticosteroids, Box A, p.556). They do not help in pure non-cancer neuropathic pain, e.g. chronic postoperative scar pain, post-herpetic neuralgia.

Treatment options for neuropathic pain refractory to antidepressants and gabapentinoid anti-epileptics are generally specialist use only. These include **methadone** (p.469), **ketamine** (p.691), **oxcarbazepine** (p.304), **valproate** (p.307), systemic **lidocaine** (p.77), or interventional anaesthesia (p.908). Their place, relative to each other, is uncertain, and selection is influenced by local availability and expertise.

The place, if any, of **capsaicin** cream 0.075% (p.651), cannabinoids (p.251), **clonidine/dexmedetomidine** (p.82), **flecainide** (p.80), transdermal **lidocaine** (p.79), **memantine** (p.691) or **mexiletine** (p.77) is uncertain.

Bone pain

Cancer-related bone pain is caused by multiple mechanisms, e.g.:[5]

- stimulation/sensitization of pain afferents by inflammatory mediators (e.g. prostaglandins) and other substances (e.g. acid/acid metabolites) produced by cancer, immune and other cells (e.g. osteoclasts)
- an increase in osteoclast number and activity → increased acidity, direct injury of sensory nerves
- mechanical stresses arising as a result of bone distension (cancer expansion) or bone instability (loss of bone mineral), triggering mechanoreceptors in the periosteum and pain on movement.

Table 1 Some considerations when selecting an adjuvant analgesic for neuropathic pain[28-32]

Drug	Supporting evidence[a]	Ease of administration			Propensity for drug interactions	Cautions (see also individual monographs)			Approximate typical monthly cost[b]	Examples of concurrent indications in palliative care
		Once daily	Oral solution[b]	Parenteral		Cardiac disease	Renal impairment	Seizure threshold		
First-line treatments for neuropathic pain										
Amitriptyline	High	Yes	Yes	No	Moderate	Arrhythmias, CHF, HB, IHD	Yes	↓	+	Depression, anxiety, bladder spasms, urgency
Duloxetine	Moderate	Yes	No	No	Moderate	Arrhythmias, CHF, HT, IHD	Avoid if GFR<30mL/min	↓	+	Depression, anxiety, stress incontinence
Gabapentin	High	No	Yes[c]	No	Low	No	↓Dose		+	Spasticity, seizures
†Nortriptyline	Moderate	Yes	No	No	Moderate	Arrhythmias, CHF, HB, IHD	Yes	↓	+	Depression
Pregabalin	High	No	Yes[c]	No	Low	CHF	↓Dose		+	Anxiety, seizures
Treatments generally reserved for use second-line or in specific situations										
Lidocaine 5% plaster[d]	Low	Yes	Topical		Low	Limited systemic absorption			+++	
Carbamazepine[e]	Low	No	Yes	No	High	HB	Yes		+	Seizures
†Clonazepam	Very low	Yes	Yes[f]	Not UK	Moderate	No	Yes		++	Spasticity, seizures, anxiety
†Oxcarbazepine	Low	No	Yes	No	Moderate	CHF, HB	↓Dose		+	Seizures
†Valproate	Low	Yes	Yes	Yes (†CSCI)	Moderate	No	Yes		+	Seizures
†Venlafaxine	Moderate	Yes (m/r)	No[f]	No	Moderate	Arrhythmias, CHF, HT, IHD	Avoid if GFR<30mL/min	↓	+	Depression, anxiety

Abbreviations: CHF = congestive heart failure; HB = heart block; HT = hypertension; IHD = ischaemic heart disease

Monthly cost: + = <£10; ++ = £10–25; +++ = >£25

a. based on RCTs vs. case reports, methodological quality, consistency within and between studies, and applicability to palliative care population. Although few RCTs have been conducted in palliative care patients, generalizability was considered more likely if benefit shown in ≥2 neuropathic pain types

b. generally, oral solutions are considerably more expensive

c. capsules can be opened and the contents dispersed in water or sprinkled on food (unauthorized use); also see Chapter 28, Table 2, p.863

d. authorized for post-herpetic neuralgia only; high cost and limited efficacy have led NHS England to discourage their use

e. first-line choice (and authorized) for trigeminal neuralgia

f. immediate-release disperses in water in 5min (unauthorized use); also see Chapter 28, Table 2, p.863.

Cancer-related bone pain is generally managed with an NSAID + opioid along with radiotherapy. Orthopaedic interventions may be needed, particularly when there is an increased risk of pathological fracture. When these fail or are inappropriate, adjuvant analgesic approaches include:

- other anti-inflammatory drugs, e.g. corticosteroids
- osteoclast inhibitors, e.g. bisphosphonates
- drugs for neuropathic pain (but see below).

Although **dexamethasone** (p.556) is widely used in this setting, benefit has *not* been confirmed in an RCT.[33]

Bisphosphonates (p.535) and **denosumab** (p.549) are osteoclast inhibitors primarily given *prophylactically* to reduce the risk of pain and other complications of bone metastases. The role of either as adjuvant analgesics for moderate–severe bone pain is unclear, because supporting data are limited/of low quality (see p.539). IV **zoledronic acid** can be considered in patients with a prognosis of >2 weeks and not already receiving prophylactic bisphosphonates or **denosumab**.

Neuropathic mechanisms have been implicated in cancer-related bone pain, including altered anatomy causing nerve entrapment and/or periosteal distension and neuroma-like hyperinnervation of the tumour/bone interface. Despite case reports of benefit from **gabapentin**,[34] results of RCTs of **pregabalin** or **gabapentin** are mixed,[35] with the most methodologically robust studies being negative.[36]

Although **calcitonin** is effective for acute pain (onset ≤10 days) associated with vertebral fractures in osteoporosis and rib fractures in cystic fibrosis,[37,38] it is *not* of benefit in chronic pain (≥3 months) associated with vertebral fractures,[37] nor cancer-related bone pain.[39]

Skeletal muscle spasm

Cramp and trigger point pains respond poorly to opioids. Generally, non-drug treatments are tried first and include local heat, massage, relaxation therapy and TENS.[40] Local treatments also include acupuncture or direct injection of local anaesthetic for myofascial trigger points or **botulinum toxin** for focal dystonias.[41,42] Most skeletal muscle relaxants act centrally (see Skeletal muscle relaxants, Table 1, p.655). Note. Generalized myofascial pain can be a manifestation of vitamin D or magnesium deficiency (see p.638).

Smooth muscle spasm (colic)

Smooth muscle relaxants act:[43,44]

- directly on smooth muscle L-type calcium channels (e.g. **mebeverine**; **nifedipine**, p.92; **peppermint oil**, p.1)
- indirectly on the transmitters that control smooth muscle tone:
  - ▷ acetylcholine (see Antimuscarinics, p.4)
  - ▷ nitric oxide (see **Glyceryl trinitrate**, p.88)
  - ▷ prostaglandins (see NSAIDs, p.341).

Peppermint oil may also influence visceral sensation and the gut microbiome.[43]

Choice is influenced by location; antimuscarinics are first-line choices for intestinal and bladder spasm, whereas NSAIDs are more effective than antimuscarinics for renal[45,46] and biliary[47,48] colic.

For intestinal spasm, PO/SC **hyoscine butylbromide** (p.15) is a common choice because, like the more expensive **glycopyrronium** (p.12), it does not cross the blood-brain barrier and, thus, lacks the central effects of **atropine** and **hyoscine *hydrobromide***. **Mebeverine** or **peppermint oil** are alternatives.

For bladder spasm, newer antimuscarinics with greater M_3-receptor selectivity are preferred (see Urinary antimuscarinics, p.611). **Hyoscine butylbromide** SC (but not PO; limited systemic absorption) is an alternative.

Glyceryl trinitrate (p.88) or **nifedipine** (p.92) are generally reserved for spasm refractory to the above approaches.

Tenesmoid pain

Cancer of the rectum or anal canal can result in tenesmoid pain. Generally, this is a mixed pain with neuropathic and smooth muscle spasm components, and skeletal muscle spasm when the anal sphincter is involved. Because RCT data are lacking, practice varies, but case series in cancer-related tenesmoid pain report benefit from, e.g. **diltiazem**, systemic **lidocaine**, **methadone**,

mexiletine, **nifedipine**, interventional techniques (lumbar sympathectomy, endoscopic laser interventions).[49] A stepwise initial approach used in some centres consists of:

- opioid + NSAID
- neuropathic adjuvants, e.g. an antidepressant + an anti-epileptic, used as per nerve pain (p.325)
- smooth muscle relaxant, e.g. **nifedipine**.

If anal sphincter spasm is contributing, consider **baclofen** or topical **glyceryl trinitrate** (p.88). Benefit from topical local anaesthetics and corticosteroids is also reported.[50]

Oesophageal spasm

This may occur with an oesophageal cancer or stent. RCT data are lacking, but smooth muscle relaxants are often tried first line, e.g. **glyceryl trinitrate** (p.88) or **nifedipine** (p.92), and **baclofen** second line (the oesophagus comprises both smooth and skeletal muscle).

Ischaemic limb pain

Critical limb ischaemic pain results from multiple mechanisms:[51,52]

- ischaemic metabolites stimulating acid-sensing channels on peripheral nociceptors, e.g. TRPV1
- inflammatory, e.g. tissue necrosis ± infection, ulceration
- neuropathic.

A routine approach has not been defined, but opioids, **gabapentin** (p.297), **ketamine** (p.691) or systemic **lidocaine** (p.77) appear beneficial.[53] A stepwise initial approach used in some centres consists of:

- opioid + NSAID
- neuropathic adjuvants, e.g. an anti-epileptic together with an antidepressant, used as per nerve pain (p.325)
- more specialist intervention, e.g. **ketamine**.

1 Paulsen O *et al.* (2014) Efficacy of methylprednisolone on pain, fatigue, and appetite loss in patients with advanced cancer using opioids: a randomized, placebo-controlled, double-blind trial. *Journal of Clinical Oncology*. **32**: 3221–3228.

2 Bennett MI (2011) Effectiveness of antiepileptic or antidepressant drugs when added to opioids for cancer pain: systematic review. *Palliative Medicine*. **25**: 553–559.

3 Gilron I et *al.* (2009) Nortriptyline and gabapentin, alone and in combination for neuropathic pain: a double-blind, randomised controlled crossover trial. *Lancet*. **374**: 1252–1261.

4 Gilron I *et al.* (2015) Combination of morphine with nortriptyline for neuropathic pain. *Pain*. **156**: 1440–1448.

5 Falk S *et al.* (2014) Cancer pain physiology. *British Journal of Pain*. **8**: 154–162.

6 Bannister K and Dickenson AH (2016) What the brain tells the spinal cord. *Pain*. **157**: 2148–2151.

7 Zhuo M (2018) Potentiation of cortical excitatory transmission in chronic pain. *Pain*. **159**: 212–213.

8 Porreca F and Navratilova E (2017) Reward, motivation, and emotion of pain and its relief. *Pain*. **158 Suppl 1**: S43–S49.

9 Leung A *et al.* (2016) Regular physical activity prevents chronic pain by altering resident muscle macrophage phenotype and increasing interleukin-10 in mice. *Pain*. **157**: 70–79.

10 Almeida C *et al.* (2015) Exercise therapy normalizes BDNF upregulation and glial hyperactivity in a mouse model of neuropathic pain. *Pain*. **156**: 504–513.

11 Patel R *et al.* (2018) Calcium channel modulation as a target in chronic pain control. *British Journal of Pharmacology*. **175**: 2173–2184.

12 Pace MC *et al.* (2018) Nociceptor plasticity: a closer look. *Journal of Cellular Physiology*. **233**: 2824–2838.

13 Finnerup NB (2019) Nonnarcotic methods of pain management. *New England Journal of Medicine*. **380**: 2440–2448.

14 Albrecht DS *et al.* (2018) Neuroinflammation of the spinal cord and nerve roots in chronic radicular pain patients. *Pain*. **159**: 968–977.

15 Boyle J *et al.* (2012) Randomized, placebo-controlled comparison of amitriptyline, duloxetine, and pregabalin in patients with chronic diabetic peripheral neuropathic pain: impact on pain, polysomnographic sleep, daytime functioning, and quality of life. *Diabetes Care*. **35**: 2451–2458.

16 Bansal D *et al.* (2009) Amitriptyline vs. pregabalin in painful diabetic neuropathy: a randomized double blind clinical trial. *Diabetic Medicine*. **26**: 1019–1026.

17 Morello CM *et al.* (1999) Randomized double-blind study comparing the efficacy of gabapentin with amitriptyline on diabetic peripheral neuropathy pain. *Archives of Internal Medicine*. **159**: 1931–1937.

18 Chandra K *et al.* (2006) Gabapentin versus nortriptyline in post-herpetic neuralgia patients: a randomized, double-blind clinical trial — the GONIP trial. *International Journal of Clinical Pharmacology and Therapeutics*. **44**: 358–363.

19 Mishra S *et al.* (2012) A comparative efficacy of amitriptyline, gabapentin, and pregabalin in neuropathic cancer pain: a prospective randomized double-blind placebo-controlled study. *American Journal of Hospice and Palliative Care*. **29**: 177–182.

20 Banerjee M *et al.* (2013) A comparative study of efficacy and safety of gabapentin versus amitriptyline as coanalgesics in patients receiving opioid analgesics for neuropathic pain in malignancy. *Indian Journal of Pharmacology*. **45**: 334–338.

21 Kelle B (2012) The efficacy of gabapentin and pregabalin in the treatment of neuropathic pain due to peripheral nerve injury. *Journal of Musculoskeletal Pain*. **20**: 300–305.

22 Razazian N *et al.* (2014) Evaluation of the efficacy and safety of pregabalin, venlafaxine, and carbamazepine in patients with painful diabetic peripheral neuropathy. A randomized, double-blind trial. *Neurosciences (Riyadh)*. **19**: 192–198.

23 Griebeler ML *et al.* (2014) Pharmacologic interventions for painful diabetic neuropathy: an umbrella systematic review and comparative effectiveness network meta-analysis. *Annals of Internal Medicine*. **161**: 639–649.

24 NICE (2013) Neuropathic pain in adults: pharmacological management in non-specialist settings. *Clinical Guideline CG173: (appendix G)*. www.nice.org.uk.
25 Treede RD (2019) The role of quantitative sensory testing in the prediction of chronic pain. *Pain*. **160 Suppl 1**: S66–S69.
26 Eisenberg E *et al.* (2006) Efficacy of mu-opioid agonists in the treatment of evoked neuropathic pain: systematic review of randomized controlled trials. *European Journal of Pain*. **10**: 667–676.
27 Eisenberg E *et al.* (2005) Efficacy and safety of opioid agonists in the treatment of neuropathic pain of nonmalignant origin: systematic review and meta-analysis of randomized controlled trials. *JAMA*. **293**: 3043–3052.
28 Wiffen PJ *et al.* (2010) Anticonvulsant drugs for acute and chronic pain. *Cochrane Database of Systematic Reviews*. **1**: CD0011133. www.cochranelibrary.com.
29 Saarto T and Wiffen PJ (2007) Antidepressants for neuropathic pain. *Cochrane Database of Systematic Reviews*. **4**: CD005454. www.cochranelibrary.com.
30 Attal N *et al.* (2010) EFNS guidelines on the pharmacological treatment of neuropathic pain: 2010 revision. *European Journal of Neurology*. **17**: 1113–e1188.
31 Dworkin RH *et al.* (2010) Recommendations for the pharmacological management of neuropathic pain: an overview and literature update. *Mayo Clinic Proceedings*. **85**: S3–S14.
32 Finnerup NB *et al.* (2016) Pharmacotherapy for neuropathic pain in adults: a systematic review and meta-analysis. *Lancet Neurology*. **14**: 162–173.
33 White P *et al.* (2018) The use of corticosteroids as adjuvant therapy for painful bone metastases: a large cross-sectional survey of palliative care providers. *American Journal of Hospice and Palliative Care*. **35**: 151–158.
34 Caraceni A *et al.* (2008) Gabapentin for breakthrough pain due to bone metastases. *Palliative Medicine*. **22**: 392–393.
35 Miller S (2017) P-126 Effectiveness of gabapentin and pregabalin for cancer-induced bone pain: a systematic review. *BMJ Supportive & Palliative Care*. **7**: A46–A47.
36 Fallon M *et al.* (2016) Randomized double-blind trial of pregabalin versus placebo in conjunction with palliative radiotherapy for cancer-induced bone pain. *Journal of Clinical Oncology*. **34**: 550–556.
37 Knopp-Sihota JA *et al.* (2012) Calcitonin for treating acute and chronic pain of recent and remote osteoporotic vertebral compression fractures: a systematic review and meta-analysis. *Osteoporos International*. **23**: 17–38.
38 Lee AC *et al.* (2018) P032 The analgesic effect of salmon calcitonin on acute rib fractures in cystic fibrosis. *Journal of Cystic Fibrosis*. **17**: S68.
39 Martinez-Zapata MJ *et al.* (2006) Calcitonin for metastatic bone pain. *Cochrane Database of Systematic Reviews*. **3**: CD003223. www.cochranelibrary.com (Last reviewed 2015)
40 Twycross R and Wilcock A (eds) (2016) *Introducing Palliative Care* (5e.)Palliativedrugs.com Ltd.
41 Sola A and Bonica J (1990) Myofascial pain syndromes. In: Bonica J (ed) *The Management of Pain* (2e). Lea and Febiger, Philadelphia, pp. 352–367.
42 Avenali M *et al.* (2018) Pain in focal dystonias — a focused review to address an important component of the disease. *Parkinsonism & Related Disorders*. **54**: 17–24.
43 Chumpitazi BP *et al.* (2018) Review article: the physiological effects and safety of peppermint oil and its efficacy in irritable bowel syndrome and other functional disorders. *Alimentary Pharmacology & Therapeutics*. **47**: 738–752.
44 Lee KJ (2015) Pharmacologic agents for chronic diarrhea. *Intestinal Research*. **13**: 306–312.
45 Gottlieb M *et al.* (2018) The evaluation and management of urolithiasis in the ED: a review of the literature. *American Journal of Emergency Medicine*. **36**: 699–706.
46 Papadopoulos G *et al.* (2014) Hyoscine N-butylbromide (Buscopan®) in the treatment of acute ureteral colic: what is the evidence? *Urologia Internationalis*. **92**: 253–257.
47 Colli A *et al.* (2012) Meta-analysis: nonsteroidal anti-inflammatory drugs in biliary colic. *Alimentary Pharmacology & Therapeutics*. **35**: 1370–1378.
48 Kumar A *et al.* (2004) Comparison of the effect of diclofenac with hyoscine-N-butylbromide in the symptomatic treatment of acute biliary colic. *ANZ Journal of Surgery*. **74**: 573–576.
49 Laoire AN *et al.* (2017) A systematic review of the effectiveness of palliative interventions to treat rectal tenesmus in cancer. *Palliative Medicine*. **31**: 975–981.
50 Ali SK and Abdulkarim S (2018) Treatment of anal cancer pain – a case report. *Journal of Pain and Symptom Management*. **56**: e1–e2.
51 Seretny M and Colvin LA (2016) Pain management in patients with vascular disease. *British Journal of Anaesthesia*. **117 Suppl 2**: ii95–ii106.
52 Rüger LJ *et al.* (2008) Characteristics of chronic ischemic pain in patients with peripheral arterial disease. *Pain*. **139**: 201–208.
53 Laoire AN and Murtagh FEM (2018) Systematic review of pharmacological therapies for the management of ischaemic pain in patients with non-reconstructable critical limb ischaemia. *BMJ Supportive & Palliative Care*. **8**: 400–410.

Updated July 2019

PARACETAMOL

Unintentional overdose from paracetamol (USAN: acetaminophen) resulting in hepatotoxicity, sometimes fatal, can occur. To reduce this risk, the dose of paracetamol must *not* exceed the maximum recommended dose and should be reduced when risk factors for hepatotoxicity exist, e.g. low body weight (Box B).

Class: Non-opioid analgesic.

Indications: mild–moderate pain, pyrexia. ***IV:*** short-term use for moderate pain or pyrexia when a rapid effect is required and/or when other routes of administration are not possible.

Contra-indications: *IV:* severe hepatic impairment (also see Dose and use).

Pharmacology

Paracetamol is a synthetic centrally acting non-opioid analgesic and antipyretic. In contrast to NSAIDs (p.341), paracetamol is only a weak inhibitor of cyclo-oxygenase, although this probably explains its antipyretic effect.[1] Although debated, its analgesic effect probably involves metabolites acting on supraspinal centres, such as the periaqueductal gray, one consequence of which is activation of descending serotoninergic inhibitory pain pathways.[2] A nerve membrane stabilizing effect, via the opening of potassium channels, may also be relevant.[3]

Across a range of painful conditions, the analgesic effect of paracetamol is inferior to that of an NSAID, e.g. **ibuprofen** (p.365).[4] Generally, paracetamol provides little or no additional analgesia when combined with either an NSAID or a strong opioid (Box A).

Box A Analgesic benefit of paracetamol in selected non-cancer pains

Acute pain

Paracetamol provides a greater degree of benefit over placebo in migraine compared with tension-type headache, with respective NNTs of 5 and 10 for no/mild pain at 2h.[5,6]

In renal colic, although relief obtained at 30min is similar for paracetamol and NSAIDs, patients receiving NSAIDs require less rescue analgesia.[7]

In postoperative pain, single doses of PO or IV paracetamol are more effective than placebo; both routes produce an NNT of about 5 for ≥50% pain relief over 4–6h.[8,9]

Chronic pain

Systematic reviews indicate that paracetamol is of little or no value in the management of osteoarthritic hip or knee pain, or low back pain.[10,11] A network meta-analysis found no clinically relevant improvement in osteoarthritic pain from paracetamol (but did with NSAIDs).[12]

Combining paracetamol with an NSAID

In acute low back pain, outcomes were no different for PO paracetamol + ibuprofen compared with ibuprofen alone.[13]

In postoperative pain, PO paracetamol + ibuprofen produced a clinically relevant opioid-sparing effect compared with paracetamol alone, but *not* compared with ibuprofen alone.[14]

Combining paracetamol with an opioid

In postoperative pain, PO or IV paracetamol combined with an opioid has a small 'opioid-sparing' effect. However, this is of uncertain clinical relevance because it does *not* translate into a meaningful reduction in opioid-related undesirable effects (which *is* seen when an NSAID is added to an opioid).[9]

PO vs IV administration

RCTs in acute pain (mostly musculoskeletal) and postoperative pain have found no clinically meaningful differences in analgesic efficacy between IV and PO paracetamol.[15-17]

In cancer pain, it is unknown if PO paracetamol adds to the analgesic effect of NSAIDs, but experience in other settings suggests this is probably unlikely (Box A). There are insufficient data to determine if PO paracetamol adds to the analgesic effect of **codeine**,[18] but when added to a strong opioid, most RCTs suggest little or no additional benefit.[19-22] On the other hand, when regular PO paracetamol was stopped in patients receiving a strong opioid with controlled cancer pain, 20% reported worsening pain sufficient to consider restarting it.[23]

The PO bio-availability of paracetamol is relatively high (60–90%), but therapeutic plasma concentrations are achieved more rapidly and consistently when it is given IV.[24] In fever, IV paracetamol provides a more rapid antipyretic effect than PO.[25,26] Because the difference in analgesic efficacy between IV and PO paracetamol is of uncertain clinical relevance (Box A), the general recommendation is to reserve IV use for situations where alternative routes are not possible (see Dose and use). PR is the slowest, most variable and most expensive route of administration, and is thus best avoided.

Most of a therapeutic dose of paracetamol is metabolized by the liver before being renally excreted; less than 5% is excreted unchanged in the urine. At therapeutic doses, ≤90% of paracetamol is metabolized to inactive glucuronide and sulfate conjugates. About 5–15% is oxidized by hepatic CYP450 enzymes to a highly reactive hepatotoxic metabolite, N-acetyl-p-benzoquinoneimine (NAPQI; Figure 1). With typical therapeutic doses (≤1g q.d.s.), NAPQI is normally inactivated by glutathione sufficiently rapidly not to cause liver damage.

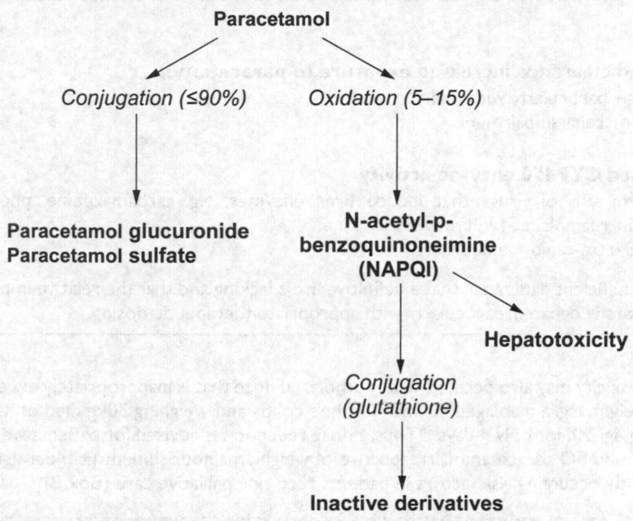

Figure 1 Metabolism of paracetamol.

CYP2E1 is responsible for ≤80% of paracetamol's oxidative metabolism to NAPQI, with ≤25% oxidized via CYP3A4 (particularly at lower doses) and CYP2D6 (particularly at higher doses).[27] Patients with genetic variations in metabolism, e.g. CYP2D6 gene duplication (ultra-rapid metabolizers), may have a greater susceptibility to hepatotoxicity, because of the increased production of NAPQI;[28,29] similarly, long-term use of drugs that induce CYP450 enzymes may also increase the risk of NAPQI production. Various other factors are associated with an increased risk of paracetamol hepatotoxicity (Box B).

Deliberate and unintentional overdose

An overdose of paracetamol overwhelms normal metabolism, shifting more paracetamol into the NAPQI pathway; the body's glutathione store becomes exhausted, and the accumulation of NAPQI leads to liver cell death. Various forms of paracetamol overdose have been defined:

- acute (deliberate ingestion of a potentially toxic dose in ≤1h)
- staggered (deliberate ingestion of a potentially toxic dose over >1h)
- therapeutic excess (unintentional ingestion of excessive paracetamol taken with intent to treat pain or fever).[30,33-36]

Serious toxicity from paracetamol is most likely with doses >150mg/kg (9g or 18 tablets in a 60kg person) taken within a 24h period, although rarely, serious toxicity has occurred with doses of 75–150mg/kg/24h. A dose <75mg/kg/24h is very unlikely to be toxic, but chronic dosing (≥2 days) increases the risk. Various factors can increase the risk of hepatotoxicity (Box B). Paracetamol overdose can also lead to acute renal failure, although this is often reversible without the need for dialysis.[37]

Box B Risk factors for paracetamol hepatotoxicity[30-32]

Low body weight
May result in an inappropriately excessive dose.
Dose reduction is advised for patients ≤50kg.
When caused by malnutrition, glutathione deficiency adds to the risk.

Glutathione deficiency
Includes patients with, e.g. malnourishment, anorexia, cachexia, chronic illness, alcohol-use disorder.

Reduced clearance/increased exposure to paracetamol
Older age, particularly with frailty.
Hepatic or renal impairment.

Increased CYP450 enzyme activity
Long-term use of drugs that induce liver enzymes, e.g. carbamazepine, phenobarbital, phenytoin, rifampicin, St John's wort.
CYP2D6 ultra-rapid metabolizers.

Note. Insufficient data mean that a definitive list is lacking and that the relative importance of risk factors is debated, particularly with appropriate therapeutic dosing.

Hepatotoxicity may also occur with an authorized dose that is inappropriately excessive for the patient's weight, e.g. a man aged 43 with Crohn's colitis and weighing 30kg died of hepatic failure after taking 4g/24h for only 4 days.[38] Thus, a dose reduction is advised for patients weighing ≤50kg for both IV and PO paracetamol. Irrespective of weight, malnourishment (± older age and frailty) are frequently occurring risk factors in patients receiving palliative care (Box B).

The dose of paracetamol must always be appropriate for the weight and circumstances of the patient, and the maximum recommended dose must not be exceeded.

Overdose can be treated with IVI **acetylcysteine**, a glutathione precursor which prevents NAPQI from reacting with liver cell proteins;[30,39] various factors are taken into account when determining its use, e.g. the amount of paracetamol taken, timing of presentation and plasma levels of paracetamol.

When considering the use of IVI **acetylcysteine** for paracetamol overdose, consult the *BNF*[39] and/or SPC.

With IV paracetamol poisoning, contact the UK National Poisons Information Service for advice (0344 892 0111).

Bio-availability 60% after 500mg PO, 90% after 1g PO; PR is about two-thirds of PO, but is higher with two 500mg suppositories than with one 1g suppository.
Onset of action 15–30min PO; 5–10min IV (pain relief), 30min IV (antipyretic effect).
Time to peak plasma concentration widely variable PO, e.g. 20min in fasting state, but 1–2h if delayed gastric emptying;[40] 15min IVI (i.e. synchronous with the end of a 15min infusion).
Plasma halflife 1–4h PO; 2–3h IV.
Duration of action 4–6h PO and IV.

Cautions

Hepatic impairment (see Dose and use, and Chapter 18, p.760), severe renal impairment (see Dose and use, and Chapter 17, p.746), patients with risk factors for paracetamol hepatotoxicity (Box B), dehydration.

Most *dispersible* and *effervescent* paracetamol-containing tablets (alone or combined with an opioid) have a high Na^+ content (≥14mmol/tablet).[41] Thus, dispersible or effervescent formulations should be avoided in patients on a salt-restricted diet, e.g. those with hypertension, renal impairment, severe hepatic impairment.[41]

Paracetamol can be taken by at least two-thirds of patients who are hypersensitive to **aspirin** or other NSAIDs.[42,43] In people with a history of **aspirin**-/NSAID-induced asthma, give a test dose of 250mg and observe for 2–3h. If no undesirable effects occur, paracetamol can safely be used in standard doses.[44]

Drug interactions

In patients taking **warfarin**, the concurrent use of regular paracetamol ≥2g/day is associated with a significant dose-dependent increase in the INR and increased risk of bleeding;[45-47] for some individuals, the INR rises to >6 in just a few days.[46,48] The underlying mechanism possibly relates to interference with the hepatic synthesis of various clotting factors. Thus, in **warfarin**-treated patients who take ≥2g/day of paracetamol for ≥3 consecutive days: the INR should be tested 3–5 days after the first dose of paracetamol, the frequency of INR monitoring should be increased and the INR tested a week after paracetamol is discontinued.[49]

5

Paracetamol 1g q.d.s. decreases **lamotrigine** plasma concentrations by about 20%, possibly by inducing glucuronidation; this may be clinically relevant for patients with **lamotrigine** concentrations at the lower end of the therapeutic range.[50]

There are conflicting reports about the impact of $5HT_3$ antagonists on the analgesic effect of paracetamol. Some report a reduction in analgesia,[51] but others an increase[52] and some no effect.[53]

Although opioids can reduce the rate of PO paracetamol absorption by delaying gastric emptying, the clinical relevance of this is unclear.[54]

Undesirable effects

Very common (>10%): dyspepsia, elevated liver enzymes (Box C).[35,55] ***IV:*** pain/erythema at the injection site.

Rare (<0.1%, >0.01%): cholestatic jaundice,[56,57] acute pancreatitis, thrombocytopenia, agranulocytosis, serious skin reactions,[58] anaphylaxis.[59,60] ***IV:*** malaise, hypotension.

Very rare (<0.01%): IV: elevated liver enzymes (Box C), thrombocytopenia, leucopenia, neutropenia.

Box C Paracetamol and elevated liver enzymes[55,61]

The plasma concentrations of liver enzymes (alanine aminotransferase (ALT), aspartate aminotransferase, γ-glutamyl transferase) can increase with normal doses of paracetamol.

For example, ALT increased >3 times the upper limit of normal in 40% of young healthy volunteers receiving paracetamol 4g/day, with the highest increase 14–16 times greater. The rise was evident after 72h and persisted for a median of 1 week after discontinuation.

These changes are probably unimportant in the absence of functional or synthetic liver impairment (e.g. indicated by an increase in plasma bilirubin or a reduction in clotting factors respectively) and possibly improve with ongoing use, although this is poorly documented.

Awareness of this phenomenon aids interpretation of abnormal LFTs and helps to avoid the erroneous assumption that rapidly worsening LFTs must indicate worsening disease within the liver, e.g. from liver metastases.

Cyclo-oxygenase inhibition may explain some of the emerging undesirable effects associated with long-term regular use. Findings of observational and interventional studies are mixed, but overall suggest a possible dose-related increased risk of hypertension (and possibly other cardiovascular events), GI haemorrhage and decrease in GFR.[62,63] Even so, despite concern, paracetamol can still generally be regarded as a safe drug for most people,[64] although, when analgesic benefit is uncertain, more careful consideration is required as to its continued use.

There is no hard evidence that paracetamol precipitates asthma in established asthmatics (also see Cautions).[63]

Dose and use

Paracetamol is a relatively weak analgesic, inferior to NSAIDs, suitable for mild–moderate pain only. Generally, paracetamol provides little or no additional analgesia when combined with an NSAID or a strong opioid (see Pharmacology). Thus, it is reasonable to trial stopping paracetamol in these settings.

In patients without risk factors for paracetamol hepatotoxicity (Box B), the standard paracetamol regimen is 1g PO q.d.s. (maximum 4g/24h).

In patients with:

- ≥1 risk factor for paracetamol hepatotoxicity (Box B), start with 500mg PO q.d.s. (maximum 3g/24h)
- severe renal impairment (creatinine clearance <30mL/min), the dose interval must be ≥q6h; in ESRF, start with 500mg PO q6–8h (maximum 3g/24h); see Chapter 17, p.746
- severe hepatic impairment *and no additional risk factors for paracetamol hepatotoxicity*, start with 500mg PO q8h (maximum 3g/24h); see Chapter 18, p.760.

Despite lower PR bio-availability, the same dose is generally used both PR and PO. However, the PR route is rarely used (see Pharmacology).

Cancer pain

Generally, PO paracetamol provides little additional benefit when combined with other analgesics (see Pharmacology) and it represents a significant tablet burden (≤8 tablets/day). Thus, a pragmatic solution might be:

- to limit the long-term use of paracetamol to patients in whom definite benefit is seen within 2 days of starting it
- if already taking paracetamol with definite past benefit, and increasing pain necessitates the *addition* of an opioid, the ongoing need for paracetamol should be determined by stopping it after 3–4 days of satisfactory pain relief with both drugs and restarting paracetamol only if the pain returns.

Parenteral administration

IV paracetamol (1g in 100mL) is given undiluted by infusion over 15min. There have been case reports of massive inadvertent iatrogenic IV overdose leading to hepatic failure, sometimes fatal, particularly in children.[65] The IV solution contains *10mg/mL*. When written just as mg, the dose has occasionally been misread and given as mL, with the result that the patient has received *10 times* the prescribed dose. To minimize the chance of this happening, a prescription for IV (or SC) paracetamol should be written in terms of *both* mg *and* mL, not just as mg.

IV paracetamol should only be used when a rapid effect is required and/or when other routes of administration are not possible (see Pharmacology).

In patients >50kg without risk factors for paracetamol hepatotoxicity (Box B), the standard paracetamol regimen is 1g up to q4h (maximum 4g/24h).

In patients with:

- weight >50kg plus ≥1 risk factor for paracetamol hepatotoxicity (Box B), restrict total maximum daily dose to 3g/24h
- weight 34–50kg, use a dose of 15mg/kg up to q4h (in practice, generally 500mg is given), total maximum daily dose 60mg/kg/24h
- severe renal impairment (creatinine clearance <30mL/min), the dose interval must be ≥q6h; see Chapter 17, p.746
- mild–moderate hepatic impairment, restrict total maximum daily dose to 3g/24h; although contra-indicated in severe hepatic impairment, it is used by some liver units in reduced doses, e.g. 500mg–1g IV t.d.s.; see Chapter 18, p.760.

†Subcutaneous administration

SC administration of paracetamol injection (1g in 100mL) has been reported with doses of 500mg (50mL) or 1000mg (100mL) given undiluted by gravity SC infusion over 30min, using the same dosing regimen as for IV paracetamol.[66]

Note. SC administration of paracetamol should *not* routinely replace PO paracetamol when the oral route is lost, particularly when analgesia will be provided by a strong opioid CSCI. Further, an NSAID that can be given once daily, e.g. SC **parecoxib** (p.373), is a more convenient analgesic/antipyretic alternative to t.d.s.–q.d.s. SC paracetamol. Thus, SC paracetamol should be reserved for selected patients, e.g. those with NSAID intolerance or who have found paracetamol to be particularly effective.

Supply

PO paracetamol is available OTC alone and in several combination products with weak opioids (see **Codeine**, p.378; **Dihydrocodeine**, p.381; **Tramadol**, p.383).

Paracetamol (generic)

Tablets and caplets 500mg, 1g, 28 days @ 1g q.d.s. = £3.

Tablets soluble and dispersible 500mg, 1g, 28 days @ 1g q.d.s. = £15; *may contain Na⁺ up to 20mmol/tablet.*

Tablets orodispersible 250mg, 28 days @ 1g q.d.s. = £77.

Capsules 500mg, 28 days @ 1g q.d.s. = £11.

Oral solution 120mg/5mL, 500mg/5mL, 28 days @ 1g q.d.s. = £101.

Oral suspension 120mg/5mL, 250mg/5mL, 28 days @ 1g q.d.s. = £30; *available sugar free. A 500mg/5mL oral suspension is available but is >5 times the cost.*

Suppositories 60mg, 80mg, 120mg, 125mg, 240mg, 250mg, 500mg, 1g, 28 days @ 1g q.d.s. = £672.

Injection (for IV infusion) 10mg/mL; 10mL (100mg) amp = £0.50, 50mL (500mg) vial or 100mL (1g) vial = £1.25.

1 Mallet C *et al.* (2017) Paracetamol: Update on its analgesic mechanism of action. *Pain relief From analgesics to alternative therapies.* InTech. Chapter 10.

2 Barrière DA *et al.* (2020) Paracetamol is a centrally acting analgesic using mechanisms located in the periaqueductal grey. *Br J Pharmacol.* **177**: 1773–1792.

3 Ray S *et al.* (2019) The paracetamol metabolite N-acetylp-benzoquinone imine reduces excitability in first- and second-order neurons of the pain pathway through actions on KV7 channels. *Pain.* **160**: 954–964.

4 Moore RA *et al.* (2015) Overview review: Comparative efficacy of oral ibuprofen and paracetamol (acetaminophen) across acute and chronic pain conditions. *European Journal of Pain.* **19**: 1213–1223.

5 Derry S and Moore RA (2013) Paracetamol (acetaminophen) with or without an antiemetic for acute migraine headaches in adults. *Cochrane Database of Systematic Reviews.* **2013**: CD008040. www.cochranelibrary.com.

6 Stephens G *et al.* (2016) Paracetamol (acetaminophen) for acute treatment of episodic tension-type headache in adults. *Cochrane Database of Systematic Reviews.* **2016**: CD011889. www.cochranelibrary.com.

7 Pathan SA *et al.* (2017) A systematic review and meta-analysis comparing the efficacy of nonsteroidal anti-inflammatory drugs, opioids, and paracetamol in the treatment of acute renal colic. *European Urology.* **73**: 583–595.

8 Toms L *et al.* (2008) Single dose oral paracetamol (acetaminophen) for postoperative pain in adults. *Cochrane Database Systematic Review.* **4**: CD004602. www.cochranelibrary.com.

9 McNicol ED *et al.* (2016) Single dose intravenous paracetamol or intravenous propacetamol for postoperative pain. *Cochrane Database of Systematic Reviews.* **5**: CD007126. www.cochranelibrary.com.

10 Leopoldino AO *et al.* (2019) Paracetamol versus placebo for knee and hip osteoarthritis. *Cochrane Database of Systematic Reviews.* **2**: CD013273. www.cochranelibrary.com.

11 Saragiotto BT *et al.* (2016) Paracetamol for low back pain. *Cochrane Database of Systematic Reviews.* **6**: CD012230. www.cochranelibrary.com.

12 Da Costa BR *et al.* (2017) Effectiveness of non-steroidal anti-inflammatory drugs for the treatment of pain in knee and hip osteoarthritis: a network meta-analysis. *The Lancet.* **390**: e21–e33.

13 Friedman BW *et al.* (2020) Ibuprofen plus acetaminophen versus ibuprofen alone for acute low back pain: an emergency department-based randomized study. *Acadamic Emergency Medicine.* **27**: 229–235.

14 Thybo KH *et al.* (2019) Effect of combination of paracetamol (acetaminophen) and ibuprofen vs either alone on patient-controlled morphine consumption in the first 24 hours after total hip arthroplasty: the PANSAID randomized clinical trial. *JAMA.* **321**: 562–571.

15 Jibril F *et al.* (2015) Intravenous versus oral acetaminophen for pain: systematic review of current evidence to support clinical decision-making. *The Canadian Journal of Hospital Pharmacy.* **68**: 238– 247.

16 Douzjian DJ and Kulik A (2017) Old drug, new route: a systematic review of intravenous acetaminophen after adult cardiac surgery. *Journal of Cardiothoracic and Vascular Anesthesia.* **31**: 694–701.

17 Furyk J *et al.* (2018) Intravenous versus oral paracetamol for acute pain in adults in the emergency department setting: a prospective, double-blind, double-dummy, randomised controlled trial. *Emergency Medicine Journal.* **35**: 179–184.

18 Straube C *et al.* (2014) Codeine, alone and with paracetamol (acetaminophen), for cancer pain. *Cochrane Database of Systematic Reviews.* **9**: CD006601. www.cochranelibrary.com.

19 Stockler M *et al.* (2004) Acetaminophen (paracetamol) improves pain and well-being in people with advanced cancer already receiving a strong opioid regimen: a randomized, double-blind, placebo-controlled cross-over trial. *Journal of Clinical Oncology.* **22**: 3389–3394.

20 Axelsson B and Christensen S (2003) Is there an additive analgesic effect of paracetamol at step 3? A double-blind randomized controlled study. *Palliative Medicine.* **17**: 724–725.

21 Israel FJ *et al.* (2010) Lack of benefit from paracetamol (acetaminophen) for palliative cancer patients requiring high-dose strong opioids: a randomized, double-blind, placebo-controlled, crossover trial. *Journal of Pain and Symptom Management.* **39**: 548–554.

22 Wiffen PJ *et al.* (2017) Oral paracetamol (acetaminophen) for cancer pain. *Cochrane Database of Systematic Reviews.* **7**: CD012637. www.cochranelibrary.com.

23 Axelsson B *et al.* (2008) Analgesic effect of paracetamol on cancer related pain in concurrent strong opioid therapy. A prospective clinical study. *Acta Oncologica.* **47**: 891–895.

24 Singla NK *et al.* (2012) Plasma and cerebrospinal fluid pharmacokinetic parameters after single-dose administration of intravenous, oral, or rectal acetaminophen. *Pain Practice.* **12**: 523–532.

25 Roy S and Simalti AK (2018) Comparison of antipyretic efficacy of intravenous (IV) acetaminophen versus oral (PO) acetaminophen in the management of fever in children. *The Indian Journal of Pediatrics*. **85**: 1–4.

26 Peacock WF *et al.* (2011) A randomized study of the efficacy and safety of intravenous acetaminophen compared to oral acetaminophen for the treatment of fever. *Academic Emergency Medicine*. **18**: 360–366.

27 Kalsi S and Wood DM (2011) Does cytochrome P450 liver isoenzyme induction increase the risk of liver toxicity after paracetamol overdose? *Open Access Emergency Medicine*. **3**: 69–76.

28 Zhao L and Pickering G (2011) Paracetamol metabolism and related genetic differences. *Drug Metabolism Reviews*. **43**: 41–52.

29 Dong H *et al.* (2000) Involvement of human cytochrome P450 2D6 in the bioactivation of acetaminophen. *Drug Metabolism and Disposition*. **28**: 1397–1400.

30 BMJ (2020) Paracetamol overdose in adults. *BMJ (British Medical Journal)*. https://bestpractice.bmj.com/

31 Caparrotta TM *et al.* (2018) Are some people at increased risk of paracetamol-induced liver injury? A critical review of the literature. *European Journal of Clinical Pharmacology*. **74**: 147–160.

32 Anonymous (2018) What dose of paracetamol for older people? *Drug and Therapeutics Bulletin*. **56(6)**: 69–72.

33 Toxbase Paracetamol. National poisons information service. https://www.toxbase.org/ (accessed December 2020)

34 MHRA (2010) Intravenous paracetamol (Perfalgan): risk of accidental overdose especially in infants and neonates. *Drug Safety Update*. www.gov.uk/drug-safety-update.

35 Larson AM *et al.* (2005) Acetaminophen-induced acute liver failure: results of a United States multicenter, prospective study. *Hepatology*. **42**: 1364–1372.

36 Krenzelok EP (2009) The FDA Acetaminophen Advisory Committee Meeting - what is the future of acetaminophen in the United States? The perspective of a committee member. *Clinical Toxicology*. **47**: 784–789.

37 von Mach MA *et al.* (2005) Experiences of a poison center network with renal insufficiency in acetaminophen overdose: an analysis of 17 cases. *Clinical Toxicology*. **43**: 31–37.

38 Claridge LC *et al.* (2010) Acute liver failure after administration of paracetamol at the maximum recommended daily dose in adults. *British Medical Journal*. **341**: c6764.

39 British National Formulary 'Emergency treatment of poisoning' and 'Acetyclcysteine' monograph. London: BMJ Group and Pharmaceutical Press www.medicinescomplete.com (accessed March 2014).

40 Prescott LF (1996) Paracetamol (Acetaminophen) A Critical Bibliographic Review. Taylor & Francis, London.

41 UK Medicines Information (2019) What is the sodium content of medicines? *Medicines Q&As*. www.evidence.nhs.uk.

42 Szczeklik A (1986) Analgesics, allergy and asthma. *Drugs*. **32**: 148–163.

43 Settipane R *et al.* (1995) Prevalence of cross-sensitivity with acetaminophen in aspirin-sensitive asthmatic subjects. *Journal of Allergy and Clinical Immunology*. **96**: 480–485.

44 Shin G *et al.* (2000) Paracetamol and asthma. *Thorax*. **55**: 882–884.

45 Caldeira D *et al.* (2015) How safe is acetaminophen use in patients treated with vitamin K antagonists? A systematic review and meta-analysis. *Thrombosis Research*. **135**: 58–61.

46 Hylek EM *et al.* (1998) Acetaminophen and other risk factors for excessive warfarin anticoagulation. *JAMA*. **279**: 657–662.

47 Launiainen T *et al.* (2010) Adverse interaction of warfarin and paracetamol: evidence from a post-mortem study. *European Journal of Clinical Pharmacology*. **66**: 97–103.

48 Gebauer MG *et al.* (2003) Warfarin and acetaminophen interaction. *Pharmacotherapy*. **23**: 109–112.

49 Lopes RD *et al.* (2011) Warfarin and acetaminophen interaction: a summary of the evidence and biologic plausibility. *Blood*. **118**: 6269–6273.

50 Gastrup S *et al.* (2016) Paracetamol decreases steady-state exposure to lamotrigine by induction of glucuronidation in healthy subjects. *British Journal of Clinical Pharmacology*. **81**: 735–741.

51 Pickering G *et al.* (2006) Analgesic effect of acetaminophen in humans: first evidence of a central serotonergic mechanism. *Clinical Pharmacology & Therapeutics*. **79**: 371–378.

52 Bhosale UA *et al.* (2015) Randomized, double-blind, placebo-controlled study to investigate the pharmacodynamic interaction of 5-HT3 antagonist ondansetron and paracetamol in postoperative patients operated in an ENT department under local anesthesia. *Journal of Basic and Clinical Physiology and Pharmacology*. **26**: 217–222.

53 Jokela R *et al.* (2010) The influence of ondansetron on the analgesic effect of acetaminophen after laparoscopic hysterectomy. *Clinical Pharmacology and Therapeutics*. **87**: 672–678.

54 Preston C Stockley's Drug Interactions. *Pharmaceutical Press*, London. www.medicinescomplete.com (accessed December 2020).

55 Watkins PB *et al.* (2006) Aminotransferase elevations in healthy adults receiving 4 grams of acetaminophen daily: a randomized controlled trial. *Journal of the American Medical Association*. **296**: 87–93.

56 Waldum H *et al.* (1992) Can NSAIDs cause acute biliary pain and cholestasis? *Journal of Clinical Gastroenterology*. **14**: 328–330.

57 Wong V *et al.* (1993) Paracetamol and acute biliary pain with cholestasis. *The Lancet*. **342**: 869.

58 Watanabe H *et al.* (2016) Toxic epidermal necrolysis caused by acetaminophen featuring almost 100% skin detachment: Acetaminophen is associated with a risk of severe cutaneous adverse reactions. *Journal of Dermatology*. **43**: 321–324.

59 Leung R *et al.* (1992) Paracetamol anaphylaxis. *Clinical and Experimental Allergy*. **22**: 831–833.

60 Morgan S and Dorman S (2004) Paracetamol (acetaminophen) allergy. *Journal of Pain and Symptom Management*. **27**: 99–101.

61 Dart RC and Bailey E (2007) Does therapeutic use of acetaminophen cause acute liver failure? *Pharmacotherapy*. **27**: 1219–1230.

62 Roberts E *et al.* (2016) Paracetamol: not as safe as we thought? A systematic literature review of observational studies. *Annals of Rheumatic Diseases*. **75**: 552–559.

63 McCrae JC *et al.* (2018) Long-term adverse effects of paracetamol – a review. *British Journal of Clinical Pharmacology*. **84**: 2218–2230.

64 Battagia A *et al.* (2016) Paracetamol: probably still a safe drug. *Annals of Rheumatic Diseases*. **10**: 1136.

65 Dart RC and Rumack BH (2012) Intravenous acetaminophen in the United States: iatrogenic dosing errors. *Pediatrics*. **129**: 349–353.

66 Leheup BF *et al.* (2018) Subcutaneous administration of paracetamol-Good local tolerability in palliative care patients: An observational study. *Palliative Medicine*. **32**: 1216–1221.

Updated February 2021

NEFOPAM

Class: Non-opioid analgesic, benzoxazocine.

Indications: Moderate pain.

Contra-indications: Concurrent use of an MAOI, epilepsy.

Pharmacology

Nefopam inhibits serotonin, noradrenaline (norepinephrine) and dopamine re-uptake transporters.[1] Thus, like analgesic-antidepressants, it enhances noradrenaline transmission in descending pain modulatory pathways (see Adjuvant analgesics, Figure 1, p.326). Nefopam also blocks voltage-gated sodium and calcium channels associated with glutamic acid, an excitatory neurotransmitter.[2,3] Antimuscarinic and sympathomimetic properties may account for some of its undesirable effects. Nefopam does *not* inhibit cyclo-oxygenase (COX) or affect platelet function,[4] thereby making it a possible alternative if NSAIDs (p.341) are contra-indicated.

In the acute pain setting, nefopam has mostly been studied in postoperative pain, with RCTs generally finding similar benefit as an NSAID or **paracetamol**. The effect is additive, with the combination of all three producing the greatest reduction in pain scores and **morphine** requirements.[5-17] On the other hand, a small RCT (n=30) in renal colic found no added benefit from combining an NSAID with nefopam.[18] The injection preparation (not UK) has been successfully given *alone* by CSCI.[19]

In chronic pain, comparisons with placebo in rheumatoid disease have given mixed results.[20,21] In osteoarthritic pain, a cross-over study (n=30) found benefit from nefopam similar to the NSAID **flurbiprofen**.[22] In neuropathic pain, RCT evidence is limited to post-herpetic neuralgia; CIVI nefopam (reduced every 3 days: 60mg/24h→40mg/24h→20mg/24h→stop) provided additional benefit while PO neuropathic adjuvants were titrated.[23]

In cancer-related pain, one RCT (n=99) found nefopam to provide similar benefit to **diclofenac**, but more participants withdrew due to undesirable effects, particularly nausea.[24] In a small placebo-controlled RCT (n=40), the addition of nefopam made no difference to overall pain relief, but there was a trend towards lower **morphine** PCA requirements.[25]

Nefopam is metabolized in the liver to an active metabolite, desmethylnefopam, which is renally eliminated.[26] In ESRF, clearance is reduced by 1/3–1/2, and peak plasma concentrations are increased 2–4 times, possibly because of secondary hepatic impairment.[27] Postoperatively, single parenteral doses provided analgesia for ≤5h.[28,29] However, pharmacological effects were seen for ≤12h after oral doses in healthy volunteers,[26] possibly reflecting the longer halflife of desmethylnefopam.

Bio-availability 36%.
Onset of action <1h.
Time to peak plasma concentration 1–3h PO, 1.5h IM.
Plasma halflife 4–5h; desmethylnefopam 10–15h.[26]
Duration of action ≤12h PO, ≤5h IV.

Cautions

Hepatic and renal impairment (see Chapter 17, p.746), prostatism, closed-angle glaucoma (antimuscarinic). Exacerbates the undesirable effects of concurrently administered antimuscarinic (see Antimuscarinics, Box C, p.5) or sympathomimetic agents.

Undesirable effects

Most common: nausea and vomiting, drowsiness, hypotension, epigastric pain.[24] In critical care, tachycardia, hypotension and sweating were reported in ≤30% of patients.[30] Sweating was also common in patients with rheumatoid arthritis.[20] However, in an RCT in cancer patients, tachycardia was noted in only 3%.[24]

Less common: diarrhoea, confusion and hallucinations (particularly in the elderly), tremor, paraesthesia, dizziness, syncope, seizures, palpitations, dry mouth, urinary retention.

Infrequent: blurred vision, insomnia, headache, pink discolouration of the urine (harmless).

Dose and use

Nefopam is generally used as an alternative to an NSAID when the latter is contra-indicated or poorly tolerated:

- start with 60mg PO t.d.s. (30mg PO t.d.s. in the elderly or ESRF; also see Chapter 17, p.746)[27] or 20mg IM q6h (not UK)
- maximum dose 90mg PO t.d.s.

Supply

Nefopam (generic)

Tablets 30mg, 28 days @ 60mg t.d.s. = £14.

Injection 10mg/mL, 2mL amp (not UK, obtainable via import; see Chapter 24, p.817).

For patients who have swallowing difficulties, nefopam tablets may be dispersed in water (see Chapter 28, Table 2, p.863).

1 Gregori-Puigjane E *et al.* (2012) Identifying mechanism-of-action targets for drugs and probes. *Proceedings of the National Academy of Sciences of the United States of America*. **109**: 11178–11183.

2 Novelli A *et al.* (2005) Nefopam inhibits calcium influx, cGMP formation, and NMDA receptor-dependent neurotoxicity following activation of voltage sensitive calcium channels. *Amino Acids*. **28**: 183–191.

3 Verleye M *et al.* (2004) Nefopam blocks voltage-sensitive sodium channels and modulates glutamatergic transmission in rodents. *Brain Research Reviews*. **1013**: 249–255.

4 Dordoni PL *et al.* (1994) Effect of ketorolac, ketoprofen and nefopam on platelet function. *Anaesthesia*. **49**: 1046–1049.

5 Martinez V *et al.* (2017) Non-opioid analgesics in adults after major surgery: systematic review with network meta-analysis of randomized trials. *British Journal of Anaesthesia*. **118**: 22–31.

6 Beloeil H *et al.* (2019) Multicentre, prospective, double-blind, randomised controlled clinical trial comparing different non-opioid analgesic combinations with morphine for postoperative analgesia: the OCTOPUS study. *British Journal of Anaesthesia*. **122**: e98–e106.

7 Son J-S *et al.* (2017) A comparison between ketorolac and nefopam as adjuvant analgesics for postoperative patient-controlled analgesia: a randomized, double-blind, prospective study. *Korean Journal of Anesthesiology*. **70**: 612–618.

8 Oh E-J *et al.* (2021) Analgesic efficacy of nefopam as an adjuvant in patient-controlled analgesia for acute postoperative pain after laparoscopic colorectal cancer surgery. *Journal of Clinical Medicine*. **10**: 270.

9 Na H *et al.* (2018) Intraoperative nefopam reduces acute postoperative pain after laparoscopic gastrectomy: a prospective, randomized study. *Journal of Gastrointestinal Surgery*. **22**: 771–777.

10 Lekprasert V *et al.* (2021) Perioperative intravenous patient-controlled analgesic efficacy of morphine with combined nefopam and parecoxib versus parecoxib in gynecologic surgery: a randomized, double-blind study. *Anesthesiology Research and Practice*. **2021**: 5461890.

11 Lee S *et al.* (2021) The analgesic efficacy of nefopam in patient-controlled analgesia after laparoscopic gynecologic surgery: a randomized, double-blind, non-inferiority study. *Journal of Clinical Medicine*. **10**: 1043.

12 Kim Y *et al.* (2018) Concurrent use of nefopam vs. ketorolac with opioid analgesic for post-operative pain management. *Korean Journal of Clinical Pharmacy*. **28**: 279–284.

13 Go Y *et al.* (2021) The effect of using nefopam in fentanyl-based intravenous patient-controlled analgesia on the incidence of postoperative nausea and vomiting in laparoscopic gynecological surgery. *Medical Biological Science and Engineering*. **4**: 20–26.

14 Eiamcharoenwit J *et al.* (2020) Analgesic efficacy of intravenous nefopam after spine surgery: a randomized, double-blind, placebo-controlled trial. *F1000 Research*. **9**: 516.

15 Cuvillon P *et al.* (2017) Opioid-sparing effect of nefopam in combination with paracetamol after major abdominal surgery: a randomized double-blind study. *Minerva Anestesiologica*. **83**: 914–920.

16 Choi E *et al.* (2019) Effects on postoperative nausea and vomiting of nefopam versus fentanyl following bimaxillary orthognathic surgery: a prospective double-blind randomized controlled trial. *Journal of Dental Anesthesia and Pain Medicine*. **19**: 55–66.

17 In C *et al.* (2019) Effects of intraoperative nefopam on catheter-related bladder discomfort in patients undergoing robotic nephrectomy: a randomized double-blind study. *Journal of Clinical Medicine*. **8**: 519.

18 Moustafa F *et al.* (2013) Usefulness of nefopam in treating pain of severe uncomplicated renal colics in adults admitted to emergency units: a randomised double-blind controlled trial. The 'INCoNU' study. *Emergency Medicine Journal*. **30**: 143–148.

19 Zhong D *et al.* (2007) Nefopam hydrochloride for postoperative subcutaneous patient controlled analgesia. *China Pharmacy*.

20 Emery P and Gibson T (1986) A double-blind study of the simple analgesic nefopam in rheumatoid arthritis. *British Journal of Rheumatology*. **25**: 72–76.

21 Swinson D *et al.* (1988) Nefopam in rheumatoid arthritis. Results of a double blind placebo controlled study. *Clinical Rheumatology*. **7**: 411–412.

22 Stamp J *et al.* (1989) A comparison of nefopam and flurbiprofen in the treatment of osteoarthrosis. *British Journal of Clinical Practice*. **43**: 24–26.

23 Joo YC *et al.* (2014) Intravenous Nefopam Reduces Postherpetic Neuralgia during the Titration of Oral Medications. *The Korean Joural of Pain*. **27**: 54–62.

24 Minotti V *et al.* (1989) Double-blind evaluation of analgesic efficacy of orally administered diclofenac, nefopam, and acetylsalicylic acid (ASA) plus codeine in chronic cancer pain. *Pain*. **36**: 177–183.

25 Pasutharnchat K *et al.* (2020) Analgesic efficacy of nefopam for cancer pain: a randomized controlled study. *F1000Research*. **9**: 378.

26 Aymard G *et al.* (2003) Comparative pharmacokinetics and pharmacodynamics of intravenous and oral nefopam in healthy volunteers. *Pharmacology and Toxicology*. **92**: 279–286.

27 Mimoz O *et al.* (2010) Nefopam pharmacokinetics in patients with end-stage renal disease. *Anaesthesia and Analgesia*. **111**: 1146–1153.

28 Beaver WT and Feise GA (1977) A comparison of the analgetic effect of intramuscular nefopam and morphine in patients with postoperative pain. *Journal of Clinical Pharmacology*. **17**: 579–591.
29 Phillips G and Vickers MD (1979) Nefopam in postoperative pain. *British Journal of Anaesthesia*. **51**: 961–965.
30 Chanques G *et al.* (2011) Analgesic efficacy and haemodynamic effects of nefopam in critically ill patients. *British Journal of Anaesthesia*. **106**: 336–343.

Updated May 2021

5

NON-STEROIDAL ANTI-INFLAMMATORY DRUGS (NSAIDS)

NSAIDs are essential drugs for cancer pain management. They are particularly useful when there is an inflammatory component, as is the case with most cancer pains.[1,2] The use of NSAIDs to relieve cancer pain is unauthorized.

Non-steroidal anti-inflammatory drugs (NSAIDs) prevent or reverse inflammation-induced hyperalgesia locally and in the CNS, thereby reducing pain.[3] There is also evidence from several RCTs that NSAIDs may be of benefit in *pure* (non-inflammatory) neuropathic pain.[4] However, neuropathic pain in cancer is typically *mixed* nociceptive–neuropathic, making benefit from an NSAID more likely.

NSAIDs also have a major role in postoperative pain.[5,6] However, there is little high-level evidence for benefit in some chronic pains, e.g. low-back pain.[7]

All NSAIDs are antipyretic.[8] It is generally accepted that inhibition of cyclo-oxygenase (COX) is their main shared mechanism of action.[9]

Cyclo-oxygenase

There are two distinct cyclo-oxygenase (COX) isoforms.[10] COX-1 is mainly 'constitutive', i.e. physiological, with near-constant levels and activity in most tissues, including the CNS. COX-2 is constitutive in parts of the CNS, renal cortex, stomach, uterus, cartilage, bone and seminal vesicles and is massively inducible within a few hours by inflammation, dehydration or trauma (Figure 1).

COX-1 also plays an indispensable role in inflammation; and COX-2, although initially producing pro-inflammatory prostaglandins, later induces anti-inflammatory PGD_2.[11] Both peptic ulcer and bone healing need COX-2.[12,13]

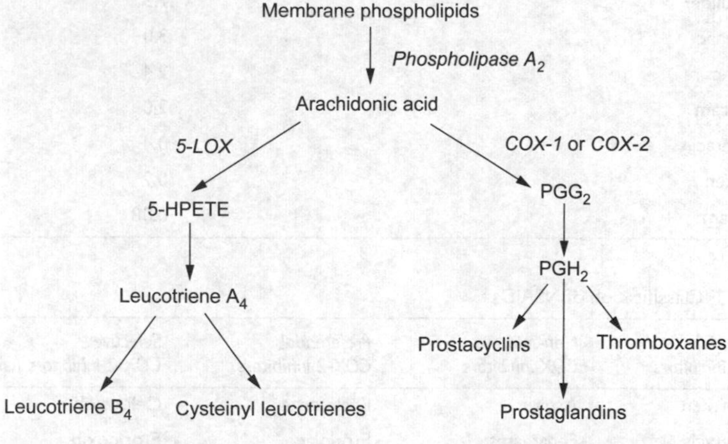

Figure 1 Products of arachidonic acid metabolism involved in inflammation.

Abbreviations: COX = cyclo-oxygenase, 5-HPETE = hydroperoxyeicosatetrenoic acid, LOX = lipoxygenase, PG = prostaglandin

Cyclo-oxygenase inhibition

Inflammation is associated with increased PG production both in the peripheral tissues and in the CNS.[14] The peripheral free nerve endings responsive to noxious stimuli become hypersensitive in the presence of inflammatory substances, increasing transduction and resulting in increased pain (*peripheral* sensitization).

Increased production of PGs in the CNS in response to a noxious stimulus leads to *central* sensitization of neurones in the dorsal horn, with further magnification of the noxious stimulus and more severe pain.[15-17] COX-2 plays a key role in central hyperalgesia.[18]

By inhibiting the production of COX, NSAIDs block the synthesis of PGs both peripherally in the tissues and in the CNS. The relative peripheral and central contributions to the total analgesic effect depend, among other things, on the NSAID in question, its pharmacokinetic details and the route of administration.[9]

NSAIDs also modify the endocannabinoid system. Endocannabinoids, like PGs, are produced *de novo* from arachidonic acid and are broken down by COX-2 (see Cannabinoids, p.251). Some NSAIDs (e.g. **ibuprofen**) inhibit other enzymes involved in endocannabinoid metabolism (e.g. fatty acid amide hydroxylase). The relative contribution of PG[19] and endocannabinoid systems to the analgesic effect of NSAIDs is uncertain.[20]

Classification

NSAIDs are now generally classified on the basis of their relative ability to inhibit COX-1 and COX-2. The degree of COX-2 selectivity varies according to the assay used[21,22] and whether the result is expressed in terms of 50% or 80% inhibition of the enzyme.[23,24] Although 80% inhibition is theoretically a better comparator, most studies use 50% (Table 1). However, the results of *in vitro* assays may not reliably reflect *in vivo* reality.[25] This is certainly the case in relation to **celecoxib**. Despite its relatively modest ranking (Table 1), no significant COX-1 inhibition is seen in volunteers taking 400mg b.d.[26] Dose and interindividual variation are the main determinants of COX-2 selectivity *in vivo*.[27]

Table 1 COX-2 selectivity ratio of IC_{50} COX-1/COX-2 (human whole-blood assays)[24]

Drug	*COX-2 selectivity ratio*
Etoricoxib	106.0
Celecoxib	7.6
Nimesulide[a]	7.3
Diclofenac	3.0
Etodolac	2.4
Meloxicam	2.0
Indometacin	0.4
Ibuprofen	0.2
Piroxicam	0.08

a. not UK.

Table 2 Classification of NSAIDs

Preferential COX-1 inhibitors	*Non-selective COX inhibitors*	*Preferential COX-2 inhibitors*	*Selective COX-2 inhibitors (coxibs)*
Flurbiprofen	Aspirin	Diclofenac	Celecoxib
Indometacin	Fenamates	Etodolac	Etoricoxib
Ketoprofen	Ibuprofen	Meloxicam	Parecoxib
Ketorolac	Nabumetone	Nimesulide (not UK)	
	Naproxen		
	Salicylates		

Although it is more correct to think of a spectrum of selectivity,[21,23] it is customary to divide NSAIDs into several seemingly disparate categories (Table 2). Inevitably, there will be differences of opinion as to where the cut-off between categories should come, particularly because selectivity is partly dose-dependent.[21] For example, with **meloxicam** 7.5mg/day, there is 70% COX-2 and 7% COX-1 inhibition but, with 15mg/day, there is 80% COX-2 and 25% COX-1 inhibition.[28] Further, thromboxane B_2 production is reduced 66% by **meloxicam** 15mg/day, the result of COX-1 inhibition.[29]

Additional sites of action

The anti-inflammatory properties of an NSAID are *not* predictive of its analgesic effect, suggesting that other mechanisms must be involved.[30] COX-independent actions are not all class effects, but include interactions with:

- synthesis and regulation of activity of dorsal horn neurotransmitters and modulators[31]
- modulation of pain transduction through spinal serotoninergic, adrenergic and cholinergic systems
- endocannabinoids
- nitric oxide production
- interleukin release
- caspase inhibition[32]
- matrix metalloproteinases (MMPs).[30]

The MMPs are a family of enzymes that cleave the various components of the extracellular matrix. MMPs are activated by tissue plasminogen activator/plasmin and are inactivated by endogenous tissue inhibitors of metalloproteinases (TIMPs). The dynamic interaction between MMPs and TIMPs determines their overall activity. MMPs can be both pro-inflammatory and anti-inflammatory, and the same MMP might have opposite roles in different circumstances.

PGs are involved in the regulation of MMP pathways. NSAIDs have different effects on MMPs and TIMPs in different inflammatory models. It is probable that the effects of NSAIDs on MMPs are both PG dependent and independent.[30]

NSAIDs also affect brain concentrations of kynurenic acid, an endogenous antagonist that acts on the glycine recognition site of the NMDA-receptor–channel complex.[33] **Diclofenac** (preferential COX-2 inhibitor) and **indometacin** (preferential COX-1 inhibitor) increase brain kynurenic acid concentrations, whereas **meloxicam** and **parecoxib** (preferential and selective COX-2 inhibitors respectively) cause a decrease. It is possible that at least some NSAIDs tonically modulate kynurenic acid metabolism and thereby impact on central nociceptive mechanisms.

Clinically, non-selective and selective COX-2 inhibitors are equally effective.[34] On the other hand, in dental pain there is a tendency for weak COX inhibitors to be superior to **aspirin**, and for strong inhibitors to be inferior, emphasizing the importance of not adopting too simplistic a view of the mode of action of these drugs (Table 3).

Table 3 Analgesic efficacy in dental pain of oral NSAIDs compared with aspirin 650mg[a, 35]

Significantly superior	*Not significantly different*	*Significantly inferior*
Azapropazone (3)[b]	Diclofenac (1)	Fenbufen (1)[b]
Diflunisal (3)[b]	Etodolac (1)	Nabumetone (1)
Flurbiprofen (1)	Sulindac (1)	Ketoprofen (2)
Ketorolac (3)[b]	Naproxen (3)	Tolmetin (3)[b]

a. numbers in brackets indicate capacity to inhibit PG synthesis: 1 = strong, 2 = moderate, 3 = weak

b. PO formulation no longer available in the UK.

NSAIDs and pyrexia

All NSAIDs are antipyretic.[8,36] Paraneoplastic fever responds to all NSAIDs, not just to **naproxen** as initially thought.[37] The response rate varies from 55–100%.[38] Although the antipyretic effect tends to wear off after a few months, further benefit may be obtained by switching to an alternative NSAID. However, the duration of benefit with second- and third-line drugs is generally shorter. For other options, see Antimuscarinics, Box E (p.9).

NSAIDs and cancer

For many years, it has been suggested that cancer-associated symptoms such as anorexia, weight loss and cachexia are manifestations of a chronic systemic inflammatory response (see Progestogens, p.599).[39] However, evidence of benefit is not robust enough to recommend the routine use of NSAIDs in these circumstances.[40,41]

On the other hand, tumour-promoting inflammation is considered one of the enabling characteristics of cancer progression.[42] COX-2 is detectable in 40–50% of adenomas and in >80% of adenocarcinomas.[43,44] It is expressed within tumour vasculature as well as in colon, breast, prostate and lung cancer cells.[45] COX-2-derived PGs contribute to tumour growth by inducing blood vessel formation (angiogenesis), which sustains tumour cell viability and growth.[45] NSAIDs suppress the production of these PGs and thus inhibit tumour development. Epidemiological data suggest that NSAIDs, particularly selective COX-2 inhibitors, may *prevent* the development of certain cancers, including colorectal, gastro-oesophageal and lung.[46-48] In an RCT of patients treated for colorectal adenoma, **celecoxib** reduced the risk of recurrence, particularly when the adenoma had either a high level of COX-2 or lacked 15-prostaglandin dehydrogenase, the enzyme metabolizing PGE_2.[49,50]

NSAIDs, mostly **celecoxib** in high doses (i.e. 400mg b.d.), have also been explored as a potential *treatment* for established cancer. In the adjuvant setting, **celecoxib** improved 3-year overall survival in patients with COX-2 positive gastric cancer treated with curative intent.[51] In advanced disease, systematic reviews found a significant increase in overall response rate to anticancer treatments in those prescribed 'add-on' **celecoxib**, although survival was unchanged.[52-54] Potentially, greater benefits (including survival) may be obtained by those with COX-2 positive cancers.[55] However, overall, the evidence is insufficient to recommend the routine use of **celecoxib** in these circumstances.

Interestingly, the pro-apoptotic (cell death) effect of **celecoxib** does *not* rely on COX-2 inhibition.[56] **Celecoxib** induces cell death, mainly by activation of an intrinsic mitochondria-dependent apoptosis pathway, independent of COX-2 inhibition.[56] With increased understanding of the specific mechanisms that regulate cancer-associated inflammation and apoptosis, it should become increasingly possible to alter the course of cancer with selective and targeted anti-inflammatory treatment without increasing the risk of CVS events.[57,58]

NSAIDs and platelet function

Platelets contain COX-1 but not COX-2. Thus, NSAIDs differ in their effect on platelet function and bleeding time (Table 4; also see p.348). Bleeding time is affected by various technical and clinical factors, is difficult to standardize[59] and is a poor predictor of bleeding in invasive procedures.[60] Although there are other methods for measuring platelet function,[61] these have not completely clarified understanding

Table 4 NSAIDs, platelet function and bleeding time

Drug	*Comment*
Aspirin	Irreversible platelet dysfunction and prolonged bleeding time as a result of acetylation of platelet COX-1
Non-acetylated salicylates, e.g. choline magnesium trisalicylate[a], salsalate[a]	No effect on platelet function or bleeding time at recommended doses
Classical NSAIDs (except diclofenac), e.g. flurbiprofen, ibuprofen, ketorolac, naproxen	Reversible platelet dysfunction and prolonged bleeding time
Diclofenac	Reversible inhibition of platelet aggregation in 2/3 of subjects.[60] IV diclofenac has a measurable effect on bleeding time, but most subjects remain within normal limits
Etodolac	No data
Meloxicam[62] Nabumetone Nimesulide[a,63] Coxibs[64]	No effect on platelet function or bleeding time

a. not UK.

about the differing effects of NSAIDs on bleeding. However, COX-2 inhibitors, because they do not affect the COX-1 in platelets and because of their associated low risk of GI bleeding, are likely to be the safest NSAIDs in people with low platelet counts.

NSAIDs and mental illness

Some mental illnesses are considered to have an inflammatory component, e.g. depression is characterized biochemically by increased levels of CRP and pro-inflammatory cytokines, including IL-6 and TNFα.[65] Thus, NSAIDs (mostly **celecoxib**) have been explored in various mental illnesses (mostly depression) as adjuvants to common treatments.

Systematic reviews have found that NSAIDs are associated with greater improvements in depression, mania (bipolar disorder) and psychosis (schizophrenia); however, most trials were small and short-term.[66-70] In RCTs, NSAIDs did not reduce the risk of Alzheimer's disease or prevent its progression.[71,72]

Undesirable effects

NSAIDs differ in their propensity to cause a range of undesirable effects. For convenience, these have been categorized as type A and type B. Generally, type A effects are mostly dose-dependent and partly predictable, whereas type B effects are mostly dose-independent and unpredictable (Table 5 and Table 6).

Table 5 Type A ('predictable') reactions to NSAIDs[74]

Organ/system	*Clinical reaction*
Blood	Decreased platelet aggregation, prolonged bleeding time (see Table 4)
GI tract	Dyspepsia Peptic ulceration, bleeding, perforation Small bowel stricture, bleeding, perforation Exacerbation of inflammatory bowel disease Protein-losing enteropathy
Kidney	Salt and water retention
Cardiovascular	Thrombosis, e.g. myocardial infarction, stroke
Lung	Bronchospasm (asthma)

Table 6 Type B ('unpredictable') reactions to NSAIDs[74]

Organ/system	*Clinical reaction*	*Most likely NSAIDs*
Immunological	Anaphylaxis	Most NSAIDs
Skin	Morbilliform rash Angioedema	Fenbufen Ibuprofen Azapropazone Piroxicam
Blood	Thrombocytopenia	Diclofenac Ibuprofen Piroxicam
	Haemolytic anaemia	Mefenamic acid Diclofenac
GI tract	Diarrhoea	Fenamates, e.g. mefenamic acid
Kidney	Interstitial nephritis	Fenoprofen[75]
Liver	Reye's syndrome (in children) Hepatotoxicity	Aspirin Diclofenac Sulindac
CNS	Aseptic meningitis	Ibuprofen

Quantitatively, the most serious undesirable effects are GI and CVS toxicity. *All* NSAIDs increase the risk of both upper GI ulceration and major CVS events (non-fatal and fatal myocardial infarction or stroke), albeit to a varying degree.[73] However, particularly in advanced progressive disease, the benefit associated with greater comfort generally far outweighs the potential harm from GI or CVS complications.

NSAIDs and the GI tract

From studies in patients with mainly rheumatoid arthritis and osteoarthritis taking an NSAID (including **aspirin**) ± gastroprotection for >2 *months*, the risk of a bleeding ulcer or perforation is about 1 in 500 patients, and the risk of dying from gastroduodenal complications is about 1 in 1,200.[76] Given the higher risk in patients with rheumatoid arthritis, and the ability of gastroprotective drugs to reduce serious ulcer complications,[77] these figures probably *overestimate* the risks in cancer and other advanced disease.

Although all NSAIDs increase the risk of GI complications, their propensity varies.[78] The most GI toxic NSAIDs are **azapropazone** (not UK), **ketorolac** (p.369) and **piroxicam**.[79] Although prescription may be justifiable in specific circumstances (see Route of administration, p.352), they should generally *not* be used.

A meta-analysis of several hundred RCTs indicated that, compared with placebo, the risk is less than doubled with **celecoxib** and **diclofenac** but quadrupled with *high-dose* **ibuprofen** (2,400mg/24h) and *high-dose* **naproxen** (1,000mg/24h).[73]

Indeed, **celecoxib** carries a significantly *lower* risk of clinically important GI events *throughout the entire GI tract*.[80] **Nabumetone** is also low risk but less widely used.[81] Combining thromboprotective **aspirin** with **celecoxib** increases the GI risk, although less than combining **aspirin** with a non-selective NSAID.[82-85]

Stomach and duodenum

The relative risk of gastric ulcer when taking an NSAID is 5–6.[86] For duodenal ulceration, the relative risk is only 1.1, although a recent population-based nested case-control study suggested it is higher.[87]

Various factors affect gastroduodenal toxicity (Box A). How much relates to COX-2 selectivity is uncertain.

Box A Factors intrinsic to NSAIDs which result in low gastroduodenal toxicity[88]	
Competitive masking of COX-1 by inactive forms, e.g. *R*-ibuprofen, *R*-etodolac.	
Weak/no uncoupling of oxidative phosphorylation Low disruption of phospholipids in protective mucus and mucous membranes	non-acidic compounds, e.g. nabumetone, coxibs.
High protein-binding (less available).	
Weak/no inhibition of platelet aggregation, e.g. non-acetylated salicylates, coxibs, meloxicam and sometimes diclofenac.	

In patients who are *Helicobacter pylori (H. pylori)* positive, the risk of developing an NSAID-related ulcer is almost doubled and the risk of bleeding is trebled.[89] The explanation for this lies in the *H. pylori*-associated chronic atrophic gastritis (mainly affecting the antrum) and makes the extracellular matrix in that part of the stomach wall vulnerable to the back-diffusion of acid. Ionized NSAID molecules, circulating in the plasma, are transported passively through leaky capillary walls into the inflamed matrix, where they become unionized in the acidic environment. In this state, the molecules are lipid-soluble and they move freely into the mucosal cells where, at a higher pH, the molecules become ionized again and consequently trapped. The local high concentration of NSAID leads to inhibition of the production of gastroprotective COX-1 in the stomach mucosa.

Eradication of *H. pylori* infection will correct the atrophic gastritis and end the sequence of events initiated by acid back-diffusion. Thus, eradication of *H. pylori* makes all COX-1-inhibiting NSAIDs safer to use, halving the incidence of peptic ulcer disease.[89] However, when trying to prevent ulcer recurrence in patients on NSAIDs, *H. pylori* eradication is less effective than a PPI.[90]

Risk factors for an NSAID-related upper GI complication (i.e. ulceration, bleeding, perforation) are listed in Box B. For example, concurrent administration of a non-selective NSAID and **warfarin** increases the risk of bleeding >10 times. This is nearly 4 times that of **warfarin** alone or with a selective COX-2 inhibitor (coxib).[91]

In rheumatoid arthritis, the risk of hospitalization and/or death from an NSAID-related upper GI complication increases progressively from 50 years.[86] Compared with those under 50, the risk is twice as great in patients aged 50–65 years, 6 times greater in patients aged 65–75 and 14 times greater in the over 75s. However, in rheumatoid arthritis, there may be other interacting risk factors. Thus, generally, 65 years is widely considered to be the appropriate point for regarding age as a risk factor.

Box B Risk factors for NSAID-related upper GI complications[86,92]

Age >65 years (see text).

Peptic ulcer ± GI bleeding in the past year confirmed by endoscopy, or strong clinical suspicion, e.g. haematemesis, melaena.

Long-term use of maximum recommended doses of an NSAID.

Serious morbidity, e.g. cancer, diabetes mellitus, hypertension, CVS disease, hepatic impairment, renal impairment.

Concurrent use of:
- a second GI irritant (e.g. corticosteroid)
- an anticoagulant
- an antiplatelet drug (e.g. aspirin, SSRI; see Important drug–drug interactions).

Platelets $<50 \times 10^9$/L.

Acid dyspepsia with an NSAID despite concurrent use of a gastroprotective drug.

Gastric infection with *H. pylori*.

Major reviews give the same ranking for gastroprotection:
- best = combination of a coxib plus PPI
- second best = coxib alone
- third best = non-selective NSAID plus PPI
- fourth best (because tolerability is poorer) = non-selective NSAID plus **misoprostol**.[93-96]

The difference among the latter three options is relatively small. One systematic review has suggested that an H_2-receptor antagonist may *not* offer significant gastroprotection.[94]

PPIs enable ulcer healing even if the NSAID is continued.[97] However, patients who develop an NSAID-related peptic ulcer should generally be switched to **celecoxib** (plus a PPI).[98]

Small bowel

NSAIDs can also cause small bowel ulceration, bleeding and perforation. In addition, they can cause protein-losing enteropathy and thin annular strictures, which may eventually reduce the bowel lumen to a pinhole.[99]

NSAID effects on the small bowel may be as important as NSAID gastropathy. In a capsule endoscopy study, macroscopic changes were found in over two-thirds of volunteers on a 2-week course of **diclofenac**. Used long-term (>3 months), similar results were seen with both non-selective COX and selective COX-2 inhibitors,[100] although the latter are probably safer in the short-term.[101,102] Other studies have given comparable results.[103-106]

Concurrent use of a PPI or H_2 antagonist is a risk factor (relative risk for PPIs = 2.7).[106] This is because, *although gastric-acid-reducing drugs reduce the risk of gastroduodenal damage, they increase enteropathy.* As more is learned about the balance between gastroduodenal and small bowel risk, the prophylactic use of PPIs in patients prescribed an NSAID may come under scrutiny.

Changes in bowel permeability may be the root cause of NSAID enteropathy.[107] PG deficiency (*not* achieved via COX inhibition) is important.[108,109] NSAIDs that undergo enterohepatic circulation (e.g. **diclofenac, indometacin, piroxicam**) are significantly more likely to damage the bowel than NSAIDs that do not (**aspirin, nabumetone, sulindac**).[110] Compared with non-selective NSAIDs, **celecoxib** is associated with a significantly lower risk of clinically important GI events *throughout the entire GI tract*.[80]

It is postulated that contact by the NSAID with the bowel wall damages the phosphatidylcholine in the mucosal cell membrane. Mitochondrial and endoplasmic reticulum damage decouples oxidative phosphorylation and leads to release of calcium and the production of free radicals. The resulting leakiness of bowel mucosal membranes leads to an ingress of Gram-negative bacteria, bile acids and proteolytic enzymes. The inflammation produced is mediated by neutrophils and causes both local and distant damage.[111] It has been suggested that this is related to the shift in intestinal microflora seen when acid is suppressed.

Prevention of intestinal damage is still in its infancy. Agents being investigated include:

- misoprostol[112,113]
- irsogladine,[114] a phosphodiesterase inhibitor
- lubiprostone,[115] which suppresses the expression of inflammatory mediators via EP4 receptors
- rebamipide,[116] a free radical scavenger
- lactoferrin,[117] a food constituent
- *Lactobacillus*
- rifaximin,[118] a broad-spectrum antibacterial.

Large bowel

Non-selective NSAIDs can cause clinical relapse of inflammatory bowel disease (IBD; i.e. Crohn's disease and ulcerative colitis) within 7–10 days of taking the drugs in about 20% of patients with IBD.[119] The mechanism of the NSAID-induced relapse appears to involve dual inhibition of COX-1 and -2, similar to the mechanism underlying NSAID damage in the small bowel.[119] In relation to IBD, **celecoxib** and **etoricoxib** do not differ from placebo and thus are first-line NSAIDs for patients with quiescent IBD.[120]

Women who use NSAIDs (but not aspirin) for >15 days a month for 6 years have an increased risk of developing *de novo* IBD.[121] NSAIDs can also cause a colitis directly and increase the risk of complications from diverticular disease.[122]

NSAIDs and the cardiovascular system

All NSAIDs increase CVS risk, particularly in patients who are hypertensive, have had a previous myocardial infarction or have undergone recent heart surgery.[123] The risk manifests in the first few weeks or months of use but appears *not* to increase long-term.[124,125]

The focus for the past 10–15 years has been on selective COX-2 inhibitors. It was reported that, with coxibs, the number of additional major CVS events would be about 3 in 1,000 per year of use and about 8 in 1,000 per year of use in high-risk patients, of which 2 would be fatal.[73] However, the analysis on which these figures were based included patients taking **rofecoxib**, withdrawn in 2004 because of an undisputed higher CVS risk.[126] Thus, these figures *overestimate* the risk with **celecoxib**. Indeed, it now appears that the risk with **celecoxib** is no higher, and may be lower, than with traditional non-selective NSAIDs.[78,125-129]

Further, another meta-analysis suggests that, in patients with an elevated CRP, *all* NSAIDs (*including* **celecoxib**) may *reduce* all-cause mortality and the risk of first myocardial infarction.[124]

Hypertension and heart failure

Except for **aspirin**, all NSAIDs have the potential to raise blood pressure and cause new or exacerbate existing hypertension; patients should be monitored accordingly. The risk may vary among NSAIDs, with **celecoxib** and **naproxen** possibly having a lower risk than **ibuprofen**.[130] The use of NSAIDs in heart failure carries a dose-dependent risk of death.[131]

NSAIDs increase the risk of heart failure necessitating hospital admission by up to 100%.[73,132] In a nested case-control study, high-dose **diclofenac** and high-dose **ibuprofen** doubled the odds, and the risk with high-dose **naproxen** was only slightly lower.[133] However, *no* increase was seen with **celecoxib** at commonly used doses (≤400mg/24h), although data are not available for high doses.[133] Thus, high-dose NSAIDs should generally be avoided in patients with CHF.

Major cardiac events (non-fatal and fatal myocardial infarction)

All NSAIDs carry a dose-dependent risk of acute myocardial infarction.[73,127,134,135] However, three recent meta-analyses have radically altered our understanding of the relative risk.[124-126] Thus, despite the conclusions of the CNT meta-analysis,[73] it now appears that **celecoxib** carries *no* greater risk of acute myocardial infarction than non-selective NSAIDs.[136]

Of interest is a Danish nationwide review that indicated that **diclofenac** and **ibuprofen** (but *not* COX-2 inhibitors or **naproxen**) are associated with an increased risk of out-of-hospital cardiac arrest.[137] Further, although it has been generally considered that high-dose **naproxen** (500mg b.d.) is safer than other non-selective NSAIDs,[73] it now seems that the risk is essentially the same for **celecoxib, diclofenac, ibuprofen** and **naproxen.**[125]

Major cerebrovascular events (non-fatal and fatal stroke)

In a large case-control study, current (compared to past) use of most NSAIDs increased the risk of *thrombotic* stroke, albeit to a varying degree, e.g. **ketorolac** (50% higher risk), **diclofenac** (25%), **ibuprofen** (15%). However, for several NSAIDs, e.g. **celecoxib, naproxen**, there was no increased risk.[138] Note. The concurrent use of an NSAID (except **celecoxib**) blocks the irreversible antiplatelet effect of low-dose **aspirin.**[139,140] Thus, in someone taking **aspirin** thromboprophylaxis, **celecoxib** is the NSAID of choice.

For *haemorrhagic* stroke, the findings of two systematic reviews of case-control and cohort studies differ in the degree of increased risk from NSAID use (OR 1.09 vs. 1.33). Both reviews found an increased risk with **diclofenac** and **meloxicam**, and one a higher risk also with **indometacin.**[141,142]

NSAIDs and the kidneys

All NSAIDs cause an increase in chloride (Cl^-) resorption from the proximal tubules and enhance ADH activity, leading to sodium (Na^+) and water retention. Thus, NSAIDs antagonize the action of diuretics and can exacerbate existing hypertension or lead to new onset hypertension.[143]

All NSAIDs can cause acute or acute-on-chronic renal impairment (Box C).[144] The risk of a first episode of acute renal impairment in NSAID users is three times that in non-users.[145] Sporadic cases of interstitial nephritis (± nephrotic syndrome or ± papillary necrosis) have been reported with most NSAIDs. The renal risks of different NSAIDs, including coxibs, are similar and thus are not a factor in determining choice.[146]

Box C Risk factors for NSAID-induced renal toxicity[147]
Age >60 years with co-morbidities.
Hypertension.
Congestive heart failure.
Dehydration, hypovolaemia.
Multiple myeloma with Bence-Jones proteinuria.[148,149]
Chronic and/or multiple NSAID use.
Concurrent use of diuretics and ACE inhibitors.
Hyponatraemia.
Cirrhosis, ascites.
Nephrotic syndrome.

In hypovolaemia, the plasma concentrations of vasoconstrictor substances such as angiotensin II, noradrenaline (norepinephrine) and vasopressin increase. This would generally lead to increased vasodilator PG secretion in the kidneys to maintain renal perfusion. However, the inhibition of renal PG production by NSAIDs prevents this, thereby precipitating renal impairment.[145,150]

Particularly in elderly patients with underlying chronic renal disease, the concurrent use of diuretics, an ACE inhibitor or angiotensin receptor antagonist and an NSAID ('triple whammy' medication) is a recognized cause of acute kidney injury (AKI).[151] Associated hypotension (e.g. intra-operative) dramatically increases the risk of AKI and has been termed 'the quadruple whammy'.[152]

Thus, except in patients expected to die in a few days, dehydrated patients should be rehydrated when starting treatment with an NSAID, or an NSAID should not be used. AKI caused by NSAIDs can be fatal. It is generally, but not always, reversible if the drug is stopped promptly.

In ESRF, NSAIDs should be avoided because of nephrotoxicity. However, in anuric patients on dialysis, they can be used in normal doses (see Chapter 17, p.746).

NSAIDs and the liver

Non-selective NSAIDs, but *not* **celecoxib**,[153] double the risk of bleeding from oesophageal varices because of their impact on platelet function (see p.344).[153]

Hepatotoxicity is a rare unpredictable effect seen with most NSAIDs, including coxibs. **Diclofenac** and **sulindac** may have the highest risk, and **ibuprofen** the lowest.[154]

Cholestasis may reduce the elimination of NSAIDs excreted in bile (**indometacin, sulindac**) and may reduce or delay absorption of fat-soluble NSAIDs, e.g. **ibuprofen**.[154]

Patients with hepatic impairment are more susceptible to NSAID-related renal impairment. Thus, most SPCs for NSAIDs include active liver disease or moderate–severe hepatic impairment as a contra-indication.[155]

For doses in hepatic impairment, see Chapter 18, p.760.

NSAIDs and bronchospasm

Some patients, with or without a history of atopic asthma, give a history of **aspirin**- or NSAID-induced asthma. In patients with asthma, about 10% report that NSAIDs exacerbate respiratory symptoms; in the general population, the figure is ≤5%.[156,157] Chronic non-aspirin NSAID users have almost double the risk of developing adult-onset asthma.[158]

Genetic polymorphisms in prostanoid receptor genes[159] and leukotriene synthase genes[160] have been described in individuals with **aspirin**-induced asthma, suggesting that the asthma is caused by an **aspirin**-induced (COX-1 inhibitory) imbalance between bronchodilator PGE_2 and bronchoconstrictor leukotrienes and is not immunologically mediated (as in atopic asthmatics).[161,162]

Aspirin-induced asthma typically occurs 30min–3h after ingestion of **aspirin**. Half of those affected react to even low-dose **aspirin** (80mg). Cross-sensitivity with other NSAIDs is normal, e.g. **diclofenac** (93%), **ibuprofen** (98%), **naproxen** (100%).[163] A history of allergic-type reactions (asthma, acute rhinitis, nasal polyps, angioedema, urticaria) with **aspirin** or another NSAID calls for extreme caution in prescribing a further NSAID (Table 7). Coxibs rarely induce asthma; the cause is probably isolated idiosyncratic allergy and *not* cross-reactivity with **aspirin** or other NSAIDs.[164]

Table 7 Use of NSAIDs in asthmatic patients

Patient characteristics	*Recommendations*
Anyone who has ever had an asthmatic reaction to aspirin or a non-coxib NSAID, or anyone with high-risk features of aspirin-induced asthma (severe asthma, nasal polyps, urticaria or chronic rhinitis)	Avoid all products containing aspirin or a non-coxib NSAID; use paracetamol instead unless also contra-indicated. *Coxibs are almost always safe*, but give the first dose under medical supervision[165]
All other asthmatic patients	Any NSAID, including aspirin, may be considered but, if any respiratory reaction occurs, stop the NSAID and manage as above

Bronchospasm has not been observed with **choline salicylate** (available only as a dental gel and ear drops in the UK), **sodium salicylate** and **azapropazone** (both not UK); it is rare with **benzydamine** (available only as a mouthwash and throat spray in the UK).[166]

The incidence of cross-sensitivity to **paracetamol** is only 7%; <2% of asthmatic patients are sensitive to both **aspirin** and **paracetamol**.[167] Further, reactions to **paracetamol** are generally less severe. Thus, **paracetamol** should always be the initial non-opioid analgesic of choice for asthmatic patients.

Management of NSAID-induced asthma is the same as for other acute asthma attacks (see Bronchodilators, p.121). Leukotriene receptor inhibitors, e.g. **montelukast**, should be considered.[168] Biological drugs (e.g. **omalizumab, mepolizumab**) may also be of benefit.[169,170]

Some patients may have been treated by **aspirin** desensitization.[171] Such patients will be on daily **aspirin**, which protects them from an attack triggered by inadvertent exposure to an NSAID. It is essential *not* to stop the **aspirin** in such patients, or sensitization may return (generally >48h after stopping).[172]

NSAIDs and bone healing

Some NSAIDs (**indometacin**, **diclofenac**, **tenoxicam**) delay bone healing in animals, but this has not been seen with others (**ibuprofen**, **ketorolac**, **piroxicam**).[173] In humans, there are concerns that NSAID use is associated with an increased risk of non-union of fractures or a decrease in heterotopic (ectopic) bone formation, commonly seen after major hip surgery.[174,175] However, although systematic reviews found no strong evidence that NSAIDs increase the risk of non-union, data are conflicting and insufficient to make a definite clinical recommendation.[176,177]

Thus, the approach taken by orthopaedic departments regarding the use of NSAIDs after fracture or orthopaedic surgery may vary. Generally, it would be sensible to use the lowest effective dose for as short a time as necessary. For example, limit the use of an NSAID to ≤14 days and then discontinue until healing is complete. However, in patients with other risk factors for delayed union or non-union (e.g. smoking, diabetes mellitus, corticosteroids), use **paracetamol** instead.[173] On the other hand, if pain relief is inadequate when using both **paracetamol** and an opioid, an NSAID should be prescribed (instead of the **paracetamol**), despite its potential negative impact.

Contra-indications for NSAIDs

Although SPCs are not completely consistent in this respect, the following is a general list of contra-indications for NSAIDs:

- hypersensitivity to **aspirin** or other NSAID (urticaria, rhinitis, asthma, angioedema)
- active GI ulceration, bleeding, perforation or inflammation
- CHF
- active liver disease or moderate–severe hepatic impairment
- severe renal impairment (creatinine clearance <30mL/min), deteriorating renal function, hyperkalemia (>5mmol/L).

These contra-indications are not necessarily absolute. There may be occasions when 'contra-indication' means 'use with great caution in the absence of a safer alternative'. **Diclofenac** and **celecoxib** are both contra-indicated in patients with established CVS disease.

Important drug–drug interactions

Pharmacodynamic

Many pharmacodynamic interactions can be predicted from the mode of action and undesirable effects of NSAIDs:

- increased risk of renal toxicity with other renally toxic drugs, e.g. aminoglycosides, **ciclosporin**
- increased risk of bleeding due to anti-platelet or anti-clotting effects, e.g. SNRIs, SSRIs, LMWH, **warfarin**
- increased risk of upper GI complications, e.g. concurrent prescription of low-dose **aspirin**, corticosteroids or **warfarin**
- antagonistic effect of NSAIDs due to Na^+ and fluid retention, e.g. antihypertensives, diuretics
- antagonistic effect of some NSAIDs with thromboprotective effect of low-dose **aspirin** (see p.348)
- antagonistic effect of NSAIDs with the uricosuric drug **probenecid**.

Compared with an SSRI alone *in low-risk patients*, concurrent use of an NSAID and an SSRI quadruples the incidence of upper GI bleeding (NNH >600)[178] and perhaps also intracranial bleeding.[179]

However, in those with additional risk factors (including many palliative care patients; Box B, p.347), the NNH is <200. Consider using a non-serotoninergic antidepressant when possible (e.g. **mirtazapine**, **nortriptyline**).[180]

Pharmacokinetic

Pharmacokinetic interactions are summarized in Tables 8 and 9 (also see Chapter 19, Table 8, p.790). Topical NSAIDs are unlikely to reach sufficient plasma concentrations to interact with other drugs.

NSAIDs can significantly affect the plasma concentrations of renally excreted drugs by causing reduced renal function and/or reduced tubular excretion. Of particular importance is the risk of toxic plasma concentrations of aminoglycosides, **ciclosporin**, **digoxin**, **lithium** and **methotrexate** (see Table 8).

Fatalities or severe renal impairment have occurred when **methotrexate** has been prescribed concurrently with an NSAID, e.g. **aspirin**, **ibuprofen**, **indometacin**, **ketoprofen**, **naproxen**, and life-threatening neutropenia has been reported with several NSAIDs.[181] However, a systematic review has suggested that, except for anti-inflammatory doses of **aspirin**, concurrent use is generally safe, although monitoring is recommended.[182]

NSAIDs can interact with **warfarin**, resulting in an increased INR; increases of up to 60% have been reported.[183,184] Patients should have their INR closely monitored during the first week after starting an NSAID and weekly for the next 3–4 weeks. The interaction may be due to CYP2C9 inhibition or competitive metabolism and may be more significant in those who are poor CYP2C9 metabolizers (see Chapter 19, Table 2, p.784).

There are few clinically significant interactions of drugs affecting the pharmacokinetics of NSAIDs (Table 9).

Choice of PO NSAID

NSAIDs are essential drugs for cancer pain management. As with all drugs, it is important to reduce risk as much as possible. Thus, for each patient, select the safest drug and, when indicated, prescribe gastroprotection.

It is unclear if some cancer patients obtain more benefit from one particular NSAID than from others, as is anecdotally reported in rheumatoid arthritis, or if any apparent differences simply relate to a relative increase in inhibition of PG synthesis.

In practice, the choice of NSAID will depend on factors such as availability, safety, cost and local guidelines. The renal risks of different NSAIDs, including coxibs, are similar and are *not* a factor in determining choice.[146]

Celecoxib

As already noted, recent reviews of CVS risk indicate that **celecoxib** ≤400mg/24h is *not* more cardiotoxic than non-selective NSAIDs (see p.348). Thus, given its undisputed low risk of upper GI complications, **celecoxib** 100–200mg b.d. is now probably *the overall NSAID of choice in palliative care* (see p.360). Generic **celecoxib** is available, and only high-GI-risk patients need a PPI concurrently (see p.346).

Celecoxib also has no effect on bleeding time and is thus a good choice in patients with thrombocytopenia (see p.344).

Other NSAIDs

Other frequently used NSAIDs include **ibuprofen** (p.365), **diclofenac** (p.362) and **naproxen** (p.371).

For high-GI-risk patients, gastroprotection, e.g. a PPI, should be prescribed concurrently (see p.346).

Although traditional advice is to take NSAIDs with food, there is no evidence that this reduces the risk of GI complications. Further, food may delay the absorption of an NSAID, which could be relevant when treating acute pain (see p.711).

Route of administration

In patients expected to die within 1–2 days, it is generally possible to discontinue NSAID use without a resurgence of pain. However, SC or PR administration can be used if an NSAID is needed and the PO route is not feasible.

Subcutaneous administration

Some centres use **diclofenac** CSCI (p.362) or **parecoxib** SC/CSCI (p.373) when the PO route is not feasible. Although its GI risk is significantly higher, **ketorolac** (p.369) is also used

Table 8 Pharmacokinetic interactions: NSAIDs affecting other drugs[181,185]

Drug affected	*Effect of NSAID*	*Clinical implications*
Aminoglycosides	May reduce renal function in susceptible individuals, thus reducing aminoglycoside clearance and increasing plasma concentration	Monitor aminoglycoside plasma concentration and renal function; adjust dose accordingly
Ciclosporin	May inhibit the renal prostacyclin synthesis needed to maintain glomerular filtration and renal blood flow. Increased and decreased ciclosporin plasma concentration reported	Monitor ciclosporin plasma concentration and renal function; adjust dose accordingly
Digoxin	May precipitate renal impairment, particularly in those with CHF, thus reducing digoxin excretion and increasing digoxin plasma concentration	Increased risk of digoxin toxicity. Monitor digoxin plasma concentration and renal function; adjust dose accordingly
Lithium	May inhibit renal excretion of lithium, increasing plasma lithium concentration	Increased risk of lithium toxicity. Avoid NSAID if possible; alternatively halve dose of lithium and monitor lithium plasma concentration. *Ketorolac is contra-indicated*
Methotrexate	Competitively inhibit the tubular excretion of methotrexate and inhibit PGE_2 synthesis, reducing renal perfusion; both increase methotrexate plasma concentration. Effect varies among NSAIDs and individuals	Increased risk of methotrexate toxicity. *Fatalities have occurred* (see text). Avoid aspirin and other salicylates during chemotherapy; probably safe between pulses. Use other NSAIDs with caution Much lower risk with low-dose chronic methotrexate treatment used in psoriasis or rheumatoid arthritis and if no pre-existing renal impairment Monitor methotrexate dose and its haematological effects
Phenytoin	May displace phenytoin from plasma proteins. May inhibit liver enzymes responsible for phenytoin metabolism	Clinical significance uncertain because the excess free phenytoin may be metabolized by the liver. However, phenytoin toxicity can develop even when the plasma concentration is within the therapeutic range
Sulfonylureas	May inhibit renal tubular excretion, increasing sulfonylurea plasma concentration and hypoglycaemic effect	Reduce sulfonylurea dose if necessary
Valproate	May displace valproate from plasma proteins, inhibit valproate metabolism and increase plasma concentration	Avoid aspirin. Importance of interaction with other NSAIDs unclear; reduce the dose of valproate if toxicity suspected
Warfarin	May inhibit metabolism of warfarin and increase INR; isolated cases reported with most NSAIDs (including coxibs)	INR increases of up to 60% have been reported; check INR closely during the first week after starting an NSAID and weekly for the next 3–4 weeks; reduce dose of warfarin if necessary; *ketorolac is contra-indicated*
Zidovudine	May increase the risk of haematological toxicity, particularly in haemophiliacs treated with ibuprofen	Monitor blood count

Table 9 Pharmacokinetic interactions: other drugs affecting NSAIDs[181,185]

Drug implicated	*NSAIDs affected*	*Effect*	*Clinical implications*
Antacids	All e/c NSAIDs	Destruction of enteric coating	Administer at different times
Antacids	Possibly all NSAIDs except celecoxib and diclofenac	Variable. Aluminium-containing antacids can *reduce* rate and/or extent of absorption of fenamates, diflunisal, indometacin and naproxen Magnesium hydroxide alone can *increase* the absorption of ibuprofen and flurbiprofen; also increases gastric toxicity of ibuprofen Sodium bicarbonate *increases* naproxen absorption	Avoid aluminium-containing antacids or use an alternative NSAID
Ciclosporin	Diclofenac	*Increased* plasma concentration of diclofenac due to reduced first-pass metabolism	Halve the dose of diclofenac
Colestyramine	All NSAIDs	Anion exchange resin binds NSAIDs in the GI tract, reducing and/or delaying absorption Binding in GI tract prevents enterohepatic recycling and increases faecal loss, even if NSAID administered IV (meloxicam, piroxicam, tenoxicam, sulindac)	Separate administration of PO NSAIDs by 4h. Colestyramine may be used to speed removal of NSAID after overdose
Fluconazole	Celecoxib Flurbiprofen Ibuprofen	*Increased* plasma concentration due to CYP2C9 inhibition by fluconazole	Halve the dose of celecoxib. Lower doses of flurbiprofen and ibuprofen may be necessary
Probenecid	Possibly all NSAIDs	Reduced metabolism and renal clearance of NSAIDs and glucuronide metabolites, which are hydrolyzed back to parent drug; NSAIDs also reduce the uricosuric effect of probenecid	Increased toxicity seen with indometacin, particularly if renal function impaired. Consider a reduction in NSAID dose but could be used therapeutically to increase the response. *Ketorolac is contra-indicated with probenecid*
Rifampicin	Celecoxib Diclofenac	*Decreased* plasma concentration due to CYP3A4 induction by rifampicin	Consider alternative NSAID if pain returns
Ritonavir	Piroxicam Possibly other NSAIDs	*Increased* plasma concentration of piroxicam with increased risk of toxicity	Manufacturer of ritonavir advises against concurrent use with piroxicam
Voriconazole	Diclofenac Flurbiprofen Ibuprofen	*Increased* plasma concentration due to CYP2C9 inhibition and reduced clearance by voriconazole	Lower doses of NSAID may be necessary

in these circumstances.[186] Further, anecdotal experience suggests that CSCI **ketorolac** may be more effective than a PO NSAID in some patients, notably (but not always) for bone pain.[187] Gastroprotection is essential.

Rectal administration

The rectal route is used less than in the past but remains an option:

- **diclofenac** suppositories (p.362)
- **indometacin** suppositories 100mg b.d.; a relatively expensive option (about five times more expensive than diclofenac).

1 McNicol E *et al.* (2004) Nonsteroidal anti-inflammatory drugs, alone or combined with opioids, for cancer pain: a systematic review. *Journal of Clinical Oncology*. **22**: 1975–1992.
2 Shah S and Hardy J (2001) Non-steroidal anti-inflammatory drugs in cancer pain: a review of the literature as relevant to palliative care. *Progress in Palliative Care*. **9**: 3–7.
3 Guindon J and Beaulieu P (2006) Antihyperalgesic effects of local injections of anandamide, ibuprofen, rofecoxib and their combinations in a model of neuropathic pain. *Neuropharmacology*. **50**: 814–823.
4 Vo T *et al.* (2009) Non-steroidal anti-inflammatory drugs for neuropathic pain: how do we explain continued widespread use? *Pain*. **143**: 169–171.
5 Jirarattanaphochai K and Jung S (2008) Nonsteroidal antiinflammatory drugs for postoperative pain management after lumbar spine surgery: a meta-analysis of randomized controlled trials. *Journal of Neurosurgery Spine*. **9**: 22–31.
6 Derry C *et al.* (2009) Single dose oral ibuprofen for acute postoperative pain in adults. *Cochrane Database of Systematic Reviews*. **3**: CD001548. www.cochranelibrary.com.
7 Enthoven WT *et al.* (2016) Non-steroidal anti-inflammatory drugs for chronic low back pain. *Cochrane Database of Systematic Reviews*. **2**: CD012087. www.cochranelibrary.com.
8 Simmons DL *et al.* (2000) Nonsteroidal anti-inflammatory drugs, acetaminophen, cyclooxygenase 2, and fever. *Clinical Infectious Diseases*. **31 (Suppl 5)**: S211–218.
9 Burian M and Geisslinger G (2005) COX-dependent mechanisms involved in the antinociceptive action of NSAIDs at central and peripheral sites. *Pharmacology and Therepeutics*. **107**: 139–154.
10 Simmons DL *et al.* (2004) Cyclooxygenase isozymes: the biology of prostaglandin synthesis and inhibition. *Pharmacological Reviews*. **56**: 387–437.
11 Kapoor M *et al.* (2005) Possible anti-inflammatory role of COX-2-derived prostaglandins: implications for inflammation research. *Current Opinion in Investigational Drugs*. **6**: 461–466.
12 Gerstenfeld LC and Einhorn TA (2004) COX inhibitors and their effects on bone healing. *Expert Opinion on Drug Safety*. **3**: 131–136.
13 Peskar BM (2005) Role of cyclooxygenase isoforms in gastric mucosal defense and ulcer healing. *Inflammopharmacology*. **13**: 15–26.
14 Schwab JM and Schluesener HJ (2003) Cyclooxygenases and central nervous system inflammation: conceptual neglect of cyclooxygenase 1. *Archives of Neurology*. **60**: 630–632.
15 Baba H *et al.* (2001) Direct activation of rat spinal dorsal horn neurons by prostaglandin E2. *Journal of Neuroscience*. **21**: 1750–1756.
16 Samad T *et al.* (2001) Interleukin-1B-mediated induction of COX-2 in the CNS contributes to inflammatory pain hypersensitivity. *Nature*. **410**: 471–475.
17 Farooqui M *et al.* (2007) COX-2 inhibitor celecoxib prevents chronic morphine-induced promotion of angiogenesis, tumour growth, metastasis and mortality, without compromising analgesia. *British Journal of Cancer*. **97**: 1523–1531.
18 Jain NK *et al.* (2008) COX-2 expression and function in the hyperalgesic response to paw inflammation in mice. *Prostaglandins Leukotrienes and Essential Fatty Acids*. **79**: 183–190.
19 Severine Vandevoorde (2008) Overview of the chemical families of fatty acid amide hydrolase and monoacylglycerol lipase inhibitors. *Current Topics in Medicinal Chemistry*. **8**: 247–267.
20 Telleria-Diaz A et *al.* (2010) Spinal antinociceptive effects of cyclooxygenase inhibition during inflammation: Involvement of prostaglandins and endocannabinoids. *Pain*. **148**: 26–35.
21 Churchill L *et al.* (1996) Selective inhibition of human cyclo-oxygenase-2 by meloxicam. *Inflammopharmacology*. **4**: 125–135.
22 Brooks P *et al.* (1999) Interpreting the clinical significance of the differential inhibition of cyclooxygenase-1 and cyclooxygenase-2. *Rheumatology*. **38**: 779–788.
23 Warner T *et al.* (1999) Nonsteroidal drug selectivities for cyclo-oxygenase-1 rather than cyclo-oxygenase-2 are associated with human gastrointestinal toxicity: a full in vitro analysis. *Proceedings of the National Academy of Science USA*. **96**: 7563–7568.
24 Riendeau D *et al.* (2001) Etoricoxib (MK-0663): Preclinical profile and comparison with other agents that selectively inhibit cyclooxygenase-2. *Journal of Pharmacology and Experimental Therapeutics*. **296**: 558–566.
25 Blain H *et al.* (2002) Limitation of the in vitro whole blood assay for predicting the COX selectivity of NSAIDs in clinical use. *British journal of clinical pharmacology*. **53**: 255–265.
26 Fries S *et al.* (2006) Marked interindividual variability in the response to selective inhibitors of cyclooxygenase-2. *Gastroenterology*. **130**: 55–64.
27 Capone ML *et al.* (2007) Pharmacodynamic of cyclooxygenase inhibitors in humans. *Prostaglandins Other Lipid Mediators*. **82**: 85–94.
28 Van Hecken A *et al.* (2000) Comparative inhibitory activity of rofecoxib, meloxicam, diclofenac, ibuprofen and naproxen on COX-2 versus COX-1 in healthy volunteers. *Journal of Clinical Pharmacology*. **40**: 1109–1120.
29 de Meijer A *et al.* (1999) Meloxicam, 15mg/day, spares platelet function in healthy volunteers. *Clinical Pharmacology and Therapeutics*. **66**: 425–430.
30 Hamza M and Dionne RA (2009) Mechanisms of non-opioid analgesics beyond cyclooxygenase enzyme inhibition. *Current Molecular Pharmacology*. **2**: 1–14.
31 McCormack K (1994) Nonsteroidal anti-inflammatory drugs and spinal nociceptive processing. *Pain*. **59**: 9–43.
32 Smith CE *et al.* (2017) Non-steroidal anti-inflammatory drugs are caspase inhibitors. *Cell Chemical Biology*. **24**: 281–292.
33 Schwieler L *et al.* (2005) Prostaglandin-mediated control of rat brain kynurenic acid synthesis - opposite actions by COX-1 and COX-2 isoforms. *Journal of Neural Transmission*. **112**: 863–872.

34 Dougados M *et al.* (2001) Evaluation of the structure-modifying effects of diacerein in hip osteoarthritis: ECHODIAH, a three-year, placebo-controlled trial. Evaluation of the Chondromodulating Effect of Diacerein in OA of the Hip. *Arthritis and Rheumatism*. **44**: 2539–2547.

35 McCormack K and Brune K (1991) Dissociation between the antinociceptive and anti-inflammatory effects of the nonsteroidal anti-inflammatory drugs: a survey of their analgesic efficacy. *Drugs*. **41**: 533–547.

36 Kathula SK *et al.* (2003) Cyclo-oxygenase II inhibitors in the treatment of neoplastic fever. *Supportive Care in Cancer*. **11**: 258–259.

37 Tsavaris N *et al.* (1990) A randomized trial of the effect of three nonsteroidal anti-inflammatory agents in ameliorating cancer-induced fever. *Journal of Internal Medicine*. **228**: 451–455.

38 Zhang H *et al.* (2019) Naproxen for the treatment of neoplastic fever: A PRISMA-compliant systematic review and meta-analysis. *Medicine (Baltimore)*. **98**: e15840.

39 Roxburgh CS and McMillan DC (2014) Cancer and systemic inflammation: treat the tumour and treat the host. *British Journal of Cancer*. **110**: 1409–1412.

40 Roeland EJ *et al.* (2020) Management of cancer cachexia: ASCO guideline. *Journal of Clinical Oncology*. **38**:2438–2453.

41 Solheim TS *et al.* (2013) Non-steroidal anti-inflammatory treatment in cancer cachexia: A systematic literature review. *Acta Oncologica*. **52**:6–17.

42 Diakos CI *et al.* (2014) Cancer-related inflammation and treatment effectiveness. *Lancet Oncology*. **15**: e493–e503.

43 Eberhart CE *et al.* (1994) Up-regulation of cyclooxygenase 2 gene expression in human colorectal adenomas and adenocarcinomas. *Gastroenterology*. **107**: 1183–1188.

44 Koki AT *et al.* (1999) Potential utility of COX-2 inhibitors in chemoprevention and chemotherapy. *Expert Opinion on Investigational Drugs*. **8**: 1623–1638.

45 Masferrer JL *et al.* (2000) Antiangiogenic and antitumor activities of cyclooxygenase-2 inhibitors. *Cancer Research*. **60**: 1306–1311.

46 Liao X *et al.* (2012) Aspirin use, tumor PIK3CA mutation, and colorectal-cancer survival. *New England Journal of Medicine*. **367**: 1596–1606.

47 Liao Z *et al.* (2007) Cyclo-oxygenase-2 and its inhibition in cancer: is there a role? *Drugs*. **67**: 821–845.

48 Huang XZ *et al.* (2017) Aspirin and non-steroidal anti-inflammatory drugs use reduce gastric cancer risk: A dose-response meta-analysis. *Oncotarget*. **8**: 4781–4795.

49 Bertagnolli MM *et al.* (2006) A Randomized Trial of celecoxib for the prevention of sporadic colorectal adenomas. *New England Journal of Medicine*. **355**: 873–884.

50 Wang J *et al.* (2018) Chemopreventive efficacy of the cyclooxygenase-2 (Cox-2) inhibitor, celecoxib, is predicted by adenoma expression of Cox-2 and 15-PGDH. *Cancer Epidemiology Biomarkers & Prevention*. **27**: 728–736.

51 Guo Q *et al.* (2017) Comprehensive evaluation of clinical efficacy and safety of celecoxib combined with chemotherapy in management of gastric cancer. *Medicine (Baltimore)*. **96**: e8857.

52 Chen J *et al.* (2014) Efficacy and safety profile of celecoxib for treating advanced cancers: a meta-analysis of 11 randomized clinical trials. *Clinical Therapeutics*. **36**: 1253–1263.

53 Yi L *et al.* (2018) Systematic review and meta-analysis of the benefit of celecoxib in treating advanced non-small-cell lung cancer. *Drug design, development and therapy*. **12**: 2455–2466.

54 Edelman MJ *et al.* (2017) Phase III Randomized, Placebo-Controlled, Double-Blind Trial of Celecoxib in Addition to Standard Chemotherapy for Advanced Non-Small-Cell Lung Cancer With Cyclooxygenase-2 Overexpression: CALGB 30801 (Alliance). *Journal of Clinical Oncology*. **35**: 2184–2192.

55 Guo Q *et al.* (2019) A comprehensive evaluation of clinical efficacy and safety of celecoxib in combination with chemotherapy in metastatic or postoperative recurrent gastric cancer patients: A preliminary, three-center, clinical trial study. *Medicine (Baltimore)*. **98**: e16234.

56 Jendrossek V (2013) Targeting apoptosis pathways by Celecoxib in cancer. *Cancer Letters*. **332**: 313–324.

57 Chavez C and Hoffman MA (2013) Complete remission of ALK-negative plasma cell granuloma (inflammatory myofibroblastic tumor) of the lung induced by celecoxib: A case report and review of the literature. *Oncol Letters*. **5**: 1672–1676.

58 Mercurio S *et al.* (2013) Evidence for new targets and synergistic effect of metronomic celecoxib/fluvastatin combination in pilocytic astrocytoma. *Acta Neuropathologica Communications*. **1**: 17.

59 Peterson P *et al.* (1998) The preoperative bleeding time test lacks clinical benefit: College of American Pathologists' and American Society of Clinical Pathologists' position article. *Archives of Surgery*. **133**: 134–139.

60 Ng KF *et al.* (2008) Comprehensive preoperative evaluation of platelet function in total knee arthroplasty patients taking diclofenac. *Journal of Arthroplasty*. **23**: 424–430.

61 Brass L (2010) Understanding and evaluating platelet function. *Hematology/ the Education Program of the American Society of Hematology Education Program*. **2010**: 387–396.

62 Guth B *et al.* (1996) Therapeutic doses of meloxicam do not inhibit platelet aggregation in man. *Rheumatology in Europe*. **25**: Abstract 443.

63 Cullen L *et al.*, editors. Selective suppression of cyclooxygenase-2 during chronic administration of nimesulide in man. Fourth International Congress on essential fatty acids and eicosanoids; 1997; Edinburgh.

64 Teerawattananon C *et al.* (2017) Risk of perioperative bleeding related to highly selective cyclooxygenase-2 inhibitors: a systematic review and meta-analysis. *Seminars in Arthritis and Rheumatism*. **46**: 520–528.

65 Maes M (2012) Targeting cyclooxygenase-2 in depression is not a viable therapeutic approach and may even aggravate the pathophysiology underpinning depression. *Metabolic Brain Disease*. **27**: 405–413.

66 Kohler O *et al.* (2014) Effect of anti-inflammatory treatment on depression, depressive symptoms, and adverse effects: a systematic review and meta-analysis of randomized clinical trials. *JAMA Psychiatry*. **71**: 1381–1391.

67 Eyre HA *et al.* (2015) A critical review of the efficacy of non-steroidal anti-inflammatory drugs in depression. *Progress in Neuropsychopharmacology and Biological Psychiatry*. **57**: 11–16.

68 Bai S *et al.* (2019) Efficacy and safety of anti-inflammatory agents for the treatment of major depressive disorder: a systematic review and meta-analysis of randomised controlled trials. *Journal of Neurology, Neurosurgery, and Psychiatry*. **91**: 21–32.

69 Zheng W *et al.* (2017) Adjunctive celecoxib for schizophrenia: A meta-analysis of randomized, double-blind, placebo-controlled trials. *Journal of Psychiatric Research*. **92**: 139–146.

70 Bavaresco DV *et al.* (2019) Efficacy of Celecoxib Adjunct Treatment on Bipolar Disorder: Systematic Review and Meta-Analysis. *CNS & Neurological Disorders - Drug Targets*. **18**: 19–28.

71 ADAPT Research Group *et al.* (2007) Naproxen and celecoxib do not prevent AD in early results from a randomized controlled trial. *Neurology*. **68**: 1800–1808.

72 Meyer PF *et al.* (2019) INTREPAD: A randomized trial of naproxen to slow progress of presymptomatic Alzheimer disease. *Neurology*. **92**: e2070–e2080.

73 CNT Collaboration (2013) Vascular and upper gastrointestinal effects of non-steroidal anti-inflammatory drugs: meta-analyses of individual participant data from randomised trials. *Lancet*. **382**: 769–779.
74 Rawlins M. Non-opioid analgesics. In: Doyle D, Hanks G, MacDonald N, editors. *Oxford Textbook of Palliative Medicine*. 2 ed. Oxford: Oxford University Press; 1997. p. 355–361.
75 Rossert J (2001) Drug-induced acute interstitial nephritis. *Kidney International*. **60**: 804–817.
76 Tramer M *et al.* (2000) Quantitative estimation of rare adverse events which follow a biological progression: a new model applied to chronic NSAID use. *Pain*. **85**: 169–182.
77 Silverstein FE *et al.* (1995) Misoprostol reduces serious gastrointestinal complications in patients with rheumatoid arthritis receiving nonsteroidal anti-inflammatory drugs. *Annals of Internal Medicine*. **123**: 241–249.
78 Arias LHM *et al.* (2019) Gastrointestinal safety of coxibs: systematic review and meta-analysis of observational studies on selective inhibitors of cyclo-oxygenase 2. *Fundamental and Clinical Pharmacology*. **33**: 134–147.
79 Castellsague J *et al.* (2012) Individual NSAIDs and upper gastrointestinal complications: a systematic review and meta-analysis of observational studies (the SOS project). *Drug Safety*. **35**: 1127–1146.
80 Moore A *et al.* (2013) Patient-level pooled analysis of adjudicated gastrointestinal outcomes in celecoxib clinical trials: meta-analysis of 51,000 patients enrolled in 52 randomized trials. *Arthritis Research and Therapy*. **15**: R6.
81 Bannwarth B (2008) Safety of the nonselective NSAID nabumetone : focus on gastrointestinal tolerability. *Drug Safety*. **31**: 485–503.
82 Strand V (2007) Are COX-2 inhibitors preferable to non-selective non-steroidal anti-inflammatory drugs in patients with risk of cardiovascular events taking low-dose aspirin? *Lancet*. **370**: 2138–2151.
83 Chan FKL *et al.* (2017) Gastrointestinal safety of celecoxib versus naproxen in patients with cardiothrombotic diseases and arthritis after upper gastrointestinal bleeding (CONCERN): an industry-independent, double-blind, double-dummy, randomised trial. *Lancet*. **389**: 2375–2382.
84 Yeomans ND *et al.* (2018) Randomised clinical trial: gastrointestinal events in arthritis patients treated with celecoxib, ibuprofen or naproxen in the PRECISION trial. *Alimentary Pharmacology & Therapeutics*. **47**: 1453–1463.
85 Reed GW *et al.* (2018) Effect of aspirin coadministration on the safety of celecoxib, naproxen, or ibuprofen. *Journal of the American College of Cardiology*. **71**: 1741–1751.
86 Fries J *et al.* (1991) Nonsteroidal anti-inflammatory drug-associated gastropathy: incidence and risk factor models. *American Journal of Medicine*. **91**: 213–222.
87 Garcia Rodriguez LA and Hernandez-Diaz S (2004) Risk of uncomplicated peptic ulcer among users of aspirin and nonaspirin nonsteroidal antiinflammatory drugs. *American Journal of Epidemiology*. **159**: 23–31.
88 Rainsford K (1999) Profile and mechanisms of gastrointestinal and other side effects of nonsteroidal anti-inflammatory drugs (NSAIDs). *American Journal of Medicine*. **107 (Suppl 6A)**: S27–S36.
89 Tang CL *et al.* (2012) Eradication of Helicobacter pylori infection reduces the incidence of peptic ulcer disease in patients using nonsteroidal anti-inflammatory drugs: a meta-analysis. *Helicobacter*. **17**: 286–296.
90 Malfertheiner P *et al.* (2007) Current concepts in the management of Helicobacter pylori infection: the Maastricht III Consensus Report. *Gut*. **56**: 772–781.
91 Cheetham TC *et al.* (2009) Gastrointestinal safety of nonsteroidal antiinflammatory drugs and selective cyclooxygenase-2 inhibitors in patients on warfarin. *Annals of Pharmacotherapy*. **43**: 1765–1773.
92 Hawkins C and Hanks G (2000) The gastroduodenal toxicity of nonsteroidal anti-inflammatory drugs. A review of the literature. *Journal of Pain and Symptom Management*. **20**: 140–151.
93 Targownik LE *et al.* (2008) The relative efficacies of gastroprotective strategies in chronic users of nonsteroidal anti-inflammatory drugs. *Gastroenterology*. **134**: 937–944.
94 Yuan JQ *et al.* (2016) Systematic review with network meta-analysis: comparative effectiveness and safety of strategies for preventing NSAID-associated gastrointestinal toxicity. *Alimentary Pharmacology and Therapeutics*. **43**: 1262–1275.
95 Chan FK *et al.* (2010) Celecoxib versus omeprazole and diclofenac in patients with osteoarthritis and rheumatoid arthritis (CONDOR): a randomised trial. *Lancet*. **376**: 173–179.
96 Chan FK *et al.* (2007) Combination of a cyclo-oxygenase-2 inhibitor and a proton-pump inhibitor for prevention of recurrent ulcer bleeding in patients at very high risk: a double-blind, randomised trial. *Lancet*. **369**: 1621–1626.
97 Hawkey C *et al.* (1998) Omeprazole compared with misoprostol for ulcers associated with nonsteroidal anti-inflammatory drugs. *New England Journal of Medicine*. **338**: 727–734.
98 NICE (2014) Dyspepsia and gastro-oesophageal reflux disease. *Clinical Guideline*. CG184. www.nice.org.uk.
99 Adebayo D and Bjarnason I (2006) Is non-steroidal anti-inflammaory drug (NSAID) enteropathy clinically more important than NSAID gastropathy? *Postgraduate Medical Journal*. **82**: 186–191.
100 Maiden L (2009) Capsule endoscopic diagnosis of nonsteroidal antiinflammatory drug-induced enteropathy. *Journal of Gastroenterology*. **44 (Suppl 19)**: 64–71.
101 Smecuol E *et al.* (2001) Acute gastrointestinal permeability responses to different non-steroidal anti-inflammatory drugs. *Gut*. **49**: 650–655.
102 Goldstein JL *et al.* (2005) Video capsule endoscopy to prospectively assess small bowel injury with celecoxib, naproxen plus omeprazole, and placebo. *Clinical Gastroenterology and Hepatology*. **3**: 133–141.
103 Maiden L *et al.* (2005) A quantitative analysis of NSAID-induced small bowel pathology by capsule enteroscopy. *Gastroenterology*. **128**: 1172–1178.
104 Fujimori S *et al.* (2010) Distribution of small intestinal mucosal injuries as a result of NSAID administration. *European Journal of Clinical Investigations*. **40**: 504–510.
105 Graham DY *et al.* (2005) Visible small-intestinal mucosal injury in chronic NSAID users. *Clinical Gastroenterology and Hepatology*. **3**: 55–59.
106 Washio E *et al.* (2016) Proton pump inhibitors increase incidence of nonsteroidal anti-inflammatory drug-induced small bowel injury: a randomized, placebo-controlled trial. *Clinical Gastroenterology and Hepatology*. **14**: 809–815.e801.
107 Bjarnason I and Takeuchi K (2009) Intestinal permeability in the pathogenesis of NSAID-induced enteropathy. *Journal of Gastroenterology*. **44 (Suppl 19)**: 23–29.
108 Wallace JL (2012) NSAID gastropathy and enteropathy: distinct pathogenesis likely necessitates distinct prevention strategies. *British Journal of Pharmacology*. **165**: 67–74.
109 Adler DH *et al.* (2009) The enteropathy of prostaglandin deficiency. *Journal of Gastroenterology*. **44 (Suppl 19)**: 1–7.
110 Hedner T *et al.* (2004) Nabumetone: Therapeutic use and safety profile in the management of osteoarthritis and rheumatoid arthritis. *Drugs*. **64**: 2315–2343; discussion 2344–2345.
111 Boelsterli UA *et al.* (2013) Multiple NSAID-induced hits injure the small intestine: underlying mechanisms and novel strategies. *Toxicol Sci*. **131**: 654–667.

112 Satoh H *et al.* (2014) Mucosal protective agents prevent exacerbation of NSAID-induced small intestinal lesions caused by antisecretory drugs in rats. *Journal of Pharmacology and Experimental Therapeutics*. **348**: 227–235.
113 Taha AS *et al.* (2018) Misoprostol for small bowel ulcers in patients with obscure bleeding taking aspirin and non-steroidal anti-inflammatory drugs (MASTERS): a randomised, double-blind, placebo-controlled, phase 3 trial. *Lancet Gastroenterology Hepatology*. **3**: 469–476.
114 Kojima Y *et al.* (2015) Effect of long-term proton pump inhibitor therapy and healing effect of irsogladine on nonsteroidal anti-inflammatory drug-induced small-intestinal lesions in healthy volunteers. *Journal of Clinical Biochemistry and Nutrition*. **57**: 60–65.
115 Hayashi S *et al.* (2014) Lubiprostone prevents nonsteroidal anti-inflammatory drug-induced small intestinal damage by suppressing the expression of inflammatory mediators via EP4 receptors. *Journal of Pharmacology Experimental Therapeutics*. **349**: 470–479.
116 Zhang S *et al.* (2013) Rebamipide helps defend against nonsteroidal anti-inflammatory drugs induced gastroenteropathy: a systematic review and meta-analysis. *Digestive Diseases and Sciences*. **58**: 1991–2000.
117 Satoh H and Takeuchi K (2012) Management of NSAID/aspirin-induced small intestinal damage by GI-sparing NSAIDs, anti-ulcer drugs and food constituents. *Current Medicinal Chemistry*. **19**: 82–89.
118 Scarpignato C *et al.* (2017) Rifaximin reduces the number and severity of intestinal lesions associated with use of nonsteroidal anti-inflammatory drugs in humans. *Gastroenterology*. **152**: 980–920.
119 Takeuchi K *et al.* (2006) Prevalence and mechanism of nonsteroidal anti-inflammatory drug-induced clinical relapse in patients with inflammatory bowel disease. *Clinical Gastroenterology and Hepatology*. **4**: 196–202.
120 Ribaldone DG *et al.* (2015) Coxib's safety in patients with inflammatory bowel diseases: a meta-analysis. *Pain Physician*. **18**: 599–607.
121 Ananthakrishnan AN *et al.* (2012) Aspirin, nonsteroidal anti-inflammatory drug use, and risk for Crohn disease and ulcerative colitis: a cohort study. *Annals of Internal Medicine*. **156**: 350–359.
122 Ballinger A (2008) Adverse effects of nonsteroidal anti-inflammatory drugs on the colon. *Current Gastroenterology Reports*. **10**: 485–489.
123 Schmidt M *et al.* (2016) Cardiovascular safety of non-aspirin non-steroidal anti-inflammatory drugs: review and position paper by the working group for Cardiovascular Pharmacotherapy of the European Society of Cardiology. *European Heart Journal*. **37**: 1015–1023.
124 Zingler G *et al.* (2016) Cardiovascular adverse events by non-steroidal anti-inflammatory drugs: when the benefits outweigh the risks. *Expert Review of Clinical Pharmacology*. **8**: 1–14.
125 Bally M *et al.* (2017) Risk of acute myocardial infarction with NSAIDs in real world use: bayesian meta-analysis of individual patient data. *British Medical Journal*. **357**: 1909.
126 Gunter BR *et al.* (2017) Non-steroidal anti-inflammatory drug-induced cardiovascular adverse events: a meta-analysis. *Journal of Clinical Pharmacy and Therapeutics*. **42**: 27–38.
127 Nissen SE *et al.* (2016) Cardiovascular safety of celecoxib, naproxen, or ibuprofen for arthritis. *New England Journal of Medicine*. **375**: 2519–2529.
128 MacDonald TM *et al.* (2017) Randomized trial of switching from prescribed non-selective non-steroidal anti-inflammatory drugs to prescribed celecoxib: the Standard care vs. Celecoxib Outcome Trial (SCOT). *European Heart Journal*. **38**: 1843–1850.
129 Barcella CA *et al.* (2018) Differences in cardiovascular safety with non-steroidal anti-inflammatory drug therapy-A nationwide study in patients with osteoarthritis. *Basic and Clinical Pharmacology and Toxicology*. **124**: 629–641.
130 Ruschitzka F *et al.* (2017) Differential blood pressure effects of ibuprofen, naproxen, and celecoxib in patients with arthritis: the PRECISION-ABPM (Prospective Randomized Evaluation of Celecoxib Integrated Safety Versus Ibuprofen or Naproxen Ambulatory Blood Pressure Measurement) Trial. *European Heart Journal*. **38**: 3282–3292.
131 Gislason GH *et al.* (2009) Increased mortality and cardiovascular morbidity associated with use of nonsteroidal anti-inflammatory drugs in chronic heart failure. *Archives of Internal Medicine*. **169**: 141–149.
132 Huerta C *et al.* (2006) Non-steroidal anti-inflammatory drugs and risk of first hospital admission for heart failure in the general population. *Heart*. **92**: 1610–1615.
133 Arfe A *et al.* (2016) Non-steroidal anti-inflammatory drugs and risk of heart failure in four European countries: nested case-control study. *British Medical Journal*. **354**: i4857.
134 Solomon SD *et al.* (2008) Cardiovascular risk of celecoxib in 6 randomized placebo-controlled trials: the cross trial safety analysis. *Circulation*. **117**: 2104–2113.
135 Trelle S *et al.* (2011) Cardiovascular safety of non-steroidal anti-inflammatory drugs: network meta-analysis. *British Medical Journal*. **342**: c7086.
136 Masclee GMC *et al.* (2018) Risk of acute myocardial infarction during use of individual NSAIDs: A nested case-control study from the SOS project. *PLoS One*. **13**: e0204746.
137 Sondergaard KB *et al.* (2017) Non-steroidal anti-inflammatory drug use is associated with increased risk of out-of-hospital cardiac arrest: a nationwide case-time-control study. *European Heart Journal Cardiovascular Pharmacotherpy*. **3**: 100–107.
138 Schink T *et al.* (2018) Risk of ischemic stroke and the use of individual non-steroidal anti-inflammatory drugs: A multi-country European database study within the SOS Project. *PLoS ONE*. **13**: e0203362.
139 Lee W *et al.* (2010) Celecoxib does not attenuate the antiplatelet effects of aspirin and clopidogrel in healthy volunteers. *Korean Circulation Journal*. **40**: 321–327.
140 Gladding PA *et al.* (2008) The antiplatelet effect of six non-steroidal anti-inflammatory drugs and their pharmacodynamic interaction with aspirin in healthy volunteers. *American Journal of Cardiology*. **101**: 1060–1063.
141 Ungprasert P *et al.* (2016) Nonaspirin nonsteroidal anti-inflammatory drugs and risk of hemorrhagic stroke: a systematic review and meta-analysis of observational studies. *Stroke*. **47**: 356–364.
142 Islam MM *et al.* (2018) Risk of hemorrhagic stroke in patients exposed to nonsteroidal anti-inflammatory drugs: a meta-analysis of observational studies. *Neuroepidemiology*. **51**: 166–176.
143 Cheng HF and Harris RC (2004) Cyclooxygenases, the kidney, and hypertension. *Hypertension*. **43**: 525–530.
144 Griffin M *et al.* (2000) Nonsteroidal antiinflammatory drugs and acute renal failure in elderly persons. *American Journal of Epidemiology*. **151**: 488–496.
145 Huerta C *et al.* (2005) Nonsteroidal anti-inflammatory drugs and risk of ARF in the general population. *American Journal of Kidney Disease*. **45**: 531–539.
146 Schneider V *et al.* (2006) Association of selective and conventional nonsteroidal antiinflammatory drugs with acute renal failure: A population-based, nested case-control analysis. *American Journal of Epidemiology*. **164**: 881–889.
147 Curiel RV and Katz JD (2013) Mitigating the cardiovascular and renal effects of NSAIDs. *Pain Medicine*. **14 (Suppl 1)**: S23–S28.
148 Winearls C (1995) Acute myeloma kidney. *Kidney International*. **48**: 1347–1361.
149 Irish AB *et al.* (1997) Presentation and survival of patients with severe renal failure and myeloma. *QJM: monthly journal of the Association of Physicians*. **90**: 773–780.
150 Harirforoosh S and Jamali F (2009) Renal adverse effects of nonsteroidal anti-inflammatory drugs. *Expert Opinion on Drug Safety*. **8**: 669–681.

151 Loboz KK and Shenfield GM (2005) Drug combinations and impaired renal function -- the 'triple whammy'. *British journal of clinical pharmacology*. **59**: 239–243.
152 Onuigbo MA and Agbasi N (2015) Intraoperative hypotension - a neglected causative factor in hospital-acquired acute kidney injury; a Mayo Clinic Health System experience revisited. *Journal of Renal Injury Prevention*. **4**: 61–67.
153 Lee YC *et al.* (2012) Non-steroidal anti-inflammatory drugs use and risk of upper gastrointestinal adverse events in cirrhotic patients. *Liver International*. **32**: 859–866.
154 North-Lewis P (ed) (2008) *Drugs and the Liver*. Pharmaceutical Press, London, pp. 178–187.
155 Delco F *et al.* (2005) Dose adjustment in patients with liver disease. *Drug Safety*. **28**: 529–545.
156 Morales DR *et al.* (2015) NSAID-exacerbated respiratory disease: a meta-analysis evaluating prevalence, mean provocative dose of aspirin and increased asthma morbidity. *Allergy*. **70**: 828–835.
157 Makowska JS *et al.* (2016) Respiratory hypersensitivity reactions to NSAIDs in Europe: the global allergy and asthma network (GA(2) LEN) survey. *Allergy*. **71**: 1603–1611.
158 Thomsen SF *et al.* (2009) Regular use of non-steroidal anti-inflammatory drugs increases the risk of adult-onset asthma: a population-based follow-up study. *Clinical Respiratory Journal*. **3**: 82–84.
159 Kim SH *et al.* (2007) Association between polymorphisms in prostanoid receptor genes and aspirin-intolerant asthma. *Pharmacogenet Genomics*. **17**: 295–304.
160 Sanak M and Szczeklik A (2001) Leukotriene C4 synthase polymorphism and aspirin-induced asthma. *Journal of Allergy and Clinical Immunology*. **107**: 561–562.
161 Mastalerz L *et al.* (2008) Prostaglandin E2 systemic production in patients with asthma with and without aspirin hypersensitivity. *Thorax*. **63**: 27–34.
162 Taniguchi M *et al.* (2008) Hyperleukotrieneuria in patients with allergic and inflammatory disease. *Allergology International*. **57**: 313–320.
163 Jenkins C *et al.* (2004) Systematic review of prevalence of aspirin induced asthma and its implications for clinical practice. *British Medical Journal*. **328**: 434.
164 Morales DR *et al.* (2014) Safety risks for patients with aspirin-exacerbated respiratory disease after acute exposure to selective nonsteroidal anti-inflammatory drugs and COX-2 inhibitors: Meta-analysis of controlled clinical trials. *Journal of Allergy and Clinical Immunology*. **134**: 40–45.
165 Celik GE *et al.* (2013) Are drug provocation tests still necessary to test the safety of COX-2 inhibitors in patients with cross-reactive NSAID hypersensitivity? *Allergologia et Immunopathologia (Madr)*. **41**: 181–188.
166 Dicpinigaitis P (2001) Effect of the cyclooxygenase-2 inhibitor celecoxib on bronchial responsiveness and cough reflex sensitivity in asthmatics. *Pulmonary Pharmacology and Therapeutics*. **14**: 93–97.
167 Settipane R *et al.* (1995) Prevalence of cross-sensitivity with acetaminophen in aspirin-sensitive asthmatic subjects. *Journal of Allergy and Clinical Immunology*. **96**: 480–485.
168 Dahlen SE *et al.* (2002) Improvement of aspirin-intolerant asthma by montelukast, a leukotriene antagonist: a randomized, double-blind, placebo-controlled trial. *American Journal Respiratory Critical Care Medicine*. **165**: 9–14.
169 Kennedy JL *et al.* (2016) Aspirin-exacerbated respiratory disease: Prevalence, diagnosis, treatment, and considerations for the future. *American Journal of Rhinology and Allergy*. **30**: 407–413.
170 Laidlaw TM (2019) Clinical updates in aspirin-exacerbated respiratory disease. *Allergy and Asthma Proceedings*. **40**: 4–6.
171 Stevenson DD (2009) Aspirin sensitivity and desensitization for asthma and sinusitis. *Current Allergy and Asthma Reports*. **9**: 155–163.
172 White AA and Stevenson DD (2018) Aspirin-Exacerbated Respiratory Disease. *The New England Journal of Medicine*. **379**: 1060–1070.
173 Boursinos LA *et al.* (2009) Do steroids, conventional non-steroidal anti-inflammatory drugs and selective Cox-2 inhibitors adversely affect fracture healing? *Journal of Musculoskeletal Neuronal Interactions*. **9**: 44–52.
174 Pountos I *et al.* (2008) Pharmacological agents and impairment of fracture healing: what is the evidence? *Injury*. **39**: 384–394.
175 Vuolteenaho K *et al.* (2008) Non-steroidal anti-inflammatory drugs, cyclooxygenase-2 and the bone healing process. *Basic & Clinical Pharmacology and Toxicology*. **102**: 10–14.
176 Borgeat A *et al.* (2018) The effect of nonsteroidal anti-inflammatory drugs on bone healing in humans: A qualitative, systematic review. *Journal of Clinical Anesthesia*. **49**: 92–100.
177 Marquez-Lara A *et al.* (2016) Nonsteroidal Anti-Inflammatory Drugs and Bone-Healing: A Systematic Review of Research Quality. *Journal of Bone and Joint Surgery Reviews*. **4**: e4.
178 Anglin R *et al.* (2014) Risk of upper gastrointestinal bleeding with selective serotonin reuptake inhibitors with or without concurrent nonsteroidal anti-inflammatory use: a systematic review and meta-analysis. *American Journal of Gastroenterology*. **109**: 811–819.
179 Shin JY *et al.* (2015) Risk of intracranial haemorrhage in antidepressant users with concurrent use of non-steroidal anti-inflammatory drugs: nationwide propensity score matched study. *British Medical Journal*. **351**: H3517.
180 de Abajo FJ and Garcia-Rodriguez LA (2008) Risk of upper gastrointestinal tract bleeding associated with selective serotonin reuptake inhibitors and venlafaxine therapy: interaction with nonsteroidal anti-inflammatory drugs and effect of acid-suppressing agents. *Archives of General Psychiatry*. **65**: 795–803.
181 Baxter K and Preston CL *Stockley's Drug Interactions*. London: Pharmaceutical Press www.medicinescomplete.com (accessed May 2017).
182 Colebatch AN *et al.* (2012) Safety of nonsteroidal antiinflammatory drugs and/or paracetamol in people receiving methotrexate for inflammatory arthritis: a Cochrane systematic review. *Journal of Rheumatology*. **90**: 62–73.
183 Brown A *et al.* (2003) An interaction between warfarin and COX-2 inhibitors: two case studies. *The Pharmaceutical Journal*. **271**: 782.
184 Verrico M *et al.* (2003) Adverse drug events involving COX-2 inhibitors. *Annals of Pharmacotherapy*. **37**: 1203–1213.
185 Tonkin A and Wing L. Interactions of nonsteroidal anti-inflammatory drugs. In: Brooks P, editor. *Bailliere's Clinical Rheumatology Anti-rheumatic drugs*. 2. London: Bailliere Tindall; 1988. p. 455–483.
186 Palliativedrugs.com (2016) Parenteral NSAIDs - which one do you use? *Latest additions: Survey results (August)*. www.palliativedrug.com.
187 Vacha ME *et al.* (2015) The role of subcutaneous ketorolac for pain management. *Hospital Pharmacy*. **50**: 108–112.

Updated (minor change) December 2021

CELECOXIB

Class: Non-opioid analgesic, NSAID, selective COX-2 inhibitor.

Indications: Pain in osteoarthritis, rheumatoid arthritis and ankylosing spondylitis, †acute pain, †cancer pain.

Contra-indications: Hypersensitivity (urticaria, rhinitis, asthma, angioedema) to **aspirin** or other NSAID, *hypersensitivity to sulfonamides*, active GI ulceration, established ischaemic heart disease, peripheral arterial disease, cerebrovascular disease, CHF (NYHA II–IV), severe hepatic impairment, severe renal impairment, deteriorating renal function, inflammatory bowel disease.

Pharmacology

Celecoxib, a sulfonamide derivative, is a selective COX-2 inhibitor. Despite only modest selectivity when tested *in vitro*,[1-3] 800mg/24h causes no significant COX-1 inhibition in healthy volunteers.[4] Non-COX-2 inhibitory properties may account for some of its activity, e.g. inhibition of endoplasmic reticulum Ca^{2+} ATPase[5] and inhibition of phosphodiesterase-5 activity.[6] The capacity to interact with non-COX-2 targets may be enhanced by accumulation of celecoxib within cells.[7] Central endogenous opioid and cannabinoid systems may also be involved.[8]

Celecoxib is the *PCF NSAID of choice in palliative care*. The risk of gastrointestinal ulceration is lower than with non-selective NSAIDs (see p.346). In all except the highest GI risk patients, celecoxib avoids the need for gastroprotection and its consequent risks (see PPIs, p.31). The risk of cardiovascular events and renal impairment is comparable to non-selective NSAIDs, including **naproxen** (see p.348).

Celecoxib is metabolized mainly via CYP2C9. *Slow (poor) metabolizers are at increased risk of undesirable effects*. In people of European ancestry, the CYP2C9*3 variant is particularly important, slowing methylhydroxylation *in vitro* by 90% and more than doubling the AUC in single-dose studies.[9] In the UK, the SPC suggests that known or suspected slow metabolizers should be treated with caution.[10] In contrast, the USA PI recommends that the dose should be *halved* in such individuals.[11] In individuals with low CYP2C9 activity, CYP2D6 may contribute to celecoxib metabolism up to 30% and consequent potential risk of CYP2D6 drug interactions in these patients.[12]

In osteoarthritis, a meta-analysis found celecoxib to be superior to placebo but not to **paracetamol** (perhaps because the authorized dose of celecoxib is restricted to 200mg/24h in this condition in the USA).[13] A Cochrane review concluded that it was unlikely that there are any clinically relevant differences in efficacy between celecoxib 200mg/24h and select other NSAIDs (e.g. **diclofenac** 150mg/24h, **naproxen** 500mg b.d.).[14] Similarly, in rheumatoid arthritis, celecoxib ≥200mg/24h is as effective as **naproxen** 500mg b.d., and celecoxib 400mg/24h is as effective as **diclofenac** 150mg/24h.[15-17]

Celecoxib is effective in postoperative pain[18] and dysmenorrhoea,[19] but *not* in renal colic.[20] There are a lack of data relating to cancer pain. Unlike opioids, celecoxib failed to control pain in mice with bone tumours.[21,22]

Celecoxib has no effect on platelet function.[23] Celecoxib does not neutralize the thromboprotective effect of low-dose **aspirin** for stroke.[24] Thus, in someone taking **aspirin** thromboprophylaxis, celecoxib is the NSAID of choice (see p.349).

Possible roles for celecoxib in cancer-related cachexia or as an adjuvant anticancer treatment (see p.344) and in various psychiatric disorders are being explored (see p.345).

Bio-availability No human data; 22–40% in dogs;[25] increased by 20% after high-fat meal.

Onset of action 60min.[26]

Time to peak plasma concentration 3h; high-fat meals delay peak by 1–2 hours; aluminium- and magnesium-containing antacids reduce peak concentration.

Plasma halflife 11h.

Duration of action 5h in single-dose post-dental-extraction pain,[26] but given that recommended frequency of administration is once daily–b.d., presumably longer when given regularly.

Cautions

Cardiovascular disease including hypertension and heart failure (risk of exacerbation, though risk may be lower than other NSAIDs);[27-29] renal and hepatic impairment (see Chapter 17, p.731

and Chapter 18, p.753). Correct hyperkalaemia before use. As with all NSAIDs, concurrent administration with an SSRI is associated with an increased risk of GI bleeding.

Drug interactions

For general interactions between NSAIDs and other drugs, see NSAIDs, Table 8, p.353 and Table 9, p.354. Of particular importance is the risk of toxic plasma levels of **digoxin**, **lithium** and **methotrexate** caused by reduced renal function and/or reduced tubular excretion. If an NSAID is prescribed, monitor the plasma drug concentration or haematological effect of these drugs as appropriate and reduce doses as necessary (see p.351).

Because they cause sodium and fluid retention, all NSAIDs can decrease the effect of diuretics, ACE inhibitors and antihypertensives.

Because an increase in INR occasionally occurs when celecoxib is prescribed for a patient already taking **warfarin**, monitor the INR weekly for 3–4 weeks and adjust the dose of **warfarin** if necessary.[30]

CYP2C9 inhibitors (see Chapter 19, Table 8, p.790) may increase plasma concentrations of celecoxib. The manufacturer recommends halving the celecoxib dose if **fluconazole** is taken concurrently.[30] In known CYP2C9 slow metabolizers, avoid concurrent administration of CYP2C9 inhibitors and celecoxib. Conversely, CYP2C9 inducers (e.g. **carbamazepine**, **phenobarbital**, **rifampicin**) may reduce plasma concentrations of celecoxib.

Celecoxib is an inhibitor of CYP2D6 and theoretically may increase the plasma concentrations of other drugs metabolized by this enzyme (see Chapter 19, Table 8, p.790) if given concurrently.

Undesirable effects

Also see NSAIDs, p.345.

Common (<10%, >1%): dyspepsia, abdominal pain, flatulence, diarrhoea (but all same as or less than other NSAIDs), pharyngitis, rhinitis, allergy, pruritus, insomnia, dizziness, hypertonia, rash, flu-like symptoms, peripheral oedema, fluid retention.

Very rare (<0.01%): aseptic meningitis in patients with SLE.

Dose and use

Gastroprotection, e.g. a PPI (p.31), needs to be prescribed only for patients at *high* risk of NSAID-related upper GI complications (see NSAIDs, Box B, p.347).

Celecoxib is the *PCF* NSAID of choice:

- start with 100mg PO b.d.
- if necessary, increase to 200mg b.d.

For patients with swallowing difficulties, the capsules can be opened and the contents sprinkled on a small amount of soft food, e.g. yoghurt, applesauce (see Chapter 28, Table 2, p.863). **Diclofenac** CSCI (p.362), **parecoxib** SC or CSCI (p.373) or **ketorolac** CSCI (p.369) are alternatives if the PO route is unavailable.

Supply

Celecoxib (generic)

Capsules 100mg, 200mg, 28 days @ 200mg b.d. = £3.25.

1 Warner TD and Mitchell JA (2008) COX-2 selectivity alone does not define the cardiovascular risks associated with non-steroidal anti-inflammatory drugs. *Lancet.* **371**: 270–273.

2 Riendeau D *et al.* (2001) Etoricoxib (MK-0663): preclinical profile and comparison with other agents that selectively inhibit cyclooxygenase-2. *Journal of Pharmacology and Experimental Therapeutics.* **296**: 558–566.

3 Schwartz JI *et al.* (2008) Comparative inhibitory activity of etoricoxib, celecoxib, and diclofenac on COX-2 versus COX-1 in healthy subjects. *Journal of Clinical Pharmacology.* **48**: 745–754.

4 Fries S *et al.* (2006) Marked interindividual variability in the response to selective inhibitors of cyclooxygenase-2. *Gastroenterology.* **130**: 55–64.

5 Alloza I *et al.* (2006) Celecoxib inhibits interleukin-12 alphabeta and beta2 folding and secretion by a novel COX2-independent mechanism involving chaperones of the endoplasmic reticulum. *Molecular Pharmacology.* **69**: 1579–1587.

6 Klein T *et al.* (2007) Celecoxib dilates guinea-pig coronaries and rat aortic rings and amplifies NO/cGMP signaling by PDE5 inhibition. *Cardiovascular Research.* **75**: 390–397.

7 Maier TJ *et al.* (2009) Cellular membranes function as a storage compartment for celecoxib. *Journal of Molecular Medicine*. **87**: 981–993.
8 Rezende RM *et al.* (2012) Endogenous opioid and cannabinoid mechanisms are involved in the analgesic effects of celecoxib in the central nervous system. *Pharmacology*. **89**: 127–136.
9 Gong L *et al.* (2012) Celecoxib pathways: pharmacokinetics and pharmacodynamics. *Pharmacogenetics and Genomics*. **22**: 310–318.
10 Pfizer (2011) Celebrex 100mg & 200mg capsules. *SPC*. www.medicines.org.uk.
11 Pfizer (2012) Celebrex capsules. *US Prescribing Information*. www.accessdata.fda.gov/scripts/cder/daf/index.cfm.
12 Siu YA *et al.* (2018) Celecoxib is a substrate of CYP2D6: impact on celecoxib metabolism in individuals with CYP2C9*3 variants. *Drug Metabolism and Pharmacokinetics*. **33**: 219–227.
13 Bannuru RR *et al.* (2015) Comparative effectiveness of pharmacologic interventions for knee osteoarthritis: a systematic review and network meta-analysis. *Annals of Internal Medicine*. **162**: 46–54.
14 Puljak L *et al.* (2017) Celecoxib for osteoarthritis. *Cochrane Database of Systematic Reviews*. **5**: CD009865. www.cochranelibrary.com.
15 Emery P *et al.* (1999) Celecoxib versus diclofenac in long-term management of rheumatoid arthritis: randomised double-blind comparison. *Lancet*. **354**: 2106–2111.
16 Fidahic M *et al.* (2017) Celecoxib for rheumatoid arthritis. *Cochrane Database of Systematic Reviews*. **6**: CD012095. www.cochranelibrary.com.
17 Simon LS *et al.* (1999) Anti-inflammatory and upper gastrointestinal effects of celecoxib in rheumatoid arthritis: a randomized controlled trial. *Journal of the American Medical Association*. **282**: 1921-1928.
18 Derry S (2009) Single dose oral celecoxib for acute postoperative pain in adults. *Cochrane Database of Systematic Reviews*. **4**: CD004234. www.thecochranelibrary.com.
19 Daniels S *et al.* (2009) Celecoxib in the treatment of primary dysmenorrhea: results from two randomized, double-blind, active- and placebo-controlled, crossover studies. *Clinical Therapeutics*. **31**: 1192–1208.
20 Phillips E *et al.* (2009) Celecoxib in the management of acute renal colic: a randomized controlled clinical trial. *Urology*. **74**: 994–999.
21 Saito O *et al.* (2005) Analgesic effects of nonsteroidal antiinflammatory drugs, acetaminophen, and morphine in a mouse model of bone cancer pain. *Journal of Anesthesia*. **19**: 218–224.
22 Mouedden ME and Meert TF (2007) Pharmacological evaluation of opioid and non-opioid analgesics in a murine bone cancer model of pain. *Pharmacology, Biochemistry, and Behavior*. **86**: 458–467.
23 Graff J *et al.* (2007) Effects of selective COX-2 inhibition on prostanoids and platelet physiology in young healthy volunteers. *Journal of Thrombosis and Haemostasis*. **5**: 2376–2385.
24 Lee W *et al.* (2010) Celecoxib does not attenuate the antiplatelet effects of aspirin and clopidogrel in healthy volunteers. *Korean Circulation Journal*. **40**: 321–327.
25 Paulson S *et al.* (2001) Pharmacokinetics of celecoxib after oral administration in dogs and humans: effects of food and site absorption. *Journal of Pharmacology and Experimental Therapeutics*. **297**: 638–645.
26 Malmstrom K *et al.* (1999) Comparison of rofecoxib and celecoxib, two cyclooxygenase-2 inhibitors, in postoperative dental pain: a randomised, placebo- and active-comparator-controlled clinical trial. *Clinical Therapeutics*. **21**: 1653–1663.
27 Chan CC *et al.* (2009) Do COX-2 inhibitors raise blood pressure more than nonselective NSAIDs and placebo? An updated meta-analysis. *Journal of Hypertension*. **27**: 2332–2341.
28 Solomon DH *et al.* (2004) Relationship between COX-2 specific inhibitors and hypertension. *Hypertension*. **44**: 140–145.
29 Arfe A *et al.* (2016) Non-steroidal anti-inflammatory drugs and risk of heart failure in four European countries: nested case-control study. *British Medical Journal*. **354**: i4857.
30 Baxter K and Preston CL *Stockley's Drug Interactions*. London: Pharmaceutical Press. www.medicinescomplete.com (accessed December 2017).

Updated (minor change) December 2021

DICLOFENAC SODIUM

Class: Non-opioid analgesic, NSAID, preferential COX-2 inhibitor.

Indications: Pain in arthritis and other musculoskeletal disorders, postoperative pain, †dysmenorrhoea, acute gout, †cancer pain, †neoplastic fever.

Contra-indications: Hypersensitivity (urticaria, rhinitis, asthma, angioedema) to **aspirin** or other NSAID, active GI ulceration, history of two or more distinct episodes of proven ulceration or bleeding, cerebrovascular bleeding or other bleeding disorders, ischaemic heart disease, peripheral arterial disease, cerebrovascular disease, CHF (NYHA II–IV), active liver disease or severe hepatic impairment, severe renal impairment, deteriorating renal function.

Pharmacology

Diclofenac is a preferential COX-2 inhibitor (see NSAIDs, Table 1 and Table 2, p.342).[1,2] The analgesic effect of diclofenac has been shown in animals to be both peripheral and central.[3-5] In addition to inhibiting COX, diclofenac:

- activates the nitric oxide–cGMP nociceptive pathway[6]
- impacts on central nociception by increasing brain concentrations of kynurenic acid, an endogenous antagonist on the glycine recognition site of the NMDA-receptor–channel complex[7]
- is a 'membrane stabilizer' (through the opening of KCNQ2/3 potassium channels; see Anti-epileptics, p.280).[8,9]

It is possible that diclofenac is more broad-spectrum in its central effects than other NSAIDs.[10] Diclofenac causes platelet dysfunction in only two-thirds of healthy volunteers.[11]

In terms of effectiveness for osteoarthritis, diclofenac is non-inferior to other NSAIDs.[12] About 10–15% of patients experience undesirable effects (mainly gastric intolerance); these are generally mild and transient; diclofenac needs to be withdrawn in only 2%.

Age[13] and renal and hepatic impairment do not have a significant effect on plasma concentrations of diclofenac. Metabolite concentrations increase in severe renal impairment, but the principal metabolite, hydroxydiclofenac, possesses little anti-inflammatory effect. However, because of a greater likelihood of (unpredictable) hepatotoxicity compared with other NSAIDs, it may be best *not* to use diclofenac in severe hepatic impairment.[14]

A meta-analysis of several hundred RCTs indicates that, compared with placebo, the risk of upper GI complications with diclofenac and *selective* COX-2 inhibitors is relatively low (about double that seen with placebo), and half that seen with high-dose **ibuprofen** and high-dose **naproxen**.[15] However, compared to **celecoxib**, diclofenac has a higher risk of upper and lower GI complications, even when combined with a PPI.[16]

Diclofenac is associated with a higher *overall* CVS risk than non-selective NSAIDs,[15,17] and is subsequently *contra-indicated* in individuals with CVS disease.[18] In a nationwide review in Denmark, diclofenac and **ibuprofen** (but *not* selective COX-2 inhibitors or **naproxen**) were associated with an increased risk of out-of-hospital cardiac arrest.[19] Other meta-analyses suggest that the risk of myocardial infarction with diclofenac is similar to other non-selective NSAIDs.[20,21] The risk of renal failure is comparable with other NSAIDs.[22]

Severe local necrosis has been described anecdotally after IM and SC use.[23] Diclofenac is available as the *sodium* and *potassium* salts. Diclofenac *potassium* is absorbed more quickly and peak plasma concentration is reached sooner. It is theoretically a better alternative in patients troubled by Na^+ and water retention. However, it is much more expensive.

Bio-availability 50% PO (both immediate-release and m/r products); suppositories about 33%.
Onset of action 20–30min.
Time to peak plasma concentration diclofenac *sodium* 2.5h e/c (fasting), 6h e/c (taken with food), ≥4h m/r, 1h suppositories; diclofenac *potassium* PO 20–60min (not significantly affected by food).
Plasma halflife 1–2h.
Duration of action 8h.

Cautions

Renal and hepatic impairment (see Chapter 17, p.731 and Chapter 18, p.753). Avoid in patients with significant CVS risk factors (i.e. hypertension, hyperlipidaemia, diabetes mellitus, smoking). Correct hyperkalaemia before use.

Because of an increased risk of bleeding (from decreased platelet aggregation), avoid concurrent prescription with **warfarin**. As with all NSAIDs, concurrent administration with an SSRI is associated with an increased risk of GI bleeding.

The thromboprotective effect of **aspirin** for stroke is compromised in people taking diclofenac concurrently.[24] Thus, in someone taking **aspirin** thromboprophylaxis, **celecoxib** is the NSAID of choice (see p.349).

Drug interactions

For general interactions between NSAIDs and other drugs, see NSAIDs, Table 8, p.353 and Table 9, p.354. Of particular importance is the risk of toxic plasma levels of **digoxin**, **lithium**, and **methotrexate** caused by reduced renal function and/or reduced tubular excretion. If diclofenac is prescribed, monitor the plasma drug concentration or haematological effect of these drugs as appropriate and reduce doses as necessary (see p.351).

Because they cause sodium and fluid retention, all NSAIDs can decrease the effect of diuretics, ACE inhibitors and antihypertensives.

In addition to the effect on platelet function (see Cautions), an increase in INR may occur when diclofenac is prescribed for a patient already taking **warfarin**; monitor the INR weekly for 3–4 weeks and adjust the dose of **warfarin** if necessary.[25]

Concurrent use of diclofenac with **ciclosporin** may increase the plasma concentration of diclofenac (up to double) and decrease the plasma concentration of **ciclosporin**. If given concurrently, the manufacturer advises halving the dose of diclofenac.

Diclofenac plasma concentration may be *increased* by **voriconazole**. This may relate to inhibition by CYP2C9; lower doses of diclofenac may be necessary. Conversely, **rifampicin** may *decrease* diclofenac plasma concentration due to CYP3A4 enzyme induction; consider an alternative NSAID if pain returns. Caution should be taken with concurrent use of other drugs that inhibit or induce these enzymes (see Chapter 19, Table 8, p.790).

Undesirable effects

Also see NSAIDs, p.345.
Common (<10%, >1%): headache, dizziness, oedema, indigestion, abdominal discomfort, nausea, constipation or diarrhoea, pruritus, rash, ecchymosis.
Very rare (<0.01%): aseptic meningitis in patients with SLE.

Dose and use

Although traditional advice is to take NSAIDs with food, there is no evidence that this reduces the risk of GI complications.

Gastroprotection, e.g. a PPI (p.31), should be prescribed concurrently for patients at *high* risk of NSAID-related upper GI complications (see NSAIDs, Box B, p.347), or **celecoxib** + PPI prescribed instead (see p.346).

PCF prefers **celecoxib** (p.360). However, diclofenac sodium is a frequently used NSAID; typical regimens are:

- immediate-release 50mg PO b.d.–t.d.s.
- m/r 75mg PO b.d. or 100mg once daily
- suppositories 50mg PR b.d.–t.d.s.

Anecdotally, some patients obtain greater benefit from 200mg/24h, e.g. m/r 100mg b.d. However, doses >150mg/24h are unauthorized.

Parenteral administration

Diclofenac is available as an injection, primarily for use in biliary and renal colic (dose 75mg IM p.r.n.; maximum 150mg/24h).[26] Injection site pain/reaction is common.

In palliative care, it is sometimes given by CSCI when the PO route is no longer possible (unauthorized use). Because PO bio-availability is 50%, a typical regimen is 75mg/24h CSCI, diluted with sodium chloride 0.9% to minimize the risk of injection site reactions. Diclofenac must be given alone via a separate syringe driver because its alkalinity makes it incompatible with other drugs (see Chapter 29, p.892).

Alternative SC/CSCI NSAIDs include **parecoxib** (p.373) and **ketorolac** (p.369).

For topical use, see p.651.

Supply

Diclofenac *sodium* (generic)
Tablets e/c 25mg, 50mg, 28 days @ 50mg t.d.s. = £4.50.
Suppositories 100mg, 28 days @ 100mg once daily = £8.50.
Oral Suspension 50mg/5mL, 28 days @ 50mg t.d.s. = £67 (unauthorized product, available as a special order; see Chapter 24, p.817). *Price based on Specials tariff in community.*

Voltarol® (Novartis)
Suppositories 12.5mg, 25mg, 50mg, 100mg; 50mg, 28 days @ 50mg t.d.s. or 100mg once daily = £17 or £9.50 respectively.
Injection 25mg/mL, 3mL amp = £1.

Akis® (Flynn)
Injection 75mg/mL, 1mL amp = £4.75.

Modified-release
Diclofenac *sodium* (generic)
Tablets m/r 75mg, 100mg, 28 days @ 75mg b.d. or 100mg once daily = £15 and £7.50.
Capsules m/r 75mg, 100mg, 28 days @ 75mg b.d. or 100mg once daily = £8.

Motifene® 75mg (Daiichi Sankyo)
Capsules (containing e/c pellets 25mg and m/r pellets 50mg) 75mg, 28 days @ 75mg b.d. = £8.

1 John V (1979) The pharmacokinetics and metabolism of diclofenac sodium (Voltarol) in animals and man. *Rheumatology and Rehabilitation.* **(Suppl 2)**: 22–37.
2 Schwartz JI *et al.* (2008) Comparative inhibitory activity of etoricoxib, celecoxib, and diclofenac on COX-2 versus COX-1 in healthy subjects. *Journal of Clinical Pharmacology.* **48**: 745–754.
3 McCormack K (1994) Nonsteroidal anti-inflammatory drugs and spinal nociceptive processing. *Pain.* **59**: 9–43.
4 Svensson CI and Yaksh TL (2002) The spinal phospholipase-cyclooxygenase-prostanoid cascade in nociceptive processing. *Annual Review of Pharmacology and Toxicology.* **42**: 553–583.
5 Ortiz MI *et al.* (2008) Additive interaction between peripheral and central mechanisms involved in the antinociceptive effect of diclofenac in the formalin test in rats. *Pharmacology, Biochemistry and Behavior.* **91**: 32–37.
6 Ortiz MI *et al.* (2003) The NO-cGMP-K+ channel pathway participates in the antinociceptive effect of diclofenac, but not of indomethacin. *Pharmacology, Biochemistry and Behavior.* **76**: 187–195.
7 Schwieler L *et al.* (2005) Prostaglandin-mediated control of rat brain kynurenic acid synthesis - opposite actions by COX-1 and COX-2 isoforms. *Journal of Neural Transmission.* **112**: 863–872.
8 Peretz A *et al.* (2005) Meclofenamic acid and diclofenac, novel templates of KCNQ2/Q3 potassium channel openers, depress cortical neuron activity and exhibit anticonvulsant properties. *Molecular Pharmacology.* **67**: 1053–1066.
9 Gan TJ (2010) Diclofenac: an update on its mechanism of action and safety profile. *Current Medical Research Opinion.* **26**: 1715–1731.
10 McCormack K and Twycross RG (2001) Are COX-2 selective inhibitors effective analgesics. *Pain Review.* **8**: 13–26.
11 Ng KF *et al.* (2008) Comprehensive preoperative evaluation of platelet function in total knee arthroplasty patients taking diclofenac. *Journal of Arthroplasty.* **23**: 424–430.
12 Pavelka K (2012) A comparison of the therapeutic efficacy of diclofenac in osteoarthritis: a systematic review of randomised controlled trials. *Current Medical Research Opinion.* **28**: 163–178.
13 Willis JV and Kendall MJ (1978) Pharmacokinetic studies on diclofenac sodium in young and old volunteers. *Scandinavian Journal of Rheumatology.* 36–41.
14 Gupta NK and Lewis JH (2008) Review article: the use of potentially hepatotoxic drugs in patients with liver disease. *Alimentary Pharmacology and Therapeutics.* **28**: 1021–1041.
15 CNT Collaboration (2013) Vascular and upper gastrointestinal effects of non-steroidal anti-inflammatory drugs: meta-analyses of individual participant data from randomised trials. *Lancet.* **382**: 769–779.
16 Chan FK *et al.* (2010) Celecoxib versus omeprazole and diclofenac in patients with osteoarthritis and rheumatoid arthritis (CONDOR): a randomised trial. *Lancet.* **376**: 173–179.
17 Schmidt M *et al.* (2018) Diclofenac use and cardiovascular risks: series of nationwide cohort studies. *BMJ.* **362**: k3426.
18 MHRA (2013) Diclofenac: new contraindications and warnings after a Europe-wide review of cardiovascular safety. *Drug Safety Update.* www.gov.uk/drug-safety-update
19 Sondergaard KB *et al.* (2017) Non-steroidal anti-inflammatory drug use is associated with increased risk of out-of-hospital cardiac arrest: a nationwide case-time-control study. *European Heart Journal Cardiovascular Pharmacotherpy.* **3**: 100–107.
20 Gunter BR *et al.* (2017) Non-steroidal anti-inflammatory drug-induced cardiovascular adverse events: a meta-analysis. *Journal of Clinical Pharmacy and Therapeutics.* **42**: 27–38.
21 Bally M *et al.* (2017) Risk of acute myocardial infarction with NSAIDs in real world use: bayesian meta-analysis of individual patient data. *British Medical Journal.* **357**: 1909.
22 Schneider V *et al.* (2006) Association of selective and conventional nonsteroidal antiinflammatory drugs with acute renal failure: A population-based, nested case-control analysis. *American Journal of Epidemiology.* **164**: 881–889.
23 Kirkpatrick G (2003) SC diclofenac. *Palliativedrugs.com.* www.palliativedrugs.com/bulletin-board.html
24 Gladding PA *et al.* (2008) The antiplatelet effect of six non-steroidal anti-inflammatory drugs and their pharmacodynamic interaction with aspirin in healthy volunteers. *American Journal of Cardiology.* **101**: 1060–1063.
25 Baxter K and Preston CL *Stockley's Drug Interactions.* London: Pharmaceutical Press. www.medicinescomplete.com (accessed May 2017).
26 Lundstam SOA *et al.* (1982) Prostaglandin-synthetase inhibition with diclofenac sodium in treatment of renal colic: comparison with use of a narcotic analgesic. *Lancet.* **1**: 1096–1097.

Updated (minor change) December 2021

IBUPROFEN

Class: Non-opioid analgesic, NSAID, non-selective COX inhibitor.

Indications: Pain in arthritic conditions and other musculoskeletal disorders, postoperative pain, dental pain, dysmenorrhoea, headache, migraine, fever, †cancer pain.

Contra-indications: Hypersensitivity (urticaria, rhinitis, asthma, angioedema) to **aspirin** or other NSAID, active GI ulceration; history of ≥2 distinct episodes of proven ulceration or bleeding; cerebrovascular bleeding or other bleeding disorders; severe CHF (NYHA IV); active liver disease or severe hepatic impairment; severe renal impairment or deteriorating renal function.

Pharmacology

Ibuprofen is a non-selective COX inhibitor (see NSAIDs, Tables 1 and 2, p.342). Like **naproxen**, it is a propionic acid derivative. The analgesic and antipyretic effects of ibuprofen are mediated by both COX inhibition and non-COX mechanisms (see p.343).[1,2]

Ibuprofen is a chiral NSAID, i.e. it is a mixture of roughly equal amounts of *S*– and *R*–enantiomers, mirror-image molecules.[3,4] The anti-inflammatory activity resides mostly in the *S*–enantiomer, but about half the *R*–enantiomer is converted to the *S*– form in the GI tract and liver.[1,5] The *S*–enantiomer reaches higher levels and persists for longer in the elderly.[6] Both enantiomers are metabolized via CYP450.

Inversion takes time, and the time frame for single doses in acute situations is too short for inversion to play an important part.[7] Even so, a single dose of ibuprofen 200–400mg PO for acute postoperative pain is highly effective, with an NNT of around 2.5.[8] In postoperative pain, ibuprofen 400mg PO q.d.s. was more effective than **paracetamol** 1g q.d.s. in reducing **morphine** requirements; although combined they led to a further reduction, the difference (**morphine** 6mg/24h) was not considered clinically relevant.[9] In arthritis, ibuprofen is concentrated at sites of inflammation, e.g. the joint synovium.[10] Doses of 200–400mg are as effective as **paracetamol** 1g, and efficacy increases as the dose increases.[11]

Low-dose ibuprofen (≤1,200mg/24h) has a relatively *low* propensity for causing upper GI complications[12,13] but, with *high-dose* ibuprofen (2,400mg/24h), the risk is quadrupled (comparable with high-dose **naproxen**; also see p.346).[14] Concern has been expressed that OTC ibuprofen may occasionally cause small bowel damage (also see p.347).[15]

Cardiovascular risk is dose related; the risk with high-dose ibuprofen (2,400mg/24h) is comparable to, or perhaps even higher than, other NSAIDs (see p.348). The risk of renal failure with ibuprofen is also comparable to other NSAIDs.[16] It is safe in overdose; few deaths attributable to ibuprofen alone have been reported involving overdoses of 36–200g.[17-21] Ibuprofen may be of benefit in cancer-related cachexia (see Progestogens, p.599).

Ibuprofen can be used topically, particularly for sprains, strains and arthritis (also see p.651).[22,23] Although application to the skin produces plasma concentrations which are only 5% of those obtained with oral administration, the underlying muscle and fascial concentrations are 25 times greater.[24,25]

Topical and PO ibuprofen have been shown to be equally effective for chronic knee pain in patients aged ≥50 years, although those with more severe or widespread pain preferred PO treatment.[26] The incidence of major undesirable effects was similar, but topical treatment led to fewer minor undesirable effects and less treatment discontinuation. Systemic undesirable effects with topical ibuprofen for acute pain are uncommon, and even local effects are not significantly different from placebo.[27]

Because it has a more rapid onset of action, IV ibuprofen (not UK) has a potential role in the management of acute pain.[28]

Bio-availability 90% PO.

Onset of action 20–30min.

Time to peak plasma concentration 1–2h.

Plasma halflife 2–3h.[1]

Duration of action 4–6h.

Cautions

Renal and hepatic impairment (see Chapter 17, p.731 and Chapter 18, p.753). Restrict dose to ≤1,800mg/24h in patients with significant CVS risk factors (i.e. hypertension, hyperlipidaemia, diabetes mellitus, smoking). Correct hyperkalaemia before use.

Because of the increased risk of bleeding (from decreased platelet aggregation), avoid concurrent prescription with **warfarin**. As with all NSAIDs, concurrent administration with an SSRI is associated with an increased risk of GI bleeding.

The thromboprotective effect of **aspirin** for stroke is compromised in people taking ibuprofen concurrently.[29-31] Thus, in someone taking **aspirin** thromboprophylaxis, **celecoxib** is the NSAID of choice (see p.349).

Drug interactions

For general interactions between NSAIDs and other drugs, see NSAIDs Table 8, p.353 and Table 9, p.354. Of particular importance is the risk of toxic plasma levels of **digoxin**, **lithium** and **methotrexate** caused by reduced renal function and/or reduced tubular excretion. If ibuprofen is prescribed, monitor the plasma drug concentration or haematological effect of these drugs as appropriate and reduce doses as necessary (see p.351).

Because they cause sodium and fluid retention, all NSAIDs can decrease the effect of diuretics, ACE inhibitors and antihypertensives.

In addition to the effect on platelet function (see Cautions), an increase in INR occasionally occurs when ibuprofen is prescribed for a patient already taking **warfarin**; monitor the INR weekly for 3–4 weeks and adjust the dose of **warfarin** if necessary.[32]

Ibuprofen is metabolized by CYP2C9. **Fluconazole** and **voriconazole** (strong CYP2C9 inhibitors) increase ibuprofen plasma concentration, and lower doses of ibuprofen may be necessary. Caution should be taken with concurrent use of other drugs that inhibit or induce this enzyme (see Chapter 19, Table 8, p.790).

Undesirable effects

Also see NSAIDs, p.345.

Common (<10%, >1%): headache, dizziness, oedema, indigestion, abdominal discomfort, nausea, constipation or diarrhoea, pruritus, rash, ecchymosis.

Very rare (<0.01%): aseptic meningitis in patients with SLE.

Dose and use

Although traditional advice is to take NSAIDs with food, there is no evidence that this reduces the risk of GI complications.

Gastroprotection, e.g. a PPI (see p.31), should be prescribed concurrently for patients at *high* risk of NSAID-related upper GI complications (see NSAIDs, Box B, p.347) or **celecoxib** + PPI prescribed instead (see p.346).

PCF prefers **celecoxib** (p.360). However, ibuprofen is a frequently used NSAID:

- typical dose ibuprofen 400mg PO t.d.s. or 200mg PO t.d.s in the frail elderly
- higher doses are associated with greater CVS risk (possibly with 600mg PO t.d.s. and definitely with 800mg PO t.d.s.).

For topical use, see p.651.

Supply

Ibuprofen tablets and capsules 200mg and 400mg, orodispersible tablets and oral suspension are available OTC.

Ibuprofen (generic)

Tablets 200mg, 400mg, 600mg, 28 days @ 400mg t.d.s. = £6.75.

Capsules 200mg, 28 days @ 400mg t.d.s. = £4.50.

Oral suspension 100mg/5mL, 200mg/5mL, 28 days @ 400mg t.d.s. = £35; *sugar-free suspension also available*.

Nurofen Meltlets® (Reckitt Benckiser)

Orodispersible tablets 200mg, 28 days @ 400mg t.d.s. = £36.

Nurofen Express® (Reckitt Benckiser)

Capsules (liquid) 200mg, 400mg, 28 days @ 400mg t.d.s. = £27.

Brufen® (Mylan)
Granules 600mg/sachet, 28 days @ 600mg b.d. = £19 *(contains 6.5mmol Na^+/sachet).*

Modified-release
Brufen Retard® (Mylan)
Tablets m/r 800mg, 28 days @ 1,600mg once daily = £8.

1 Rainsford KD (2009) Ibuprofen: pharmacology, efficacy and safety. *Inflammopharmacology.* **17**: 275–342.
2 Soares DM *et al.* (2011) Cyclooxygenase-independent mechanism of ibuprofen-induced antipyresis: the role of central vasopressin V(1) receptors. *Fundamental and Clinical Pharmacology.* **25**: 670–681.
3 Rudy AC et *al.* (1991) Stereoselective metabolism of ibuprofen in humans: administration of R-, S- and racemic ibuprofen. *Journal of Pharmacology and Experimental Therapeutics.* **259**: 1133–1139.
4 Jamali F et *al.* (1992) Human pharmacokinetics of ibuprofen enantiomers following different doses and formulations: intestinal chiral inversion. *Journal of Pharmaceutical Sciences.* **81**: 221–225.
5 Ding G et *al.* (2007) Effect of absorption rate on pharmacokinetics of ibuprofen in relation to chiral inversion in humans. *Journal of Pharmacy and Pharmacology.* **59**: 1509–1513.
6 Tan SC et *al.* (2003) Influence of age on the enantiomeric disposition of ibuprofen in healthy volunteers. *British Journal of Clinical Pharmacology.* **55**: 579–587.
7 Evans AM (2001) Comparative pharmacology of S(+)-ibuprofen and (RS)-ibuprofen. *Clinical Rheumatology.* **20 (Suppl 1)**: S9–14.
8 Derry C et *al.* (2009) Single dose oral ibuprofen for acute postoperative pain in adults. *Cochrane Database of Systematic Reviews.* **3**: CD001548. www.thecochranelibrary.com
9 Thybo KH et *al.* (2019) Effect of combination of paracetamol (acetaminophen) and ibuprofen vs either alone on patient-controlled morphine consumption in the first 24 hours after total hip arthroplasty: the PANSAID randomized clinical trial. *Jama.* **321**: 562–571.
10 Glass RC and Swannell AJ (1978) Concentrations of ibuprofen in serum and synovial fluid from patients with arthritis [proceedings]. *British Journal of Clinical Pharmacology.* **6**: 453–454.
11 McQuay HJ and Moore RA (2007) Dose-response in direct comparisons of different doses of aspirin, ibuprofen and paracetamol (acetaminophen) in analgesic studies. *British Journal of Clinical Pharmacology.* **63**: 271–278.
12 Masso Gonzalez EL et *al.* (2010) Variability among nonsteroidal antiinflammatory drugs in risk of upper gastrointestinal bleeding. *Arthritis and Rheumatism.* **62**: 1592–1601.
13 Michels SL et *al.* (2012) Over-the-counter ibuprofen and risk of gastrointestinal bleeding complications: a systematic literature review. *Current Medical Research Opinion.* **28**: 89–99.
14 CNT Collaboration (2013) Vascular and upper gastrointestinal effects of non-steroidal anti-inflammatory drugs: meta-analyses of individual participant data from randomised trials. *Lancet.* **382**: 769–779.
15 Sidhu R et *al.* (2010) Undisclosed use of nonsteroidal anti-inflammatory drugs may underlie small-bowel injury observed by capsule endoscopy. *Clinical Gastroenterology and Hepatology.* **8**: 992–995.
16 Schneider V et *al.* (2006) Association of selective and conventional nonsteroidal antiinflammatory drugs with acute renal failure: A population-based, nested case-control analysis. *American Journal of Epidemiology.* **164**: 881–889.
17 Wood DM et *al.* (2006) Fatality after deliberate ingestion of sustained-release ibuprofen: a case report. *Critical Care.* **10**: R44.
18 Krenova M and Pelclova D (2005) Fatal poisoning with ibuprofen. *Clinical Toxicology.* **43**: 537.
19 Volans G et *al.* (2003) Ibuprofen overdose. *International Journal of Clinical Practice Supplement.* 54–60.
20 Holubek W et *al.* (2007) A report of two deaths from massive ibuprofen ingestion. *Journal of Medical Toxicology.* **3**: 52–55.
21 Lodise M et *al.* (2012) Acute Ibuprofen intoxication: report on a case and review of the literature. *American Journal of Forensic Medicine and Pathology.* **33**: 242–246.
22 Chlud K and Wagener H (1987) Percutaneous nonsteroidal anti-inflammatory drug (NSAID) therapy with particular reference to pharmacokinetic factors. *EULAR Bulletin.* **2**: 40–43.
23 Predel HG et *al.* (2018) Efficacy and tolerability of a new ibuprofen 200mg plaster in patients with acute sports-related traumatic blunt soft tissue injury/contusion. *Postgraduate Medicine.* **130**: 24–31.
24 Mondino A et *al.* (1983) Kinetic studies of ibuprofen on humans. Comparative study for the determination of blood concentrations and metabolites following local and oral administration. *Medizinische Welt.* **34**: 1052–1054.
25 Kageyama T (1987) A double blind placebo controlled multicenter study of piroxicam 0.5% gel in osteoarthritis of the knee. *European Journal of Rheumatology and Inflammation.* **8**: 114–115.
26 Underwood M et *al.* (2008) Topical or oral ibuprofen for chronic knee pain in older people. The TOIB study. *Health Technology Assessment.* **12**: iii–155.
27 Massey T et *al.* (2010) Topical NSAIDS for acute pain in adults. *Cochrane Database of Systematic Reviews.* **6**: CD007402. www.thecochranelibrary.com
28 Smith HS and Voss B (2012) Pharmacokinetics of intravenous ibuprofen: implications of time of infusion in the treatment of pain and fever. *Drugs.* **72**: 327–337.
29 Awa K et *al.* (2012) Prediction of time-dependent interaction of aspirin with ibuprofen using a pharmacokinetic/pharmacodynamic model. *Journal of Clinical Pharmacy and Therapeutics.* **37**: 469–474.
30 Gladding PA et *al.* (2008) The antiplatelet effect of six non-steroidal anti-inflammatory drugs and their pharmacodynamic interaction with aspirin in healthy volunteers. *American Journal of Cardiology.* **101**: 1060–1063.
31 Gengo FM et *al.* (2008) Effects of ibuprofen on the magnitude and duration of aspirin's inhibition of platelet aggregation: clinical consequences in stroke prophylaxis. *Journal of Clinical Pharmacology.* **48**: 117–122.
32 Baxter K and Preston CL *Stockley's Drug Interactions.* London: Pharmaceutical Press. www.medicinescomplete.com (accessed May 2017).

Updated (minor change) December 2021

*KETOROLAC TROMETAMOL

Class: Non-opioid analgesic, NSAID, preferential COX-1 inhibitor.

Indications: Short-term management of moderate–severe acute postoperative pain, †intractable cancer pain unresponsive to usual measures.

Contra-indications: Hypersensitivity (urticaria, rhinitis, asthma, angioedema) to **aspirin** or other NSAID; syndrome of nasal polyps, angioedema and bronchospasm; history of asthma; history of or active GI perforation, ulceration or bleeding (particularly NSAID-related); cerebrovascular bleeding, bleeding disorders, severe CHF, severe hepatic impairment, moderate or severe renal impairment (eGFR <60mL/min/1.73m^2), deteriorating renal function.

Concurrent prescription with **warfarin**, **heparin**, **aspirin**, other NSAID, **pentoxifylline** (increased risk of bleeding), **lithium** (increased plasma concentration and toxicity) and **probenecid** (increased ketorolac plasma concentration and halflife).

Pharmacology

Ketorolac is a cyclic propionate structurally related to the acetate NSAIDs, e.g. **indometacin**.[1] It inhibits both COX-1 and COX-2, but has higher COX-1 selectivity than many NSAIDs. Other mechanisms include the activation, in the periphery, of the nitric oxide–cGMP pathway.[2] This may help to explain why ketorolac's analgesic effect is far greater than its anti-inflammatory and antipyretic properties: in animal studies, ketorolac is about 350 times more potent than **aspirin** as an analgesic, but only 20 times more potent as an antipyretic.[1] As an anti-inflammatory, ketorolac is about half as potent as **indometacin** and twice as potent as **naproxen**. Like most COX-1 inhibitors, ketorolac inhibits platelet aggregation.

Ketorolac trometamol is more water-soluble than the parent substance. Over 99% of the oral dose is absorbed; about 75% of a dose is excreted in the urine within 7h, and over 90% within 2 days, over half as unmodified ketorolac.[3] The rest is excreted in the faeces. The analgesic and anti-inflammatory activity of ketorolac resides mainly in the *S*-enantiomer, which is cleared more rapidly than the less active *R*-enantiomer.

Of all the NSAIDs, ketorolac (PO or parenteral) carries the highest risk for gastritis and duodenitis, and upper GI complications (ulceration, bleeding, perforation).[4,5] A meta-analysis calculated a 15-times increase in risk with ketorolac, which is several times the risk of non-selective NSAIDs generally.[6]

Likewise, ketorolac (PO or parenteral) possibly carries the highest risk of acute myocardial infarction of any NSAID.[7,8] A retrospective case-crossover study of 38,000 people with strokes found PO ketorolac to be associated with only a moderate increase in the risk of stroke (odds ratio 1.9), but parenterally the risk of ischaemic or haemorrhagic stroke was increased 4–6 times.[9]

However, other postoperative studies indicate that, compared with opioids, the *short-term* use of ketorolac is associated with only a small increased risk of GI and operative site bleeding.[10,11] The risk increases with age and a treatment duration >1 week.[10,12] Thus, authorization for ketorolac is restricted to short-term (≤2 days) postoperative use. In some countries, authorization has been withdrawn, e.g. France and Germany.

Although individual doses ≤30mg are recommended in acute pain, in a study in patients attending an emergency department with moderate–severe pain (mean score 7–8 out of 10), no difference was detected after 2h between doses of 10mg, 15mg and 30mg (mean scores 5 out of 10).[13] Further, in cancer pain, in a week-long RCT, *PO* ketorolac 10mg q.d.s. was no better than **paracetamol** 600mg + **codeine** 60mg q.d.s.;[14] it was also found to be no better than PO **diclofenac**.[15]

However, anecdotal palliative care reports suggest that CSCI ketorolac may be effective in some patients who fail to obtain satisfactory relief with a PO NSAID (+ opioid), mostly in bone pain but also neuropathic pain.[15] It has been used for periods of up to 8 months,[16] but always with a gastroprotective drug. Nonetheless, because of their lower GI and CVS risk, **diclofenac** (p.362) or **parecoxib** (p.373) are generally preferred in comparable situations.

Bio-availability >99% PO.

Onset of action 30min PO; 10–30min IM/IV.

Time to peak plasma concentration 30–45min PO.

Plasma halflife 5h; 7h in the elderly;[17] 6–19h with renal impairment.[12]

Duration of action 6h PO; 4–6h IM.

Cautions

Renal and hepatic impairment (see Chapter 17 and Chapter 18, p.731 and p.753). Avoid in patients with significant CVS risk factors (i.e. hypertension, hyperlipidaemia, diabetes mellitus, smoking). Correct hyperkalaemia before use.

Aspirin thromboprotection should be discontinued. Concurrent administration with an SSRI is associated with an increased risk of GI bleeding.

Drug interactions

For general interactions between NSAIDs and other drugs, see NSAIDs Table 8, p.353 and Table 9, p.354. Of particular importance is the risk of toxic plasma levels of **digoxin**, **lithium** and **methotrexate** caused by reduced renal function and/or reduced tubular excretion (see p.351). See above for drugs contra-indicated with ketorolac.

Because they cause sodium and fluid retention, all NSAIDs can decrease the effect of diuretics, ACE inhibitors and antihypertensives.

Undesirable effects

Also see NSAIDs, p.345.

Very common (>10%): headache, dyspepsia, nausea, abdominal pain.

Common (<10%, >1%): dizziness, drowsiness, tinnitus, oedema, hypertension, anaemia, stomatitis, vomiting, bloating, flatulence, GI ulceration, diarrhoea, constipation, abnormal renal function, pruritus, purpura, rash, bleeding and pain at injection site (less with CSCI).

Very rare (<0.01%): aseptic meningitis in patients with SLE.

Dose and use

Because ketorolac carries the highest risk of upper GI ulceration, bleeding and perforation, generally its use is reserved for patients unresponsive to usual measures, including a PO NSAID. Gastroprotection, e.g. a PPI (p.31), must always be given.

CSCI: because ketorolac is irritant, dilute to the largest volume possible, and preferably use sodium chloride 0.9% as the diluent (see Chapter 29, p.887).

Use is generally *short-term* while arranging and awaiting benefit from more definitive therapy, e.g. radiotherapy. However, in the absence of other options, ketorolac has been used for extended periods without causing serious GI events.[18]

Although only authorized for IV or IM use, ketorolac can be given by intermittent injections 15–30mg SC t.d.s. Because these can be uncomfortable, for regular use it is better given by CSCI:

- start with ketorolac 60mg/24h by CSCI; *this is also the recommended maximum dose in people >65 years or <50kg*
- if necessary, increase in 15mg/24h increments to 90mg/24h (authorized maximum dose)
- occasionally, 120mg/24h is used.[18]

During titration, some centres also allow p.r.n. doses of 15mg SC as long as the permitted maximum 24h dose is not exceeded (e.g. a patient <65 years permitted a maximum of 90mg/24h but receiving 60mg/24h CSCI would be allowed ≤2 p.r.n. doses of 15mg SC/24h). If using for an extended period, maintain on the lowest effective dose.

Alternative SC/CSCI NSAIDs include **diclofenac** (p.362) and **parecoxib** (p.373).

CSCI compatibility with other drugs: ketorolac is alkaline in solution, and there is a high risk of *incompatibility* when mixed with acidic drugs (see Chapter 29, p.892). There are 2-drug compatibility data for ketorolac in sodium chloride 0.9% with **diamorphine** and **oxycodone**.[19]

Incompatibility has been reported with **cyclizine**, **glycopyrronium**, **haloperidol**, **hydromorphone**, **levomepromazine**, **midazolam** and **morphine**.

For more details, 3-drug compatibility data, and compatibility data for mixing drugs in WFI, see Appendix 3, p.933 and www.palliativedrugs.com Syringe Driver Survey Database (SDSD).

Supply

There is no PO ketorolac product available in the UK.

Ketorolac trometamol (generic)
Injection 30mg/mL, 1mL amp = £1, *vehicle contains alcohol.*

1 Gillis J and Brogden R (1997) Ketorolac: a reappraisal of its pharmacodynamic and pharmacokinetic properties and therapeutic use in pain management. *Drugs*. **53**: 139–188.
2 Lazaro-Ibanez GG *et al.* (2001) Participation of the nitric oxide-cyclic GMP-ATP-sensitive K(+) channel pathway in the antinociceptive action of ketorolac. *European Journal of Pharmacology*. **426**: 39–44.
3 Litvak K and McEvoy G (1990) Ketorolac: an injectable nonnarcotic analgesic. *Clinical Pharmacy*. **9**: 921–935.
4 Chang CH *et al.* (2011) Risk of hospitalization for upper gastrointestinal adverse events associated with nonsteroidal anti-inflammatory drugs: a nationwide case-crossover study in Taiwan. *Pharmacoepidemiology and Drug Safety*. **20**: 763–771.
5 Castellsague J *et al.* (2012) Individual NSAIDs and upper gastrointestinal complications: a systematic review and meta-analysis of observational studies (the SOS project). *Drug Safety*. **35**: 1127–1146.
6 Masso Gonzalez EL *et al.* (2010) Variability among nonsteroidal anti-inflammatory drugs in risk of upper gastrointestinal bleeding. *Arthritis and Rheumatism*. **62**: 1592–1601.
7 Shau WY *et al.* (2012) Risk of new acute myocardial infarction hospitalization associated with use of oral and parenteral non-steroidal anti-inflammation drugs (NSAIDS): a case crossover study of Taiwan's National health Insurance claims database and review of current evidence. *BMC Cardiovascular Disorders*. **12**: 4.
8 Masclee GMC *et al.* (2018) Risk of acute myocardial infarction during use of individual NSAIDs: a nested case-control study from the SOS project. *PLoS One*. **13**: e0204746.
9 Chang CH *et al.* (2010) Increased risk of stroke associated with nonsteroidal anti-inflammatory drugs: a nationwide case-crossover study. *Stroke*. **41**: 1884–1890.
10 Strom B *et al.* (1996) Parenteral ketorolac and risk of gastrointestinal and operative site bleeding. A postmarketing surveillance study. *Journal of the American Medical Association*. **275**: 376–382.
11 Rainer T *et al.* (2000) Cost effectiveness analysis of intravenous ketorolac and morphine for treating pain after limb injury: double blind randomised controlled trial. *British Medical Journal*. **321**: 1247–1251.
12 Reinhart D (2000) Minimising the adverse effects of ketorolac. *Drug Safety*. **22**: 487–497.
13 Motov S *et al.* (2016) Comparison of intravenous ketorolac at three single-dose regimens for treating acute pain in the emergency department: a randomized controlled trial. *Annals of Emergency Medicine*. **70**: 177–184.
14 Carlson RW *et al.* (1990) A multiinstitutional evaluation of the analgesic efficacy and safety of ketorolac tromethamine, acetaminophen plus codeine, and placebo in cancer pain. *Pharmacotherapy*. **10**: 211–216.
15 Pannuti F *et al.* (1999) A double-blind evaluation of the analgesic efficacy and toxicity of oral ketorolac and diclofenac in cancer pain. The TD/10 recordati Protocol Study Group. *Tumori*. **85**: 96–100.
16 Vacha ME *et al.* (2015) The role of subcutaneous ketorolac for pain management. *Hospital Pharmacy*. **50**: 108–112.
17 Greenwald R (1992) Ketorolac: an innovative nonsteroidal analgesic. *Drugs of Today*. **28**: 41–61.
18 Gaines M *et al.* (2015) Long-term continuous subcutaneous infusion of ketorolac in hospice patients. *Journal of Palliative Medicine*. **18**: 317.
19 Dickman A and Schneider J (2016) *The Syringe Driver: Continuous Subcutaneous Infusions in Palliative Care*, (4e). Oxford University Press, Oxford.

Updated (minor change) December 2021

NAPROXEN

Class: Non-opioid analgesic, NSAID, non-selective COX inhibitor.

Indications: Pain in arthritic conditions and other musculoskeletal disorders, dysmenorrhoea, acute gout, †cancer pain, †fever.

Contra-indications: Hypersensitivity (urticaria, rhinitis, asthma, angioedema) to **aspirin** or other NSAID; active GI ulceration, history of ≥2 distinct episodes of proven ulceration or bleeding; cerebrovascular bleeding, bleeding disorders, severe CHF, active liver disease or severe hepatic impairment, severe renal impairment or deteriorating renal function.

Pharmacology

Naproxen is a non-selective COX inhibitor. It is a propionic acid derivative (like **ibuprofen**). Absorption is not affected by food or antacids. A steady state is achieved after 4–5 days of b.d. administration. It is extensively metabolized in the liver to 6-*O*-desmethylnaproxen and then conjugated. Excretion is almost entirely urinary (95%), with <1% unchanged drug. Plasma concentrations do not increase with doses >500mg b.d., because of rapid urinary excretion.[1]

A meta-analysis of several hundred RCTs indicates that, compared with placebo, the risk of upper GI complications is quadrupled with high-dose naproxen (500mg b.d.), comparable with high-dose **ibuprofen** (2,400mg/24h).[2]

Like other NSAIDs, naproxen increases the risk of CVS events (see p.348).

Naproxen increases the mean arterial pressure by 5–6 mmHg in patients with established hypertension.[3] As with all NSAIDs, naproxen should be avoided in severe CHF.[4] Naproxen carries a similar risk of inducing acute renal failure as other NSAIDs.[5]

Although generally given b.d., a single dose of naproxen 500mg at bedtime was equal in efficacy to 250mg b.d. in patients with osteoarthritis[6] and with rheumatoid arthritis.[7]

Naproxen *sodium* 275mg (not UK) is equivalent to 250mg naproxen. It is more rapidly absorbed, resulting in plasma concentrations about 1.5–2 times higher than those of naproxen over the first hour, and better analgesia from 4h onwards.[8]

Bio-availability 95% PO.

Onset of action 20–30min.

Time to peak plasma concentration 1.5–5h depending on dose and formulation.[9,10]

Plasma halflife 12–15h.

Duration of action 6–8h single dose; >12h multiple doses.

Cautions

Renal and hepatic impairment (see Chapter 17 and Chapter 18, p.731 and p.753). Correct hyperkalaemia before use.

Because of an increased risk of bleeding (from decreased platelet aggregation), avoid concurrent prescription with **warfarin**. As with all NSAIDs, concurrent administration with an SSRI is associated with an increased risk of GI bleeding.

The thromboprotective effect of **aspirin** for stroke is compromised in people taking naproxen concurrently.[11] Thus, in someone taking **aspirin** thromboprophylaxis, **celecoxib** is the NSAID of choice (see p.349).

Drug interactions

For general interactions between NSAIDs and other drugs, see NSAIDs, Table 8, p.353 and Table 9, p.354. Of particular importance is the risk of toxic plasma levels of **digoxin**, **lithium** and **methotrexate** caused by reduced renal function and/or reduced tubular excretion. If naproxen is prescribed, monitor the plasma drug concentration or haematological effect of these drugs as appropriate and reduce doses as necessary (see p.351).

Naproxen plasma concentrations are increased by **probenecid**.

Because they cause sodium and fluid retention, all NSAIDs can decrease the effect of diuretics, ACE inhibitors and antihypertensives.

In addition to the effect on platelet function (see Cautions), an increase in INR occasionally occurs when naproxen is prescribed for a patient already taking **warfarin**; monitor the INR weekly for 3–4 weeks and adjust the dose of **warfarin** if necessary.[12]

Undesirable effects

Also see NSAIDs, p.345.

Common (<10%, >1%): confusion, dizziness, drowsiness, fatigue, headache, visual disturbance, tinnitus, oedema, indigestion, abdominal discomfort, nausea, constipation or diarrhoea, pruritus, rash, ecchymosis.

Dose and use

Although traditional advice is to take NSAIDs with food, there is no evidence that this reduces the risk of GI complications.

In patients at *high* risk of NSAID-related upper GI complications (see NSAIDs, Box B, p.347), ideally, naproxen should *not* be used; **celecoxib** + PPI is preferable (see p.360). If naproxen is unavoidable, prescribe gastroprotection, e.g. a PPI (p.31) concurrently.

PCF prefers **celecoxib** (p.360). However, naproxen is a frequently used NSAID:
- typically naproxen 250–500mg PO b.d.
- can be taken as a single daily dose, either each morning or each evening
- occasionally, with careful monitoring, it may be worth titrating up to a total dose of 1.5g/24h (i.e. 500mg t.d.s.); this is higher than the manufacturer's recommended maximum dose of 1–1.25g/24h (depending on indication) and should normally be done for only a limited period. This is comparable to doses used for severe rheumatoid arthritis.

Supply

Naproxen 250mg tablets are available OTC for dysmenorrhoea.

Naproxen (generic)
Tablets 250mg, 500mg, 28 days @ 500mg b.d. = £2.50.
Tablets e/c 250mg, 375mg, 500mg, 28 days @ 500mg b.d. = £5.50.
Oral suspension (sugar-free) 125mg/5mL, 250mg/5mL, 28 days @ 500mg b.d. = £252.
Oral suspension (sugar-free) 200mg/5mL, 28 days @ 500mg b.d. = £38 (unauthorized product, available as a special order; see Chapter 24, p.817). *Price based on specials tariff in community.*

Stirlescent® (Stirling Anglian)
Tablets effervescent 250mg, 28 days @ 500mg b.d. = £295.

With **esomeprazole**
Vimovo® (Grunenthal)
Tablets m/r naproxen 500mg e/c + **esomeprazole** 20mg, 28 days @ 1 tablet b.d. = £14.

1 Simon L and Mills J (1980) Nonsteroidal anti-inflammatory drugs. Part 2. *New England Journal of Medicine*. **302**: 1237–1243.
2 CNT Collaboration (2013) Vascular and upper gastrointestinal effects of non-steroidal anti-inflammatory drugs: meta-analyses of individual participant data from randomised trials. *Lancet*. **382**: 769–779.
3 Johnson AG *et al.* (1994) Do nonsteroidal anti-inflammatory drugs affect blood pressure? A meta-analysis. *Annals of Internal Medicine*. **121**: 289–300.
4 Gislason GH *et al.* (2009) Increased mortality and cardiovascular morbidity associated with use of nonsteroidal anti-inflammatory drugs in chronic heart failure. *Archives of Internal Medicine*. **169**: 141–149.
5 Schneider V *et al.* (2006) Association of selective and conventional nonsteroidal antiinflammatory drugs with acute renal failure: a population-based, nested case-control analysis. *American Journal of Epidemiology*. **164**: 881–889.
6 Mendelsohn S (1991) Clinical efficacy and tolerability of naproxen in osteoarthritis patients using twice-daily and once-daily regimens. *Clinical Therapy*. **13 (Suppl A)**: 8–15.
7 Graziano F (1991) Once-daily or twice-daily administration of naproxen in patients with rheumatoid arthritis. *Clinical Therapy*. **13 (Suppl A)**: 20–25.
8 Sevelius H *et al.* (1980) Bioavailability of naproxen sodium and its relationship to clinical analgesic effects. *British Journal of Clinical Pharmacology*. **10**: 259–263.
9 Kelly J *et al.* (1989) Pharmacokinetic properties and clinical efficacy of once-daily sustained-release naproxen. *European Journal of Clinical Pharmacology*. **36**: 383–388.
10 Davies N and Anderson K (1997) Clinical pharmacokinetics of naproxen. *Clinical Pharmacokinetics*. **32**: 268–293.
11 Gladding PA *et al.* (2008) The antiplatelet effect of six non-steroidal anti-inflammatory drugs and their pharmacodynamic interaction with aspirin in healthy volunteers. *American Journal of Cardiology*. **101**: 1060–1063.
12 Baxter K and Preston CL *Stockley's Drug Interactions*. London: Pharmaceutical Press. www.medicinescomplete.com (accessed December 2017).

Updated (minor change) December 2021

PARECOXIB

Class: Non-opioid analgesic, NSAID, selective COX-2 inhibitor.

Indications: Short-term treatment of postoperative pain in adults, †intractable cancer pain unresponsive to usual measures.

Contra-indications: Hypersensitivity (urticaria, rhinitis, asthma, angioedema) to **aspirin** or other NSAIDs, *hypersensitivity to sulfonamides*, previous serious cutaneous drug reaction, active GI ulceration, established ischaemic heart disease, peripheral arterial disease, cerebrovascular disease, CHF (NYHA II–IV), postoperative pain after coronary artery bypass graft surgery, severe hepatic impairment, severe renal impairment (but see Dose and use), deteriorating renal function, inflammatory bowel disease.

Pharmacology

Parecoxib is an injectable pro-drug of **valdecoxib**, a selective COX-2 inhibitor.[1] In 2005, PO **valdecoxib** was withdrawn from the EU/USA by the manufacturer because of concerns about the risk of serious skin reactions (including Stevens–Johnson Syndrome and toxic epidermal necrolysis) and the increased risk of cardiovascular events associated with **rofecoxib** (see NSAIDs, p.348).[2] Parecoxib was withdrawn at the same time in the USA but not the EU.[3]

Serious cutaneous reactions are reported with other COX-2 inhibitors, e.g. **celecoxib**, but rates are highest with **valdecoxib** (3–4 times that of **celecoxib**).[2] Nonetheless, the incidence appears to be very rare.[4] For parecoxib, no serious cutaneous reactions were seen in 28 RCTs and only 17 (2 fatal) in >10 years post-authorization data.[5]

Parecoxib is used for postoperative pain.[5-8] In parenteral comparisons, parecoxib 40mg IV provides similar relief to **ketorolac** 30mg IV;[8-10] in PO comparisons, parecoxib 20–50mg IM/IV has similar analgesic efficacy as **celecoxib** 400mg, **diclofenac** 100mg and **naproxen** 500mg.[7]

Generally, parecoxib is well tolerated in the postoperative setting. Compared with placebo, there is a greater risk of mostly mild–moderate hypotension (3% vs. 2%) and renal impairment (1.3% vs 0.6%).[5] However, after coronary artery bypass graft surgery, there is four times the risk of thrombo-embolic events, i.e. myocardial infarction, cardiac arrest, pulmonary embolism and stroke (2% vs. 0.5%), and, consequently, parecoxib is contra-indicated in this setting.[11,12] There is no increased risk in non-cardiac surgery.[13]

Like other selective COX-2 inhibitors, parecoxib (80mg/24h for 1 week) has no significant effect on platelet function or bleeding time[14] and its use does not appear to increase the risk of postoperative bleeding.[15]

Short-term, parecoxib 40mg IV b.d. is associated with significantly less upper GI toxicity than **ketorolac** 15mg IV q.d.s.[16] Similarly, over 4 weeks, compared to non-selective NSAIDs, the risk of upper GI toxicity was significantly less with PO **valdecoxib**, with rates no different from placebo.[17]

In a palliative care setting, parecoxib is used SC as an alternative to other injectable NSAIDs (e.g. **diclofenac**, **ketorolac**). Published experience is limited and mostly relates to its use for cancer-related bone pain that persists despite opioids and adjuvant analgesics. In a pilot study of 19 such patients, improved analgesia was seen in 17 out of 24 (70%) courses of parecoxib (40mg SC once daily for up to 3 days; 20mg for those <50kg).[18] In a retrospective case series (n=80), parecoxib CSCI (mostly 40–60mg/24h over a median of 11 days) appeared effective. Pain was not formally rated consistently, but there was a significant reduction in the number of p.r.n. opioid doses.[19] Infusion site reactions were the most common undesirable effect (about 20%). When monitored, a reduction in renal function was relatively common (11 out of 66, 17%) and was of sufficient concern to warrant discontinuation in three patients.[19]

Parecoxib is rapidly hydrolyzed to **valdecoxib** in the liver. Elimination of **valdecoxib** is via extensive hepatic metabolism, largely by CYP3A4 and CYP2C9 to produce mostly inactive metabolites that are excreted in the urine.

Onset of action 10–15min (IV/IM).

Time to peak plasma concentration 30min (IV); 1h (IM).

Plasma halflife 22min (parecoxib); 8h (**valdecoxib**).

Duration of action 6–12h.

Cautions

Renal and moderate hepatic impairment (see Dose and use, and Chapter 17 and Chapter 18, p.731 and p.753). Patients with significant CVS risk factors (i.e. hypertension, hyperlipidaemia, diabetes mellitus, smoking).

GI risk factors (see NSAIDs, Box B, p.347).

Drug interactions

For general interactions among NSAIDs and other drugs, see NSAIDs, Table 8, p.353 and Table 9, p.354. Of particular importance is the risk of toxic plasma levels of **digoxin**, **lithium** and **methotrexate** caused by reduced renal function and/or reduced tubular excretion. If an NSAID is prescribed, monitor the plasma drug concentration or haematological effect of these drugs as appropriate and reduce doses as necessary (see p.351).

Because they cause sodium and fluid retention, all NSAIDs can decrease the effect of diuretics, ACE inhibitors and antihypertensives.

There is no direct pharmacokinetic interaction between parecoxib and **warfarin**. However, because patients taking anticoagulants are at an increased risk of bleeding complications, they should be closely monitored.

The manufacturers of parecoxib report that **fluconazole** (moderate/potent inhibitor of both CYP3A4 and CYP2C9) increased the plasma levels of **valdecoxib** by 20% and raised its AUC by 60%, and recommend reducing the dose of parecoxib in patients receiving **fluconazole**.

Valdecoxib is a moderate inhibitor of CYP2C19 and CYP2D6 and theoretically may increase the plasma concentrations of other drugs metabolized by these enzymes (see Chapter 19, Table 8, p.790).

5

Undesirable effects

Also see NSAIDs, p.345.

Very common (>10%): nausea.

Common (<10%, >1%): hypertension, hypotension, oliguria, peripheral oedema, dyspepsia, abdominal pain, flatulence, vomiting, hyperhidrosis.

The SPC contains a longer list of common undesirable effects, but many relate to the postoperative experience of patients; when compared with placebo in this setting, there are few differences (see Pharmacology). In a palliative care setting, SC/CSCI site reactions and deterioration in renal function appear common (see Pharmacology).

Serious undesirable effects are uncommon or rare and include cardiovascular (e.g. myocardial infarction, severe hypotension), hypersensitivity (e.g. anaphylaxis, angioedema) and severe skin reactions (see Pharmacology).

Dose and use

Gastroprotection, e.g. a PPI (p.31), should be prescribed concurrently for patients at *high* risk of NSAID-related upper GI complications (see NSAIDs, Box B, p.347).

Discontinue parecoxib at the first sign of a rash involving the skin ± mucous membranes.

Postoperative pain

For adults ≥50kg and normal renal function:

- give 40mg IM/IV stat followed by 20–40mg q6–12h p.r.n.
- maximum dose 80mg/24h.

For adults <50kg, or in the presence of moderate hepatic impairment or severe renal impairment (also see below):

- give 20mg IM/IV stat followed by 20mg q12h p.r.n.
- maximum dose 40mg/24h.

†Cancer pain

Generally used when a parenteral NSAID is needed; alternatives include **diclofenac** (p.362) and **ketorolac** (p.369). Mostly used for cancer-related bone pain inadequately controlled despite PO NSAIDs, opioids and adjuvant analgesics. Once daily–b.d. dosing is generally sufficient, and SC use has been reported:

- start with 40mg SC once daily
- if necessary, increase to 40mg b.d.
- halve the above doses in adults <50kg or in the presence of moderate hepatic impairment or severe renal impairment (see below).

Because of the long duration of action of parecoxib, CSCI administration is not necessary. Nonetheless, parecoxib has been used CSCI 40–80mg/24h in a 30mL syringe diluted with sodium chloride 0.9%.[19] Because of the lack of compatibility data, it should not be mixed with other drugs.

Renal and hepatic impairment

Generally, NSAIDs are not recommended in severe renal impairment (CrCl <30mL/min) because of their effects on the kidney (see p.349). However, parecoxib is authorized for use in severe renal impairment at a reduced dose (see above).

Because **valdecoxib** exposure is increased by 130% in moderate hepatic impairment, the dose of parecoxib must be reduced (see above); in severe hepatic impairment, parecoxib is contra-indicated.

Supply

Parecoxib (generic)

Injection (powder for reconstitution) 40mg, 1 vial = £5. *Reconstitute a 40mg vial with 2mL sodium chloride 0.9% or glucose 5% to give a final concentration of 20mg/mL; do not use WFI.*

1 Cheer SM and Goa KL (2001) Parecoxib (parecoxib sodium). *Drugs*. **61**: 1133–1141.
2 EMEA (2005) Public statement on the suspension of the marketing authorisation for Bextra (valdecoxib) in the European Union. *EMEA Post-Authorisation Evaluation of Medicines for Human Use*. www.ema.europa.eu.
3 Sonawane KB *et al.* (2018) Serious adverse drug events reported to the FDA: analysis of the FDA Adverse Event Reporting System 2006-2014 database. *Journal of Managed Care & Specialty Pharmacy*. **24**: 682–690.
4 Layton D *et al.* (2006) Serious skin reactions and selective COX-2 inhibitors: a case series from prescription-event monitoring in England. *Drug Safety*. **29**: 687–696.
5 Schug SA *et al.* (2017) The safety profile of parecoxib for the treatment of postoperative pain: a pooled analysis of 28 randomized, double-blind, placebo-controlled clinical trials and a review of over 10 years of postauthorization data. *Journal of Pain Research*. **10**: 2451–2459.
6 Huang JM *et al.* (2018) Efficacy and safety of postoperative pain relief by parecoxib injection after laparoscopic surgeries: a systematic review and meta-analysis of randomized controlled trials. *Pain Practice*. **18**: 597–610.
7 Lloyd R *et al.* (2009) Intravenous or intramuscular parecoxib for acute postoperative pain in adults. *Cochrane Database of Systematic Reviews*. **2**: CD004771. www.cochranelibrary.com.
8 Kranke P *et al.* (2004) Patients' global evaluation of analgesia and safety of injected parecoxib for postoperative pain: a quantitative systematic review. *Anesthesia & Analgesia*. **99**: 797–806.
9 Bikhazi GB *et al.* (2004) A clinical trial demonstrates the analgesic activity of intravenous parecoxib sodium compared with ketorolac or morphine after gynecologic surgery with laparotomy. *American Journal of Obstetrics and Gynecology*. **191**: 1183–1191.
10 Siribumrungwong K *et al.* (2015) Comparing parecoxib and ketorolac as preemptive analgesia in patients undergoing posterior lumbar spinal fusion: a prospective randomized double-blinded placebo-controlled trial. *BMC Musculoskeletal Disorders*. **16**: 59.
11 Ott E *et al.* (2003) Efficacy and safety of the cyclooxygenase 2 inhibitors parecoxib and valdecoxib in patients undergoing coronary artery bypass surgery. *Journal of Thoracic and Cardiovascular Surgery*. **125**: 1481–1492.
12 Nussmeier NA *et al.* (2005) Complications of the COX-2 inhibitors parecoxib and valdecoxib after cardiac surgery. *New England Journal of Medicine*. **352**: 1081–1091.
13 Schug SA *et al.* (2009) Cardiovascular safety of the cyclooxygenase-2 selective inhibitors parecoxib and valdecoxib in the postoperative setting: an analysis of integrated data. *Anesthesia and Analgesia*. **108**: 299–307.
14 Noveck R *et al.* (2001) Parecoxib sodium does not impair platelet function in healthy elderly and non-elderly individuals: two randomised, controlled trials. *Clinical Drug Investigation*. **21**: 465–476.
15 Teerawattananon C *et al.* (2017) Risk of perioperative bleeding related to highly selective cyclooxygenase-2 inhibitors: a systematic review and meta-analysis. *Seminars in Arthritis and Rheumatism*. **46**: 520–528.
16 Stoltz RR *et al.* (2002) Upper GI mucosal effects of parecoxib sodium in healthy elderly subjects. *American Journal of Gastroenterology*. **97**: 65–71.
17 Rostom A *et al.* (2007) Gastrointestinal safety of cyclooxygenase-2 inhibitors: a Cochrane Collaboration systematic review. *Clinical Gastroenterology and Hepatology*. **5**: 818–828.
18 Kenner DJ *et al.* (2015) Daily subcutaneous parecoxib injection for cancer pain: an open label pilot study. *Journal of Palliative Medicine*. **18**: 366–372.
19 Armstrong P *et al.* (2018) Use of parecoxib by continuous subcutaneous infusion for cancer pain in a hospice population. *BMJ Supportive & Palliative Care*. **8**: 25–29.

Updated (minor change) December 2021

WEAK OPIOIDS

There is no pharmacological need for weak opioids in cancer pain (see p.321). Low doses of **morphine** (or an alternative strong opioid) generally provide quicker and better relief from cancer pain than a weak opioid.[1,2] Moving directly from a non-opioid to a strong opioid is increasingly preferred in adults, and is the norm in children, in whom weak opioids are generally contra-indicated. However, in some countries, weak opioids remain a practical necessity because of the restricted availability (or non-availability) of oral **morphine** and other strong opioids.

Codeine is the archetypical weak opioid (and **morphine** the archetypical strong opioid).[3] However, the division of opioids into 'weak' and 'strong' is to a certain extent arbitrary. In reality, opioids manifest a range of strengths, which is not fully reflected in two discrete categories. **Dihydrocodeine** and **tramadol** can be considered as equipotent to **codeine** and are also generally classified as weak opioids (Table 1).

By IM injection, weak opioids can all provide analgesia equivalent, or almost equivalent, to **morphine** 10mg IM. High-dose **codeine** (or alternative) is comparable to low-dose **morphine** (or alternative), and vice versa.

Table 1 Weak opioids; dihydrocodeine and tramadol can be considered equipotent to codeine

Drug	*PO bio-availability (%)*	*Time to peak plasma concentration (h)*	*Plasma halflife (h)*	*Duration of analgesia (h)*[a]
Codeine	40 (12–84)	1–2	2.5–3.5	4–6
Dihydrocodeine	20	1.6–1.8	3.5–4.5	3–6
Tramadol	75[b]	2	6[c]	4–9

a. when used in typical doses for mild–moderate pain
b. multiple doses >90%
c. active metabolite (M1) 7.5h; both figures double in cirrhosis and severe renal failure.

Weak opioids are said to have a 'ceiling' effect for analgesia. This is an oversimplification; although mixed agonist–antagonists (e.g. **pentazocine**) have a true ceiling effect, the maximum effective dose of weak opioid agonists is arbitrary. At higher doses, there are progressively more undesirable effects, e.g. nausea and vomiting, which outweigh any additional analgesic effect. Other dose-limiting factors are the number of tablets which patients will readily accept and, in some combination products, the dose of the non-opioid, e.g. **paracetamol**.

There is little to choose between **codeine** and its alternatives in terms of efficacy,[4] but there is no consensus about which is the weak opioid of choice. All weak opioids can produce the whole range of opioid undesirable effects (see p.394). The following should be noted:

- **codeine** has little or no analgesic effect until metabolized to **morphine**, mainly via CYP2D6. Thus, in poor metabolizers, it is essentially ineffective. In contrast, in ultra-rapid metabolizers, it is potentially toxic; in children this has led to rare postoperative deaths, leading to restrictions on its use (see p.378)
- **dihydrocodeine**, like **codeine**, is a substrate for CYP2D6 and its partial metabolism is limited in poor metabolizers and blocked by CYP2D6 inhibitors. However, unlike **codeine**, there is no evidence that such inhibition reduces its analgesic effect, i.e. **dihydrocodeine** is an active substance, not a pro-drug like **codeine** (see p.381)
- **tramadol** is less constipating than **codeine** and **dihydrocodeine**, but causes more vomiting, dizziness and anorexia. Further, if used with another drug which affects serotonin metabolism or availability, it can lead to serotonin toxicity, particularly in the elderly. It lowers seizure threshold. Unless metabolized to O-desmethyltramadol (M1) via CYP2D6, **tramadol** has a much-reduced analgesic effect; it is thus practically ineffective in poor metabolizers. In contrast, in ultra-rapid metabolizers it is potentially toxic, and similar restrictions exist on its use in children as for **codeine** (see p.383)
- **pentazocine** should *not* be used; it often causes psychotomimetic effects (e.g. dysphoria, depersonalization, frightening dreams, hallucinations).[5]

Weak opioids differ in their potential to cause toxicity when renal function is impaired. For general information on the choice of opioids and use in ESRF see Chapter 17, p.743. All weak opioids should be avoided in severe hepatic impairment (see Chapter 18, p.762). When there is an *acute* deterioration in renal or hepatic function, an opioid may rapidly accumulate because of reduced excretion or metabolism (see p.393).

Whichever weak opioid is used, the following general rules should be observed:

- a weak opioid should be added to, not substituted for, a non-opioid analgesic
- it is generally inappropriate to switch from one weak opioid to another weak opioid
- if a weak opioid is inadequate when given regularly, change to **morphine** (or an alternative strong opioid).

Patients using opioids must be monitored for undesirable effects (see Strong opioids, Box B, p.394), particularly nausea and vomiting, and constipation. Depending on individual circumstances, an anti-emetic should be prescribed for regular or p.r.n. use (see QCG: Nausea and vomiting, p.264) and, routinely, a laxative prescribed (see QCG: Opioid-induced constipation, p.45).

Opioids can impair driving ability, and patients should be counselled accordingly (see Chapter 22, p.809).

Concurrent treatment with ≥2 CNS depressants (e.g. benzodiazepines, gabapentinoids, opioids) increases the risk of respiratory depression, particularly in susceptible groups, e.g. the elderly and those with renal or hepatic impairment.[6]

1 Caraceni A *et al.* (2012) Use of opioid analgesics in the treatment of cancer pain: evidence-based recommendations from the EAPC. *Lancet Oncology*. **13**: e58–e68.
2 Bandieri E *et al.* (2016) Randomized trial of low-dose morphine versus weak opioids in moderate cancer pain. *Journal of Clinical Oncology*. **34**: 436–442.
3 WHO (1986) *Cancer Pain Relief.* World Health Organization, Geneva.
4 Moore RA and McQuay HJ (1997) Single-patient data meta-analysis of 3453 postoperative patients: oral tramadol versus placebo, codeine and combination analgesics. *Pain*. **69**: 287–294.
5 Woods A *et al.* (1974) Medicines evaluation and monitoring group: central nervous system effects of pentazocine. *British Medical Journal*. **1**: 305–307.
6 MHRA (2020) Benzodiazepines and opioids: reminder of risk of potentially fatal respiratory depression. *Drug Safety Update*. www.gov.uk/drug-safety-update.

Updated September 2021

CODEINE PHOSPHATE

Class: Opioid analgesic.

Indications: Moderate pain, cough, diarrhoea.

There is no pharmacological need for weak opioids in cancer pain (see p.321). Low doses of **morphine** (or an alternative strong opioid) generally provide quicker and better relief from cancer pain than a weak opioid.[1,2] Moving directly from a non-opioid to a strong opioid is increasingly preferred in adults and is the norm in children, in whom weak opioids are generally contra-indicated. However, in some countries, weak opioids remain a practical necessity because of the restricted availability (or non-availability) of oral **morphine** and other strong opioids.

Contra-indications: None absolute if titrated carefully to effect. Avoid use in children and adolescents (see below).[3-5]

Pharmacology

Codeine (methylmorphine) is an opium alkaloid, about one tenth as potent as **morphine**. An increasing analgesic response has been reported with IM doses up to 360mg.[6] However, in practice, codeine is generally used PO in doses of 15–60mg, often in combination with a non-opioid. Although widely prescribed, there are a lack of RCT data on the efficacy and tolerability of fixed-dose **paracetamol**–codeine combinations in cancer pain.

Codeine is metabolized mainly (80%) by conjugation to codeine-6-glucuronide, which may contribute to its analgesic effect.[7,8] However, most of its analgesic effect results from the ≤10% of codeine which is converted to **morphine** by O-demethylation via CYP2D6.[9,10] If this pathway is blocked by CYP2D6 inhibitors (see Chapter 19, Table 8, p.790), codeine lacks significant analgesic activity. However, because of genetic polymorphism (see Chapter 19, Table 3, p.785), there is wide interindividual variation in the production of **morphine**, which results in a wide range of responses to codeine.[11-15]

Compared with the general population (extensive metabolizers), poor metabolizers produce little or no **morphine** and obtain little or no pain relief from codeine. On the other hand, undesirable effects are comparable in both groups.[14,16] In contrast, ultra-rapid metabolizers produce more **morphine**, which can lead to opioid intoxication. Rarely, in children, this has been fatal, and has led to severe restrictions on its use in children (see Cautions).[3,17–20]

Like **morphine**, codeine is antitussive and also slows GI transit.[21] Given that opioids can cause pruritus, it is noteworthy that a patient with primary biliary cholangitis obtained relief with regular PO codeine (also see Chapter 26, p.825).[22] Because of constipation, codeine was stopped and the pruritus returned. When codeine was restarted together with a laxative, the patient again obtained relief.
Bio-availability 40% (12–84%) PO.[9]
Onset of action 30–60min for analgesia; 1–2h for antitussive effect.
Time to peak plasma concentration 1–2h.
Plasma halflife 2.5–3.5h.[9]
Duration of action 4–6h.

Cautions

Codeine use in children and adolescents is *contra-indicated* in those:
- <12 years for pain, cough or diarrhoea
- <18 years for pain after surgery to remove tonsils and/or adenoids.

Further, the MHRA advises that codeine:[4,5]
- is not recommended in those 12–18 years whose breathing might be compromised, e.g. by neuromuscular disorders, severe cardiac or respiratory conditions, chest infection, multiple trauma, extensive surgical procedures
- should only be used in children >12 years for acute moderate pain if **paracetamol** or **ibuprofen** alone is ineffective and that:
  - ▷ the maximum total daily dose is ≤240mg/24h given in divided doses ≥q6h
  - ▷ treatment duration is ≤3 days and stopped if ineffective
  - ▷ information on recognizing **morphine** toxicity is given to caregivers.

Although not specifically covered by the MHRA advice, similar cautions can be applied to the use of codeine for diarrhoea in those 12–18 years old.

Codeine is *contra-indicated* in adults and children who are *known* CYP2D6 ultra-rapid metabolizers. Although generally unknown in routine clinical practice, the prevalence is higher in some ethnic populations (see Chapter 19, Table 3, p.785).

Driving ability may be impaired by a dose of 50mg (see Chapter 22, p.809).[23,24] Like **morphine** and **dihydrocodeine**, codeine is more toxic in severe renal impairment and should be avoided. This is because of accumulation of **morphine** and other active metabolites (see Chapter 17, p.743).

Codeine is generally best not used in patients with moderate–severe hepatic impairment; reduced metabolism could result in less being transformed into **morphine**, thereby reducing its analgesic effect (see Chapter 18, p.762).[25]

Drug interactions

Concurrent treatment with ≥2 CNS depressants (e.g. benzodiazepines, gabapentinoids, opioids) increases the risk of respiratory depression, particularly in susceptible groups, e.g. the elderly and those with renal or hepatic impairment.[26]

CYP2D6 inhibitors (e.g. **fluoxetine**, **paroxetine**, **quinidine**) block the biotransformation of codeine to **morphine** and will render codeine ineffective as an analgesic; see Chapter 19, Table 8, p.790 for more details.

Undesirable effects

Codeine can produce the whole range of opioid undesirable effects (see Strong opioids, Box B, p.394).

Dose and use

Note. Low-dose PO **morphine** (20–30mg/24h) generally provides quicker and better relief from cancer pain than codeine.[2]

Patients using opioids must be monitored for undesirable effects, particularly nausea and vomiting, and constipation. Depending on individual circumstances, an anti-emetic should be prescribed for regular or p.r.n. use (see QCG: Nausea and vomiting, p.264) and, routinely, a laxative prescribed (see QCG: Opioid-induced constipation, p.45).

*It is bad practice to prescribe codeine to patients already taking **morphine** or any other strong opioid; if a greater effect is needed, the regular and p.r.n. doses of **morphine** (or another strong opioid) should be increased.*

Pain relief

Codeine is often given PO in a combination product with a non-opioid. Prices can vary significantly between different combination products, codeine content and the individual formulations, e.g. tablets vs capsules or dispersible or effervescent tablets (see Supply). The codeine content of these products is generally 8mg, 15mg or 30mg (lower strengths, e.g. 8–12mg, are present in some

OTC combination products containing **aspirin, ibuprofen** or **paracetamol**). Thus, patients with inadequate relief may benefit by changing to a higher strength product. When given alone, the dose of codeine is generally 30–60mg PO q4h. Higher doses can be given, but equivalent analgesic PO doses of **morphine** (one tenth of the dose of codeine) may be less constipating.

Cough

Codeine is effective as an antitussive by any route. The dose is tailored to the patient's need, e.g. 15–30mg PO p.r.n. up to q4h. Administration as an oral linctus or solution/syrup is *not* necessary (see Antitussives, p.158).

Diarrhoea

To control diarrhoea, a dose of 30–60mg PO is used both p.r.n. and regularly up to q4h. However, **loperamide** (p.36) may be preferable.

Supply

Codeine phosphate (generic)
Tablets 15mg, 30mg, 60mg, 28 days @ 30mg q.d.s. = £4.25.
Oral linctus 15mg/5mL, 28 days @ 30mg q.d.s. = £9; *sugar-free formulations are available.*
Oral solution 25mg/5mL, 28 days @ 25mg q.d.s. = £7.50.
Injection 60mg/mL, 1mL amp = £2.75. Schedule 2 **CD**.

Codeine with **aspirin** (co-codaprin; generic)
Tablets dispersible codeine phosphate 8mg, **aspirin** 500mg, 28 days @ 2 q.d.s. = £23.

Codeine with **paracetamol** (co-codamol 8mg/500mg; generic)
Capsules codeine phosphate 8mg, **paracetamol** 500mg, 28 days @ 2 q.d.s. = £55.
Tablets codeine phosphate 8mg, **paracetamol** 500mg, 28 days @ 2 q.d.s. = £6.
Tablets effervescent codeine phosphate 8mg, **paracetamol** 500mg, 28 days @ 2 q.d.s. = £14.

Codeine with **paracetamol** (co-codamol 15mg/500mg; generic)
Capsules codeine phosphate 15mg, **paracetamol** 500mg, 28 days @ 2 q.d.s. = £16.
Tablets codeine phosphate 15mg, **paracetamol** 500mg, 28 days @ 2 q.d.s. = £9.
Tablets effervescent codeine phosphate 15mg, **paracetamol** 500mg, 28 days @ 2 q.d.s. = £18.

Codeine with **paracetamol** (co-codamol 30mg/500mg; generic)
Capsules codeine phosphate 30mg, **paracetamol** 500mg, 28 days @ 2 q.d.s. = £13.
Tablets codeine phosphate 30mg, **paracetamol** 500mg, 28 days @ 2 q.d.s. = £7.50.
Tablets effervescent codeine phosphate 30mg, **paracetamol** 500mg, 28 days @ 2 q.d.s. = £16.
Oral solution (sugar-free) codeine phosphate 30mg, **paracetamol** 500mg/5mL, 28 days @ 10mL q.d.s. = £90.

This is not a complete list; see BNF for more information.

Note: Dispersible or effervescent formulations may contain Na+ up to 20mmol/tablet or sachet. Check individual brand SPC and avoid high-Na+ formulations in renal impairment.

1 Caraceni A *et al.* (2012) Use of opioid analgesics in the treatment of cancer pain: evidence-based recommendations from the EAPC. *Lancet Oncology*. **13**: e58–e68.

2 Bandieri E *et al.* (2016) Randomized trial of low-dose morphine versus weak opioids in moderate cancer pain. *Journal of Clinical Oncology*. **34**: 436–442.

3 Racoosin JA *et al.* (2013) New evidence about an old drug - risk with codeine after adenotonsillectomy. *New England Journal of Medicine*. **368**: 2155–2157.

4 MHRA (2013) Codeine: restricted use as an analgesic in children and adolescents after European safety review. *Drug Safety Update*. www.gov.uk/drug-safety-update.

5 MHRA (2015) Codeine for cough and cold: restricted use in children. *Drug Safety Update*. www.gov.uk/drug-safety-update.

6 Beaver W (1966) Mild analgesics: a review of their clinical pharmacology (Part II). *American Journal of Medical Science*. **251**: 576–599.

7 Lotsch J *et al.* (2006) Evidence for morphine-independent central nervous opioid effects after administration of codeine: contribution of other codeine metabolites. *Clinical Pharmacology and Therapeutics*. **79**: 35–48.

8 Vree TB *et al.* (2000) Codeine analgesia is due to codeine-6-glucuronide, not morphine. *International Journal of Clinical Practice*. **54**: 395–398.

9 Persson K *et al.* (1992) The postoperative pharmacokinetics of codeine. *European Journal of Clinical Pharmacology*. **42**: 663–666.

10 Findlay JWA *et al.* (1978) Plasma codeine and morphine concentrations after therapeutic oral doses of codeine-containing analgesics. *Clinical Pharmacology and Therapeutics*. **24**: 60–68.
11 Sindrup SH and Brosen K (1995) The pharmacogenetics of codeine hypoalgesia. *Pharmacogenetics*. **5**: 335–346.
12 Caraco Y *et al.* (1996) Pharmacogenetic determination of the effects of codeine and prediction of drug interactions. *Journal of Pharmacology and Experimental Therapeutics*. **278**: 1165–1174.
13 Lurcott G (1999) The effects of the genetic absence and inhibition of CYP2D6 on the metabolism of codeine and its derivatives, hydrocodone and oxycodone. *Anesthesia Progress*. **45**: 154–156.
14 Eckhardt K *et al.* (1998) Same incidence of adverse drug events after codeine administration irrespective of the genetically determined differences in morphine formation. *Pain*. **76**: 27–33.
15 Lotsch J *et al.* (2004) Genetic predictors of the clinical response to opioid analgesics: clinical utility and future perspectives. *Clinical Pharmacokinetics*. **43**: 983–1013.
16 Susce MT *et al.* (2006) Response to hydrocodone, codeine and oxycodone in a CYP2D6 poor metabolizer. *Progress in Neuropsychopharmacology and Biological Psychiatry*. **30**: 1356–1358.
17 Gasche Y *et al.* (2004) Codeine intoxication associated with ultrarapid CYP2D6 metabolism. *New England Journal of Medicine*. **351**: 2827–2831.
18 Koren G *et al.* (2006) Pharmacogenetics of morphine poisoning in a breastfed neonate of a codeine-prescribed mother. *Lancet*. **368**: 704.
19 Kirchheiner J *et al.* (2007) Pharmacokinetics of codeine and its metabolite morphine in ultra-rapid metabolizers due to CYP2D6 duplication. *Pharmacogenomics Journal*. **7**: 257–265.
20 Williams DG *et al.* (2002) Pharmacogenetics of codeine metabolism in an urban population of children and its implications for analgesic reliability. *British Journal of Anaesthesia*. **89**: 839–845.
21 Anonymous (1989) Drugs in the management of acute diarrhoea in infants and young children. *Bulletin of the World Health Organization*. **67**: 94–96.
22 Zylicz Z and Krajnik M (1999) Codeine for pruritus in primary biliary cirrhosis. *Lancet*. **353**: 813.
23 Linnoila M and Hakkinen S (1974) Effects of diazepam and codeine, alone and in combination with alcohol, on simulated driving. *Clinical Pharmacology and Therapeutics*. **15**: 368–373.
24 Linnoila M and Mattila MJ (1973) Proceedings: Drug interaction on driving skills as evaluated by laboratory tests and by a driving simulator. *Pharmakopsychiatric Neuropsychopharmakologie*. **6**: 127–132.
25 Tegeder I *et al.* (1999) Pharmacokinetics of opioids in liver disease. *Clinical Pharmacokinetics*. **37**: 17–40.
26 MHRA (2020) Benzodiazepines and opioids: reminder of risk of potentially fatal respiratory depression. *Drug Safety Update*. www.gov.uk/drug-safety-update.

Updated September 2021

5

DIHYDROCODEINE TARTRATE

Class: Opioid analgesic.

Indications: Moderate–severe pain.

There is no pharmacological need for weak opioids in cancer pain (see p.321). Low doses of **morphine** (or an alternative strong opioid) generally provide quicker and better relief from cancer pain than a weak opioid.[1,2] Moving directly from a non-opioid to a strong opioid is increasingly preferred in adults and is the norm in children, in whom weak opioids are generally contra-indicated. However, in some countries, weak opioids remain a practical necessity because of the restricted availability (or non-availability) of oral **morphine** and other strong opioids.

Contra-indications: None absolute if titrated carefully to effect.

Pharmacology

Dihydrocodeine is a semisynthetic analogue of **codeine**. It relieves pain and cough[3,4] and causes constipation.[5] Like **codeine**, dihydrocodeine is a substrate for CYP2D6. Its partial metabolism to dihydromorphine is limited in poor metabolizers and is blocked by CYP2D6 inhibitors (see Chapter 19, Table 8, p.790).[6] However, unlike **codeine**, there is no evidence that inhibition reduces the analgesic effect of dihydrocodeine.[7] In other words, dihydrocodeine is an active substance, not a pro-drug like **codeine**.[8,9]

By injection (not UK), dihydrocodeine 60mg IM is comparable to **morphine** 10mg IM.[10,11] Dihydrocodeine is about twice as potent as **codeine** by injection but, because its oral bio-availability is low, the two drugs are essentially equipotent by mouth.[12]

Bio-availability 20% PO.
Onset of action 30min.
Time to peak plasma concentration 1.7h.
Plasma halflife 3.5–4.5h.
Duration of action 4h.

Cautions

May impair the ability to perform skilled tasks, e.g. driving (see Chapter 22, p.809). Prolonged erections have occurred when **sildenafil** was taken concurrently with dihydrocodeine, possibly because abnormally high concentrations of cyclic guanosine monophosphate were produced in peripheral nerve endings.[13]

Like **morphine** and **codeine**, the risk of toxicity with dihydrocodeine is higher in severe renal impairment, probably because of accumulation of an active glucuronide, and should be avoided (also see Chapter 17, p.743).[14] Dihydrocodeine is best avoided in moderate–severe hepatic impairment (see Chapter 18, p.762).

Drug interactions

Concurrent treatment with ≥2 CNS depressants (e.g. benzodiazepines, gabapentinoids, opioids) increases the risk of respiratory depression, particularly in susceptible groups, e.g. the elderly and those with renal or hepatic impairment.[15]

Undesirable effects

Dihydrocodeine can produce the whole range of opioid undesirable effects (see Strong opioids, Box B, p.394).

Dose and use

Note. Low-dose PO **morphine** (20–30mg/24h) generally provides quicker and better relief from cancer pain than a Step 2 analgesic.[1]

Patients using opioids must be monitored for undesirable effects, particularly nausea and vomiting, and constipation. Depending on individual circumstances, an anti-emetic should be prescribed for regular or p.r.n. use (see QCG: Nausea and vomiting, p.264) and, routinely, a laxative prescribed (see QCG: Opioid-induced constipation, p.45).

*It is bad practice to prescribe dihydrocodeine to patients already taking **morphine** or any other strong opioid; if a greater effect is needed, the regular and p.r.n. doses of **morphine** (or another strong opioid) should be increased.*

As a single agent:
- start with 30mg PO q4–6h
- if necessary, increase to 60mg q4–6h.

The higher dose is associated with a significant increase in undesirable effects.[16]

Supply

Dihydrocodeine tartrate (generic)
Tablets 30mg, 28 days @ 30mg q.d.s. = £6.

DF118 Forte® (Martindale)
Tablets dihydrocodeine tartrate 40mg, 28 days @ 40mg t.d.s. = £9.50.

Dihydrocodeine with **paracetamol** (co-dydramol; generic)
Tablets dihydrocodeine tartrate 10mg, **paracetamol** 500mg, 28 days @ 2 q.d.s. = £12.
Tablets dihydrocodeine tartrate 20mg, **paracetamol** 500mg, 28 days @ 2 q.d.s. = £23.
Tablets dihydrocodeine tartrate 30mg, **paracetamol** 500mg, 28 days @ 2 q.d.s. = £27.

Modified-release

As for all m/r opioids, brand prescribing is recommended to reduce the risk of confusion and error in dispensing and administration (see p.xvii).

Modified-release 12-hourly oral products
DHC Continus® (Napp)
Tablets m/r dihydrocodeine tartrate 60mg, 90mg, 120mg, 28 days @ 60mg b.d. = £5.

1 Bandieri E *et al.* (2015) Randomized trial of low-dose morphine versus weak opioids in moderate cancer pain. *Journal of Clinical Oncology*. **34**: 436–442.
2 Caraceni A *et al.* (2012) Use of opioid analgesics in the treatment of cancer pain: evidence-based recommendations from the EAPC. *Lancet Oncology*. **13**: e58–e68.
3 Weiss B (1959) Dihydrocodeine. A pharmacologic review. *American Journal of Pharmacy*. **August**: 286–301.
4 Luporini G *et al.* (1998) Efficacy and safety of levodropropizine and dihydrocodeine on nonproductive cough in primary and metastatic lung cancer. *European Respiratory Journal*. **12**: 97–101.
5 Freye E *et al.* (2001) Dose-related effects of controlled release dihydrocodeine on oro-cecal transit and pupillary light reflex. A study in human volunteers. *Arzneimittelforschung*. **51**: 60–66.
6 Fromm M *et al.* (1995) Dihydrocodeine: A new opioid substrate for the polymorphic CYP2D6 in humans. *Clinical Pharmacology and Therapeutics*. **58**: 374–382.
7 Wilder-Smith CH *et al.* (1998) The visceral and somatic antinociceptive effects of dihydrocodeine and its metabolite, dihydromorphine. A cross-over study with extensive and quinidine-induced poor metabolizers. *British Journal of Clinical Pharmacology*. **45**: 575–581.
8 Webb JA *et al.* (2001) Contribution of dihydrocodeine and dihydromorphine to analgesia following dihydrocodeine administration in man: a PK-PD modelling analysis. *British Journal of Clinical Pharmacology*. **52**: 35–43.
9 Schmidt H *et al.* (2003) The role of active metabolites in dihydrocodeine effects. *International Journal of Clinical Pharmacology and Therapeutics*. **41**: 95–106.
10 Seed JC *et al.* (1958) A comparison of the analgesic and respiratory effects of dihydrocodeine and morphine in main. *Archives Internationales de Pharmacodynamie et de Therapie*. **116**: 293–339.
11 Palmer RN *et al.* (1966) Incidence of unwanted effects of dihydrocodeine bitartrate in healthy volunteers. *Lancet*. **2**: 620–621.
12 Anonymous. Dihydrocodeine (tartrate). In: Dollery C, editor. *Therapeutic Drugs*. Edinburgh: Churchill Livingstone; 1991. p. 133–136.
13 Goldmeier D and Lamba H (2002) Prolonged erections produced by dihydrocodeine and sildenafil. *British Medical Journal*. **324**: 1555.
14 Barnes J *et al.* (1985) Dihydrocodeine in renal failure: further evidence for an important role in the kidney in the handling of opioid drugs. *British Medical Journal*. **290**: 740–742.
15 MHRA (2020) Benzodiazepines and opioids: reminder of risk of potentially fatal respiratory depression. *Drug Safety Update*. www.gov.uk/drug-safety-update.
16 McQuay H *et al.* (1993) A multiple dose comparison of ibuprofen and dihydrocodeine after third molar surgery. *British Journal of Oral and Maxillofacial Surgery*. **31**: 95–100.

Updated September 2021

5

TRAMADOL

Class: Opioid analgesic (but see Pharmacology).

Indications: Moderate–severe pain.

There is no pharmacological need for weak opioids in cancer pain (see p.321). Low doses of **morphine** (or an alternative strong opioid) generally provide quicker and better relief from cancer pain than a weak opioid.[1,2] Moving directly from a non-opioid to a strong opioid is increasingly preferred in adults and is the norm in children in whom weak opioids are generally contra-indicated. However, in some countries, weak opioids remain a practical necessity because of the restricted availability (or non-availability) of oral **morphine** and other strong opioids.

Contra-indications: Use of MAOIs concurrently or within 14 days, severe hepatic impairment, ESRF (creatinine clearance <10mL/min), uncontrolled epilepsy. Avoid use in children (see Cautions).

Pharmacology

Tramadol, like **tapentadol** (p.487), is a synthetic centrally acting analgesic with both non-opioid and opioid properties.[3,4] Its efficacy is comparable to **codeine** (p.378), and it is often used in preference.[5–7] High quality data specific to cancer pain is lacking.[8]

Tramadol is derived from **codeine** (p.378) and is structurally similar to **venlafaxine** (p.236). It exists as a racemic mixture and stimulates neuronal serotonin and noradrenaline (norepinephrine) release. It also inhibits presynaptic re-uptake: serotonin mainly via (+) tramadol and noradrenaline mainly via (–) tramadol. This enhances the impact of the descending inhibitory pathways associated with pain transmission, acting synergistically with tramadol's weak opioid effect (Table 1 and Table 2).[4] In animal models, tramadol also has an anti-inflammatory effect independent of PG inhibition.[9]

Table 1 μ-opioid receptor affinities: K_i (micromol) values[a,10]

	Receptor affinity
Morphine	0.009
Tapentadol	0.16
Tramadol[b]	2.4

a. the lower the K_i value, the greater the receptor affinity
b. much lower for (+) M1, i.e. 0.003.

Table 2 Inhibition of monoamine uptake: K_i (micromol) values[a,10]

	Noradrenaline	*Serotonin*
Morphine	>100	>100
Tapentadol	0.48	2.4
Tramadol	0.59[b]	0.87[c]

a. the lower the K_i value, the greater the functional uptake inhibition
b. (–) tramadol
c. (+) tramadol.

Tramadol is converted in the liver, mainly via CYP2D6, to the active metabolite O-desmethyltramadol (M1), which is several times more potent than tramadol itself. Thus, tramadol (like **codeine**) can be considered a pro-drug. Further biotransformation of M1 results in inactive metabolites which are excreted by the kidneys.

Although **naloxone** (an opioid antagonist, see p.490) can only partially reverse the effects of tramadol, in a series of 11 patients with a tramadol overdose, seven had a good response to **naloxone**, and only one had no response.[11]

Changes in CYP2D6 activity, both acquired (e.g. drug-induced) and constitutional (≤10% of Caucasians are either CYP2D6 poor or ultra-rapid metabolizers)[12] can affect the response to tramadol. Decreased CYP2D6 activity will result in decreased response/higher dose requirements. Conversely, increased CYP2D6 has resulted in life-threatening respiratory depression in a child (see Cautions and Drug interactions, and Chapter 19, p.781).[13–17]

Although in RCTs tramadol significantly relieved neuropathic pain of various aetiologies (e.g. diabetic neuropathy, post-herpetic neuralgia, polyneuropathy), a systematic review concluded that the overall evidence was of low quality and the NNT of 4.4 a likely overestimate of benefit.[18] Thus, at best, tramadol is comparable with several anti-epileptics, but not as good as TCAs (NNT = 2.3; see Adjuvant analgesics, p.325), or as **oxycodone** in post-herpetic neuralgia (NNT = 2.5).[19]

Tramadol is as effective as **codeine** as a cough suppressant.[20,21] Postoperatively, it causes less respiratory depression than equi-analgesic doses of **morphine**.[22] It also causes less constipation than **codeine**, **dihydrocodeine** and **morphine**,[23–25] but more vomiting, dizziness and anorexia than **codeine** and **dihydrocodeine**.[26] In contrast to **morphine**, tramadol reduces the basal pressure in the sphincter of Oddi (for <20min after IM administration) and does not increase the pressure in the common bile duct.[27]

Although the risk of dependence and misuse is less compared with **morphine** and other opioids,[28] tramadol is a Schedule 3 **CD**. Like other opioids, tramadol is associated with the development of physical dependence (see Dose and use)[29] and, in overdose, CNS depression, respiratory depression and death.[30] There are also case reports of possible opioid-induced hyperalgesia (also see Strong opioids, p.398).

By injection, tramadol is generally regarded as one tenth as potent as **morphine** injection (i.e. tramadol 100mg IV is equivalent to **morphine** 10mg IV).[31] In fact, various pre- and postoperative studies give a range between one tenth and one twentieth as potent as **morphine**.[32,33] Thus, the figure of one tenth is more of a 'convenient to remember' number than a scientifically precise one. Some of the postoperative studies also suggest that, to produce adequate analgesia, tramadol needs to be administered more frequently than **morphine** over the first few hours (by IV PCA), after which doses become less frequent. The need for the equivalent of a loading dose with tramadol may reflect its different mode of action from **morphine**. A delayed maximum effect has also been reported in an RCT of oral tramadol and **morphine**.[34]

By mouth, RCTs indicate tramadol is one fifth to one quarter as potent as **morphine** (i.e. tramadol 100mg PO is equivalent to **morphine** 20–25mg PO).[35,36] However, extensive clinical experience has led many physicians to regard PO tramadol as one tenth as potent as PO **morphine** (i.e. tramadol 100mg PO is equivalent to **morphine** 10mg PO), i.e. the same as by injection.[37–39]

When converting from tramadol PO to SC/IM/IV, generally the same dose can be used.

Bio-availability 65–75% PO; 90% with multiple doses;[40] 77% PR.[41,42]

Onset of action 30min–1h.

Time to peak plasma concentration 2h; 4–8h m/r.

Plasma halflife 6h; active metabolite 7.4h; these more than double in cirrhosis and severe renal failure.

Duration of action 4–9h.

Cautions

Genetic polymorphism in CYP2D6 affects the metabolism of tramadol, like **codeine**. In 2017, following a safety review, the FDA placed similar restrictions on the use of tramadol in children and adolescents as for **codeine** (p.379).[43] In the UK, a similar review has not been undertaken, but tramadol is not recommended or authorized for use in children <12 years. If tramadol is unavoidable in children 12–18 years, apply the same contra-indications and cautions as for **codeine** (p.379).

Renal and hepatic impairment (see Dose and use, and also Chapter 17, p.743 and Chapter 18, p.762).

Tramadol has been associated with seizures, notably when the total daily dose exceeds 400mg or when tramadol is used concurrently with other medications that lower the seizure threshold, e.g. TCAs, SSRIs, antipsychotics and other opioids.[11,44,45] Seizures have also been reported in patients after rapid IV injection of tramadol. Treat with standard measures, e.g. benzodiazepines (p.170). Resolution generally occurs in <1 day.[11] Fatalities resulting from tramadol-induced seizures are rare.[46] Use with caution in controlled epilepsy, head trauma or raised intracranial pressure.

Serotonin toxicity has occasionally occurred when tramadol has been taken concurrently with a second drug that also interferes with presynaptic serotonin re-uptake (see Antidepressants, Box A, p.217). Risk factors include the use of higher doses, old age, the second drug being a CYP2D6 inhibitor, CYP2D6 poor-metabolizer status, and hepatic impairment.[47]

Tramadol (like **methadone**, p.469) is associated with hypoglycaemia;[48–50] in a large population cohort study, it occurred mostly within 10 days of starting and more frequently in the elderly.[48]

The FDA has warned of an increased risk of suicide in emotionally unstable patients taking tramadol, particularly if they are also taking antidepressants or tranquillizers.

May impair the ability to perform skilled tasks, e.g. driving (see Chapter 22, p.809).

Drug interactions

Concurrent treatment with ≥2 CNS depressants (e.g. benzodiazepines, gabapentinoids, opioids) increases the risk of respiratory depression, particularly in susceptible groups, e.g. the elderly and those with renal or hepatic impairment.[51]

Because of the increased risk of seizures and serotonin toxicity, concurrent use of tramadol with an MAOI is contra-indicated, and its use with other antidepressants, particularly SSRIs or TCAs, requires caution (see Cautions and below).[47,52]

Carbamazepine and **rifampicin**[53] increase the metabolism of tramadol and M1, and thus may decrease analgesia (see Chapter 19, p.781). CYP2D6 inhibitors, e.g. **fluoxetine**, **paroxetine**, **quinidine**, and **ritonavir**, inhibit the conversion of tramadol to M1 and may decrease analgesia while increasing the risk of serotonin toxicity.[47,54]

Tramadol occasionally prolongs the INR of patients taking **warfarin**.[55,56] Monitor the INR closely for 3–4 weeks if tramadol is prescribed for a patient already taking **warfarin**.

There are mixed reports of the analgesic effect of tramadol being reduced by **ondansetron** (possibly by blocking the action of serotonin at presynaptic $5HT_3$-receptors on primary afferent nociceptive neurones in the spinal dorsal horn).[57] In one postoperative pain study, the dose of tramadol needed by IV PCA was 2–3 times greater in patients receiving **ondansetron**,[58] but was unaffected in another.[59]

Undesirable effects

Tramadol can produce the whole range of opioid undesirable effects (see Strong opioids, Box B, p.394) in addition to those attributed to monoamine re-uptake inhibition (see Antidepressants, Table 3, p.218). The incidence and nature of undesirable effects (monoamine re-uptake inhibition vs. opioid) may vary with activity of CYP2D6 (see Pharmacology). Urinary incontinence.[60]
Rare (<0.1%): seizures (dose-dependent; see Cautions).

Dose and use

Note. Low-dose PO **morphine** (20–30mg/24h) generally provides quicker and better relief from cancer pain than tramadol.[2]

Patients using opioids must be monitored for undesirable effects, particularly nausea and vomiting, and constipation. Depending on individual circumstances, an anti-emetic should be prescribed for regular or p.r.n. use (see QCG: Nausea and vomiting, p.264) and, routinely, a laxative prescribed (see QCG: Opioid-induced constipation, p.45).

Most cancer patients prescribed tramadol will already be taking a non-opioid:
- start with tramadol 50mg PO q.d.s *or* an equivalent daily dose using a q12h or once daily m/r product (see Supply); for very frail patients, dose as in renal impairment (see below)
- if necessary, increase the dose in stages to a maximum recommended total daily dose of 400mg
- higher doses have been given, e.g. 600mg/24h and sometimes more[37,38]
- for break-through pain when taking m/r tramadol, consider immediate-release tramadol or immediate-release **morphine** (p.404).

Renal or hepatic impairment

In severe renal impairment, because of impaired metabolism or elimination:
- *halve* the starting dose by reducing the frequency to 50mg PO q12h using immediate-release products; likewise in very frail patients[3]
- if necessary, increase the dose in stages to a maximum recommended total daily dose of 200mg.

Despite ESRF (creatinine clearance <10mL/min) being a contra-indication, some centres have successfully used tramadol in this setting (see Chapter 17, p.743).[61]

Tramadol is contra-indicated in severe hepatic impairment. In moderate hepatic impairment, because of impaired metabolism to the active metabolite, tramadol is best avoided; if unavoidable, dose as in severe renal impairment (see Chapter 18, p.762).

Stopping tramadol

Abruptly stopping tramadol, even after only a few days of use, can result in typical symptoms of opioid withdrawal (e.g. anxiety, restlessness, abdominal cramps, diarrhoea, goose flesh, sweating), and tapering the dose over several days is recommended.

However, opioid withdrawal should not occur when tramadol is being substituted by another μ-opioid agonist, e.g. **morphine**. Nonetheless, abruptly stopping tramadol has also sometimes resulted in symptoms *not* typical of opioid withdrawal (e.g. severe anxiety/panic attacks, delirium, paranoia, hallucinations, paraesthesia), particularly with doses >400mg/24h.[62,63] This suggests the potential for a discontinuation reaction similar to that seen with antidepressants (see p.223)[62] and is another reason why tapering the dose over several days is recommended.

Supply

All products are Schedule 3 **CD** (with storage exemption).

Tramadol (generic)
Capsules 50mg, 28 days @ 100mg q.d.s. = £4.75.
Orodispersible tablets 50mg, 28 days @ 100mg q.d.s. = £27.
Oral drops 100mg/mL (2.5mg/drop), 10mL, 28 days @100mg (40 drops) q.d.s. = £280. *Mix with water before taking.*
Injection 50mg/mL, 2mL amp = £0.75.

Tramadol with **paracetamol** (generic)
Tablets tramadol hydrochloride 37.5mg, **paracetamol** 325mg, 28 days @ 2 q.d.s. = £7.

Tramacet® 37.5mg/325mg (Grünenthal)
Tablets effervescent tramadol hydrochloride 37.5mg, **paracetamol** 325mg, 28 days @ 2 q.d.s. = £36.

Modified-release products

A large number of tramadol m/r products are available, administered either q12h or once daily, and prescribers should clearly specify which one they require. As for all m/r opioids, brand prescribing is recommended to reduce the risk of confusion and error in dispensing and administration (see p.xvii).

Modified-release 12-hourly oral products
Zydol® SR (Grünenthal)
Tablets m/r 50mg, 100mg, 150mg, 200mg, 28 days @ 200mg b.d. = £32. *Other brands include Brimisol® PR, Invodol® SR, Mabron®, Marol®, Tilodol® SR, Tramulief® SR; some may be significantly cheaper but do not have the full range of strengths available.*

Zamadol® SR (Mylan)
Capsules m/r 50mg, 100mg, 150mg, 200mg, 28 days @ 200mg b.d. = £27.
Other brands include Maxitram® SR, Tramquel® SR.

Modified-release 24-hourly oral products
Zamadol® 24h (Mylan)
Tablets m/r 150mg, 200mg, 300mg, 400mg, 28 days @ 400mg once daily = £29. *Other brands include Tradorec® XL, Zydol® XL; not all have the full range of strengths available.*

1 Caraceni A *et al.* (2012) Use of opioid analgesics in the treatment of cancer pain: evidence-based recommendations from the EAPC. *Lancet Oncology.* **13**: e58–e68.
2 Bandieri E *et al.* (2016) Randomized trial of low-dose morphine versus weak opioids in moderate cancer pain. *Journal of Clinical Oncology.* **34**: 436–442.
3 Grond S and Sablotzki A (2004) Clinical pharmacology of tramadol. *Clinical Pharmacokinetics.* **43**: 879–923.
4 Dickman A (2007) Tramadol: a review of this atypical opioid. *European Journal of Palliative Care.* **14**: 181–185.
5 Jadad AR and Browman GP (1995) The WHO analgesic ladder for cancer pain management. *Journal of the American Medical Association.* **274**: 1870–1873.
6 Tassinari D *et al.* (2011) The second step of the analgesic ladder and oral tramadol in the treatment of mild to moderate cancer pain: a systematic review. *Palliative Medicine.* **25**: 410–423.
7 Goncalves JA *et al.* (2015) Does tramadol have a role in pain control in palliative care? *American Journal of Hospice and Palliative Care.* **32**: 631–633.
8 Wiffen PJ *et al.* (2017) Tramadol with or without paracetamol (acetaminophen) for cancer pain. *Cochrane Database of Systematic Reviews.* **5**: CD012508. www.cochranelibrary.com.
9 Buccellati C *et al.* (2000) Tramadol anti-inflammatory activity is not related to a direct inhibitory action on prostaglandin endoperoxide synthases. *European Journal of Pain.* **4**: 413–415.
10 Tzschentke TM *et al.* (2014) The mu-opioid receptor agonist/noradrenaline reuptake inhibition (MOR-NRI) concept in analgesia: the case of tapentadol. *CNS Drugs.* **28**: 319–329.
11 Marquardt KA *et al.* (2005) Tramadol exposures reported to statewide poison control system. *Annals of Pharmacotherapy.* **39**: 1039–1044.
12 Sachse C *et al.* (1997) Cytochrome P450 2D6 variants in a Caucasian population: allele frequencies and phenotypic consequences. *American Journal of Human Genetics.* **60**: 284–295.
13 Stamer UM *et al.* (2003) Impact of CYP2D6 genotype on postoperative tramadol analgesia. *Pain.* **105**: 231–238.
14 Poulsen L *et al.* (1996) The hypoalgesic effect of tramadol in relation to CYP2D6. *Clinical Pharmacology and Therapeutics.* **60**: 636–644.
15 Kim E *et al.* (2010) Adverse events in analgesic treatment with tramadol associated with CYP2D6 extensive-metaboliser and OPRM1 high-expression variants. *Annals of the Rheumatic Diseases.* **69**: 1889–1890.

16 Elkalioubie A *et al.* (2011) Near-fatal tramadol cardiotoxicity in a CYP2D6 ultrarapid metabolizer. *European Journal of Clinical Pharmacology*. **67**: 855–858.
17 Orliaguet G *et al.* (2015) A case of respiratory depression in a child with ultrarapid CYP2D6 metabolism after tramadol. *Pediatrics*. **135**: e753–e755.
18 Duehmke RM (2017) Tramadol for neuropathic pain in adults. *Cochrane Database of Systematic Reviews*. **6**: CD003726. www.cochranelibrary.com.
19 Watson C and Babul N (1998) Efficacy of oxycodone in neuropathic pain: a randomized trial in postherpetic neuralgia. *Neurology*. **50**: 1837–1841.
20 Szekely SM and Vickers MD (1992) A comparison of the effects of codeine and tramadol on laryngeal reactivity. *European Journal of Anaesthesiology*. **9**: 111–120.
21 Louly PG *et al.* (2009) N-of-1 double-blind, randomized controlled trial of tramadol to treat chronic cough. *Clinical Therapeutics*. **31**: 1007–1013.
22 Houmes R *et al.* (1992) Efficacy and safety of tramadol versus morphine for moderate and severe postoperative pain with special regard to respiratory depression. *Anesthesia and Analgesia*. **74**: 510–514.
23 Wilder-Smith C and Bettiga A (1997) The analgesic tramadol has minimal effect on gastrointestinal motor function. *British Journal of Clinical Pharmacology*. **43**: 71–75.
24 Wilder-Smith CH *et al.* (1999) Effect of tramadol and morphine on pain and gastrointestinal motor function in patients with chronic pancreatitis. *Digestive Diseases and Sciences*. **44**: 1107–1116.
25 Wilder-Smith C *et al.* (2001) Treatment of severe pain from osteoarthritis with slow-release tramadol or dihydrocodeine in combination with NSAID's: a randomised study comparing analgesia, antinociception and gastrointestinal effects. *Pain*. **91**: 23–31.
26 Rodriguez RF *et al.* (2007) Incidence of weak opioids adverse events in the management of cancer pain: a double-blind comparative trial. *Journal of Palliative Medicine*. **10**: 56–60.
27 Wu SD *et al.* (2004) Effects of narcotic analgesic drugs on human Oddi's sphincter motility. *World Journal of Gastroenterology*. **10**: 2901–2904.
28 Preston K *et al.* (1991) Abuse potential and pharmacological comparison of tramadol and morphine. *Drug and Alcohol Dependency*. **27**: 7–18.
29 Soyka M *et al.* (2004) Tramadol use and dependence in chronic noncancer pain patients. *Pharmacopsychiatry*. **37**: 191–192.
30 FDA (2010) Safety alerts for human medical products Ultram (tramadol hydrochloride), Ultracet (tramadol hydrochloride/ acetaminophen). www.fda.gov (accessed 10th Aug 2010)
31 Vickers M *et al.* (1992) Tramadol: pain relief by an opioid without depression of respiration. *Anaesthesia*. **47**: 291–296.
32 Naguib M *et al.* (1998) Perioperative antinociceptive effects of tramadol. A prospective, randomized, double-blind comparison with morphine. *Canadian Journal of Anaesthesia*. **45**: 1168–1175.
33 Pang WW *et al.* (1999) Comparison of patient-controlled analgesia (PCA) with tramadol or morphine. *Canadian Journal of Anaesthesia*. **46**: 1030–1035.
34 Leppert W (2001) Analgesic efficacy and side effects of oral tramadol and morphine administered orally in the treatment of cancer pain. *Nowotwory*. **51**: 257–266.
35 Wilder-Smith CH *et al.* (1994) Oral tramadol, a mu-opioid agonist and monoamine reuptake-blocker, and morphine for strong cancer-related pain. *Annals of Oncology*. **5**: 141–146.
36 Tawfik MO *et al.* (1990) Tramadol hydrochloride in the relief of cancer pain: a double blind comparison against sustained release morphine. *Pain*. **41 (Suppl 1)**: S377.
37 Leppert W and Luczak J (2005) The role of tramadol in cancer pain treatment--a review. *Supportive Care in Cancer*. **13**: 5–17.
38 Grond S *et al.* (1999) High-dose tramadol in comparison to low-dose morphine for cancer pain relief. *Journal of Pain and Symptom Management*. **18**: 174–179.
39 Palliativedrugs.com (2008) Tramadol - What is your experience? *March/April Survey*. www.palliativedrugs.com.
40 Gibson T (1996) Pharmacokinetics, efficacy, and safety of analgesia with a focus on tramadol HCl. *American Journal of Medicine*. **101 (Suppl 1A)**: 47s–53s.
41 Mercadante S *et al.* (2005) Randomized double-blind, double-dummy crossover clinical trial of oral tramadol versus rectal tramadol administration in opioid-naive cancer patients with pain. *Supportive Care in Cancer*. **13**: 702–707.
42 Lintz W *et al.* (1998) Pharmacokinetics of tramadol and bioavailability of enteral tramadol formulations. 3rd Communication: suppositories. *Arzneimittelforschung*. **48**: 889–899.
43 FDA (2017) FDA restricts use of prescription codeine pain and cough medicines and tramadol pain medicines in children; recommend against use in breastfeeding women. *Drug Safety Communication*. www.fda.gov/drugs/drugsafety.
44 Boyd IW (2005) Tramadol and seizures. *Medical Journal of Australia*. **182**: 595–596.
45 Spiller HA *et al.* (1997) Prospective multicenter evaluation of tramadol exposure. *Journal of Toxicology and Clinical Toxicology*. **35**: 361–364.
46 Close BR (2005) Tramadol: does it have a role in emergency medicine? *Emergency Medicine Australasia*. **17**: 73–83.
47 Park SH *et al.* (2014) Serotonin syndrome: is it a reason to avoid the use of tramadol with antidepressants? *Journal of Pharmacy Practice*. **27**: 71–78.
48 Fournier JP *et al.* (2015) Tramadol use and the risk of hospitalization for hypoglycemia in patients with noncancer pain. *JAMA Internal Medicine*. **175**: 186–193.
49 Odonkor CA and Chhatre A (2016) What's tramadol got to do with it? A case report of rebound hypoglycemia, a reappraisal and review of potential mechanisms. *Pain Physician*. **19**: e1215–e1220.
50 Makunts T *et al.* (2019) Retrospective analysis reveals significant association of hypoglycemia with tramadol and methadone in contrast to other opioids. *Scientific Reports*. **9**: 12490.
51 MHRA (2020) Benzodiazepines and opioids: reminder of risk of potentially fatal respiratory depression. *Drug Safety Update*. www.gov.uk/drug-safety-update.
52 Pilgrim JL *et al.* (2011) Deaths involving contraindicated and inappropriate combinations of serotonergic drugs. *International Journal of Legal Medicine*. **125**: 803–815.
53 Saarikoski T *et al.* (2013) Rifampicin markedly decreases the exposure to oral and intravenous tramadol. *European Journal of Clinical Pharmacology*. **69**: 1293–1301.
54 Laugesen S *et al.* (2005) Paroxetine, a cytochrome P450 2D6 inhibitor, diminishes the stereoselective O-demethylation and reduces the hypoalgesic effect of tramadol. *Clinical Pharmacology and Therapeutics*. **77**: 312–323.
55 Sabbe JR *et al.* (1998) Tramadol-warfarin interaction. *Pharmacotherapy*. **18**: 871–873.
56 Juel J *et al.* (2013) Administration of tramadol or ibuprofen increases the INR level in patients on warfarin. *European Journal of Clinical Pharmacology*. **69**: 291–292.

57 De Witte JL *et al.* (2001) The analgesic efficacy of tramadol is impaired by concurrent administration of ondansetron. *Anesthesia and Analgesia*. **92**: 1319–1321.
58 Arcioni R *et al.* (2002) Ondansetron inhibits the analgesic effects of tramadol: a possible 5-HT(3) spinal receptor involvement in acute pain in humans. *Anesthesia and Analgesia*. **94**: 1553–1557.
59 Rauers NI *et al.* (2010) Antagonistic effects of ondansetron and tramadol? A randomized placebo and active drug controlled study. *Journal of Pain*. **11**: 1274–1281.
60 Gautam SK *et al.* (2013) Urinary incontinence induced by tramadol. *Indian Journal of Palliative Care*. **19**: 76–77.
61 King S *et al.* (2011) A systematic review of the use of opioid medication for those with moderate to severe cancer pain and renal impairment: A European palliative care research collaborative opioid guidelines project. *Palliative Medicine*. **25**: 525–552.
62 Senay EC *et al.* (2003) Physical dependence on Ultram (tramadol hydrochloride): both opioid-like and atypical withdrawal symptoms occur. *Drug Alcohol Dependence*. **69**: 233–241.
63 Rajabizadeh G *et al.* (2009) Psychosis following Tramadol Withdrawal. *Addiction and Health*. **1**: 58–61.

Updated September 2021

STRONG OPIOIDS

This chapter focuses on the use of opioids in advanced cancer, where most (but not all) pains are opioid-responsive.[1] The management of chronic non-cancer pain is *not* covered.

Contra-indications: Provided the dose of an opioid is carefully titrated against the patient's pain, there are generally no absolute contra-indications to the use of strong opioids for cancer pain. However, there are circumstances, e.g. renal or hepatic impairment, when it may be better to avoid the use of certain opioids and/or positively choose certain other ones (also see Chapter 17, p.743 and Chapter 18, p.762).

Chemical classes

Opioids can be divided into four chemical classes (Table 1). Knowledge of the different chemical classes is of value when dealing with cases of intolerance to a particular opioid, e.g. cutaneous histamine release causing a rash and pruritus. However, in many situations switching from one phenanthrene to another phenanthrene is satisfactory, e.g. neurotoxicity (see p.398).

Table 1 Chemical classification of opioids

Phenanthrenes	*Benzomorphans*	*Phenylpiperidines*	*Diphenylheptanes*
Codeine	Diphenoxylate	Fentanils	Dextropropoxyphene
Dextromethorphan	Loperamide	Pethidine[a]	Methadone
Dihydrocodeine	Pentazocine[a]		
Hydrocodone			
Tramadol			
Morphine			
Diamorphine			
Buprenorphine			
Hydromorphone			
Oxycodone			
Oxymorphone			
Tapentadol			

a. *not* recommended for use in palliative care.

Opioid receptors

There are four main opioid receptors (μ, κ, δ and nociceptin opioid peptide, NOP) distributed in varying densities throughout the body, particularly in nervous tissue. Their naturally occurring ligands are opioid peptides, and together they contribute to various physiological functions including the modulation of pain, hormones and the immune system (Table 2).[2,3]

In nervous tissue, opioid peptides function as neurotransmitters. Like other peptides, they are synthesized as large inactive precursors in the neuronal cell body, and are then cleaved while being transported to the nerve terminals. The active fragment is released into the synapse and binds to one or more receptors.

Opioid receptors are found both pre- and post-synaptically, with the former predominating, controlling the release of several neurotransmitters. Endogenous peptides are rapidly degraded and have a relatively short duration of action. In contrast, exogenous opioids such as **morphine** have a prolonged effect. They produce analgesia primarily by interacting with μ-opioid receptors in the CNS, e.g. in the dorsal horn of the spinal cord and peri-aqueductal grey area of the midbrain.

Opioid receptors, synthesized in the dorsal root ganglion, are transported to peripheral as well as central nerve terminals. In the presence of tissue injury and inflammation, the number of peripheral opioid receptors increases, and exogenous and endogenous opioids (released by activated inflammatory cells in close proximity to nerve fibres) thereby exert a peripheral analgesic action. Conversely, in bone and neuropathic pain, opioid receptor expression is reduced, contributing towards a reduced response to opioids.[4,5]

All clinically important opioid analgesics act as agonists at the μ-opioid receptor, which is also responsible for typical opioid undesirable effects (Table 2). In an attempt to reduce the latter, broad-spectrum opioid agonists, active at two or more receptor subtypes, are in development. One that has reached clinical trials, **cebranopadol** (a μ-opioid and NOP-receptor agonist), is yet to demonstrate a clear advantage beyond a possible ceiling effect for respiratory depression (similar to **buprenorphine**).[6–8]

Some opioids are mixed agonist–antagonists, e.g. **buprenorphine** is a *partial agonist* at the μ-opioid and NOP receptors, and an *antagonist* at the κ- and δ-opioid receptors.[9,10] (Note. At usual analgesic doses, **buprenorphine** acts as a *full* μ agonist; see p.428.)

Undesirable effects generally relate to both central and peripheral μ-opioid receptor activation, mainly in the CNS and GI tract.

Some opioids also possess non-opioid activity. Thus, **methadone** (p.469) blocks the pre-synaptic re-uptake of serotonin and the NMDA-receptor–channel, **tapentadol** (p.487) blocks re-uptake of noradrenaline (norepinephrine), and **tramadol** (p.383) blocks re-uptake of both serotonin and noradrenaline.

Opioid receptors are G-protein-coupled receptors. In the absence of a ligand, the receptor constantly oscillates through a range of possible active and inactive states. Once an opioid agonist binds to the receptor, conformational changes occur allowing interaction with a G protein which subsequently dissociates into its various subunits responsible for multiple 'downstream' effects. For example, in opioid-related analgesia, the G protein is inhibitory ($G_{i/o}$) and its subunits close Ca^{2+} and other ion channels, open rectifying K^+ channels, and reduce cyclic adenosine monophosphate production, thereby reducing neurotransmitter release and nerve impulse transmission. Several kinase cascades are also activated, e.g. signal-regulated kinase (ERK1/2), c-Jun N-terminal kinases (JNKs) and AKT/protein kinase B, which have a wide impact on cell function, e.g. through changes in protein expression and receptor activation. Conversely, some G proteins (G_s) have stimulatory (pronociceptive) effects, which may play a role in opioid-induced hyperalgesia (see p.398).

Following agonist binding and G-protein activation, the opioid receptor is phosphorylated, enhancing the binding of the protein β-arrestin2. This prevents G-protein coupling and facilitates receptor internalization (for recycling or destruction), desensitizing the receptor and contributing towards the development of tolerance. Further, β-arrestin2 also independently modulates cell signalling and this may also contribute towards tolerance and other undesirable effects of opioids, e.g. constipation, respiratory depression (based on receptor knock-out studies in rodents, but findings inconsistent).[11,12] This has led to the development of μ-opioid biased agonists which show functional selectivity: i.e. although activating the same receptor, they evoke different signalling cascades, probably through the induction of different receptor conformations.[13] Thus, **oliceridine** stimulates μ-opioid receptor coupling with G proteins as usual, but subsequently less phosphorylation and recruitment of β-arrestin2. Developed as an IV formulation, **oliceridine** is a potent opioid with a rapid onset but short duration of effect, best suited to PCA delivery (improved tolerability seen via PCA, but not with regular bolus dosing).[14,15] It is authorized in the USA for acute severe pain.

Thus, the pharmacology of opioid receptors is complex. Further, opioid receptors have additional (allosteric) binding sites which can modulate their function, and they can exist as:

- homodimers, e.g. two μ-opioid receptors
- heterodimers, with another opioid receptor, e.g. μ–δ, δ–κ, or non-opioid receptor, e.g. μ–$5HT_{1A}$, μ–D_1, δ–CB_1, μ–σ_1
- 'splice variants' of the μ-opioid receptor, with one, six and seven transmembrane proteins.

Table 2 Opioid receptors, ligands[16] and effects[a]

Receptors	*Mu (μ)*	*Delta (δ)*	*Kappa (κ)*	*Nociceptin opioid peptide (NOP)*
Endogenous opioid	β-Endorphin Endormorphins	Enkephalins	Dynorphins	Nociceptin
Exogenous agonist	Morphine Buprenorphine[b] Codeine Dextropropoxphene Diamorphine Dihydrocodeine Fentanils Hydromorphone Methadone[c] Oxycodone Pethidine Tapentadol[c] Tramadol[c]	DSTBULET	U50488H Pentazocine	Buprenorphine[b]
Antagonists	Naloxone Naltrexone Pentazocine	Buprenorphine Naloxone	Buprenorphine Naloxone	
Effector mechanism	G protein opens K^+ channel	G protein opens K^+ channel	G protein closes Ca^{++} channel	G protein opens K^+ channel
Effects[d]	*Hyperpolarization of neurons, inhibition of neurotransmitter release*			
	Analgesia Euphoria Nausea Constipation Cough suppression Dependence Respiratory depression Miosis	Similar to μ but less marked	Analgesia Aversion Diuresis Dysphoria	Mixed analgesia (spinal) and anti-analgesia (brain)

a. also see individual drug monographs
b. partial agonist. Note. At usual analgesic doses, buprenorphine behaves as a full μ agonist; see p.428
c. non-opioid effects also contribute towards analgesia (see text)
d. not an exhaustive list; other roles include hormone and immune system regulation.

All are considered potential targets for novel analgesic approaches.[13]

Finally, genetic variation in the μ-opioid receptor gene may contribute to inter-individual response to opioids (see Chapter 19, p.781).

Clinical use

The focus of this section of *PCF* is on the use of strong opioids for *cancer* pain. Because the use of strong opioids for chronic *non-cancer* pain is generally associated with lower benefits and higher risks,[17,18] specialist advice should be followed (e.g. Faculty of Pain Medicine)[19] and/or sought from chronic pain teams.

Based on familiarity, availability and cost, **morphine** (p.404) is the strong opioid of choice for moderate–severe cancer pain management.[20-24] Other strong opioids are used mostly when:

- **morphine** is not readily available
- the TD route is preferable (**buprenorphine, fentanyl**)
- the patient has severe renal impairment or ESRF (see p.743)
- the patient has unacceptable undesirable effects with **morphine** (e.g. use **oxycodone**).[20]

Some patients report better pain relief after switching opioids (see p.400). Similarly, the pattern and severity of undesirable effects may be altered, e.g. when switching from **morphine** to **oxycodone** (p.480) or TD **fentanyl** (p.440). Explanations for these observations include differences between opioids in their pharmacology, intrinsic activity at different opioid receptor subtypes, and the plasticity of the response of the opioid receptor to different ligands (see p.389).

Methadone (p.469), **tapentadol** (p.487) and **tramadol** (p.383) have opioid and non-opioid effects which, in the case of **tapentadol** and **tramadol**, are analgesically synergistic.

Strong opioids are not the panacea for cancer pain; effective analgesia generally requires the use of both a strong opioid and a non-opioid. Further, even combined use does not guarantee success, particularly with neuropathic pain or if the psychosocial dimension of pain and suffering is ignored. Other reasons for poor relief include:

- underdosing (failure to titrate the dose upwards or dose at the correct interval)
- poor patient adherence (patient not taking medication)
- poor alimentary absorption (e.g. because of vomiting).

Pentazocine should *not* be used; it is a weak opioid by mouth[25,26] and often causes undesirable psychotropic effects (dysphoria, depersonalization, frightening dreams, hallucinations).[27] **Pethidine** also should *not* be used (Box A).

The dose of strong opioid should be individualized by careful titration against the patient's pain. Once an effective dose is determined, the regular dose should be rationalized as far as possible, e.g. by conversion to m/r products. P.r.n. doses should also be prescribed for break-through pain (see p.323). Both the pain and use of p.r.n. medications should be reviewed regularly.

Although branded and generic versions of the same PO opioid formulations are often bio-equivalent, names and appearances vary. In addition, for some opioids, a wide range of different formulations are available, some of which are not interchangeable or have different durations of action (see Cautions). Consequently, to reduce the risk of error and avoid confusing patients and carers, prescribing by brand for oral m/r products, transmucosal and transdermal products is recommended.[28,29]

Cautions

Because of reports of serious incidents and the potential for toxicity with strong opioids, diligent prescribing, dispensing, administration, monitoring and counselling are required to reduce the risk of error and/or confusion, particularly between:

- immediate-release and m/r products
- products with different durations of action, e.g. 12-hourly vs. 24-hourly m/r products, 7-day vs. 3- or 4-day transdermal patches
- products with both low- and high-strength concentrates, e.g. oral solutions, injections
- products with different bio-availabilities that are not interchangeable, e.g. **fentanyl** transmucosal products.

Also see individual monographs.

Because of the wide number of different formulations and brands available, prescribing by brand for PO m/r, transmucosal and transdermal products is recommended to reduce the risk of error and/or avoid confusing patients and carers.

All opioids can impair driving ability, and patients should be counselled accordingly. Further, **morphine**, **diamorphine** and **methadone** are included in a law in England, Scotland and Wales relating to driving with certain drugs above specified plasma concentrations (see Chapter 22, p.809).

Box A Pethidine

The use of pethidine is actively discouraged in palliative care.

Pethidine is a synthetic μ agonist. In typical doses PO, it is little more than a weak opioid (Table 3, p.401). It has a relatively short duration of action (2–3h) and is thus a bad choice for round-the-clock analgesia.

Pethidine has a toxic metabolite, norpethidine, which accumulates when pethidine is given regularly. Particularly in renal impairment, norpethidine causes tremors, multifocal myoclonus, agitation and, occasionally, seizures.[30]

Pethidine:

- is not antitussive
- is less constipating than morphine but causes more vomiting
- causes less smooth muscle spasm (e.g. sphincter of Oddi)
- is antimuscarinic (anticholinergic)
- is associated with a higher risk of postoperative delirium compared with other opioids[31]
- does not cause constriction of the pupils.

Drug–drug interaction with:

- phenobarbital
- chlorpromazine
- MAOIs

} increased production of norpethidine.

Serotonin toxicity

Pethidine must not be given concurrently with an MAOI because of the risk of serotonin toxicity (see Antidepressants, Box A, p.217).[32-34]

Overdose and effect of naloxone

Overdose is a mixed picture of CNS depression (pethidine) and excitation (norpethidine), with both stupor and seizures. Naloxone will reverse the pethidine-induced stupor but not the stimulant effects of norpethidine. Seizures should be treated with a benzodiazepine (see p.170).

Renal or hepatic impairment

Opioids differ in their potential to cause toxicity when renal or hepatic function is impaired. For general information on the choice of opioids and use in severe renal impairment and ESRF, or severe hepatic impairment, see Chapter 17, p.743 and Chapter 18, p.762.

When there is an *acute* deterioration in renal or hepatic function, an opioid may rapidly accumulate because of reduced excretion or metabolism (see individual monographs, also p.731 and p.753); consider a dose reduction pre-emptively, and always when there is evidence of toxicity, e.g. sedation, myoclonus, delirium. When toxicity is moderate–severe, e.g. marked sedation, respiratory depression (see QCG: Reversal of opioid-induced respiratory depression, p.498), discontinue the regular opioid and allow only a reduced p.r.n. dose. Subsequently, if the situation stabilizes/improves, a regular dose can be restarted based on p.r.n. use. Alternatively, consider a switch to a renally/hepatically safer opioid according to circumstances.

Drug interactions

Concurrent treatment with ≥2 CNS depressants (e.g. benzodiazepines, gabapentinoids, opioids) increases the risk of respiratory depression, particularly in susceptible groups, e.g. the elderly and those with renal or hepatic impairment.[35]

Many opioids are metabolized by the CYP450 enzyme pathway (see Chapter 19, Table 1, p.783), and interactions may occur with drugs that induce or inhibit these enzymes (see the individual monographs and also Chapter 19, Table 8, p.790).

For opioids associated with serotonin toxicity, see below.

Undesirable effects

Strong opioids tend to cause the same undesirable effects (Box B), although to a varying degree. Strategies are necessary to deal with them, particularly nausea and vomiting (see QCG: Nausea and vomiting, p.264) and constipation (see QCG: Opioid-induced constipation, p.45).[36] For opioid-induced pruritus, see Chapter 26, p.825.

Box B Undesirable effects of opioids when used for cancer pain

Common initial
Nausea and vomiting[a]
Drowsiness
Light-headedness/unsteadiness
Delirium (acute confusional state)

Common ongoing
Constipation
Nausea and vomiting[a]
Dry mouth

Possible ongoing
Suppression of hypothalamic–pituitary axis
Suppression of immune system

Less common
Neurotoxicity:
- hyperalgesia
- allodynia
- myoclonus
- cognitive failure/delirium
- hallucinations

Sweating
Urinary retention
Postural hypotension
Spasm of the sphincter of Oddi
Pruritus (see Chapter 26, p.825)

Rare
Respiratory depression
Psychological dependence
Allergy[b]

a. generally, opioid-related nausea and vomiting is transient and improves after 5–7 days; if persistent despite an anti-emetic (see QCG: Nausea and vomiting, p.264), consider other possible causes before switching to another opioid (see p.400)

b. true IgE-mediated anaphylaxis is very rare and many reports of 'allergy' are an intolerance to an undesirable effect. However, opioids can directly trigger the release of histamine from mast cells, leading to, e.g. pruritus, rash.

Respiratory depression

When appropriately titrated against the patient's pain, strong opioids do not cause clinically important respiratory depression in patients in pain.[37-39] Strong opioids also relieve moderate–severe breathlessness at rest at doses which do not cause respiratory depression (see p.412).

Naloxone, a specific opioid antagonist, is rarely needed in palliative care (see p.490). In contrast to postoperative patients, cancer patients with pain:

- may have been receiving a weak opioid for some time, i.e. are not opioid-naïve
- generally take opioids PO (slower absorption, lower peak concentration)
- titrate the dose upwards step by step (less likelihood of an excessive dose being given).

The relationship of the therapeutic dose to the lethal dose of a strong opioid (the therapeutic ratio) is greater than commonly supposed. For example, patients who take a double dose of immediate-release **morphine** at bedtime are no more likely to die during the night than those who do not.[40]

Nonetheless, there is an association between the use of opioids and sleep-disordered breathing, e.g. nocturnal apnoeas resulting in hypoxaemia.[41] Opioids cause this by reducing the central respiratory drive and/or relaxing the upper airway. It appears to be common, with central apnoeas affecting half of patients in one study (all receiving a **morphine**-equivalent dose >100mg/24h PO), which resolved completely when the opioid was stopped.[41] The SPCs of several opioids now caution about the increased risk of causing or worsening sleep-disordered breathing. Although the full clinical relevance is unknown, it has been suggested as an explanation for the increased deaths and cardiovascular events reported in patients receiving opioids, and as another reason to avoid opioids when possible in chronic non-cancer pain.[41]

Tolerance and dependence

Generally, tolerance to strong opioids is not a practical problem in pain due to advanced cancer.[42,43] In the absence of cancer progression, doses tend to remain stable (an increasing requirement should raise the possibility of either opioid-poorly responsive pain and/or opioid-induced hyperalgesia, see below). The development of physical dependence does not prevent a reduction in the dose if the patient's pain ameliorates, e.g. as a result of radiotherapy or a nerve block.[44]

Psychological dependence (addiction) to **morphine** is rare in patients with cancer pain.[39,45,46] Greatest caution in this respect should be reserved for patients with a present or past history of substance abuse; even then, strong opioids should be used when there is clinical need.[47] Nonetheless, sensible precautions include the provision of opioid by a single prescriber, close liaison with addiction medicine services and the use of an opioid contract (Box C).

On the other hand, preliminary data from a cancer centre in the USA found that about one fifth of patients with cancer pain exhibited behaviours associated with non-medical opioid use (i.e. the use of opioids without a prescription or in ways other than medically prescribed), e.g. frequent early requests for repeat prescriptions, excessive self-escalation of dose. The extent to which this is explained by pre-existing substance abuse is unclear.[48]

However, with the dramatic increase in the use of opioids for chronic *non-cancer* pain, there have been corresponding increases in rates of misuse, abuse and addiction, along with fatal overdose, particularly with concurrent benzodiazepine use.[35,50–52] Further, deaths from causes other than overdose are also increased.[53] These concerns have led to a re-appraisal of the place of opioids in chronic non-cancer pain and to the introduction of opioid products that reduce abuse potential. For example, some m/r products form insoluble precipitates if an attempt is made to crush and dissolve them, preventing their injection.[54] Others contain a sequestered opioid antagonist which, if the tablet is crushed or dissolved, is released in sufficient amounts to antagonize the opioid and prevent a 'high' (see p.490).

For the use of strong opioids for chronic non-cancer pain, specialist advice should be followed (e.g. Faculty of Pain Medicine)[19] and/or sought from chronic pain teams.

Opioid-related serotonin toxicity

Serotonin toxicity results from the ingestion of drug(s) which increase brain serotonin above a critical level (see Antidepressants, Box A, p.217). Toxicity manifests as a triad of neuro-excitatory features:

- *autonomic hyperactivity:* sweating, fever, mydriasis, tachycardia, hypertension, tachypnoea, sialorrhoea, diarrhoea
- *neuromuscular hyperactivity:* tremor, clonus, myoclonus, hyperreflexia, pyramidal rigidity (advanced stage)
- *altered mental status:* agitation, hypomania, delirium (advanced stage).

Clonus (inducible, spontaneous or ocular), agitation, sweating, tremor and hyperreflexia are essential features.

Opioids are relatively weak serotonin re-uptake inhibitors and only cause symptoms in higher doses or susceptible individuals or when used concurrently with a second drug with serotoninergic potency, notably an MAOI but also with many other antidepressants and some psychostimulants (see Antidepressants, Box A, p.217).

Fatalities from serotonin toxicity have occurred with **dextromethorphan**, **pethidine** (Box A), **tramadol**, and possibly **fentanyl** when used in conjunction with an MAOI.[55] Non-fatal serotonin toxicity has also been observed with other fentanils, **dextropropoxyphene**, **methadone**, **pentazocine** and **tapentadol**. Concurrent administration of these opioids with an MAOI (or within 2 weeks of cessation of an MAOI) is generally best avoided (also see Antidepressants, Box A, p.217).

Box C Example of a contract for controlled substance prescriptions with addicts[a]

Controlled substance medications (narcotics, tranquillizers and barbiturates) are very useful, but have high potential for misuse and are therefore closely controlled by the local, state, and federal government. They are intended to relieve pain, to improve function and/or ability to work, not simply to feel good. Because my physician is prescribing such medication for me to help manage my condition, I agree to the following conditions:

1 I am responsible for my controlled substance medications. If the prescription of medication is lost, misplaced, or stolen, or if I use it up sooner than prescribed, I understand that it will not be replaced.

2 I will not request or accept controlled substance medication from any other physicians or individual while I am receiving such medication from Dr.________________. Besides being illegal to do so, it may endanger my health. The only exception is if it is prescribed while I am admitted in a hospital.

3 Refills of controlled substance medication:

- Will be made only during Dr.________________ regular office hours, in person, once each month during a scheduled office visit. Refills will not be made at night, on holidays, or weekends.
- Will not be made if I "run out early". I am responsible for taking the medication in the dose prescribed and for keeping track of the amount remaining.
- Will not be made as an "emergency", such as on Friday afternoon because I suddenly realize I will "run out tomorrow". I will call at least seventy-two hours ahead if I need assistance with a controlled substance medication prescription.

4 I will bring in the containers of all medications prescribed by Dr.________________ each time I see him even if there is no medication remaining. These will be in the original containers from the pharmacy for each medication.

5 I understand that if I violate any of the above conditions, my controlled substances prescription and/or treatment with Dr.________________ may be ended immediately. If the violation involves obtaining controlled substances from another individual, as described above, I may also be reported to my physician, medical facilities, and other authorities.

6 I understand that the main treatment goal is to improve my ability to function and/or work. In consideration of that goal and the fact that I am being given potent medication to help me reach that goal, I agree to help myself by the following better health habits: exercise, weight control, and the non-use of tobacco and alcohol. I understand that only through following a healthier life-style can I hope to have the most successful outcome to my treatment.

I have been fully informed by Dr.________________ and his staff regarding psychological dependence (addiction) of a controlled substance, which I understand is rare. I know that some persons may develop a tolerance, which is the need to increase the dose of the medication to achieve the same effect of pain control, and I do know that I will become physically dependent on the medication. This will occur if I am on the medication for several weeks, and, when I stop the medication, I must do so slowly and under medical supervision or I may have withdrawal symptoms.

I have read this contract and it has been explained to me by Dr.________________ and/ or his staff. In addition, I fully understand the consequences of violating said contract.

Patient's Signature	Date	Witness	Date

a. reproduced with permission from Hansen 1999.[49] © Southern Medical Association.

The onset of toxicity is generally rapid and progressive, typically as the second drug reaches effective blood levels (one or two doses). Occasionally, recurrent mild symptoms may occur for weeks before the development of severe toxicity. The patient is often alert or agitated, with tremor (sometimes severe), myoclonus and hyperreflexia. Ankle clonus is generally demonstrable or, in severe toxicity, occurs spontaneously. Neuromuscular signs are initially greater in the lower limbs then become more generalized as toxicity increases. Other symptoms include shaking, shivering (often including chattering of the teeth), and sometimes trismus. Pyramidal rigidity is a late development in severe cases and can impair respiration. Rigidity, a fever of >38.5°C or deteriorating blood gases indicate life-threatening toxicity.

Opioid-induced endocrinopathy

Opioids are associated with wide-ranging dose-related endocrine effects, including interference with the production of various hypothalamic, pituitary, gonadal and adrenal hormones, e.g.:[56-61]

- inhibition of gonadotrophin-releasing hormone from the hypothalamus:
  - ▷ ↓ luteinizing hormone (LH) release from the pituitary → ↓ production of testosterone (testes) or oestrogen (ovaries)
  - ▷ ↓ follicle-stimulating hormone (FSH) release from the pituitary → ↓ production of sperm or ovarian follicles
  - ▷ associated with loss of libido, impotence, irregular menses or amenorrhoea, subfertility and other consequences of hypogonadism, e.g. reduced muscle mass, osteoporosis, fatigue
- inhibition of adrenocorticotrophic hormone (ACTH) from the pituitary:
  - ▷ ↓ cortisol production and release (adrenals)
  - ▷ ↓ androgen release (adrenals); an important source in women, also converted to oestrogens
  - ▷ associated with symptoms such as fatigue, weight loss, anorexia, vomiting, diarrhoea, abdominal pain, hypoglycaemia, hypotension, and those caused by sex hormone deficiency (see above)
- inhibition of growth hormone from the pituitary:
  - ▷ associated with decreased cognitive function and possibly other effects.

In patients with chronic non-cancer pain, hormone suppression is evident after 1 week of opioid administration and appears dose-related. In one study, abnormally low levels of sex hormones were found in three-quarters of men receiving opioids equivalent to **morphine** <150mg/24h PO, and in all receiving >150mg/24h PO.[62] The risk appears greater with m/r compared with immediate-release formulations; it is hypothesized that the greater fluctuation in plasma opioid level with the latter results in only intermittent inhibition of endocrine function.[63] Adrenal insufficiency also appears dose-related; in one study, it was absent in patients taking an opioid equivalent to **morphine** <60mg/24h PO, increasing to 50% of those receiving >200mg/24h PO.[64] Hypocortisolism sufficient to cause Addisonian crisis has been reported with opioids given PO, TD and IT.[65]

IT **morphine** (mean doses 5–12mg/24h) produced hypogonadism in most subjects, both men and women.[66–68] In one study, one third of patients also developed hypocortisolism ± growth hormone deficiency, leading to an Addisonian crisis in one patient.[66] Thus, in patients due to receive long-term IT opioids, it is recommended to measure sex hormone levels at baseline and annually thereafter (see Chapter 32, Table 4, p.914).

The clinical implications of opioid-induced endocrinopathy in those with advanced life-limiting illnesses is unclear. However, when any patient receiving long-term opioids has symptoms suggestive of an endocrinopathy, it may be necessary to refer to an endocrinologist for investigation and possible replacement hormone therapy.[66] In men receiving opioids for chronic non-cancer pain, sexual function, mood, bone density and pain tolerance can benefit from testosterone replacement.[61,69]

Compared with **morphine** and other opioids, **buprenorphine** (p.428) appears less likely to suppress the gonadal axis or testosterone levels.

If the opioid treatment is stopped, although testosterone levels generally increase within 24–72h, hypogonadism may persist for months–years.

Opioids and immune function

Opioids modulate immune cell function directly (by binding to opioid and Toll-like receptors on immune cells) and indirectly via activation of the hypothalamic–pituitary–adrenal (HPA) axis and the sympathetic nervous system.[70] Immune function is suppressed by the opioid-induced release of glucocorticoids and catecholamines (e.g. adrenaline (epinephrine), noradrenaline (norepinephrine)) from the adrenal medulla, and the release of catecholamines and neuropeptide Y from sympathetic nerve fibres which innervate lymphoid tissue (e.g. lymph nodes, spleen).[70] Thus, in some studies, **morphine** depresses natural killer cell activity, T-lymphocyte proliferation, monocyte/macrophage function and cytokine release function (e.g. interleukin-2, interferon-γ), potentially reducing host resistance to bacterial, fungal and viral infections and impeding cancer immunosurveillance.[71–75] Further, partly through its effects on the immune system, **morphine** can influence cancer cell growth and metastasis. However, it is unclear if the overall effect is beneficial or deleterious.[70] Cancer cells also express opioid receptors, further complicating this area of research. In animal models of cancer, their overexpression is associated with cancer growth and metastasis, with contrasting reports of exogenous opioids either stimulating or inhibiting angiogenesis.[70,76]

Compared with **morphine** (and **diamorphine**), other opioids appear less immunosuppressive.[77–80] In patients with cancer pain, although one small retrospective study found the incidence of infections to be less in those receiving **oxycodone** compared to **morphine**, another found no difference between **fentanyl**, **morphine** and **oxycodone**.[81,82] Nonetheless, there was a dose relationship, with the risk of infection increasing by 2% per 10mg increase in daily oral **morphine**-equivalent dose.[82] Large-cohort studies in a wider population of patients also suggest a dose-related increase in the risk of pneumonia with immunosuppressive opioids (e.g. **morphine**, **fentanyl**).[83]

However, overall, data are limited and inconsistent, and the clinical implications of these effects are uncertain.[79,83] Nonetheless, they may help to explain the increased susceptibility to infection seen in opioid abusers.[84] On the other hand, because pain is immunosuppressive, opioid analgesia may improve immune function in patients with pain.[70,85]

Opioid-induced hyperalgesia

Opioid-induced hyperalgesia (OIH) is an increased response to a painful stimulus, associated with exposure to opioids. Although well demonstrated in animals, the findings in human studies are inconsistent and their relevance debated. In part, this may relate to differences in assessments used and populations studied.[86]

OIH has been shown in both acute and chronic pain and appears to result from sustained sensitization of the nervous system, in which excitatory neurotransmitters and the NMDA-receptor–channel complex play important roles.[87] The exact cause is unclear, but possibly includes the following opioid-related mechanisms:[87–90]

- activation of glial cells (via, e.g. Toll-like (TLR4) receptors), which play a role in inflammation, pain signal transmission, pain hypersensitivity and opioid tolerance
- activation of excitatory pathways, e.g.:
  - ▷ adenylyl cyclase and cyclic adenosine monophosphate levels increase, resulting in greater protein kinase activity, ultimately facilitating pain signal transmission, e.g. through activation of the NMDA-receptor–channel complex
  - ▷ μ-opioid receptors are G-protein-coupled receptors, generally containing 7-transmembrane (7TM) domains and binding with $G_{i/o}$, which leads to an inhibitory effect. Ongoing opioid exposure increases the expression of the splice variant 6TM μ-opioid receptor; this couples to G_s, which leads to an excitatory effect
  - ▷ increased expression/sensitivity of transient receptor potential vanilloid 1 (TRPV1) receptors
- in the case of **morphine**, accumulation of morphine-3-glucuronide, which can activate glial cells via TLR4.

Susceptibility to OIH appears to vary widely, and genetic make-up probably plays an important part in its development.[87,88]

Clinical features

In surgical pain, OIH may contribute to exaggerated levels of pain in the immediate postoperative period and the development of a chronic pain state. In patients with cancer, OIH may manifest in various ways:

- rapidly developing tolerance to opioids
- short-lived benefit from increased doses
- a change of pain pattern (Box D).

OIH probably also contributes towards narcotic bowel syndrome, which presents with chronic or frequently recurring abdominal pain, unexplained by GI pathology; additional features include continuing/progressive pain despite increasing doses of opioids.[91]

Box D Clinical features of opioid-induced hyperalgesia[92]

What the patient says
- increased sensitivity to pain stimulus (hyperalgesia)
- worsening pain despite increasing doses of opioids
- pain which becomes more diffuse, extending beyond the distribution of the pre-existing pain.

What the doctor finds
- any dose of any opioid, but particularly with high-dose morphine or hydromorphone, and in renal impairment
- pain elicited from ordinary non-painful stimuli, e.g. stroking skin with cotton (allodynia)
- presence of other manifestations of opioid-induced neural hyperexcitability, e.g. myoclonus, seizures, delirium.

The extreme upper end of the spectrum may be those patients who manifest evidence of severe neural hyperexcitability (e.g. myoclonus, allodynia, and/or hyperalgesia), particularly when taking high doses of **morphine** or an alternative strong opioid. This may be accompanied by sedation and delirium (when it is often described as opioid neurotoxicity). However, OIH:
- is *not* limited to very high doses or to any one opioid
- is probably under-diagnosed
- is more common than generally thought.

Severe pain that does not respond to increasing doses of opioids, or is complicated by severe undesirable effects, should raise the *possibility* of OIH.[92]

Evaluation

A diagnosis of OIH is generally made on the basis of a high level of clinical suspicion, probability, and pattern recognition. OIH must be differentiated from increased pain caused by disease progression or the development of opioid tolerance, both of which may be managed by increasing the opioid dose.

Management

Management is based largely on theoretical grounds and clinical observation.[87]

Prophylaxis

Use a multimodal approach to analgesia, e.g.:
- an NSAID may help to reduce inflammation and production of excitatory amino acid neurotransmitters which activate the pronociceptive and anti-opioid systems
- **pregabalin** may block calcium channels which may contribute to hyperalgesia in nerve pain.

Treatment
- progressively and rapidly reduce the dose of the causal opioid to about 25% of the peak dose
- switch conservatively (as a dose reduction will likely be needed) to an opioid with less risk of OIH, i.e. **fentanyl** (highest) → **morphine** → **methadone** → **buprenorphine** (lowest)[93]; see Opioid switching below
- (rarely) if OIH occurs at very low doses (e.g. **morphine** <10mg/24h PO), discontinue the opioid completely
- use a multimodal approach to analgesia, i.e. use non-opioids, e.g. **paracetamol** or an NSAID, and adjuvant analgesics, e.g. **pregabalin**
- consider **ketamine** (p.691) an NMDA-receptor–channel blocker.[94]

When switching from **morphine** because of severe neural hyperexcitability, a lower than expected dose of the alternative opioid is likely to be needed unless the dose of **morphine** has recently been much reduced (as suggested above).[95,96]

If these steps do not lead to a resolution of the OIH:

- consider spinal, regional or local analgesia (with local anaesthetics), and tail off systemic opioids completely
- check for hypomagnesaemia because this can aggravate OIH (also see p.638)[97,98]
- consider treatment with ultralow doses of an opioid antagonist (see p.490).[99,100]

Opioid switching ('rotation')

It is crucial to appreciate that conversion ratios are *never* more than an approximate guide. Thus, careful monitoring during conversion is necessary to avoid both underdosing and excessive dosing. For general considerations when switching opioids, see Appendix 2, p.925.

Generally, switching from **morphine** (or another strong opioid) to an alternative is undertaken in an attempt to improve analgesia and/or reduce undesirable effects. It is reported necessary in about 10–44% of patients.[1,101,102] Before switching, it is worth considering if other options may be more appropriate, e.g. the use of adjuvant analgesics or modifying the management of the undesirable effects.

There are a lack of high-quality RCT data to support switching. One open-label prospective study which randomized patients to either **morphine** or **oxycodone** first-line found that about one third required a switch to the alternative opioid, generally for undesirable effects (e.g. drowsiness, nausea/vomiting, confusion/hallucinations); these improved in similar proportions, such that overall, 95% of patients found an effective and tolerable dose of either **morphine** or **oxycodone**. Apart from supporting the use of **morphine** over **oxycodone** first-line (i.e. similar efficacy and tolerability at a lower cost), these findings suggest that only a small proportion of patients (~5%) will require multiple switches in opioid.[103]

Examples of when more specific switches may be appropriate include:

- poor adherence or *intractable* constipation (→ TD **fentanyl**)
- significant decline in the patient's renal function (**morphine** → **alfentanil**, **buprenorphine**, **fentanyl**, **methadone**; see Chapter 17, p.743)
- opioid-induced hyperalgesia or other manifestations of neurotoxicity, e.g. cognitive failure/ delirium, hallucinations, myoclonus, allodynia.

In cases of neurotoxicity, **fentanyl**, **hydromorphone**, **oxycodone** and **methadone** have all been substituted successfully for **morphine**.[104–107] Similarly, in the presence of inadequate pain relief and intolerable undesirable effects, TD **buprenorphine** has been substituted successfully for TD **fentanyl**, and vice versa.[108]

When converting from **morphine** to an alternative strong opioid, or vice versa, the initial dose depends on the relative potency of the two drugs (Table 3; also see Appendix 2, p.925).

However, relative potencies and thus conversion ratios are *never* more than an approximate guide because of:[110–113]

- wide interindividual variation in opioid pharmacokinetics; influencing factors include age, ethnicity, and renal or hepatic impairment
- other variables, including dose and duration of opioid treatment, direction of switch in opioid, nutritional status and concurrent medications
- their method of derivation, e.g. single dose rather than chronic dose studies, using typical doses.

Thus, careful monitoring during conversion is necessary to avoid both underdosing and excessive dosing.

Providing explicit guidance on switching opioids is difficult because the reasons for switching are varied, as are the patients' circumstances. One guideline, based on expert consensus, recommends routinely reducing the calculated equivalent dose of the new opioid by 25–50%.[114] Various patient factors are then taken into account to modify the reduction, which potentially could see it removed (e.g. young patient, no undesirable effects, in severe pain, switching at low dose) or increased further (e.g. older patient, delirious, in moderate pain, switching at high dose).

Certainly, a dose reduction of at least 50% would seem prudent when switching at high doses (e.g. **morphine** or equivalent doses of ≥1g/24h PO), in elderly or frail patients, because of intolerable undesirable effects (e.g. delirium), or when there has been a recent rapid escalation of the first opioid (possibly due to opioid-induced hyperalgesia). In such circumstances, p.r.n. doses can be relied on to make up any deficit while re-titrating to a satisfactory dose of the new opioid.

A separate strategy is necessary for **methadone** (p.469).

5

Table 3 Approximate potency of opioids relative to morphine; PO and immediate-release formulations unless stated otherwise[a]

Analgesic	*Potency relative to morphine*	*Duration of action (h)*[b]
Codeine	1/10	4–6
Dihydrocodeine	1/10	3–6
Tramadol	1/10	4–9
Pethidine	1/8	2–4
Tapentadol	1/3	4–6
Hydrocodone (not UK)	2/3	4–8
Papaveretum	2/3[c]	3–5
Oxycodone	1.5 (2)[d]	4–6
Methadone	5–10[e]	8–12
Hydromorphone	4–5 (5–7.5)[d]	4–5
Buprenorphine (SL)	80	6–8
Buprenorphine (TD)	100 (75–115)[d]	Formulation dependent (72–168)
Fentanyl (TD)	100 (150)[d]	72

a. multiply dose of opioid in first column by relative potency in the second column to determine the equivalent dose of morphine sulfate/hydrochloride; conversely, divide morphine dose by the relative potency to determine the equivalent dose of another opioid

b. dependent in part on severity of pain and on dose; often longer lasting in very elderly and those with renal impairment

c. papaveretum (strong opium) is standardized to contain 50% morphine base; potency expressed in relation to morphine sulfate

d. the numbers in parenthesis are the manufacturers' preferred relative potencies; for explanation of divergence, see individual drug monographs

e. a single 5mg dose of methadone is equivalent to morphine 7.5mg, but a variable long plasma halflife and broad-spectrum receptor affinity result in a much higher than expected relative potency when administered regularly, sometimes much higher than the range given above; *it is essential to read the methadone monograph*, p.469.[95,109]

Combining strong opioids

It is generally considered bad practice to prescribe more than one strong opioid for simultaneous use. Thus, for example, regular **morphine** is best backed up by p.r.n **morphine** for break-through pain (see p.323).

However, there are circumstances when more than one strong opioid may be necessary, for example TD **fentanyl** backed up by p.r.n. **morphine** (see QCG: Use of transdermal fentanyl patches, p.448). Also, someone with good pain relief from a regular weak opioid may have a supply of **morphine** for back-up use in case of severe break-through pain.

There are reports of two strong opioids being used successfully in combination, e.g. providing better pain relief at relatively lower doses and reduced undesirable effects.[115–117] For example, in one, regular **oxycodone** plus p.r.n. **morphine** was more beneficial than regular **morphine** plus p.r.n. **morphine**.[115] In another, patients on regular **morphine** benefited from the addition of a second regular opioid at low dose (either **methadone** or TD **fentanyl**).[116] However, the quality of the evidence is low or very low.[118] Thus, despite such reports, because of the increased complexity and scope for error, unless under specialist supervision, patients should *not* normally have two strong opioids prescribed concurrently on a regular basis.[119,120]

1 Wiffen PJ *et al.* (2017) Opioids for cancer pain - an overview of Cochrane reviews. *Cochrane Database of Systematic Reviews*. **7**: CD012592. www.cochranelibrary.com.

2 Mika J (2008) The opioid systems and the role of glial cells in the effects of opioids. *Advances in Palliative Medicine*. **7**: 185–196.

3 Sauriyal DS *et al.* (2011) Extending pharmacological spectrum of opioids beyond analgesia: Multifunctional aspects in different pathophysiological states. *Neuropeptides*. **45**: 175–188.

4 Zhu C *et al.* (2017) Neuron-restrictive silencer factor-mediated downregulation of mu-opioid receptor contributes to the reduced morphine analgesia in bone cancer pain. *Pain*. **158**: 879–890.

5 Sun L *et al.* (2017) Nerve injury-induced epigenetic silencing of opioid receptors controlled by DNMT3a in primary afferent neurons. *Pain*. **158**: 1153–1165.

6 Eerdekens MH *et al.* (2019) Cancer-related chronic pain: Investigation of the novel analgesic drug candidate cebranopadol in a randomized, double-blind, noninferiority trial. *European Journal of Pain*. **23**: 577–588.

7 Christoph A *et al.* (2017) Cebranopadol, a novel first-in-class analgesic drug candidate: first experience in patients with chronic low back pain in a randomized clinical trial. *Pain*. **158**: 1813–1824.

8 Dahan A *et al.* (2017) Respiratory effects of the nociceptin/orphanin FQ peptide and opioid receptor agonist, cebranopadol, in healthy human volunteers. *Anesthesiology*. **126**: 697–707.

9 Lutfy K *et al.* (2003) Buprenorphine-induced antinociception is mediated by mu-opioid receptors and compromised by concomitant activation of opioid receptor-like receptors. *Journal of Neuroscience*. **23**: 10331–10337.

10 Virk MS *et al.* (2009) Buprenorphine is a weak partial agonist that inhibits opioid receptor desensitization. *Journal of Neuroscience*. **29**: 7341–7348.

11 Siuda ER *et al.* (2017) Biased mu-opioid receptor ligands: a promising new generation of pain therapeutics. *Current Opinion in Pharmacology*. **32**: 77–84.

12 Kliewer A *et al.* (2020) Morphine-induced respiratory depression is independent of ß-arrestin2 signalling. *British Journal of Pharmacology*. **177**: 2923–2931.

13 Olson KM *et al.* (2017) Novel molecular strategies and targets for opioid drug discovery for the treatment of chronic pain. *Yale Journal of Biology and Medicine*. **90**: 97–110.

14 Singla N *et al.* (2017) A randomized, Phase IIb study investigating oliceridine (TRV130), a novel micro-receptor G-protein pathway selective (mu-GPS) modulator, for the management of moderate to severe acute pain following abdominoplasty. *Journal of Pain Research*. **10**: 2413–2424.

15 Viscusi ER *et al.* (2019) APOLLO-1: a randomized placebo and active-controlled phase III study investigating oliceridine (TRV130), a G protein-biased ligand at the micro-opioid receptor, for management of moderate-to-severe acute pain following bunionectomy. *Journal of Pain Research*. **12**: 927–943.

16 McDonald J and Lambert DG (2005) Opioid receptors. Continuing education in anaesthesia. *Critical Care and Pain*. **5**: 22–25.

17 Manchikanti L *et al.* (2017) Responsible, safe, and effective prescription of opioids for chronic non-cancer pain: American Society of Interventional Pain Physicians (ASIPP) guidelines. *Pain Physician*. **20**: S3–S92.

18 Els C *et al.* (2018) Adverse events associated with medium- and long-term use of opioids for chronic non-cancer pain: an overview of Cochrane Reviews. *Cochrane Database of Systematic Reviews*. **10**: CD012509. www.cochranelibrary.com.

19 Faculty of Pain Medicine. Opioids aware: a resource for patients and healthcare professionals to support prescribing of opioid medicines for pain. Available from: www.fpm.ac.uk (accessed February 2022).

20 Caraceni A *et al.* (2012) Use of opioid analgesics in the treatment of cancer pain: evidence-based recommendations from the EAPC. *Lancet Oncology*. **13**: e58–e68.

21 Quigley C (2005) The role of opioids in cancer pain. *British Medical Journal*. **331**: 825–829.

22 NICE (2012) Opioids in palliative care: safe and effective prescribing of strong opioids for pain in palliative care adults. *Clinical Guideline*. CG140 (update 2016) www.nice.org.uk.

23 Fallon M *et al.* (2018) Management of cancer pain in adult patients: ESMO Clinical Practice Guidelines. *Annals of Oncology*. **29 (Suppl 4)**: iv166–iv191.

24 WHO (2019) WHO guidelines for the pharmacological and radiotherapeutic management of cancer pain in adults and adolescents. *World Health Organization*, Geneva. www.who.int.

25 Hoskin P and Hanks G (1991) Opioid agonist-antagonist drugs in acute and chronic pain states. *Drugs*. **41**: 326–344.

26 Twycross RG. Pentazocine. *Pain Relief in Advanced Cancer*. Edinburgh: Churchill Livingstone; 1994. p. 247–248.

27 Woods A *et al.* (1974) Medicines evaluation and monitoring group: central nervous system effects of pentazocine. *British Medical Journal*. **1**: 305–307.

28 Smith J (2004) Building a safer NHS for patients - Improving medication safety. A Report by the Chief Pharmaceutical Officer. Gateway ref 1459. 105–111 Department of Health, London .

29 Care Quality Commission and NHS England (2013) Safer use of controlled drugs - preventing harms from fentanyl and buprenorphine transdermal patches. *Use of controlled drugs supporting information*. www.cqc.org.uk.

30 Plummer JL *et al.* (2001) Norpethidine toxicity. *Pain Reviews*. **8**: 159–170.

31 Swart LM *et al.* (2017) The comparative risk of delirium with different opioids: a systematic review. *Drugs and Aging*. **34**: 437–443.

32 Shee JC (1960) Dangerous potentiation of pethidine by iproniazid, and its treatment. *British Medical Journal*. **ii**: 507–509.

33 Taylor D (1962) Alarming reaction to pethidine in patients on phenelzine. *Lancet*. **2**: 401–402.

34 Rogers KJ and Thornton JA (1969) The interaction between monoamine oxidase inhibitors and narcotic analgesics in mice. *British Journal of Pharmacology*. **36**: 470–480.

35 MHRA (2020) Benzodiazepines and opioids: reminder of risk of potentially fatal respiratory depression. *Drug Safety Update*. www.gov.uk/drug-safety-update.

36 Cherny N *et al.* (2001) Strategies to manage the adverse effects of oral morphine: an evidence-based report. *Journal of Clinical Oncology*. **19**: 2542–2554.

37 Borgbjerg FM *et al.* (1996) Experimental pain stimulates respiration and attenuates morphine-induced respiratory depression: a controlled study in human volunteers. *Pain*. **64**: 123–128.

38 Estfan B *et al.* (2007) Respiratory function during parenteral opioid titration for cancer pain. *Palliative Medicine*. **21**: 81–86.

39 Sykes NP (2007) Morphine kills the pain, not the patient. *Lancet*. **369**: 1325–1326.

40 Regnard CFB and Badger C (1987) Opioids, sleep and the time of death. *Palliative Medicine*. **1**: 107–110.

41 Schwarzer A *et al.* (2015) Sleep-disordered breathing decreases after opioid withdrawal: results of a prospective controlled trial. *Pain*. **156**: 2167–2174.

42 Collin E *et al.* (1993) Is disease progression the major factor in morphine 'tolerance' in cancer pain treatment? *Pain*. **55**: 319–326.

43 Portenoy RK (1994) Tolerance to opioid analgesics: clinical aspects. *Cancer Surveys*. **21**: 49–65.

44 Twycross RG and Wald SJ. Longterm use of diamorphine in advanced cancer. In: Bonica JJ, Albe-Fessard D, editors. *Advances in Pain Research and Therapy*. 1. New York: Raven Press; 1976. p. 653–661.

45 Passik S and Portenoy R. Substance abuse issues in palliative care. In: Berger A, editor. *Principles and Practice of Supportive Oncology*. Philadelphia: Lippincott-Raven; 1998. p. 513–529.

46 Joranson D *et al.* (2000) Trends in medical use and abuse of opioid analgesics. *Journal of the American Medical Association*. **283**: 1710–1714.
47 Arthur J and Bruera E (2019) Balancing opioid analgesia with the risk of nonmedical opioid use in patients with cancer. *Nature Reviews Clinical Oncology*. **16**: 213–226.
48 Yennurajalingham S *et al.* (2021) Frequency of and factors associated with nonmedical opioid use behavior among patients with cancer receiving opioids for cancer pain. *JAMA Oncology*. **7**: 404–411.
49 Hansen H (1999) Treatment of chronic pain with antiepileptic drugs. *Southern Medical Journal*. **92**: 642–649.
50 Babalonis S and Walsh SL (2015) Warnings unheeded: the risks of co-prescribing opioids and benzodiazepines. *Pain: Clinical Updates*. **23**: 6.
51 Ballantyne JC *et al.* (2016) WHO analgesic ladder: a good concept gone astray. *British Medical Journal*. **352**: i20.
52 MHRA (2020) Opioids: risk of dependence and addiction. *Drug Safety Update*. www.gov.uk/drug-safety-update.
53 Ray WA *et al.* (2016) Prescription of long-acting opioids and mortality in patients with chronic noncancer pain. *Journal of the American Medical Association*. **315**: 2415–2423.
54 Cicero TJ *et al.* (2012) Effect of abuse-deterrent formulation of OxyContin. *New England Journal of Medicine*. **367**: 187–189.
55 Gillman PK (2005) Monoamine oxidase inhibitors, opioid analgesics and serotonin toxicity. *British Journal of Anaesthesia*. **95**: 434–441.
56 McWilliams K *et al.* (2014) A systematic review of opioid effects on the hypogonadal axis of cancer patients. *Supportive Care in Cancer*. **22**: 1699–1704.
57 Debono M *et al.* (2011) Tramadol-induced adrenal insufficiency. *European Journal of Clinical Pharmacology*. **67**: 865–867.
58 Rhodin A *et al.* (2014) Recombinant human growth hormone improves cognitive capacity in a pain patient exposed to chronic opioids. *Acta Anaesthesiologica Scandinavica*. **58**: 759–765.
59 NICE (2003) Human growth hormone (somatropin) in adults with growth hormone deficiency. *Technology appraisal guidance*. TA64. www.nice.org.uk.
60 Wehbeh L and Dobs AS (2020) Opioids and the hypothalamic-pituitary-gonadal (HPG) axis. *Journal of Clinical Endocrinology and Metabolism*. **105**(9): dgaa417.
61 deVries F *et al.* (2020) Opioids and their endocrine effects: A systematic review and meta-analysis. *Journal of Clinics in Endocrinology and Metabolism*. **105**: 1020–1029.
62 Daniell HW (2002) Hypogonadism in men consuming sustained-action oral opioids. *The Journal of Pain*. **3**: 377–384.
63 Rubinstein A and Carpenter DM (2014) Elucidating risk factors for androgen deficiency associated with daily opioid use. *American Journal of Medicine*. **127**: 1195–1201.
64 Lamprecht A *et al.* (2018) Secondary adrenal insufficiency and pituitary dysfunction in oral/transdermal opioid users with non-cancer pain. *European Journal of Endocrinology*. **179**: 353–362.
65 Donegan D (2019) Opioid induced adrenal insufficiency: what is new? *Current Opinion in Endocrinology, Diabetes and Obesity*. **26**: 133–138.
66 Abs R *et al.* (2000) Endocrine consequences of long-term intrathecal administration of opioids. *Journal of Clinical Endocrinology and Metabolism*. **85**: 2215–2222.
67 Finch PM *et al.* (2000) Hypogonadism in patients treated with intrathecal morphine. *Clinical Journal of Pain*. **16**: 251–254.
68 Roberts LJ *et al.* (2002) Sex hormone suppression by intrathecal opioids: a prospective study. *Clinical Journal of Pain*. **18**: 144–148.
69 O'Rourke TK, Jr. and Wosnitzer MS (2016) Opioid-induced androgen deficiency (OPIAD): diagnosis, management, and literature review. *Current Urology Reports*. **17**: 76.
70 Boland JW and Pockley AG (2017) Influence of opioids on immune function in patients with cancer pain: from bench to bedside. *British Journal of Pharmacology*. In press.
71 Sacerdote P *et al.* (1997) Antinociceptive and immunosuppressive effects of opiate drugs: a structure-related activity study. *British Journal of Pharmacology*. **121**: 834–840.
72 Risdahl JM *et al.* (1998) Opiates and infection. *Journal of Neuroimmunology*. **83**: 4–18.
73 McCarthy L *et al.* (2001) Opioids, opioid receptors, and the immune response. *Drug and Alcohol Dependence*. **62**: 111–123.
74 Boland JW *et al.* (2014) Effects of opioids on immunologic parameters that are relevant to anti-tumour immune potential in patients with cancer: a systematic literature review. *British Journal of Cancer*. **111**: 866–873.
75 Diasso PD *et al.* (2019) The effects of long-term opioid treatment on the immune system in chronic non-cancer pain patients: a systematic review. *European Journal of Pain*. **24**: 481–496.
76 Carli M *et al.* (2020) Opioid receptors beyond pain control: the role in cancer pathology and the debated importance of their pharmacological modulation. *Pharmacological Research*. **159**: 104938.
77 Sacerdote P *et al.* (2000) The effects of tramadol and morphine on immune responses and pain after surgery in cancer patients. *Anesthesia and Analgesia*. **90**: 1411–1414.
78 Budd K and Shipton E (2004) Acute pain and the immune system and opioimmunosuppression. *Acute Pain*. **6**: 123–135.
79 Plein LM and Rittner HL (2018) Opioids and the immune system - friend or foe? *British Journal of Pharmacology*. **175**: 2717–2725.
80 Sacerdote P *et al.* (2008) Buprenorphine and methadone maintenance treatment of heroin addicts preserves immune function. *Brain, Behavior, and Immunity*. **22**: 606–613.
81 Suzuki M *et al.* (2013) Correlation between the administration of morphine or oxycodone and the development of infections in patients with cancer pain. *American Journal of Hospice and Palliative Care*. **30**: 712–716.
82 Shao YJ *et al.* (2017) Contribution of opiate analgesics to the development of infections in advanced cancer patients. *Clinical Journal of Pain*. **33**: 295–299.
83 Khosrow-Khavar F *et al.* (2019) Opioids and the risk of infection: A critical appraisal of the pharmacologic and clinical evidence. *Expert Opinion on Drug Metabolism and Toxicology*. **15**: 565–575.
84 Alonzo NC and Bayer BM (2002) Opioids, immunology, and host defenses of intravenous drug abusers. *Infectious Disease Clinics of North America*. **16**: 553–569.
85 Page GG (2005) Immunologic effects of opioids in the presence or absence of pain. *Journal of Pain and Symptom Management*. **29**: S25–S31.
86 Higgins C *et al.* (2019) Evidence of opioid-induced hyperalgesia in clinical populations after chronic exposure: a systematic review and meta-analysis. *British Journal of Anaesthesia*. **122**: e114–e126.
87 Edwards DA and Chen L (2014) The evidence for opioid-induced hyperalgesia today. *Austin Journal of Anesthesia and Analgesia*. **2**: 12.
88 Roeckel LA *et al.* (2016) Opioid-induced hyperalgesia: Cellular and molecular mechanisms. *Neuroscience*. **338**: 160–182.
89 Shah M and Choi S (2017) Toll-like receptor-dependent negative effects of opioids: a battle between analgesia and hyperalgesia. *Frontiers in Immunology*. **8**: 642.
90 Lacagnina MJ *et al.* (2018) Toll-like receptors and their role in persistent pain. *Pharmacology and Therapeutics*. **184**: 145–158.

91 Keefer L *et al.* (2016) Centrally mediated disorders of gastrointestinal pain. *Gastroenterology.* **150**: 1408–1419.
92 Zylicz Z and Twycross R (2008) Opioid-induced hyperalgesia may be more frequent than previously thought. *Journal of Clinical Oncology.* **26**: 1564.
93 Koppert W (2007) Opioid-induced hyperalgesia. Pathophysiology and clinical relevance. *Acute Pain.* **9**: 21–24.
94 Walker SM and Cousins MJ (1997) Reduction in hyperalgesia and intrathecal morphine requirements by low-dose ketamine infusion. *Journal of Pain and Symptom Management.* **14**: 129–133.
95 Bruera E *et al.* (1996) Opioid rotation in patients with cancer pain. *Cancer.* **78**: 852–857.
96 Lawlor P *et al.* (1998) Dose ratio between morphine and methadone in patients with cancer pain. *Cancer.* **82**: 1167–1173.
97 Dubray C *et al.* (1997) Magnesium deficiency induces an hyperalgesia reversed by the NMDA receptor antagonist MK801. *Neuroreport.* **8**: 1383–1386.
98 Begon S *et al.* (2002) Magnesium increases morphine analgesic effect in different experimental models of pain. *Anesthesiology.* **96**: 627–632.
99 Gan T *et al.* (1997) Opioid-sparing effects of a low-dose infusion of naloxone in patient-administered morphine sulfate. *Anesthesiology.* **87**: 1075–1081.
100 Chindalore VL *et al.* (2005) Adding ultralow-dose naltrexone to oxycodone enhances and prolongs analgesia: a randomized, controlled trial of Oxytrex. *Journal of Pain.* **6**: 392–399.
101 Corli O *et al.* (2016) Are strong opioids equally effective and safe in the treatment of chronic cancer pain? A multicenter randomized phase IV 'real life' trial on the variability of response to opioids. *Annals of Oncology.* **27**: 1107–1115.
102 Mercadante S and Bruera E (2016) Opioid switching in cancer pain: From the beginning to nowadays. *Critical Reviews in Oncology/Hematology.* **99**: 241–248.
103 Riley J *et al.* (2015) Morphine or oxycodone for cancer-related pain? A randomized, open-label, controlled trial. *Journal of Pain and Symptom Management.* **49**: 161–172.
104 Sjogren P *et al.* (1994) Disappearance of morphine-induced hyperalgesia after discontinuing or substituting morphine with other opioid agonists. *Pain.* **59**: 313–316.
105 Hagen N and Swanson R (1997) Strychnine-like multifocal myoclonus and seizures in extremely high-dose opioid administration: treatment strategies. *Journal of Pain and Symptom Management.* **14**: 51–58.
106 Ashby M *et al.* (1999) Opioid substitution to reduce adverse effects in cancer pain management. *Medical Journal of Australia.* **170**: 68–71.
107 Morita T *et al.* (2005) Opioid rotation from morphine to fentanyl in delirious cancer patients: an open-label trial. *Journal of Pain and Symptom Management.* **30**: 96–103.
108 Aurilio C *et al.* (2009) Opioids switching with transdermal systems in chronic cancer pain. *Journal of Experimental and Clinical Cancer Research.* **28**: 61.
109 Nixon AJ (2005) Methadone for cancer pain: a case report. *American Journal of Hospice and Palliative Care.* **22**: 337.
110 Anderson R *et al.* (2001) Accuracy in equianalgesic dosing: conversion dilemmas. *Journal of Pain and Symptom Management.* **21**: 397–406.
111 Pasternak G (2001) Incomplete cross tolerance and multiple mu opioid peptide receptors. *Trends in Pharmacological Sciences.* **22**: 67–70.
112 Pereira J *et al.* (2001) Equianalgesic dose ratios for opioids: a critical review and proposals for long-term dosing. *Journal of Pain and Symptom Management.* **22**: 672–687.
113 Knotkova H *et al.* (2009) Opioid rotation: the science and the limitations of the equianalgesic dose table. *Journal of Pain and Symptom Management.* **38**: 426–439.
114 Fine PG and Portenoy RK (2009) Establishing "best practices" for opioid rotation: conclusions of an expert panel. *Journal of Pain and Symptom Management.* **38**: 418–425.
115 Lauretti GR *et al.* (2003) Comparison of sustained-release morphine with sustained-release oxycodone in advanced cancer patients. *British Journal of Cancer.* **89**: 2027–2030.
116 Mercadante S *et al.* (2004) Addition of a second opioid may improve opioid response in cancer pain: preliminary data. *Supportive Care Cancer.* **12**: 762–766.
117 Kotlinska-Lemieszek A (2010) Rotation, partial rotation (semi-switch), combining opioids, and titration. Does "opioid plus opioid" strategy make a step forward on our way to improving the outcome of pain treatment? *Journal of Pain and Symptom Management.* **40**: e10–e12.
118 Fallon MT and Laird BJA (2011) A systematic review of comination strong opioid therapy in cancer pain (in press). *Palliative Medicine.*
119 Davis MP *et al.* (2005) Look before leaping: combined opioids may not be the rave. *Supportive Care in Cancer.* **13**: 769–774.
120 Strasser F (2005) Promoting science in a pragmatic world: not (yet) time for partial opioid rotation. *Supportive Care in Cancer.* **13**: 765–768.

Updated (minor change) February 2022

MORPHINE

Class: Strong opioid analgesic.

Indications: Severe or †moderate pain, †diarrhoea, †cough, †breathlessness.

Contra-indications: None absolute if titrated carefully against a patient's pain (also see Strong opioids, p.389).

Pharmacology

Morphine is the main pharmacologically active constituent of opium. Its effects are mediated by specific opioid receptors both within the CNS and peripherally. Under normal circumstances, its main peripheral action is on smooth muscle. However, in the presence of tissue injury and inflammation, the number of opioid receptors at the peripheral end of a nociceptive afferent nerve fibre increases, and exogenous and endogenous opioids (released by activated inflammatory cells in close proximity to the nerve fibre) thereby exert a peripheral analgesic action.[1] Thus, there is increasing interest in the role of topical morphine (see Dose and use). Conversely, in bone and neuropathic pain, opioid receptor expression is reduced, contributing towards a reduced response to opioids. Nonetheless, in pooled data from RCTs in pure neuropathic pain states, morphine provided a 25–33% improvement in pain in two-thirds of patients (NNT = 3.7 (95% CI 2.6–6.5)). However, this is considered very low quality evidence, mostly because of the small number of participants (≤152).[2] In practice, a multimodal approach to pain relief is followed (see p.321).

5

Morphine, like all μ-opioid receptor agonists (μ agonists) increases intestinal transit time by decreasing propulsive activity and increasing non-propulsive activity via its effect on the myenteric plexus in the longitudinal muscle layer. This causes predictable opioid-induced constipation, which requires prophylactic regular laxatives when morphine is used regularly for pain (see Dose and use). Conversely, it can also be used for diarrhoea, although generally **loperamide** (p.36), a peripherally acting μ agonist, is preferred. All opioids can be used for cough and act by suppressing the cough reflex centre in the brain stem (see Antitussives, p.158). Morphine is also used to relieve breathlessness (see Dose and use).

The liver is the principal site of morphine metabolism.[3] Metabolism also occurs in other organs,[4] including the CNS.[5] Glucuronidation, the main metabolic pathway, is rarely impaired except in severe hepatic impairment, and morphine is well tolerated in patients with mild–moderate hepatic impairment.[6] However, with impairment severe enough to prolong the prothrombin time, the plasma halflife of morphine may be increased (see Chapter 18, p.762).[4]

The major metabolites of morphine are morphine-3-glucuronide (M3G; 55–80%) and morphine-6-glucuronide (M6G; 10–15%), which are excreted by the kidneys.[7] M6G binds to opioid receptors and contributes substantially to the effects of morphine, both desirable (e.g. analgesia) and undesirable (e.g. nausea and vomiting, sedation and respiratory depression).[8-10] In renal impairment, the plasma halflife of M6G increases from 2.5h to ≤50h, and is likely to lead to accumulation and enhanced toxicity (see Chapter 17, p.743). Similarly, in the last week of life, M6G accumulates as renal function deteriorates, increasing the risk of opioid toxicity and thereby delirium;[11] this may also explain why some RCTs of IV hydration at the end of life found a reduced incidence of sedation, myoclonus and delirium.[12] M3G will also accumulate, but the significance of this is unclear; it binds poorly to opioid receptors and is considered devoid of an analgesic effect. Although animal studies suggest a neuro-excitatory effect, this has not been clearly demonstrated in humans.[13]

Morphine is administered by a range of routes. Systemic absorption from topical application to ulcers or inflamed surfaces varies with the amount and concentration of the gel used; bio-availability ranges from negligible (with 0.06–0.125% gel) to almost the same as SC (0.125–0.5% gel applied to large ulcers).[14-17]

Because of the wide range in PO bio-availability, when switching from PO to SC/IM/IV morphine, the dose required is generally 1/2–1/3 of the PO dose.[18,19] In practice, for morphine, most centres use a conversion ratio of PO:SC/IM/IV of 2:1. Conversely, when switching from SC/IM/IV to PO, the PO dose should be 2–3 times greater than the SC/IM/IV dose. In a recent observational study, about 80% of patients achieved a satisfactory 24h PO dose at 3 times the previous 24h IV dose, rounded down to convenient-strength m/r tablets.[20]

Bio-availability 35% PO, ranging from 15–64%; 25% PR.
Peak effect ≤60min PO (immediate-release tablets); 20min IV; 30–60min IM; 50–90min SC.
Time to peak plasma concentration 15–60min PO (immediate-release tablets), 1–6h m/r (product dependent); 10–20min IM; 15min SC; 45–60min PR.
Plasma halflife 1.5–4.5h PO; 1.5h IV.
Duration of action 3–6h; 12–24h m/r (product dependent).

Cautions

Renal impairment and severe hepatic impairment (see Dose and use, and Chapter 17, p.743 and Chapter 18, p.762).

Drug interactions

Concurrent treatment with ≥2 CNS depressants (e.g. benzodiazepines, gabapentinoids, opioids) increases the risk of respiratory depression, particularly in susceptible groups, e.g. the elderly and those with renal or hepatic impairment.[21]

The following have been reported with PO morphine, although their clinical relevance is unknown:

- **rifampicin** may reduce plasma levels of morphine, possibly via the induction of p-glycoprotein in the GI tract
- **quinidine** may increase plasma levels of morphine via the inhibition of p-glycoprotein in the GI tract
- morphine may increase plasma levels of **gabapentin** by slowing GI transit time
- **metoclopramide** may increase the rate of absorption of morphine via increased gastric emptying. (Conversely, morphine can also reduce the pro-kinetic effects of **metoclopramide** on gastric emptying.)

Undesirable effects

See Table 1, and Strong opioids, Box B, p.394.

Dose and use

Patients using opioids must be monitored for undesirable effects, particularly nausea and vomiting, and constipation. Depending on individual circumstances, an anti-emetic should be prescribed for regular or p.r.n. use (see QCG: Nausea and vomiting, p.264) and, routinely, a laxative prescribed (see QCG: Opioid-induced constipation, p.45).

Opioids can impair driving ability, and patients should be counselled accordingly. Morphine is included in a law in England, Wales and Scotland relating to driving with certain drugs above specified plasma concentrations (see Chapter 22, p.809).

Based on familiarity, availability and cost, morphine is the strong opioid of choice for moderate–severe cancer pain.[23,24] However, in terms of efficacy and undesirable effects, morphine, **hydromorphone** and **oxycodone** are essentially similar.[25] Morphine is generally prescribed with a non-opioid when the non-opioid + a weak opioid does not provide adequate relief (see p.321).

There is no pharmacological need for weak opioids in cancer pain (see p.321). Low doses of morphine (or an alternative strong opioid) generally provide quicker and better relief from cancer pain than a weak opioid.[23,26] Moving directly from a non-opioid to a strong opioid is increasingly preferred in adults, and is the norm in children, in whom weak opioids are generally contra-indicated (see p.728).

Oral

Morphine is available as immediate-release tablets and solutions, and m/r tablets, capsules and suspensions (the latter recently discontinued in the UK). Most m/r products are administered b.d., some once daily. Because the pharmacokinetic profiles of m/r products differ,[27-29] it is best to keep individual patients on the same brand. M/r tablets should be swallowed whole; crushing or chewing them will lead to a rapid release of an overdose of morphine. For administration of immediate-release and m/r morphine to patients with swallowing difficulties or enteral feeding tubes (see Chapter 28, p.853).

Patients can be started on either an ordinary (immediate-release) or an m/r formulation (Box A).[30,31] An observational study supports a starting dose of 5mg q4h as generally safe for opioid-naïve patients, and 10mg q4h for those being switched from a regular weak opioid.[32] However, slight variation exists between guidelines, e.g. in the recommended starting dose.[33] It is important to recognize that guidelines are just guidelines; for each patient, when deciding the starting dose, it is necessary to consider the individual circumstances, e.g. severity of the pain, current analgesia, presence of renal impairment, increasing age or frailty. In every case, the patient must be monitored closely and the dose titrated as necessary.

Traditionally, to make things easier for patients, morphine q4h has been given on waking, 1000h, 1400h, 1800h with a double dose at bedtime. Despite contrary results in a non-blinded study,[34] RCT evidence has shown that this approach results in less pain through the night, better sleep, and no increase in early morning pain.[35]

Table 1 Potential intolerable effects of morphine

Type	Effects	Initial action	Comment
For general undesirable effects of opioid analgesics, see Strong opioids, Box B, p.394.			
Gastric stasis	Epigastric fullness, flatulence, anorexia, hiccup, persistent nausea	Prescribe a prokinetic, e.g. metoclopramide 10mg PO/SC t.d.s. (see p.268)	If the problem persists, change to an alternative opioid with less impact on the GI tract
Sedation	Intolerable persistent sedation	Reduce dose of morphine; consider a psychostimulant, e.g. methylphenidate 5mg PO b.d. (see p.246)	Sedation may be caused by other factors; stimulant rarely appropriate
Cognitive failure	Hyperactive delirium with hallucinations	Prescribe an antipsychotic, e.g. haloperidol 500microgram PO/SC stat & q2h p.r.n. (see p.198); reduce dose of morphine and, if no improvement, switch to an alternative opioid	Some patients develop intractable delirium with one opioid but not with an alternative opioid
Myoclonus	Multifocal twitching ± jerking of limbs	Prescribe a benzodiazepine, e.g. diazepam 5mg PO or midazolam 2.5mg SC stat & q1h p.r.n. (see p.171); reduce dose of morphine but increase again if pain recurs	Uncommon with typical oral doses; more common with high dose IV and spinal morphine
Neurotoxicity	Abdominal muscle spasms, symmetrical jerking of legs; whole-body allodynia, hyperalgesia (manifests as excruciating pain)	Prescribe a benzodiazepine, e.g. diazepam 5mg PO or midazolam 2.5mg SC stat & q1h p.r.n. (see p.171); reduce dose of morphine; consider changing to an alternative opioid	A rare syndrome in patients receiving intrathecal or high dose IV morphine; occasionally seen with typical oral and SC doses
Vestibular stimulation	Movement-induced nausea and vomiting	Prescribe an antihistaminic antimuscarinic anti-emetic, e.g. cyclizine 50mg PO or 25mg SC b.d.–t.d.s. (see p.273)	If intractable, try levomepromazine (p.201) or switch to an alternative opioid
Pruritus	Whole-body itch with systemic morphine; localized to upper body or face/nose with spinal morphine	With systemic opioids, prescribe PO H_1-antihistamine (e.g. chlorphenamine 4mg PO stat; if beneficial continue with 4mg t.d.s. or q4h p.r.n. for 2–3 days). Possibly switch opioids, e.g. morphine → oxycodone. For spinal opioids, see p.908.	Pruritus after systemic opioids is uncommon. It can sometimes be caused by cutaneous histamine release and be self-limiting, but the most distressing cases are chronic and antihistamine-resistant. Centrally acting opioid antagonists also relieve the pruritus but will also antagonize analgesia[22]
Histamine release	Life-threatening compromise in airway/ breathing and/or circulation	For treatment of anaphylaxis, see p.920. Change to a chemically distinct opioid immediately, e.g. methadone	Very rare

Box A Starting a patient on PO morphine

The starting dose of morphine is calculated to give a greater analgesic effect than the medication already in use:

- if the patient was previously receiving a weak opioid regularly (e.g. codeine 240mg/24h or equivalent), give morphine 10mg q4h or m/r 20–30mg q12h, but less if suspected to be a poor codeine metabolizer (see p.378)
- if changing from an alternative strong opioid (e.g. fentanyl, methadone), a much higher dose of morphine may be needed
- if the patient is frail and elderly, or opioid-naïve, a lower dose helps to reduce initial drowsiness, confusion and unsteadiness, e.g. morphine 5mg q4h or m/r 10–15mg q12h
- because of accumulation of an active metabolite, a lower and/or less frequent regular dose may suffice in mild–moderate renal impairment, e.g. morphine 5–10mg q6–8h (but the use of a renally safer opioid is generally advisable with moderate–severe renal impairment (see Dose and use, p.409 and Chapter 17, p.743)).

When adjusting the dose of morphine, p.r.n. use should be taken into account; increments should not exceed 33–50% every 24h. As a general rule, the p.r.n. dose must be increased when the regular dose is increased.

Patients using opioids must be monitored for undesirable effects, particularly nausea and vomiting, and constipation (see Strong opioids, Box B, p.394). Depending on individual circumstances, an anti-emetic should be prescribed for regular or p.r.n. use (see QCG: Nausea and vomiting, p.264) and, routinely, a laxative prescribed (see QCG: Opioid-induced constipation, p.45).

Opioids can impair driving ability, and patients should be counselled accordingly. Morphine is included in a law in England, Wales and Scotland relating to driving with certain drugs above specified plasma concentrations (see Chapter 22, p.809).

Upward titration of the dose of morphine should stop when either the pain is relieved or unacceptable undesirable effects occur. In the latter case, it is generally necessary to consider alternative measures. The aim is to have the patient free of pain and mentally alert after the initial drowsiness has cleared.

Because of poor absorption, m/r morphine may not be satisfactory in patients troubled by frequent vomiting or those with diarrhoea or an ileostomy.

Scheme 1: immediate-release morphine oral solution or tablets

- give morphine q4h 'by the clock' with p.r.n. doses 1/10–1/6 of the 24h dose
- after 1–2 days, recalculate q4h dose by dividing the total used in previous 24h (regular + p.r.n. use) by 6
- continue q4h and p.r.n. doses
- increase the regular dose until there is adequate relief throughout each 4h period, taking p.r.n. use into account
- a double dose at bedtime obviates the need to wake the patient for a dose during the night
- >90% of patients achieve satisfactory pain relief within 5 days.

Scheme 2: immediate-release morphine and modified-release (m/r) morphine

- begin as for Scheme 1
- when the q4h dose is stable, replace with m/r morphine q12h, or once daily if a 24h product is prescribed
- the q12h dose will be three times the previous q4h dose; a q24h dose will be six times the previous q4h dose, rounded to a convenient number of tablets or capsules
- continue to provide immediate-release morphine solution or tablets for p.r.n. use; give 1/10–1/6 of the 24h dose q2–4h.

Scheme 3: m/r morphine and immediate-release morphine

- generally start with m/r morphine 20–30mg q12h, or 10–15mg q12h in frail elderly patients
- use immediate-release morphine solution or tablets for p.r.n. medication; give 1/10–1/6 of the 24h dose q2–4h
- if necessary, increase the dose of m/r morphine every 2–3 days until there is adequate relief throughout each 12h period, guided by p.r.n. use.

When adjusting the dose of morphine, p.r.n. use should be taken into account; increments should not exceed 33–50% every 24h.[36] Instructions must be clear: extra p.r.n. morphine does not mean that the next regular dose is omitted.

P.r.n. doses of morphine for break-through cancer pain are typically 1/10–1/6 of the regular 24h dose but, as with the regular dose, individual titration is required to find the optimal dose. In practice, satisfactory p.r.n. doses vary from 1/20 (5%) to 1/5 (20%) of the 24h dose.[37,38]

As a general rule, the p.r.n. dose should be increased when the regular dose is increased. A p.r.n. dose is generally permitted every q2–4h as required (up to q1h when pain severe, or in the last days of life). However, frequent use of p.r.n. doses, i.e. ≥2 a day, should prompt a review of pain management. The mean time to onset of effect is 15min with a solution of morphine compared with 30min after an immediate-release tablet, suggesting that morphine solution is the better option for p.r.n. use (see also p.450).

An anti-emetic, e.g. **haloperidol** 500microgram PO, should be supplied for p.r.n. use during the first week or prescribed regularly if the patient has had nausea with a weak opioid (see QCG: Nausea and vomiting, p.264). Warn patients about the possibility of initial drowsiness. A laxative should be prescribed routinely unless there is a definite reason for not doing so, e.g. the patient has an ileostomy (see QCG: Opioid-induced constipation, p.45). *Constipation may be more difficult to manage than the pain.* Laxative suppositories and enemas continue to be necessary in about one third of patients.[39]

Subcutaneous administration

In the UK, if the PO route becomes an unreliable means of administering regular morphine, e.g. because of vomiting or difficulty swallowing, generally the CSCI route is used (see Chapter 29, p.887).

In strong opioid-naïve patients:

- start with 20mg/24h CSCI and 5mg SC p.r.n. (halve both doses in the frail elderly or mild–moderate renal impairment)
- if necessary, titrate the dose upwards, guided by p.r.n. use.

For general considerations when switching routes, see Appendix 2, p.925. When switching morphine PO to CSCI, most centres divide the total daily PO dose by 2 and re-titrate as necessary, e.g.:

- patient taking m/r morphine 30mg PO b.d. = 60mg/24h PO
- divide 60mg/24h by 2 = 30mg/24h CSCI
- the p.r.n. dose is 1/10–1/6 of the 24h dose, i.e. 3–5mg SC p.r.n.

For CSCI dilute with WFI, sodium chloride 0.9% or glucose 5%.

CSCI compatibility with other drugs: there are 2-drug compatibility data for morphine sulfate in WFI with **clonazepam**, **cyclizine**, **glycopyrronium**, **hyoscine *butylbromide***, **hyoscine *hydrobromide***, **ketamine**, **levomepromazine**, **metoclopramide** and **octreotide**.

Morphine sulfate is *incompatible* with **ketorolac** and may be *incompatible* with higher concentrations of **haloperidol** or **midazolam**.

For more details and 3-drug compatibility data, see Appendix 3, Chart 1 (p.936) and Chart 5 (p.944).

Compatibility charts for mixing drugs in sodium chloride 0.9% can be found in the extended appendix section of the on-line *PCF* on www.medicinescomplete.com.

Renal or hepatic impairment

Because of the risk of impaired metabolism or elimination:

- lower than usual starting doses are advised in mild–moderate renal impairment, e.g. 5–10mg PO q6–8h, and severe hepatic impairment (see Chapter 18, p.762)
- the use of a renally safer opioid is generally advisable with severe renal impairment or ESRF. If the use of morphine is unavoidable, start with 1.25–2.5mg PO/SC p.r.n., and once the pain is controlled consider switching to an equivalent dose of **buprenorphine** or **fentanyl** TD (see Chapter 17, p.743).

For a general approach when renal or hepatic function deteriorates rapidly, see p.393.

Intravenous administration

IV morphine is widely used for the rapid relief of severe pain caused by acute trauma or medical emergencies.

In opioid-naïve patients:

- give a prophylactic anti-emetic IV, e.g. **metoclopramide** 10mg
- over 5–10min, give a total of morphine 5–10mg (2.5–5mg in the elderly) IV
- when insufficient, give additional morphine at a rate not exceeding 1–2mg/min until satisfactory relief obtained; monitor for undesirable effects, e.g. excessive sedation, respiratory depression
- the dose can be repeated q2–4h as required.

Although uncommon in UK, CIVI morphine and/or p.r.n. IV morphine are used in palliative care units in Europe and North America.[40,41] Generally, this is in the context of the first few days of an inpatient admission for pain control. Subsequently, patients can be switched from IV to PO (see Pharmacology).

Rapid IV/SC titration of morphine dose for severe cancer pain

Although rapid IV/SC titration of morphine is generally *not* necessary, it can be useful in patients with severe acute pain, whether already taking opioids ('opioid-tolerant') or opioid-naïve.[42,43] Further, because of difficulties in relation to follow-up, rapid IV titration is the norm at some centres in India for new patients presenting with pain of ≥5 out of 10.

Two IV methods are included here: the first with 10min and the second with 1min intervals between each IV bolus (Box B and Box C).[43-47] In India, a single cumulative IV dose is given, followed immediately by PO medication (Box B). About 80% of patients obtain relief with 10mg or less.[44,45] At the Cleveland Clinic (USA), patients are maintained on CIVI for several days before conversion to PO medication (Box C). Although these methods have been used safely in many patients, **naloxone** should be readily available (see QCG: Reversal of opioid-induced respiratory depression, p.498).

IV patient-controlled analgesia (PCA) can also be used but is more costly, requires inpatient admission and may take >10h to achieve relief.[48,49] Some centres use a more rapidly acting strong opioid, e.g. IV **fentanyl**, with subsequent doses given after pauses of only 5–10min.[50]

Note. Patients who have required a rapid escalation in opioid requirements must be monitored closely. The underlying cause may be transient, e.g. haemorrhage into a liver metastasis, and a subsequent reduction in dose will be necessary.

Buccal morphine

Morphine is only slowly absorbed through the buccal mucosa.[51,52] Thus, most of a morphine solution given sublingually or into the gingival gutter will be swallowed and absorbed from the GI tract. Nonetheless, in the past, this route was successfully used in moribund patients.

Rectal morphine

Morphine is absorbed from suppositories.[53] From the lower and middle rectum, it will enter the systemic circulation bypassing the liver. From the upper rectum, it will undergo hepatic first-pass metabolism after it enters the portal circulation. However, there are extensive anastomoses between the rectal veins which make it impossible to predict how much will enter the portal circulation.[54,55] Despite the uncertainty, in practice the same dose is given PR as PO and titrated as necessary.

Morphine suppositories are no longer commercially available in the UK. Although not authorized for this route and not generally recommended, m/r morphine oral tablets have been used PR to provide analgesia in moribund patients, generally while organizing a more reliable delivery method.[56]

Spinal morphine

In the UK, <5% of cancer patients needing morphine receive it spinally, i.e. ED or IT. This route of administration (see p.908) is normally undertaken by an anaesthetist. Particularly with neuropathic pain, morphine is generally combined with a local anaesthetic (e.g. **bupivacaine**), and sometimes with **clonidine**.

Topical morphine

The number of peripheral opioid receptors increases in nociceptive afferent nerve fibres in the presence of local inflammation.[1,15,57] This property is exploited in joint surgery, where morphine is given intra-articularly at the end of the operation.[58] Topical morphine has also been used successfully to relieve otherwise intractable pain associated with cutaneous ulceration, often

Box B Rapid titration of morphine dose in opioid-naïve patients (Institute of Palliative Medicine, India)[44,45]

Prerequisites

Pain ≥5/10 on a numerical scale.

Probability of a partial or complete response to morphine.[a]

Method

Obtain venous access with a butterfly cannula.

Give metoclopramide 10mg IV routinely, if no contra-indications.

Dilute the contents of 15mg morphine ampoule in a 10mL syringe.[b]

Inject 1.5mg (1mL) every 10min until the patient is pain-free or complains of undue sedation.[c]

If patients experience nausea, give additional metoclopramide 5mg IV.

Results

Dose required (with approximate percentages):

- 1.5–4.5mg (40%)
- 6–9mg (40%)
- 10.5–15mg (15%)
- >15mg (5%).

Complete relief in 80%; none in 1%.

Drop-outs 2%.

Undesirable effects: sedation 32%; other 3%.

Ongoing treatment

Prescribe a dose of oral morphine q4h similar to the IV dose, rounded to nearest 5mg, e.g. needed morphine 3–6mg IV → 5mg PO; the minimum dose is 5mg.

Advise about p.r.n. doses and, if >2/24h needed, to increase the dose the next day.

In practice, 20% of patients need a dose increase within 3 days.

a. most patients will already be taking an NSAID

b. ampoule strengths varies from country to country; use local standard

c. if ampoule = 10mg/mL (diluted to 10mg in 10mL), a bolus dose of 2mg would be reasonable.

Box C Rapid titration of morphine dose in both opioid-tolerant and opioid-naïve patients (based on practice at Cleveland Clinic, Ohio, USA)[42,46,47]

Sequence	*IV*	*SC*
Dose	1mg/min up to 10mg	2mg q5min up to 10mg
Pause	5min	10min
Dose	1mg/min up to 10mg	2mg q5min up to 10mg
Pause	5min	10min
Dose	1mg/min up to 10mg[a]	2mg q5min up to 10mg[a]

Maintenance IV/SC dose

Regard cumulative effective dose as the equivalent of a q4h dose, and prescribe accordingly.

Example

Cumulative effective IV dose = 9mg.

If giving intermittent injections, dose = 9mg q4h, rounded to 10mg.

If CIVI, total daily IV dose = 9mg x 6 = 54mg/24h.

Round this up or down to convenient number of ampoules, i.e. 50mg or 60mg.

P.r.n. dose = 5–10mg q1h.

a. review cause if relief inadequate after a total of 30mg.

decubitus ulcers.[59-62] It is often given as a 0.1% (1mg/mL) gel, using IntraSite®. If prepared under sterile conditions, morphine sulfate is stable for at least 28 days when mixed with IntraSite® gel at a concentration of 0.125% (1.25mg/mL). This preparation can be made by thoroughly mixing 1mL of morphine sulfate 10mg/mL injection with 8g of IntraSite® gel.[63] A fact sheet with further information can be obtained from the www.palliativedrugs.com Document library. Morphine 0.1% and 0.2% in Intrasite® gel is also available as a special order product.

Higher concentrations, namely 0.3–0.5%, have been used when managing pain associated with:

- vaginal inflammation associated with a fistula
- rectal ulceration.[60]

The amount of gel applied varies according to the size and the site of the ulcer, but is typically 5–10mL applied b.d.–t.d.s. The topical morphine is kept in place with either a non-absorbable pad or dressing, e.g. Opsite® or Tegaderm®, or gauze coated with petroleum jelly. Other morphine 0.2% ointments and gels have been locally prepared.[64] Other opioids, e.g. **diamorphine** or **methadone**, and other carriers, e.g. Stomahesive® paste or **metronidazole** gel, have also been used.[62,65]

For cancer-treatment-related oral mucositis, an oral morphine solution *without alcohol* of 2mg/mL can be used (special order, see Supply). Use 15mL to rinse the mouth for 2min q2–3h (see p.669). It provides better pain relief than a placebo mouthwash or one containing **co-magaldrox** + **lidocaine** + **diphenhydramine**.[66,67] Significant relief occurs after about 30min, and lasts about 3.5h.[68]

In vitro and animal studies suggest that topical morphine may also aid wound healing by stimulating angiogenesis.[69] However, no such benefit was seen in an RCT of patients with ulcerative oral lichen planus.[70]

†Morphine for breathlessness

Opioids are used for breathlessness which persists despite optimal treatment of the underlying cause, along with non-drug approaches relevant to the performance status and prognosis of the patient.[71] Most experience is with morphine.

Current evidence and clinical experience supports the use of regular opioids for patients who are breathless at rest, but not for those breathless only on exertion.[72] For the latter group, a p.r.n. dose of an opioid also has limited utility because exertional breathlessness generally recovers within 5–20min, much quicker than the time it takes to locate, administer and obtain benefit from an opioid.[73] Thus, non-drug measures are of primary importance in this circumstance.[71]

Systematic reviews ± meta-analyses of RCTs mostly in COPD, CHF and cancer support the use of opioids by the oral and parenteral but *not* the nebulized route.[74-76] A specific review of nebulized (and nasal) opioids concluded the same, and these should not be used outside of a clinical trial.[71,77]

Data from larger RCTs of oral opioids are emerging, mostly in COPD, cancer and CHF.[78-80] **Oxycodone** was ineffective,[78] and benefit from morphine limited to those with more severe functional limitation (i.e. modified MRC breathlessness grade ≥3).[79,81] However, because of slow recruitment, some trials were stopped early (and are consequently underpowered)[78,80,82] or abandoned completely.[83] Most authors concluded that further trials are required.

Morphine and other opioids reduce the ventilatory response to hypercapnia, hypoxia and exercise, decreasing respiratory effort and breathlessness.[71] Improvements are seen at doses that do *not* cause respiratory depression.[81,84,85]

Generally, small doses are sufficient, typically PO morphine 10–30mg/24h, but sometimes less, and only rarely more.[81,86-91] For opioid-naïve patients, some advocate starting with an m/r product, others an immediate-release one (Box D). Both approaches have specific advantages, e.g. the m/r approach is simpler, provides relief more quickly for some patients, and opioid plasma concentrations fluctuate less over a 24h period; the immediate-release approach identifies those patients who benefit from doses <10mg/24h and appears to be associated with fewer withdrawals because of undesirable effects.[90,91] RCT supporting evidence is greater for the m/r approach. Only Australia has a morphine product authorized for chronic breathlessness, a once daily m/r product (Kapanol®).

Box D Starting PO morphine for breathlessness in opioid-naïve patients[90,91]

Approaches using either m/r or immediate-release morphine products have been described for patients with moderate–severe breathlessness, mostly with COPD or lung cancer. Whichever is used, because of the risk of undesirable effects, it is important to provide appropriate explanation, laxatives, anti-emetics and monitoring. In studies of 3–6 months' duration, benefit is generally maintained at the same dose after the initial titration.

M/r approach

- start with MST Continus® 5mg PO b.d. for 1 week
- if baseline VAS/NRS breathlessness is not reduced ≥10%, increase by 10mg/24h weekly
- usual maximum 30mg/24h.

In one study using this approach,[91] about 60% of patients benefited from morphine, most at 10mg/24h. However, undesirable effects, e.g. drowsiness, confusion, nausea and vomiting, and constipation, were a common cause of discontinuation during initial titration (20%).

Immediate-release approach

Mostly in an attempt to minimize the risk of undesirable effects and maintain the confidence of patients who may be wary of taking an opioid, others advocate slower initial titration, with immediate-release morphine solution increased until breathlessness is tolerable, e.g.:

- in the first week, start with 500microgram PO b.d. and increase at 48h intervals → 500microgram q.d.s. → 1mg q4h
- then, at weekly intervals, increase the q4h dose to 2mg → 3mg → 5mg
- if necessary, continue to adjust each week using 30–50% dose increments
- reduce dose if undesirable effects occur; if persistent, consider a switch to an alternative opioid
- when the dose is unchanged for 2 weeks, consider switching to an m/r formulation.

In one study using this approach,[90] a similar overall response rate of 60% was obtained, with most of those switched to a m/r formulation requiring 10–15mg/24h (only one required 20mg/24h). However, 40% remained on an immediate-release formulation requiring doses ≤10mg/24h.

Undesirable effects were a less frequent cause of discontinuation during initial titration (7%). However, unlike in the m/r study, a switch to an alternative opioid was permitted in cases of intolerance, and was necessary in about 10%.

In patients already taking morphine for pain, there are limited data to guide practice. One study suggests a reasonable starting point to be:[92]

- divide the 24h dose by 6 (e.g. morphine 60mg/24h ÷ 6 = 10mg q4h)
- start with p.r.n. doses equivalent to 25% of what would be the q4h analgesic dose (e.g. 10mg ÷ 4 = 2.5mg); this may suffice in those with mild–moderate breathlessness at rest
- if necessary, increase to 50% of the q4h analgesic dose (e.g. 10mg ÷ 2 = 5mg)
- if frequent p.r.n. doses are needed, the regular background opioid dose should be increased accordingly.

As with pain, individual titration is required for optimal benefit, and p.r.n. doses equal to or higher than the q4h analgesic dose may be required. In some patients, morphine by CSCI is better tolerated and provides greater relief, possibly by avoiding the peaks (with undesirable effects) and troughs (with loss of effect) of oral medication. If using an alternative opioid to morphine, adopt the same approach.

Generally, the average reduction in breathlessness as assessed by NRS (0–10) or VAS (0–100mm) is relatively small, e.g. about 1 point/10mm respectively. Nonetheless, this represents a change that is clinically important.[93]

Several adverse effects (e.g. excess exacerbations, emergency department visits, hospitalizations, deaths) have been associated with the use of opioids and/or benzodiazepines in patients with COPD.[75,94] Although some found a relationship with any opioid dose, others reported no excess deaths or hospitalizations with lower opioid doses (± benzodiazepines) equivalent to morphine ≤30mg/24h PO.[75] This supports limiting the dose of morphine to within this dose range in this group of patients.

Breathlessness in the last days of life

The incidence of breathlessness increases as death approaches. For severe breathlessness in the last days of life:

- patients often fear suffocating to death, and a positive approach to the patients, their family and colleagues about the relief of terminal breathlessness is important
- no patient should die with distressing breathlessness
- failure to relieve terminal breathlessness is a failure to utilize drug treatment correctly.

Because of the distress, inability to sleep and exhaustion, patients and their carers generally accept that drug-related drowsiness may need to be the price paid for greater comfort. However, unless there is overwhelming distress, sedation is not the primary aim of treatment, and some patients become mentally brighter when their breathlessness is reduced.

Even so, because increasing drowsiness also generally reflects the deteriorating clinical condition, it is important to stress the gravity of the situation and the aim of treatment to the relatives. Drug treatment typically comprises:

- parenteral administration of an opioid and a sedative-anxiolytic; e.g. for opioid-naive patients, start with:
  - ▷ morphine 5–10mg/24h + **midazolam** 10mg/24h by CSCI *and*
  - ▷ morphine 2.5mg + **midazolam** 2.5mg SC p.r.n. q1h
  - ▷ for those already receiving PO morphine or another opioid, convert to the equivalent parenteral 24h and p.r.n. doses
  - ▷ titrate both p.r.n. and regular doses to obtain satisfactory relief
- **haloperidol** or **levomepromazine** if the patient develops a hyperactive delirium; see p.172 (may be aggravated by a benzodiazepine).[95-97]

Supply

Unless indicated otherwise, all products are Schedule 2 **CD**.

Immediate-release oral products

Morphine oral solution is available in two strengths, 2mg/mL and a high potency concentrate of 20mg/mL supplied with a calibrated syringe. *Deaths have occurred from accidental overdose with the concentrated solution*, mostly when doses prescribed in *mg* were administered as *mL*. Prescribing should be in *mg* not mL to minimize the risk of *20 times* the prescribed dose being given.[98]

Sevredol® (Napp)
Tablets 10mg, 20mg, 50mg; 10mg and 100mg dose = £0.10 and £1 respectively.

Morphine sulfate (generic)
Oral solution 2mg/mL (**PoM**); 10mg dose = £0.10; *may contain alcohol.*
Oral solution (alcohol-free) 2mg/mL (**PoM**), 10mg dose = Price unavailable, (unauthorized product, available as a special order; see Chapter 24, p.817).

Oramorph® (Glenwood GmbH)
Oral solution 2mg/mL (**PoM**); 10mg dose = £0.10; *contains alcohol.*
Concentrated oral solution 20mg/mL, 100mg dose = £0.75.

Modified-release products

As for all m/r opioids, brand prescribing is recommended to reduce the risk of confusion and error in dispensing and administration (see p.xvii).

Modified-release 12-hourly oral products
Morphgesic® SR (Advanz Pharma)
Tablets m/r 10mg, 30mg, 60mg, 100mg, 28 days @ 30mg q12h = £8.50.

MST Continus® (Napp)
Tablets m/r 5mg, 10mg, 15mg, 30mg, 60mg, 100mg, 200mg, 28 days @ 30mg q12h = £12.

Zomorph® (Ethypharm)
Capsules containing m/r granules 10mg, 30mg, 60mg, 100mg, 200mg, 28 days @ 30mg q12h = £8.
May be swallowed whole or opened and the granules sprinkled on cold soft food and swallowed whole. Can also be given via gastric or gastrostomy tubes >16Fr with an open distal end or lateral pores (see SPC and p.863).

Modified-release 24-hourly oral products
MXL® (Napp)
Capsules containing m/r granules 30mg, 60mg, 90mg, 120mg, 150mg, 200mg, 28 days @ 60mg *once daily* = £15. *May be swallowed whole or opened and the granules sprinkled on cold soft food and swallowed whole.*

Parenteral products
Morphine *sulfate* (generic)
Injection 1mg/mL (1mL, 5mL and 10mL amp = £3.75, £4.75 and £1.50); 10mg/mL and 15mg/mL (1mL amp = £1); 20mg/mL (1mL amp = £8); 30mg/mL (1mL and 2mL amps = £1.25 and £2).
Infusion 1mg/mL 50mL vial = £4.50, 2mg/mL 50mL vial = £6.50.

5

1 Smith HS (2008) Peripherally-acting opioids. *Pain Physician*. **11**: S121–132.
2 Cooper TE *et al.* (2017) Morphine for chronic neuropathic pain in adults. *Cochrane Database of Systematic Reviews*. **5**: CD011669. www.cochranelibrary.com.
3 Hasselstrom J *et al.* (1986) The metabolism and bioavailability of morphine in patients with severe liver cirrhosis. *British Journal of Clinical Pharmacology*. **29**: 289–297.
4 Mazoit J-X *et al.* (1987) Pharmacokinetics of unchanged morphine in normal and cirrhotic subjects. *Anesthesia and Analgesia*. **66**: 293–298.
5 Sandouk P *et al.* (1991) Presence of morphine metabolites in human cerebrospinal fluid after intracerebroventricular administration of morphine. *European Journal of Drug Metabolism and Pharmacology*. **16**: 166–171.
6 Regnard CFB and Twycross RG (1984) Metabolism of narcotics (letter). *British Medical Journal*. **288**: 860.
7 McQuay HJ *et al.* (1990) Oral morphine in cancer pain: influences on morphine and metabolite concentration. *Clinical Pharmacology and Therapeutics*. **48**: 236–244.
8 Osborne RJ *et al.* (1986) Morphine intoxication in renal failure: the role of morphine-6-glucuronide. *British Medical Journal*. **292**: 1548–1549.
9 Thompson P *et al.* (1992) Mophine-6-glucuronide: a metabolite of morphine with greater emetic potency than morphine in the ferret. *British Journal of Pharmacology*. **106**: 3–8.
10 Klimas R and Mikus G (2014) Morphine-6-glucuronide is responsible for the analgesic effect after morphine administration: a quantitative review of morphine, morphine-6-glucuronide, and morphine-3-glucuronide. *British Journal of Anaesthesia*. **113**: 935–944.
11 Franken LG *et al.* (2016) Pharmacokinetics of morphine,morphine-3-glucuronide and morphine-6-glucuronide in terminally ill adult patients. *Clinical Pharmacokinetics*. **55**: 697–709.
12 Good P *et al.* (2014) Medically assisted hydration for adult palliative care patients. *Cochrane Database of Systematic Reviews*. **4**: CD006273. www.cochranelibrary.com.
13 Gretton S and Riley J (2008) Morphine metabolites: a review of their clinical effects. *European Journal of Palliative Care*. **15**: 110–114.
14 Westerling D *et al.* (1994) Transdermal administration of morphine to healthy subjects. *British Journal of Clinical Pharmacology*. **37**: 571–576.
15 Ribeiro MD *et al.* (2004) The bioavailability of morphine applied topically to cutaneous ulcers. *Journal of Pain and Symptom Management*. **27**: 434–439.
16 Watterson G *et al.* (2004) Peripheral opioids in inflammatory pain. *Archives of Disease in Childhood*. **89**: 679–681.
17 Jansen M (2006) Morphine gel. Palliativedrugs.com bulletin board message.; Available from: www.palliativedrugs.com.
18 Hanks G *et al.* (2001) Morphine and alternative opioids in cancer pain: the EAPC recommendations. *British Journal of Cancer*. **84**: 587–593.
19 Takahashi M *et al.* (2003) The oral-to-intravenous equianalgesic ratio of morphine based on plasma concentrations of morphine and metabolites in advanced cancer patients receiving chronic morphine treatment. *Palliative Medicine*. **17**: 673–678.
20 Lasheen W *et al.* (2010) The intravenous to oral relative milligram potency ratio of morphine during chronic dosing in cancer pain. *Palliative Medicine*. **24**: 9–16.
21 MHRA (2020) Benzodiazepines and opioids: reminder of risk of potentially fatal respiratory depression. *Drug Safety Update*. www.gov.uk/drug-safety-update.
22 Twycross RG *et al.* (2003) Itch: scratching more than the surface. *Quarterly Journal of Medicine*. **96**: 7–26.
23 Caraceni A *et al.* (2012) Use of opioid analgesics in the treatment of cancer pain: evidence-based recommendations from the EAPC. *Lancet Oncology*. **13**: e58–e68.
24 Fallon M *et al.* (2018) Management of cancer pain in adult patients: ESMO Clinical Practice Guidelines. *Annals of Oncology*. **29 (Suppl 4)**: iv166–iv191.
25 Caraceni A *et al.* (2011) Is oral morphine still the first choice opioid for moderate to severe cancer pain? A systematic review within the European Palliative Care Research Collaborative guidelines project. *Palliative Medicine*. **25**: 402–409.
26 Bandieri E *et al.* (2016) Randomized trial of low-dose morphine versus weak opioids in moderate cancer pain. *Journal of Clinical Oncology*. **34**: 436–442.
27 Bloomfield S *et al.* (1993) Analgesic efficacy and potency of two oral controlled-release morphine preparations. *Clinical Pharmacology and Therapeutics*. **53**: 469–478.
28 Gourlay G *et al.*, editors. A comparison of Kapanol (a new sustained-release morphine formulation), MST Continus and morphine solution in cancer patients: pharmacokinetic aspects. The Seventh World Congress on Pain; 1993; Seattle: IASP Press.
29 West R and Maccarrone C, editors. Single dose pharmacokinetics of a new oral sustained-release morphine formulation, Kapanol capsules. The Seventh World Congress on Pain; 1993; Seattle: IASP Press.
30 Mercadante S (2007) Opioid titration in cancer pain: a critical review. *European Journal of Pain*. **11**: 823–830.
31 De Conno F *et al.* (2008) The MERITO Study: a multicentre trial of the analgesic effect and tolerability of normal-release oral morphine during 'titration phase' in patients with cancer pain. *Palliative Medicine*. **22**: 214–221.
32 Ripamonti CI *et al.* (2009) Normal-release oral morphine starting dose in cancer patients with pain. *Clinical Journal of Pain*. **25**: 386–390.
33 Taubert M *et al.* (2010) Re: Update on cancer pain guidelines. *Journal of Pain and Symptom Management*. **24**: 1–5.

34 Todd J *et al.* (2002) An assessment of the efficacy and tolerability of a 'double dose' of normal-release morphine sulphate at bedtime. *Palliative Medicine*. **16**: 507–512.

35 Dale O *et al.* (2009) A double-blind, randomized, crossover comparison between single-dose and double-dose immediate-release oral morphine at bedtime in cancer patients. *Journal of Pain and Symptom Management*. **37**: 68–76.

36 Carver AC and Foley KM (2001) Symptom assessment and management. *Neurologic Clinics*. **19**: 921–947.

37 Currow DC *et al.* (2020) A randomized, double-blind, crossover, dose ranging study to determine the optimal dose of oral opioid to treat breakthrough pain for patients with advanced cancer already established on regular opioids. *European Journal of Pain*. **24**: 983–991.

38 Donnelly S *et al.* (2002) Morphine in cancer pain management: a practical guide. *Supportive Care in Cancer*. **10**: 13–35.

39 Twycross RG and Harcourt JMV (1991) The use of laxatives at a palliative care centre. *Palliative Medicine*. **5**: 27–33.

40 Mercadante S *et al.* (2008) Intravenous morphine for breakthrough (episodic-) pain in an acute palliative care unit: a confirmatory study. *Journal of Pain and Symptom Management*. **35**: 307–313.

41 Mercadante S (2010) Intravenous morphine for management of cancer pain. *Lancet Oncology*. **11**: 484–489.

42 Hagen N *et al.* (1997) Cancer pain emergencies: a protocol for management. *Journal of Pain and Symptom Management*. **14**: 45–50.

43 Davis MP *et al.* (2004) Opioid dose titration for severe cancer pain: a systematic evidence-based review. *Journal of Palliative Medicine*. **7**: 462–468.

44 Kumar K *et al.* (2000) Intravenous morphine for emergency treatment of cancer pain. *Palliative Medicine*. **14**: 183–188.

45 Harris JT *et al.* (2003) Intravenous morphine for rapid control of severe cancer pain. *Palliative Medicine*. **17**: 248–256.

46 Davis MP (2004) Acute pain in advanced cancer: an opioid dosing strategy and illustration. *American Journal of Hospice and Palliative Care*. **21**: 47–50.

47 Davis MP (2005) Rapid opioid titration in severe cancer pain. *European Journal of Palliative Care*. **12**: 11–14.

48 Radbruch L *et al.* (1999) Intravenous titration with morphine for severe cancer pain: report of 28 cases. *Clinical Journal of Pain*. **15**: 173–178.

49 Schiessl C *et al.* (2010) Rhythmic pattern of PCA opioid demand in adults with cancer pain. *European Journal of Pain*. **14**: 372–379.

50 Soares LG *et al.* (2003) Intravenous fentanyl for cancer pain: a "fast titration" protocol for the emergency room. *Journal of Pain and Symptom Management*. **26**: 876–881.

51 Coluzzi P (1998) Sublingual morphine: efficacy reviewed. *Journal of Pain and Symptom Management*. **16**: 184–192.

52 Dyal BW *et al.* (2019) Sublingual versus swallowed morphine: a comparison. *Cancer Nursing*. **44**: e13–e22.

53 deBoer AG *et al.* (1982) Rectal drug administration: clinical pharmacokinetic considerations. *Clinical Pharmacokinetics*. **7**: 285–311.

54 Johnson AG and Lux G (1988) Progress in the Treatment of Gastrointestinal Motility Disorder. The role of cisapride. Excerpta Medica, Amsterdam.

55 Ripamonti C and Bruera E (1991) Rectal, buccal and sublingual narcotics for the management of cancer pain. *Journal of Palliative Care*. **7**: 30–35.

56 Wilkinson T *et al.* (1992) Pharmacokinetics and efficacy of rectal versus oral sustained-release morphine in cancer patients. *Cancer Chemotherapy and Pharmacology*. **31**: 251–254.

57 Krajnik M and Zylicz Z (1997) Topical opioids - fact or fiction? *Progress in Palliative Care*. **5**: 101–106.

58 Likar R *et al.* (1999) Dose-dependency of intra-articular morphine analgesia. *British Journal of Anaesthesia*. **83**: 241–244.

59 Back NI and Finlay I (1995) Analgesic effect of topical opioids on painful skin ulcers. *Journal of Pain and Symptom Management*. **10**: 493.

60 Krajnik M *et al.* (1999) Potential uses of topical opioids in palliative care - report of 6 cases. *Pain*. **80**: 121–125.

61 Twillman R *et al.* (1999) Treatment of painful skin ulcers with topical opioids. *Journal of Pain and Symptom Management*. **17**: 288–292.

62 Gutierrez Y *et al.* (2021) Topical opioid use in dermatologic disease: a systematic review. *Dermatologic Therapy*. **34**: e15150.

63 Zeppetella G and Ribeiro MD (2005) Morphine in intrasite gel applied topically to painful ulcers. *Journal of Pain and Symptom Management*. **29**: 118–119.

64 Ciałkowska-Rysz A and Dzierżanowski T (2019) Topical morphine for treatment of cancer-related painful mucosal and cutaneous lesions: a double-blind, placebo-controlled cross-over clinical trial. *Archives of medical science : AMS*. **15**: 146–151.

65 Le Bon B *et al.* (2009) Effectiveness of topical administration of opiods inpalliative care a systematic review. *Journal of Pain and Symptom Management*. **37**: 913–917.

66 Cerchietti LC *et al.* (2002) Effect of topical morphine for mucositis-associated pain following concomitant chemoradiotherapy for head and neck carcinoma. *Cancer*. **95**: 2230–2236.

67 Vayne-Bossert P *et al.* (2010) Effect of topical morphine (mouthwash) on oral pain due to chemotherapy- and/or radiotherapy-induced mucositis: a randomized double-blinded study. *Journal of Palliative Medicine*. **13**: 125–128.

68 Cerchietti LC *et al.* (2003) Potential utility of the peripheral analgesic properties of morphine in stomatitis-related pain: a pilot study. *Pain*. **105**: 265–273.

69 Ondrovics M *et al.* (2017) Opioids: Modulators of angiogenesis in wound healing and cancer. *Oncotarget*. **8**: 25783–25796.

70 Zaslansky R *et al.* (2018) Topical application of morphine for wound healing and analgesia in patients with oral lichen planus: a randomized, double-blind, placebo-controlled study. *Clinical Oral Investigations*. **22**: 305–311.

71 Twycross *et al.* (2016) *Introducing Palliative Care*. (6e). Pharmaceutical Press, London. pp. 149–159.

72 Johnson MJ *et al.* (2016) Opioids, exertion, and dyspnea: a review of the evidence. *American Journal of Hospital Palliative Care*. **33**: 194–200.

73 Mercadante S *et al.* (2016) Epidemiology and characteristics of episodic breathlessness in advanced cancer patients: an observational study. *Journal of Pain and Symptom Management*. **51**: 17–24.

74 Barnes H *et al.* (2019) Opioids for the palliation of refractory breathlessness in adults with advanced disease and terminal illness. *Cochrane Database of Systematic Reviews*. **3**: CD011008. www.cochranelibrary.com.

75 Ekstrom M *et al.* (2018) One evidence base; three stories: do opioids relieve chronic breathlessness? *Thorax*. **73**: 88–90.

76 Kohberg C *et al.* (2016) Opioids: an unexplored option for treatment of dyspnea in IPF. *European Clinical Respiratory Journal*. **3**: 30629.

77 Bausewein C and Simon ST (2014) Inhaled nebulized and intranasal opioids for the relief of breathlessness. *Current Opinion in Supportive and Palliative Care*. **8**: 208–212.

78 Ferreira DH *et al.* (2020) Controlled-release oxycodone versus placebo in the treatment of chronic breathlessness - a multi-site randomised placebo controlled trial. *Journal of Pain and Symptom Management*. **59**: 581–589.
79 Currow D *et al.* (2020) Regular, sustained-release morphine for chronic breathlessness: a multicentre, double-blind, randomised, placebo-controlled trial. *Thorax*. **75**: 50–56.
80 Johnson MJ *et al.* (2019) Oral modified release morphine for breathlessness in chronic heart failure: a randomized placebo-controlled trial. *ESC Heart Failure*. **6**: 1149–1160.
81 Verberkt CA *et al.* (2020) Effect of sustained-release morphine for refractory breathlessness in chronic obstructive pulmonary disease on health status: a randomized clinical trial. *JAMA Internal Medicine*. **180**: 1306–1314.
82 Ferreira DH *et al.* (2018) Extended-release morphine for chronic breathlessness in pulmonary arterial hypertension-a randomized, double-blind, placebo-controlled, crossover study. *Journal of Pain and Symptom Management*. **56**: 483–492.
83 Kochovska S *et al.* (2019) A randomized, double-blind, multisite, pilot, placebo-controlled trial of regular, low-dose morphine on outcomes of pulmonary rehabilitation in COPD. *Journal of Pain and Symptom Management*. **58**: e7–e9.
84 Lopez-Saca JM and Centeno C (2014) Opioids prescription for symptoms relief and the impact on respiratory function: updated evidence. *Current Opinion in Supportive and Palliative Care*. **8**: 383–390.
85 Verberkt CA *et al.* (2017) Respiratory adverse effects of opioids for breathlessness: a systematic review and meta-analysis. *European Respiratory Journal*. **50**: 1701153.
86 Cohen M *et al.* (1991) Continuous intravenous infusion of morphine for severe dyspnoea. *Southern Medical Journal*. **84**: 229–234.
87 Boyd K and Kelly M (1997) Oral morphine as symptomatic treatment of dyspnoea in patients with advanced cancer. *Palliative Medicine*. **11**: 277–281.
88 Abernethy AP *et al.* (2003) Randomised, double blind, placebo controlled crossover trial of sustained release morphine for the management of refractory dyspnoea. *British Medical Journal*. **327**: 523–528.
89 Allen S *et al.* (2005) Low dose diamorphine reduces breathlessness without causing a fall in oxygen saturation in elderly patients with end-stage idiopathic pulmonary fibrosis. *Palliative Medicine*. **19**: 128–130.
90 Rocker GM *et al.* (2013) Opioid therapy for refractory dyspnea in patients with advanced chronic obstructive pulmonary disease: patients' experiences and outcomes. *Canadian Medical Association Journal Open*. **1**: e27–e36.
91 Currow DC *et al.* (2011) Once-daily opioids for chronic dyspnea: a dose increment and pharmacovigilance study. *Journal of Pain and Symptom Management*. **42**: 388–399.
92 Allard P *et al.* (1999) How effective are supplementary doses of opioids for dyspnea in terminally ill cancer patients? A randomized continuous sequential clinical trial. *Journal of Pain and Symptom Management*. **17**: 256–265.
93 Johnson MJ *et al.* (2013) Clinically important differences in the intensity of chronic refractory breathlessness. *Journal of Pain and Symptom Management*. **46**: 957–963.
94 Vozoris NT *et al.* (2016) Incident opioid drug use and adverse respiratory outcomes among older adults with COPD. *European Respiratory Journal*. **48**: 683–693.
95 Navigante AH *et al.* (2006) Midazolam as adjunct therapy to morphine in the alleviation of severe dyspnea perception in patients with advanced cancer. *Journal of Pain and Symptom Management*. **31**: 38–47.
96 Matsuda Y *et al.* (2017) Low-dose morphine for dyspnea in terminally ill patients with idiopathic interstitial pneumonias. *Journal of Palliative Medicine*. **20**: 879–883.
97 Mori M *et al.* (2021) How successful is parenteral oxycodone for relieving terminal cancer dyspnea compared with morphine? A multicenter prospective observational study. *Journal of Pain and Symptom Management*. **62**: 336–345.
98 FDA (2011) Medwatch safety alert. Morphine sulfate oral solution 100mg per 5mL (20mg/mL): medication use error - reports of accidental overdose. Available from: www.fda.gov/Safety/MedWatch/SafetyInformation (archived).

Updated January 2022

DIAMORPHINE

Class: Strong opioid analgesic (available only in the UK).

Indications: As for **morphine**; used in the UK instead of parenteral **morphine** because of its greater solubility, particularly when large doses are necessary.

Contra-indications: None absolute if titrated carefully against a patient's pain (also see Strong opioids, p.389 and p.395).

Pharmacology

Diamorphine (di-acetylmorphine, heroin) is available for medicinal analgesic use only in the UK. It is generally considered to be a pro-drug without intrinsic activity.[1] *In vivo*, it is rapidly de-acetylated (plasma halflife 3min) to an active metabolite, 6-mono-acetylmorphine (6-MAM) (plasma halflife 20min), and then to **morphine** itself.[2] Thus, similar considerations as for **morphine** apply regarding the use of diamorphine in patients with renal or hepatic impairment/failure (see p.409).[3]

IM diamorphine is more than twice as potent as IM **morphine**.[4-6] The greater potency of parenteral diamorphine could be because 6-MAM is more potent than **morphine**[7] or because diamorphine and 6-MAM cross the blood–brain barrier more readily than **morphine**. However, by mouth the two opioids are almost equipotent.[8]

IM diamorphine acts more quickly than IM **morphine**,[6,9] but IV, the converse is true.[10] This paradox is not easily explained, but it could relate to differences in plasma protein-binding (diamorphine 40%, **morphine** 20%).

In terms of analgesic efficacy and effect on mood, diamorphine has no clinical advantage over **morphine** by oral or SC/IM routes.[4,5,8] Diamorphine hydrochloride is much more water-soluble than **morphine** sulfate/hydrochloride and, in the UK, is the strong opioid of choice when high-dose injections are needed (Table 1). In some countries, **hydromorphone** (p.466) is used instead.

Table 1 Solubility of selected opioids[11]

Preparation	*Amount of water needed to dissolve 1g at 25°C (mL)*
Morphine	5,000
Morphine hydrochloride	24
Morphine sulfate	21
Diamorphine hydrochloride	1.6[a]
Hydromorphone	3

a. 1g of diamorphine hydrochloride dissolved in 1.6mL has a volume of 2.4mL.

Like **morphine**, diamorphine can be given by many different routes, including spinally. However, the PO tablet product is no longer available. The buccal and intranasal routes are used mostly in children for acute pain or breakthrough pain,[12,13] although the only authorized nasal spray (Ayendi®) has recently been discontinued. Diamorphine can be used for the same range of indications as **morphine**, including bladder spasms (intravesical administration)[14,15] and painful decubitus ulcers (topically in IntraSite® gel).[16,17]

Bio-availability (as 6-MAM) no data.

Onset of action 5–10min SC.

Time to peak plasma concentration 1.5–2h PO as 6-MAM and **morphine**.

Plasma halflife 3min IV; metabolized to active metabolites.

Duration of action 4h.

Cautions

Renal impairment and severe hepatic impairment (see Dose and use, and Chapter 17, p.743 and Chapter 18, p.762).

Drug interactions

Concurrent treatment with ≥2 CNS depressants (e.g. benzodiazepines, gabapentinoids, opioids) increases the risk of respiratory depression, particularly in susceptible groups, e.g. the elderly and those with renal or hepatic impairment.[18]

Stability

Diamorphine hydrochloride is stable indefinitely when stored as a powder,[19] but de-acetylates when in solution, first to 6-mono-acetylmorphine (6-MAM) and then to **morphine**. The rate of de-acetylation is situation-dependent. Thus, *in vivo*, diamorphine is converted to 6-MAM in minutes, whereas the stability of diamorphine hydrochloride in simple solution is much longer. Further, because 6-MAM is the primary active agent, there is no loss of potency until 6-MAM is degraded to **morphine**.[7]

In one study, after 3 months in simple solution, 30% of the diamorphine had degraded to 6-MAM, but it was only at 12 months that a trace of **morphine** became detectable.[20] A second study looked at the effect of ambient temperature.[21,22] The loss of 10% of diamorphine to 6-MAM took 8 weeks when kept at 22°C, but only 2 weeks at 37°C. Other studies have produced comparable results.[23,24]

Undesirable effects

See Strong opioids, p.394 and **Morphine**, Table 1, p.407.

Dose and use

Patients using opioids must be monitored for undesirable effects, particularly nausea and vomiting, and constipation. Depending on individual circumstances, an anti-emetic should be prescribed for regular or p.r.n. use (see QCG: Nausea and vomiting, p.264) and, routinely, a laxative prescribed (see QCG: Opioid-induced constipation, p.45).

Opioids can impair driving ability, and patients should be counselled accordingly. Diamorphine is included in a law in England, Wales and Scotland relating to driving with certain drugs above specified plasma concentrations (see Chapter 22, p.809).

5

In the UK, diamorphine is used for all the same indications as **morphine**. Although previously diamorphine was given by a wide range of routes, it is now generally reserved for SC/CSCI use (see Chapter 29, p.890).

SC/CSCI

In strong opioid-naïve patients:

- start with 15mg/24h CSCI and 2.5mg SC p.r.n. (halve doses in the frail elderly or mild–moderate renal impairment)
- if necessary, titrate the dose upwards, guided by p.r.n. use; conventionally, p.r.n. SC doses are 1/10–1/6 of the total 24h CSCI dose.

For general considerations when switching opioids, see Appendix 2, p.925. The following are practical clinical conversion ratios:

- PO **morphine** to CSCI diamorphine, give one third of the 24h dose, e.g. **morphine** 60mg/24h PO = diamorphine 20mg/24h CSCI
- CSCI **morphine** to CSCI diamorphine, divide the 24h dose by 1.5 (i.e. decrease by one third), e.g. **morphine** 30mg/24h CSCI = diamorphine 20mg/24h CSCI
- if necessary, titrate the dose upwards, guided by p.r.n. use; conventionally, p.r.n. SC doses are 1/10–1/6 of the total 24h CSCI dose.

For CSCI dilute with WFI, concentration-dependent *incompatibility* occurs with sodium chloride 0.9% at higher doses (see Chapter 29, p.889).

CSCI compatibility with other drugs: there are 2-drug compatibility data for diamorphine in WFI with **clonazepam**, **dexamethasone**, **glycopyrronium**, **hyoscine *butylbromide***, **hyoscine *hydrobromide***, **ketorolac**, **levomepromazine**, **metoclopramide**, **midazolam**, **octreotide** and **ondansetron**.

Concentration-dependent *incompatibility* occurs with **cyclizine** or **haloperidol** at higher concentrations. For more details and 3-drug compatibility data, see Appendix 3, Chart 1 (p.936) and Chart 3 (p.940).

Compatibility charts for mixing drugs in sodium chloride 0.9% can be found in the extended appendix section of the on-line PCF on *www.medicinescomplete.com*.

Renal or hepatic impairment

Because of the risk of impaired metabolism or elimination:

- halve the usual starting doses in mild–moderate renal impairment
- use cautiously in severe hepatic impairment; reduce the starting dose to 1.25–2.5mg SC q2–4h p.r.n or 5mg/24h CSCI (also see Chapter 18, p.762)
- the use of a renally safer opioid is generally advisable with severe renal impairment or ESRF. If use of diamorphine is unavoidable, see Chapter 17, p.743.

For a general approach when renal or hepatic function deteriorates rapidly, see p.393.

Supply

Because diamorphine ampoules cost about three times more than **morphine** ampoules, **morphine** should be considered the first-line parenteral strong opioid of choice, unless the need for high doses makes diamorphine more convenient because of its greater solubility.[25,26] All preparations are Schedule 2 **CD**.

Diamorphine (generic)
Injection (powder for reconstitution) 5mg amp = £2.50; 10mg amp = £3.25; 30mg amp = £3.25; 100mg amp = £8.50; 500mg amp = £38.

1 Inturrisi CE *et al.* (1984) The pharmacokinetics of heroin in patients with chronic pain. *New England Journal of Medicine*. **310**: 1213–1217.
2 Barrett DA *et al.* (1992) The effect of temperature and pH on the deacetylation of diamorphine in aqueous solution and in human plasma. *Journal of Pharmacy and Pharmacology*. **44**: 606–608.
3 King S *et al.* (2011) A systematic review of the use of opioid medication for those with moderate to severe cancer pain and renal impairment: A European palliative care research collaborative opioid guidelines project. *Palliative Medicine*. **25**: 525–552.
4 Kaiko RF *et al.* (1981) Analgesic and mood effects of heroin and morphine in cancer patients with postoperative pain. *New England Journal of Medicine*. **304**: 1501–1505.
5 Beaver WT *et al.* (1981) Comparison of the analgesic effect of intramuscular heroin and morphine in patients with cancer pain. *Clinical Pharmacology and Therapeutics*. **29**: 232.
6 Reichle CW *et al.* (1962) Comparative analgesic potency of heroin and morphine in postoperative patients. *Journal of Pharmacology and Experimental Therapeutics*. **136**: 43–46.
7 Wright CI and Barbour FA (1935) The respiratory effects of morphine, codeine and related substances. *Journal of Pharmacology and Experimental Therapeutics*. **54**: 25–33.
8 Twycross RG (1977) Choice of strong analgesic in terminal cancer: diamorphine or morphine? *Pain* **3**: 93–104.
9 Dundee JW *et al.* (1966) Studies of drugs given before anaesthesia XI: diamorphine (heroin) and morphine. *British Journal of Anaesthesia*. **38**: 610–619.
10 Morrison L *et al.* (1991) Comparison of speed of onset of analgesic effect of diamorphine and morphine. *British Journal of Anaesthesia*. **66**: 656–659.
11 Hanks GW and Hoskin PJ (1987) Opioid analgesics in the management of pain in patients with cancer: a review. *Palliative Medicine*. **1**: 1–25.
12 Kendall J *et al.* (2015) A novel multipatient intranasal diamorphine spray for use in acute pain in children: pharmacovigilance data from an observational study. *Emergency Medical Journal*. **32**: 269–273.
13 Jamieson L *et al.* (2021) Healthcare professionals' views of the use of oral morphine and transmucosal diamorphine in the management of paediatric breakthrough pain and the feasibility of a randomised controlled trial: A focus group study (DIPPER). *Palliative Medicine*. **35**: 1118–1125.
14 McCoubrie R and Jeffrey D (2003) Intravesical diamorphine for bladder spasm. *Journal of Pain and Symptom Management*. **25**: 1–3.
15 Duckett J (1997) Intravesical morphine analgesia after bladder surgery. *Journal of Urology*. **157**: 1407–1409.
16 Abbas SQ (2004) Diamorphine-Intrasite dressings for painful pressure ulcers. *Journal of Pain and Symptom Management*. **28**: 532–534.
17 Flock P (2003) Pilot study to determine the effectiveness of diamorphine gel to control pressure ulcer pain. *Journal of Pain and Symptom Management*. **25**: 547–554.
18 MHRA (2020) Benzodiazepines and opioids: reminder of risk of potentially fatal respiratory depression. *Drug Safety Update*. www.gov.uk/drug-safety-update.
19 Lerner M and Mills A (1963) Some modern aspects of heroin analysis. *Bulletin on Narcotics*. **15**: 37–42.
20 Rizzotti G (1935) Contributo allo studio delle alterazioni delle soluzioni acquose di eroina. *Archives Internationales de Pharmacodynamie et de Therapie*. **52**: 87–96.
21 Twycross RG and Gilhooley RA (1973) Euporiant elixirs. *British Medical Journal*. **4**: 552.
22 Twycross RG (1974) Diamorphine and cocaine elixir BPC. *Pharmaceutical Journal*. **212**: 153 & 159.
23 Kleinberg ML *et al.* (1990) Stability of heroin hydrochloride in infusion devices and containers for intravenous administration. *American Journal of Hospital Pharmacy*. **47**: 377–381.
24 Omar OA *et al.* (1989) Diamorphine stability in aqueous solution for subcutaneous infusion. *Journal of Pharmacy and Pharmacology*. **41**: 275–277.
25 Scottish Government (2020 update) Diamorphine hydrochloride powder for reconstitution and injection 5mg & 10mg ampoules. *Medicine Supply Alert Notice*. www.sehd.scot.nhs.uk.
26 Palliativedrugs.com (2010) Diamorphine essential opioid or time to say goodbye? www.palliativedrugs.com.

Updated November 2021

*ALFENTANIL

Class: Strong opioid analgesic.

Indications: Intra-operative analgesia; analgesia and procedure-related pain in mechanically ventilated patients on ICUs; †an alternative in cases of intolerance to other strong opioids, particularly in renal failure;[1] †procedure-related pain in non-ventilated patients;[2-4] †break-through pain.[5]

Contra-indications: Do not administer concurrently with MAOIs or within 2 weeks of their discontinuation. Generally, none absolute if titrated carefully against a patient's pain (see also Strong opioids, p.389).

Pharmacology

Alfentanil is a synthetic lipophilic μ-opioid receptor agonist in the same class as **fentanyl** and **sufentanil** (see p.389). Compared with these, it has a more rapid onset of action and time to peak effect, and a shorter duration of action (Table 1). Its potency is approximately one quarter to one tenth that of **fentanyl**[6] (and 10–20 times more than parenteral **morphine**).

Alfentanil is less lipophilic than **fentanyl** and is 90% bound to mainly α_1-acid glycoprotein.[7] However, because most of the unbound alfentanil is un-ionized, it rapidly enters the CNS. Alfentanil is metabolized in the liver by CYP3A4 to inactive metabolites that are excreted in the urine. Alfentanil can accumulate with chronic administration, particularly in the elderly and the obese, and even with only mild hepatic impairment.[8,9] Renal impairment does not significantly alter the clearance of alfentanil, and, consequently, alfentanil is used at some centres when a parenteral opioid is required in severely reduced renal function or ESRF. Lower doses may be sufficient because of changes in protein binding (see p.743).[1] However, unless the volume is prohibitive, **fentanyl** is generally recommended as the first-line parenteral opioid in ESRF at the end of life (see p.743).[1]

It has been suggested that analgesic tolerance occurs rapidly with alfentanil,[10] but this has been refuted.[11] However, tolerance does not seem to be a problem in palliative care.[12]

Because alfentanil is available in a more concentrated form (500microgram/mL) than **fentanyl** (50microgram/mL), a smaller equivalent dose volume is needed, and this facilitates administration by CSCI or SL. For similar reasons, in countries where alfentanil is not available, **sufentanil** is used instead (Table 1 and Box A).[13]

Alfentanil has been used successfully by short-term PCA, CSCI or SL for procedure-related pain, e.g. dressing changes in burns or trauma patients.[2,4,14] It has also been used SL and nasally for break-through pain, including severe intractable angina in inoperable coronary artery disease.[5,15,16] In the UK, an unauthorized spray for buccal or nasal use, containing alfentanil 5mg/5mL, can be obtained via special order. It is expensive compared with using the injection formulation (see Supply). A dose of 140microgram/0.14mL spray is delivered. Details and instructions for use can be downloaded from the Document library of palliativedrugs.com. In an audit of patients already on regular strong opioids, about three-quarters benefited from SL alfentanil in doses of 560–1,680microgram (4–12 sprays; titrated as necessary). Pain relief was seen within 10min. However, such use has diminished since transmucosal **fentanyl** products have become available (p.450).

Spinal administration of lipophilic opioids remains controversial because of the rapid clearance into the systemic circulation (see Chapter 32, p.908).[17]

Opioid withdrawal symptoms can occur when switching from **morphine** (or other less lipophilic/less potent opioid) to CSCI alfentanil.[18] These manifest with symptoms like gastric flu and last for a few days; p.r.n. doses of the original opioid will relieve troublesome symptoms.

Table 1 Pharmacokinetics of single IV doses of fentanils[19-21]

	Alfentanil	*Sufentanil*	*Fentanyl*
Onset of action (min)	0.75[a]	1	1.5[b]
Time to peak effect (min)	1.5	2.5	4.5
Plasma halflife (min)	95	165	220
Duration of action (min)	30[a]	60	60

a. if given IM, onset slower (<5min), and duration of action longer (60min)
b. if given IM, onset slower (7–15min), and duration of action longer (1–2h).

Box A Sufentanil injection (not UK)

A lipophilic opioid with a strong affinity for the μ-opioid receptor. Time to onset of action and to peak effect is mid-way between that of alfentanil and fentanyl (Table 1).[20]

Sufentanil is about 7.5–10 times more potent than fentanyl,[22,23] and this allows a smaller volume to be given by injection. Divide the parenteral dose of fentanyl by 10 to obtain an easy-to-calculate starting dose.

Example
Fentanyl 1,000microgram/24h CSCI (i.e. 20mL of 50microgram/mL)
→ sufentanil 100microgram/24h CSCI (i.e. 2mL of 50microgram/mL).

Sufentanil can be administered SC, IV or spinally.[24] By CSCI, it is compatible with other commonly prescribed drugs.[25]

The injection formulation has been given intranasally (using an atomizer) for, e.g. moderate–severe acute trauma pain, break-through cancer pain;[26,27] specific 15microgram and 30microgram SL tablet formulations have been developed for use in postoperative pain (as part of a PCA system) and moderate–severe acute pain.[28,29]

Accumulates in fat tissue when given continuously;[30] monitor carefully when switching to another opioid.

Is not dependent on renal function for elimination, and is thus useful in renal impairment.

Cautions

Hepatic or renal impairment (also see Chapter 17, p.743 and Chapter 18, p.762).

Drug interactions

Concurrent treatment with ≥2 CNS depressants (e.g. benzodiazepines, gabapentinoids, opioids) increases the risk of respiratory depression, particularly in susceptible groups, e.g. the elderly and those with renal or hepatic impairment.[31]

Alfentanil is metabolized by CYP3A4. Caution is required with concurrent use of drugs that inhibit or induce this enzyme (see Chapter 19, Table 8, p.790). Reports of interactions where closer monitoring ± dose adjustment are required are listed in Box B.[32]

Box B Interactions between alfentanil and other drugs involving CYP450[a]

Plasma concentrations of alfentanil	
***Increased* by**	***Decreased* by**
Aprepitant[b]	Apalutamide[c]
Azoles, e.g. fluconazole, itraconazole, voriconazole	Aprepitant[b]
Cimetidine	Enzalutamide
Diltiazem	Carbamazepine[c]
Macrolides, e.g. clarithromycin, erythromycin	Fosphenytoin[c]
	Phenobarbital[c]
	Phenytoin[c]
	Rifampicin

a. not an exhaustive list; limited to drugs most likely to be encountered in palliative care and excludes anticancer, antiviral, HIV and immunosuppressive drugs (seek specialist advice)
b. aprepitant can increase the exposure to CYP3A4 substrates in the short-term and then reduce their exposure within 2 weeks
c. based on theoretical extrapolation.

Undesirable effects

See Strong opioids, p.394.

Dose and use

Patients using opioids must be monitored for undesirable effects, particularly nausea and vomiting, and constipation. Depending on individual circumstances, an anti-emetic should be prescribed for regular or p.r.n. use (see QCG: Nausea and vomiting, p.264) and, routinely, a laxative prescribed (see QCG: Opioid-induced constipation, p.45).

Opioids can impair driving ability, and patients should be counselled accordingly (see Chapter 22, p.809).

†Procedure-related pain (see QCG, p.426)

- give 250–500microgram alfentanil SL (using the 500microgram/mL injection formulation), or SC/IV.

CSCI as an alternative to morphine

Used mostly for patients with severe renal impairment/ESRF in whom there is evidence of **morphine** neurotoxicity (see p.398), or when volume restrictions prevent the use of **fentanyl**.

For general considerations when switching opioids, see Appendix 2 (p.925). Given the shorter duration of action of alfentanil, it is difficult to give a single precise dose conversion ratio. However, the following are safe practical conversion ratios:

- PO **morphine** to CSCI alfentanil: give one thirtieth of the 24h dose, e.g. **morphine** 60mg/24h PO = alfentanil 2mg/24h CSCI
- CSCI **morphine** to CSCI alfentanil: give one fifteenth of the 24h dose, e.g. **morphine** 30mg/24h = alfentanil 2mg/24h
- CSCI **diamorphine** to CSCI alfentanil: give one tenth of the 24h dose, e.g. **diamorphine** 30mg/24h = alfentanil 3mg/24h.

Conventionally, p.r.n. SC doses of alfentanil are 1/10–1/6 of the total 24h CSCI dose. Because of the short duration of action of alfentanil (≤30min), even with an optimally titrated p.r.n. dose frequent dosing may be required; this is one reason why **fentanyl** is recommended first-line in these circumstances (see Pharmacology).

The CSCI dose of alfentanil should be reviewed at least daily and titrated accordingly. For CSCI dilute with WFI, sodium chloride 0.9% or glucose 5%.

CSCI compatibility with other drugs: there are 2-drug compatibility data for alfentanil in WFI with **clonazepam**, **dexamethasone**, **glycopyrronium**, **haloperidol**, **hyoscine** ***butylbromide***, **levomepromazine**, **metoclopramide**, **midazolam**, **octreotide** and **ondansetron**.

Concentration-dependent *incompatibility* occurs with **cyclizine**. For more details and 3-drug compatibility data, see Appendix 3, Chart 1 (p.936) and Chart 2 (p.938).

Compatibility charts for mixing drugs in sodium chloride 0.9% can be found in the extended appendix section of the on-line *PCF* on *www.medicinescomplete.com*.

Alternative CSCI dosing schedules

The recommendations above may well be too conservative for some patients. It is important to review sooner rather than later, and increase the dose if necessary. Some centres have used other conversion ratios with apparent success:

- CSCI **morphine** to CSCI alfentanil: give one tenth of the 24h dose, e.g. **morphine** 30mg/24h = alfentanil 3mg/24h[12]
- CSCI **diamorphine** to CSCI alfentanil: give one sixth of the 24h dose, e.g. **diamorphine** 30mg/24h = alfentanil 5mg/24h.[33,34]

For the latter, p.r.n. SC **diamorphine/morphine** is given to supplement CSCI alfentanil, giving the same p.r.n. dose as used before the switch to alfentanil. When the switch has been prompted by opioid neurotoxicity, a recurrence has not been observed with 1–2 p.r.n. doses/24h of **diamorphine/morphine**.

†Break-through cancer pain, SL administration

Given the variability in the intensity of break-through pains, p.r.n. recommendations are best expressed as a range of doses rather than a single fixed dose. There is a poor relationship between the effective SL p.r.n. dose and regular CSCI dose. Individual dose titration is necessary, e.g. starting with 1/10–1/6 of the daily alfentanil CSCI dose and titrating upwards if necessary. The alfentanil 500microgram/mL injection formulation can be used SL (Table 2). However, retaining even 2mL in the mouth (sublingually or buccally) for 5–10min is difficult. Generally, authorized **fentanyl** transmucosal products are now used (p.450).

Table 2 Equivalent volumes of parenteral formulations of alfentanil, fentanyl and sufentanil for SL use[a]

Alfentanil 500microgram/mL		*Fentanyl 50microgram/mL*		*Sufentanil 50microgram/mL (not UK)*	
Dose (microgram)	*Volume (mL)*	*Dose (microgram)*	*Volume (mL)*	*Dose (microgram)*	*Volume (mL)*
100	0.2	25	0.5	2.5	N/A
200	0.4	50	1	5	0.1
300	0.6	75	1.5	7.5	0.15
400	0.8	100[b]	2	10	0.2
500	1	125	N/O	12.5	0.25
600	1.2	150	N/O	15	0.3
800	1.6	200[b]	N/O	20	0.4
1,000	2	250	N/O	25	0.5

Abbreviations: N/A = not applicable; NO = not optimal, because ≥2mL

a. this is *not* a true dose conversion chart. Alfentanil, fentanyl and sufentanil have differing properties (Table 1). As always with analgesics, individual patient dose titration is required

b. fentanyl SL product commercially available (see p.450); generally use in preference.

Supply

All preparations are Schedule 2 **CD**.

Alfentanil (generic)

Nasal spray (with attachment for buccal/SL use) 140microgram/spray, 5mg/5mL bottle = £55–£99. (Unauthorized product, available as a special order from the pharmacy manufacturing unit, Torbay hospital; see Chapter 24, p.817. *Telephone number for enquiries: 01803 664707; email: torbaypharmaceuticals@nhs.net. The solution is stable for 1 year unopened and for 28 days after opening.*)

Injection 500microgram/mL, 2mL amp = £0.75, 10mL amp = £2.75, 50mL vial = £15.

Injection (for dilution and use as a continuous infusion) 5mg/mL, 1mL amp = £2.50.

The high-strength 5mg/mL injection is used at some centres when the CSCI/CIVI dose is >5mg/24h. However, to avoid the risk of the high-strength injection being administered by mistake, in many hospitals its availability is restricted to the ICU.

1 King S *et al.* (2011) A systematic review of the use of opioid medication for those with moderate to severe cancer pain and renal impairment: A European palliative care research collaborative opioid guidelines project. *Palliative Medicine*. **25**: 525–552.

2 Gallagher G *et al.* (2001) Target-controlled alfentanil analgesia for dressing change following extensive reconstructive surgery for trauma. *Journal of Pain and Symptom Management*. **21**: 1–2.

3 Miner JR *et al.* (2011) Alfentanil for procedural sedation in the emergency department. *Annals of Emergency Medicine*. **57**: 117-121.

4 Fontaine M *et al.* (2016) Feasibility of monomodal analgesia with IV alfentanil during burn dressing changes at bedside (in spontaneously breathing non-intubated patients). *Burns*. **43**: 337–342.

5 Duncan A (2002) The use of fentanyl and alfentanil sprays for episodic pain. *Palliative Medicine*. **16**: 550.

6 Larijani G and Goldberg M (1987) Alfentanil hydrochloride: a new short acting narcotic analgesic for surgical procedures. *Clinical Pharmacy*. **6**: 275–282.

7 Bernards C. Clinical implications of physicochemical properties of opioids. In: Stein C, editor. *Opioids in Pain Control: basic and clinical aspects*. Cambridge: Cambridge University Press; 1999. pp. 166–187.

8 Bodenham A and Park GR (1988) Alfentanil infusions in patients requiring intensive care. *Clinical Pharmacokinetics*. **15**: 216–226.

9 Bosilkovska M *et al.* (2012) Analgesics in patients with hepatic impairment: pharmacology and clinical implications. *Drugs*. **72**: 1645–1669.

10 Kissin I *et al.* (2000) Acute tolerance to continuously infused alfentanil: the role of cholecystokinin and N-methyl-D-aspartate-nitric oxide systems. *Anesthesia and Analgesia*. **91**: 110–116.

11 Schraag S *et al.* (1999) Lack of rapid development of opioid tolerance during alfentanil and remifentanil infusions for postoperative pain. *Anesthesia and Analgesia*. **89**: 753–757.
12 Ferraz Gonçalves J *et al.* (2020) Use of alfentanil in palliative care. *Pharmacy (Basel)*. **8**: 240.
13 Gardner-Nix J (2001) Oral transmucosal fentanyl and sufentanil for incident pain. *Journal of Pain and Symptom Management*. **22**: 627–630.
14 Kwon YS *et al.* (2016) A comparison of oxycodone and alfentanil in intravenous patient-controlled analgesia with a time-scheduled decremental infusion after laparoscopic cholecystectomy. *Pain Research and Management*. Epub DOI: 10.1155/2016/7868152.
15 Osborn H and Jefferson M (2010) Intranasal alfentanil for severe intractable angina in inoperable coronary artery disease. *Palliative Medicine*. **24**: 94–95.
16 Brenchley J and Ramlakhan S (2006) Intranasal alfentanil for acute pain in children. *Emergency Medical Journal*. **23**: 488.
17 Bujedo BM (2014) Spinal opioid bioavailability in postoperative pain. *Pain Practice*. **14**: 350–364.
18 Carmichael JP and Lee MA (2010) Symptoms of opioid withdrawal syndrome after switch from oxycodone to alfentanil. *Journal of Pain and Symptom Management*. **40**: e4–6.
19 Willens JS and Myslinski NR (1993) Pharmacodynamics, pharmacokinetics, and clinical uses of fentanyl, sufentanil, and alfentanil. *Heart Lung*. **22**: 239–251.
20 Scholz J *et al.* (1996) Clinical pharmacokinetics of alfentanil, fentanyl and sufentanil. An update. *Clinical Pharmacokinetics*. **31**: 275–292.
21 Hall T and Hardy J. (2005) The lipophilic opioids: fentanyl, alfentanil, sufentanil and remifentanil. In: Davis M *et al.*, editors. *Opioids in Cancer Pain*. Oxford: Oxford University Press.
22 Reynolds L *et al.* (2004) Relative analgesic potency of fentanyl and sufentanil during intermediate-term infusions in patients after long-term opioid treatment for chronic pain. *Pain*. **110**: 182–188.
23 Scott JC *et al.* (1991) Electroencephalographic quantitation of opioid effect: comparative pharmacodynamics of fentanyl and sufentanil. *Anesthesiology*. **74**: 34–42.
24 Waara-Wolleat KL *et al.* (2006) A review of intrathecal fentanyl and sufentanil for the treatment of chronic pain. *Pain Medicine*. **7**: 251–259.
25 White C *et al.* (2008) Subcutaneous sufentanil for palliative care patients in a hospital setting. *Palliative Medicine*. **22**: 89–90.
26 Lemoel F *et al.* (2019) Intranasal sufentanil given in the emergency department triage zone for severe acute traumatic pain: a randomized double-blind controlled trial. *Internal and Emergency Medicine*. **14**: 571–579.
27 Good P *et al.* (2009) Intranasal sufentanil for cancer-associated breakthrough pain. *Palliative Medicine*. **23**: 54–58.
28 Thangaraju P *et al.* (2021) Efficacy and safety of sufentanil sublingual tablet system in postoperative pain management: a systematic review and meta-analysis. *BMJ Supportive & Palliative Care*. Epub. Online ahead of print. DOI: 10.1136/bmjspcare-2020-002693.
29 Deeks ED (2019) Sufentanil 30 microgram sublingual tablet: A review in acute pain. *Clinical Drug Investigation*. **39**: 411–418.
30 Alazia M *et al.* (1992) Pharmacokinetics of long term sufentanil infusion (72 hours) used for sedation in ICU patients. *Anesthesiology*. **77**: A364 (abstract).
31 MHRA (2020) Benzodiazepines and opioids: reminder of risk of potentially fatal respiratory depression. *Drug Safety Update*. www.gov.uk/drug-safety-update.
32 Preston C. *Stockley's Drug Interactions*. London: Pharmaceutical Press www.medicinescomplete.com (accessed July 2021).
33 Cran A *et al.* (2017) Opioid rotation to alfentanil: comparative evaluation of conversion ratios. *BMJ Supportive and Palliative Care*. **7**: 265–266.
34 Dorman S (2017) *Personal communication*.

Updated July 2021

Quick Clinical Guide: Procedure-related pain

1 Palliative care patients may experience pain while undergoing procedures, e.g.:
- position change
- investigation, e.g. MRI
- wound dressing change
- venous cannulation
- urethral catheterization
- removing impacted faeces
- insertion of nasogastric tube
- insertion/removal of central line
- insertion/removal of spinal line
- drainage of chest/abdomen
- treatment, e.g. radiation therapy.

2 The goal is adequate pain relief without undesirable effects. What is appropriate depends on the anticipated pain severity, procedure duration, current opioid use, and the patient's past personal experience. Thus, severe procedure-related pain may necessitate parenteral analgesia and sedation as first-line therapy.

3 Always include non-drug approaches:
- discuss past experiences of procedure-related pain, identify what was helpful or unhelpful, and clarify present concerns
- explain the procedure thoroughly before starting
- assure that you will stop immediately if requested
- as far as possible, choose the most comfortable position for the patient
- distract and relax, e.g. through talking, music, hypnosis and other relaxation techniques.

4 Use a local anaesthetic for:
- venous cannulation; if needle-phobic or if requested, e.g. EMLA® cream (wait 60min)
- urethral catheterization; use lidocaine 2% gel, e.g. Instillagel® (wait 5min)
- chest aspiration; infiltrate tissue with lidocaine injection, e.g. 5mL of 1% (wait 5min).

5 If available, consider nitrous oxide–oxygen (Entonox®) inhalation if only mild–moderate pain anticipated, the procedure is short and the patient is able to use the mask or mouthpiece effectively.

6 Give analgesia from the appropriate step of the ladder (also see Box A).
Note. General anaesthetic approaches are beyond the scope of these guidelines.

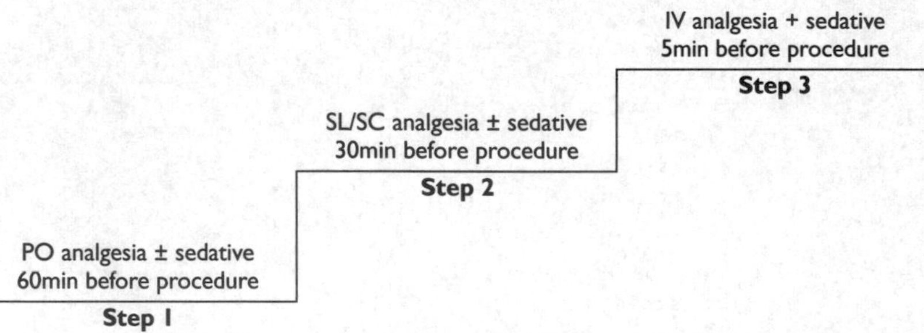

7 If pain relief inadequate, give a repeat dose and wait again; if still inadequate, move to the next step.

8 When a sedative or sedative analgesic is used, practitioners must be competent in airway management. Monitor the patient to ensure that the airway remains patent, and intervene if the patient becomes cyanosed because of severely depressed respiration.

Box A Examples of analgesia for procedure-related pain in adults

Use lower doses in older or frail patients and those with renal or hepatic impairment.

Step 1: If anticipating mild–moderate pain
Give 60min before the procedure:
PO morphine; give the patient's usual rescue dose for break-through pain.
If necessary, combine with:
- PO diazepam 5mg *or*
- SL lorazepam 500microgram–1mg *or*
- an alternative sedative.

Step 2: If anticipating moderate–severe pain
Give 30min before procedure:
SC morphine; give 50% of the patient's usual PO morphine rescue dose.
If necessary, combine with:
- SC midazolam 2.5–5mg *or*
- SL lorazepam 500microgram–1mg *or*
- an alternative sedative.

Step 3: If anticipating severe–excruciating pain
Give 5min before procedure:
IV morphine; give 50% of the patient's usual PO morphine rescue dose. Alternatively, give IV ketamine 0.5–1mg/kg (typically 25–50mg).
Combine with:
- IV midazolam 2mg over 1–2min, followed by 1mg every 2min until adequate sedation *or*
- an alternative sedative.

Note. There is a risk of marked sedation when ketamine and a sedative such as midazolam are combined in this way; use only if competent in airway management.

Alternatives to SC/IV morphine
- fentanyl 50–100microgram or more transmucosally using an authorized product (p.450) or SC/IV
- alfentanil 250–500microgram SL (*from ampoule for injection or spray*) or SC/IV
- sufentanil 12.5–25microgram SL (*from ampoule for injection; not UK*) or SC/IV.

9 An opioid antagonist (naloxone) and a benzodiazepine antagonist (flumazenil) should be available in case of need. To prevent the complete reversal of any background regular opioid analgesic therapy, use naloxone 100microgram IV, repeated every 2min until the respiratory rate and cyanosis have improved. The initial dose of flumazenil is 200microgram IV over 15 seconds; if the desired level of consciousness is not obtained after 1 minute, further 100microgram doses can be given at 1 minute intervals p.r.n. up to a maximum total dose of 1mg.

10 If the procedure is to be repeated, give analgesia based on previous experience, e.g. drugs used and the patient's comments.

BUPRENORPHINE

Buprenorphine is experiencing a renaissance in the management of chronic cancer and non-cancer pain and opioid dependence.[1-4] Preliminary data suggest that compared to **morphine** and other opioids, buprenorphine appears to cause less hyperalgesia (see p.398) and tolerance, and has less effect on the immune and endocrine systems. However, clinical trials are needed to find out whether such differences represent real clinical advantages.

Class: Strong opioid analgesic.

Indications: *SL tablet (200 and 400microgram) and injection* moderate–severe pain, premedication and peri-operative analgesia, †intolerance to other strong opioids.
TD patches (5–20microgram/h) moderate non-cancer pain; †intolerance to other strong opioids.
TD higher-dose patches (35–70microgram/h) severe non-cancer pain; moderate–severe cancer pain, †intolerance to other strong opioids.
SL higher-dose tablet (400microgram, 2mg, 8mg) withdrawal and maintenance therapy for opioid addicts, (also available as a combined formulation with **naloxone**, to prevent parenteral misuse); oromucosal and SC depot injection products are also available (see Supply).

Contra-indications: None absolute if titrated carefully against a patient's pain (also see Strong opioids, p.389). TD buprenorphine should not be used for acute (transient, intermittent or short-term) pain, e.g. postoperative, or when there is need for rapid dose titration for severe uncontrolled pain.

Pharmacology

Buprenorphine is a partial μ-opioid receptor and opioid-receptor-like (ORL-1) *agonist* and a κ- and δ-opioid receptor *antagonist*.[5] It has high affinity at the μ-, κ- and δ-opioid receptors, but affinity at the ORL-1 receptor is 500-fold less. It associates and dissociates slowly from receptors.[6] Analgesia is via the μ-opioid receptor, and subjective and physiological effects are generally similar to **morphine**. A common polymorphism of the μ-opioid receptor (N40D), present in ≤50% of people, reduces the efficacy of buprenorphine at the receptor (but not **fentanyl** (p.440), **methadone** (p.469), **morphine** (p.404) or **oxycodone** (p.480)) and may contribute towards a reduced clinical effect.[7]

Buprenorphine is effective in cancer pain, but because of very low quality evidence, particularly for the TD patch, the authors of a systematic review positioned its use after **morphine** and the common alternatives, **oxycodone** and **fentanyl**.[8]

Studies, mostly in volunteers, suggest that compared with **morphine** and other opioids, buprenorphine exerts a more prominent antihyperalgesic than analgesic effect;[9-11] however, this is not a consistent finding.[12] Animal studies, case reports and one RCT (in diabetic neuropathy) suggest that buprenorphine may be of particular benefit in neuropathic pain.[2,13-18] However, high-quality RCTs are needed to confirm this.[19] The co-administration of an ultra-low dose of an opioid antagonist potentiated the analgesic effect of buprenorphine (as with other opioids) in healthy volunteers but not patients (also see p.490).[20,21]

Antagonist effects at the κ-opioid receptor may limit spinal analgesia, hyperalgesia, sedation and psychotomimetic effects.[4,22] This may also explain the antidepressant effect of buprenorphine.[23,24]

In animal studies, buprenorphine shows a ceiling effect or a bell-shaped dose-response curve for analgesic (>1mg/kg) and respiratory effects (0.1mg/kg). This is thought to be due to its partial agonist effect at the μ-opioid receptor. An agonist effect at the pronociceptive supraspinal ORL-1 receptor may also contribute.[25] In humans, a ceiling effect has been shown for respiratory depression (~200microgram/70kg IV)[26,27] and other effects, e.g. euphoria (4–8mg SL),[28,29] but *not* for analgesia.[27] Total daily doses up to 32mg SL are reported to provide effective analgesia.[30] Thus, the ceiling dose for analgesia in humans is much higher than the 'maximum' TD dose recommended by the UK manufacturers, namely 3.36mg/24h (70microgram/h patches x 2).

Studies of buprenorphine TD or SL up to 1.6mg/24h have confirmed that it is possible to use **morphine** (or other μ agonist) for break-through pain,[31,32] and to switch either way between buprenorphine and **morphine** (or other μ agonist) without loss of analgesia.[33,34]

However, greater difficulties are experienced when switching patients on higher doses of opioids, using larger doses of buprenorphine.[35] When patients on various opioids (oral **morphine** equivalent 15–450mg/24h) were switched using doses of buprenorphine 2mg SL (resulting in maximum post-switch doses of 6–24mg/24h), over half experienced intolerable undesirable effects and abandoned the switch. Generally, undesirable effects related to opioid excess in patients receiving low doses of oral **morphine** equivalent (≤20mg/24h) and opioid withdrawal in those receiving high doses (>300mg/24h). This experience guided the development of a clinical protocol, although the dosing algorithm has not yet been tested formally.[35]

The use of other μ agonists for break-through pain in patients on higher doses of buprenorphine may also be less straightforward (see Opioid-maintenance therapy and pain management in addicts). Nonetheless, various μ agonists have been used in patients on SL buprenorphine 2–32mg/24h, although higher doses than usual may be required.[36,37]

Buprenorphine has either no effect or a smaller effect than **morphine** on pressure within the biliary and pancreatic ducts.[38,39] Buprenorphine does slow intestinal transit, but possibly less than **morphine**.[40,41] Constipation may be less severe.[42]

Compared with **morphine** and other opioids, buprenorphine appears less likely to suppress the gonadal axis or testosterone levels (see p.397).[43] This may relate to its antagonist effect at the κ-opioid receptor.[44] Because hypogonadism is associated with reduced sexual desire and function, mood disturbance, fatigue and other physiological effects, e.g. muscle wasting and osteoporosis, this may become an important consideration in patients requiring long-term opioid therapy.[45-47]

Compared with **morphine** and other opioids, buprenorphine has little or no immunosuppressive effect (see p.397).[2,48-51]

Compared with **methadone**, buprenorphine has no clinically relevant effect on the QT interval, even at high doses used for opioid-maintenance therapy (see Chapter 20, p.797).[52-55]

In an anecdotal report, 2 out of 5 patients with cholestatic pruritus responded to treatment with buprenorphine.[56,57] However, there are insufficient data at present to recommend its use in this circumstance.

TD buprenorphine

Buprenorphine is highly lipid-soluble, making it suitable for TD delivery. It is available in the UK in formulations delivering lower and higher doses, i.e. 5, 10, 15 or 20microgram/h as 7-day patches[58-60] and 35, 52.5 or 70microgram/h as 3- or 4-day patches (see Dose and use).[61] Like other strong opioids, buprenorphine is an alternative to both weak opioids and **morphine**.[62] Buprenorphine is evenly distributed in a drug-in-adhesive matrix. Its release is controlled by the physical characteristics of the matrix and is proportional to the surface area of the patch. Absorption of the buprenorphine through the skin and into the systemic circulation is influenced by the stratum corneum and blood flow. Thus, if the skin is warm and vasodilated, the rate of absorption increases.

There are few practical differences in the use of the buprenorphine or **fentanyl** matrix patches, and similar safety considerations apply (see Cautions). Compared with **fentanyl**, TD buprenorphine (as Transtec®) adheres better. However, after patch removal, it is associated with more persistent erythema (± localized pruritus) and sometimes a more definite dermatitis.[63] This is generally caused by the adhesive, but occasionally buprenorphine itself causes a contact dermatitis ± more widespread skin rash.[64]

Retrospective analysis suggests that, compared with TD **fentanyl**, patients receiving TD buprenorphine (as Transtec®) have a slower rate of dose increase and longer periods of dose stability.[65] This requires confirmation in an RCT. Indeed, systematic reviews have highlighted a lack of high quality studies of TD buprenorphine.[66,67]

Opioid-maintenance therapy and pain management in addicts

Buprenorphine binds to the μ-opioid receptor with a higher affinity than other μ-opioid agonists. Studies in addicts indicate that buprenorphine ≥16mg SL is required to suppress illicit opioid use;[68] at this dose level, ≥80% of the μ-opioid receptors in the brain are occupied by buprenorphine, which is sufficient to antagonize the subjective and respiratory depressant effects of **hydromorphone**, a μ agonist.[6,69] This has implications for the management of acute pain in these patients, e.g. postoperative or traumatic pain (see Chapter 25, p.821), and potentially for patients on higher-dose buprenorphine for chronic pain (see above). Nonetheless, there are reports of supplemental opioids providing adequate postoperative pain relief in patients receiving buprenorphine ≥16mg SL.[70]

Similar considerations will apply to patients receiving other buprenorphine products authorized for opioid-maintenance therapy, i.e. oromocosal tablets and SC depot injection products (see Supply).

Respiratory depression

Buprenorphine demonstrates a ceiling effect for respiratory depression. Thus, unlike other opioids where progressive doses reduce ventilation to the point of apnoea, with buprenorphine, the level of respiratory depression plateaus once a certain dose is reached. In a healthy volunteer study, this equated to a maximum reduction of 50% in minute ventilation at doses >3microgram/kg IV.[26] Although significant respiratory depression is rarely seen with clinically recommended doses, *it can still occur, particularly in opioid-naïve patients in the acute pain setting.*[71]

A lower risk of respiratory depression may explain why buprenorphine (mainly SL ± **naloxone**) appears to have a better safety profile than **methadone**.[72] However, serious or fatal respiratory depression has occurred in addicts misusing buprenorphine, generally in high-dose IV and in combination with benzodiazepines or other CNS depressants, e.g. alcohol.[73,74] Because buprenorphine has both high receptor affinity and prolonged receptor binding, **naloxone** in standard doses does not reverse the effects of buprenorphine, and higher doses must be used (Box A).[2,75] The non-specific respiratory stimulant **doxapram** can also be used, 1–1.5mg/kg IV over 30sec, repeated if necessary at hourly intervals, or 1.5–*4mg/min* CIVI.[75-77]

Box A Reversal of buprenorphine-induced respiratory depression	
1	Discontinue buprenorphine (stop CSCI/CIVI, remove TD patch).
2	Give oxygen by mask.
3	Give IV naloxone *2mg* stat over 90sec.
4	Commence naloxone *4mg/h* by CIVI.
5	Continue CIVI until the patient's condition is satisfactory (probably <90min).
6	Monitor the patient frequently for the next 24h, and restart CIVI if respiratory depression recurs.
7	If the patient's condition remains satisfactory, restart buprenorphine at a reduced dose, e.g. half the previous dose.

Potency

Buprenorphine has a longer duration of action than **morphine**. In postoperative single-dose studies, buprenorphine provided analgesia for 6–7h, compared with 4–5h with **morphine**.[78] This is reflected in the recommended dose frequency (q6–8h vs. q4h for **morphine**). However, the longer duration of action of buprenorphine almost certainly means *single-dose* studies *underestimate* the relative potency of buprenorphine. Thus, the following should *not* be regarded as 'cast iron'. They merely provide a rough guide for use when switching route or opioids (also see Appendix 2, p.925):

- SL buprenorphine is about half as potent as IV/IM/SC buprenorphine; thus, in round figures, 200microgram SL is equivalent to 100microgram by injection[79,80]
- SL buprenorphine is about 80 times more potent than PO **morphine**;[33] thus, in round figures, 200microgram SL buprenorphine is equivalent to 15mg PO **morphine**
- IV/IM/SC buprenorphine is 30–40 times more potent than IV/IM/SC **morphine**;[81] thus, in round figures, 300microgram IV buprenorphine is equivalent to 10mg IV **morphine**
- TD buprenorphine is 70–115 times more potent than PO **morphine**; the lower limit is based on a small prospective study, and the upper limit a large retrospective chart review.[82-84]

Thus, *PCF* considers TD buprenorphine to be 100 times more potent than PO **morphine**, a convenient compromise. A PO **morphine** to TD buprenorphine conversion ratio of 100:1 makes a 5microgram/h TD buprenorphine patch equivalent to about 12mg/24h PO **morphine**. (Note. A lack of definitive data explains the wide variation seen in recommendations and clinical practice.[85-87])

A conversion ratio of PO **morphine** to TD buprenorphine of 100:1 also means that TD buprenorphine and TD **fentanyl** can be considered essentially equipotent (see Appendix 2, Table 2, p.928). However, others suggest that TD **fentanyl** is 1.4 times more potent than TD buprenorphine,[34,84] making TD **fentanyl** 25 and 50microgram/h patches equivalent to buprenorphine 35 and 70microgram/h patches respectively. Even so, when switching opioids because of possible opioid-induced hyperalgesia, it is prudent to reduce the calculated equivalent dose of the new opioid by 25–50% (see Strong opioids, Opioid switching ('rotation'), p.400).

Switching opioids

When making any opioid switch, patients changing from another opioid to buprenorphine may experience worsening pain and/or opioid-withdrawal symptoms. Careful monitoring and titration of buprenorphine is required to ensure any worsening pain is dealt with promptly.

Opioid withdrawal manifests with GI and flu-like symptoms, e.g. abdominal pain, diarrhoea, arthralgia and myalgia, and lasts for a few days. With TD and lower doses of SL buprenorphine, p.r.n. doses of the previous opioid will relieve troublesome symptoms.

However, in addiction medicine, when switching generally involves high-dose SL buprenorphine, the practice is to discontinue the first opioid, await the development of withdrawal symptoms, and only then commence buprenorphine. In this way, opioid withdrawal will not be precipitated by buprenorphine (because of its greater affinity for the μ-opioid receptor) but, rather, once withdrawal symptoms are present, they should be relieved by it.

Pharmacokinetics

The bio-availability of PO buprenorphine is low (15%); it undergoes extensive first-pass metabolism in the GI mucosa and liver, where it is almost completely converted by CYP3A4 to norbuprenorphine. Norbuprenorphine has similar opioid-receptor-binding affinities to buprenorphine but does not readily cross the blood–brain barrier and has little, if any, central effect.[88] Both buprenorphine and norbuprenorphine undergo glucuronidation to what have traditionally been considered inactive metabolites, although animal work has questioned this.[89,90]

The bio-availability of SL buprenorphine is about 50%; it is rapidly absorbed into the oral mucosa (2–3min), followed by a slower absorption into the systemic circulation (t_{max} 30min–3.5h after a single dose; 1–2h with repeat dosing).[88] This, together with a duration of action of 6–8h, suggests that SL buprenorphine is *not* ideal for the treatment of break-through pain. Nonetheless, onset of analgesia in 10–20min is reported for SL buprenorphine,[40] and it has been successfully used as a rescue analgesic in patients receiving higher dose TD buprenorphine (i.e. Transtec®).[91] After parenteral and SL administration, 70% of buprenorphine is excreted unchanged in the faeces, and some enterohepatic recirculation is likely, whereas norbuprenorphine is mainly excreted in the urine.[92] Vomiting is more common with SL administration than IM or TD.

Buprenorphine has a large volume of distribution and is highly protein-bound (96%; α- and β-globulins).[88] It does not accumulate in renal impairment nor is it generally removed by haemodialysis, and thus analgesia is unaffected.[93,94] Although accumulation of norbuprenorphine can occur, this is of uncertain clinical relevance given its lack of central effect.[88,93] Thus, buprenorphine is potentially a reasonable option for patients with renal impairment (see p.743).

There is an increase in overall exposure to buprenorphine in moderate (1.6-fold) and severe (3-fold) hepatic impairment, sufficient to advise smaller starting doses and careful titration with the latter (see p.762). Buprenorphine crosses the placenta and enters breast milk. The incidence, severity and duration of the neonatal abstinence syndrome appears to be less than with **methadone**.[95,96]

The bio-availability of IV buprenorphine is by definition 100%, and that of SC essentially the same. Bio-availability is irrelevant in relation to TD patches; the stated delivery rates reflect the mean amount of drug delivered to patients throughout the patch's recommended duration of use. Inevitably, there will be interindividual variation in the amount delivered. Extrapolating from data relating to TD fentanyl, the absorption of TD buprenorphine could also be impaired in patients with cachexia, possibly because of a loss of skin hydration.[97] Pharmacokinetic data are summarized in Table 1.

Table 1 Pharmacokinetic details for buprenorphine

	IV	*TD (Hapoctasin®)*	*TD (Transtec®)*	*TD (BuTrans®)*	*SL*
Onset of action	5–15min[78]	4–12h	21h for 35microgram/h patch; 11h for 70microgram/h patch	18–24h	10–20min[40]
Time to peak plasma concentration	5min	34h for 35microgram/h patch; 29h for 70microgram/h patch	60h	3 days	30min–3.5h single dose; 1–2h multiple doses[22,88]
Plasma halflife	20–25h	24–27h[a]	25–36h[a]	13–35h[a]	24–69h[88]
Duration of action	6–8h	3 days	4 days	7 days	6–8h

a. the halflife after a patch has been removed and not replaced.

Cautions

Although most of the safety warnings and cautions from the regulatory authorities regarding the use of TD patches have been issued for **fentanyl** (p.441), adverse events have also occurred with the use of buprenorphine TD patches.[98] Thus, the same cautions are applicable, i.e. health professionals and patients/carers must be made aware:[99]

- that buprenorphine is a strong opioid analgesic
- that buprenorphine TD patches are inappropriate for short-term, intermittent or postoperative pain in patients who had not previously been receiving a strong opioid
- of directions for safe use, storage and disposal
- of the signs of an overdose and when to seek attention
- that the rate of absorption of buprenorphine may be increased if the skin under the patch becomes vasodilated, e.g. in febrile patients, at high ambient temperatures, or by an external heat source, e.g. electric blanket, heat lamps, saunas, hot tubs or MRI scans
- of drug interactions which can increase buprenorphine levels.

Additional errors reported for TD patches include the failure to remove old patches, the dispensing and application of higher-strength patches than prescribed, and incorrect disposal. The latter is associated with accidental exposure and deaths in others, particularly children.

Hepatic impairment (for severe hepatic impairment, see Chapter 18, p.762), or severe renal impairment (see Chapter 17, p.743). For a general approach when renal or hepatic function deteriorates rapidly, see Strong opioids, p.393.

The combination of high-dose buprenorphine SL with antiretrovirals, particularly **delavirdine** and **ritonavir**, increases the QT interval, but the clinical significance of this is uncertain.[100] Although the SPC contra-indicates the use of buprenorphine within 14 days of MAOI use and warns of the potential for serotonin toxicity, both appear to be blanket precautions (see Strong opioids, p.395).

Drug interactions

Concurrent treatment with ≥2 CNS depressants (e.g. benzodiazepines, gabapentinoids, opioids) increases the risk of respiratory depression, particularly in susceptible groups, e.g. the elderly and those with renal or hepatic impairment.[101]

A single case report describes respiratory depression when IM **ketorolac** was added to epidural buprenorphine.[102]

Buprenorphine is mainly a substrate of CYP3A4, and the manufacturers and others advise caution if prescribed concurrently with CYP3A4 inhibitors (e.g. **clarithromycin**, **erythromycin**, **itraconazole**, protease inhibitors), or avoiding concurrent use, because of the potential to increase buprenorphine levels. Although for most CYP3A4 inhibitors this is a theoretical concern, **atazanavir**, **ritonavir** and **delavirdine** (not UK) have been shown to significantly increase buprenorphine plasma levels in patients receiving high doses of SL buprenorphine (8–16mg/24h).[103] Accordingly, it is recommended that the dose of buprenorphine is halved in patients receiving high-dose buprenorphine SL if used concurrently with a CYP3A4 inhibitor (see Chapter 19, Table 8, p.790).[103]

Conversely, CYP3A4 inducers (e.g. **carbamazepine**, **phenobarbital**, **phenytoin**, **rifampicin**) could reduce buprenorphine levels. For **rifampicin**, reduced levels are seen following SL but not IV buprenorphine.[104]

Undesirable effects

Also see Strong opioids, Box B (p.394).

Very common (>10%): nausea; erythema and pruritus at the patch application site.

Common (<10%, >1%): asthenia, drowsiness, dizziness, headache, oedema, vomiting, constipation, sweating.

Dose and use

Patients using opioids must be monitored for undesirable effects, particularly nausea and vomiting, and constipation. Depending on individual circumstances, an anti-emetic should be prescribed for regular or p.r.n. use, (see QCG: Nausea and vomiting, p.264) and, routinely, a laxative prescribed (see QCG: Opioid-induced constipation, p.45).

Opioids can impair driving ability, and patients should be counselled accordingly (see Chapter 22, p.809).

TD

The use of TD buprenorphine patches is summarized in the Quick Clinical Guide (see QCG: Use of transdermal buprenorphine patches, p.438). This is based on a dose conversion ratio of PO **morphine** to TD buprenorphine of 100:1. Prescribers using the manufacturer's ratio of 75–115:1 should follow the dose conversion guidelines in the SPC (see Appendix 2, Box A, p.929).

In 2013, in response to large numbers of safety incident reports about buprenorphine and **fentanyl** TD patches, the Care Quality Commission highlighted the need to ensure that:

- use is appropriate, e.g. chronic *not* acute pain
- dose is appropriate, i.e. in line with published conversion charts
- dose is titrated appropriately, i.e. by no more than 50% of the previous daily dose
- date and site of application are recorded to avoid inadvertent dose omission or duplication.

Further, to avoid confusing patients and carers, prescribing by brand was recommended.[98] Subsequently, others have highlighted the importance of specifying the dose-rate and frequency of patch replacement on the prescription and pharmacy label.[105]

TD patches and MRI scans: buprenorphine patches should be removed before the patient enters the scan room, due to the risks from heating. Patients should be advised to bring a replacement patch with them to facilitate this (also see Chapter 30, p.901).

In Europe, TD patches are the commonest formulation of buprenorphine used in chronic cancer and non-cancer pain. Particularly for patients unable to swallow or take PO/SL products reliably, TD buprenorphine provides an alternative non-invasive route for opioid administration.[85]

Compared to the SL and parenteral routes, the TD patches permit smaller initial doses of buprenorphine to be delivered more consistently (without large peaks and troughs) and are thus better tolerated.[106] In the UK, TD buprenorphine patches are available:

- as 5, 10, 15 and 20microgram/h 7-day patches
- as 35, 52.5 and 70microgram/h 3-day or 4-day patches; the 4-day patches can be replaced on fixed days in the week, i.e. after 3 and 4 days alternately.

Because of the wide number of different formulations and brands available (see Supply), prescribing by brand is recommended to avoid confusing patients and carers.[98]

For patients who have not already been taking an opioid, a low patch strength should be prescribed, i.e. 5microgram/h (equivalent to **morphine** 12mg/24h PO). For patients switching from another strong opioid, see QCG: Use of transdermal buprenorphine patches (p.438). General advice and recommended starting doses are also detailed in the manufacturer's SPC.

Absorption of buprenorphine through the skin and into the systemic circulation is influenced by both the condition of the skin and cutaneous blood flow. Thus, if the skin is warm and vasodilated, the rate of absorption will be increased.

It is important to give adequate rescue doses of **morphine** (see QCG: Use of transdermal buprenorphine patches, p.438) or another strong opioid. Adjusting the patch strength on a daily basis is not recommended. With inpatients, the use of a monitoring chart is recommended (see Document library, www.palliativedrugs.com).[107]

SL

The tablet should not be chewed or swallowed, as this will reduce efficacy:

- manufacturer's recommended starting dose 200microgram SL (equivalent to approximately **morphine** 15mg PO) q8h; this may be too much for some patients
- moisten the mouth with a sip of water beforehand if the mouth is dry
- use an appropriate dose of a strong opioid as a rescue analgesic. Note. SL buprenorphine is *not* an ideal rescue analgesic but, if used, allow one tenth of the total daily dose, rounded to a convenient tablet size, q3h p.r.n.; some limit this to a maximum of 4 doses per 24h
- titrate the dose every 4–5 days, based on p.r.n. use
- typical dose 800–1,200microgram/24h, given as 200–400microgram q6–8h
- doses of 2–24*mg*/24h have been reported in chronic pain patients switched from other opioids.[35,108]

SC/IM/IV

- manufacturer's recommended starting dose 300microgram (equivalent to approximately **morphine** 10mg SC/IM/IV) q8h; this may be too much for some patients
- give IV over ≥2min
- if necessary, titrate to 600microgram q6–8h (the recommended maximum in acute pain; in chronic pain higher doses may be required).

CSCI/CIVI

- buprenorphine has been given CIVI diluted in sodium chloride 0.9% at a concentration of 15microgram/mL; there are no compatibility data for mixing with other drugs used in palliative care
- for patients receiving CSCI/CIVI buprenorphine, p.r.n. injections of about one tenth of the total daily dose can be used for break-through pain.

Supply

All preparations are Schedule 3 **CD**.

Buprenorphine (generic)
Tablets SL 200microgram, 400microgram, 28 days @ 200microgram t.d.s. = £7.

Transdermal products
Buprenorphine (generic)
Matrix patches (for 7 days) 5microgram/h, 10microgram/h, 15microgram/h, 20microgram/h, 1 = £1.50, £2.50, £3.75 and £4.50 respectively.
Brands include Bupramyl®, Butec®, Butrans®, Panitaz®, Reletrans® and Sevodyne®.
Matrix patches (for 3 or 4 days) 35microgram/h, 52.5microgram/h, 70microgram/h, 1 = £2.25, £3.50 and £4.50 respectively.
Brands include Hapoctasin® (3 days only), Bupeaze®, Carlosafine®, Relevtec®, Transtec®.

Parenteral products
Temgesic® (Indivior UK)
Injection 300microgram/mL, 1mL amp = £0.50.

Higher-dose products

The following buprenorphine products are authorized for opioid withdrawal and maintenance therapy for addicts:

- SL tablets 400microgram, 2mg and 8mg
- SL tablets and SL films with **naloxone** (in a combination ratio of 4:1); these two products are *not interchangeable*
- oromucosal (oral lyophilisate) tablets 2mg and 8mg (Espranor®); these are *not interchangeable with SL tablets*
- modified-release SC depot injection 8mg–128mg (Buvidal®) given weekly or monthly.

See BNF for full details and range of products.

1 Resnick RB (2003) Food and Drug Administration approval of buprenorphine-naloxone for office treatment of addiction. *Annals of Internal Medicine*. **138**: 360.

2 Budd K and Raffa R, (eds) (2005) Buprenorphine - the unique opioid analgesic. Georg Thieme Verlag, Stuttgart, Germany, pp. 134.

3 Gowing L *et al.* (2017) Buprenorphine for the management of opioid withdrawal. *Cochrane Database Systematic Reviews*. **5**: CD002025. www.cochranelibrary.com.

4 Davis MP et *al.* (2018) Treating chronic pain: An overview of clinical studies centered on the buprenorphine option. *Drugs*. **78**: 1211–1228.

5 Infantino R *et al.* (2021) Buprenorphine: far beyond the "ceiling". *Biomolecules*. **11**: 816.

6 Greenwald M *et al.* (2007) Buprenorphine duration of action: mu-opioid receptor availability and pharmacokinetic and behavioral indices. *Biological Psychiatry*. **61**: 101–110.

7 Knapman A *et al.* (2014) Buprenorphine signalling is compromised at the N40D polymorphism of the human mu opioid receptor in vitro. *British Journal of Pharmacology*. **171**: 4273–4288.

8 Schmidt-Hansen M *et al.* (2015) Buprenorphine for treating cancer pain. *Cochrane Database of Systematic Reviews*. **3**: CD009596. www.cochranelibrary.com.

9 Koppert W *et al.* (2005) Different profiles of buprenorphine-induced analgesia and antihyperalgesia in a human pain model. *Pain*. **118**: 15–22.

10 Simonnet G (2005) Opioids: from analgesia to anti-hyperalgesia? *Pain*. **118**: 8–9.

11 Mercieri M *et al.* (2017) Low-dose buprenorphine infusion to prevent postoperative hyperalgesia in patients undergoing major lung surgery and remifentanil infusion: a double-blind, randomized, active-controlled trial. *British Journal of Anaesthesia*. **119**: 792–802.

12 Ravn P *et al.* (2013) Morphine- and buprenorphine-induced analgesia and antihyperalgesia in a human inflammatory pain model: a double-blind, randomized, placebo-controlled, five-arm crossover study. *Journal of Pain Research*. **6**: 23–38.

13 Kress HG (2009) Clinical update on the pharmacology, efficacy and safety of transdermal buprenorphine. *European Journal of Pain*. **13**: 219–230.

14 Hans G (2007) Buprenorphine--a review of its role in neuropathic pain. *Journal of Opioid Management*. **3**: 195–206.

15 Sanchez-Blazquez P and Garzon J (1988) Pertussis toxin differentially reduces the efficacy of opioids to produce supraspinal analgesia in the mouse. *European Journal of Pharmacology*. **152**: 357–361.

16 Likar R and Sittl R (2005) Transdermal buprenorphine for treating nociceptive and neuropathic pain: four case studies. *Anesthesia and Analgesia*. **100**: 781–785.

17 Penza P *et al.* (2008) Short- and intermediate-term efficacy of buprenorphine TDS in chronic painful neuropathies. *Journal of the Peripheral Nervous System*. **13**: 283–288.

18 Simpson RW and Wlodarczyk JH (2016) Transdermal buprenorphine relieves neuropathic pain: a randomized, double-blind, parallel-group, placebo-controlled trial in diabetic peripheral neuropathic pain. *Diabetes Care*. **39**: 1493–1500.

19 Wiffen PJ *et al.* (2017) Opioids for cancer pain - an overview of Cochrane reviews. *Cochrane Database of Systematic Reviews*. **7**: CD012592. www.cochranelibrary.com.

20 Hay JL *et al.* (2011) Potentiation of buprenorphine antinociception with ultra-low dose naltrexone in healthy subjects. *European Journal of Pain*. **15**: 293–298.

21 Ling W *et al.* (2012) Comparisons of analgesic potency and side effects of buprenorphine and buprenorphine with ultra-low-dose naloxone. *Journal of Addiction Medicine*. **6**: 118–123.

22 Johnson RE *et al.* (2005) Buprenorphine: considerations for pain management. *Journal of Pain and Symptom Management*. **29**: 297–326.

23 Falcon E *et al.* (2016) Antidepressant-like effects of buprenorphine are mediated by kappa opioid receptors. *Neuropsychopharmacology*. **41**: 2344–2351.

24 Serafini G *et al.* (2018) The Efficacy of Buprenorphine in Major Depression, Treatment-Resistant Depression and Suicidal Behavior: A Systematic Review. *International Journal of Molecular Sciences*. **19**: (8).

25 Lutfy K *et al.* (2003) Buprenorphine-induced antinociception is mediated by mu-opioid receptors and compromised by concomitant activation of opioid receptor-like receptors. *Journal of Neuroscience*. **23**: 10331–10337.

26 Dahan A *et al.* (2005) Comparison of the respiratory effects of intravenous buprenorphine and fentanyl in humans and rats. *British Journal Anaesthesia*. **94**: 825–834.

27 Dahan A *et al.* (2006) Buprenorphine induces ceiling in respiratory depression but not in analgesia. *British Journal of Anaesthesia*. **96**: 627–632.

28 Budd K (2002) Buprenorphine: a review. Evidence Based Medicine in Practice. Hayward Medical Communications, Newmarket.

29 Walsh S *et al.* (1994) Clinical pharmacology of buprenorphine: ceiling effects at high doses. *Clinical Pharmacology and Therapeutics*. **55**: 569–580.

30 Cote J and Montgomery L (2014) Sublingual buprenorphine as an analgesic in chronic pain: a systematic review. *Pain Medicine*. **15**: 1171–1178.

31 Mercadante S *et al.* (2006) Safety and effectiveness of intravenous morphine for episodic breakthrough pain in patients receiving transdermal buprenorphine. *Journal of Pain and Symptom Management*. **32**: 175–179.

32 van Niel JC *et al.* (2016) Efficacy of full micro-opioid receptor agonists is not impaired by concomitant buprenorphine or mixed opioid agonists/antagonists - preclinical and clinical evidence. *Drug Research*. **66**: 562–570.

33 Atkinson R *et al.* The efficacy in sequential use of buprenorphine and morphine in advanced cancer pain. In: Doyle D, editor. *Opioids in the treatment of cancer pain*. London: Royal Society of Medicine Services; 1990. p. 81–87.
34 Mercadante S *et al.* (2007) Switching from transdermal drugs: an observational "N of 1" study of fentanyl and buprenorphine. *Journal of Pain and Symptom Management*. **34**: 532–538.
35 Rosenblum A *et al.* (2012) Sublingual buprenorphine/naloxone for chronic pain in at-risk patients: development and pilot test of a clinical protocol. *Journal of Opioid Management*. **8**: 369–382.
36 Kornfeld H and Manfredi L (2010) Effectiveness of full agonist opioids in patients stabilized on buprenorphine undergoing major surgery: a case series. *American Journal of Therapeutics*. **17**: 523–528.
37 Heit HA and Gourlay DL (2008) Buprenorphine: new tricks with an old molecule for pain management. *Clinical Journal of Pain*. **24**: 93–97.
38 Pausawasdi S *et al.* (1984) The effect of buprenorphine and morphine on intraluminal pressure of the common bile duct. *Journal of the Medical Association of Thailand*. **67**: 329–333.
39 Staritz M *et al.* (1986) Effect of modern analgesic drugs (tramadol, pentazocine, and buprenorphine) on the bile duct sphincter in man. *Gut*. **27**: 567–569.
40 Robbie DS (1979) A trial of sublingual buprenorphine in cancer pain. *British Journal of Clinical Pharmacology*. **7 (Suppl 3)**: S315–S317.
41 Bach V *et al.* (1991) Buprenorphine and sustained release morphine - effect and side-effects in chronic use. *The Pain Clinic*. **4**: 87–93.
42 Pace MC *et al.* (2007) Buprenorphine in long-term control of chronic pain in cancer patients. *Frontiers in Bioscience*. **12**: 1291–1299.
43 Hallinan R *et al.* (2009) Hypogonadism in men receiving methadone and buprenorphine maintenance treatment. *International Journal of Andrology*. **32**: 131–139.
44 Bliesener N *et al.* (2005) Plasma testosterone and sexual function in men receiving buprenorphine maintenance for opioid dependence. *Journal of Clinical Endocrinology and Metabolism*. **90**: 203–206.
45 Daniell HW (2002) Hypogonadism in men consuming sustained-action oral opioids. *The Journal of Pain*. **3**: 377–384.
46 Rajagopal A *et al.* (2004) Symptomatic hypogonadism in male survivors of cancer with chronic exposure to opioids. *Cancer*. **100**: 851–858.
47 Hallinan R *et al.* (2008) Erectile dysfunction in men receiving methadone and buprenorphine maintenance treatment. *Journal of Sexual Medicine*. **5**: 684–692.
48 Sacerdote P *et al.* (2000) The effects of tramadol and morphine on immune responses and pain after surgery in cancer patients. *Anesthesia and Analgesia*. **90**: 1411–1414.
49 Budd K and Shipton E (2004) Acute pain and the immune system and opioimmunosuppression. *Acute Pain*. **6**: 123–135.
50 Sacerdote P *et al.* (2008) Buprenorphine and methadone maintenance treatment of heroin addicts preserves immune function. *Brain, Behavior, and Immunity*. **22**: 606–613.
51 Canneti A *et al.* (2013) Safety and efficacy of transdermal buprenorphine and transdermal fentanyl in the treatment of neuropathic pain in AIDS patients. *Minerva Anestesiologica*. **79**: 871–883.
52 Wedam EF *et al.* (2007) QT-interval effects of methadone, levomethadyl, and buprenorphine in a randomized trial. *Archives of Internal Medicine*. **167**: 2469–2475.
53 Esses JL *et al.* (2008) Successful transition to buprenorphine in a patient with methadone-induced torsades de pointes. *Journal of Interventional Cardiac Electrophysiology*. **23**: 117–119.
54 Isbister GK *et al.* (2017) QT interval prolongation in opioid agonist treatment: analysis of continuous 12-lead electrocardiogram recordings. *British Journal of Clinical Pharmacology*. **83**: 2274–2282.
55 Harris SC *et al.* (2017) Effects of buprenorphine on QT intervals in healthy subjects: results of 2 randomized positive- and placebo-controlled trials. *Postgraduate Medicine*. **129**: 69–80.
56 Juby L *et al.* (1994) Buprenorphine and hepatic pruritus. *British Journal of Clinical Practice*. **48**: 331.
57 Reddy L *et al.* (2007) Transdermal buprenorphine may be effective in the treatment of pruritus in primary biliary cirrhosis. *Journal of Pain and Symptom Management*. **34**: 455–456.
58 Steiner DJ *et al.* (2011) Efficacy and safety of the seven-day buprenorphine transdermal system in opioid-naive patients with moderate to severe chronic low back pain: an enriched, randomized, double-blind, placebo-controlled study. *Journal of Pain and Symptom Management*. **42**: 903–917.
59 Conaghan PG *et al.* (2011) Transdermal buprenorphine plus oral paracetamol vs an oral codeine-paracetamol combination for osteoarthritis of hip and/or knee: a randomised trial. *Osteoarthritis and Cartilage*. **19**: 930–938.
60 Steiner D *et al.* (2011) Efficacy and safety of buprenorphine transdermal system (BTDS) for chronic moderate to severe low back pain: a randomized, double-blind study. *Journal of Pain and Symptom Management*. **12**: 1163–1173.
61 Llkar R *et al.* (2007) Transdermal buprenorphine patches applied in a 4-day regimen versus a 3-day regimen: a single-site, Phase III, randomized, open-label, crossover comparison. *Clinical Therapeutics*. **29**: 1591–1606.
62 Davis MP (2005) Buprenorphine in cancer pain. *Supportive Care in Cancer*. **13**: 878–887.
63 Schmid-Grendelmeier P *et al.* (2006) A comparison of the skin irritation potential of transdermal fentanyl versus transdermal buprenorphine in middle-aged to elderly healthy volunteers. *Current Medical Research Opinion*. **22**: 501–509.
64 Vander Hulst K *et al.* (2008) Allergic contact dermatitis from transdermal buprenorphine. *Contact Dermatitis*. **59**: 366–369.
65 Sittl R *et al.* (2006) Patterns of dosage changes with transdermal buprenorphine and transdermal fentanyl for the treatment of noncancer and cancer pain: a retrospective data analysis in Germany. *Clinical Therapeutics*. **28**: 1144–1154.
66 Deandrea S *et al.* (2009) Managing severe cancer pain: the role of transdermal buprenorphine: a systematic review. *Therapeutics and Clinical Risk Management*. **5**: 707–718.
67 Tassinari D *et al.* (2011) Transdermal opioids as front line treatment of moderate to severe cancer pain: a systemic review. *Palliative Medicine*. **25**: 478–487.
68 Mattick RP et al. (2014) Buprenorphine maintenance versus placebo or methadone maintenance for opioid dependence. *Cochrane Database of Systematic Reviews*. **2**: CD002207. www.cochranelibrary.com.
69 Greenwald MK *et al.* (2003) Effects of buprenorphine maintenance dose on mu-opioid receptor availability, plasma concentrations, and antagonist blockade in heroin-dependent volunteers. *Neuropsychopharmacology*. **28**: 2000–2009.
70 Goel A *et al.* (2019) The perioperative patient on buprenorphine: a systematic review of perioperative management strategies and patient outcomes. *Canadian Journal of Anesthesia*. **66**: 201–217.
71 Richards S *et al.* (2017) Buprenorphine-related complications in elderly hospitalised patients: a case series. *Anaesthesia and Intensive Care*. **45**: 256–261.
72 Dasgupta N *et al.* (2010) Post-marketing surveillance of methadone and buprenorphine in the United States. *Pain Medicine*. **11**: 1078–1091.
73 Kintz P (2001) Deaths involving buprenorphine: a compendium of French cases. *Forensic Science International*. **121**: 65–69.

74 Hakkinen M *et al.* (2012) Benzodiazepines and alcohol are associated with cases of fatal buprenorphine poisoning. *European Journal of Clinical Pharmacology*. **68**: 301–309.
75 Dahan A *et al.* (2010) Incidence, reversal, and prevention of opioid-induced respiratory depression. *Anesthesiology*. **112**: 226–238.
76 British National Formulary Section 3.5.1 Respiratory stimulants London: BMJ Group and Pharmaceutical Press. www.medicinescomplete.com (accessed October 2021).
77 Orwin JM (1977) The effect of doxapram on buprenorphine induced respiratory depression. *Acta anaesthesiologica Belgica*. **28**: 93–106.
78 Heel RC *et al.* (1979) Buprenorphine: a review of its pharmacological properties and therapeutic efficiency. *Drugs*. **17**: 81–110.
79 Ellis R *et al.* (1982) Pain relief after abdominal surgery-a comparison of i.m. morphine, sublingual buprenorphine and self-administered i.v. pethidine. *British Journal of Anaesthesia*. **54**: 421–428.
80 ullingham RE *et al.* (1984) Mandatory sublingual buprenorphine for postoperative pain. *Anaesthesia*. **39**: 329–334.
81 Cuschieri RJ et *al.* (1984) Comparison of morphine and sublingual buprenorphine following abdominal surgery. *British Journal of Anaesthesia*. **56**: 855–859.
82 Sittl R *et al.* (2005) Equipotent doses of transdermal fentanyl and transdermal buprenorphine in patients with cancer and noncancer pain: results of a retrospective cohort study. *Clinical Therapeutics*. **27**: 225–237.
83 Likar R *et al.* (2008) Challenging the equipotency calculation for transdermal buprenorphine: four case studies. *International Journal of Clinical Practice*. **62**: 152–156.
84 Mercadante S *et al.* (2009) Equipotent doses to switch from high doses of opioids to transdermal buprenorphine. *Supportive Care in Cancer*. **17**: 715–718.
85 Caraceni A *et al.* (2012) Use of opioid analgesics in the treatment of cancer pain: evidence-based recommendations from the EAPC. *Lancet Oncology*. **13**: e58–68.
86 NICE (2016) Palliative care for adults: strong opioids for pain relief. *Clinical Guideline*. CG104. www.nice.org.uk.
87 Palliativedrugs.com (2013) The oral morphine equivalent of buprenorphine TD patches - What conversion do you use? Survey Results. *Additions Archive*. **March**: www.palliativedrugs.com.
88 Elkader A and Sproule B (2005) Buprenorphine: clinical pharmacokinetics in the treatment of opioid dependence. *Clinical Pharmacokinetics*. **44**: 661–680.
89 McQuay H and Moore R (1995) Buprenorphine kinetics in humans. In: Cowan A, Lewis J, editors. *Buprenorphine: combatting drug abuse with a unique opioid*. New York: Wiley-Liss; p. 137–147.
90 Brown SM *et al.* (2011) Buprenorphine metabolites, buprenorphine-3-glucuronide and norbuprenorphine-3-glucuronide, are biologically active. *Anesthesiology*. **115**: 1251–1260.
91 Poulain P *et al.* (2008) Efficacy and safety of transdermal buprenorphine: a randomized, placebo-controlled trial in 289 patients with severe cancer pain. *Journal of Pain and Symptom Management*. **36**: 117–125.
92 Cone EJ *et al.* (1984) The metabolism and excretion of buprenorphine in humans. *Drug Metabolism and Disposition*. **12**: 577–581.
93 Hand CW *et al.* (1990) Buprenorphine disposition in patients with renal impairment: single and continuous dosing, with special reference to metabolites. *British Journal of Anaesthesia*. **64**: 276–282.
94 Filitz J *et al.* (2006) Effect of intermittent hemodialysis on buprenorphine and norbuprenorphine plasma concentrations in chronic pain patients treated with transdermal buprenorphine. *European Journal of Pain*. **10**: 743–748.
95 Fischer G (2000) Treatment of opioid dependence in pregnant women. *Addiction*. **95**: 1141–1144.
96 Lacroix I *et al.* (2004) Buprenorphine in pregnant opioid-dependent women: first results of a prospective study. *Addiction*. **99**: 209–214.
97 Heiskanen T *et al.* (2009) Transdermal fentanyl in cachectic cancer patients. *Pain*. **144**: 218–222.
98 Care Quality Commission and NHS England (2013) Safer use of controlled drugs - preventing harms from fentanyl and buprenorphine transdermal patches. *Use of controlled drugs supporting information*. www.cqc.org.uk.
99 All Wales Medicine Strategy Group (2016) Safeguarding users of opioid patches by standardising patient/caregiver counselling. www.awmsg.org.
100 Baker JR *et al.* (2006) Effect of buprenorphine and antiretroviral agents on the QT interval in opioid-dependent patients. *Annals of Pharmacotherpy*. **40**: 392–396.
101 MHRA (2020) Benzodiazepines and opioids: reminder of risk of potentially fatal respiratory depression. *Drug Safety Update*. www.gov.uk/drug-safety-update.
102 Jain PN and Shah SC (1993) Respiratory depression following combination of epidural buprenorphine and intramuscular ketorolac. *Anaesthesia*. **48**: 898–899.
103 Preston CL. *Stockley's Drug Interactions*. London: Pharmaceutical Press. www.medicinescomplete.com (accessed October 2021).
104 Hagelberg NM *et al.* (2016) Rifampicin decreases exposure to sublingual buprenorphine in healthy subjects. *Pharmacology Research and Perspectives*. **4**: e00271.
105 UKMI (2019) Buprenorphine patches – how can you minimise the risk of medication errors? *Medicines Q&As*. www.sps.nhs.uk.
106 James IG *et al.* (2010) A randomized, double-blind, double-dummy comparison of the efficacy and tolerability of low-dose transdermal buprenorphine (BuTrans seven-day patches) with buprenorphine sublingual tablets (Temgesic) in patients with osteoarthritis pain. *Journal of Pain and Symptom Management*. **40**: 266–278.
107 Nottingham University Hospitals and Palliativedrugs.com (2021) Strong opioid transdermal patch monitoring chart. *Document Library*. Pain (strong opioids): www.palliativedrugs.com.
108 Malinoff HL *et al.* (2005) Sublingual buprenorphine is effective in the treatment of chronic pain syndrome. *American Journal of Therapeutics*. **12**: 379–384.

Updated November 2021

Quick Clinical Guide: Use of transdermal buprenorphine patches

1 Indications for using transdermal (TD) buprenorphine instead of morphine include:
- intolerable undesirable effects with morphine, e.g. nausea and vomiting, constipation, hallucinations, dysphagia
- end-stage renal failure (no centrally active metabolites)
- 'tablet phobia' or poor compliance with oral medication
- high risk of tablet misuse/diversion (although the patch can still be abused).

2 TD buprenorphine is contra-indicated in patients with acute (short-term) pain and in those who need rapid dose titration for severe uncontrolled pain.

3 TD buprenorphine patches are available:
- as 5, 10, 15 and 20microgram/h 7-day patches
- as 35, 52.5 and 70microgram/h 3-day or 4-day patches.

The patch brand, dose-rate and frequency of patch replacement should be stated on the prescription to avoid confusion. The maximum authorized dose is two 70microgram/h patches.

Use Table 1 below to decide a safe starting dose for TD buprenorphine and an appropriate rescue dose of morphine. These recommendations are based on a PO morphine to TD buprenorphine dose conversion ratio of 100:1 derived from published data, which is in keeping with the manufacturer's dose ratio range of 75–115:1 (see SPC). It is an approximation, and inevitably there will be individual variation. If switching to buprenorphine because of possible opioid-induced hyperalgesia, reduce the calculated equivalent dose by 25–50%.

4 Patients not previously receiving opioids should start on a 5microgram/h patch; patients with unrelieved pain despite maximum dose of a weak opioid should commence on 20 or 35microgram/h patches, according to circumstances.

5 For patients taking a dose of morphine that is not the exact equivalent of a buprenorphine patch, it will be necessary to opt for a patch that is either slightly more or slightly less than the morphine dose. Thus, if the patient still has pain, round up to a higher patch strength; if pain-free and frail, round down.

Table 1 Comparative doses based on dose conversion ratio 100:1

PO morphine[a]		*SC/IV morphine*[a]		*TD buprenorphine*	
mg/24h	*p.r.n. mg*[b]	*mg/24h*[c]	*p.r.n. mg*[b]	*microgram/h*	*microgram/24h*
					7-day patch
12	2[d]	6	1	5	120
24	5[d]	12	2.5	10	240
36	6[d]	18	3	15	360
48	10	24	5	20	480
					3- or 4-day patches
84	15	42	7.5	35	840
126	20	63	10	52.5	1,260
168	30	84	15	70[e]	1,680

a. an alternative strong opioid can be used, calculated using the appropriate conversion factor. Note. SL buprenorphine is *not* an ideal rescue medication, but some centres use an initial dose of 200microgram SL q3h, up to 4 doses per 24h, for patients receiving any strength of the 3- or 4-day patches

b. using traditional one sixth of total daily dose as p.r.n. dose and rounded to a convenient dose; give up to q1h; some centres opt for one tenth of total daily dose

c. assuming conversion ratio of PO morphine to SC/IV morphine of 2:1

d. at these doses, p.r.n. codeine/dihydrocodeine (30–60mg) or tramadol (50mg) may suffice

e. for combinations of patches, add the p.r.n. doses together, e.g. 70microgram/h + 52.5microgram/h patches = 15mg + 10mg morphine SC/IV = 25mg morphine SC/IV, but can round up to 30mg or down to 20mg for convenience.

6 The date of application and/or the date for renewal should be written in a consistent manner on the patch. Apply to dry, non-inflamed, non-irradiated, hairless skin on the upper trunk or arm. Body hair may be clipped with scissors but not shaved. If the skin is washed beforehand, use only water; do not use soap and do not apply oils, cream or ointment to the area. Press patch firmly in place for at least 30 seconds; adhesive tape (e.g. Micropore®) can be applied to the edges to aid adherence. Careful removal of the patch helps to minimize local skin irritation.

7 Systemic analgesic concentrations are generally reached within 12–24h, but levels continue to rise for 32–54h. If converting from:
- 4-hourly PO morphine, give regular doses for the first 12h after applying the patch
- 12-hourly m/r morphine, apply the patch and the final m/r dose at the same time
- 24-hourly m/r morphine, apply the patch 12h after the final m/r dose
- CSCI/CIVI opioids, continue the infusion for about 12h after applying the patch.

8 Steady-state plasma concentrations of buprenorphine are reached after 9 days (1–2 days with patch strength of ≤20microgram/h); the patient should use p.r.n. doses liberally, particularly during the first 24h, of either the previously used weak opioid, or morphine/other strong opioid, or buprenorphine (see Table 1 above).

9 After 72h, if a patient continues to need 2 or more rescue doses of analgesic/day, the next-strength patch should be used.

10 Patients could experience opioid-withdrawal symptoms when changed from another opioid (particularly large doses) to TD buprenorphine. These manifest with symptoms like gastric flu and last for a few days; p.r.n. doses of the previous opioid will relieve troublesome symptoms.

11 Buprenorphine is less constipating than morphine; halve the dose of laxatives when starting buprenorphine and re-titrate.

12 Buprenorphine may cause nausea and vomiting; if necessary, prescribe an anti-emetic, e.g. haloperidol 500microgram–1.5mg PO stat & at bedtime.

13 In febrile patients, the rate of absorption of buprenorphine increases and may cause toxicity, e.g. drowsiness. Absorption is also enhanced by an external heat source over the patch, e.g. electric blanket or hot-water bottle; patients should be warned about this. Patients may swim or shower with a patch, but should not soak in a hot bath. Remove patches before MRI scans.

14 Remove and replace patches once (7-day patch) or twice (3- and 4-day patches) a week. The 4-day patch can be replaced on fixed days in the week, i.e. after 3 and 4 days alternately. Change the site of application each time to avoid enhanced absorption; do not reuse an application site for at least 1 week (3- and 4-day patches) or 3 weeks (7-day patch). The use of a monitoring chart is recommended for inpatients.

15 A reservoir of buprenorphine accumulates in the body, particularly in adipose tissue, and significant plasma levels persist for at least 24h after discontinuing TD buprenorphine.

16 TD buprenorphine is unsatisfactory in <5% of patients.

17 In moribund patients, continue TD buprenorphine and give additional SC morphine p.r.n. (see Table 1 above). If >2 p.r.n. doses are required/24h, give morphine by CSCI, starting with a dose equal to the sum of the p.r.n. doses over the preceding 24h. If necessary, adjust the p.r.n. dose taking into account the total opioid dose (i.e. TD buprenorphine + CSCI morphine).

18 Used patches still contain buprenorphine; after removal, fold the patch with the adhesive side inwards, and then discard in a sharps container (hospital) or dustbin (home), and wash hands. Ultimately, any unused patches should be returned to a pharmacy.

Updated December 2021

FENTANYL

For transmucosal fentanyl for cancer-related break-through pain or procedure-related pain, see p.450.

Class: Strong opioid analgesic.

Indications: ***TD:*** severe, chronic (persistent, long-term) pain, including cancer, †AIDS,[1,2] †intolerance to other strong opioids.[3]
Injection: severe pain, premedication and peri-operative analgesia, analgesic/respiratory depressant in patients requiring assisted ventilation, neuroleptanalgesia (i.e. in combination with an antipsychotic/neuroleptic), †an alternative in cases of intolerance to other strong opioids, or in severe renal impairment and/or severe hepatic impairment (see p.744 and p.763).

Contra-indications: ***TD:*** acute (transient, intermittent or short-term) pain, e.g. postoperative, or when there is need for rapid dose titration for severe uncontrolled pain; opioid-naïve patients (but see Dose and use); severe respiratory depression.
Injection: within 14 days of using an MAOI.

Pharmacology

Fentanyl (*like* **morphine**) is a strong μ-opioid receptor agonist. It has a relatively low molecular weight and (*unlike* **morphine**) is lipophilic. This makes it suitable for TD and transmucosal administration (see p.450). As with **morphine** (p.404), there is limited very low quality evidence of benefit of fentanyl in pure neuropathic pain states.[4] Like **buprenorphine**, fentanyl appears to have little effect on the sphincter of Oddi.[5]

TD fentanyl is used in the management of chronic severe pain,[6-8] particularly cancer-related.[9-14] Generally, TD fentanyl is used only when PO strong opioids, e.g. **morphine**, **oxycodone**, are not tolerated. In some patients, TD fentanyl may be the preferred strong opioid, e.g. those unable to swallow (see Dose and use).[3] SC/CSCI fentanyl is a reasonable option when a strong opioid is required in patients with ESRF or severe hepatic impairment (see below).

Fentanyl is sequestrated in body fats, including epidural fat and the white matter of the CNS.[15] Thus, by any route (including spinally), after systemic redistribution, fentanyl acts supraspinally mainly in the thalamus (white matter). Any effect in the dorsal horn (grey matter) is probably minimal.

The lipophilic nature of fentanyl also provides one explanation for the difference in undesirable effects compared with **morphine**. When converting from PO or parenteral **morphine** to TD or parenteral fentanyl, there is a massive decrease in opioid molecules outside the CNS,[16] with, in consequence, less constipation (the dose of laxatives should be halved in anticipation).[14,17-19] This also explains why peripherally mediated withdrawal symptoms (e.g. diarrhoea, colic, nausea, sweating) are also sometimes seen. Such symptoms are easily treatable by using p.r.n. doses of **morphine** until they resolve after a few days.

Elimination of fentanyl mainly involves biotransformation in the liver by CYP3A4 to inactive norfentanyl, which is excreted in the urine. Less than 7% is excreted unchanged. The SPCs generally advise caution in patients with renal or hepatic impairment. Nonetheless, because it does not have active metabolites, fentanyl is a reasonable option for patients with renal impairment or failure and is generally recommended as the first-line SC/CSCI opioid in ESRF at the end of life (see Dose and use, and also p.743). Because the plasma clearance of fentanyl is mostly affected by changes in hepatic blood flow rather than reduced metabolism, fentanyl is also generally the SC/CSCI opioid of choice in severe hepatic impairment (see p.762).

Matrix and reservoir TD fentanyl patches are available from several manufacturers. All the SPCs contain dose conversion recommendations from PO **morphine** which, although broadly similar, do vary. The original manufacturer in the UK initially recommended a dose conversion ratio for PO **morphine** to TD fentanyl of 150:1. However, several RCTs support a smaller ratio, ranging 70:1–125:1. Indeed, at the same time in Germany, the original manufacturer promoted 100:1. Consequently, *PCF* has opted for a conversion ratio for PO **morphine** to TD fentanyl of 100:1, as have others.[20-23]

The original manufacturer's SPC now contains conversion tables based on both 150:1 and 100:1, with the former recommended for patients who have a need for opioid rotation (e.g. because of undesirable effects) or who are less clinically stable, and the latter for patients on a stable and well-tolerated opioid regimen (see Appendix 2, Box B, p.930). It is unclear on what evidence this distinction is made. Studies exploring patient factors that may influence conversion ratios, e.g. reason for switching or prior dose of opioid, show inconsistent findings.[24,25]

PCF also favours a PO **morphine** to TD **buprenorphine** conversion ratio of 100:1, and this means that TD **buprenorphine** and TD fentanyl can be considered essentially equipotent (see Appendix 2, Table 2, p.928). However, others suggest that fentanyl is 1.4 times more potent than TD **buprenorphine**,[26,27] which would make TD fentanyl 25microgram/h and 50microgram/h patches equivalent to **buprenorphine** 35microgram/h and 70microgram/h patches respectively. Even so, when switching opioids because of possible opioid-induced hyperalgesia, it is prudent to reduce the calculated equivalent dose of the new opioid by 25–50% (see p.400).

At one PCU, it was noted that patients admitted on TD fentanyl were receiving relatively higher equivalent opioid doses than other patients.[28] The reasons for this are not clear but may include a failure to appreciate the potency of fentanyl, and the induction of opioid-induced hyperalgesia by inappropriately high doses.[29] It is noteworthy that TD fentanyl was successfully reduced or discontinued in 60% of patients.[28]

Pharmacokinetic data are summarized in Table 1. Bio-availability is irrelevant in relation to TD patches; the stated delivery rates reflect the mean amount of drug delivered to patients throughout the patch's recommended duration of use. Inevitably, there will be interindividual variation in the amount delivered, e.g. for the 100microgram/h patch, the mean (±SD) delivery is 97 (±15) microgram/h,[30] and the amount of unused fentanyl in the patch after 3 days can vary from 30–85% of the original contents.[31] Generally, steady-state plasma concentrations of fentanyl are reached by the end of the second patch application period (i.e. ≤144h).

TD fentanyl patches are formulated to last for 3 days, but for some patients the duration of pain relief is less. As long as poor adhesion of the patch is not to blame, this is an end-of-dose phenomenon; as fentanyl in the patch is used, the concentration gradient driving fentanyl absorption reduces, thereby resulting in lower plasma concentrations. The correct response is to increase the patch strength. Even so, a minority of patients (<10%) do best if the patch is changed every 2 days.[13,32,33]

Changes in skin temperature under a TD fentanyl patch can significantly increase the absorption of the fentanyl into the systemic circulation, increasing plasma fentanyl concentrations by ≤60% (see Cautions).

Compared to patients with a normal weight (mean BMI 23kg/m^2), TD fentanyl patches produce plasma fentanyl concentrations 1/3–1/2 lower in those with cachexia (mean BMI 16kg/m^2).[34] The reason for this is unclear; a difference in plasma albumin levels is one possible explanation.[34-36]

Table 1 Pharmacokinetic data for fentanyl

	TD	*SC/IM*	*IV*
Onset of action	3–23h[37]	7–15min IM	1.5min
Time to peak plasma concentration	12–24h[a]	Median 15min, range 10–30min[38]	<5min
Plasma halflife	13–22h[b,39]	Median 10h, range 6–16h[38]	4h
Duration of action	72h; for some patients, 48h[40]	1–2h IM	60min

a. following application of the first patch. Because of accumulation, plasma concentrations are about 40% higher with subsequent same strength patches; steady state is reached in ≤144h

b. the halflife after a patch has been removed and not replaced.

Cautions

Reports of serious adverse events (overdoses and deaths) have prompted UK and international regulatory authorities to issue safety warnings about the use of TD fentanyl patches.[41] Factors contributing to adverse drug events include:

- lack of appreciation that fentanyl is a strong opioid analgesic
- inappropriate use for short-term, intermittent or postoperative pain in patients who had not previously been receiving a strong opioid

continued

- lack of patient education regarding directions for safe use, storage and disposal
- lack of awareness of the signs of an overdose and when to seek attention
- lack of awareness that the rate of absorption of fentanyl may be increased if the skin under the patch becomes vasodilated, e.g. in febrile patients, at high ambient temperatures,[42] or by an external heat source, e.g. electric blanket, heat lamps, saunas, hot tubs or MRI scans
- lack of awareness of drug interactions that can increase fentanyl levels.

Deaths continue to occur from incorrect use.[43,44] Additional errors include the failure to remove old patches, the dispensing and application of higher-strength patches than prescribed, and incorrect disposal (used patches contain significant amounts of fentanyl). The latter is associated with accidental exposure and deaths in others, particularly children.[45]

Reservoir patches should *not* be cut, because damage to the rate-controlling membrane can lead to a rapid release of fentanyl and overdose. Although cutting matrix patches is theoretically safer, it is strongly discouraged because of similar concerns.[41] Further, cutting has become generally unnecessary since the introduction of a 12microgram/h patch.

Patients with COPD or other medical conditions that predispose to respiratory depression (e.g. myasthenia gravis) or who are susceptible to the intracranial effects of hypercapnia (e.g. those with raised intracranial pressure). Caution is also needed if bradyarrhythmic (symptomatic bradycardia can occur),[46] elderly, cachectic, debilitated, with moderate–severe renal or hepatic impairment (also see p.743 and p.762), hypovolaemic or hypotensive.

Addicts misuse TD fentanyl patches in various ways, e.g. heating the patch, applying buccally, chewing, ingesting, inhaling and IV injection of patch contents, sometimes with fatal consequences.[47] There is increasing abuse (and deaths) from illicit fentanyl.[47]

Drug interactions

Concurrent treatment with ≥2 CNS depressants (e.g. benzodiazepines, gabapentinoids, opioids) increases the risk of respiratory depression, particularly in susceptible groups, e.g. the elderly and those with renal or hepatic impairment.[48]

Fentanyl is metabolized by CYP3A4. Caution is required with concurrent use of drugs that inhibit or induce these enzymes (see Chapter 19, Table 8, p.790). Interactions where closer monitoring ± dose adjustment are required are listed in Box A.[36,49-52]

Box A Interactions between fentanyl and other drugs involving CYP450[a]

Plasma concentrations of fentanyl	
***Increased* by**	***Decreased* by**
Aprepitant[b]	Apalutamide
Azoles[c], e.g. fluconazole, itraconazole, voriconazole	Aprepitant[b]
Cimetidine	Carbamazepine
Macrolides, e.g. clarithromycin, erythromycin	Enzalutamide[53]
	Fosphenytoin
	Phenobarbital
	Phenytoin
	Rifampicin

a. not an exhaustive list; limited to drugs most likely to be encountered in palliative care and *excludes* anticancer, antiviral, HIV and immunosuppressive drugs (seek specialist advice)

b. aprepitant can increase exposure to CYP3A4 substrates in the short-term, then reduce their exposure within 2 weeks

c. case reports of interactions with fatal (PO fluconazole) or serious (PO itraconazole) consequences with TD fentanyl patches.

IV fentanyl has been reported to reduce the metabolism of IV **midazolam**, reducing the clearance by 30% and extending the halflife by 50%.[49]

Fentanyl is not recommended in patients who have used an MAOI within the past 2 weeks (injection is contra-indicated). Although they have been used safely together, serotonin toxicity (sometimes fatal) has occurred (also see Antidepressants, Box A, p.217); manufacturers' SPCs warn of a risk of serotonin toxicity when fentanyl is *used in combination* with other serotoninergic drugs, e.g. SSRIs.[49]

Undesirable effects

Also see Strong opioids, Box B, p.394.
Very common (>10%): drowsiness, dizziness, headache, insomnia, nausea, vomiting, constipation, muscle rigidity (including thoracic muscles) when given IV (see p.491).
Common (<10%, >1%): anxiety, visual disturbance, palpitations, dry mouth, anorexia, dyspepsia, abdominal pain, diarrhoea, sweating, vasodilation.
Topical effects: Occasional skin irritation, hypersensitivity.

Dose and use

Patients using opioids must be monitored for undesirable effects, particularly nausea and vomiting, and constipation. Depending on individual circumstances, an anti-emetic should be prescribed for regular or p.r.n. use (see QCG: Nausea and vomiting, p.264) and, routinely, a laxative prescribed (see QCG: Opioid-induced constipation, p.45).

Opioids can impair driving ability, and patients should be counselled accordingly (see Chapter 22, p.809).

TD

In response to large numbers of safety incident reports about TD fentanyl patches, the Care Quality Commission highlighted the need to ensure that:

- use is appropriate, e.g. chronic *not* acute pain
- dose is appropriate, i.e. in line with published conversion charts
- dose is titrated appropriately, i.e. by no more than 50% of the previous daily dose
- date and site of application are recorded to avoid inadvertent dose omission or duplication
- TD patches are prescribed by brand, to avoid confusing patients and carers.[54]

Generally, the use of TD fentanyl patches in opioid-naïve patients is discouraged (see below) and in *non-cancer pain* is now contra-indicated.[55]

Under no circumstances should a *reservoir* patch be cut in an attempt to reduce the dose (see Cautions).

TD patches and MRI scans: fentanyl patches should be removed before the patient enters the scan room, due to the risks from heating. Patients should be advised to bring a replacement patch with them to facilitate this (also see p.901).

The use of TD fentanyl patches is summarized in the QCG: Use of transdermal fentanyl patches (p.448). The QCG and the comments in this section are based on a dose conversion ratio of PO **morphine** to TD fentanyl of 100:1. Prescribers using the manufacturer's ratio of 150:1 should follow the dose conversion guidelines in the SPC (also see Appendix 2, Box B, p.930).

Two different TD fentanyl patch formulations are currently available:

- *matrix* patch (e.g. Durogesic DTrans®, Matrifen Matrix®): the fentanyl is evenly distributed throughout a drug-in-adhesive matrix, and the release of fentanyl is controlled by the physical characteristics of the matrix
- *reservoir* patch (e.g. Fentalis Reservoir®): the fentanyl is contained within a reservoir, and the release of fentanyl is controlled by a rate-limiting membrane.

Absorption of the fentanyl through the skin and into the systemic circulation is influenced by both the condition of the skin and cutaneous blood flow. Thus, if the skin is warm and vasodilated, the rate of absorption can be significantly increased (see Pharmacology, and Cautions).

Bio-equivalence has been demonstrated between two different makes of *matrix* patches, and between *matrix* and *reservoir* patches.[56-58] However, the matrix patch is thinner (because there is no reservoir) and, for equal strengths, more than one third smaller. Consequently, to avoid confusing patients and carers, prescribing by brand is recommended.[54]

In the UK, most manufacturers and the Care Quality Commission/NHS England recommend against use of TD fentanyl patches in opioid-naïve patients, advising initial titration with immediate-release **morphine**.[54] The MHRA has contra-indicated the use of TD fentanyl patches in opioid-naïve patients with non-cancer pain.[55] In North America, the manufacturer stresses that TD fentanyl patches should be commenced *only* in patients who have been receiving strong opioids in a dose at least equivalent to a 25microgram/h patch for ≥1 week, such as:

- **morphine** 60mg/24h PO
- **oxycodone** 30mg/24h PO
- **hydromorphone** 8mg/24h PO.

In palliative care, TD fentanyl is generally considered a second-line strong opioid, and only considered for use when:

- PO strong opioids, e.g. **morphine**, **oxycodone**, are not tolerated, *or*
- patients with *stable strong opioid requirements* are no longer able to swallow and CSCI is not readily available.[3,59]

Nonetheless, there are reports where TD fentanyl has been used satisfactorily as a first-line strong opioid (± previous weak opioid use), e.g. in patients with severe dysphagia, renal failure, or who are living in social circumstances where there is a high risk of diversion and tablet misuse.[60-63] (Note. Misuse of TD fentanyl patches can also occur; see Cautions.) However, because the lowest strength of fentanyl patch (12microgram/h) is about equivalent to 30mg/24h of **morphine**, prescribers considering the use of TD fentanyl as a first-line strong opioid, particularly in opioid-naïve patients, should be sufficiently experienced and able to closely monitor the patient; otherwise specialist advice should be sought.

Undesirable effects, e.g. nausea and vomiting, are more frequent in strong opioid-naïve patients and in one study resulted in one sixth of patients discontinuing TD fentanyl 12microgram/h.[64]

It is important to give adequate p.r.n. doses of **morphine** or another strong opioid for break-through pain. The patch strength can be increased by 12–25microgram/h *no more than once a week* (see QCG: Use of transdermal fentanyl patches, p.448).

With inpatients, the use of a monitoring chart is recommended (for an example, see www.palliativedrugs.com Document library).[65]

SC/IM/IV

- start with a stat dose of 50–200microgram, and subsequently 50microgram p.r.n.
- reduce the starting dose in the elderly and frail, or in severe renal or severe hepatic impairment, e.g. 12.5–25microgram SC p.r.n.
- traditionally, p.r.n. dosing intervals are q1h, but more frequent dosing with close monitoring may be required in severe acute pain
- give IV doses by slow injection; this reduces the risk of muscular rigidity.

CSCI

In the UK, this route is recommended mostly in the setting of severe and end-stage renal impairment (eGFR <30mL/min/1.73m^2) or severe hepatic impairment (see p.743 and p.762):

- *opioid-naïve*
  - ▷ initial dose 100–150microgram/24h CSCI
  - ▷ allow 12.5–25microgram SC p.r.n. q1h
- *converting from another opioid*
  - ▷ calculate equivalent dose (see Appendix 2, p.925)
  - ▷ reduce by 25–50% and use as initial dose
  - ▷ allow a suitable p.r.n. SC dose (conventionally, 1/10–1/6 of the total 24h CSCI dose).

For CSCI, dilute with WFI, sodium chloride 0.9% or glucose 5%. Volume constraints for a syringe driver can limit the use of higher doses of fentanyl and/or the ability to combine it with other drugs.

***CSCI compatibility with other drugs*:** limited clinical experience suggests that fentanyl in doses <500microgram is compatible with **haloperidol**, **levomepromazine** or **midazolam**, using WFI as diluent (also see Chapter 29, p.892). For further information, see www.palliativedrugs.com Syringe Driver Survey Database (SDSD).

Health professionals are encouraged to add details of any successful or unsuccessful combinations to the existing list of fentanyl combinations on the www.palliativedrugs.com SDSD).

If the required dose of CSCI fentanyl causes volume issues, consider using **alfentanil** (p.420) instead. However, because **alfentanil** has a shorter halflife, continue to use fentanyl SC p.r.n. for break-through pain.

Transmucosal fentanyl formulations (p.450) could be used as an alternative p.r.n. analgesic, but only when the patient has sufficient time and ability to co-operate with the necessary titration. When increasing the background CSCI dose according to transmucosal fentanyl p.r.n. use, because of the lower (and variable) bio-availability of transmucosal fentanyl products, apply an appropriate reduction to the calculated CSCI increment and monitor the patient closely for signs of toxicity. Example: three p.r.n. doses of Effentora® (bio-availability 65%) 200microgram are required/24h → total dose/24h (600microgram) is reduced by one third → CSCI dose increment ≤400microgram/24h (also see Fentanyl (transmucosal), Table 1 and Table 2, p.450).

If the patient is not in the last days of life, a switch to TD fentanyl may be possible once stable pain control is achieved. Select a patch that delivers a similar rate of fentanyl in microgram/h as the CSCI, continuing the infusion unchanged for 6h after applying the patch, then discontinue (see QCG: Use of transdermal fentanyl patches, p.448).

5

CIVI

Fentanyl CIVI is used in some centres (generally *not* UK) for initial control of cancer pain. When an effective stable dose is found, the route is switched to TD. Select a patch that delivers a similar rate of fentanyl in microgram/h as the CIVI; continue the infusion unchanged for 6h after applying the patch, then discontinue (see QCG: Use of transdermal fentanyl patches, p.448).[66] This appears satisfactory for most patients; other methods exist but are more complex.[66]

Supply

All preparations are Schedule 2 **CD**.

Transdermal products
Fentanyl (generic)
Matrix patches (for 3 days) 12microgram/h, 25microgram/h, 37.5microgram/h (Mezolar Matrix® only), 50microgram/h, 75microgram/h, 100microgram/h, 1 = £2.50, £3.50, £3, £6.50, £9.50 and £12 respectively.
Brands include Durogesic DTrans®, Fencino®, Matrifen®, Mezolar Matrix®, Opiodur®, Victanyl®, Yemex®.
Reservoir patches (for 3 days) 25microgram/h, 50microgram/h, 75microgram/h, 100microgram/h, 1 = £3.50, £6.50, £9.50 and £12 respectively.
Brands include Fentalis Reservoir®.

Parenteral products
Fentanyl citrate (generic)
Injection 50microgram/mL, 2mL amp = £1.25, 10mL amp = £1.50.
Infusion 50microgram/mL, 50mL vial = £5.50.

1 Newshan G and Lefkowitz M (2001) Transdermal fentanyl for chronic pain in AIDS: a pilot study. *Journal of Pain and Symptom Management*. **21**: 69–77.
2 Canneti A *et al.* (2013) Safety and efficacy of transdermal buprenorphine and transdermal fentanyl in the treatment of neuropathic pain in AIDS patients. *Minerva Anestesiologica*. **79**: 871–883.
3 Tassinari D *et al.* (2011) Transdermal opioids as front line treatment of moderate to severe cancer pain: a systemic review. *Palliative Medicine*. **25**: 478–487.
4 Derry S *et al.* (2016) Fentanyl for neuropathic pain in adults. *Cochrane Database of Systematic Reviews*. **10**: CD011605. www.cochranelibrary.com.
5 Koo HC *et al.* (2010) Effect of transdermal fentanyl patches on the motility of the sphincter of oddi. *Gut and Liver*. **4**: 368–372.
6 Simpson R *et al.* (1997) Transdermal fentanyl as treatment for chronic low back pain. *Journal of Pain and Symptom Management*. **14**: 218–224.
7 Milligan K and Campbell C (1999) Transdermal fentanyl in patients with chronic, nonmalignant pain: a case study series. *Advances in Therapy*. **16**: 73–77.
8 Allan L *et al.* (2001) Randomised crossover trial of transdermal fentanyl and sustained release oral morphine for treating chronic non-cancer pain. *British Medical Journal*. **322**: 1154–1158.
9 Yeo W *et al.* (1997) Transdermal fentanyl for severe cancer-related pain. *Palliative Medicine*. **11**: 233–239.
10 Payne R *et al.* (1998) Quality of life and cancer pain: satisfaction and side effects with transdermal fentanyl versus oral morphine. *Journal of Clinical Oncology*. **16**: 1588–1593.
11 Sloan P *et al.* (1998) A clinical evaluation of transdermal therapeutic system fentanyl for the treatment of cancer pain. *Journal of Pain and Symptom Management*. **16**: 102–111.
12 Nugent M *et al.* (2001) Long-term observations of patients receiving transdermal fentanyl after a randomized trial. *Journal of Pain and Symptom Management*. **21**: 385–391.
13 Radbruch L *et al.* (2001) Transdermal fentanyl for the management of cancer pain: a survey of 1005 patients. *Palliative Medicine*. **15**: 309–321.

14 Hadley G *et al.* (2013) Transdermal fentanyl for cancer pain. *Cochrane Database of Systematic Reviews.* **10**: CD010270. www.cochranelibrary.com.
15 Ummenhofer W *et al.* (2000) Comparative spinal distribution and clearance kinetics of intrathecally administered morphine, fentanyl, alfentanil, and sufentanil. *Anesthesiology.* **92**(3): 739–753.
16 Herz A and Teschemacher H-J (1971) Activities and sites of antinociceptive action of morphine-like analgesics and kinetics of distribution following intravenous, intracerebral and intraventricular application. *Advances in Drug Research.* **6**: 79–119.
17 Wang DD *et al.* (2018) Transdermal fentanyl for cancer pain: Trial sequential analysis of 3406 patients from 35 randomized controlled trials. *Journal of Cancer Research & Therapeutics.* **14**: S14–S21.
18 Tassinari D *et al.* (2008) Adverse effects of transdermal opiates treating moderate-severe cancer pain in comparison to long-acting morphine: a meta-analysis and systematic review of the literature. *Journal of Palliative Medicine.* **11**: 492–501.
19 Hannon B *et al.* (2013) The role of fentanyl in refractory opioid-related acute colonic pseudo-obstruction. *Journal of Pain and Symptom Management.* **45**: e1–e3.
20 Caraceni A *et al.* (2012) Use of opioid analgesics in the treatment of cancer pain: evidence-based recommendations from the EAPC. *Lancet Oncology.* **13**: e58–68.
21 Donner B *et al.* (1996) Direct conversion from oral morphine to transdermal fentanyl: a multicenter study in patients with cancer pain. *Pain.* **64**: 527–534.
22 Mercadante S and Caraceni A (2011) Conversion ratios for opioid switching in the treatment of cancer pain: a systematic review. *Palliative Medicine.* **25**: 504–515.
23 Reddy A *et al.* (2016) The opioid rotation ratio of strong opioids to transdermal fentanyl in cancer patients. *Cancer.* **122**: 149–156.
24 Jia SS *et al.* (2015) Modified Glasgow prognostic score predicting high conversion ratio in opioid switching from oral oxycodone to transdermal fentanyl in patients with cancer pain. *International Journal of Clinical Experimental Medicine.* **8**: 7606–7612.
25 Matsumura C *et al.* (2016) Indication of adequate transdermal fentanyl dose in opioid switching from oral cxycodone in patients with cancer. *American Journal of Hospice and Palliative Care.* **33**: 109–114.
26 Mercadante S *et al.* (2007) Switching from transdermal drugs: an observational "N of 1" study of fentanyl and buprenorphine. *Journal of Pain and Symptom Management.* **34**: 532–538.
27 Mercadante S *et al.* (2009) Equipotent doses to switch from high doses of opioids to transdermal buprenorphine. *Supportive Care in Cancer.* **17**: 715–718.
28 Botterman J and Criel N (2011) Inappropriate use of high doses of transdermal fentanyl at admission to a palliative care unit. *Palliative Medicine.* **25**: 111–116.
29 Mauermann E *et al.* (2016) Does fentanyl lead to opioid-induced hyperalgesia in healthy volunteers? a double-blind, randomized, crossover trial. *Anesthesiology.* **124**: 453–463.
30 Van Nimmen NF *et al.* (2010) Fentanyl transdermal absorption linked to pharmacokinetic characteristics in patients undergoing palliative care. *Journal of Clinical Pharmacology.* **50**: 667–678.
31 Marquardt KA *et al.* (1995) Fentanyl remaining in a transdermal system following three days of continuous use. *Annals of Pharmacotherapy.* **29**: 969–971.
32 Donner B *et al.* (1998) Long-term treatment of cancer pain with transdermal fentanyl. *Journal of Pain and Symptom Management.* **15**: 168–175.
33 Arnet I *et al.* (2016) Poor adhesion of fentanyl transdermal patches may mimic end-of-dosage failure after 48 hours and prompt early patch replacement in hospitalized cancer pain patients. *Journal of Pain Research.* **9**: 993–999.
34 Heiskanen T *et al.* (2009) Transdermal fentanyl in cachectic cancer patients. *Pain.* **144**: 218–222.
35 Hadgraft J and Lane ME (2005) Skin permeation: the years of enlightenment. *International Journal of Pharmaceutics.* **305**: 2–12.
36 Kuip EJ *et al.* (2017) A review of factors explaining variability in fentanyl pharmacokinetics; focus on implications for cancer patients. *British Journal of Clinical Pharmacology.* **83**: 294–313.
37 Gourlay GK et *al.* (1989) The transdermal administration of fentanyl in the treatment of post-operative pain: pharmacokinetics and pharmacodynamic effects. *Pain.* **37**: 193–202.
38 Capper SJ *et al.* (2010) Pharmacokinetics of fentanyl after subcutaneous administration in volunteers. *European Journal of Anaesthesiology.* **27**: 241–246.
39 Portenoy RK *et al.* (1993) Transdermal fentanyl for cancer pain. *Anesthesiology.* **78**: 36–43.
40 Smith J and Ellershaw J (1999) Improvement in pain control by change of fentanyl patch after 48 hours compared with 72 hours. *Poster EAPC Congress, Geneva.* PO1/1376.
41 MHRA (2018) Transdermal fentanyl patches: life-threatening and fatal opioid toxicity from accidental exposure, particularly in children. *Drug Safety Update.* www.gov.uk/drug-safety-update.
42 Sindali K *et al.* (2012) Life-threatening coma and full-thickness sunburn in a patient treated with transdermal fentanyl patches: a case report. *Journal of Medical Case Reports.* **6**: 220.
43 Jumbelic MI (2010) Deaths with transdermal fentanyl patches. *American Journal of Forensic Medicine and Pathology.* **31**: 18–21.
44 Nara A *et al.* (2019) A fatal case of poisoning with fentanyl transdermal patches in Japan. *Journal of Forensic Sciences.* **64**: 1936–1942.
45 MHRA (2014) Transdermal fentanyl "patches": reminder of potential for life-threatening harm from accidental exposure, particularly in children. *Drug Safety Update.* www.gov.uk/drug-safety-update.
46 Hawley P (2013) Case report of severe bradycardia due to transdermal fentanyl. *Palliative Medicine.* **27**: 793–795.
47 Kuczyńska K *et al.* (2018) Abuse of fentanyl: An emerging problem to face. *Forensic Science International.* **289**: 207–214.
48 MHRA (2020) Benzodiazepines and opioids: reminder of risk of potentially fatal respiratory depression. *Drug Safety Update.* www.gov.uk/drug-safety-update.
49 Baxter K and Preston CL *Stockley's Drug Interactions.* London: Pharmaceutical Press www.medicinescomplete.com (accessed May 2020).
50 Takane H *et al.* (2005) Rifampin reduces the analgesic effect of transdermal fentanyl. *Annals of Pharmacotherapy.* **39**: 2139–2140.
51 Sasson M and Shvartzman P (2006) Fentanyl patch sufficient analgesia for only one day. *Journal of Pain and Symptom Management.* **31**: 389–391.
52 Morii H et *al.* (2007) Failure of pain control using transdermal fentanyl during rifampicin treatment. *Journal of Pain and Symptom Management.* **33**: 5–6.
53 Westdorp H *et al.* (2018) Difficulties in pain management using oxycodone and fentanyl in enzalutamide-treated patients with advanced prostate cancer. *Journal of Pain and Symptom Management.* **55**: e6–e8.
54 Care Quality Commission and NHS England (2013) Safer use of controlled drugs - preventing harms from fentanyl and buprenorphine transdermal patches. *Use of controlled drugs supporting information.* www.cqc.org.uk.

55 MHRA (2020) Transdermal fentanyl patches for non-cancer pain: do not use in opioid-naive patients. *Drug Safety Update*. www.gov.uk/drug-safety-update.

56 Freynhagen R *et al.* (2005) Switching from reservoir to matrix systems for the transdermal delivery of fentanyl: a prospective, multicenter pilot study in outpatients with chronic pain. *Journal of Pain and Symptom Management*. **30**: 289–297.

57 Marier JF *et al.* (2006) Pharmacokinetics, tolerability, and performance of a novel matrix transdermal delivery system of fentanyl relative to the commercially available reservoir formulation in healthy subjects. *Journal of Clinical Pharmacology*. **46**: 642–653.

58 Kress HG *et al.* (2010) Transdermal fentanyl matrix patches Matrifen and Durogesic DTrans are bioequivalent. *European Journal of Pharmceutics and Biopharmaceutics*. **75**: 225–231.

59 NICE (2016) Palliative care for adults: strong opioids for pain relief. *Clinical Guideline*. CG104 www.nice.org.uk.

60 Vielvoye-Kerkmeer A *et al.* (2000) Transdermal fentanyl in opioid-naive cancer pain patients: an open trial using transdermal fentanyl for the treatment of chronic cancer pain in opioid-naive patients and a group using codeine. *Journal of Pain and Symptom Management*. **19**: 185–192.

61 van Seventer R *et al.* (2003) Comparison of TTS-fentanyl with sustained-release oral morphine in the treatment of patients not using opioids for mild-to-moderate pain. *Current Medical Research Opinion*. **19**: 457–469.

62 Tawfik MO *et al.* (2004) Use of transdermal fentanyl without prior opioid stabilization in patients with cancer pain. *Current Medical Research Opinion*. **20**: 259–267.

63 Othman AH *et al.* (2016) Transdermal fentanyl for cancer pain management in opioid-naive pediatric cancer patients. *Pain Medicine*. **17(7)**: 1329–1336.

64 Mercadante S *et al.* (2010) Low doses of transdermal fentanyl in opioid-naive patients with cancer pain. *Current Medical Research Opinion*. **26**: 2765–2768.

65 Palliativedrugs.com (2019) Strong opioid transdermal patch monitoring chart. *Document Library*. Pain (strong opioids): www.palliativedrugs.com.

66 Samala RV *et al.* (2014) Efficacy and safety of a six-hour continuous overlap method for converting intravenous to transdermal fentanyl in cancer pain. *Journal of Pain and Symptom Management*. **48**: 132–136.

Updated March 2021

Quick Clinical Guide: Use of transdermal fentanyl patches

These recommendations use only a dose conversion ratio for PO morphine to TD fentanyl of 100:1 and, as such, differ from those in UK SPCs. It is an approximation, and inevitably there will be individual variation.

Note. Pain not relieved by morphine will generally not be relieved by fentanyl. If in doubt, seek specialist advice before prescribing TD fentanyl.

1 Indications for using TD fentanyl instead of morphine include:
- intolerable undesirable effects with morphine, e.g. nausea and vomiting, constipation, hallucinations
- renal or hepatic failure (fentanyl has no active metabolite)
- dysphagia, 'tablet phobia' or poor compliance with oral medication
- high risk of tablet misuse/diversion.

2 TD fentanyl is contra-indicated in patients with acute (short-term) pain and in those who need rapid dose titration for severe uncontrolled pain. Generally, it is *not* recommended in opioid-naïve patients or as a first-line strong opioid (seek specialist advice). Thus, TD fentanyl is most appropriate for patients already on a stable dose of morphine (or another strong opioid) for ≥1 week.

3 TD fentanyl patches are available in six strengths: 12, 25, 37.5, 50, 75 and 100microgram/h for 3 days. The patch brand, dose and duration should be stated on the prescription to avoid confusion.

4 Use Table 1 below to decide a safe starting dose for TD fentanyl and an appropriate p.r.n. dose of morphine. The starting dose for patients previously taking a weak opioid should be 12microgram/h.

5 For patients taking a dose of morphine that is not the exact equivalent of a fentanyl patch, it will be necessary to opt for a patch that is either slightly more or slightly less than the morphine dose. Thus, if the patient still has pain, round up to a higher patch strength; if pain-free and frail, round down. However, if switching because of possible opioid-induced hyperalgesia, reduce the calculated equivalent dose by 25–50%.

Table 1 Comparative doses of PO morphine and TD fentanyl (based on dose conversion ratio 100:1)

PO morphine		*SC/IV morphine*		*TD fentanyl*	
mg/24h	*p.r.n. mg*[a]	*mg/24h*[b]	*p.r.n. mg*[a]	*microgram/h*	*mg/24h*
30	5	15	2.5	12	0.3
60	10	30	5	25	0.6
90	15	45	7.5	37.5	0.9
120	20	60	10	50	1.2
180	30	90	15	75	1.8
240	40	120	20	100[c]	2.4

a. using traditional 1/6 of total daily dose as p.r.n. dose

b. assuming morphine SC/IV is twice as potent as PO

c. for combinations of patches, add the p.r.n. doses together, e.g. 100microgram/h + 75microgram/h patches = 20mg + 15mg morphine SC/IV = 35mg morphine SC/IV, but can round up to 40mg or down to 30mg for convenience.

6 The date of application and/or the date for renewal should be written on the patch. Apply to dry, non-inflamed, non-irradiated, hairless skin on the upper trunk or arm. Body hair may be clipped with scissors but not shaved. If the skin is washed beforehand, use only water; do not use soap and do not apply oils, cream or ointment to the area. Press patch firmly in place for at least 30 seconds; adhesive tape (e.g. Micropore®) can be applied to the edges to aid adherence. Careful removal of the patch helps to minimize local skin irritation.

7 Effective systemic analgesic concentrations are reached in 12–24h. When converting from:
- 4-hourly PO morphine, give regular doses for the first 12h after applying the patch
- 12-hourly m/r morphine, apply the patch and the final m/r dose at the same time
- 24-hourly m/r morphine, apply the patch 12h after the final m/r dose
- CSCI/CIVI morphine, continue the infusion unchanged for 8–12h after applying the patch, then discontinue
- CSCI/CIVI fentanyl, continue the infusion unchanged for 6h after applying the patch, then discontinue.

8 The patient should use p.r.n. doses liberally during the first 3 days, particularly the first 24h. Safe rescue doses of PO morphine are given in Table 1 above.

9 If pain relief is insufficient (>2 p.r.n. doses of morphine required/24h), the patch strength can be increased by 12–25microgram/h. Because steady-state plasma concentrations take ≤6 days to achieve, this should be *no more than once a week* (i.e. after assessing the response to two 72h applications); the only exception is following the very first patch application, when the patch strength can be increased after 72h if necessary.

10 About 10% of patients experience opioid withdrawal symptoms when changed from morphine to TD fentanyl. These manifest with symptoms like gastric flu and last for a few days; p.r.n. doses of morphine will relieve troublesome symptoms.

11 Fentanyl is less constipating than morphine; halve the dose of laxatives when starting fentanyl and re-titrate.

12 Fentanyl may cause nausea and vomiting; if necessary, prescribe an anti-emetic, e.g. haloperidol 500microgram–1.5mg stat & at bedtime.

13 In febrile patients, the rate of absorption of fentanyl increases and may cause toxicity, e.g. drowsiness. Absorption is also enhanced by high ambient temperatures or external heat sources over the patch, e.g. electric blanket or hot-water bottle; patients should be warned about this. Patients may shower with a patch but should not soak in a hot bath. Remove patches before MRI scans.

14 Remove patches after 72h; use a different skin site position for the new patches to rest the underlying skin for 3–6 days. The use of a monitoring chart is recommended for inpatients.

15 A reservoir of fentanyl accumulates in the body, and significant blood concentrations persist for at least 24h after discontinuing TD fentanyl.

16 TD fentanyl is unsatisfactory in <5% of patients. However, discontinuation is more common when TD fentanyl is used in strong opioid-naïve patients.

17 Additional or alternative analgesic approaches should be considered when the dose exceeds 300microgram/h.

18 In moribund patients, continue TD fentanyl and give additional SC morphine p.r.n. (see Table 1). If >2 p.r.n. doses are required/24h, give morphine by CSCI, starting with a dose equal to the sum of the p.r.n. doses over the preceding 24h. If necessary, adjust the p.r.n. dose, taking into account the total opioid dose (i.e. TD fentanyl + CSCI morphine).

19 Used patches still contain fentanyl; after removal, fold the patch with the adhesive side inwards and discard in a sharps container (hospital) or dustbin (home), and wash hands. Ultimately, any unused patches should be returned to a pharmacy.

Updated March 2021

FENTANYL (TRANSMUCOSAL)

For information on transdermal and parenteral use of fentanyl, see p.440.

Relative to PO opioids, transmucosal fentanyl products are expensive (about £5–12/episode). They are more effective than placebo, but direct comparison with PO **morphine** or each other is limited. Careful patient selection, training, titration and monitoring are required to ensure optimum use. They are *not* interchangeable.

Medicine advisory boards (Scottish Medicines Consortium, All Wales Medicines Strategy Group) have recommended restricting their use to patients unsuitable for other short-acting opioids, e.g. PO **morphine**.

Class: Strong opioid analgesic.

Indications: Break-through cancer pain in patients on regular strong opioids. The use of fentanyl injection SL or nasally is off-label.

Contra-indications: Use in strong opioid-naïve patients, acute non-cancer pain (e.g. postoperative pain, migraine), severe obstructive airways disease. *Instanyl®*: previous facial radiotherapy, recurrent epistaxis.

Pharmacology

Fentanyl (*like* **morphine**) is a strong μ-opioid receptor agonist. It has a relatively low molecular weight and (*unlike* **morphine**) is lipophilic, which makes it suitable for TD (p.440) and transmucosal administration. Multiple formulations are authorized for the treatment of break-through cancer pain. In the UK, these include SL tablets (Abstral®), a lozenge (Actiq®), a buccal/SL tablet (Effentora®) and nasal sprays (Instanyl®, PecFent®). Elsewhere, other formulations available may include an SL tablet (Recivit®), an SL spray (Subsys®) and a buccal film (Breakyl®).

Break-through cancer pain generally has a relatively rapid onset (median 5–10min) and short duration (45–60min), but can range from <1min to 4–6h in duration (see p.323).[1] By comparison, PO opioids such as **morphine** on average take about 30–40min to achieve meaningful pain relief, and have a longer duration of effect (3–6h).[2] Thus, transmucosal fentanyl products aim to provide rapid-onset pain relief which better matches the time course of a typical break-through pain.

Pharmacokinetics

The transmucosal formulations range from an aqueous solution of fentanyl (Instanyl®) to combinations which include bio-adhesive substances, e.g. croscarmellose (Abstral®), pectin (PecFent®). The pharmacokinetic characteristics of the products vary and the products are *not* interchangeable (Tables 1 and 2). Fentanyl is readily absorbed transmucosally, and the bio-adhesive substances tend to *slow* its rate of absorption. Various justifications are given (e.g. to aid mucosal adherence, to attenuate the peak plasma concentration), but the fact that a novel delivery system can be patented (although not fentanyl itself) is also relevant.

With the buccal/SL products, the amount of fentanyl absorbed directly across the mucosa or swallowed varies with formulation and route of administration. A lack of saliva will impede dissolution of tablet formulations, and patients with a dry mouth should moisten their mouth with water beforehand. About two-thirds of any swallowed fentanyl will be eliminated by intestinal or hepatic first-pass metabolism. Nonetheless, significant amounts of swallowed fentanyl are absorbed, e.g. about 25% and 15% of the systemically available Actiq® and Effentora® respectively is via GI absorption.[6,11,12] The effects of the GI absorption on the plasma concentration of fentanyl include producing a 'double peak', maintaining high levels for longer (e.g. >2h) and contributing to the wide range in T_{max}.[5]

The rate and degree of absorption of fentanyl from the nasal cavity is dependent on mucosal perfusion. Vasoconstrictive nasal decongestants, e.g. **oxymetazoline** (not UK), double the time to maximum plasma concentration and halve the maximum plasma concentration of a dose of nasal fentanyl. Thus, the concurrent use of vasoconstrictive nasal decongestants, e.g **pseudoephedrine**, with Instanyl® or PecFent® should be avoided.

Once absorbed, fentanyl is rapidly distributed to the best-perfused tissues, i.e. brain, heart and lungs, and then to fat, muscle and other tissues. Subsequently, fentanyl is redistributed between

Table 1 Selected characteristics and pharmacokinetic data for *oromucosal* fentanyl products available in the UK[a,b]

	Abstral®	*Actiq®* [c]	*Effentora®* [d]
Formulation	SL tablet	Buccal lozenge	Buccal/SL tablet
Dose range and presentation	100, 200, 300, 400, 600, 800microgram Different shapes; packs of 10 or 30	200, 400, 600, 800, 1,200, 1,600microgram On a stick, marked with dose and different colours; packs of 3 or 30	100, 200, 400, 600, 800microgram 100 smaller in size; embossed 1, 2, etc.; packs of 4 or 28
Maximum dose/episode	800microgram	1,600microgram	800microgram
Maximum frequency of use	Maximum 4 episodes/24h, ideally ≥4h apart (see Dose and use)	Maximum 4 episodes/24h, ideally ≥4h apart (see Dose and use)	Maximum 4 episodes/24h, ≥4h apart
Approximate cost per dose (also see Supply)	£5	£7	£5
Time to dissolution	<2min	Applied over 15min	Buccal 14–25min; SL quicker
Onset of action[e]	10min	15min	10min
Time to peak plasma concentration, median (range)	30–60min (15–240min) Longer with highest dose	Across dose range 90min (30–480min)[3,4] Longer with highest dose	Pooled data 53min (20–240min)[5] Longer with highest dose
Plasma halflife (range)	Mean 5–14h	Median 18h (7–49h) 800microgram[3]	Median 12h (2–44h), pooled data[5]
Duration of action	≥1h	≥1h (≤3.5h reported with higher doses)[6]	≥2h
Bio-availability	55%	50% (25% transmucosal, 25% PO)[6]	65% (50% transmucosal, 15% PO)
Comments		Requires continual movement around the mouth; less effective if finished <15min as more is swallowed	Absorption not affected by mild (grade 1) mucositis[7]

a. the source (i.e. healthy volunteers vs. patients) and quality (e.g. small number of subjects, whole dose range not studied, use of massage over buccal tablet) of the data vary widely
b. data based on venous blood sampling; with arterial sampling, a higher maximum concentration is achieved about 15min quicker[8]
c. an equivalent product, Cynril®, is available as a branded generic
d. pharmacokinetics are similar for either buccal or SL placement
e. earliest *statistically significant* difference between fentanyl product and placebo in mean pain intensity difference; a *clinically meaningful* difference has been variably defined and generally takes longer (see Pharmacodynamics).

Table 2 Selected characteristics and pharmacokinetic data for intranasal fentanyl products[a]

	Instanyl®	*PecFent®*
Formulation	Nasal spray	Nasal spray
Dose range and presentation	50, 100, 200microgram/spray (100microL) 1 dose repeated once after 10min p.r.n.; colour-coded and in single doses (6 dose pack)	100, 200, 400 and 800microgram; given as 1 or 2 doses of 100 or 400microgram/spray (100microL); colour-coded and in 8 and 32 dose bottles
Maximum dose/episode	400microgram	800microgram
Maximum frequency of use	Maximum 4 episodes/24h, ≥4h apart	Maximum 4 episodes/24h, ≥4h apart
Approximate cost per spray (also see Supply)	£6; up to half require 2 doses, thus average cost up to £9	£4.50; about half require 200 or 800microgram dose, thus average cost = £7
Time to dissolution	N/A	N/A
Onset of action[b]	5min	10min
Time to peak plasma concentration, median (range)	Across dose range 12–15min (6–90min)[9]	Across dose range 15–21min (5–180min)[4]
Plasma halflife (range)	Median 19h (8–30h); 200microgram, 2 doses 10min apart[10]	Mean 15–25h
Duration of action	≥1h	≥1h
Bio-availability	90%	No data
Comments	Non-preserved solution, pH 6.6, osmolality ~ sodium chloride 0.9%	Preserved solution containing pectin, adjusted for pH and osmolality C_{max} is about one third that of Instanyl® Audible click denotes dose administered; visual priming guide and dose counter, end-of-use lock

a. the source (i.e. healthy volunteers vs. patients) and quality (e.g. small number of subjects, whole dose range not studied) of the data vary widely

b. earliest *statistically significant* difference between fentanyl product and placebo in mean pain intensity difference; a *clinically meaningful* difference has been variably defined and can take longer (see text).

the deep tissue compartment and plasma. This pattern of rapid distribution followed by a slower redistribution explains why fentanyl has a relatively short duration of action despite a long halflife (Table 1 and Table 2). However, with repeat administration, saturation of the deep tissue compartment can occur, resulting in higher peak plasma concentrations of fentanyl and a more prolonged effect.

Up to 85% of fentanyl is protein-bound, mainly to α_1-acid glycoprotein, but also to albumin and lipoproteins. Elimination mainly involves biotransformation in the liver by CYP3A4 to inactive norfentanyl, which is excreted in the urine. Less than 7% is excreted unchanged. The SPCs of all of the transmucosal fentanyl products advise caution in their use in patients with moderate–severe hepatic or renal impairment, but this is based on limited data which suggest a reduced clearance of fentanyl, e.g. via alterations in metabolic clearance and plasma protein binding. Nonetheless, fentanyl is a reasonable option for patients with renal impairment or failure (also see p.440 and p.743),[13] including those with hepatorenal syndrome (see p.762).[14]

Pharmacokinetic studies of repeat/chronic dosing of the transmucosal products are limited. Repeating a dose of PecFent® after an interval of 1h or 2h significantly increases the maximum plasma concentration, but not when doses are given 4h apart.[4] Accumulation of fentanyl can occur with regular use; when Abstral® (whole of dose range) or Effentora® (400microgram) are given q6h, steady state is reached after about 3–5 days, and the maximum plasma concentration becomes double that of the initial dose.[15,16] Thus, even when an effective and tolerable dose is identified through titration, with subsequent regular use, accumulation and undesirable effects could occur.

Pharmacodynamics

Generally, patients recruited to the development studies for the fentanyl transmucosal products were relatively young (mean age 50–60 years), had a good performance status (ECOG PS 0–2), no clinically relevant renal or hepatic impairment and were taking regular scheduled doses of an opioid equivalent to PO **morphine** 160–280mg/24h. Thus, additional caution is required when giving these products to patients with characteristics that differ from this group, particularly those who are elderly. A sober critique of the published papers is also required for various reasons, including:

- many studies are sponsored by the manufacturer and thus lack impartiality
- although similar methods of evaluation are used across studies, the criteria used to define a response vary, making direct comparison difficult (see below)
- some approaches undertaken in the studies do not reflect recommended clinical practice, e.g.:
  - ▷ only single doses of Abstral® were used for titration and maintenance in the study on which its safety data is based, with the effective dose confirmed over several consecutive episodes; by comparison, in the SPC, a second dose is permitted during titration, with no mention of confirmation of the effective dose[17]
  - ▷ Effentora® tablet remnants were 'massaged' after 10–15min in the pharmacokinetic and some efficacy studies, potentially artificially enhancing absorption and efficacy data[18]
  - ▷ patients who had already used Instanyl® were enrolled into an efficacy study, artificially enhancing the proportion achieving successful titration (>90% vs. more usual 60–70%)[10]
  - ▷ in some instances the regulatory authorities expressed concerns about the amount and/or quality of data, e.g. Abstral® pharmacokinetic data, Instanyl® safety reporting.[10,19]

For speed of onset of analgesia, generally what is promoted is the earliest *statistically significant* difference in pain intensity between the fentanyl product and placebo (generally 5–15min). Although some patients report a reduction in pain intensity which is considered *clinically meaningful* by this time, this generally takes longer for most products. Reliable comparison of the different products is difficult because the definition and calculation of a clinically meaningful change varies, e.g. reduction in pain intensity score from baseline of ≥2/10 or 30–33%, by episode (at least one or all) or by patient. Further, applying different criteria to the same data can produce different times; e.g. for PecFent®, half of the patients experience a reduction in pain intensity score of ≥2 by 15min, but a ≥33% reduction takes 30min.[4,20] (Note. It has been suggested that a ≥50% improvement in pain intensity is required for it to be of *substantial* clinical importance.[21]) However, data suggest that for half of the episodes, an improvement in pain intensity of at least moderate clinical importance appears by about 10min (Instanyl®[22]), 15min (PecFent®[20]) or 30min (Abstral®,[23] Actiq®,[24] Effentora®[25]). Even so, in up to a quarter of episodes, an alternative rescue analgesic is needed because of an inadequate response to the fentanyl product. Clinicians must provide careful explanation to ensure the patient uses both rescue analgesics correctly.

High-quality comparative data, either between products or with PO analgesics, are limited. Generally, the transmucosal products perform statistically significantly better than the immediate-release PO formulations tested, but the absolute differences in outcomes are relatively small, making their clinical relevance uncertain (Box A).

Given the mismatch between the time–action relationship of PO **morphine** and the typical time course of a break-through pain, it is interesting how well PO **morphine** performs in these studies. Unlike the fentanyl product, the PO **morphine** was not optimized in a titration phase and was given as *tablets* rather than as a *solution*, which is absorbed and acts more quickly. Studies have reported a median (range) T_{max} of 60min (20–90min) vs. 125min (40–240min), and mean time to meaningful pain relief of about 15min vs. 30min for morphine solution vs. tablets respectively.[32,33] Only an inadequate comparison of Abstral® with PO **morphine** *solution* is currently available.[34]

Box A Higher-quality active comparator studies of transmucosal fentanyl products

Abstral® vs. SC morphine[26]

A fixed dose of Abstral® 100microgram SL has been compared with morphine 5mg SC in patients receiving regular opioids (oral morphine equivalent 20–120mg/24h). Abstral® failed to show non-inferiority. Although the absolute differences were small (and statistically non-significant), when compared at 30min SC morphine provided better pain relief (mean (95% CI) pain intensity difference -0.5 (-1.1 to 0.1)), achieved a ≥50% reduction in pain intensity in more patients (57% vs. 52%) and fewer required further analgesia (37% vs. 51%). Nonetheless, >90% of patients preferred the SL route.

Actiq® vs. PO morphine tablets[24]

Actiq®, titrated to an effective dose, has been compared with morphine *tablets* (previously identified effective dose, encapsulated to maintain blinding) in a double-blind, double-dummy, multiple cross-over study. For the primary and secondary outcomes, Actiq® was statistically superior to PO morphine tablets. However, the differences were small and their clinical relevance uncertain.

For example, for Actiq® vs. PO morphine tablets, the proportion of episodes after 15min with clinical meaningful pain relief (defined as a ≥33% reduction in pain intensity) was 42% vs. 32%. Nonetheless, >90% of patients chose to continue with Actiq®.

Effentora® vs. PO oxycodone tablets[27,28]

Effentora® titrated to an effective dose has been compared with oxycodone *tablets* (titrated to an effective dose and encapsulated to maintain blinding) in double-blind, double-dummy, cross-over studies in opioid-tolerant patients mostly with non-cancer break-through pain (only two had cancer pain). Findings were similar in both studies: for primary and most secondary outcomes, Effentora® was statistically superior to PO oxycodone tablets. However, the differences were small and their clinical relevance uncertain.

For example, in the larger of the two studies,[27] for Effentora® vs. PO oxycodone tablets:

- mean (SD) pain intensity difference at 15min (primary outcome) was 0.8 (1.1) vs. 0.6 (0.9)
- percentage of episodes with a reduction in pain intensity of ≥33% was 13% vs. 9% (15min) and 41% vs. 32% (30min); for a reduction ≥50%, it was 6% vs. 4% (15min) and 21% vs. 16% (30min)
- patients rated the overall medication performance as 'good' to 'excellent' in 41% vs. 26% of episodes at 30min, and 79% vs. 71% at 60min.

PecFent® vs. PO morphine tablets[29,30]

PecFent®, titrated to an effective dose, has been compared with encapsulated morphine *tablets* (one sixth of the total daily dose, or previously identified effective dose) in a double-blind, double-dummy, multiple cross-over study. For the primary and most secondary outcomes, PecFent® was statistically superior to PO morphine tablets. However, the differences were small and their clinical relevance uncertain.

For example, for PecFent® vs. PO morphine tablets:

- mean (SD) pain intensity difference at 15min (primary outcome) was 3.0 (0.2) vs. 2.7 (0.2)
- percentage of episodes with clinical meaningful pain relief (defined as a ≥2 reduction in pain intensity) was 25% vs. 23% (5min); 52% vs. 45% (10min) and 76% vs. 69% (15min).

Instanyl® vs. Actiq®[10,31]

Instanyl® and Actiq® (both titrated to an effective dose) have been compared in an open-label RCT. The primary outcome was time to meaningful pain relief, measured by stop-watch. The fastest time to meaningful pain relief was significantly more likely with Instanyl® than Actiq®, with a median difference of 5min (11min vs. 16min respectively). A second dose of Instanyl® or Actiq® was required in about 60% and 30% of episodes respectively. For Instanyl® this was permitted 10min after the first dose, and for Actiq® 15min after fully consuming the first dose, i.e. at least 30min after starting the first dose. Usual rescue analgesia was required in 5–8% of episodes. Patients found the administration of Instanyl® easier and overall preferred Instanyl® (75%) to Actiq® (25%).

Abstral® 100microgram has been compared with SC **morphine** 5mg in a single-dose, double-blind, double-dummy RCT.[26] The SL route was preferred by >90% of patients. Although pain relief over 30–60min was similar, the results favoured **morphine**, with fewer patients requiring a second dose compared to Abstral® (35% vs. 50%). Notably, for 70% of patients their regular opioid dose was equivalent to PO **morphine** 20–60mg/24h, i.e. lower than the minimum recommended by the manufacturer (see Dose and use).

The lack of high-quality comparative data among the transmucosal products prevents conclusions about the best product to use. However, the practical aspects of using some of the products have been compared in a patient satisfaction survey.[35] Following instruction, 30 patients were asked to use a single *placebo* version of Abstral®, Effentora® and Instanyl® and to rate factors such as ease of access from packaging, ease of administration and palatability; they also rated their current rescue analgesic (generally PO **morphine** or **oxycodone**) similarly. They were asked to indicate if they would be prepared to use the transmucosal product and, if so, which they felt was the best and why. Several themes emerged:

- *ease of access:* the fentanyl products were generally more difficult to access than usual rescue analgesia, particularly the child-proof container for Instanyl®
- *ease of use:* Abstral® and the usual rescue analgesia were equal best
- *palatability:* Abstral® was rated best
- *patients willing to use:* Abstral® (90%) vs. Effentora® and Instanyl® (about 60% each); three patients would not use any (did not like the product or could not open the packaging)
- *which is best and why:*
  - ▷ Abstral® (~70%); easy to access and use, dissolved quickly
  - ▷ Instanyl® (~20%); quick to use (once you get into package), route familiar
  - ▷ Effentora® (~10%); liked sensation in the mouth
  - ▷ one could not choose between Abstral® and Effentora®.

The use of placebos means that overall satisfaction with the products could not be compared. Nonetheless, taking these practical issues and other factors into account, the *PCF* suggests the following in patients with cancer taking regular strong opioids and experiencing break-through cancer pain:

- use immediate-release PO strong opioids first-line and titrate accordingly (include a trial of a PO solution if tablets not adequate); only when inadequate with regards to speed of onset of action or prolonged undesirable effects should the transmucosal products be considered (echoed in NICE guidance)[36]
- a patient's circumstances should be considered carefully to ensure the patient fulfils the necessary requirements for use of a transmucosal product, e.g. current opioid dose, ability to access, use, store and dispose of the product reliably (see Dose and use)
- decide which route and product are the most appropriate, i.e.:
  - ▷ *nasal:* generally works more quickly and is shorter lasting (less PO absorption) than the SL/buccal route; PecFent® works slightly more slowly than Instanyl®, but has a safer accountable delivery system and is cheaper
  - ▷ *SL/buccal:* there is little difference in terms of efficacy; Abstral® dissolves the quickest, making it the most convenient to use.

There may be other, more specific, reasons that guide choice of route, e.g. patient preference, presence of severe dry mouth or mucositis (use nasal), or frequent nose bleeds (use SL/buccal).

In contrast to *PCF* and NICE guidance,[36] European guidelines recommend that either PO or transmucosal fentanyl products can be used for break-through cancer pain without clearly distinguishing a first-line preference.[37]

There are limited data on the wider impact of the transmucosal fentanyl products, e.g. on quality of life, mood, physical function and healthcare utilization.[38–40]

Unauthorized alternatives

Some palliative care services use the parenteral formulation of various fentanils for SL administration, e.g. fentanyl (50microgram/mL), **sufentanil** (50microgram/mL, not UK) and **alfentanil** (500microgram/mL and 5mg/mL).[41,42] Onset of analgesic effect may be broadly similar (5–10min), but duration of effect is likely to differ (fentanyl>**sufentanil**>**alfentanil**) (see **Alfentanil**, p.420). Although the availability of authorized transmucosal fentanyl products has largely rendered this practice unnecessary, it may still have a role when either the authorized products are unavailable or only small doses are required.

Using a 1mL graduated oral syringe:

- start with fentanyl 25–50microgram SL (0.5–1mL of 50microgram/mL injection formulation)
- if necessary, increase to 50–100microgram SL; many patients do not need more than this
- doses >100microgram are impractical because 2mL is the maximum volume that can be reliably kept in the mouth for transmucosal absorption (see **Alfentanil**, Table 2, p.424).[42]

The 50microgram/mL fentanyl injection solution has also been administered as a nasal spray. In adults, this approach is limited by the large dose volume. However, it has provided effective analgesia in children 1–18 years old presenting pre-hospital or to the emergency department with acute moderate–severe pain.[43-45] A 1mL syringe attached to a mucosal atomizer device permits the appropriate amount of fentanyl to be converted into a spray. The initial dose is generally 1–2microgram/kg, administered in divided doses to a maximum of 1mL in each nostril, with some centres permitting a second dose of 0.5microgram/kg after 10min if required.[46]

To overcome the dose/volume issues, higher-concentration fentanyl solutions up to 300microgram/mL have also been used. However, compared with the standard solution, they are less readily available, more expensive and, at least in children <50kg, no more effective.[43,47] Obviously, the authorized products avoid the dose/volume issue, and the use of Instanyl® 50–100microgram by paramedics for acute severe pain has been reported.[48]

Further dilution of the 50microgram/mL fentanyl injection solution to produce 10microgram/mL and 25microgram/mL solutions has permitted 1microgram/0.1mL and 2.5microgram/0.1mL doses to be administered intranasally to dying neonates and infants with respiratory distress;[49] others have nebulized the injection formulation.[50] However, evidence supporting the use of transmucosal fentanyl to relieve breathlessness in other circumstances is limited.[50-56]

Cautions

All companies provide additional information for prescribers, pharmacists and patients; these include check-lists to ensure proper patient selection and education around use, signs of opioid overdose, safe storage and disposal. Store out of reach of children (accidental deaths have occurred).

In 2007, after reports of serious overdoses and deaths in the USA, the FDA issued a safety warning about the use of Fentora® (Effentora®). Factors which contributed to the adverse drug events included improper:

- patient selection, e.g. non-opioid tolerant, acute (non-cancer) pain
- dosing, e.g. wrong dose prescribed, exceeding recommended maximum use
- product substitution, e.g. like-for-like swap from Actiq® to Fentora®.

Thus, these products need to be used correctly, specifically:

- do *not* use in opioid-naïve (non-tolerant) patients, including those who only take strong opioids p.r.n.
- they are contra-indicated in the management of acute or postoperative pain, including headache/migraine
- they are not interchangeable; do *not* convert patients on a microgram per microgram basis from one to another; it is necessary to titrate the new formulation
- when dispensing, do *not* substitute one product for another.

Use with caution in patients with COPD or other medical conditions predisposing them to respiratory depression (e.g. myasthenia gravis) or susceptible to the intracranial effects of hypercapnia (e.g. those with raised intracranial pressure). Also use with caution in bradyarrhythmia, elderly, cachectic, debilitated, moderate–severe hepatic or renal impairment (also see Chapter 17, p.743 and Chapter 18, p.762), hypovolaemia or hypotension, and if a history or high risk of abuse or diversion.

Mouth wounds, mucositis (may enhance absorption); nasal vasoconstrictive decongestants (reduce the effect); other nasal medications (the SPC for Instanyl® recommends avoiding because of lack of data, whereas that for PecFent® advises avoiding within 15min of a dose); epistaxis.

Actiq® contains 2g of sugars; inform diabetic patients, also risk of tooth decay (uncommon).

Drug interactions

Concurrent treatment with ≥2 CNS depressants (e.g. benzodiazepines, gabapentinoids, opioids) increases the risk of respiratory depression, particularly in susceptible groups, e.g. the elderly and those with renal or hepatic impairment.[57]

Fentanyl is metabolized by CYP3A4. Caution is required with concurrent use of drugs that inhibit or induce these enzymes (see Chapter 19, Table 8, p.790). Interactions where closer monitoring ± dose adjustment are required are listed in Box B.[58–62]

Box B Interactions between fentanyl and other drugs involving CYP450[a]

Plasma concentrations of fentanyl	
***Increased* by**	***Decreased* by**
Aprepitant[b]	Apalutamide
Azoles[c], e.g. fluconazole, itraconazole, voriconazole	Aprepitant[b]
Cimetidine	Carbamazepine
Macrolides, e.g. clarithromycin, erythromycin	Enzalutamide[63]
	Fosphenytoin
	Phenobarbital
	Phenytoin
	Rifampicin

a. not an exhaustive list; limited to drugs most likely to be encountered in palliative care and excludes anticancer, antiviral, HIV and immunosuppressive drugs (seek specialist advice)
b. aprepitant can increase the exposure to CYP3A4 substrates in the short-term, then reduce their exposure within 2 weeks
c. case reports of interactions with fatal (PO fluconazole) or serious (PO itraconazole) consequences with TD fentanyl patches.

IV fentanyl has been reported to reduce the metabolism of IV **midazolam**, reducing the clearance by 30% and extending the halflife by 50%.[62]

Fentanyl is not recommended in patients who have used an MAOI within the past 2 weeks. Although both have been used safely together, serotonin toxicity (sometimes fatal) has occurred (also see Antidepressants, Box A, p.217); manufacturers' SPCs warn of a risk of serotonin toxicity when fentanyl is *used in combination* with other serotoninergic drugs, e.g. SSRIs.[62]

Undesirable effects

Also see Strong opioids, p.394.

Very common (>1/10): drowsiness, dizziness, headache, confusion, nausea, vomiting, sweating.

Topical effects: less common and formulation-dependent, but include: oral and nasal discomfort, inflammation or ulceration, rhinorrhoea, epistaxis, sore throat, dysgeusia, dental caries with Actiq® (uncommon).

Dose and use

Patients using opioids must be monitored for undesirable effects, particularly nausea and vomiting, and constipation. Depending on individual circumstances, an anti-emetic should be prescribed for regular or p.r.n. use, (see QCG: Nausea and vomiting, p.264) and, routinely, a laxative prescribed (see QCG: Opioid-induced constipation, p.45).

Opioids can impair driving ability, and patients should be counselled accordingly (see Chapter 22, p.809).

Prescribers of transmucosal fentanyl products should:

- be experienced in the management of opioid therapy in cancer patients
- limit use to opioid-tolerant patients who can adhere to the instructions regarding indication, administration, storage and returns
- provide ongoing supervision
- keep in mind the potential for fentanyl to be misused[64-67]
- understand that the formulations are *not* bio-equivalent and *not* directly interchangeable, and thus:
  - ▷ prescribe by brand[68]
  - ▷ when switching transmucosal products, *de novo* titration from the lowest available dose is required; the only exception is Effentora®, when a starting dose higher than 100microgram may be considered (Box E).

Transmucosal fentanyl products should be used only in adults on a regular strong opioid for chronic cancer pain for ≥1 week:

- **morphine** 60mg/24h PO
- fentanyl 25microgram/h TD (50microgram/h required in some studies)
- **hydromorphone** 8mg/24h PO
- **oxycodone** 30mg/24h PO
- an equivalent dose of another opioid.

Individual titration is required because the effective dose cannot be reliably predicted from the maintenance dose of opioid.[18,27,31,69-71] Despite this, the use of doses proportional to the maintenance dose has been suggested.[72-75]

Careful monitoring is required during initial or subsequent titration; the complexity of the titration schedules varies between products (Boxes C–G). Even so, transmucosal fentanyl products are unsatisfactory in about 1/4–1/3 of patients, either because they fail to provide relief at the highest practical dose or they cause unacceptable undesirable effects.

The optimal dose found during successful titration (Boxes C–G) can be used to treat up to a maximum of 4 episodes/24h. The recommended minimum interval between treatments is generally ≥4h. This varies between products (e.g. Abstral® specifies ≥2h, Instanyl® allows a minimum interval of 2h in 'exceptional circumstances', and Actiq® does not specify a minimum) and even for the same product between countries (e.g. PecFent® in the UK and USA). However, applying the ≥4h apart rule across all products would be reasonable, because it was used by most studies and more frequent dosing than q4h appears to increase the maximum plasma concentration achieved with the subsequent dose of fentanyl.[4] Thus, an alternative p.r.n. analgesic, e.g. **morphine** PO, will be required to treat any additional more frequent episodes. Further, in about 5–25% of episodes, the transmucosal products fail to provide adequate relief, and an alternate analgesic is required.[71,76]

Supply

All formulations are fentanyl citrate and schedule 2 **CD**. All costs per dose for each transmucosal product are independent of strength or pack size and are NHS list price. Not all pack sizes are available for every strength.

Oromucosal formulations
Abstral® (Kyowa Kirin)
Tablets sublingual 100microgram, 200microgram, 300microgram, 400microgram, 600microgram, 800microgram, pack sizes 10 and 30, 1 tablet = £4.99.

Actiq® (Teva UK)
Lozenge buccal with oromucosal applicator 200microgram, 400microgram, 600microgram, 800microgram, 1,200microgram and 1,600microgram, pack sizes 3 and 30, 1 lozenge = £7.01.
Note. An equivalent product, Cynril®, is available as a branded generic.

Effentora® (Teva UK)
Tablets buccal 100microgram, 200microgram, 400microgram, 600microgram, 800microgram, pack sizes 4 and 28, 1 tablet = £4.99.

Intranasal formulations
Instanyl® (Takeda)
Nasal spray 50micrograms/metered dose spray, 100microgram/metered dose spray and 200microgram/metered dose spray, single dose (6 dose pack), 1 spray = £5.95.

PecFent® (Kyowa Kirin)
Nasal spray 100microgram/metered dose spray, 400microgram/metered dose spray, 8 or 32 dose, 1 spray = £4.56; the dose required may consist of 1 or 2 sprays.

Parenteral formulations
Fentanyl (generic)
Injection 50microgram/mL, 2mL amp = £1.25, 10mL amp = £1.50.

Box C Abstral® dose and use

Follow the manufacturer's guidance on administration, titration, storage and disposal in the SPC, prescriber's guide, dose titration guide and PIL. A hospital/hospice referral pad for GPs is also available.

Abstral® is an SL tablet, placed in the deepest part under the tongue. The tablets must not be chewed or sucked, and patients should not eat or drink until they have dissolved. Those with a dry mouth should moisten their mouth with water beforehand.[77] The tablet generally dissolves quickly (<5min), with the particles produced adhering to the oral mucosa, from which the fentanyl is subsequently absorbed.

Evaluate each dose after 15–30min and, if effective, i.e. a *single* dose provides adequate analgesia with few or no undesirable effects, this is the maintenance dose. If unsuccessful, during titration, a further dose can be given and subsequently a higher dose used for the next episode:

- start with 100microgram; if unsuccessful, give an additional 100microgram dose
- for the next episode give 200microgram; if unsuccessful, give an additional 100microgram tablet
- for the next episode give 300microgram; if unsuccessful, give an additional 100microgram tablet
- for the next episode give 400microgram; if unsuccessful, give an additional 200microgram tablet
- for the next episode give 600microgram; if unsuccessful, give an additional 200microgram tablet
- for the next episode give 800microgram, the maximum dose.

The SPC suggests that intermediate doses of 500microgram and 700microgram can be considered if there is adequate analgesia but undesirable effects at either the 600microgram or 800microgam doses. However, in practice, such doses are rarely used. It requires the use of a 100microgram tablet plus a 400microgram or 600microgram tablet, and doubles the cost of treating an episode (~£10).

Note. In the study on which its safety data are based, only single doses of Abstral® were used for titration and maintenance, with the effective dose confirmed over several consecutive episodes.[17]

More than two-thirds of patients find an effective and tolerable dose; about one quarter require 800microgram.[78] However, because of inadequate relief after 30min, an alternative rescue analgesic is needed in about 10% of episodes.[17]

The maximum frequency of use is 4 episodes/24h. In studies, doses had to be ≥2h apart (each pain episode was limited to treatment with a single dose),[17,79] and is the recommended interval in the SPC; nonetheless, ≥4h apart is ideal (see text). Regular daily use of medication for break-through pain (traditionally ≥2/24h) should prompt a review and possible increase in the dose of the regular strong opioid. Subsequently, if a single dose of Abstral® fails to provide consistent relief, the dose should be further titrated as above.

Abstral® is generally well tolerated and remains effective. Use of a median dose of 600microgram treating a mean of 3 episodes/day for 5–6 months showed that:

- opioid-related undesirable effects (e.g. nausea) are common but not a major cause of discontinuation
- application site irritation rarely occurred
- about 75% of patients were satisfied or very satisfied with its use.[17,79]

Although Abstral® is only authorized for break-through cancer pain, some data exist for its use in non-cancer pain.[80]

Box D Actiq® dose and use

Follow the manufacturer's guidance on administration, titration, storage and disposal in the SPC, patient's and caregiver's guide, PIL and health professional's guide.

Actiq® is a 'lozenge on a stick' containing fentanyl in a hard-sweet matrix. In order to achieve maximum mucosal exposure to the fentanyl, the lozenge should be placed between the cheek and the gum and moved constantly up and down, and changed at intervals from one cheek to the other. It should not be chewed. The lozenge should be consumed completely over 15min; quicker than this, and more fentanyl is swallowed. Patients with xerostomia (dry mouth) may find it hard to consume it in this time period.[81] If necessary, moisten the mouth with water beforehand. Initially, prescribe 6 doses of one strength at a time:

- start with fentanyl 200microgram and consume over 15min; drinking or eating is not permitted during administration
- wait 15min; if there is inadequate analgesia, use a second 200microgram lozenge
- not more than two lozenges should be used for any one episode of pain
- continue with 200microgram for a further two episodes of pain, allowing a second lozenge when necessary
- if on review, the break-through pain is not controlled satisfactorily with a single 200microgram dose, increase to 400microgram
- wait 15min; use a second 400microgram lozenge if necessary
- continue this upwards titration through the available dose strengths until a *single* dose provides adequate analgesia with little or no undesirable effects; this is the maintenance dose
- the maximum dose is 1,600microgram.

The lozenge should be removed from the mouth once the pain is relieved; partly consumed lozenges should be dissolved under hot running water and the handle discarded in a waste container out of reach of children.

About three-quarters of patients find an effective and tolerable dose. An alternative rescue analgesic is required in 5–15% of episodes (permitted if inadequate response 15min after Actiq® dose fully completed).

The maximum frequency of use is 4 episodes/24h. In studies, doses generally had to be ≥2h apart (each pain episode was limited to treatment with a single dose);[24] ≥4h apart is ideal (see text). Regular daily use of medication for break-through pain (traditionally ≥2/24h) should prompt a review and possible increase in the dose of the regular strong opioid. Subsequently, if a single dose of Actiq® fails to provide consistent relief, the dose should be further titrated as detailed above.

Actiq® is generally well tolerated and remains effective. Follow-up over a mean of about 3 months showed that:

- opioid-related undesirable effects are common (e.g. nausea) but not a major cause of discontinuation
- a single dose is effective in 85–90% of episodes
- about 1/2–3/4 of patients require a dose adjustment, mostly upwards, but sometimes downwards
- patient ratings of global medication performance remain the same (generally 'very good').[82,83]

Box E Effentora® dose and use

Follow the manufacturer's guidance on administration, titration, storage and disposal in the SPC, patient's and caregiver's guide and PIL.

Effentora® is a tablet which can be placed either buccally (between the cheek and gum near a molar tooth) or SL. Absorption is similar from both sites, but the tablet dissolves more quickly SL.[84] A dry mouth should be moistened with water beforehand. Mild mucositis (grade 1) does not affect absorption,[7] but avoid use in more severe grades because the impact on absorption has not been examined.

The tablets must not be chewed or sucked, and patients should not eat or drink until they have dissolved. The time to dissolution is generally 15–25min but can be longer. However, any tablet remnants should be swallowed after 30min with a glass of water.

Evaluate each dose after 30min and, if effective, this is the maintenance dose. If unsuccessful, during the titration phase, a further dose can be given and subsequently a higher dose used for the next episode. Titration packs, each containing 4 tablets, are available; prescribing 1 pack of 100microgram and 3 packs of 200microgram is sufficient to escalate through the dose range over 5 episodes:

- start with 100microgram; if unsuccessful, give an additional 100microgram dose
- for the next episode give 200microgram (2 × 100microgram tablets); if unsuccessful, give an additional 200microgram tablet
- for the next episode give 400microgram (2 × 200microgram tablets); if unsuccessful, give an additional 200microgram tablet
- for the next episode give 600microgram (3 × 200microgram tablets); if unsuccessful, give an additional 200microgram tablet
- for the next episode give the maximum dose of 800microgram (4 × 200microgram tablets).

If switching from another transmucosal fentanyl product, although titration is still necessary, a starting dose higher than 100microgram may be considered.

About two-thirds of patients find an effective and tolerable dose. Subsequently only a *single* dose of the appropriate strength tablet is used per episode, which can be prescribed in 28 tablet packs. An alternative rescue analgesic is required in about 10–25% of episodes.

The maximum frequency of use is 4 episodes/24h, with at least 4h between doses (including any other rescue analgesic used). Regular daily use of medication for break-through pain (traditionally ≥2/24h) should prompt a review and possible increase in the dose of the regular strong opioid. Subsequently, if a single dose of Effentora® fails to provide consistent relief, the dose may require further titration as above.

Effentora® is generally well tolerated and remains effective. Follow-up over a mean of 6 months showed that:

- opioid-related undesirable effects are common (e.g. nausea) but not a major cause of discontinuation
- application site problems (e.g. pain, irritation, ulceration) are seen in 6% and lead to discontinuation in <2%
- 70% of patients continue on the same dose
- patient ratings of global medication performance remain the same (generally 'good').[85]

Although Effentora® is only authorized for ≤800microgram in break-through cancer pain in patients receiving oral morphine equivalent of ≥60mg/24h, data exist for its use in:

- highly opioid-tolerant cancer patients (oral morphine equivalent >700mg/24h) in doses of 1,200–3,200microgram[86]
- opioid-tolerant Japanese cancer patients receiving an oral morphine equivalent of 30–59mg/24h using a 50microgram tablet (not UK) as the starting dose[87]
- opioid-tolerant patients with non-cancer break-through pain, e.g. degenerative back pain, complex regional pain syndrome[27,64,88-90]
- opioid-naïve patients with severe pain attending emergency departments with possible or definite fractures or dislocations (single dose of 100microgram) or undergoing invasive procedures.[91,92]

The use of Effentora® in non-cancer patients is controversial, and concerns exist around safety and the potential for misuse.[64-66]

Box F Instanyl® dose and use

Follow the guidance on priming, administration, storage and disposal in the manufacturer's SPC, physician's guides and patient brochure/PIL.

Instanyl® is a nasal spray. Not all patients feel the spray and they should be warned not to repeat the dose because of this. There is no dose counter in multi-dose bottles (not UK).

Evaluate each dose after 10min and, if effective, this is the maintenance dose; if unsuccessful, a maximum of one further dose can be given.

Evaluate each dose strength over 3–4 episodes; increase to the next higher strength if there is frequent need for a second dose:
- start with 50microgram in one nostril; if unsuccessful, give an additional 50microgram in the other nostril
- if unsuccessful over several episodes, give 100microgram in one nostril; if necessary, give an additional 100microgram in the other nostril
- if unsuccessful over several episodes, give 200microgram in one nostril; if necessary, give an additional 200microgram in the other nostril; this is the *maximum* dose.

About 2/3–3/4 of patients find an effective and tolerable dose. Although the aim is to use only one dose per episode, 30–50% require a second dose. An alternative rescue analgesic is required in about 15% of episodes; this is given after waiting ≥10min after a dose of Instanyl®.

The maximum frequency of use is 4 episodes/24h, with at least 4h between doses (including any other rescue analgesic used). Although the SPC states that Instanyl® can be used after 2h 'in exceptional circumstances', ≥4h apart is ideal (see text). Regular daily use of medication for break-through pain (traditionally ≥2/24h) should prompt a review and possible increase in the dose of the regular strong opioid. The dose of Instanyl® may subsequently need to be re-titrated.

Instanyl® is generally well tolerated and remains effective; opioid-related undesirable effects are common (e.g. nausea) but not a major cause of discontinuation. Follow-up for ≤3 months showed that:
- 65% of patients continue on the same dose
- <3% of patients drop out because of drug-related undesirable effects
- 15% of patients drop out because of a lack of efficacy.[93]

The multi-dose bottles (not UK) should be stored upright in the child-resistant container for safety; if not used for >1 week, they need to be primed again by spraying a single dose in the air.

Box G PecFent® dose and use

Follow the guidance on priming, administration, storage and disposal in the manufacturer's SPC, physician's and pharmacist's guides and patient brochure/PIL.

PecFent® is a nasal spray. Not all patients feel the spray, but there is an audible click when the dose is administered, and the dose counter advances by one. Advise patients not to blow their nose for 1h after administration:

- start with 100microgram in one nostril
- if unsuccessful, for the next episode, give 200microgram (100microgram in each nostril)
- if unsuccessful, for the next episode, prescribe higher concentration formulation and give 400microgram in one nostril
- if unsuccessful, for the next episode, increase to the maximum dose of 800microgram (400microgram in each nostril).

Evaluate each dose after 30min and, if ineffective, an alternative rescue analgesic can be given.

If any of the above doses are effective, this should be confirmed in the next episode. About three-quarters of patients find an effective and tolerable dose; an alternative rescue analgesic is needed in about 5–10% of episodes. Subsequently, if a previously effective dose fails to provide relief over several episodes, consider titration to a higher dose.

The maximum frequency of use is 4 episodes/24h, with at least 4h between doses (including any other rescue analgesic used). Regular daily use of medication for break-through pain (traditionally ≥2/24h) should prompt a review and a possible increase in the dose of the regular strong opioid. The dose of PecFent® may subsequently need to be re-titrated.

PecFent® is generally well tolerated and remains effective.[20,76] Follow-up over a mean of about 10 months showed that:

- 70% continue on the same dose
- <7% of patients drop out because of drug-related undesirable effects
- <3% of patients drop out because of a lack of efficacy.[94]

Preliminary data exist on the pre-emptive use of PecFent® in opioid-tolerant patients to relieve predictable break-through pain related to cancer treatment (e.g. positioning/immobilization required for radiotherapy), odynophagia or painful defaecation due to mucositis;[95,96] the dose is administered 20–30min prior to the activity.

The bottles should be kept in the child-resistant container for safety; if not used for >5 days, they need to be primed again by spraying a single dose in the air. Discard 60 days after first opening.

1 Davies A *et al.* (2013) Breakthrough cancer pain: an observational study of 1000 European oncology patients. *Journal of Pain and Symptom Management*. **46**: 619–628.

2 Zeppetella G (2008) Opioids for cancer breakthrough pain: a pilot study reporting patient assessment of time to meaningful pain relief. *Journal of Pain and Symptom Management*. **35**: 563–567.

3 Darwish M *et al.* (2007) Absolute and relative bioavailability of fentanyl buccal tablet and oral transmucosal fentanyl citrate. *Journal of Clinical Pharmacology*. **47**: 343–350.

4 European Medicines Agency (2010) Assessment report for Pecfent. Procedure No. EMA/H/C/001164.

5 European Medicines Agency (2008) Effentora: EPAR - Scientific discussion.

6 Lichtor J *et al.* (1999) The relative potency of oral transmucosal fentanyl citrate compared with intravenous morphine in the treatment of moderate to severe postoperative pain. *Anesthesia and Analgesia*. **89**: 732–738.

7 Darwish M *et al.* (2007) Absorption of fentanyl from fentanyl buccal tablet in cancer patients with or without oral mucositis: a pilot study. *Clinical Drug Investigation*. **27**: 605–611.

8 Darwish M *et al.* (2006) Comparison of equivalent doses of fentanyl buccal tablets and arteriovenous differences in fentanyl pharmacokinetics. *Clinical Pharmacokinetics*. **45**: 843–850.

9 Kaasa S *et al.* (2010) Pharmacokinetics of intranasal fentanyl spray in patients with cancer and breakthrough pain. *Journal of Opioid Management*. **6**: 17–26.

10 European Medicines Agency (2009) Assessment report for Instanyl. Procedure No. EMEA/H/C/959. London.

11 Vasisht N *et al.* (2010) Single-dose pharmacokinetics of fentanyl buccal soluble film. *Pain Medicine*. **11**: 1017–1023.

12 Darwish M *et al.* (2006) Pharmacokinetic properties of fentanyl effervescent buccal tablets: a phase I, open-label, crossover study of single-dose 100, 200, 400, and 800 microgram in healthy adult volunteers. *Clinical Therapeutics*. **28**: 707–714.
13 King S *et al.* (2011) A systematic review of the use of opioid medication for those with moderate to severe cancer pain and renal impairment: A European palliative care research collaborative opioid guidelines project. *Palliative Medicine*. **25**: 525–552.
14 Bosilkovska M *et al.* (2012) Analgesics in patients with hepatic impairment: pharmacology and clinical implications. *Drugs*. **72**: 1645–1669.
15 Darwish M *et al.* (2007) Single-dose and steady-state pharmacokinetics of fentanyl buccal tablet in healthy volunteers. *Journal of Clinical Pharmacology*. **47**: 56–63.
16 Lister N *et al.* (2011) Pharmacokinetics, safety, and tolerability of ascending doses of sublingual fentanyl, with and without naltrexone, in Japanese subjects. *Journal of Clinical Pharmacology*. **51**: 1195–1204.
17 Rauck RL *et al.* (2009) Efficacy and long-term tolerability of sublingual fentanyl orally disintegrating tablet in the treatment of breakthrough cancer pain. *Current Medical Research Opinion*. **25**: 2877–2885.
18 Slatkin NE *et al.* (2007) Fentanyl buccal tablet for relief of breakthrough pain in opioid-tolerant patients with cancer-related chronic pain. *Journal of Supportive Oncology*. **5**: 327–334.
19 European Medicines Agency (2008) Committee for medicinal products for human use (CHMP). Opinion following article 29(4) referral for Rapinyl.
20 Portenoy RK *et al.* (2010) A multicenter, placebo-controlled, double-blind, multiple-crossover study of Fentanyl Pectin Nasal Spray (FPNS) in the treatment of breakthrough cancer pain. *Pain*. **151**: 617–624.
21 Dworkin RH *et al.* (2008) Interpreting the clinical importance of treatment outcomes in chronic pain clinical trials: IMMPACT recommendations. *Journal of Pain*. **9**: 105–121.
22 Kress HG *et al.* (2009) Efficacy and tolerability of intranasal fentanyl spray 50 to 200 microg for breakthrough pain in patients with cancer: a phase III, multinational, randomized, double-blind, placebo-controlled, crossover trial with a 10-month, open-label extension treatment period. *Clinical Therapeutics*. **31**: 1177–1191.
23 Prostraken (2010) *Personal communication*.
24 Coluzzi P *et al.* (2001) Breakthrough cancer pain: a randomized trial comparing oral transmucosal fentanyl citrate (OTFC) and morphine sulfate immediate release (MSIR). *Pain*. **91**: 123–130.
25 Zeppetella G *et al.* (2010) Consistent and clinically relevant effects with fentanyl buccal tablet in the treatment of patients receiving maintenance opioid therapy and experiencing cancer-related breakthrough pain. *Pain Practice*. **10**: 287–293.
26 Zecca E *et al.* (2017) Fentanyl sublingual tablets versus subcutaneous morphine for the management of severe cancer pain episodes in patients receiving opioid treatment: A double-blind, randomized, noninferiority trial. *Journal of Clinical Oncology*. **35**: 759–765.
27 Ashburn MA *et al.* (2011) The efficacy and safety of fentanyl buccal tablet compared with immediate-release oxycodone for the management of breakthrough pain in opioid-tolerant patients with chronic pain. *Anesthesia and Analgesia*. **112**: 693–702.
28 Webster LR *et al.* (2013) Fentanyl buccal tablet compared with immediate-release oxycodone for the management of breakthrough pain in opioid-tolerant patients with chronic cancer and noncancer pain: a randomized, double-blind, crossover study followed by a 12-week open-label phase to evaluate patient outcomes. *Pain Medicine*. **14**: 1332–1345.
29 Fallon M *et al.* (2011) Efficacy and safety of fentanyl pectin nasal spray compared with immediate-release morphine sulfate tablets in the treatment of breakthrough cancer pain: a multicenter, randomized, controlled, double-blind, double-dummy multiple-crossover study. *Journal of Supportive Oncology*. **9**: 224–231.
30 Davies A *et al.* (2011) Consistency of efficacy, patient acceptability, and nasal tolerability of fentanyl pectin nasal spray compared with immediate-release morphine sulfate in breakthrough cancer pain. *Journal of Pain and Symptom Management*. **41**: 358–366.
31 Mercadante S *et al.* (2009) A comparison of intranasal fentanyl spray with oral transmucosal fentanyl citrate for the treatment of breakthrough cancer pain: an open label, randomised, crossover trial. *Current Medical Research Opinion*. **25**: 2805–2815.
32 Sawe J *et al.* (1983) Steady-state kinetics and analgesic effect of oral morphine in cancer patients. *European Journal of Clinical Pharmacology*. **24**: 537–542.
33 Freye E *et al.* (2007) Effervescent morphine results in faster relief of breakthrough pain in patients compared to immediate release morphine sulfate tablet. *Pain Practice*. **7**: 324–331.
34 Velazquez Rivera I *et al.* (2014) Efficacy of sublingual fentanyl vs. oral morphine for cancer-related breakthrough pain. *Advances in Therapy*. **31**: 107–117.
35 England R *et al.* (2011) How practical are transmuscosal fentanyl products for breakthrough cancer pain? Novel use of placebo formulations to survey user opinion. *BMJ Supportive and Palliative Care*. **1**: 349–351.
36 NICE (2016) Opioids in palliative care: safe and effective prescribing of strong opioids for pain in palliative care adults. *Clinical Guideline*. CG104. www.nice.org.uk.
37 Caraceni A *et al.* (2012) Use of opioid analgesics in the treatment of cancer pain: evidence-based recommendations from the EAPC. *Lancet Oncology*. **13**: e58–e68.
38 Guitart J *et al.* (2015) Sublingual fentanyl tablets for relief of breakthrough pain in cancer patients and association with quality-of-life outcomes. *Clinical Drug Investigation*. **35**: 815–822.
39 Davies A *et al.* (2015) Improved patient functioning after treatment of breakthrough cancer pain: an open-label study of fentanyl buccal tablet in patients with cancer pain. *Supportive Care in Cancer*. **23**: 2135–2143.
40 Ueberall MA *et al.* (2016) Efficacy, safety, and tolerability of fentanyl pectin nasal spray in patients with breakthrough cancer pain. *Journal of Pain Research*. **9**: 571–585.
41 Gardner-Nix J (2001) Oral transmucosal fentanyl and sufentanil for incident pain. *Journal of Pain and Symptom Management*. **22**: 627–630.
42 Zeppetella G (2001) Sublingual fentanyl citrate for cancer-related breakthrough pain: a pilot study. *Palliative Medicine*. **15**: 323–328.
43 Murphy A *et al.* (2014) Intranasal fentanyl for the management of acute pain in children. *Cochrane Database Systematic Reviews*. **10**: CD009942. www.cochranelibrary.com.
44 Fein DM *et al.* (2017) Intranasal fentanyl for initial treatment of vaso-occlusive crisis in sickle cell disease. *Pediatric Blood Cancer*. **64**:
45 Hansen MS and Dahl JB (2013) Limited evidence for intranasal fentanyl in the emergency department and the prehospital setting--a systematic review. *Danish Medical Journal*. **60**: A4563.
46 Cole J *et al.* (2009) Intranasal fentanyl in 1-3-year-olds: a prospective study of the effectiveness of intranasal fentanyl as acute analgesia. *Emergency Medicine Australasia*. **21**: 395–400.
47 Borland M *et al.* (2011) Equivalency of two concentrations of fentanyl administered by the intranasal route for acute analgesia in children in a paediatric emergency department: a randomized controlled trial. *Emergency Medicine Australasia*. **23**: 202–208.
48 Karlsen AP *et al.* (2014) Safety of intranasal fentanyl in the out-of-hospital setting: a prospective observational study. *Annals of Emergency Medicine*. **63**: 699–703.
49 Harlos MS *et al.* (2013) Intranasal fentanyl in the palliative care of newborns and infants. *Journal of Pain and Symptom Management*. **46**: 265–274.

50 Pieper L *et al.* (2018) Intranasal fentanyl for respiratory distress in children and adolescents with life-limiting conditions. *BMC Palliative Care*. **17**: 106.

51 Simon ST *et al.* (2013) Fentanyl for the relief of refractory breathlessness: a systematic review. *Journal of Pain and Symptom Management*. **46**: 874–886.

52 Pinna MA *et al.* (2015) A randomized crossover clinical trial to evaluate the efficacy of oral transmucosal fentanyl citrate in the treatment of dyspnea on exertion in patients with advanced cancer. *American Journal of Hospice and Palliative Care*. **32**: 298–304.

53 Simon ST *et al.* (2016) EffenDys-Fentanyl buccal tablet for the relief of episodic breathlessness in patients with advanced cancer: a multicenter, open-label, randomized, morphine-controlled, crossover, phase II trial. *Journal of Pain and Symptom Management*. **52**: 617–625.

54 Hui D *et al.* (2016) Impact of prophylactic fentanyl pectin nasal spray on exercise-induced episodic dyspnea in cancer patients:A double-blind, randomized controlled trial. *Journal of Pain and Symptom Management*. **52**: 459–468.

55 Pilkey J *et al.* (2019) The use of intranasal fentanyl for the palliation of incident dyspnea in advanced congestive heart failure:A pilot study. *Journal of Palliative Care*. **34**: 96–102.

56 Hui D *et al.* (2019) Prophylactic fentanyl sublingual spray for episodic exertional dyspnea in cancer patients: A pilot double-blind randomized controlled trial. *Journal of Pain and Symptom Management*. **58**: 605–613.

57 MHRA (2020) Benzodiazepines and opioids: reminder of risk of potentially fatal respiratory depression. *Drug Safety Update*. www.gov.uk/drug-safety-update.

58 Kharasch ED *et al.* (2004) Influence of hepatic and intestinal cytochrome P4503A activity on the acute disposition and effects of oral transmucosal fentanyl citrate. *Anesthesiology*. **101**: 729–737.

59 Takane H *et al.* (2005) Rifampin reduces the analgesic effect of transdermal fentanyl. *Annals of Pharmacotherpy*. **39**: 2139–2140.

60 Sasson M and Shvartzman P (2006) Fentanyl patch sufficient analgesia for only one day. *Journal of Pain and Symptom Management*. **31**: 389–391.

61 Morii H *et al.* (2007) Failure of pain control using transdermal fentanyl during rifampicin treatment. *Journal of Pain and Symptom Management*. **33**: 5–6.

62 Preston CL *Stockley's Drug Interactions*. London: Pharmaceutical Press www.medicinescomplete.com (accessed May 2020).

63 Westdorp H *et al.* (2018) Difficulties in pain management using oxycodone and fentanyl in enzalutamide-treated patients with advanced prostate cancer. *Journal of Pain and Symptom Management*. **55**: e6–e8.

64 Fine PG *et al.* (2010) Long-term safety and tolerability of fentanyl buccal tablet for the treatment of breakthrough pain in opioid-tolerant patients with chronic pain: an 18-month study. *Journal of Pain and Symptom Management*. **40**: 747–760.

65 Markman JD (2008) Not so fast: the reformulation of fentanyl and breakthrough chronic non-cancer pain. *Pain*. **136**: 227–229.

66 Passik SD *et al.* (2011) Aberrant Drug-Related Behavior Observed During Clinical Studies Involving Patients Taking Chronic Opioid Therapy for Persistent Pain and Fentanyl Buccal Tablet for Breakthrough Pain. *Journal of Pain and Symptom Management*. **41**: 116–125.

67 Nunez-Olarte JM and Alvarez-Jimenez P (2011) Emerging opioid abuse in terminal cancer patients taking oral transmucosal fentanyl citrate for breakthrough pain. *Journal of Pain and Symptom Management*. **42**: e6–e8.

68 NHS PrescQipp (2016) Immediate release fentanyl (DROP-List). *Bulletin*. **132**: www.prescqipp.info.

69 Christie J *et al.* (1998) Dose-titration, multicenter study of oral transmucosal fentanyl citrate for the treatment of breakthrough pain in cancer patients using transdermal fentanyl for persistent pain. *Journal of Clinical Oncology*. **16**: 3238–3248.

70 Portenoy R *et al.* (1999) Oral transmucosal fentanyl citrate (OTFC) for the treatment of breakthrough pain in cancer patients: a controlled use titration study. *Pain*. **79**: 303–312.

71 Portenoy RK *et al.* (2006) A randomized, placebo-controlled study of fentanyl buccal tablet for breakthrough pain in opioid-treated patients with cancer. *Clinical Journal of Pain*. **22**: 805–811.

72 Mercadante S *et al.* (2014) Intranasal fentanyl versus fentanyl pectin nasal spray for the management of breakthrough cancer pain in doses proportional to basal opioid regimen. *Journal of Pain*. **15**: 602–607.

73 Shimoyama N *et al.* (2015) Efficacy and safety of sublingual fentanyl orally disintegrating tablet at doses determined from oral morphine rescue doses in the treatment of breakthrough cancer pain. *Japanese Journal of Clinical Oncology*. **45**: 189–196.

74 Mercadante S *et al.* (2016) Fentanyl pectin nasal spray versus oral morphine in doses proportional to the basal opioid regimen for the management of breakthrough cancer pain: a comparative study. *Journal of Pain and Symptom Management*. **52**: 27–34.

75 Mercadante S *et al.* (2015) Fentanyl buccal tablet vs. oral morphine in doses proportional to the basal opioid regimen for the management of breakthrough cancer pain: a randomized, crossover, comparison study. *Journal of Pain and Symptom Management*. **50**: 579–586.

76 Portenoy RK *et al.* (2010) Long-term safety, tolerability, and consistency of effect of fentanyl pectin nasal spray for breakthrough cancer pain in opioid-tolerant patients. *Journal of Opioid Management*. **6**: 319–328.

77 Davies A *et al.* (2016) The influence of low salivary flow rates on the absorption of a sublingual fentanyl citrate formulation for breakthrough cancer pain. *Journal of Pain and Symptom Management*. **51**: 538–545.

78 Nalamachu SR *et al.* (2012) Successful dose finding with sublingual fentanyl tablet: Combined results from 2 open-label titration studies. *Pain Practice*. **12**: 449–456.

79 Nalamachu S *et al.* (2011) Long-term effectiveness and tolerability of sublingual fentanyl orally disintegrating tablet for the treatment of breakthrough cancer pain. *Current Medical Research Opinion*. **27**: 519–530.

80 Guitart J *et al.* (2013) Efficacy and safety of sublingual fentanyl orally disintegrating tablets in patients with breakthrough pain: multicentre prospective study. *Clinical Drug Investigation*. **33**: 675–683.

81 Davies AN and Vriens J (2005) Oral transmucosal fentanyl citrate and xerostomia. *Journal of Pain and Symptom Management*. **30**: 496–497.

82 Payne R *et al.* (2001) Long-term safety of oral transmucosal fentanyl citrate for breakthrough cancer pain. *Journal of Pain and Symptom Management*. **22**: 575–583.

83 Hanks GW *et al.* (2004) Oral transmucosal fentanyl citrate in the management of breakthrough pain in cancer: an open, multicentre, dose-titration and long-term use study. *Palliative Medicine*. **18**: 698–704.

84 Darwish M *et al.* (2008) Bioequivalence following buccal and sublingual placement of fentanyl buccal tablet 400 microg in healthy subjects. *Clinical Drug Investigation*. **28**: 1–7.

85 Weinstein SM *et al.* (2009) Fentanyl buccal tablet for the treatment of breakthrough pain in opioid-tolerant patients with chronic cancer pain:A long-term, open-label safety study. *Cancer*. **115**: 2571–2579.

86 Mercadante S *et al.* (2011) Fentanyl buccal tablets for breakthrough pain in highly tolerant cancer patients: preliminary data on the proportionality between breakthrough pain dose and background dose. *Journal of Pain and Symptom Management*. **42**: 464–469.

87 Kosugi T *et al.* (2014) A randomized, double-blind, placebo-controlled study of fentanyl buccal tablets for breakthrough pain: efficacy and safety in Japanese cancer patients. *Journal of Pain and Symptom Management*. **47**: 990–1000.

88 Simpson DM *et al.* (2007) Fentanyl buccal tablet for the relief of breakthrough pain in opioid-tolerant adult patients with chronic neuropathic pain: a multicenter, randomized, double-blind, placebo-controlled study. *Clinical Therapy*. **29**: 588–601.
89 Portenoy RK *et al.* (2007) Fentanyl buccal tablet (FBT) for relief of breakthrough pain in opioid-treated patients with chronic low back pain: a randomized, placebo-controlled study. *Current Medical Research Opinion*. **23**: 223–233.
90 Farrar JT *et al.* (2010) A novel 12-week study, with three randomized, double-blind placebo-controlled periods to evaluate fentanyl buccal tablets for the relief of breakthrough pain in opioid-tolerant patients with noncancer-related chronic pain. *Pain Medicine*. **11**: 1313–1327.
91 Shear ML *et al.* (2010) Transbuccal fentanyl for rapid relief of orthopedic pain in the ED. *American Journal of Emergency Medicine*. **28**: 847–852.
92 Bortolussi R *et al.* (2016) A phase II study on the efficacy and safety of procedural analgesia with fentanyl buccal tablet in cancer patients for the placement of indwelling central venous access systems. *Supportive Care in Cancer*. **24**: 1537–1543.
93 Kongsgaard UE *et al.* (2014) The use of Instanyl® in the treatment of breakthrough pain in cancer patients: a 3-month observational, prospective, cohort study. *Support Care Cancer*. **22**: 1655–1662.
94 Taylor D *et al.* (2014) A report on the long-term use of fentanyl pectin nasal spray in patients with recurrent breakthrough pain. *Journal of Pain and Symptom Management*. **47**: 1001–1007.
95 Mazzola R *et al.* (2017) Fentanyl pectin nasal spray for painful mucositis in head and neck cancers during intensity-modulated radiation therapy with or without chemotherapy. *Clinical and Translational Oncology*. **19**: 593–598.
96 Bell BC and Butler EB (2013) Management of predictable pain using fentanyl pectin nasal spray in patients undergoing radiotherapy. *Journal of Pain Research*. **6**: 843–848.

Updated December 2021

HYDROMORPHONE

Class: Strong opioid analgesic.

Indications: Severe or †moderate pain in cancer; †an alternative in cases of intolerance to other strong opioids;[1,2] †cough.

Contra-indications: None absolute if titrated carefully against a patient's pain. (Also see Cautions, and Strong opioids, p.389.)

Pharmacology

Hydromorphone is an analogue of **morphine** with similar pharmacokinetic and pharmacodynamic properties.[3] Thus, it is both analgesic and antitussive. Hydromorphone, **morphine** and **oxycodone** are comparable in terms of analgesic efficacy, although differ in potency.[1,2] Undesirable effects are similar but, as with all opioids, these can vary in severity between individuals. Hydromorphone can be used as an alternative in cases of intolerance to **morphine** or another opioid.[1]

PO hydromorphone is absorbed mainly in the small intestine. As with **morphine**, bioavailability is subject to wide inter-individual variation.[4] Hydromorphone is metabolized in the liver by 6-ketoreduction with subsequent glucuronidation. The main metabolite is hydromorphone-3-glucuronide (H3G). All the metabolites are renally excreted and can accumulate in renal impairment.[5] Nonetheless, with appropriate caution, hydromorphone is used in this setting (see Dose and use).[6]

H3G has no analgesic activity but, like morphine-3-glucuronide (see p.404), it is a CNS neuro-excitant, producing dose-dependent behavioural excitation in animals, e.g. agitation, myoclonus, seizures.[7] Thus, H3G is probably responsible for features of neuro-excitation described in case reports and clinical studies, e.g. hyperalgesia, cognitive impairment, delirium, tremor, myoclonus, seizures.[6] Toxic CNS levels of H3G may result from high doses of hydromorphone and/or accumulation in renal impairment.[6,8]

Hydromorphone is available in PO (immediate-release, modified-release) and injectable formulations. When switching from PO hydromorphone to SC/IV hydromorphone, the UK manufacturer recommends a conversion ratio of 3:1. However, this may be too conservative for some patients, and clinical experience is that a conversion ratio of 2:1 can be used, i.e. the hydromorphone SC/IV 24h dose should be half of the hydromorphone PO 24h dose. (Also see Strong opioids, p.400 and Appendix 2, Table 3, p.931.) For switching from other oral opioids to CSCI hydromorphone, see Dose and use.

Compared with **morphine**, hydromorphone costs more. However, hydromorphone is more soluble than **morphine**, and is available as a high-concentration injection (50mg/mL). Because hydromorphone is more potent than morphine (see below), this permits a high dose to be delivered in a small volume. Thus, in countries where **diamorphine** (p.417) is not available, hydromorphone is used CSCI, particularly when higher doses are required.

According to the UK manufacturer, PO hydromorphone is about 7.5 times more potent than PO **morphine**,[9,10] and this accounts for the choice of capsule content (1.3mg and 2.6mg; stated to be equivalent to PO **morphine** 10mg and 20mg respectively). However, independent reviews and guidelines recommend that when switching from PO **morphine** to PO hydromorphone, a conversion ratio of 5:1 is used; i.e. the hydromorphone dose should be one fifth of the **morphine** dose.[2,11] A conversion ratio of 5:1 is also appropriate for switching from CSCI **morphine** to CSCI hydromorphone. (Also see Strong opioids, p.400 and Appendix 2, Table 1, p.927 and Table 4, p.932.) Nonetheless, a double-blind RCT that converted patients with satisfactory pain control with 60mg or 90mg/24h of PO **morphine** to PO hydromorphone, found 5:1 and 8:1 conversion ratios equally effective and tolerated.[12]

Bio-availability 37–62% PO.[4]

Onset of action <5min IV;[13] 15min SC/IM; 30min PO.[14]

Time to peak plasma concentration 45min PO.[15]

Plasma halflife 2.5h early phase, with a prolonged late phase.

Duration of action 4–5h immediate-release; 12–24h m/r (product-dependent).[16-18]

Cautions

In 2005, the FDA warned that the concurrent ingestion of alcohol could hasten the release of hydromorphone from one m/r product, resulting in 'dose dumping', i.e. a rapid rise in plasma concentrations. In 2011, the EMA reported the results of a review of the interaction between alcohol and opioid m/r mechanisms, and concluded that the risk is minor for most m/r products except those using polymethylmethacrylate-triethylcitrate (none in the UK).[19]

Moderate–severe renal or hepatic impairment (see Dose and use, and Chapter 17, p.743 and Chapter 18, p.762).

Drug interactions

Concurrent treatment with ≥2 CNS depressants (e.g. benzodiazepines, gabapentinoids, opioids) increases the risk of respiratory depression, particularly in susceptible groups, e.g. the elderly and those with renal or hepatic impairment.[20]

Undesirable effects

Also see Strong opioids, p.394.

Dose and use

Patients using opioids must be monitored for undesirable effects, particularly nausea and vomiting, and constipation. Depending on individual circumstances, an anti-emetic should be prescribed for regular or p.r.n. use (see QCG: Nausea and vomiting, p.264) and, routinely, a laxative prescribed (see QCG: Opioid-induced constipation, p.45).

Opioids can impair driving ability, and patients should be counselled accordingly (see Chapter 22, p.809).

Oral

PO hydromorphone is used in the same way as PO **morphine**, generally q4h as immediate-release capsules or q12h as m/r capsules; both formulations can be swallowed whole or, if necessary, opened and the contents sprinkled on a small amount of soft food, e.g. yoghurt. The m/r granules should not be crushed or chewed, because this could lead to a rapid release of an overdose (see Chapter 28, Box A, p.857).

In the UK, hydromorphone is unlikely to be used primarily as an antitussive, but theoretically could be (see Antitussives, p.158).

Continuous subcutaneous administration

For general considerations when switching routes ± converting opioids, see Appendix 2, p.925.

A large case series suggests the following calculations are suitable across a range of doses:

- PO hydromorphone to CSCI hydromorphone: give half of the 24h dose, e.g. hydromorphone 32mg/24h PO = hydromorphone 16mg/24h CSCI
- PO **morphine** to CSCI hydromorphone: give a tenth of the 24h dose, e.g. **morphine** 60mg/24h PO = hydromorphone 6mg/24h CSCI
- PO **oxycodone** to CSCI hydromorphone: give an eighth of the 24h dose, e.g. **oxycodone** 40mg/24h PO = hydromorphone 5mg/24h CSCI.[21]

When switching from CSCI **morphine** to CSCI hydromorphone, *PCF* recommends a conversion ratio of 5:1 (see Pharmacology):

- CSCI **morphine** to CSCI hydromorphone: give a fifth of the 24h dose, e.g. **morphine** 30mg/24h CSCI = hydromorphone 6mg/24h CSCI.

For CSCI dilute with WFI, sodium chloride 0.9% or glucose 5%. Conventionally, p.r.n. SC doses of hydromorphone are 1/10–1/6 of the total 24h CSCI dose.

CSCI compatibility with other drugs: although most data are for dilution in sodium chloride 0.9%, there are 2-drug compatibility data for hydromorphone in WFI with **glycopyrronium**, **hyoscine *butylbromide***, **hyoscine *hydrobromide***, **ketamine**, **levomepromazine**, **metoclopramide** and **midazolam**.

Concentration-dependent *incompatibility* may occur with **cyclizine**, **dexamethasone**, **haloperidol** and **ketorolac**. For more details and 3-drug compatibility data, see Appendix 3, Chart 1 (p.936) and Chart 4 (p.942).

Compatibility charts for mixing drugs in sodium chloride 0.9% can be found in the extended appendix section of the on-line *PCF* on *www.medicinescomplete.com.*

Renal or hepatic impairment

Because of the risk of impaired metabolism or elimination:[22-24]

- lower than usual starting doses are advised in moderate–severe renal impairment or moderate hepatic impairment
- avoid if possible in severe hepatic impairment; if unavoidable, lower the usual starting dose *and* increase the dosing interval of immediate-release products to q8h (see Chapter 18, p.762)
- hydromorphone is advised against in hepatorenal syndrome.

Despite the risk of accumulation of H3G and other glucuronide metabolites, hydromorphone is successfully used in some centres in severe renal impairment and ESRF (see Chapter 17, p.743).

For a general approach when renal or hepatic function deteriorates rapidly, see Strong opioids, p.393.

Supply

All products are Schedule 2 **CD**.

Palladone® (Napp)

Capsules 1.3mg, 2.6mg, 1.3mg dose = £0.16.

Injection 2mg/mL, 10mg/mL, 20mg/mL and 50mg/mL, 1mL amp = £1.50, £13, £26 and £34 respectively.

Modified-release oral formulation

As for all m/r opioids, brand prescribing is recommended to reduce the risk of confusion and error in dispensing and administration (see p.xvii).

Palladone® SR (Napp)

Capsules enclosing m/r granules 2mg, 4mg, 8mg, 16mg, 24mg, 28 days @ 2mg, 8mg or 24mg every 12h = £21, £56 and £160 respectively.

1 Bao YJ *et al.* (2016) Hydromorphone for cancer pain. *Cochrane Database of Systematic Reviews.* **10**: CD011108. www.cochranelibrary.com.

2 Caraceni A *et al.* (2012) Use of opioid analgesics in the treatment of cancer pain: evidence-based recommendations from the EAPC. *Lancet Oncology.* **13**: e58–e68.

3 Quigley C and Glare P. Hydromorphone. In: Davis M, Glare P, Quigley C, Hardy J, editors. *Opioids in Cancer Pain*. 2 ed. Oxford: Oxford University Press; 2009. pp. 245–252.
4 Vallner J *et al.* (1981) Pharmacokinetics and bioavailability of hydromorphone following intravenous and oral administration to human subjects. *Journal of Clinical Pharmacology*. **21**: 152–156.
5 King S *et al.* (2011) A systematic review of the use of opioid medication for those with moderate to severe cancer pain and renal impairment: A European palliative care research collaborative opioid guidelines project. *Palliative Medicine*. **25**: 525–552.
6 Lee KA *et al.* (2016) Evidence for neurotoxicity due to morphine or hydromorphone use in renal impairment: a systematic review. *Journal of Palliative Medicine*. **19**: 1179–1187.
7 Wright AW *et al.* (2001) Hydromorphone-3-glucuronide: a more potent neuro-excitant than its structural analogue, morphine-3-glucuronide. *Life Sciences*. **69**: 409–420.
8 Babul N *et al.* (1995) Hydromorphone metabolite accumulation in renal failure. *Journal of Pain and Symptom Management*. **10**: 184–186.
9 McDonald C and Miller A (1997) A comparative potency study of a controlled release tablet formulation of hydromorphone with controlled release morphine in patients with cancer pain. *European Journal of Palliative Care Abstracts of the Fifth Congress*.
10 Moriarty M *et al.* (1999) A randomised crossover comparison of controlled release hydromorphone tablets with controlled release morphine tablets in patients with cancer pain. *Journal of Clinical Research*. **2**: 1–8.
11 Mercadante S and Caraceni A (2011) Conversion ratios for opioid switching in the treatment of cancer pain: a systematic review. *Palliative Medicine*. **25**: 504–515.
12 Inoue S *et al.* (2018) A double-blind, randomized comparative study to investigate the morphine to hydromorphone conversion ratio in Japanese cancer patients. *Japanese Journal of Clinical Oncology*. **48**: 442–449.
13 Coda B *et al.* (1997) Hydromorphone analgesia after intravenous bolus administration. *Pain*. **71**: 41–48.
14 Benedetti CB and Butler SH. Systemic analgesics. In: Bonica JJ, ed. *The Management of Pain*. Philedelphia: Lea and Febiger; 1990.
15 Durnin C *et al.* (2001) Pharmacokinetics of oral immediate-release hydromorphone (Dilaudid IR) in young and elderly subjects. *Proceedings of the Western Pharmacology Society*. **44**: 79-80.
16 Hagen N *et al.* (1995) Steady-state pharmacokinetics of hydromorphone and hydromorphone-3-glucuronide in cancer patients after immediate and controlled-release hydromorphone. *Journal of Clinical Pharmacology*. **35**: 37–44.
17 Bruera E *et al.* (1996) A randomized, double-blind, double-dummy, crossover trial comparing the safety and efficacy of oral sustained-release hydromorphone with immediate-release hydromorphone in patients with cancer pain. Canadian Palliative Care Clinical Trials Group. *Journal of Clinical Oncology*. **14**: 1713–1717.
18 Hays H *et al.* (1994) Comparative clinical efficacy and safety of immediate release and controlled release hydromorphone for chronic severe cancer pain. *Cancer*. **74**: 1808–1816.
19 European Medicines Agency (2010) EMA concludes review of modified-release oral opioids of the WHO level III scale management of pain. *Press release* 23 July 2010: www.ema.europa.eu.
20 MHRA (2020) Benzodiazepines and opioids: reminder of risk of potentially fatal respiratory depression. *Drug Safety Update*. www.gov.uk/drug-safety-update.
21 Reddy A *et al.* (2017) The conversion ratio from intravenous hydromorphone to oral opioids in cancer patients. *Journal of Pain and Symptom Management*. **54**: 280–288.
22 Durnin C *et al.* (2001) Pharmacokinetics of oral immediate-release hydromorphone (Dilaudid IR) in subjects with moderate hepatic impairment. *Proceedings of the Western Pharmacology Society*. **44**: 83–84.
23 Bosilkovska M *et al.* (2012) Analgesics in patients with hepatic impairment: pharmacology and clinical implications. *Drugs*. **72**: 1645–1669.
24 Durnin C *et al.* (2001) Pharmacokinetics of oral immediate-release hydromorphone (Dilaudid IR) in subjects with renal impairment. *Proceedings of the Western Pharmacology Society*. **44**: 81–82.

Updated June 2021

*METHADONE

Class: Strong opioid analgesic.

Methadone should be used as a strong opioid analgesic only by those fully conversant with its pharmacology.[1] It is generally best reserved for patients who fail to respond well to **morphine** or another μ-opioid receptor agonist. Important facts about methadone include:

- wide interindividual variation in pharmacokinetics
- a large volume of distribution and high protein-binding resulting in a long plasma halflife and a greater risk of accumulation; long intervals are needed between dose adjustments
- metabolism is modified to a clinically important extent by other drugs that may be used in oncology or palliative care
- no single conversion ratio between **morphine** and methadone; the relative potency is highly variable and dose-dependent
- it is associated with potentially fatal cardiac arrhythmias (see Cautions and Chapter 20, p.797).

Also, because methadone is used to treat opioid addiction, there is a social stigma attached to its use.

Indications: Moderate–severe pain, †an alternative in cases of intolerance to other strong opioids, †pain poorly responsive to **morphine**, †pain relief in ESRF.[2] Also treatment of opioid addiction.

Contra-indications: None absolute if titrated carefully against a patient's pain (also see Strong opioids, p.389).

Pharmacology

Methadone is a synthetic strong opioid with mixed properties. Thus, it is a μ-opioid receptor agonist, an NMDA-receptor–channel blocker[2] and a presynaptic blocker of serotonin and noradrenaline (norepinephrine) re-uptake.[3] However, the analgesic relevance of the non-opioid effects is debated.[4] Differential effects at the μ-opioid receptor may alone explain the reported benefit from switching one opioid to another. Thus, compared with **morphine**, methadone (like **fentanyl**) is associated with higher levels of receptor internalization, β-arrestin recruitment and little or no stimulation of Na^+, K^+-ATPase activity (also see p.389).[4,5] Although some suggest that the non-opioid effects make methadone of particular benefit in neuropathic pain,[6–8] RCT evidence is limited, of very low quality and insufficient to make any reliable conclusion.[9]

Methadone is a racemic mixture (*R*- and *S*-enantiomers); *R*-methadone is responsible for most of the analgesic and undesirable effects, whereas *S*-methadone is antitussive and has a more potent effect on cardiac conduction (see Chapter 20, p.800). Methadone is a non-acidic and lipophilic drug that is generally well absorbed from all routes of administration. However, PO bio-availability shows wide variation, in part explained by methadone being a substrate for P-glycoprotein (see Chapter 19, p.781).

Partly because of its lipid solubility, methadone has a high volume of distribution, with only about 1% of the drug in the blood.[10] Methadone accumulates in tissues when given repeatedly, creating an extensive reservoir.[11] Protein-binding (principally to a glycoprotein) is 60–90%;[12] this is double that of **morphine**. Both volume of distribution and protein-binding contribute to the long plasma halflife (it takes 4–7 days to achieve steady state), and accumulation is a potential problem. Methadone is metabolized mainly in the liver by CYP450 isoenzymes to inactive metabolites (see Drug interactions).[13] About half of the drug and its metabolites are excreted by the intestines and half by the kidneys, most of the latter unchanged.[14] Renal and hepatic impairment do not affect methadone clearance;[15,16] even so, caution is needed (see Dose and use).

IM methadone is about equivalent to half the PO methadone dose (i.e. a PO:IM conversion ratio of 2:1).[17] In single doses, IM methadone is marginally more potent than IM **morphine**. However, with repeated doses, methadone is several times more potent and longer acting; analgesia lasts 8–12h and sometimes more.[18,19] There is no single conversion ratio between methadone and **morphine**. When patients with inadequate pain relief or undesirable effects with **morphine** are switched, the eventual 24h dose of methadone *is typically 5–10 times smaller than the previous dose of **morphine**, but sometimes 20–30 times smaller, and occasionally even smaller.*[20–23] The relative potency of methadone tends to increase as the dose of **morphine** increases, i.e. proportionately less methadone is needed as the **morphine** dose increases.[21–23]

When considering the use of methadone, the difficulty of a subsequent switch from methadone to another opioid should also be borne in mind. For such switches, typically the PO **morphine** equivalent dose will be 5–10 times greater than the PO methadone dose, with a wide range again reported, e.g. from 1–75 times.[24] Thus, it is prudent to use conservative dose calculations and monitor the patient closely.

Methadone is used in several different settings in adults and children:[25,26]

First-line strong opioid

Because it is relatively inexpensive, it is a popular first-line opioid in resource-poor countries. RCT evidence is limited for both cancer and non-cancer pain, and insufficient for meta-analysis.[27–29] Nonetheless, when used first-line in cancer pain, methadone appears to provide similar analgesia to **morphine** but, in some studies, more undesirable effects.[29] For example, in one RCT, 20% of patients allocated to methadone 7.5mg PO b.d. discontinued treatment, compared with 5% of those who received **morphine** m/r 15mg PO b.d. Half of the withdrawals occurred in the first week, and most were because of sedation or nausea. For patients remaining in the study, there was no difference in efficacy or undesirable effects.[19] This suggests that a smaller starting dose of PO methadone (e.g. 2.5–5mg b.d. or even 1–2mg b.d.) would have been more appropriate.[30,31] Indeed, in one large case series of patients with cancer and non-cancer pain receiving methadone first-line, the median effective PO dose was 2.5mg b.d., with only 20% needing ≥10mg/24h.[32] A potential advantage of methadone over other opioids for cancer-related neuropathic pain needs confirmation.[33] The oral solution of methadone is used as a long-acting opioid for patients with difficulty swallowing tablets reliably, e.g. children.[2]

Second-line strong opioid

Patients who experience unacceptable undesirable effects, e.g. nausea, vomiting, hallucinations, sedation, or more specific neurotoxicity with **morphine**, e.g. hyperalgesia, allodynia and/or myoclonus ± sedation and delirium, generally benefit from switching to methadone. However, switching to another opioid also helps.[34–37] Thus, when switching from **morphine** in these circumstances, it would seem sensible to choose an opioid that is easier and safer to use than methadone, e.g. **oxycodone, fentanyl**.

Some patients who experience inadequate analgesia with **morphine** (or another opioid), when switched to relatively low-dose methadone can obtain good relief.[38–41] However, in these circumstances, adjuvant use is generally preferred to a complete switch.

Adjuvant analgesic

Because of the difficulties associated with a complete switch from **morphine** to methadone, a preferred approach in many centres in patients with opioid poorly-responsive pain is to add a small dose of methadone (as per first-line use) alongside **morphine** (or another strong opioid).[42,43] The dose of **morphine** is progressively reduced if opioid toxicity occurs. Although simpler, this approach does *not* avoid the need for close supervision. Only low-level evidence (grade D) exists to support this approach.[44]

Other uses

Methadone is an alternative strong opioid for patients with ESRF at risk of excessive drowsiness ± delirium with **morphine** because of accumulation of morphine-6-glucuronide.[2] Methadone is poorly removed by haemodialysis.[45] However, **alfentanil** or **fentanyl** are easier to use and generally preferred in this setting (see p.743).

Methadone can also be used as a strong opioid analgesic in former opioid addicts who are being maintained on methadone.[46,47] The once daily maintenance dose (typically 60–120mg PO) is halved and given q12h and subsequently titrated as necessary. An alternate strategy is to add another strong opioid and titrate this to achieve analgesia, leaving the methadone maintenance dose unchanged.[48]

Methadone has been successfully used for cancer break-through pain, either PO or SL (≤1mL of locally prepared solutions ranging from 5mg/mL to 40mg/mL held for 2min); the average time to meaningful pain relief is 30min and 10min respectively.[49,50] However, given that the time to peak plasma concentration is ≤4h, together with a long halflife and duration of action, this approach is unsuitable for patients with frequent short-lasting occurrences of break-through pain (see p.323).

Bio-availability 80% (range 40–100%) PO.

Onset of action <30min PO; 15min IM.

Time to peak plasma concentration 4h PO; 1h IM.

Plasma halflife highly variable; mean 20–35h (range 5–130h);[51] longer in older patients; acidifying the urine results in a shorter halflife (20h), and raising the pH with sodium bicarbonate results in a longer halflife (>40h).[52]

Duration of action 4–5h PO and 3–5h IM single dose; 8–12h repeated doses.

Cautions

In 2006, after a review of deaths and life-threatening adverse events (e.g. respiratory depression, cardiac arrhythmia) associated with unintentional overdose, drug interactions and prolongation of the QT interval, the FDA in the USA issued a safety warning about the use of methadone. This highlighted the need for:

- physicians to be fully aware of the pharmacology of methadone
- close monitoring of the patient when starting methadone, particularly when switching from a high dose of another opioid
- slow dose titration and close monitoring of the patient when changing the dose of methadone
- patients to be warned not to exceed the prescribed dose.

Because methadone generally has a long plasma halflife, accumulation to a variable extent should be anticipated, particularly in the frail elderly or in renal or hepatic impairment (see Dose and use). Drowsiness and respiratory depression may develop after several days/weeks on a steady dose. *PCF* recommends careful titration and ongoing close monitoring by specialists to minimize the risk of this occurring (see Dose and use).[53]

QT interval prolongation and, rarely, a serious ventricular arrhythmia (*torsade de pointes*) have been observed during treatment with methadone. Generally, the latter is associated with, but not limited to, higher-dose treatment (>120mg/24h PO) (see Chapter 20, p.800).[54] The SPC recommends that methadone is administered with caution to patients at risk of developing QT prolongation, e.g. those with:

- a history of cardiac conduction abnormalities
- a family history of sudden death
- advanced heart disease or ischaemic heart disease
- liver disease
- electrolyte abnormalities
- concurrent treatment with drugs that:
  - ▷ may cause electrolyte abnormalities
  - ▷ have a potential to prolong QT
  - ▷ inhibit CYP3A4.

Note. The injectable formulation of methadone in the USA (but *not* the UK) contains a preservative, chlorobutanol, which has an additive QT-prolonging effect.[55]

The risk that this rare but potentially fatal cardiac complication poses must be considered in the context of the patient's circumstances. A common sense approach should prevail, and ECG monitoring will be largely irrelevant in the last days of life. On the other hand, for a patient with a prognosis of several months or longer, it may be appropriate to identify any risk factors for QT prolongation and consider ECG ± electrolyte monitoring, particularly if exceeding 100mg/24h PO (see Chapter 20, p.797).[56]

Even so, research is needed to establish the magnitude of the risk of *torsade de pointes* with methadone, and the overall value of monitoring in the palliative care setting.[54]

Plasma levels of methadone are increased in CYP2D6 poor metabolizers, resulting in a greater risk of undesirable effects, including fatal overdose.[57] Similarly, plasma levels of *S*-methadone are increased in CYP2B6 poor metabolizers which, because *S*-methadone is a more potent blocker of the potassium channels in the cardiac myocytes than *R*-methadone, may increase the patient's risk of prolonged QTc and arrhythmia (also see Chapter 19, p.781).[58]

Drug interactions

Concurrent treatment with ≥2 CNS depressants (e.g. benzodiazepines, gabapentinoids, opioids) increases the risk of respiratory depression, particularly in susceptible groups, e.g. the elderly and those with renal or hepatic impairment.[59]

Because of the long halflife of methadone and time taken to reach steady state, closely monitor for respiratory depression for at least 2 weeks after initiation or changes to prescribing because the respiratory effect of methadone may be delayed.

Methadone is metabolized mostly by CYP3A4 and CYP2B6, with CYP2D6, CYP2C9, CYP2C19 and CYP1A2 involved to a lesser degree. This varies with the enantiomer. Caution is needed with concurrent use of drugs that inhibit or induce these enzymes (see Chapter 19, Table 8, p.790). Clinically important pharmacokinetic drug interactions are listed in Box A. Note particularly that enzyme inducers, e.g. **carbamazepine**, **phenobarbital**, **phenytoin**, **rifampicin**, **St John's wort**, increase the metabolism of methadone and may reverse previously satisfactory pain relief or even precipitate withdrawal symptoms.[60,61] Conversely, methadone overdose has occurred when such inducers have been stopped, including after cessation of smoking (polycyclic aromatic hydrocarbons in tobacco smoke are CYP1A2 inducers).[62] Methadone may double **desipramine** plasma concentrations.

Avoid concurrent use with other drugs that prolong the QT interval, see Chapter 20, Box B, p.799.

Risk of serotonin toxicity when used together with other serotoninergic drugs, e.g. **selegiline**, SSRIs (see Antidepressants, Box A, p.217). The concurrent use of MAOIs and methadone is contra-indicated in the SPC; however, see Strong opioids (p.395).

Symptomatic bradycardia has been reported in a patient on **thalidomide** given methadone.[64]

Undesirable effects

Also see Strong opioids, Box B, p.394. Methadone may occasionally cause neurotoxicity, e.g. myoclonus,[65] or more florid opioid-induced hyperalgesia.[66–68] Local erythema and induration when given by CSCI.[69]

Box A Interactions between methadone and other drugs involving CYP450[a, 2,56,60,63]

Plasma concentrations of methadone	
***Increased* by**	***Decreased* by**
Aprepitant[b]	Apalutamide[b]
Azoles (all)	Carbamazepine
Cannabidiol	Enzalutamide[b]
Ciprofloxacin	Fosphenytoin
Diltiazem[b]	Phenobarbital
Macrolides[b], e.g. clarithromycin, erythromycin	Phenytoin
SSRIs (all)	Rifampicin
Verapamil[b]	St John's wort
	Tobacco smoking

a. not an exhaustive list; limited to drugs most likely to be encountered in palliative care and *excludes* anticancer, antiviral, HIV and immunosuppressive drugs (seek specialist advice)

b. based on theoretical extrapolation.

Rarely, hypoglycaemia (particularly with IV methadone and PO doses >40mg/24h, possibly by stimulating insulin release),[70] sensorineural hearing loss (generally after overdose; can be permanent),[71] and encephalopathy (after overdose).[72]

Dose and use

Patients using opioids must be monitored for undesirable effects, particularly nausea and vomiting, and constipation. Depending on individual circumstances, an anti-emetic should be prescribed for regular or p.r.n. use (see QCG: Nausea and vomiting, p.264) and, routinely, a laxative prescribed (see QCG: Opioid-induced constipation, p.45).

Opioids can impair driving ability, and patients should be counselled accordingly. Methadone is included in the law in England, Wales and Scotland relating to driving with certain drugs above specified plasma concentrations (see Chapter 22, p.809).

Regardless of how methadone is used, practitioners must be experienced in its use and the importance of ongoing close supervision cannot be overemphasized. Because of methadone's large volume of distribution, during the first few days of use the body tissues become saturated; once saturation is complete the plasma concentration of methadone can disproportionately increase, risking sedation, and possibly respiratory depression or even death.[73,74] For this reason, caution is needed at the start of treatment and after any dose increase.

First-line strong opioid

Uncommon in the UK (see Pharmacology). See QCG: Use of methadone for cancer pain, p.478.

Second-line strong opioid ('switching')

When there is a need to switch from **morphine** because of undesirable effects, an opioid that is easier and safer to use than methadone is preferred, e.g. **oxycodone**. For opioid poorly-responsive pain, the adjuvant use of methadone (see below) is less complicated than attempting a complete switch.

Several methods exist for switching from **morphine** to methadone, e.g.:[56,75–84]

- *3-day switch:* **morphine** is tailed off and the methadone progressively introduced over 3 days (sometimes longer); methadone dose based on conversion ratios, which differ according to **morphine** dose
- *stop and go, regular dose:* **morphine** is abruptly stopped and switched to a regular dose of methadone based on conversion ratios, which differ according to **morphine** dose
- *stop and go, p.r.n. dose:* **morphine** is abruptly stopped and, for the first week, p.r.n. doses of methadone are used to establish the regular dose needed thereafter.

Direct comparisons are limited; some or no differences have been found between methods.[84,85] *However, a systematic review considered the last approach likely to be the safest and most effective*[82] and is the one favoured by the *PCF* (see QCG: Use of methadone for cancer pain, p.478). The QCG evolved by incorporating feedback to www.palliativedrugs.com from clinicians.[20,86] The single loading dose aids tissue saturation and helps to reduce the number of p.r.n. doses needed in the first 48h.[20] The recommendations may be overcautious, but are safer, particularly in the elderly and for those switching from large doses of **morphine**. Although a complete switch is generally undertaken as inpatients, there are reports of carefully managed outpatient regimens; in some, pain relief can take weeks rather than days to achieve.[41,87,88]

Caution is also needed when there has been rapid dose escalation of the pre-switch opioid; in these circumstances it is probably safer to calculate the initial dose of methadone using the pre-escalation dose.[89]

Maintenance doses vary considerably, but most are <80mg/24h PO.[90] *Subsequent switching from methadone to another opioid can be difficult. In one series, 12 of 13 patients experienced increased pain ± dysphoria.*

Adjuvant analgesic ('adding')

The addition of a relatively small dose of methadone is reported to benefit patients who have failed to obtain adequate relief from an appropriately titrated dose of **morphine** or other strong opioid (see QCG: Use of methadone for cancer pain, p.478). About one half to two thirds of patients respond, with benefit generally apparent within 1–2 weeks and/or at doses ≤15mg/24h PO.[42,43,91]

Renal or hepatic impairment

In ESRF (i.e. eGFR <15mL/min/1.73m²), start with 50% of the usual dose (see QCG: Use of methadone for cancer pain, p.478, and Chapter 17, p.743).

In severe hepatic impairment, methadone is best avoided (see Chapter 18, p.762).

Routes of administration

Methadone can be given PO, buccally, SL, PR, SC/CSCI, IM, IV or CIVI ± PCA.[92–95] It has also been used as a topical analgesic for mouth ulcers (as a mouthwash),[96] and for open wounds and ulcers (in powder form mixed with Stomahesive®).[97] Successful use of a locally prepared TD gel has been described in patients unable to tolerate administration by other routes.[98]

When changing from methadone PO to SC (or IM/IV), a safe conversion is to halve the methadone PO dose, i.e. a conversion ratio of 2:1. For some patients, subsequent upwards dose titration may be needed.[99]

When switching from another PO/TD or parenteral strong opioid, see QCG: Use of methadone for cancer pain, p.478.

Methadone SC (generally doses >25mg) or CSCI can cause marked local inflammation, necessitating site rotation and possibly other measures (see QCG: Use of methadone for cancer pain, p.478).[99,100] For CSCI, dilute with WFI, sodium chloride 0.9% or glucose 5%.

CSCI compatibility with other drugs: limited clinical experience suggests that methadone is compatible with **alfentanil, clonazepam, dexamethasone, haloperidol, hydromorphone, hyoscine *butylbromide*, ketamine, levomepromazine, metoclopramide, midazolam, morphine *sulfate*** and **oxycodone**.

For more details, see the www.palliativedrugs.com Syringe Driver Survey Database (SDSD).

Supply

All products are Schedule 2 **CD**.

Ensure the correct concentration is prescribed; incidents have occurred because of confusion between methadone oral solution 1mg/mL and methadone oral concentrates 10mg/mL and 20mg/mL (authorized for opioid dependence), which need further dilution with Methadose® diluent to the required strength.[101]

Physeptone® (Martindale)
Tablets 5mg, 28 days @ 5mg b.d. = £3.
Oral solution 1mg/mL, 28 days @ 5mg b.d. = £3; *sugar-free available*.
Injection 10mg/mL, 1mL amp = £0.75; 50mg/mL, 1mL amp = £1.50.

1 Caraceni A *et al.* (2012) Use of opioid analgesics in the treatment of cancer pain: evidence-based recommendations from the EAPC. *Lancet Oncology*. **13**: e58–e68.
2 Edmonds K *et al.* (2020) Emerging challenges to the safe and effective use of methadone for cancer-related pain in paediatric and adult patient populations. *Drugs*. **80**: 115–130.
3 Codd E *et al.* (1995) Serotonin and norepinephrine uptake inhibiting activity of centrally acting analgesics: structural determinants and role in antinociception. *Journal of Pharmacology and Experimental Therapeutics*. **274**: 1263–1270.
4 Doi S *et al.* (2016) Characterization of methadone as a beta-arrestin-biased mu-opioid receptor agonist. *Molecular Pain*. **12**: 1–9.
5 Masocha W *et al.* (2016) Distinguishing subgroups among mu-opioid receptor agonists using Na(+),K(+)-ATPase as an effector mechanism. *European Journal of Pharmacology*. **774**: 43–49.
6 Takase N *et al.* (2015) Methadone for patients with malignant psoas syndrome: case series of three patients. *Journal of Palliative Medicine*. **18**: 645–652.
7 Sugiyama Y *et al.* (2016) A retrospective study on the effectiveness of switching to oral methadone for relieving severe cancer-related neuropathic pain and limiting adjuvant analgesic use in Japan. *Journal of Palliative Medicine*. **19**: 1051–1059.
8 Rigo F *et al.* (2017) Management of neuropathic pain with methadone combined with ketamine: A randomized, double blind, active-controlled clinical trial. *Pain Physician*. **20**: 207–215.
9 McNicol ED *et al.* (2017) Methadone for neuropathic pain in adults. *Cochrane Database of Systematic Reviews*. **5**: CD012499. www.cochranelibrary.com.
10 Ferrari A *et al.* (2004) Methadone-metabolism, pharmacokinetics and interactions. *Pharmacological Research*. **50**: 551–559.
11 Robinson AE and Williams FM (1971) The distribution of methadone in man. *Journal of Pharmacy and Pharmacology*. **23**: 353–358.
12 Eap CB *et al.* (1990) Binding of D-methadone, L-methadone and DL-methadone to proteins in plasma of healthy volunteers: role of variants of X1-acid glycoprotein. *Clinical Pharmacology and Therapeutics*. **47**: 338–346.
13 Fainsinger R *et al.* (1993) Methadone in the management of cancer pain: clinical review. *Pain*. **52**: 137–147.
14 Inturrisi CE and Verebely K (1972) The levels of methadone in the plasma in methadone maintenance. *Clinical Pharmacology and Therapeutics*. **13**: 633–637.
15 King S *et al.* (2011) A systematic review of the use of opioid medication for those with moderate to severe cancer pain and renal impairment: A European palliative care research collaborative opioid guidelines project. *Palliative Medicine*. **25**: 525–552.
16 Bosilkovska M *et al.* (2012) Analgesics in patients with hepatic impairment: pharmacology and clinical implications. *Drugs*. **72**: 1645–1669.
17 Beaver WT *et al.* (1967) A clinical comparison of the analgesic effects of methadone and morphine administered intramuscularly, and of orally and parenterally administered methadone. *Clinical Pharmacology and Therapeutics*. **8**: 415–426.
18 Sawe J *et al.* (1981) Patient-controlled dose regimen of methadone for chronic cancer pain. *British Medical Journal*. **282**: 771–773.
19 Bruera E *et al.* (2004) Methadone versus morphine as a first-line strong opioid for cancer pain: a randomized, double-blind study. *Journal of Clinical Oncology*. **22**: 185–192.
20 Cornish CJ and Keen JC (2003) An alternative low-dose ad libitum schedule for conversion of other opioids to methadone. *Palliative Medicine*. **17**: 643–644.
21 Benitez-Rosario MA *et al.* (2009) Morphine-methadone opioid rotation in cancer patients: analysis of dose ratio predicting factors. *Journal of Pain and Symptom Management*. **37**: 1061–1068.
22 Mercadante S and Caraceni A (2011) Conversion ratios for opioid switching in the treatment of cancer pain: a systematic review. *Palliative Medicine*. **25**: 504–515.
23 Chatham MS *et al.* (2013) Dose ratios between high dose oral morphine or equivalents and oral methadone. *Journal of Palliative Medicine*. **16**: 947–950.
24 Walker PW *et al.* (2008) Switching from methadone to a different opioid: what is the equianalgesic dose ratio? *Journal of Palliative Medicine*. **11**: 1103–1108.
25 Madden K *et al.* (2018) Methadone as the initial long-acting opioid in children with advanced cancer. *Journal of Palliative Medicine*. **21**: 1317–1321.
26 Habashy C *et al.* (2018) Methadone for pain management in children with cancer. *Paediatric Drugs*. **20**: 409–416.
27 Nicholson AB *et al.* (2017) Methadone for cancer pain. *Cochrane Database of Systematic Reviews*. **2**: CD003971. www.cochranelibrary.com.
28 Haroutiunian S *et al.* (2012) Methadone for chronic non-cancer pain in adults. *Cochrane Database of Systematic Reviews*. **11**: CD008025. www.cochranelibrary.com.
29 Mercadante S and Bruera E (2018) Methadone as a first-line opioid in cancer pain management: A systematic review. *Journal of Pain and Symptom Management*. **55**: 998–1003.
30 Mercadante S *et al.* (2008) Sustained-release oral morphine versus transdermal fentanyl and oral methadone in cancer pain management. *European Journal of Pain*. **12**: 1040–1046.
31 Gallagher R (2009) Methadone: an effective, safe drug of first choice for pain management in frail older adults. *Pain Medicine*. **10**: 319–326.
32 Salpeter SR *et al.* (2013) The use of very-low-dose methadone for palliative pain control and the prevention of opioid hyperalgesia. *Journal of Palliative Medicine*. **16**: 616–622.
33 Haumann J *et al.* (2016) Methadone is superior to fentanyl in treating neuropathic pain in patients with head-and-neck cancer. *European Journal of Cancer*. **65**: 121–129.
34 Sjogren P *et al.* (1994) Disappearance of morphine-induced hyperalgesia after discontinuing or substituting morphine with other opioid agonists. *Pain*. **59**: 313–316.
35 Hagen N and Swanson R (1997) Strychnine-like multifocal myoclonus and seizures in extremely high-dose opioid administration: treatment strategies. *Journal of Pain and Symptom Management*. **14**: 51–58.
36 Ashby M *et al.* (1999) Opioid substitution to reduce adverse effects in cancer pain management. *Medical Journal of Australia*. **170**: 68–71.
37 Morita T *et al.* (2005) Opioid rotation from morphine to fentanyl in delirious cancer patients: an open-label trial. *Journal of Pain and Symptom Management*. **30**: 96–103.
38 Tse DM *et al.* (2003) An ad libitum schedule for conversion of morphine to methadone in advanced cancer patients: an open uncontrolled prospective study in a Chinese population. *Palliative Medicine*. **17**: 206–211.
39 Mercadante S *et al.* (2001) Switching from morphine to methadone to improve analgesia and tolerability in cancer patients: a prospective study. *Journal of Clinical Oncology*. **19**: 2898–2904.
40 Mercadante S *et al.* (1999) Rapid switching from morphine to methadone in cancer patients with poor response to morphine. *Journal of Clinical Oncology*. **17**: 3307–3312.
41 Porta-Sales J *et al.* (2016) Efficacy and safety of methadone as a second-line opioid for cancer pain in an outpatient clinic: a prospective open-label study. *Oncologist*. **21**: 981–987.

42 Courtemanche F *et al.* (2016) Methadone as a coanalgesic for palliative care cancer patients. *Journal of Palliative Medicine.* **19**: 972–978.
43 Fürst P *et al.* (2018) Improved pain control in terminally ill cancer patients by introducing low-dose oral methadone in addition to ongoing opioid treatment. *Journal of Palliative Medicine.* **21**: 177–181.
44 Fallon MT and Laird BJ (2011) A systematic review of combination step III opioid therapy in cancer pain: an EPCRC opioid guideline project. *Palliative Medicine.* **25**: 597–603.
45 Furlan V *et al.* (1999) Methadone is poorly removed by haemodialysis. *Nephrology, Dialysis, Transplantation.* **14**: 254–255.
46 Manfredi P *et al.* (2001) Methadone analgesia in cancer pain patients on chronic methadone maintenance therapy. *Journal of Pain and Symptom Management.* **21**: 169–174.
47 Rowley D *et al.* (2011) Review of cancer pain management in patients receiving maintenance methadone therapy. *American Journal of Hospice and Palliative Care.* **28**: 183–187.
48 Taveros MC and Chuang EJ (2016) Pain management strategies for patients on methadone maintenance therapy: a systematic review of the literature. *BMJ Supportive and Palliative Care.* 1–7.
49 Fisher K *et al.* (2004) Characterization of the early pharmacodynamic profile of oral methadone for cancer-related breakthrough pain: a pilot study. *Journal of Pain and Symptom Management.* **28**: 619–625.
50 Hagen NA *et al.* (2010) A formal feasibility study of sublingual methadone for breakthrough cancer pain. *Palliative Medicine.* **24**: 696–706.
51 Lugo RA *et al.* (2005) Pharmacokinetics of methadone. *Journal of Pain and Palliative Care Pharmacotherapy.* **19**: 13–24.
52 Nilsson MI *et al.* (1982) Pharmacokinetics of methadone during maintenance treatment: adaptive changes during the induction phase. *European Journal of Clinical Pharmarcology.* **22**: 343–349.
53 Hendra T *et al.* (1996) Fatal methadone overdose. *British Medical Journal.* **313**: 481–482.
54 Wilcock A and Beattie JM (2009) Prolonged QT interval and methadone: implications for palliative care. *Current Opinion in Supportive and Palliative Care.* **3**: 252–257.
55 Kornick CA *et al.* (2003) QTc interval prolongation associated with intravenous methadone. *Pain.* **105**: 499–506.
56 McPherson M *et al.* (2019) Safe and appropriate use of methadone in hospice and palliative care: expert consensus white paper. *Journal of Pain and Symptom Management.* **57**: 635–645.
57 Bunten H *et al.* (2011) CYP2B6 and OPRM1 gene variations predict methadone-related deaths. *Addiction Biology.* **16**: 142–144.
58 Eap CB *et al.* (2007) Stereoselective block of hERG channel by (S)-methadone and QT interval prolongation in CYP2B6 slow metabolizers. *Clinical Pharmacology and Therapeutics.* **81**: 719–728.
59 MHRA (2020) Benzodiazepines and opioids: reminder of risk of potentially fatal respiratory depression. *Drug Safety Update.* www.gov.uk/drug-safety-update.
60 Preston C. *Stockley's Drug Interactions.* London: Pharmaceutical Press www.medicinescomplete.com (accessed May 2021).
61 Kreek MJ *et al.* (1976) Rifampin-induced methadone withdrawal. *New England Journal of Medicine.* **294**: 1104–1106.
62 Wahawisan J *et al.* (2011) Methadone toxicity due to smoking cessation--a case report on the drug-drug interaction involving cytochrome P450 isoenzyme 1A2. *Annals of Pharmacotherapy.* **45**: e34.
63 Madden K *et al.* (2020) Clinically significant drug-drug interaction between methadone and cannabidiol. *Pediatrics.* **145**: e20193256.
64 Buchanan D (2010) Sinus bradycardia related to methadone in a patient with myeloma receiving thalidomide therapy. *Palliative Medicine.* **24**: 742–743.
65 Sarhill N *et al.* (2001) Methadone-induced myoclonus in advanced cancer. *American Journal of Hospice and Palliative Care.* **18**: 51–53.
66 Davis MP *et al.* (2007) When opioids cause pain. *Journal of Clinical Oncology.* **25**: 4497–4498.
67 El Osta B *et al.* (2007) Intractable pain: intoxication or undermedication? *Journal of Palliative Medicine.* **10**: 811–814.
68 Hoff AM *et al.* (2017) Methadone-induced neurotoxicity in advanced cancer: a case report. *Journal of Palliative Medicine.* **20**: 1042–1044.
69 Bruera E *et al.* (1991) Local toxicity with subcutaneous methadone. Experience of two centers. *Pain.* **45**: 141–143.
70 Masharani U and Alba D (2018) Methadone-associated hypoglycemia in chronic renal failure masquerading as an insulinoma. *Pain Medicine.* **19**: 1876–1878.
71 Ghasemi S *et al.* (2019) Methadone associated long term hearing loss and nephrotoxicity; a case report and literature review. *Substance Abuse Treatment, Prevention, and Policy.* **14**: 48.
72 Haghighi-Morad M *et al.* (2020) Methadone-induced encephalopathy: a case series and literature review. *BMC Medical Imaging volume.* **20**: 6.
73 Twycross RG (1977) A comparison of diamorphine with cocaine and methadone. *British Journal of Clinical Pharmacology* **4**: 691–692.
74 Lipman AG (2005) Methadone: effective analgesia, confusion, and risk. *Journal of Pain and Palliative Care Pharmacotherapy.* **19** 3–5.
75 Santiago-Palma J *et al.* (2001) Intravenous methadone in the management of chronic cancer pain: safe and effective starting doses when substituting methadone for fentanyl. *Cancer.* **92**: 1919–1925.
76 Blackburn D *et al.* (2002) Methadone: an alternative conversion regime. *European Journal of Palliative Care.* **9**: 93–96.
77 Blackburn D (2005) Methadone: the analgesic. *European Journal of Palliative Care.* **12**: 188–191.
78 Bruera E *et al.* (1996) Opioid rotation in patients with cancer pain. *Cancer.* **78**: 852–857.
79 Auret K *et al.* (2006) Pharmacokinetics and pharmacodynamics of methadone enantiomers in hospice patients with cancer pain. *Therapeutic Drug Monitoring.* **28**: 359–366.
80 Moksnes K *et al.* (2011) How to switch from morphine or oxycodone to methadone in cancer patients? a randomised clinical phase II trial. *European Journal of Cancer.* **47**: 2463–2470.
81 Moksnes K *et al.* (2012) Serum concentrations of opioids when comparing two switching strategies to methadone for cancer pain. *European Journal of Clinical Pharmacology.* **68**: 1147–1156.
82 McLean S and Twomey F (2015) Methods of rotation from another strong opioid to methadone for the management of cancer pain: a systematic review of the available evidence. *Journal of Pain and Symptom Management.* **50**: 248–259.
83 Hawley P *et al.* (2017) Clinical outcomes of start-low, go-slow methadone initiation for cancer-related pain: What's the hurry? *Journal of Palliative Medicine.* **20**: 1244–1251.
84 Lukin B *et al.* (2020) Conversion of other opioids to methadone: a retrospective comparison of two methods. *BMJ Supportive & Palliative Care.* **10**: 201–204.
85 Poulain P *et al.* (2016) Efficacy and safety of two methadone titration methods for the treatment of cancer-related pain: The EQUIMETH2 trial (methadone for cancer-related pain). *Journal of Pain and Symptom Management.* **52**: 626–636.
86 Morley J and Makin M (1998) The use of methadone in cancer pain poorly responsive to other opioids. *Pain Reviews.* **5**: 51–58.
87 Soares LG (2005) Methadone for cancer pain: what have we learned from clinical studies? *American Journal of Hospice and Palliative Care.* **22**: 223–227.
88 Hagen N and Wasylenko E (1999) Methadone: outpatient titration and monitoring strategies in cancer patients. *Journal of Pain and Symptom Management.* **18**: 369–375.

89 Zimmermann C *et al.* (2005) Rotation to methadone after opioid dose escalation: How should individualization of dosing occur? *Journal of Pain and Palliative Care Pharmacotherapy*. **19**: 25–31.
90 Scholes C *et al.* (1999) Methadone titration in opioid-resistant cancer pain. *European Journal of Cancer Care*. **8**: 26–29.
91 Wallace E *et al.* (2013) Addition of methadone to another opioid in the management of moderate to severe cancer pain. A case series. *Journal of Palliative Medicine*. **16**: 305–309.
92 Davis M and Walsh D (2001) Methadone for relief of cancer pain: a review of pharmacokinetics, pharmacodynamics, drug interactions and protocols of administration. *Supportive Care in Cancer*. **9**: 73–83.
93 Manfredi PL and Houde RW (2003) Prescribing methadone, a unique analgesic. *Journal of Supportive Oncology*. **1**: 216–220.
94 Spaner D (2014) Effectiveness of the buccal mucosa route for methadone administration at the end of life. *Journal of Palliative Medicine*. **17**: 1262–1265.
95 Elsass K *et al.* (2018) Nonoral routes of methadone for analgesia in palliative care #358. *Journal of Palliative Medicine*. **21**: 1357–1358.
96 Gallagher R (2004) Methadone mouthwash for the management of oral ulcer pain. *Journal of Pain and Symptom Management*. **27**: 390–391.
97 Gallagher RE *et al.* (2005) Analgesic effects of topical methadone: a report of four cases. *Clinical Journal of Pain*. **21**: 190–192.
98 Love R and Bourgeois K (2014) Topical methadone: an alternative for pain control in end-of-life management. *Journal of Palliative Medicine*. **17**: 128.
99 Centeno C and Vara F (2005) Intermittent subcutaneous methadone administration in the management of cancer pain. *Journal of Pain and Palliative Care Pharmacotherapy*. **19**: 7–12.
100 Mathew P and Storey P (1999) Subcutaneous methadone in terminally ill patients: manageable local toxicity. *Journal of Pain and Symptom Management*. **18**: 49–52.
101 Care Quality Commission (2014) Safer use of controlled drugs — preventing harms from methadone. *Use of controlled drugs supporting information*. www.cqc.org.uk.

Updated July 2021

Quick Clinical Guide: Use of methadone for cancer pain

The *PCF* methadone monograph must be read before using this guide; it details the necessary considerations for using methadone. Ongoing close supervision by specialists fully conversant with methadone's pharmacology is essential.

Methadone has both opioid and non-opioid properties and a long, variable halflife (range 5–130h vs. 2.5h for morphine). Inevitable accumulation is the reason for the week-long intervals between dose adjustments.

There is no single conversion ratio for methadone and other opioids. When switching from morphine, the eventual 24h dose of methadone is typically 5–10 times smaller than the dose of morphine, sometimes 20–30 times smaller, and occasionally even smaller.

Indications for use

- *first-line strong opioid*: uncommon in the UK
- *second-line strong opioid* (when it is not possible to switch to another easier-to-use opioid) in the following circumstances:
  - ▷ neurotoxicity with morphine (e.g. myoclonus, allodynia, hyperalgesia) that does not respond to a reduction in dose
  - ▷ end-stage renal failure (ESRF; not first-line choice)
- *adjuvant analgesic*: morphine poorly-responsive pain, e.g. mixed nociceptive–neuropathic pain despite additional use of NSAID + adjuvant analgesics. Probably the commonest indication in palliative care.

Dose titration

First-line strong opioid

When prescribing PO methadone as first-line strong opioid:

- start with methadone 2.5mg (1–2mg in the elderly/ESRF) q12h regularly and q3h p.r.n.:
  - ▷ if necessary, titrate the *regular dose* upwards *once a week*, guided by p.r.n. use, but generally by no more than 5mg/24h
  - ▷ continue with 2.5mg (1–2mg in the elderly/ESRF) q3h p.r.n.
- for most patients, relatively small doses will be sufficient (i.e. ≤10mg/24h)
- for doses ≥15mg q12h:
  - ▷ if necessary, titrate the *regular dose* upwards *once a week*, guided by p.r.n. use, but generally by no more than 10mg/24h; keep p.r.n. dose unchanged
- for doses ≥30mg q12h:
  - ▷ consider increasing the p.r.n. dose to 1/10–1/6 of the q24h dose rounded to a convenient tablet size or volume.

For the corresponding SC/CSCI doses, halve the above doses; also see Box A.

Box A Converting from PO methadone to SC or CSCI methadone

To convert PO methadone to SC (or IM/IV) methadone, halve the PO dose. This is a safe conversion ratio and is satisfactory for most patients; some need dose titration.

Because of its long halflife, methadone (10mg/mL injection) can be given SC q8–12h. If SC injection is painful or causes local inflammation, give by CSCI instead.

If CSCI methadone causes a skin reaction:

- administer as a more dilute solution in a 20–30mL syringe
- change the site daily
- consider applying hydrocortisone cream 1% topically around the needle entry site (under an occlusive dressing)
- consider adding dexamethasone (e.g. 0.66mg) to the diluted combination of drugs (compatibility data permitting).

Note. SC/IM are the only authorized routes for methadone injection in the UK.

Adjuvant analgesic

When using PO methadone alongside an existing strong opioid, follow dose initiation as for first-line use above, *but also*:

- reduce the regular and p.r.n. doses of the original strong opioid *before* starting methadone if there is opioid-related toxicity or there has been a recent rapid and ineffective increase in doses, e.g. to the last tolerated or pre-escalation doses
- continue to use the original opioid for p.r.n. rescue doses. If completely ineffective, consider alternatives (e.g. PO/SC ketamine, SC methadone; generally as an inpatient)
- benefit is generally apparent within 1–2 weeks and/or at doses ≤15mg/24h; some centres stop methadone if no benefit from 20–30mg/24h
- if pain improves, consider reducing the dose of the original opioid.

5

Second-line strong opioid

1 If switching from PO morphine to PO methadone, use the method in Box B.

Box B Switching from PO morphine to PO methadone

For morphine poorly-responsive pain, the adjuvant use of methadone is less complicated and thus safer than attempting a complete switch.

Morphine is stopped abruptly when methadone is started.

If switching from:

- immediate-release morphine: give the first dose of methadone ≥2h (pain present) or 4h (pain-free) after last dose of morphine
- m/r morphine: give the first dose of methadone ≥6h (pain present) or 12h (pain-free) after the last dose of a 12h product, or ≥12h (pain present) or 24h (pain-free) after the last dose of a 24h product.

Give a single loading dose of PO methadone 1/10 of the previous total 24h PO morphine dose, up to a maximum of 30mg.

Give q3h p.r.n. doses of PO methadone 1/30 of the previous total 24h PO morphine dose, rounded to a convenient tablet size or volume, up to a maximum of 30mg per dose.

Example 1: Morphine 300mg/24h PO = loading dose of methadone 30mg PO, and 10mg q3h p.r.n.

Example 2: Morphine 1,200mg/24h PO = loading dose of methadone 120mg PO, and 40mg q3h p.r.n.; however, both are limited to the maximum of 30mg.

For patients in severe pain and who need more analgesia in <3h, see point 4 below.

On day 6, the amount of methadone taken *in total* over the previous 2 days is noted and divided by 4 to give a regular q12h dose, with 1/10–1/6 of the 24h dose q3h p.r.n., *e.g. methadone 80mg PO in previous 48h → 20mg q12h and 5mg PO q3h p.r.n.*

If ≥2 doses/day of p.r.n. methadone continue to be needed, the *regular* dose of methadone should be increased *once a week*, guided by p.r.n. use.

Note. For patients who need SC (or IM/IV) methadone halve the above PO methadone doses.

2 If switching from another PO/TD or parenteral strong opioid, calculate the morphine-equivalent 24h *PO* dose and then follow the guidelines in Box B.

3 If there has been recent rapid escalation of the pre-switch opioid dose, calculate the initial dose of methadone using the pre-escalation dose of the opioid.

4 For patients in severe pain and who need more analgesia in <3h, options include:
   - taking the previously used opioid q1h p.r.n. (50–100% of the p.r.n. dose used before switching)
   - if neurotoxicity with the pre-switch opioid, use an appropriate dose of an alternative strong opioid.

5 The switch to methadone is successful (i.e. improved pain relief and/or reduced toxicity) in about 75% of patients.

6 If a patient:
   - becomes oversedated, reduce the dose generally by 33–50% (some centres monitor the level of consciousness and respirations q4h for 24h)
   - develops opioid abstinence symptoms, give p.r.n. doses of the previous opioid to control these.

Updated July 2021

OXYCODONE

Class: Strong opioid analgesic.

Indications: Moderate–severe cancer and post-operative pain, severe non-cancer pain, †an alternative in cases of intolerance to other strong opioids,[1,2] restless legs syndrome (Targinact®; see Box A).

Contra-indications: Moderate–severe hepatic impairment. Otherwise none absolute if titrated carefully against a patient's pain (also see Strong opioids, p.389).

Pharmacology

Oxycodone is a strong opioid with similar properties to **morphine** (p.404).[3-5] Its main effects are the result of activity at the μ-opioid receptor, although this may involve different G-protein subunits and thereby different downstream effects to **morphine** (also see Strong opioids, p.389).[6-9] Studies in rodents suggest oxycodone may also possess activity at δ- and κ-opioid receptors.[10,11]

Like **morphine**, oxycodone shows efficacy in pure neuropathic pain states (diabetic and postherpetic neuropathy), with an NNT of 5.7 (95% CI 4.0–9.9) for moderate benefit. However, as with **morphine**, the evidence is considered very low quality.[12]

Oxycodone appears to be less immunosuppressive than **morphine**. In patients with cancer pain, although one small retrospective study found the incidence of infections to be less in those receiving oxycodone compared to **morphine**, another found no difference between **fentanyl**, **morphine** and oxycodone, with the risk of infection increasing with dose (see Strong opioids, p.397).

Most of the analgesic effect arises from oxycodone itself.[13] The main metabolite, noroxycodone (via CYP3A4), is active at the μ-opioid receptor but to a much lesser degree. Another metabolite, **oxymorphone** (via CYP2D6), is produced in relatively small amounts but has ≥10 times the affinity and activity of oxycodone.[13] However, studies in postoperative and cancer pain found no differences between CYP2D6 ultra-rapid, extensive or poor metabolizers in the dose requirements or analgesic efficacy of oxycodone, suggesting **oxymorphone** contributes little overall.[14,15] Nonetheless, case reports suggest that opioid-naïve CYP2D6 ultra-rapid metabolizers may be at greater risk of undesirable CNS effects when starting oxycodone, because of an enhanced production of **oxymorphone** (also see Chapter 19, p.781).[16] (Note. **Oxymorphone** is commercially available in some countries (not UK) and is 3 times and 10 times more potent than PO and parenteral **morphine** respectively.)[17]

By mouth, oxycodone has a mean bio-availability of 75%, whereas **morphine**'s is about half this (p.404). This partly explains why PO oxycodone is more potent than PO **morphine** (i.e. *fewer* mg of oxycodone are needed than **morphine** to have a comparable analgesic effect).[18-23]

For general considerations when converting opioids ± switching routes, see Appendix 2, p.925. According to the UK manufacturer, oxycodone PO is twice as potent as **morphine** PO. Although reasonable in terms of caution and safety, this almost certainly exaggerates the actual potency of oxycodone, and a conversion ratio of **morphine** to oxycodone of 1.5:1 is generally used in clinical practice, i.e. the dose of oxycodone PO should be two-thirds of the **morphine** PO dose (e.g. oxycodone 10mg PO is equivalent to **morphine** 15mg PO).

Parenterally, when the bio-availability of **morphine** and oxycodone are comparable, the situation is different. Despite a short-term (2h) postoperative PCA study which suggested that **morphine** is less potent parenterally than oxycodone (i.e. *more* mg of **morphine** will be needed, as with PO administration),[24] earlier single-dose studies and two more recent longer PCA studies (1–2 days) suggest that by injection **morphine** is more potent than oxycodone, in the region of 4:3. Thus, *fewer* mg of **morphine** will be needed (**morphine** 10mg being approximately equivalent to oxycodone 13mg).[17,18,25] However, given the modest difference in potency together with the constraints of ampoule size, it is reasonable in clinical practice to use a conversion ratio of 1:1, i.e. when converting from **morphine** injection to oxycodone injections (or vice versa), regard SC/IV **morphine** 10mg as equivalent to SC/IV oxycodone 10mg.

When switching from PO oxycodone to SC/IV oxycodone, although the UK manufacturer recommends a conversion ratio of 2:1, because mean PO bio-availability is 75%, this may be too conservative for some patients. Thus, some centres use a conversion ratio of 1.5:1, i.e. the oxycodone SC/IV 24h dose should be two-thirds of the oxycodone PO 24h dose. For switching from PO **morphine** to CSCI oxycodone, see Dose and use.

About 20% of oxycodone is excreted unchanged in the urine. In mild–moderate hepatic impairment, oxycodone and noroxycodone concentrations increase by 50% and 20% respectively (but the **oxymorphone** concentration decreases), and the elimination halflife increases by about 2h. In renal impairment, the clearance of oxycodone, noroxycodone and conjugated **oxymorphone** are reduced. Oxycodone plasma concentration increases by 50% and the halflife lengthens by 1h.[19,26] Nonetheless, oxycodone is used as an alternative to **morphine** in mild–moderate renal impairment and is used cautiously in some centres in severe renal impairment for initial pain management (see Dose and use, and Chapter 17, p.743).

The clearance of oxycodone reduces with increasing age, probably because of the age-related decline in renal and hepatic function. Consequently, compared with younger adults, plasma concentration, overall exposure and halflife increase in the elderly.[27] In the presence of systemic inflammation sufficient to increase C-RP and IL-6 levels, there is inhibition of CYP3A, resulting in higher plasma levels of oxycodone.[28]

Bio-availability 75% PO, ranging from 60–87%.[29,30]
Onset of action 20–30min PO.
Time to peak plasma concentration 1–1.5h; 3h m/r.
Plasma halflife 2–4h (4.5h m/r); 3–5h (5.5h m/r) in ESRF
Duration of action 4–6h; 12h m/r.

Cautions

Renal and mild hepatic impairment (see Dose and use, and Chapter 17, p.743 and Chapter 18, p.762).

Drug interactions

Concurrent treatment with ≥2 CNS depressants (e.g. benzodiazepines, gabapentinoids, opioids) increases the risk of respiratory depression, particularly in susceptible groups, e.g. the elderly and those with renal or hepatic impairment.[31,32]

Inhibitors of CYP3A4 (e.g. **clarithromycin**, **erythromycin**, **fluconazole**, **itraconazole**, **voriconazole**, see p.790) can inhibit oxycodone metabolism and may enhance its effects.[33-37] However, inhibition of CYP2D6 (e.g. with **quinidine**) appears to have no detectable clinical impact.[38]

Inducers of CYP3A4 (e.g. **rifampicin**, **St John's wort**, see p.790) decrease plasma concentrations of oxycodone.[33,39,40] Case reports suggest that the enzyme inducer **enzalutamide** reduces the analgesic efficacy of oxycodone.[41]

Undesirable effects

See Strong opioids, Box B, p.394. Various studies have suggested possible differences in the undesirable effect profiles of oxycodone and **morphine**.[42] However, systematic reviews comparing efficacy and tolerability of oxycodone versus **morphine** and other opioids found no strong evidence of any overall difference in their undesirable effect profiles.[4,5]

Dose and use

Patients using opioids must be monitored for undesirable effects, particularly nausea and vomiting, and constipation. Depending on individual circumstances, an anti-emetic should be prescribed for regular or p.r.n. use (see QCG: Nausea and vomiting, p.264) and, routinely, a laxative prescribed (see QCG: Opioid-induced constipation, p.45).

Opioids can impair driving ability, and patients should be counselled accordingly (see Chapter 22, p.809).

Although oxycodone is similar to **morphine** (and **hydromorphone**) in terms of efficacy and undesirable effects,[2] because it is more expensive it should generally be reserved for patients who cannot tolerate **morphine**. In Scotland, oxycodone injections are restricted to cancer patients who cannot tolerate **diamorphine** or **morphine** injections.

A combination product of oxycodone with **naloxone** is available (Targinact®; Box A).

Remains of m/r tablets (e.g. Oxycontin®, Longtec®, Targinact®) may appear in the patient's faeces ('ghost tablets'), but these are inert residues and do not affect the efficacy of the products.

Oral

Immediate-release oxycodone products are available as capsules, oral solutions and now tablets (see Supply). When both immediate-release and m/r tablets are used, appropriate caution must be used to avoid unnecessary confusion.

Immediate-release oxycodone is generally given q4h but, in some patients, q6h is satisfactory. Oxycodone 12-hourly m/r tablets are biphasic in their release of oxycodone; i.e. there is an initial fast release which leads to the early onset of analgesia, and a slow release which provides a prolonged duration of action. Modified-release tablets should be swallowed whole; crushing or chewing them will lead to a rapid release of an overdose of oxycodone. Most m/r products are administered b.d., some once daily (see Supply).

For strong opioid-naïve patients:

- start with 5mg q4–6h for immediate-release products (see Supply)
- start with 10mg b.d. for 12-hourly m/r tablets
- halve the above doses in elderly/frail patients or those with mild–moderate renal impairment or mild hepatic impairment (also see below)
- if necessary, titrate the dose upwards, guided by p.r.n. use; conventionally, p.r.n. PO doses are 1/10–1/6 of the total 24h PO dose.

For patients switching from PO **morphine** to PO oxycodone, *PCF* recommends a conversion ratio of 1.5:1 (see Pharmacology):

- PO **morphine** to PO oxycodone: decrease the dose by one third, e.g. **morphine** 15mg PO → oxycodone 10mg PO.

For general considerations when converting opioids, see Appendix 2, p.925.

Box A Oxycodone combined with naloxone (Targinact®)

Targinact® is marketed as a range of tablets containing m/r formulations of oxycodone and naloxone in a fixed dose ratio of 2:1, i.e. oxycodone/naloxone 5mg/2.5mg, 10mg/5mg, 20mg/10mg and 40mg/20mg. The addition of naloxone is to antagonize the constipating effect of oxycodone. The desire to develop a formulation that deters misuse (e.g. by crushing and injecting IV) is also relevant.

Targinact® is authorized for severe pain. Evidence to support claims of improved pain control, better GI tolerability, and improved quality of life are based mostly on uncontrolled observational studies.[43,44]

RCTs have mostly involved relatively young non-cancer (mid–late 50s) and cancer patients (early 60s) with either moderate or severe pain, and with no significant hepatic or renal impairment. Reported use in older non-cancer (early 80s) and cancer patients (mean age 70) is mostly limited to open-label studies.[45–48]

In most of the non-cancer studies, those unwilling or unable to tolerate a 'restricted laxative regimen' were excluded, i.e. the most severely constipated. Although Targinact® improved bowel function and reduced the number of patients requiring laxatives, the absolute differences were small (e.g., on average, one extra bowel action/week and a reduction of 0.6mg/24h in bisacodyl dose). However, laxatives were taken only p.r.n.[49-52]

In RCTs including cancer patients, Targinact® improved bowel function and there was a trend towards a reduction in laxative use. However, absolute differences were of similar magnitudes as above, and laxatives were taken only p.r.n.[51,53]

Targinact® is significantly more expensive than the equivalent dose of m/r oxycodone alone or an equivalent dose of morphine + regular laxatives. Because the benefit of Targinact® in patients taking laxatives *regularly* is uncertain, the Scottish Medicines Consortium, the *Drug and Therapeutics Bulletin* and *PCF* do *not* recommend its use.[54]

Although Targinact® is also authorized as a second-line treatment for restless legs syndrome refractory to dopaminergic therapy, the available evidence is limited.[55,56]

continued

Box A Continued

If clinicians choose to prescribe Targinact®, its use should be restricted to occasions when the upward titration of regularly administered laxatives is ineffective (see Laxatives, p.40).[57] Because constipation is generally multifactorial in origin, Targinact® is likely to augment rather than replace laxatives.[49,50]

The m/r formulation of naloxone avoids a 'bolus dose', and >97% is removed by first-pass metabolism in the liver. Thus, the main effect of naloxone is on the GI tract, with insufficient amounts reaching the systemic circulation to adversely affect analgesia.[58,59] However, plasma concentrations of naloxone can increase significantly in:

- *hepatic impairment:* use of Targinact® requires caution in mild impairment and is contra-indicated in moderate–severe impairment
- *portosystemic shunt:* collateral circulation bypasses the liver, caused by, e.g. chronic liver disease, portal vein thrombosis[60,61]
- *renal impairment:* use Targinact® with caution.

The increase in naloxone can antagonize the analgesic effect of oxycodone, resulting in either frank opioid withdrawal or the need to increase to an artificially higher dose.[62] Thus, in a patient with progressive hepatic impairment, a switch from Targinact® to the same dose of oxycodone m/r, resulted in opioid-induced respiratory depression within 12h.[62]

Dose recommendations:

- in opioid-naïve patients, generally start with oxycodone/naloxone 10mg/5mg b.d.
- in elderly/frail patients, start with 5mg/2.5mg b.d.
- in those already taking strong opioids, switch to the equivalent dose of oxycodone
- maximum dose 80mg/40mg b.d.

When higher analgesic doses are required, the manufacturer recommends supplemental oxycodone m/r tablets, taken at the same time as the m/r combination tablets. However, this reduces the impact of the naloxone, and oxycodone:naloxone ratios >4:1 have no significant effect on bowel function.[50,63] However, a recent study used doses ≤90mg/45mg b.d.[64]

Common undesirable effects include nausea, vomiting, abdominal pain and diarrhoea. The manufacturer warns that patients on long-term opioids may develop opioid-withdrawal symptoms when switched to Targinact®.

Subcutaneous administration

Oxycodone injection may be given SC as a bolus or by CSCI (and also IV by bolus and by CIVI). For CSCI, dilute with WFI, sodium chloride 0.9% or glucose 5%.

For strong opioid-naïve patients:

- start with 7.5mg/24h CSCI
- if necessary, titrate the dose upwards, guided by p.r.n. use; conventionally, p.r.n. SC doses are 1/10–1/6 of the total 24h CSCI dose.

For general considerations when switching routes ± converting opioids, see Appendix 2, p.925. The following are practical clinical conversion ratios:

- PO oxycodone to CSCI oxycodone: decrease the dose by one third, e.g. oxycodone 30mg/24h PO → oxycodone 20mg/24h CSCI (see Pharmacology)
- PO **morphine** to CSCI oxycodone: decrease the dose by half, e.g. **morphine** 60mg/24h PO → oxycodone 30mg/24h CSCI.

When switching from **morphine** CSCI to oxycodone CSCI, *PCF* recommends a dose conversion ratio of 1:1 (see Pharmacology):

- CSCI **morphine** to CSCI oxycodone: give the same dose, e.g. **morphine** 30mg/24h CSCI → oxycodone 30mg/24h CSCI
- if necessary, titrate the dose upwards, guided by p.r.n. use.

Two strengths of injection are available, 10mg/mL and high-strength 50mg/mL. The latter may be useful in situations where high doses cause volume difficulties for CSCI. However, there is an increased risk of serious mistakes being made when more than one strength is readily available.[65,66] There are also differences in compatibility with other drugs (see below) and, on a mg for mg basis, the high-strength injection costs about twice as much.

CSCI with oxycodone 10mg/mL

There are 2-drug compatibility data for mixtures in WFI with **clonazepam**, **dexamethasone**, **glycopyrronium**, **haloperidol**, **hyoscine *butylbromide***, **hyoscine *hydrobromide***, **levomepromazine**, **metoclopramide**, **midazolam** and **octreotide**.

Concentration-dependent incompatibility may occur when oxycodone (hydrochloride) is mixed with **cyclizine** (lactate); for more details see Appendix 3, Chart 1, p.936.

CSCI with oxycodone 50mg/mL

Differences in compatibility with other drugs for the 10mg/mL and 50mg/mL formulations of oxycodone have been reported.[67,68] This may be due to the different ratios of excipients in each formulation (see Appendix 3, Table 1, p.936). It is important *not* to extrapolate compatibility information from one formulation to the other.

More details

For 2-drug and 3-drug compatibility data for oxycodone 10mg/mL in WFI, and for currently available data for oxycodone 50mg/mL, see Appendix 3, Chart 1 (p.936), Chart 6 (p.946) and Table 1 (p.950).

Information on compatibility in sodium chloride 0.9% can be found in the extended appendix section of the on-line *PCF* on *www.medicinescomplete.com*.

Renal or hepatic impairment

Because of the risk of impaired metabolism or elimination:

- lower than usual starting doses are advised in mild–moderate renal impairment or mild hepatic impairment, i.e. start with a maximum of 10mg/24h PO as for frail/elderly patients
- in severe renal impairment or ESRF, start with 1–2mg PO q6–8h and p.r.n.; once pain is controlled, consider switching to an equivalent dose of TD fentanyl (see Chapter 17, p.743)
- oxycodone is contra-indicated in moderate–severe hepatic impairment. If unavoidable, lower the usual starting dose *and* increase the dosing interval of immediate-release products to q8h (see Chapter 18, p.762).

For a general approach when renal or hepatic function deteriorates rapidly, see Strong opioids, p.393.

Supply

All preparations are Schedule 2 CD.

Immediate-release oral products

Oxycodone oral solution is available in two strengths, 1mg/mL and a high potency concentrate of 10mg/mL; incidents have occurred from confusion between the two formulations.[69,70] Prescribing should be in *mg* not mL to minimize the risk of 10 times the intended dose being given.

Oxycodone (generic)
Capsules 5mg, 10mg, 20mg, 5mg dose = £0.12.
Oral solution 5mg/5mL, 5mg dose = £0.17.
Concentrated oral solution 10mg/mL, 5mg dose = £0.20.
Injection 10mg/mL, 1mL and 2mL amp = £1.25 and £2.75 respectively.
High-strength injection 50mg/mL, 1mL amp = £12.

Oxyact® (Kent)
Tablets 5mg, 10mg, 20mg, 5mg dose = £0.10.

Modified-release 12-hourly oral products

As for all m/r opioids, brand prescribing is recommended to reduce the risk of confusion and error in dispensing and administration (see p.xvii).[70]

Oxycodone (generic)
Tablets m/r 5mg, 10mg, 15mg, 20mg, 30mg, 40mg, 60mg, 80mg, 120mg, 28 days @ 5mg or 120mg b.d. = £5.50 and £155 respectively. *Note. The 15mg, 30mg, 60mg and 120mg tablets are not available for all brands; only Longtec® and OxyContin® have the full range of strengths available.*
Brands include Abtard®, Leveraxo®, Longtec®, Oxeltra®, OxyContin®, Oxylan®, Reltebon®.

Modified-release 24-hourly oral products
Onexila® XL (Aspire Pharma)
Tablets m/r 10mg, 20mg, 40mg, 80mg, 28 days @ 10mg once daily = £13.

Oxycodone/naloxone combined
Targinact® (Napp)
Tablets m/r containing oxycodone/naloxone in a fixed ratio of 2:1, 5mg/2.5mg, 10mg/5mg, 20mg/10mg, 40mg/20mg, 28 days @10mg/5mg b.d. = £42.

5

1 King S *et al.* (2011) A systematic review of the use of opioid medication for those with moderate to severe cancer pain and renal impairment: A European palliative care research collaborative opioid guidelines project. *Palliative Medicine*. **25**: 525–552.

2 Caraceni A *et al.* (2012) Use of opioid analgesics in the treatment of cancer pain: evidence-based recommendations from the EAPC. *Lancet Oncology*. **13**: e58–e68.

3 Kalso E (2005) Oxycodone. *Journal of Pain and Symptom Management*. **29 (Suppl 5)**: S47–S56.

4 Schmidt-Hansen M *et al.* (2017) Oxycodone for cancer-related pain. *Cochrane Database of Systematic Reviews*. **8**: CD003870. www.cochranelibrary.com.

5 Ma H (2016) The adverse events of oxycodone in cancer-related pain. *Medicine*. **95**: 1–9.

6 Gaspari S *et al.* (2017) RGS9-2 Modulates responses to oxycodone in pain-free and chronic pain states. *Neuropsychopharmacology*. **42**: 1548–1556.

7 Lemberg KK *et al.* (2006) Antinociception by spinal and systemic oxycodone: why does the route make a difference? In vitro and in vivo studies in rats. *Anesthesiology*. **105**: 801–812.

8 Kalso E *et al.* (1990) Morphine and oxycodone in the management of cancer pain: plasma levels determined by chemical and radioreceptor assays. *Pharmacology and Toxicology*. **67**: 322–328.

9 Nakamura A *et al.* (2013) Differential activation of the mu-opioid receptor by oxycodone and morphine in pain-related brain regions in a bone cancer pain model. *British Journal of Pharmacology*. **168**: 375–388.

10 Yang PP *et al.* (2016) Activation of delta-opioid receptor contributes to the antinociceptive effect of oxycodone in mice. *Pharmacological Research*. **111**: 867–876.

11 Ross F and Smith M (1997) The intrinsic antinociceptive effects of oxycodone appear to be kappa-opioid receptor mediated. *Pain*. **73**: 151–157.

12 Gaskell H *et al.* (2016) Oxycodone for neuropathic pain in adults. *Cochrane Database of Systematic Reviews*. **7**: CD010692. www.cochranelibrary.com.

13 Ruan X *et al.* (2017) Revisiting oxycodone analgesia: a review and hypothesis. *Anesthesiology Clinics*. **35**: e163–e174.

14 Zwisler ST *et al.* (2010) Impact of the CYP2D6 genotype on post-operative intravenous oxycodone analgesia. *Acta Anaesthesiologica Scandinavica*. **54**: 232–240.

15 Andreassen TN *et al.* (2012) Do CYP2D6 genotypes reflect oxycodone requirements for cancer patients treated for cancer pain? A cross-sectional multicentre study. *European Journal of Clinical Pharmacology*. **68**: 55–64.

16 de Leon J *et al.* (2003) Adverse drug reactions to oxycodone and hydrocodone in CYP2D6 ultrarapid metabolizers. *Journal of Clinical Psychopharmacology*. **23**: 420–421.

17 Beaver WT *et al.* (1978) Analgesic studies of codeine and oxycodone in patients with cancer. II. Comparisons of intramuscular oxycodone with intramuscular morphine and codeine. *Journal Pharmacology and Experimental Therapeutics*. **207**: 101–108.

18 Kalso E and Vainio A (1990) Morphine and oxycodone in the management of cancer pain. *Clinical Pharmacology and Therapeutics*. **47**: 639–646.

19 Heiskanen T and Kalso E (1997) Controlled-release oxycodone and morphine in cancer related pain. *Pain*. **73**: 37–45.

20 Bruera E *et al.* (1998) Randomized, double-blind, cross-over trial comparing safety and efficacy of oral controlled-release oxycodone with controlled-release morphine in patients with cancer pain. *Journal of Clinical Oncology*. **16**: 3222–3229.

21 Mucci-LoRusso P *et al.* (1998) Controlled-release oxycodone compared with controlled-release morphine in the treatment of cancer pain: a randomized, double-blind, parallel-group study. *European Journal of Pain*. **2**: 239–249.

22 Curtis GB *et al.* (1999) Relative potency of controlled-release oxycodone and controlled-release morphine in a postoperative pain model. *European Journal of Clinical Pharmacology*. **55**: 425–429.

23 Lauretti GR *et al.* (2003) Comparison of sustained-release morphine with sustained-release oxycodone in advanced cancer patients. *British Journal of Cancer*. **89**: 2027–2030.

24 Kalso E *et al.* (1991) Intravenous morphine and oxycodone for pain after abdominal surgery. *Acta anaesthesiologica Scandinavica*. **35**: 642–646.

25 Silvasti M *et al.* (1998) Comparison of analgesic efficacy of oxycodone and morphine in postoperative intravenous patient-controlled analgesia. *Acta anaesthesiologica Scandinavica*. **42**: 576–580.

26 Glare P and Davis MP. Oxycodone. In: MP Davis, P Glare, C Quigley, Hardy J, editors. *Opioids in Cancer Pain*. 2 ed. Oxford: Oxford University Press; 2009. p. 155–173.

27 Huddart R *et al.* (2018) PharmGKB summary: oxycodone pathway, pharmacokinetics. *Pharmacogenetics and Genomics* **28**: 230–237.

28 Sato H and Naito T (2016) Relationships between oxycodone pharmacokinetics, central symptoms, and serum interleukin-6 in cachectic cancer patients. *European Journal of Clinical Pharmacology*. **72**: 1463–1470.

29 Leow K *et al.* (1992) Single-dose and steady-state pharmacokinetics and pharmacodynamics of oxycodone in patients with cancer. *Clinical Pharmacology and Therapeutics*. **52**: 487–495.

30 Poyhia R *et al.* (1992) The pharmacokinetics and metabolism of oxycodone after intramuscular and oral administration to healthy subjects. *British Journal of Clinical Pharmacology*. **33**: 617–621.

31 MHRA (2020) Benzodiazepines and opioids: reminder of risk of potentially fatal respiratory depression. *Drug Safety Update*. www.gov.uk/drug-safety-update.

32 MHRA (2021) Pregabalin (Lyrica): reports of severe respiratory depression. *Drug Safety Update*. www.gov.uk/drug-safety-update.

33 Preston CL. *Stockley's Drug Interactions*. London: Pharmaceutical Press http://www.medicinescomplete.com (accessed August 2021).

34 Hagelberg NM *et al.* (2009) Voriconazole drastically increases exposure to oral oxycodone. *European Journal of Clinical Pharmacology*. **65**: 263–271.

35 Nieminen TH *et al.* (2010) Oxycodone concentrations are greatly increased by the concomitant use of ritonavir or lopinavir/ritonavir. *European Journal of Clinical Pharmacology*. **66**: 977–985.
36 Hagelberg NM *et al.* (2011) Interaction of oxycodone and voriconazole-a case series of patients with cancer pain supports the findings of randomised controlled studies with healthy subjects. *European Journal of Clinical Pharmacology*. **67**: 863–864.
37 Charpiat B *et al.* (2017) Respiratory depression related to multiple drug-drug interactions precipitated by a fluconazole loading dose in a patient treated with oxycodone. *European Journal of Clinical Pharmacology*. **73**: 787–788.
38 Kleine-Bruggeney (2010) Pharmacogenetics in palliative care. *Forensic Science International*. **203**: 63–70.
39 Nieminen TH *et al.* (2009) Rifampin greatly reduces the plasma concentrations of intravenous and oral oxycodone. *Anesthesiology*. **110**: 1371–1378.
40 Nieminen TH *et al.* (2010) St John's wort greatly reduces the concentrations of oral oxycodone. *European Journal of Pain*. **14**: 854–859.
41 Westdorp H *et al.* (2018) Difficulties in pain management using oxycodone and fentanyl in enzalutamide-treated patients with advanced prostate cancer. *Journal of Pain and Symptom Management*. **55**: e6–e8.
42 Leppert W (2010) Role of oxycodone and oxycodone/naloxone in cancer pain management. *Pharmacological Reports*. **62**: 578–591.
43 Morlion BJ *et al.* (2018) Oral prolonged-release oxycodone/naloxone for managing pain and opioid-induced constipation: A review of the evidence. *Pain Practice*. **18**: 647–665.
44 Bantel C *et al.* (2018) Prolonged-release oxycodone/naloxone reduces opioid-induced constipation and improves quality of life in laxative-refractory patients: results of an observational study. *Clinical and Experimental Gastroenterology*. **11**: 57–67.
45 Lazzari M *et al.* (2016) Switching to low-dose oral prolonged-release oxycodone/naloxone from WHO-Step I drugs in elderly patients with chronic pain at high risk of early opioid discontinuation. *Clinical Interventions in Aging*. **11**: 641–649.
46 Petro E *et al.* (2016) Low-dose oral prolonged-release oxycodone/naloxone for chronic pain in elderly patients with cognitive impairment: an efficacy-tolerability pilot study. *Neuropsychiatric Disease and Treatment*. **12**: 559–569.
47 Clemens KE *et al.* (2011) Bowel function during pain therapy with oxycodone/naloxone prolonged-release tablets in patients with advanced cancer. *International Journal of Clinical Practice*. **65**: 472–478.
48 Candy B *et al.* (2018) Mu-opioid antagonists for opioid-induced bowel dysfunction in people with cancer and people receiving palliative care. *Cochrane Database of Systematic Reviews*. **6**: CD006332. www.cochranelibrary.com.
49 Simpson K *et al.* (2008) Fixed-ratio combination oxycodone/naloxone compared with oxycodone alone for the relief of opioid-induced constipation in moderate-to-severe noncancer pain. *Current Medical Research Opinion*. **24**: 3503–3512.
50 Lowenstein O *et al.* (2009) Combined prolonged-release oxycodone and naloxone improves bowel function in patients receiving opioids for moderate-to-severe non-malignant chronic pain: a randomised controlled trial. *Expert Opinion in Pharmacotherapy*. **10**: 531–543.
51 Dupoiron D *et al.* (2017) A phase III randomized controlled study on the efficacy and improved bowel function of prolonged-release (PR) oxycodone-naloxone (up to 160/80 mg daily) vs oxycodone PR. *European Journal of Pain*. **21**: 1528–1537.
52 Xiaomei L *et al.* (2020) Prolonged-release (PR) oxycodone/naloxone improves bowel function compared with oxycodone PR and provides effective analgesia in Chinese patients with non-malignant pain: a randomized, double-blind trial. *Advances in Therapy*. **37**: 1188–1202.
53 Ahmedzai SH *et al.* (2012) A randomized, double-blind, active-controlled, double-dummy, parallel-group study to determine the safety and efficacy of oxycodone/naloxone prolonged-release tablets in patients with moderate/severe, chronic cancer pain. *Palliative Medicine*. **26**: 50–60.
54 Anonymous (2010) Targinact - opioid relief without constipation? *Drugs and Therapeutics Bulletin*. **48**: 138–141.
55 de Oliveira CO *et al.* (2016) Opioids for restless legs syndrome. *Cochrane Database of Systematic Reviews*. **6**: CD006941. www.cochranelibrary.com.
56 Anonymous (2016) Targinact for restless legs syndrome. *Drugs and Therapeutics Bulletin*. **54**: 42.
57 Larkin PJ *et al.* (2018) Diagnosis, assessment and management of constipation in advanced cancer: ESMO Clinical Practice Guidelines. *Annals of Oncology*. **29 (Suppl 4)**: 111–125.
58 Vondrackova D *et al.* (2008) Analgesic efficacy and safety of oxycodone in combination with naloxone as prolonged release tablets in patients with moderate to severe chronic pain. *Journal of Pain*. **9**: 1144–1154.
59 Sandner-Kiesling A *et al.* (2010) Long-term efficacy and safety of combined prolonged-release oxycodone and naloxone in the management of non-cancer chronic pain. *International Journal of Clinical Practice*. **64**: 763–774.
60 Lau F and Gardiner M (2017) Oxycodone/naloxone: An unusual adverse drug reaction. *Australian Family Physician*. **46**: 42–43.
61 Kang JH *et al.* (2013) Opioid withdrawal syndrome after treatment with low-dose extended-release oxycodone and naloxone in a gastric cancer patient with portal vein thrombosis. *Journal of Pain and Symptom Management*. **46**: e15–e17.
62 Franklin AE *et al.* (2017) A case of opioid toxicity on conversion from extended-release oxycodone and naloxone to extended-release oxycodone in a patient with liver dysfunction. *Journal of Pain and Symptom Management*. **53**: e1–e2.
63 Meissner W *et al.* (2009) A randomised controlled trial with prolonged-release oral oxycodone and naloxone to prevent and reverse opioid-induced constipation. *European Journal of Pain*. **13**: 56–64.
64 Dupoiron D *et al.* (2017) Long-term efficacy and safety of oxycodone-naloxone prolonged-release formulation (up to 180/90 mg daily) - results of the open-label extension phase of a phase III multicenter, multiple-dose, randomized, controlled study. *European Journal of Pain*. **21**: 1485–1494.
65 National Patient Safety Agency (2008) Reducing risk of overdose with midazolam injection in adults. *Rapid Response Report*. NPSA/2008/RRR2011.
66 National Patient Safety Agency (2006) Ensuring safer practice with high dose ampoules of diamorphine and morphine. *Safer Practice Notice*. NPSA/2006/2012. www.nrls.npsa.nhs.uk.
67 Gardiner P (2003) Compatibility of an injectable oxycodone formulation with typical diluents, syringes, tubings, infusion bags and drugs for potential co-administration. *Hospital Pharmacist* **10**: 354–361.
68 Hines S and Pleasance S (2009) Compatibility of an injectable high strength oxycodone formulation with typical diluents, syrings, tubings and infusion bags and drugs for potential co-administration. *European Journal of Hospital Pharmacy Practice*. **15**: 32–38.
69 National Pharmacy Association (2015) Potential risk of error in selecting incorrect oxycodone strength. www.npa.co.uk.
70 Care Quality Commission and NHS England (2013) Safer use of controlled drugs - preventing harms from oral oxycodone medicines. *Use of controlled drugs supporting information*. www.cqc.org.uk.

Updated August 2021

TAPENTADOL

Class: Strong opioid analgesic (but see below).

Indications: Moderate–severe acute pain (immediate-release products); severe chronic pain (m/r products).

Contra-indications: None absolute if titrated carefully against a patient's pain. (Also see Cautions below, and Strong opioids, p.389).

Pharmacology

Tapentadol is a centrally acting analgesic which is both a μ agonist and an inhibitor of synaptic re-uptake of noradrenaline (norepinephrine); the latter enhances the action of the descending pain-inhibitory pathway, contributing to a synergistic analgesic effect.[1-3] This possibly explains why tapentadol is only about ≤3 times less potent than **morphine**, despite an affinity for the μ-opioid receptor some ≥18 times lower (see **Tramadol**, Table 1, p.384).[1-3] Tapentadol also has some serotoninergic activity, but this is not considered relevant to its analgesic effect.

Tramadol, like tapentadol, is also a synthetic centrally acting analgesic with both non-opioid and opioid properties. However, at recommended maximum doses, tapentadol is equivalent to a much higher dose of PO **morphine** than **tramadol** (p.383), namely 150mg/24h vs. 40mg/24h. Thus, for practical purposes, **tramadol** is best considered a weak opioid (alongside **codeine**), and tapentadol a strong opioid (alongside **morphine**; see p.321).

RCTs of tapentadol, using mainly **oxycodone** as the comparator, have been conducted in both acute (e.g. postoperative orthopaedic, low back pain)[4-6] and chronic pain (e.g. osteoarthritis, low back pain, diabetic neuropathy, cancer-related).[2] These have shown tapentadol to be superior to placebo and/or non-inferior to **oxycodone** *at the lower end of its dose range*; i.e. in the RCTs used to obtain regulatory approval for tapentadol m/r, the maximum comparative dose was **oxycodone** m/r ≤50mg b.d. Further, median doses in the cancer pain study were only tapentadol m/r 25mg b.d. and **oxycodone** m/r 5mg b.d.[7]

Tapentadol is comparable in cost to **oxycodone**. However, a lack of comparative studies with other cheaper strong opioid products resulted in recommendations *against* its use in acute pain[8] and its restriction in chronic pain to patients who fail to get satisfactory analgesia from **morphine**.[9,10] Subsequent studies have found the analgesic effect of tapentadol m/r non-inferior to **oxycodone** + **naloxone** m/r (Targinact®; see p.480) in chronic pain, and to **morphine** m/r in cancer pain.[2]

Undesirable effects include those typical of an opioid agonist. However, during initial titration, GI effects are generally less than with **oxycodone** (e.g. less nausea, vomiting, constipation).[2] In non-cancer chronic pain studies, drug-related treatment withdrawals were about 20% for tapentadol vs. 30–40% for **oxycodone**.[2] In cancer pain studies, compared with **oxycodone** (median dose 5mg m/r b.d.), rates of constipation and nausea were about 7% lower with tapentadol;[7] compared with **morphine** (median dose 60mg m/r b.d.), rates of nausea and vomiting were 10% lower with tapentadol, but only during intital titration.[11] There were similar rates of treatment withdrawal for all three drugs (≤9%). Data are mixed over whether tapentadol m/r is associated with similar or greater degrees of constipation compared with **oxycodone + naloxone** m/r.[2]

A Cochrane review of tapentadol in chronic musculoskeletal pain concluded it was associated with better pain relief than placebo or **oxycodone** (although the difference with the latter is of uncertain clinical significance) and fewer undesirable effects.[12] A similar review in cancer pain was unable to pool RCT data and concluded that analgesic efficacy and undesirable effects were similar between tapentadol, **oxycodone** and **morphine**.[13] A systematic review of treatments for neuropathic pain considered the evidence insufficient to make a conclusive recommendation for tapentadol, but noted an NNT of 10.2, much higher than, e.g., tricyclic antidepressants (3.6), other strong opioids (4.3) or **tramadol** (4.7).[14,15]

Food does not alter absorption to a clinically relevant degree. Tapentadol is extensively metabolized in the liver to inactive metabolites by glucuronidation, with ≤15% of a dose metabolized via CYP450 (mostly 2C9 and 2C19), thus reducing the likelihood of pharmacokinetic drug–drug interactions; only 3% is excreted unchanged in the urine. Systemic exposure to tapentadol is increased by hepatic but not renal impairment, although in the latter, levels of tapentadol-O-glucuronide (considered inactive) are increased. It has no effect on the QT interval (see Chapter 20, p.797).

By mouth, it is about 5 times *less* potent than **oxycodone** (e.g. tapentadol 50mg is approximately equivalent to **oxycodone** 10mg). By extrapolation, this suggests that it is about 3 times *less* potent than PO **morphine** (e.g. tapentadol 50mg is approximately equivalent to **morphine** 15mg), and study data support this.[11,16] Thus, the maximum recommended m/r dose of tapentadol 250mg b.d. is approximately equivalent to **oxycodone** 50mg b.d. or **morphine** 75mg b.d.
Bio-availability 32% PO.
Onset of action <1h immediate-release.
Time to peak plasma concentration 75min immediate-release; 3–6h m/r.
Plasma halflife 4h immediate-release; 5–6h m/r.
Duration of action 4–6h immediate-release; 12h m/r.

Cautions

Renal or hepatic impairment (see Dose and use). Epilepsy or risk of seizures (lack of clinical trial data). Switching from another μ agonist (e.g. **morphine**, **oxycodone**) to tapentadol may cause low-grade opioid withdrawal (see Dose and use).

Abrupt discontinuation of tapentadol may result in symptoms of opioid withdrawal, and the SPC advises tapering gradually. On the other hand, the SPC also notes that even with ≤12 months of use, withdrawal symptoms were either absent or mild.

Tapentadol has the potential for abuse and addiction.

Drug interactions

Concurrent treatment with ≥2 CNS depressants (e.g. benzodiazepines, gabapentinoids, opioids) increases the risk of respiratory depression, particularly in susceptible groups, e.g. the elderly and those with renal or hepatic impairment.[17]

Avoid concurrent administration with an MAOI or within 2 weeks of the cessation of one, due to potential additive effects on synaptic noradrenaline concentrations.

Tapentadol is not completely devoid of serotoninergic activity. There have been reports of serotonin toxicity involving the use of tapentadol in conjunction with serotoninergic drugs (e.g. SSRIs);[18] also see Antidepressants, Box A, p.217.

Undesirable effects

See Strong opioids, Box B, p.394.

Dose and use

Patients using opioids must be monitored for undesirable effects, particularly nausea and vomiting, and constipation. Depending on individual circumstances, an anti-emetic should be prescribed for regular or p.r.n. use (see QCG: Nausea and vomiting, p.264) and, routinely, a laxative prescribed (see QCG: Opioid-induced constipation, p.45).

Opioids can impair driving ability, and patients should be counselled accordingly (see Chapter 22, p.809).

Moderate–severe acute pain

Use immediate-release products:

- start with 50mg PO q4–6h if moderate pain/strong opioid-naïve
- a higher starting dose may be necessary for severe pain/previous strong opioid use
- if the first dose is inadequate, a second dose can be taken after 1h (once only)
- if required, increase progressively to 100mg q4h or 150mg q6h
- maximum dose 600mg/24h (700mg in first 24h of use).

Severe chronic pain

Use m/r products:

- start with 50mg PO q12h if strong opioid-naïve
- a higher starting dose may be necessary when switching from another strong opioid; recommendations vary widely,[19] but the following is adapted from a cancer pain trial based on existing oral **morphine** equivalent (OME) use:[20]
  - ▷ OME ≤30mg/24h → tapentadol 50mg b.d.
  - ▷ 31–40mg/24h → tapentadol 75mg b.d.
  - ▷ 41–60mg/24h → tapentadol 100mg b.d.
  - ▷ 61–90mg/24h → tapentadol 150mg b.d.

- ▷ 91–120mg/24h → tapentadol 200mg b.d.
- ▷ 121–150mg/24h → tapentadol 250mg b.d.
- ▷ within the first week, 30% required a dose increase and 8% a decrease
- if necessary, increase by 50mg b.d. every 3 days
- maximum dose 250mg b.d.

In the cancer pain studies, break-through pain was treated with appropriate doses of immediate-release **morphine** or **oxycodone** p.r.n.; conventionally, p.r.n. PO doses are 1/10–1/6 of the total 24h PO dose (see Pharmacology for dose equivalents).[19]

Modified-release tablets should be swallowed whole; crushing or chewing them will lead to a rapid release of an overdose of tapentadol (see Chapter 28, Box A, p.857).

5

Remains of m/r tablets may appear in the patient's faeces ('ghost tablets'), but these are inert residues and do not affect the efficacy of the products.

Renal or hepatic impairment

Dose reduction is not required in mild–moderate renal impairment.

In moderate hepatic impairment, systemic exposure to tapentadol is increased >4 times. The SPC recommended starting doses are:

- immediate release: 25–50mg q8h, *or*
- m/r: 25–50mg once daily.

Because of a lack of clinical trial data, the SPC recommends against the use of tapentadol in patients with severe hepatic or renal impairment.

For a general approach when renal or hepatic function deteriorates rapidly, see p.393.

Supply

All products are Schedule 2 **CD**.

Immediate-release oral products

Palexia® (Grünenthal)

Tablets 50mg, 75mg, 50mg dose = £0.50

Oral solution 20mg/mL, 50mg dose = £0.50; *can be diluted in water or a non-alcoholic cold drink, and is suitable for administration via EFT.*

Modified-release oral products

As for all m/r opioids, brand prescribing is recommended to reduce the risk of confusion and error in dispensing and administration (see p.xvii).

Ationdo® SR (Grünenthal)

Tablets m/r 25mg, 50mg, 100mg, 150mg, 200mg, 250mg, 28 days @ 100mg q12h = £50.

1 Tzschentke TM *et al.* (2014) The mu-opioid receptor agonist/noradrenaline reuptake inhibition (MOR-NRI) concept in analgesia: the case of tapentadol. *CNS Drugs*. **28**: 319–329.

2 Deeks ED (2018) Tapentadol prolonged release: a review in pain management. *Drugs* **78**:1805–1816.

3 Schroder W *et al.* (2011) Synergistic interaction between the two mechanisms of action of tapentadol in analgesia. *Journal of Pharmacology and Experimental Therapeutics*. **337**: 312–320.

4 Frampton JE (2010) Tapentadol immediate release: a review of its use in the treatment of moderate to severe acute pain. *Drugs*. **70**: 1719–1743.

5 Biondi D *et al.* (2013) Tapentadol immediate release versus oxycodone immediate release for treatment of acute low back pain. *Pain Physician*. **16**: e237–e246.

6 Vorsanger GJ *et al.* (2013) Immediate-release tapentadol or oxycodone for treatment of acute postoperative pain after elective arthroscopic shoulder surgery: a randomized, phase IIIb study. *Journal of Opioid Management*. **9**: 281–290.

7 Imanaka K *et al.* (2013) Efficacy and safety of oral tapentadol extended release in Japanese and Korean patients with moderate to severe, chronic malignant tumor-related pain. *Current Medical Research and Opinion*. **29**: 1399–1409.

8 Anonymous (2012) Tapentadol (Palexia) for moderate to severe acute pain. *Drug and Therapeutics Bulletin*. **50**: 30–33.

9 Scottish Medicines Consortium (2011) Tapentadol prolonged-release tablets (Palexia SR). www.scottishmedicines.org.uk.

10 All Wales Medicine Strategy Group (2011) Tapentadol prolonged-release tablets (Palexia SR). www.awmsg.nhs.wales.

11 Kress HG *et al.* (2014) Tapentadol prolonged release for managing moderate to severe, chronic malignant tumor-related pain. *Pain Physician*. **17**: 329–343.

12 Santos J *et al.* (2015) Tapentadol for chronic musculoskeletal pain in adults. *Cochrane Database of Systematic Reviews*. **5**: CD009923. www.cochranelibrary.com.

13 Wiffen PJ *et al.* (2015) Oral tapentadol for cancer pain. *Cochrane Database of Systematic Reviews.* **9**: CD011460. www.cochranelibrary.com.
14 Finnerup NB *et al.* (2016) Pharmacotherapy for neuropathic pain in adults: a systematic review and meta-analysis. *Lancet Neurology.* **14**: 162–173.
15 Finnerup NB and Attal N (2015) Tapentadol prolonged release in the treatment of neuropathic pain related to diabetic polyneuropathy-authors' reply. *Lancet Neurology.* **14**: 685–686.
16 Galvez R *et al.* (2013) Tapentadol prolonged release versus strong opioids for severe, chronic low back pain: results of an open-label, phase 3b study. *Advances in Therapy.* **30**: 229–259.
17 MHRA (2020) Benzodiazepines and opioids: reminder of risk of potentially fatal respiratory depression. *Drug Safety Update.* www.gov.uk/drug-safety-update.
18 MHRA (2019) Tapentadol (Palexia): risk of seizures and reports of serotonin syndrome when co-administered with other medicines. *Drug Safety Update.* www.gov.uk/drug-safety-update.
19 Sanchez Del Aguila MJ *et al.* (2015) Practical considerations for the use of tapentadol prolonged release for the management of severe chronic pain. *Clinical Therapeutics.* **37**: 94–113.
20 Imanaka K *et al.* (2014) Ready conversion of patients with well-controlled, moderate to severe, chronic malignant tumor-related pain on other opioids to tapentadol extended release. *Clinical Drug Investigation.* **34**: 501–511.

Updated October 2021

OPIOID ANTAGONISTS (THERAPEUTIC TARGET WITHIN THE CNS)

For *Opioid antagonists (therapeutic target outside the CNS)*, see p.500; these are authorized for opioid-induced constipation, with effects limited to the periphery and leaving CNS opioid analgesic effects unaltered. Generally, this is because of an inability to penetrate the blood–brain barrier. The exception is **naloxone** in Targinact®, where use of an m/r formulation limits systemic absorption (see p.482) and thereby limits central antagonism.

Indications: Reversal of opioid-induced respiratory depression (**naloxone**), acute opioid overdose (**naloxone**), prevention of relapse in opioid addiction (**naltrexone**) and alcohol addiction (**nalmefene, †naltrexone**), †pruritus caused by cholestasis (**naloxone, naltrexone, nalmefene**) or spinal opioids (**naloxone**).

Contra-indications: Naloxone: none when used to reverse life-threatening opioid-induced respiratory depression or acute opioid overdose.
Naltrexone, nalmefene: patients physically dependent on opioids (i.e. after 2 weeks of regular PO use), acute hepatitis, severe hepatic impairment, severe renal impairment (eGFR <30mL/min/1.73m^2).

Pharmacology

For **naloxone, naltrexone** and **nalmefene**, the main therapeutic target is within the CNS. They reversibly block access to opioid receptors and, if given after an opioid agonist, they displace the latter because of their higher receptor affinity.

Although generally thought of as pure antagonists (i.e. having a high affinity for opioid receptors but no intrinsic activity), the reality is more complex. High doses of opioid antagonists reverse opioid analgesia (as expected), but *ultra-low* doses potentiate the opioid analgesic effect and/or reduce opioid undesirable effects (e.g. nausea and vomiting, and pruritus). This has mostly been explored using *ultra-low*-dose **naloxone** (e.g. 0.25microgram/kg/h IVI) in postoperative pain.[1-9] In other settings, *ultra-low*-dose **naltrexone** (e.g. ≤1mg/24h PO) has shown similar effects.[10-13]

These phenomena are best explained by opioid antagonists having other effects in addition to classical opioid receptor antagonism. These may include interfering with G-protein coupling and/or acting as antagonists at Toll-like receptor 4 (TLR4).

Interfering with G-protein coupling: a ligand binding to an opioid receptor can trigger either an inhibitory or excitatory response, dependent on the type of G-protein coupled to the receptor, either G_I/G_O (inhibitory) or G_s (excitatory). Typically, with an opioid agonist, the G_I/G_O (inhibitory) activity predominates, resulting in analgesia and other opioid effects. In such circumstances, a typical clinical dose of an opioid antagonist like **naloxone** will displace the opioid agonist from the receptor and thereby reverse its effects. However, the G_s excitatory response can increase in various circumstances, e.g. chronic opioid use, nerve damage.[14] This may contribute to opioid tolerance and, when predominant, to opioid-induced hyperalgesia (p.398).[15] *Ultra-low* levels of **naloxone** are sufficient to bind to and prevent the scaffolding protein (filamin A) from coupling the G_s protein to the opioid receptor, and thereby reduces the excitatory response.[16]

TLR4 antagonism: **naloxone** and **naltrexone** are TLR4 antagonists.[17] The TLR4 receptor is expressed in dorsal root ganglion neurones and widely in the CNS, particularly glial cells. Its activation promotes inflammation and other changes, and it is an important mediator of CNS sensitization and thereby inflammatory and neuropathic pain (and also drug reward and reinforcement). Apart from products released in nerve damage, opioids also activate TLR4, which may counteract their analgesic effect and contribute towards tolerance and, when predominant, opioid-induced hyperalgesia (p.398).[18] Thus, in animal models of nerve injury, ultra-low dose **naloxone** enhanced the analgesic effect of **morphine**, and ultra-low dose (+)-**naltrexone** prevented mechanical allodynia and its potentiation by **morphine**.[18-20]

5

Compared with **naloxone**, **naltrexone** has a higher PO bio-availability and a longer duration of action; it undergoes extensive first-pass metabolism.[21,22] The major metabolite of **naltrexone**, 6-β-naltrexol, is a *neutral* antagonist, i.e. it inhibits activation of opioid receptors but, unlike **naloxone** and **naltrexone**, it does not suppress basal receptor signalling, thereby reducing the risk of severe withdrawal.

Pharmacokinetic details are summarized in Table 1.

Table 1 Pharmacokinetic details for naloxone and naltrexone

	Naloxone	*Naltrexone*
Bio-availability (%)	6 PO	5–40 PO
Onset of action	1–2min IV; 2–5min SC/IM	May precipitate withdrawal symptoms in <5min in opioid-dependent patients
Time to peak plasma concentration		1–2h PO
Plasma halflife	About 1h	4h; 13h for 6-β-naltrexol[23]

Reversal of opioid-induced respiratory depression

The most important clinical property of **naloxone** is reversal of opioid-induced respiratory depression (and other opioid effects). In addition to a deliberate overdose, accidental overdose can occur in those misusing opioids and, less commonly, in patients requiring opioids for analgesia.

Increasingly, traditional doses of **naloxone** (e.g. 400microgram IV stat) are recommended only for use in *immediately life-threatening situations*, i.e. unconscious patient with minimal/no respiratory effort. In other circumstances, careful titration using lower doses of **naloxone** (e.g. 20–100microgram) is recommended to avoid precipitating a severe acute withdrawal syndrome and, in those receiving opioids for analgesia, severe pain and hyperalgesia (see QCG: Reversal of opioid-induced respiratory depression, p.498).[24-27] Acute opioid withdrawal causes the release of catecholamines, which can result in vomiting, shivering, sweating, tremor, agitation, anxiety, aggression, tachycardia, hypertension and, rarely, life-threatening pulmonary oedema (also see below) and cardiac arrhythmia.

However, compared with other opioids, antagonism of **buprenorphine** requires higher doses of **naloxone**, because **buprenorphine** has both high receptor affinity and prolonged receptor binding (see QCG: Reversal of opioid-induced respiratory depression, p.498 and also p.428). **Naloxone** has been reported to be only partially effective in reversing the effects of **tramadol**.[28,29] However, in a series of 11 patients with a **tramadol** overdose, seven had a good response to **naloxone**, and only one had no response.[30]

An apparent lack of response to adequate doses of **naloxone** following an IV opioid overdose should raise the possibility of 'wooden chest' syndrome. The greatest risk is with the illicit use of large/rapid IV doses of potent fentanils, although it has occurred following anaesthetic induction with IV **fentanyl**. Features include laryngospasm and rigidity of the chest, diaphragm and abdominal wall muscles, necessitating muscle paralysis, intubation and ventilation. Non-opioid effects of fentanils are probably responsible, e.g. adrenergic and dopaminergic receptor agonism, monoamine re-uptake inhibition.[31,32]

Patients with opioid overdose may develop pulmonary oedema. Because pulmonary oedema has been seen both in older patients with typical doses of **naloxone**, e.g. 200–400microgram IV, and in healthy teenagers with doses as low as 40–80microgram IV, it has been suggested that **naloxone** can trigger the release of central and peripheral catecholamines which leads to vasoconstriction of the pulmonary vasculature followed by pulmonary oedema.[33] Alternatively, because pulmonary oedema is almost universal in fatal opioid overdose,[34,35] **naloxone**, by increasing respiratory rate and tidal volume, may simply unmask pulmonary oedema which has developed secondary to severe hypoxaemia and acidaemia.[36]

Delayed-onset pulmonary oedema (48h after overdose treated with **naloxone**) due to acute cardiomyopathy has also been reported, possibly the result of cardiac muscle damage caused by hypoxaemia.[37]

Prevention of relapse in opioid addiction

Naltrexone 100mg ***PO blocks the effect of a*** challenge of IV **diamorphine** 25mg by 96% at 24h, and 46% at 72h.[38] Thus, **naltrexone** is primarily used to prevent relapse in opioid addiction by blocking opioid 'highs'. It is also used PO off-label to reduce the relapse rate in alcohol addiction. **Naltrexone** is given PO either once daily or three times per week. It is also available as a long-acting depot IM injection (duration of action >1 month; for use in alcohol and opioid addiction) and an SC pellet implant (duration of action weeks–months).[39] Both injectable products are unauthorized in the UK, but are available through private addiction clinics.

Opioid combination products to deter opioid abuse

In an attempt to reduce the risk of opioid abuse, PO/SL formulations containing both a strong opioid and an opioid antagonist have been developed, e.g.:

- Suboxone® (**buprenorphine + naloxone**) given SL for opioid dependency
- Targinact® (**oxycodone + naloxone**) for PO use (see p.480)
- Embeda® (**morphine + naltrexone**) for PO use (not UK)
- Troxyca® ER (**oxycodone + naltrexone**) for PO use (not UK).

When administered as indicated, the opioid antagonist either remains sequestered (Embeda®, Troxyca® ER) or the amount absorbed is insufficient to antagonize the analgesic effect of the opioid (Suboxone®, Targinact®). However, if abused (e.g. the tablets crushed and administered by insufflation or IV), the opioid antagonist is then released and available in sufficient amounts to antagonize the opioid.

Pruritus

Cholestatic pruritus

This is partly a consequence of increased opioidergic tone caused by a raised plasma enkephalin concentration.[40] Centrally acting opioid antagonists are thought to counteract the increased tone within the CNS, and thereby improve the pruritus (also see Chapter 26, p.825).

Benefit from CIVI/CSCI **naloxone**,[41-43] PO **naltrexone**[44,45] and PO **nalmefene**[46] is seen in cholestatic pruritus caused by chronic liver disease, e.g. primary biliary cholangitis. However, opioid antagonists are generally considered a third-line treatment in this setting, because they are less effective than either bile sequestrants (e.g. **cholestyramine**) or **rifampicin** (p.518).[47,48] **Sertraline** also provides a simpler alternative treatment option in this setting and in cholestasis due to biliary obstruction in cancer (see Chapter 26, Table 1, p.829).

Opioid antagonists can precipitate an opioid-withdrawal-like reaction in patients with cholestasis, including hallucinations and dysphoria.[49,50] To avoid or minimize such a reaction, treatment must be started cautiously with a low dose (see Dose and use). Further, the use of **naltrexone** to relieve cholestatic jaundice may sometimes unmask or exacerbate underlying pain, necessitating discontinuation of **naltrexone**.[51] Thus, patients with cholestatic jaundice and pruritus and severe pain should *not* be treated with a centrally acting opioid antagonist.[52] However, case reports suggest benefit from **methylnaltrexone**, a peripherally acting opioid antagonist which avoids the risk of opioid withdrawal and/or reversal of opioid analgesia, making it a reasonable option to trial in patients receiving opioids (see p.500 and p.831). For other treatments for cholestatic pruritus, see Chapter 26, Table 1, p.829.

There are reports of patients with cholestatic pruritus who have responded to **buprenorphine** (p.428) alone or in combination with ultra-low doses of **naloxone**.[53-56] Sometimes ultra-low doses of **naloxone** or **naltrexone** improved both the pruritus and the pain.[57] However, there are insufficient data at present to recommend this approach.

Uraemic pruritus

This situation is more complex because there are several causal mechanisms, both peripheral (cutaneous) and central (neural).[58] The opioid system is involved, but in uraemia there is no increase in opioidergic tone (and thus no danger of a withdrawal syndrome if an opioid antagonist is given). Instead, the ratio between μ-opioid (pruritus-inducing) and κ-opioid (pruritus-suppressing) receptors alters in favour of the former, predisposing to the onset or exacerbation of pruritus.[59,60] Thus, both μ antagonists, e.g. **naltrexone**, and κ *agonists*, e.g. **nalfurafine** (not UK), have been explored in this setting. Only the latter provide consistent benefit, although to a lesser degree than that achieved with **gabapentin** or **pregabalin** (see Chapter 26, Table 1, p.829).[61,62]

Ultra-low-dose **naloxone** is also used to relieve pruritus caused by spinal opioids, when other treatments have failed (see Chapter 32, p.915).

Miscellaneous

Naloxone is reported to benefit patients with septic shock,[63] **morphine**-induced peripheral vasodilation,[64] ischaemic central neurological deficits[65,66] and post-stroke central pain.[67]

Endogenous opioids inhibit cell proliferation, an effect which intermittent low-dose **naltrexone** appears to augment by provoking a compensatory elevation in opioid growth factor (OGF; an enkephalin) and OGF receptor (a non-classical opioid receptor). This interaction impacts upon the cell cycle, inhibiting proliferation. The potential roles of low-dose **naltrexone** and OGF in cancer and auto-immune diseases (e.g. multiple sclerosis, Crohn's disease) are being explored.[68-70]

In the past, PO **naloxone** and **naltrexone** have been used to correct delayed gastric emptying and constipation. However, because both act centrally as well as peripherally, there is a risk of analgesic reversal and systemic withdrawal. Consequently, opioid antagonists that do not readily cross the blood–brain barrier are preferable (p.500).

Cautions

In patients receiving opioids for pain relief, **naloxone** should *not* be used for drowsiness and/or delirium which is not life-threatening, because of the danger of reversing the opioid analgesia and precipitating a major physical withdrawal syndrome. Instead, omit or reduce the next regular opioid dose, and subsequently continue at a reduced dose.

The use of **naltrexone** will also impede opioid analgesia (see Box A),[71] and can also precipitate an opioid-withdrawal-like syndrome in patients with cholestatic pruritus who are not taking opioids (see Pharmacology). **Naltrexone** may cause occasional hepatotoxicity.[72] The manufacturer advises checking LFTs before and at intervals during treatment.

Undesirable effects

Naloxone: nausea and vomiting; occasionally severe hypertension, pulmonary oedema (see above); rarely tachycardia, arrhythmias and even cardiac arrest.[73]

Naltrexone: *very common (>10% in detoxifying opioid addicts):* insomnia, headaches, anxiety, nausea and vomiting, intestinal colic, lack of energy, joint and muscle pain.

The long-term use of **naltrexone** increases the concentration of opioid receptors in the CNS and results in a temporary enhanced response to the subsequent administration of opioid analgesics.[74] The management of severe acute and postoperative pain in patients receiving long-term **naltrexone** requires careful consideration (Box A).[71,75,76] Similar caution is needed for **nalmefene** (see SPC).

Box A Management of acute pain in patients receiving naltrexone

Elective surgery

The use of naltrexone must be identified well before the operation.

Ensure effective liaison between the substance misuse and acute pain teams.

Consider switching patients on naltrexone IM depot injections to PO tablets before surgery.

For minor surgery, when non-opioids are considered sufficient to manage the postoperative pain, leave naltrexone SC pellet *in situ*; if severe postoperative pain anticipated, remove SC pellet.

Discontinue PO naltrexone 72h before the operation.

Maximize the use of non-opioid analgesics, e.g. IV paracetamol, NSAID.

Note. If an opioid analgesic is required, a bigger than usual dose may be needed but, conversely, there may be an increased response to opioids (see Pharmacology and Undesirable effects).

To avoid precipitating opioid withdrawal, do not restart naltrexone until 3–7 days after the last dose of opioid, depending on the duration of use and halflife of the opioid.

Unexpected severe acute pain, e.g. trauma, emergency surgery

If possible, use non-opioid analgesics, e.g.:

- IV paracetamol and/or NSAID
- ketamine 100microgram/kg IV every 5min until satisfactory analgesia obtained, plus a single dose of midazolam 20–40microgram/kg IV to minimize dysphoria; may be repeated after 30min; give further midazolam only if dysphoria present.

Note. There is a risk of marked sedation when ketamine and midazolam are combined in this way; to be used only by those competent in airway management.

If venous access is difficult, ketamine can be given SC; use the same doses as for IV, but allow 15min between doses.

The above are generally used to achieve rapid pain relief until other measures can be instituted, e.g.:

- local anaesthetic blocks
- epidural analgesia (local anaesthetic ± clonidine).

Dose and use

Reversal of opioid-induced respiratory depression (naloxone)

Naloxone is best given IV but, if not practical, may be given IM or SC. An intranasal spray product is authorized for use in circumstances where IV access is not immediately available.[77,78]

Dose recommendations vary.[24,25] For *PCF* recommendations, see QCG: Reversal of opioid-induced respiratory depression, p.498.

†Cholestatic pruritus (naloxone, naltrexone, nalmefene)

Rifampicin is a more effective alternative, as is probably **sertraline** (see p.518). Opioid antagonists are unsuitable for patients who are physically dependent on opioids.

To try and avoid or minimize an opioid-withdrawal-like syndrome, start with a low dose. Although some recommend the initial use of **naloxone** CIVI, others have successfully used **naltrexone** *de novo* 12.5–25mg PO b.d. and subsequently titrated as below:

- start with a low dose of **naloxone** by CIVI, e.g. 0.002microgram/kg/min (about 160–200microgram/24h)[50]; long-term administration by CSCI has also been reported[43]
- if no withdrawal-like symptoms occur, the rate can be doubled every 3–4h; but if symptoms occur, continue with the current dose until resolved
- after 18–24h, when a rate known to be associated with opioid antagonistic effects is reached (0.2microgram/kg/min), *stop* the **naloxone** infusion and *start* **naltrexone** 12.5–25mg PO b.d.[44,49,50]

- increase the dose every few days until a satisfactory clinical response is obtained; at this stage, consolidate the effective dose into a single daily maintenance dose
- the effective dose range for PO **naltrexone** is 25–250mg once daily.[50]

For **nalmefene**, start with 2mg PO b.d.; double the dose every 2 days until pruritus is relieved or no further improvement; individual maximum doses 30–120mg b.d..[79] Note. The only authorized **nalmefene** product available in the UK is unsuitable for this dosing regimen (see Supply).

Supply

Naloxone

Naloxone hydrochloride (generic)

Injection 20microgram/mL, 2mL amp = £5.50; 400microgram/mL, 1mL amp = £4, (2mL prefilled syringe also available); 1mg/mL, 2mL prefilled syringe = £17.

Nyxoid® (Napp)

Nasal spray 18mg/mL, 0.1mL (1.8mg) dose = £26 (2 dose pack).

Naltrexone

Naltrexone hydrochloride (generic)

Tablets *(scored)* 50mg, 28 days @ 50mg once daily = £23.

Capsules 0.5mg, 1mg, 1.5mg, 3mg, 4mg, 4.5mg; price unobtainable (unauthorized products, available as a special order; see Chapter 24, p.817).

Oral solution or suspension 5mg/5mL, 28 days @ 50mg once daily = £226 or £119 (unauthorized, available as a special order; see Chapter 24, p.817); *price based on specials tariff in community.*

Nalmefene

Tablets 18mg, 28 = £85 (authorized for alcohol addiction only). *Do not divide or crush, because of the risk of skin sensitization.*

1 Firouzian A *et al.* (2016) Ultra-low-dose naloxone as an adjuvant to patient controlled analgesia (PCA) with morphine for postoperative pain relief following lumber discectomy: a double-blind, randomized, placebo-controlled trial. *Journal of Neurosurgical Anesthesiology.* **30**: 26–31.

2 Xiao Y *et al.* (2015) A randomized clinical trial of the effects of ultra-low-dose naloxone infusion on postoperative opioid requirements and recovery. *Acta Anaesthesiologica Scandinavica.* **59**: 1194–1203.

3 He F *et al.* (2016) The effect of naloxone treatment on opioid-induced side effects: a meta-analysis of randomized and controlled trails. *Medicine (Baltimore).* **95**: e4729.

4 Largent-Milnes TM *et al.* (2008) Oxycodone plus ultra-low-dose naltrexone attenuates neuropathic pain and associated mu-opioid receptor-Gs coupling. *Journal of Pain.* **9**: 700–713.

5 Hay JL *et al.* (2011) Potentiation of buprenorphine antinociception with ultra-low dose naltrexone in healthy subjects. *European Journal of Pain.* **15**: 293–298.

6 Cepeda MS *et al.* (2004) Addition of ultralow dose naloxone to postoperative morphine PCA: unchanged analgesia and opioid requirement but decreased incidence of opioid side effects. *Pain.* **107**: 41–46.

7 Maxwell LG *et al.* (2005) The effects of a small-dose naloxone infusion on opioid-induced side effects and analgesia in children and adolescents treated with intravenous patient-controlled analgesia: a double-blind, prospective, randomized, controlled study. *Anesthesia and Analgesia.* **100**: 953–958.

8 Murphy JD *et al.* (2011) Analgesic efficacy of intravenous naloxone for the treatment of postoperative pruritus: a meta-analysis. *Journal of Opioid Management.* **7**: 321–327.

9 Joshi G *et al.* (1999) Effects of prophylactic nalmefene on the incidence of morphine-related side effects in patients receiving intravenous patient-controlled analgesia. *Anesthesiology.* **90**: 1007–1011.

10 Cruciani RA *et al.* (2003) Ultra-low dose oral naltrexone decreases side effects and potentiates the effect of methadone. *Journal of Pain and Symptom Management.* **25**: 491–494.

11 Hamann S and Sloan P (2007) Oral naltrexone to enhance analgesia in patients receiving continuous intrathecal morphine for chronic pain: a randomized, double-blind, prospective pilot study. *Journal of Opioid Management.* **3**: 137–144.

12 Chindalore VL *et al.* (2005) Adding ultralow-dose naltrexone to oxycodone enhances and prolongs analgesia: a randomized, controlled trial of Oxytrex. *Journal of Pain.* **6**: 392–399.

13 Raffaeli W and Indovina P (2015) Low-dose naltrexone to prevent intolerable morphine adverse events: a forgotten remedy for a neglected, global clinical need. *Pain Medicine.* **16**: 1239–1242.

14 Crain S and Shen K (2000) Antagonists of excitatory opioid receptor functions enhance morphine's analgesic potency and attenuate opioid tolerance/dependence liability. *Pain.* **84**: 121–131.

15 Sjogren P *et al.* (1994) Disappearance of morphine-induced hyperalgesia after discontinuing or substituting morphine with other opioid antagonists. *Pain.* **59**: 313–316.

16 Wang HY and Burns LH (2009) Naloxone's pentapeptide binding site on filamin A blocks Mu opioid receptor-Gs coupling and CREB activation of acute morphine. *PLoS ONE.* **4**: e4282.

17 Wang X *et al.* (2016) Pharmacological characterization of the opioid inactive isomers (+)-naltrexone and (+)-naloxone as antagonists of toll-like receptor 4. *British Journal of Pharmacology.* **173**: 856–869.

18 Ellis A *et al.* (2016) Morphine amplifies mechanical allodynia via TLR4 in a rat model of spinal cord injury. *Brain Behaviour and Immunity.* **58**: 348–356.

19 Yang CP *et al.* (2013) Intrathecal ultra-low dose naloxone enhances the antihyperalgesic effects of morphine and attenuates tumour necrosis factor-α and tumour necrosis factor-α receptor 1 expression in the dorsal horn of rats with partial sciatic nerve transection. *Anesthesia and Analgesia.* **117**: 1493–1502.

20 Ellis A *et al.* (2014) Systemic administration of propentofylline, ibudilast, and (+)-naltrexone each reverses mechanical allodynia in a novel rat model of central neuropathic pain. *Journal of Pain.* **15**: 407–421.

21 Gonzalez J and Brogden R (1988) Naltrexone: a review of its pharmacodynamic and pharmacokinetic properties and therapeutic efficacy in the management of opioid dependence. *Drugs.* **35**: 192–213.

22 Crabtree B (1984) Review of naltrexone: a long-acting opiate antagonist. *Clinical Pharmacy.* **3**: 273–280.

23 Gutstein H and Akil H. (2001) Opioid analgesics. In: Hardman JG and Limbird LE (eds). *Goodman & Gilman's The Pharmacological Basis of Therapeutics.* 10th edn. New York, London: McGraw-Hill.

24 Connors NJ and Nelson LS (2016) The evolution of recommended naloxone dosing for opioid overdose by medical specialty. *Journal of Medical Toxicology.* **12**: 276–281.

25 UK Medicines Information (2019) What naloxone doses should be used in adults to reverse urgently the effects of opioids? *Medicines Q&A.* www.sps.nhs.uk.

26 NHS England (2014) Risk of distress and death from inappropriate doses of naloxone in patients on long-term opioid/opiate treatment. *Patient Safety Alert.* NHS/PSA/W/2014/2016. www.england.nhs.uk.

27 NHS England (2015) Support to minimise the risk of distress and death from inappropriate doses of naloxone. *Patient Safety Alert.* NHS/PSA/Re/2015/2009. www.england.nhs.uk.

28 Raffa RB *et al.* (1992) Opioid and nonopioid components independently contribute to the mechanism of action of tramadol, an 'atypical' opioid analgesic. *Journal of Pharmacology and Therapeutics.* **260**: 275–285.

29 Shipton EA (2000) Tramadol - present and future. *Anaesthesia and Intensive Care.* **28**: 363–374.

30 Marquardt KA *et al.* (2005) Tramadol exposures reported to statewide poison control system. *Annals of Pharmacotherapy.* **39**: 1039–1044.

31 Torralva R and Janowsky A (2019) Noradrenergic mechanisms in fentanyl-mediated rapid death explain failure of naloxone in the opioid crisis. *Journal of Pharmacology Experimental Therapeutics.* **374**: 453–475.

32 Torralva R *et al.* (2020) Fentanyl but not morphine interacts with nonopioid recombinant human neurotransmitter receptors and transporters. *Journal of Pharmacology Experimental Therapeutics.* **374**: 376–391.

33 Patti R *et al.* (2019) Naloxone-induced noncardiogenic pulmonary oedema. *American Journal of Therapeutics.* **0**: 1–2.

34 Ridgway ZA and Pountney AJ (2007) Acute respiratory distress syndrome induced by oral methadone managed with non-invasive ventilation. *Emergency Medicine Journal.* **24**: 681.

35 Feeney C *et al.* (2011) Morphine-induced cardiogenic shock. *Annals of Pharmacotherpy.* **45**: e30.

36 Clarke SF *et al.* (2005) Naloxone in opioid poisoning: walking the tightrope. *Emergency Medicine Journal.* **22**: 612–616.

37 Paranthaman SK and Khan F (1976) Acute cardiomyopathy with recurrent pulmonary edema and hypotension following heroin overdosage. *Chest.* **69**: 117–119.

38 Verebey K (1981) The clinical pharmacology of naltrexone: pharmacology and pharmacodynamics. *NIDA Research Monograph.* **28**: 147–158.

39 Sudakin D (2016) Naltrexone: Not just for opioids anymore. *Journal of Medical Toxicology.* **12**: 71–75.

40 Davis M (2007) Cholestasis and endogenous opioids: liver disease and exogenous opioid pharmacokinetics. *Clinical Pharmacokinetics.* **46**: 825–850.

41 Bergasa N *et al.* (1992) A controlled trial of naloxone infusions for the pruritus of chronic cholestasis. *Gastroenterology.* **102**: 544–549.

42 Bergasa N *et al.* (1995) Effects of naloxone infusions in patients with the pruritus of cholestasis. *Annals of Internal Medicine.* **123**: 161–167.

43 Kumar N *et al.* (2013) Opiate receptor antagonists for treatment of severe pruritus associated with advanced cholestatic liver disease. *Journal of Palliative Medicine.* **16**: 122–123.

44 Terg R *et al.* (2002) Efficacy and safety of oral naltrexone treatment for pruritus of cholestasis, a crossover, double blind, placebo-controlled study. *Journal of Hepatology.* **37**: 717–722.

45 Wolfhagen F *et al.* (1997) Oral naltrexone treatment for cholestatic pruritus: a double-blind, placebo-controlled study. *Gastroenterology.* **113**: 1264–1269.

46 Bergasa N *et al.* (1999) Oral nalmefene therapy reduces scratching activity due to the pruritus of cholestasis: a controlled study. *Journal of the American Academy of Dermatology.* **41**: 431–434.

47 Tandon P *et al.* (2007) The efficacy and safety of bile acid binding agents, opioid antagonists, or rifampin in the treatment of cholestasis-associated pruritus. *American Journal of Gastroenterology.* **102**: 1528–1536.

48 Hirschfield GM *et al.* (2018) The British Society of Gastroenterology/UK-PBC primary biliary cholangitis treatment and management guidelines. *Gut.* **67**: 1568–1594.

49 Jones E and Dekker L (2000) Florid opioid withdrawal-like reaction precipitated by naltrexone in a patient with chronic cholestasis. *Gastroenterology.* **118**: 431–432.

50 Jones E *et al.* (2002) Opiate antagonist therapy for the pruritus of cholestasis: the avoidance of opioid withdrawal-like reactions. *Quarterly Journal of Medicine.* **95**: 547–552.

51 McRae CA *et al.* (2003) Pain as a complication of use of opiate antagonists for symptom control in cholestasis. *Gastroenterology.* **125**: 591–596.

52 Lonsdale-Eccles AA and Carmichael AJ (2009) Opioid antagonist for pruritus of cholestasis unmasking bony metastases. *Acta Dermato Venereologica.* **89**: 90.

53 Juby L *et al.* (1994) Buprenorphine and hepatic pruritus. *British Journal of Clinical Practice.* **48**: 331.

54 Reddy L *et al.* (2007) Transdermal buprenorphine may be effective in the treatment of pruritus in primary biliary cirrhosis. *Journal of Pain and Symptom Management.* **34**: 455–456.

55 Marinangeli F *et al.* (2009) Intravenous naloxone plus transdermal buprenorphine in cancer pain associated with intractable cholestatic pruritus. *Journal of Pain and Symptom Management.* **38**: e5–e8.

56 Zylicz Z *et al.* (2005) Severe pruritus of cholestasis in disseminated cancer: developing a rational treatment strategy. A case report. *Journal of Pain and Symptom Management.* **29**: 100–103.

57 Jones EA and Zylicz Z (2005) Treatment of pruritus caused by cholestasis with opioid antagonists. *Journal of Palliative Medicine.* **8**: 1290–1294.

58 Manenti L *et al.* (2009) Uraemic pruritus: clinical characteristics, pathophysiology and treatment. *Drugs.* **69**: 251–263.

59 Kumagai H *et al.* (2000) Endogenous opioid system in uraemic patients. Joint Meeting of the Seventh World Conference on Clinical Pharmacology and IUPHAR - Division of Clinical Pharmacology and the Fourth Congress of the European Association for Clinical Pharmacology and Therapeutics.
60 Odou P *et al.* (2001) A hypothesis for endogenous opioid peptides in uraemic pruritus: role of enkephalin. *Nephrology, Dialysis, Transplantation*. **16**: 1953–1954.
61 Hercz D *et al.* (2020) Interventions for itch in people with advanced chronic kidney disease. *Cochrane Database Systematic Reviews*. **12**: CD011393. www.cochranelibrary.com.
62 Fishbane S *et al.* (2020) A Phase 3 trial of Difelikefalin in hemodialysis patients with pruritus. *New England Journal of Medicine*. **382**: 222–232.
63 Peters WP *et al.* (1981) Pressor effect of naloxone in septic shock. *Lancet*. **i**: 529–532.
64 Cohen RA and Coffman JD (1980) Naloxone reversal of morphine-induced peripheral vasodilatation. *Clinical Pharmacology and Therapeutics*. **28**: 541–544.
65 Baskin DS and Hosobuchi Y (1981) Naloxone reversal of ischaemic neurological deficits in man. *Lancet*. **ii**: 272–275.
66 Bousigue J-Y *et al.* (1982) Naloxone reversal of neurological deficit. *Lancet*. **ii**: 618–619.
67 Ray D and Tai Y (1988) Infusions of naloxone in thalamic pain. *British Medical Journal*. **296**: 969–970.
68 Li Z *et al.* (2018) Low-dose naltrexone (LDN): A promising treatment in immune-related diseases and cancer therapy. *International Immunopharmacology*. **61**: 178–184.
69 Patten D *et al.* (2018) The safety and efficacy of low-dose naltrexone in the management of chronic pain and inflammation in multiple sclerosis, fibromyalgia, Crohn's disease, and other chronic pain disorders. *Pharmacotherapy*. **38**: 382–389.
70 Liubchenko K *et al.* (2020) Naltrexone's impact on cancer progression and mortality: A systematic review of studies in humans, animal models, and cell cultures. *Advances in Therapy*. Online ahead of print. DOI 10.1007/s12325-12320-01591-12329.
71 Vickers AP and Jolly A (2006) Naltrexone and problems in pain management. *British Medical Journal*. **332** (7534): 132–133.
72 Mitchell J (1986) Naltrexone and hepatotoxicity. *Lancet*. **1**: 1215.
73 Partridge BL and Ward CF (1986) Pulmonary oedema following low-dose naloxone administration. *Anesthesiology*. **65**: 709–710.
74 Yoburn BC *et al.* (1988) Upregulation of opioid receptor subtypes correlates with potency changes of morphine and DADLE. *Life Sciences*. **43**: 1319–1324.
75 WHO (2009) Guidelines for the psychosocially assisted pharmacological treatment of opioid dependence. www.who.int.
76 Petri C and Richards J (2020) Management of sedation and analgesia in critically ill patients receiving long-acting naltrexone therapy for opioid use disorder. *Annals of the American Thoracic Society*. **17**: 1352–1357.
77 Sabzghabaee AM *et al.* (2014) Naloxone therapy in opioid overdose patients: intranasal or intravenous? A randomized clinical trial. *Archives of Medical Science*. **10**: 309–314.
78 Dietze P and Cantwell K (2016) Intranasal naloxone soon to become part of evolving clinical practice around opioid overdose prevention. *Addiction*. **111**: 584–586.
79 Bergasa N *et al.* (1998) Open-label trial of oral nalmefene therapy for the pruritus of cholestasis. *Hepatology*. **27**: 679–684.

Updated July 2021

Quick Clinical Guide: Reversal of opioid-induced respiratory depression

Traditional IV doses of naloxone (e.g. 400microgram stat) should be used only in immediately life-threatening situations (i.e. unresponsive patient with/near respiratory arrest).

In other circumstances, careful titration using lower doses of naloxone (e.g. 20–100microgram IV) should be used to avoid a severe acute withdrawal syndrome and, in those receiving opioids for analgesia, severe pain and hyperalgesia.

The dose should be titrated against level of consciousness (i.e. patient easily rousable; they do not have to be fully alert) and satisfactory respiratory function (i.e. respiratory rate ≥8 breaths/min and no cyanosis).

Because buprenorphine has both high receptor affinity and prolonged receptor binding, naloxone in standard doses does not reverse the effects of buprenorphine, and higher doses must be used (see Box A).

Diagnosis

Seek relevant clinical history (see below). Most episodes are preceded by a progressive reduction in consciousness. When the respiratory rate is <8 breaths/min and:

- patient unresponsive or responsive only to painful stimuli, give naloxone: *use lower doses*, unless episode is immediately life-threatening (see below)
- patient is alert/easily rousable (opens eyes in response to verbal command): adopt a policy of close 'watchful waiting'; consider omitting or reducing the next regular dose of opioid and then continuing at the lower dose.

Note:

- criteria vary; e.g. some use respiratory rates ≤10 breaths/min, include hypoxaemia (e.g. SpO_2 <90% on air) and/or hypercapnia
- assessment of SpO_2 can be confounded by comorbid conditions and supplemental oxygen. It may be normal even in severe hypercapnia (particularly with supplemental oxygen), only declining rapidly when near respiratory arrest
- pupil size is an unreliable indicator of opioid overdose in patients taking regular opioids
- naloxone should not be given to patients on opioids when death is expected and imminent; a slow respiratory rate is a normal occurrence.

Initial treatment

General approaches include:

- maintain airway
- administer oxygen to maintain SpO_2 >95% (88–92% if pre-existing hypercapnic respiratory failure)
- discontinue opioid (e.g. stop CSCI/CIVI, remove TD patch)
- obtain IV access
- administer naloxone IV (if not practical, can be given IM or SC; a nasal spray product is available for use in immediately life-threatening respiratory depression).

Immediately life-threatening respiratory depression

In this situation, i.e. unresponsive patient with/near respiratory arrest (no/minimal respiratory effort), traditional doses of naloxone are used. Administer each dose over 30 seconds. Assess after 1min and, if no response, move to the next dose:

- start with 400microgram IV → 800microgram → 800microgram → 2–4mg
- if no response to 2–4mg, consider an alternate diagnosis, including the possibility of 'wooden chest' syndrome.

A nasal spray product (Nyxoid®) is available for use in circumstances where IV access is not immediately available:

- give 1.8mg (one spray) into one nostril and wait 2–3min
- if there is no response (or if respiratory depression recurs), repeat the dose, alternating nostrils.

Severe but not immediately life-threatening respiratory depression

This is written from the perspective of an iatrogenic overdose in a patient receiving opioid analgesia, but it can also be applied to overdose from drug misuse.

When naloxone is indicated (see Diagnosis):
- dilute a 1mL ampoule containing naloxone 400microgram to 4mL with sodium chloride 0.9% for injection
- administer 1mL (100microgram) IV every 2min until respirations are satisfactory.

Even lower doses may be used:
- administer 20microgram IV every 2min until respirations are satisfactory
- if a 20microgam/mL naloxone ampoule is not available, dilute a 1mL ampoule containing naloxone 400microgram to 10mL with sodium chloride 0.9% for injection and administer 0.5mL (20microgram).

Ongoing treatment

After the last dose of naloxone, monitor level of consciousness and respiratory rate every 15min for 2h, then hourly for 6h after an immediate-release opioid; monitor for longer after a modified-release opioid or an opioid with a long halflife, e.g. 12h after a 12-hourly modified-release opioid, 24h after methadone.

Further boluses are likely to be necessary, because naloxone is shorter acting than morphine and other opioids. If more than three repeat bolus doses are required, consider IVI naloxone for up to 24h, sometimes longer:
- dilute 10 ampoules containing naloxone 400microgram in 1mL to 20mL with sodium chloride 0.9% or glucose 5% to produce a 200microgram/mL solution
- administer via a large peripheral vein or central venous catheter
- use an IVI device (e.g. syringe pump) to deliver an hourly dose which is 60% of the stat dose that had previously maintained satisfactory ventilation for ≥15min
- titrate the IVI as necessary.

Naloxone IVI requires close monitoring; some centres recommend use only within a critical care unit.

Rarely, an opioid overdose is complicated by pulmonary oedema, but the signs may be absent until naloxone improves the respiratory rate and tidal volume. Consider if there is unexpected breathlessness and persistent hypoxaemia despite oxygen. Treat with oxygen, IV furosemide, IVI nitrates and ventilation as necessary. Generally, the pulmonary oedema responds to these approaches in 24–48h.

Review opioid regimen

Consider:
- possible causes for the opioid overdose, e.g.:
  - ▷ excessive dosing (e.g. opioid poorly responsive pain, prescription/administration error)
  - ▷ drug–drug interaction (e.g. fentanyl and clarithromycin)
  - ▷ drug accumulation because of an opioid with a long halflife (e.g. methadone)
  - ▷ reduced elimination because of renal impairment (e.g. morphine)
- only when there is sustained respiratory improvement, restarting on a lower dose of opioid
- switching to another opioid; seek specialist advice.

Box A Reversal of buprenorphine-induced respiratory depression

1. Discontinue buprenorphine (stop CSCI/CIVI, remove TD patch).
2. Give oxygen by mask.
3. Give IV naloxone *2mg* stat over 90sec.
4. Commence naloxone *4mg/h* by CIVI.
5. Continue CIVI until the patient's condition is satisfactory (probably <90min).
6. Monitor the patient frequently for the next 24h, and restart CIVI if respiratory depression recurs.
7. If the patient's condition remains satisfactory, restart buprenorphine at a reduced dose, e.g. half the previous dose.

The non-specific respiratory stimulant doxapram can also be used, 1–1.5mg/kg IV over 30sec, repeated if necessary at hourly intervals, or 1.5–*4mg/min* CIVI.

Updated July 2021

OPIOID ANTAGONISTS (THERAPEUTIC TARGET OUTSIDE THE CNS)

For *Opioid antagonists (therapeutic target within the CNS)*, see p.490; these are authorized for reversal of opioid-induced respiratory depression and acute opioid overdose. Because they reverse opioid-induced analgesia, their use for reversing the peripheral effects of opioids (e.g. constipation) is restricted. The exception is **naloxone** in Targinact®, where use of an m/r formulation limits systemic absorption (see p.482) and thereby limits central antagonism.

Indications: Opioid-induced constipation in adults whose response to laxatives is inadequate; post-operative ileus (**alvimopan** PO (not UK)).[1,2]

Contra-indications: Methylnaltrexone: known or suspected bowel obstruction; acute surgical abdomen.
Naldemedine: known or suspected bowel obstruction or perforation; increased risk of GI perforation (i.e. those at risk of recurrent bowel obstruction); concurrent use of a *potent CYP3A4 inhibitor* (see Drug interactions).
Naloxegol: known or suspected bowel obstruction; increased risk of GI perforation (i.e. those at risk of recurrent bowel obstruction; recurrent or advanced ovarian cancer; other cancers of the GI tract or peritoneum; concurrent use of a vascular endothelial growth factor inhibitor); concurrent use of a *potent CYP3A4 inhibitor* (see Drug interactions).

Pharmacology

Alvimopan (not UK), **methylnaltrexone**, **naldemedine** and **naloxegol** do not readily cross the blood–brain barrier, and thus act as peripheral opioid antagonists. Although referred to as PAMORA (peripherally acting mu-opioid receptor antagonists), they also bind to other types of opioid receptor, albeit with lower and differing levels of affinity. All are more effective than placebo in improving aspects of opioid-induced constipation, e.g. time to bowel movement, weekly bowel frequency, symptom scores.[3] However, none has been directly compared with *optimized* conventional laxatives.[3]

For patients with cancer and/or those receiving palliative care, there is moderate-quality evidence supporting the use of SC **methylnaltrexone** and PO **naldemedine**.[1]

Methylnaltrexone (SC)

A methyl derivative of noroxymorphone, authorized for use in adults to treat opioid-induced constipation when there has been an insufficient response to laxatives. A PO product (not UK) is authorized for opioid-induced constipation in adults with chronic pain.[4,5]

RCTs have been undertaken in those with advanced illness (palliative care patients) using doses based on body weight, and in those with chronic pain (mostly back pain) using a fixed dose of 12mg SC.[6,7]

In patients with advanced illness, **methylnaltrexone** was used alongside existing laxative therapy, whereas in patients with chronic pain, only p.r.n. rescue laxatives were permitted. Systematic reviews based on these RCTs report an overall NNT of 3 (95% CI 3–6) and an NNH (for diarrhoea) of 30 (95% CI 18–111);[6,8] another found only the risk of abdominal pain to be significantly higher than placebo, and a serious adverse event rate of 0.2%.[7]

Off-label uses of SC **methylnaltrexone** include opioid-induced constipation in children[9-11] and post-operative[12-14] or non-surgical critical care patients,[15] and opioid-related acute colonic pseudo-obstruction.[16] **Methylnaltrexone** may also improve other peripheral effects of opioids, e.g. delayed gastric emptying, urinary retention.[12] Case reports also suggest benefit in cholestatic pruritus (see p.831).[17]

After SC **methylnaltrexone**, peak plasma concentration is reached in about 30min. Elimination is mostly as unchanged drug (85%), via the urine (50%) and faeces. The main metabolites (methylnaltrexone sulfate, methyl-6-naltrexol) are inactive. Mild–moderate hepatic impairment does not affect the metabolism of **methylnaltrexone** to a clinically relevant degree; the effect of severe hepatic impairment has not been evaluated.

The clearance of **methylnaltrexone** reduces with increasing renal impairment. When severe, overall exposure (AUC) is doubled, and dose reduction is required (see Dose and use). For pharmacokinetic data see Table 1.

Naldemedine

Naldemedine is an amide derivative of **naltrexone** and is authorized for opioid-induced constipation in adults previously treated with a laxative.

RCTs of **naldemedine** 200microgram PO once daily have been undertaken in patients with cancer pain and chronic non-cancer pain.[18-20] Across the studies, patients with severe constipation were excluded, e.g. no bowel movement for 7 consecutive days. Participants were outpatients with mean ages of 65 (cancer) and 55 (non-cancer). Mostly, cancer patients had a good performance status (0–1), lung or breast cancer (cancers affecting GI function were excluded) and extensive disease (~90%). Most were taking **oxycodone** (mean oral **morphine**-equivalent dose 60mg/24h vs. about 115mg/24h in non-cancer pain patients). Existing laxative therapy was continued in some but not other studies. In the long-term studies, if distressing GI undesirable effects occurred, the **naldemedine** could be temporarily stopped and restarted at a lower dose (100microgram once daily); this was necessary in about 10% and 2% of cancer patients respectively. However, the authorized 200microgram product is film-coated and not scored, and such a dose reduction will not be possible.

In patients with cancer, there has been a short-term (2 weeks) RCT followed by a 12 week open-label extension.[18,21] **Naldemedine** was used alongside existing laxative therapy (mostly **magnesium oxide** or **senna**). About 70% responded to **naldemedine** (compared with one third to placebo), defined as achieving ≥3 spontaneous bowel movements (SBM)/week and an increase in ≥1 SBM/week from baseline, equating to an NNT of 3 (95% CI 2–4). The weekly frequencies of SBM overall (5 vs. 2), with complete evacuation (3 vs. 1) and without straining (4 vs. 1) were all significantly higher with **naldemedine**, and the need for rescue laxatives significantly lower (3 vs. 1 fewer uses/week). Median time to first SBM was significantly shorter with **naldemedine** (5h vs. 27h). Despite this, no differences were seen in change in overall scores for constipation-related symptoms and quality of life, although some domains were significantly improved in patients receiving **naldemedine** (e.g. stool symptom score), and more could be considered responders for symptoms (~10% vs. 3%) and in the dissatisfaction domain (~34% vs. 20%). However, baseline scores were low, suggesting that the constipation had a relatively low level of severity/impact. Compared to placebo, more patients experienced adverse events with **naldemedine** (44% vs. 26%), particularly diarrhoea (20% vs. 7%); although mostly mild–moderate, they resulted in more discontinuations (9% vs. 1%).[18,21]

In chronic non-cancer pain studies lasting 12 weeks, about half of patients responded to **naldemedine** (compared with one third to placebo) as defined above and sustained for ≥75% of weeks of follow-up. This equated to about one additional bowel movement/week that was complete/without straining.[19] However, patients were either not taking laxatives or were willing to discontinue them at screening. Thus, laxatives (**bisacodyl** ± enemas) were only used p.r.n. No details of laxative use during the 2–4 week screening period were given, but the frequency of use was reduced by about one/week by both **naldemedine** and placebo.[19]

In a long-term RCT in chronic non-cancer pain, about half of patients enrolled were on regular laxative treatment (defined as use ≥1/week). In this group, compared to placebo, there was an increase in frequency of bowel movements with **naldemedine** (mean difference 1.2/week) sustained over 12 months. In patients not on regular laxative therapy, a significant difference was evident over the first 3 months only, in part because of a greater placebo response in this group.[20] This suggests constipation was relatively mild, particularly as there was a low use of p.r.n. 'rescue' laxatives; at most, only 15% of patients receiving placebo (± regular laxatives) required them.[20] Nonetheless, a greater and sustained improvement in constipation-related symptoms and quality of life were seen with **naldemedine** ± regular laxatives.[20]

A systematic review based on these short- and long-term RCTs in chronic pain patients report an overall NNT for **naldemedine** of 5 (95% CI 4–8).[8] Overall, **naldemedine** appeared well tolerated in this population, with a tolerability and safety profile similar to placebo, with the exception of about doubling the incidence of diarrhoea (e.g. ~11% vs. 5%), abdominal pain (~8% vs. 3%) and vomiting (~6% vs. 3%); these were mostly mild–moderate in severity and only occasionally necessitated discontinuation (4% vs. 2%).[19,20]

PO absorption of **naldemedine** is rapid and not affected by food to a clinically relevant degree. Naldemedine is primarily metabolized via hepatic CYP3A and enterobacteria in the GI tract, with elimination via the urine and faeces.

Mild–moderate hepatic impairment does not affect the metabolism of **naldemedine** to a clinically relevant degree, and no dose adjustment is required. The effect of severe hepatic impairment has not been evaluated.

Renal impairment does not affect the pharmacokinetics of **naldemedine** to a clinically relevant degree. No dose adjustment is required with any degree of renal impairment, including ESRF requiring haemodialysis. For pharmacokinetic data see Table 1.

Naloxegol

A pegylated form of **naloxone**, authorized for opioid-induced constipation in adults when there has been an inadequate response to laxatives.

In RCTs, **naloxegol** 25mg PO consistently improved bowel function and symptoms, but *only* in the subset of patients defined as having an inadequate response to laxatives, i.e. those with moderate symptoms of opioid-induced constipation (≥1 of: hard or lumpy stools, straining, or a sensation of incomplete bowel movement or anorectal obstruction) despite taking ≥1 type of laxative for ≥4 days during the previous 2 weeks. In this group, about half respond to **naloxegol** (compared with one third to placebo), with an NNT of 5–7.[22]

However, laxatives were only taken p.r.n. and in small amounts, i.e. on average **bisacodyl** ≤10mg *weekly*.[22,23] This suggests a very different population to that typically seen in palliative care. Further, severely constipated patients were excluded from the RCTs, i.e. those with faecal impaction or no bowel movement for 2 weeks.

RCTs involved relatively young patients (early 50s; only 10% ≥65, 2% ≥75) with non-cancer pain (mostly back pain) and, at most, mild hepatic/renal impairment with a mean oral **morphine**-equivalent dose of 140mg/day.[22] *Thus, RCT data to support the use of **naloxegol** in patients with cancer-related pain are lacking.* Consequently, in the USA, authorization is limited to patients with chronic non-cancer pain. The highest level evidence in cancer-related pain is a prospective observational study involving mostly oncology outpatients, many receiving chemotherapy.[24]

Direct comparisons with *optimized* conventional laxatives are lacking. However, in patients with chronic non-cancer pain with opioid-induced constipation, an open-label cross-over comparison of **naloxegol** 25mg vs. a fixed-dose of a **macrogol** (17g/day) found no difference in patient preference (about half each), improvement in bowel function or symptoms, and use of rescue laxatives. During the **macrogol** phase, there were fewer adverse events (17% vs. 24%), serious adverse events (0.4% vs. 1%) and treatment discontinuations (1% vs. 3%).[25]

PO absorption of **naloxegol** is rapid and enhanced by food (a high-fat meal increases C_{max} and AUC by about 30% and 45% respectively). A secondary plasma concentration peak occurs 0.5–3h after the first, probably reflecting enterohepatic recirculation. Metabolism is mostly via CYP3A, and elimination via the faeces (70%). Mild–moderate hepatic impairment does not affect the metabolism of **naloxegol** to a clinically relevant degree; the effect of severe hepatic impairment has not been evaluated.

Generally, because renal excretion is a minor route of elimination (≤5% unchanged **naloxegol**), pharmacokinetics are not significantly altered by renal impairment. Nonetheless, unpredictable increases in exposure to **naloxegol** can occur, possibly because of the effect of renal impairment on other clearance pathways (e.g. liver, GI wall). Consequently, a lower initial dose is recommended in patients with moderate–severe renal impairment. Haemodialysis has no effect on the pharmacokinetics of **naloxegol**. For pharmacokinetic data see Table 1.

Table 1 Pharmacokinetic details for selected peripheral opioid antagonists

	Methylnaltrexone	*Naldemedine*	*Naloxegol*
Bio-availability (%)	80% (SC)	20–55% (PO, estimate)	60% (PO, estimate)
Onset of action	Can be rapid (within 30min); median time to bowel movement ranges 1–6h	Median time to bowel movement ranges 5–18h	Median time to bowel movement ranges 5–21h
Time to peak plasma concentration	0.5h (SC)	0.75h	≤2h
Plasma halflife	8h	11h	6–11h
Duration of action	<24h	<24h	<24h

5

Cautions

Methylnaltrexone (SC): known or suspected lesions of the GI tract; patients with colostomy, active diverticular disease, faecal impaction, peritoneal catheter (excluded from studies), increased risk of perforation (e.g. GI cancer, peptic ulcer, pseudo-obstruction). Experience with a large series of patients with peritoneal carcinomatosis (n=333) suggests SC **methylnaltrexone** can be used in this group; only one patient (0.3%) was considered to have developed a related perforation, 1 day after dosing.[26]
Naldemedine: increased risk of GI perforation from other causes not constituting a contra-indication, e.g. Crohn's disease, active/recurrent diverticulitis, infiltrative GI cancers or peritoneal metastases, severe peptic ulcer disease; potential disruption of the blood–brain barrier (trials excluded patients with Alzheimer's disease, brain tumours or multiple sclerosis); cardiovascular disease (trials excluded patients with recent myocardial infarction, symptomatic CHF or overt cardiovascular disease).
Naloxegol: increased risk of GI perforation from other causes not constituting a contra-indication, e.g. Crohn's disease, active/recurrent diverticulitis, infiltrative GI cancers or peritoneal metastases, severe peptic ulcer disease; potential disruption of the blood–brain barrier (trials excluded patients with Alzheimer's disease, brain tumours or multiple sclerosis); use of **methadone** or high doses of opioid (i.e. ≥200mg/day oral **morphine** equivalent) increases risk of GI symptoms, e.g. abdominal pain and diarrhoea; cardiovascular disease (trials excluded patients with recent myocardial infarction, symptomatic CHF, overt cardiovascular disease).

Drug interactions

Exposure to **naldemedine** and **naloxegol** is increased 3 and 10 times respectively by concurrent use of a *potent CYP3A4 inhibitor*, e.g. **clarithromycin**, grapefruit juice (specifically large quantities), **itraconazole**, protease inhibitors, **telithromycin**, **voriconazole** (see Chapter 19, Table 8, p.790). The manufacturers consider concurrent use a contra-indication (**naloxegol**) or recommend against it (**naldemedine**).

A lower initial starting dose of **naloxegol** is recommend with concurrent use of a *moderate CYP3A4 inhibitor*, e.g. **diltiazem**, **erythromycin**, **fluconazole**, **verapamil** (see Dose and use, and Chapter 19, Table 8, p.790). For **naldemedine**, monitor for undesirable effects with concurrent use.

Both **naldemedine** and **naloxegol** are rendered ineffective by *potent CYP3A4 inducers*, which reduce their exposure by ≥75%, e.g. **carbamazepine**, **rifampicin**, **St. John's wort** (see Chapter 19, Table 8, p.790).

Ciclosporin, a *potent P-glycoprotein inhibitor*, doubles the exposure to **naldemedine**; monitor for undesirable effects with concurrent use.

Undesirable effects

Methylnaltrexone (SC)

Very common (≥10%): abdominal pain (generally mild–moderate),[27] diarrhoea, flatulence, nausea (these generally resolve after a bowel movement).
Common (<10%, >1%): vomiting, dizziness, mild peripheral opioid-withdrawal symptoms (see **naloxegol** below), injection site reactions.
Not known: GI perforation (stomach, small and large bowel).[28]

Naldemedine

Common (<10%, >1%): abdominal pain, diarrhoea (≤25% of cancer patients), nausea, vomiting. Generally mild–moderate and resolve without stopping treatment.
Uncommon (<1%, >0.1%): opioid-withdrawal symptoms (see **naloxegol** below).[29]

Naloxegol

Very common (≥10%): abdominal pain and diarrhoea. GI symptoms are most likely in the first ≤4 weeks of treatment.
Common (<10%, >1%): headache, nasopharyngitis, flatulence, nausea, vomiting, hyperhidrosis.
Uncommon (<1%, >0.1%): opioid-withdrawal syndrome (defined as ≥3 of the following: diarrhoea, dysphoria, fever, insomnia, lacrimation or rhinorrhoea, muscle aches, nausea or vomiting, pupillary dilation or piloerection or sweating, yawning). Generally, occurs in the first few days of treatment and is mild–moderate in intensity.

Dose and use

Naloxegol has been approved by NICE[30] and the Scottish Medicines Consortium,[31] but both the *Drug and Therapeutics Bulletin* and *PCF* consider **naloxegol** to be of very limited value clinically.[32] Its benefit compared with an optimized laxative regimen is unknown, and there are a lack of RCT data in patients with cancer. It is much more expensive than even high doses of stimulant laxatives.

By comparison, **methylnaltrexone**, although an SC injection and more expensive, has the advantages of a higher response rate (≤70% vs. ≤50%) and a lower NNT (3 vs. 5–7), and has been widely used in palliative care.

Thus, if a clinician chooses to prescribe **naloxegol**, its use should be restricted (as with **methylnaltrexone**) to occasions when upward titration of regularly administered laxatives is ineffective, poorly tolerated or not adhered to (see p.40).[33]

Naldemedine has been approved by NICE and the SMC.[34] Although the benefit of **naldemedine** compared to an optimized laxative regimen is unknown, there are RCT data in cancer patients, albeit relatively fit oncology outpatients. Compared to **naloxegol**, it is cheaper, has the advantage of dosing that does not have to be timed around food, and dose adjustment is not necessary in renal impairment.

Because constipation in advanced disease is generally multifactorial in origin, peripheral opioid antagonists will augment rather than replace laxatives.

Methylnaltrexone

Injection sites should be rotated, using soft, non-bruised areas of the abdomen or upper legs/arms.

Between 1/3–2/3 of patients given **methylnaltrexone** defaecate within 30min–4h.[35-40] Patients should be warned of the possibility of a rapid effect; those with reduced mobility should have immediate access to a commode.

Patients should discontinue **methylnaltrexone** and seek advice if they develop severe, persistent or worsening symptoms, e.g. abdominal pain, diarrhoea.

Patients with advanced illness (palliative care patients)

- continue all other laxative treatment
- the dose is based on the patient's weight:
  - ▷ 38–61kg: start with 8mg SC on alternate days
  - ▷ 62–114kg: start with 12mg SC on alternate days
  - ▷ outside this range: give *0.15mg/kg (150microgram/kg*) on alternate days
- for dose adjustment in renal impairment, see below
- the interval between administrations can be varied, either extended or reduced, but not more than once daily; in open-label extension studies, the median (range) interval between doses was 3 (1–39) days.

Trial data do not extend beyond 4 months in patients with advanced illness.

Patients with chronic pain but not advanced illness

- stop all other laxative treatment until the response to **methylnaltrexone** is known
- start with 12mg SC on alternate days, irrespective of the patient's weight
- if after 3 days there is an insufficient response, resume laxatives
- otherwise, follow guidance as above.

Trial data do not extend beyond 12 months in patients with chronic pain.

In severe renal impairment (creatinine clearance <30mL/min), reduce the dose:

- for patients weighing 62–114kg, reduce to 8mg
- outside this range, reduce to *0.075mg/kg* (*75microgram/kg*), rounding up the dose volume to the nearest 0.1mL.

Methylnaltrexone has not been studied in patients requiring dialysis and is not recommended in this setting.

Naldemedine

Half of subjects experience a bowel action after 5–18h. In studies, compared to patients with chronic non-cancer pain, a higher proportion of patients with cancer pain respond, and to a greater degree. Possible explanations include differences in opioid dose and body weight or continued use of regular vs. only p.r.n. laxatives. There is also a higher incidence of undesirable effects. Thus, although the SPC states that **naldemedine** can be taken with or without laxatives, it may be prudent to adopt a similar approach as with **naloxegol**, i.e. stop all other laxative treatment until the response to **naldemedine** is known, and resume laxatives after 3 days if there is an insufficient response.

Patients should discontinue **naldemedine** and seek advice if they develop severe, persistent or worsening symptoms, e.g. abdominal pain, diarrhoea:

- start with 200microgram PO once daily
- it can be taken at any time of day, but timing should be consistent.

Naloxegol

Half of subjects experience a bowel action after 6–12h, and about two-thirds within 24h.[22,41] Patients should discontinue **naloxegol** and seek advice if they develop severe, persistent or worsening symptoms, e.g. abdominal pain, diarrhoea:

- stop all other laxative treatment until the response to **naloxegol** is known
- start with **naloxegol** 25mg PO once daily, taken in the morning on an empty stomach, i.e. 30min before or 2h after breakfast
- ideally, the tablet should be swallowed whole; if necessary, it can be crushed to a powder, mixed in half a glass of water (120mL) and drunk immediately; refer to the SPC for administration via an NG tube
- if there is unacceptable abdominal pain/diarrhoea, reduce the dose to 12.5mg once daily
- if after 3 days there is an insufficient response, resume laxatives (necessary in about half of trial participants)
- use a starting dose of 12.5mg PO once daily if:
  - ▷ moderate–severe renal impairment (CrCl <60mL/min)
  - ▷ concurrent use of a *moderate* CYP3A4 *inhibitor* (see Drug interactions).

If tolerated and if necessary, increase after 2 days to 25mg once daily.

Supply

Methylnaltrexone

Relistor® (Bausch & Lomb)

Injection methylnaltrexone bromide 12mg/0.6mL, one vial = £21.

Naldemedine

Rizmoic® (Shionogi)

Tablets 200microgram, 28 days @ 200microgram once daily = £42.

Naloxegol

Moventig® (Kyowa Kirin)

Tablets naloxegol 12.5mg, 25mg, 28 days @ 12.5mg or 25mg each morning = £50.

---

1 Candy B *et al.* (2018) Mu-opioid antagonists for opioid-induced bowel dysfunction in people with cancer and people receiving palliative care. *Cochrane Database of Systematic Reviews*. **6**: CD006332. www.cochranelibrary.com

2 Becker G and Blum HE (2009) Novel opioid antagonists for opioid-induced bowel dysfunction and postoperative ileus. *Lancet*. **373**: 1198–1206.

3 Nusrat S *et al.* (2019) Pharmacological treatment of opioid-induced constipation is effective but choice of endpoints affects the therapeutic gain. *Digestive Diseases and Sciences*. **64**: 39–49.

4 Rauck R *et al.* (2017) Randomized, double-blind trial of oral methylnaltrexone for the treatment of opioid-induced constipation in patients with chronic noncancer pain. *Pain Practice*. **17**: 820–828.

5 Rauck RL *et al.* (2019) Safety of oral methylnaltrexone for opioid-induced constipation in patients with chronic noncancer pain. *Journal of Pain Research*. **12**: 139–150.

6 Ford AC *et al.* (2013) Efficacy of pharmacological therapies for the treatment of opioid-induced constipation: systematic review and meta-analysis. *American Journal of Gastroenterology*. **108**: 1566–1574.

7 Siemens W and Becker G (2016) Methylnaltrexone for opioid-induced constipation: review and meta-analyses for objective plus subjective efficacy and safety outcomes. *Therapeutics and Clinical Risk Management*. **12**: 401–412.

8 Nee J *et al.* (2018) Efficacy of treatments for opioid-induced constipation: systematic review and meta-analysis. *Clinical Gastroenterology and Hepatology*. **16**: 1569–1584.

9 Lopez J *et al.* (2016) Methylnaltrexone for the treatment of constipation in critically ill children. *Journal of Clinical Gastroenterology*. **50**: 351–352.

10 Flerlage JE and Baker JN (2015) Methylnaltrexone for opioid-induced constipation in children and adolescents and young adults with progressive incurable cancer at the end of life. *Journal of Palliative Medicine*. **18**: 631–633.
11 Rodrigues A *et al.* (2013) Methylnaltrexone for opioid-induced constipation in pediatric oncology patients. *Pediatric Blood and Cancer*. **60**: 1667–1670.
12 Deibert P *et al.* (2010) Methylnaltrexone: the evidence for its use in the management of opioid-induced constipation. *Core Evidence*. **4**: 247–258.
13 Anissian L *et al.* (2012) Subcutaneous methylnaltrexone for treatment of acute opioid-induced constipation: phase 2 study in rehabilitation after orthopedic surgery. *Journal of Hospital Medicine*. **7**: 67–72.
14 Zand F *et al.* (2015) The effect of methylnaltrexone on the side effects of intrathecal morphine after orthopedic surgery under spinal anesthesia. *Pain Practice*. **15**: 348–354.
15 Patel PB *et al.* (2020) Methylnaltrexone for the treatment of opioid-induced constipation and gastrointestinal stasis in intensive care patients. Results from the MOTION trial. *Intensive Care Medicine*. **46**: 747–755.
16 Weinstock LB and Chang AC (2011) Methylnaltrexone for treatment of acute colonic pseudo-obstruction. *Journal of Clinical Gastroenterology*. **45**: 883–884.
17 Hohl CM *et al.* (2015) Methylnaltrexone to palliate pruritus in terminal hepatic disease. *Journal of Palliative Care*. **31**: 124–126.
18 Katakami N *et al.* (2017) Randomized phase III and extension studies of naldemedine in patients with opioid-induced constipation and cancer. *Journal of Clinical Oncology*. **35**: 3859–3866.
19 Hale M *et al.* (2017) Naldemedine versus placebo for opioid-induced constipation (COMPOSE-1 and COMPOSE-2): two multicentre, phase 3, double-blind, randomised, parallel-group trials. *Lancet Gastroenterolgoy and Hepatology*. **2**: 555–564.
20 Webster LR *et al.* (2018) Long-term use of naldemedine in the treatment of opioid-induced constipation in patients with chronic noncancer pain: a randomized, double-blind, placebo-controlled phase 3 study. *Pain*. **159**: 987–994.
21 Katakami N *et al.* (2018) Randomized phase III and extension studies: efficacy and impacts on quality of life of naldemedine in subjects with opioid-induced constipation and cancer. *Annals of Oncology*. **29**: 1461–1467.
22 Chey WD *et al.* (2014) Naloxegol for opioid-induced constipation in patients with noncancer pain. *New England Journal of Medicine*. **370**: 2387–2396.
23 Astra Zeneca (2016) Personal communication.
24 Cobo Dols M *et al.* (2021) Efficacy of naloxegol on symptoms and quality of life related to opioid-induced constipation in patients with cancer: a 3-month follow-up analysis. *BMJ Supportive & Palliative Care*. **11**: 25–31.
25 Brenner DM *et al.* (2019) A randomized, multicenter, prospective, crossover, open-label study of factors associated with patient preferences for naloxegol or PEG 3350 for opioid-induced constipation. *American Journal of Gastroenterology*. **114**: 954–963.
26 Nelson KK *et al.* (2019) Methylnaltrexone is safe in cancer patients with peritoneal carcinomatosis. *Scientific Reports*. **9**: 9625.
27 Slatkin NE *et al.* (2011) Characterization of abdominal pain during methylnaltrexone treatment of opioid-induced constipation in advanced illness: a post hoc analysis of two clinical trials. *Journal of Pain and Symptom Management*. **42**: 754–760.
28 Mackey AC *et al.* (2010) Methylnaltrexone and gastrointestinal perforation. *Journal of Pain and Symptom Management*. **40**: e1–e3.
29 Ishii K *et al.* (2020) Naldemedine-induced opioid withdrawal syndrome in a patient with breast cancer without brain metastasis. *Internal Medicine*. **59**: 293–296.
30 NICE (2015) Naloxegol for opioid-induced constipation. *Technology Appraisal*. TA345. www.nice.org.uk.
31 Scottish Medicines Consortium (2015) Naloxegol (1106/15).
32 Anonymous (2015) Naloxegol for opioid-induced constitpation. *Drugs and Therapeutics Bulletin*. **53**: 138–140.
33 Larkin PJ *et al.* (2018) Diagnosis, assessment and management of constipation in advanced cancer: ESMO Clinical Practice Guidelines. *Annals of Oncology*. **29 (Suppl 4)**: 111–125.
34 NICE (2020) Naldemedine for treating opioid-induced constipation. *Technology Appraisal*. TA651. www.nice.org.uk.
35 Portenoy RK *et al.* (2008) Subcutaneous methylnaltrexone for the treatment of opioid-induced constipation in patients with advanced illness: a double-blind, randomized, parallel group, dose-ranging study. *Journal of Pain and Symptom Management*. **35**: 458–468.
36 Thomas J *et al.* (2008) Methylnaltrexone for opioid-induced constipation in advanced illness. *New England Journal of Medicine*. **358**: 2332–2343.
37 Slatkin N *et al.* (2009) Methylnaltrexone for treatment of opioid-induced constipation in advanced illness patients. *Journal of Supportive Oncology*. **7**: 39–46.
38 Michna E *et al.* (2011) Subcutaneous methylnaltrexone for treatment of opioid-induced constipation in patients with chronic, nonmalignant pain: a randomized controlled study. *Journal of Pain*. **12**: 554–562.
39 Candy B *et al.* (2011) Laxatives or methylnaltrexone for the management of constipation in palliative care patients. *Cochrane Database of Systematic Reviews*. **19**: CD003448. www.cochranelibrary.com.
40 Bull J *et al.* (2015) Fixed-dose subcutaneous methylnaltrexone in patients with advanced illness and opioid-induced constipation: results of a randomized, placebo-controlled study and open-label extension. *Journal of Palliative Medicine*. **18**: 593–600.
41 Webster L *et al.* (2014) Randomised clinical trial: the long-term safety and tolerability of naloxegol in patients with pain and opioid-induced constipation. *Alimentary Pharmacology and Therapeutics*. **40**: 771–779.

Updated (minor change) October 2021

6: INFECTIONS

6

ANTIBACTERIALS IN PALLIATIVE CARE

Remember: always ask about drug allergies before prescribing an antibacterial.

The dose and frequency of many antibacterials are reduced in renal impairment.

The *BNF* contains a comprehensive account of antibacterial use,[1] and many hospitals have antibacterial policies that govern local infection control and treatment, e.g. prevention of methicillin-resistant *Staphylococcus aureus* (MRSA) infection, prevention of *Clostridium difficile* infection. Thus, any specific recommendations about antibacterials in *PCF* should be considered together with local policy. When in doubt, seek advice from a local medical microbiologist.

Be aware that rigorously applied screening and infection control protocols will impose significant burdens at the end of life.[2]

Penicillin allergy

Allergic reactions to penicillins occur in 1–10% of exposed individuals, and anaphylaxis in <0.05%. Those with a history of urticaria, rash or anaphylaxis immediately after starting a course of a penicillin should not be prescribed a penicillin, a cephalosporin or other beta-lactam antibacterial.

Those with a history of a minor rash (e.g. non-confluent, non-pruritic rash restricted to a small area of the body) or a rash that occurs >72h after a penicillin is started are probably *not* allergic to penicillin, and a penicillin need not be withheld if indicated. However, the possibility of an allergic reaction should be kept in mind. Other beta-lactam antibacterials (including cephalosporins) can be used in these patients.[1]

Stop and think!

In a moribund patient with progressive incurable disease, are you justified in giving antibacterials for an intercurrent infection that may be the natural endpoint of the dying process?

Antibacterials in end-stage disease should have the primary purpose of ameliorating distressing symptoms (including fever and malaise) and not simply delaying inevitable death. It is important to *stop and think:* if antibacterials are automatically prescribed when infection is diagnosed, they may simply serve to prolong suffering.[3-5]

The potential for antibacterials to impact the survival of patients with advanced cancer varies with the type of infection and setting of the patient. For example, in hospital inpatients referred to a palliative care service, a prolonged survival was associated with the recent use of antibacterials for sepsis but not focal infection.[6] Overall, compared with patients with infections who did not receive antibacterials, this amounted to a difference in median survival of about 2–3 weeks. However, median survival differed by about 5 months (sepsis) and 2 months (focal infection) between patients deemed to have had a good vs. a poor initial response to the antibacterials, with the latter surviving only about 1 and 3 weeks respectively.[6] On the other hand, in a community-based hospice programme, the presence of infection or the use of antibacterials made no difference to the median survival of patients of about 30 days.[7]

Nonetheless, whatever the setting, in addition to symptom relief, clinicians should balance the potential for any benefit from extra time gained by the use of antibacterials with the burden of irreversible progressive physical deterioration. Thus, antibacterials are generally appropriate for a patient with advanced cancer who develops a chest infection while still relatively active and independent. However, in someone who has become bedbound as a result of general progressive deterioration and who seems close to death, pneumonia should still be allowed to be 'the old person's friend'. In such circumstances, it is generally appropriate *not* to prescribe antibacterials and to 'give death a chance'.

Although some terminally ill patients recover from a chest infection without an antibacterial, others progress to a 'grumbling pneumonia'. A continuing wet cough may cause much distress and possibly loss of sleep. If this is the case, an antibacterial may be indicated for symptom relief.

When it is difficult to make a decision, a '2-day rule' could be invoked: if after 2 days of general symptom management the patient is clinically stable, prescribe an antibacterial, but, if the patient is clearly much worse, do not. Conversely, given the poor survival of those who fail to have a good initial response to antibacterials,[6] there is also a need for a reverse '2-day rule': namely, discontinue antibacterials after a few days if there is no apparent response, particularly if the patient is now moribund.

General considerations

Evidence for symptom improvement with antibacterials at the end of life remains patchy. Only 8 of 11 studies in a systematic review of antibacterial use in hospice patients considered symptom response as an outcome following antibacterial therapy.[8]

Several surveys give similar prevalence rates for *symptomatic* infection in palliative care patients, namely about 40%,[7] and show that the response to antibacterials varies according to the type of infection (Table 1). Provided a patient does not have an indwelling urinary catheter, UTIs should generally be treated routinely unless there is an overriding reason for not doing so (see p.521).[6,9] Cough caused by infection is also significantly reduced by antibacterials.[9] On the other hand, in patients with end-stage progressive disease being cared for at home, the use of antibacterials to treat sepsis is generally futile (Table 1).

Table 1 Response to antimicrobials[a] in >600 home-care patients[7]

Type of infection	*Number*	*Response (%)*[b]
UTI	265	79
RTI	221	43
Oral cavity[a]	63	46
Skin or SC	59	41
Sepsis	25	0

a. includes the use of antibacterials for infections at all sites, and of antifungals for oral candidosis

b. reduction of fever ± amelioration of site-specific symptoms within 3 days.

Specific recommendations

The specific information given in this chapter is limited to selected situations that may occur in palliative care:

- local infection causing severe pain
- ascending cholangitis associated with a biliary stent
- infection associated with an airway stent
- respiratory tract infection in the dying patient
- cellulitis in patients with lymphoedema (p.529).

Note. Generally, to ensure adequate plasma concentrations, it is recommended that antibacterials are prescribed at consistent regular intervals, e.g. q6h, q8h or q12h, and this should be adhered to in patients with severe infection, particularly those needing IV antibacterials. However, in patients approaching the last days of life, particularly those taking PO antibacterials, a more pragmatic and less rigorous administration, e.g. q.d.s., t.d.s., b.d., can be considered.

Antibacterials to relieve infection-related pain

Antibacterials are essential in some patients for the relief of severe pain associated with infection around a malignant tumour in, e.g., the neck, the gluteal muscles underlying an ulcerated cancer, or the perineum.[10] Sometimes there is a history of a rapid increase in pain intensity over several days that is poorly responsive to escalating doses of a strong opioid. The pain is often associated with fever and malaise and may be complicated by delirium. Commonly, there will be a mixture of more superficial aerobic infection with deeper anaerobic infection. Treatment is similar to that recommended for ascending cholangitis (see below).

Ascending cholangitis

Ascending cholangitis may occur in patients with a partially obstructed or stented common bile duct. It often causes severe systemic disturbance and should be treated promptly:

- **piperacillin/tazobactam** 4.5g IVI over 30min q8h *or*
- if a minor rash with a penicillin in the past (see p.507), **cefuroxime** 1.5g IV q8h plus **metronidazole** 500mg IVI over 20–60min q8h
- if the patient is in septic shock, also give a single dose of **gentamicin** 5mg/kg (maximum dose 500mg) IV over 20–30min
- if a risk of multiresistant Gram-negative bacilli, serious penicillin allergy or in any doubt, consult a medical microbiologist.

When IV administration is difficult, authorized alternatives include:

- **ceftazidime** 1–2g IM q8h; a maximum of 1g is given per injection site, reconstituted with 3mL **lidocaine** 0.5–1% solution (total injection volume about 3.8mL)
- **ceftriaxone** 1–2g IM once daily; a maximum of 1g is given per injection site, reconstituted with 3.5mL **lidocaine** 1% solution (total injection volume about 4mL); SC use also reported (off-label; see below).

The doses and/or frequency of **cefuroxime**, **ceftazidime**, **piperacillin/tazobactam** and **gentamicin** should be reduced in renal impairment.

Infection associated with an airway stent

The presence of an airway stent, whether for cancer or other obstruction, increases the risk of serious respiratory tract infection.[11] In a systematic review of 500 patients, mortality rate was almost 70%.[12] Commonest pathogens are *Staphylococcus aureus* and *Pseudomonas aeruginosa*. Treatment should be commenced promptly and guided by the advice of a medical microbiologist.

Respiratory tract infection in the imminently dying patient

Occasionally, death rattle (noisy respiratory secretions) is caused by profuse purulent sputum from a chest infection, and an antibacterial is prescribed in the hope that it will reduce the copious purulent, malodorous discharge from the mouth.[13] In this circumstance, the IV route is generally the best. However, if not practical, the IM or SC routes can be used instead.[14-17]

Some centres use single doses of **ceftriaxone**; either 1–2g IV or 1g IM reconstituted with 3.5mL **lidocaine** 1% (total injection volume about 4mL).[13] **Ceftriaxone** is a broad-spectrum antibacterial and has a long duration of action. Patients who responded did so within hours (marked reduction in purulent sputum and resolution of associated halitosis). Non-responders appeared not to benefit from a second dose after 24h.

Other centres give **ceftriaxone** by SC injection (off-label)[16-19] and administer multiple doses if a patient survives >1 day, e.g. **ceftriaxone** 250mg–1g SC once daily (prepared from 1g vial reconstituted with 2.2mL **lidocaine** 1%; total injection volume about 2.8mL). If the authorized larger volume of 3.5mL **lidocaine** 1% is added (total injection volume about 4mL), the mixture can be administered as a divided dose, given at the same time but using two or more separate SC/IM sites.[20]

Survey results suggest that the above is reasonably well tolerated, and it has been used for ≤10 days when patients have not been imminently dying.[14,16]

The bio-availability (in volunteers) of SC **cefepime** is comparable with IM.[21] Further, when 1g is infused over 30min, pain at the injection site is absent or minimal. Thus, **cefepime** could be a useful option. Concern about the safety of **cefepime**[22] has been shown to be groundless.[23]

Although other antimicrobials have also been given SC, supporting data, except for **ertapenem**,[24] are generally lacking.[17]

Supply

Cefuroxime (generic)

Injection (powder for reconstitution) 250mg, 750mg, 1.5g (IV only), 2 days @ 1.5g t.d.s. = £30.

Ceftazidime (generic)

Injection (powder for reconstitution) 1g, 2g, 2 days @ 1g t.d.s. = £47.

Ceftriaxone (generic)

Injection (powder for reconstitution) 1g vial = £10, 2g vial = £20.

Gentamicin sulfate (generic)

Injection 40mg/mL, 2mL amp or vial = £1.50.

Piperacillin/tazobactam (generic)

Injection (powder for reconstitution) piperacillin 2g/tazobactam 250mg, piperacillin 4g/tazobactam 500mg, 2 days @ 4.5g t.d.s = £30.

Also see **metronidazole**, p.515.

1 British National Formulary, Chapter 5 Infections: Antibacterials. London: BMJ Group and Pharmaceutical Press. www.medicinescomplete.com (accessed October 2019).
2 Bukki J *et al.* (2013) Methicillin-resistant *Staphylococcus aureus* (MRSA) management in palliative care units and hospices in Germany: a nationwide survey on patient isolation policies and quality of life. *Palliative Medicine*. **27**: 84–90.
3 Lam PT *et al.* (2005) Retrospective analysis of antibiotic use and survival in advanced cancer patients with infections. *Journal of Pain and Symptom Management*. **30**: 536–543.
4 Thompson AJ *et al.* (2012) Antimicrobial use at the end of life among hospitalized patients with advanced cancer. *American Journal of Hospice and Palliative Care*. **29**: 599–603.
5 Albrecht JS *et al.* (2013) A nationwide analysis of antibiotic use in hospice care in the final week of life. *Journal of Pain and Symptom Management*. **46**: 483–490.
6 Thai V *et al.* (2012) Impact of infections on the survival of hospitalized advanced cancer patients. *Journal of Pain and Symptom Management*. **43**: 549–557.
7 Reinbolt RE *et al.* (2005) Symptomatic treatment of infections in patients with advanced cancer receiving hospice care. *Journal of Pain and Symptom Management*. **30**: 175–182.
8 Rosenberg JH *et al.* (2013) Antimicrobial use for symptom management in patients receiving hospice and palliative care: a systematic review. *Journal of Palliative Medicine*. **16**: 1568–1574.
9 Mirhosseini M *et al.* (2006) The role of antibiotics in the management of infection-related symptoms in advanced cancer patients. *Journal of Palliative Care*. **22**: 69–74.
10 Bruera E and MacDonald N (1986) Intractable pain in patients with advanced head and neck tumors: a possible role of local infection. *Cancer Treatment Reports*. **70**: 691–692.
11 Grosu HB *et al.* (2013) Stents are associated with increased risk of respiratory infections in patients undergoing airway interventions for malignant airways disease. *Chest*. **144**: 441–449.
12 Agrafiotis M *et al.* (2009) Infections related to airway stenting: a systematic review. *Respiration*. **78**: 69–74.
13 Spruyt O and Kausae A (1998) Antibiotic use for infective terminal respiratory secretions. *Journal of Pain and Symptom Management*. **15**: 263–264.
14 palliativedrugs.com (2010) Survey: SC/IM antibiotics – do you use this route? www.palliativedrugs.com.
15 Azevedo EF (2012) Administration of antibiotics subcutaneously: an integrative literature review. *Acta Paulista de Enfermagem*. **25**: 817–822.
16 Gauthier D *et al.* (2014) Subcutaneous and intravenous ceftriaxone administration in patients more than 75 years of age. *Medicine et Maladies Infectieuses*. **44**: 275–280.
17 Roubaud-Baudron C *et al.* (2017) Tolerance of subcutaneously administered antibiotics: a French national prospective study. *Age and ageing*. **46**: 151–155.
18 Borner K *et al.* (1985) Comparative pharmacokinetics of ceftriaxone after subcutaneous and intravenous administration. *Chemotherapy*. **31**: 237–245.
19 Bricaire F *et al.* (1988) Pharmacokinetics and tolerance of ceftriaxone after subcutaneous administration. *Pathologie Biologie (Paris)*. **36**: 702–705.
20 Tahmasebi M S/C injection of antibiotics. *Bulletin board (August 2005)*. http://www.palliativedrugs.com.
21 Walker P *et al.* (2005) Subcutaneous administration of cefepime. *Journal of Pain and Symptom Management*. **30**: 170–174.
22 Yahav D *et al.* (2007) Efficacy and safety of cefepime: a systematic review and meta-analysis. *The Lancet Infectious Diseases*. **7**: 338–348.
23 FDA (2009) Cefepime (marketed as Maxipime) update of ongoing safety review. www.fda.gov/drugs/drugsafety (Archived).
24 Ferry T *et al.* (2012) Prolonged subcutaneous high dose (1 g bid) of Ertapenem as salvage therapy in patients with difficult-to-treat bone and joint infection. *Journal of Infection*. **65**: 579–582.

Updated October 2019

ORAL CANDIDOSIS

Oral yeast carriage is present in about one third of the general population. The prevalence in patients with advanced cancer is significantly higher (about 50–90%).[1] Thus, it is not surprising that oral candidosis is a common fungal infection in the palliative care population of patients (13–30%).[2-4]

Many patients with oral candidosis have concurrent oesophageal infection,[5] and some patients develop systemic fungal infections. Oral candidosis is associated with:

- poor performance status
- dry mouth
- poor denture hygiene
- topical antibacterials and/or corticosteroids
- in AIDS, with CD4 cell count <200cells/mm^3.[1,2]

Oral candidosis is *not* associated with the use of oral/parenteral antibacterials, and most data suggest that it is *not* associated with the use of oral/parenteral corticosteroids.[6]

Non-*Candida albicans* species are increasingly being isolated from patients with oral candidosis.[2,3] The reason for this is thought to be related to increased use of antifungal drugs; the consequence of this change is an increased incidence of azole drug resistance (many non-*Candida albicans* species exhibit inherent azole drug resistance).[4,7]

Management strategy

Correct the correctable

Underlying causal factors must be considered and corrected if possible, particularly dry mouth and poor denture hygiene.

Dentures must be thoroughly cleaned at least once daily, brushing the denture with a toothbrush, nailbrush or denture brush, and using soap and water or an appropriate commercial product.[8] Dentures should also be soaked for several minutes in an appropriate antiseptic, e.g. **chlorhexidine** or dilute **sodium hypochlorite**. The latter should not be used for dentures with metal parts. Failure to sterilize the denture will lead to failure of antifungal treatment. The dentures should be thoroughly rinsed before re-insertion.

Drug treatment

A systematic review concluded that there was limited evidence about the efficacy of antifungal drugs in patients with cancer, but that there was some evidence that drugs absorbed from the GI tract are more effective than drugs not absorbed from the GI tract.[9]

Nystatin suspension is a good choice for mild oral candidosis in non-immunocompromised patients.[10] Success requires sufficient drug contact with the lesions; the use of larger dose volumes, e.g. 4–6mL, increases efficacy.[11] **Miconazole** oral gel is a topical alternative.[12]

Fluconazole is the preferred choice for moderate–severe infections, oesophageal candidosis, patients who are immunocompromised, and in those who cannot use **nystatin**.[11] **Itraconazole** is generally reserved for those with **fluconazole**-resistant infection; drug interactions are more likely (see below), and PO bio-availability is variable. Other alternatives in this setting are **posaconazole** and **voriconazole**.

The non-fasting PO bio-availability of **itraconazole** is around 55%. Because an acidic environment is needed to obtain maximal absorption from *capsules*, administration with food is recommended. Hypochlorhydria and acid-reducing drugs decrease absorption (also see Drug interactions). In contrast, the *oral solution* is not dependent on an acidic environment for absorption, and the PO bio-availability is >80% when administered on an empty stomach. Because of the difference in bio-availability, the formulations are *not* interchangeable. (Note. The capsules are authorized for oral candidosis generally, but the higher bio-available oral solution only for use in oral/oesophageal candidosis in immunocompromised patients.)

Cross-resistance and cross-infection do occur and, if there is a high prevalence of azole resistance within the local patient population, then even azole-naïve patients may be infected with azole-resistant organisms.[13] Local treatment protocols must take this into account, and alternative antifungals may be required.

Potential topical treatments in resistant cases (or other special circumstances) include **chlorhexidine**,[1] **gentian violet** (e.g. 0.5–1%, 1.5mL applied twice daily)[14] and tea tree oil.[15]

Cautions

Because of a teratogenic risk with **fluconazole** and **itraconazole**, the manufacturers advise that women of child-bearing potential should use contraceptive precautions until the next menstrual period after completing treatment. Because of similar toxicological findings in animal studies with other azoles, it would be wise to extend this precaution to **miconazole**.

Itraconazole may cause or worsen left ventricular dysfunction or CHF and is contra-indicated unless its use is necessitated by life-threatening infection.
Renal impairment: reduce dose of **fluconazole** by 50% if creatinine clearance is <50mL/min; the bio-availability of oral **itraconazole** may be reduced in renal impairment (also see Chapter 17, p.731).
Hepatic impairment: serious or fatal hepatotoxicity may occur with **fluconazole** and **itraconazole**. The manufacturers advise monitoring liver function in patients receiving large doses and/or prolonged courses, and in patients with known liver dysfunction. With both drugs, treatment should be discontinued if symptoms suggestive of hepatotoxicity develop, e.g. jaundice, dark urine.

MHRA has issued an alert for products or medical devices containing **chlorhexidine**, following reports of anaphylaxis.[16]

Drug interactions

Azole antifungals have a strong inhibitory effect on human cytochrome P450 enzymes, particularly CYP3A4 (see Chapter 19, p.781). This results in inhibition of adrenal steroid synthesis (cortisol, testosterone, oestrogens and progesterone) and the metabolism of many drugs.

Drug interactions are most likely with **itraconazole**. They are generally less likely and less pronounced with **fluconazole** (a weaker CYP inhibitor), although several clinically important interactions have been reported.[17] With maximum doses of **miconazole** oromucosal gel, systemic absorption can be sufficient to cause significant interactions, e.g. with **warfarin**.[18]

Avoid concurrent administration of **fluconazole**, **itraconazole** or **miconazole** with:

- drugs metabolized by CYP3A4 which are known to prolong the QT interval, e.g. **amiodarone**, **astemizole** (not UK), **domperidone**, **erythromycin**, **methadone**, **pimozide** or **quinidine**, because of a risk of fatal cardiac arrhythmias (also see Chapter 20, p.797)
- statins metabolized by CYP3A4, e.g. **atorvastatin**, **lovastatin** and **simvastatin**
- ergot alkaloids, e.g. **ergotamine**
- **eletriptan**, **naloxegol**, **triazolam** (not UK) and PO **midazolam** (not UK).

Fluconazole, **itraconazole** or **miconazole** may increase the plasma concentration of all drugs metabolized by CYP3A4 (see Chapter 19, Table 8, p.790), and thus increase undesirable effects or toxicity. Box A lists drugs used in palliative care where increased plasma concentrations have been reported.

Box A Drugs which may require dose reduction if used concurrently with an azole[a,17]

Alfentanil	Haloperidol
Alprazolam	Loperamide
Aprepitant	Methylprednisolone
Budesonide (inhaled)	Midazolam
Carbamazepine	Nifedipine
Dexamethasone	Phenytoin
Digoxin	Risperidone
Fentanyl	Theophylline
Fluticasone (inhaled)	TCAs
Glibenclamide	Warfarin
Glipizide	

a. generally, drug interactions are more likely with itraconazole>fluconazole>miconazole; significant interactions can occur with miconazole gel (see text).

Strong CYP3A4 inducers, e.g. **carbamazepine**, **phenytoin**, **phenobarbital**, **rifampicin**, **rifabutin** and possibly *Hypericum perforatum* (**St John's wort**), reduce **fluconazole** and **itraconazole** plasma concentrations, which may result in antifungal treatment failure.

The absorption of **itraconazole** (but not **fluconazole**) is affected by antacids, **sucralfate**, H_2-receptor antagonists, PPIs or food (see above).

Table 1 Antifungal treatment[11,20]

Class	*Drug*	*Recommended regimen*	*Comments*	*Cost for lowest dose for 7 days*
Polyene group	Nystatin[a]	***Oral suspension*** 100,000 units/mL; 4–6mL q.d.s. for 7–14 days (continue for 48h after lesions disappear)	For mild infection. Smaller volumes make it more difficult to hold against lesions	£7
	Amphotericin[a] (not UK)	***Lozenges*** 10mg; 1 lozenge q.d.s. for 10–15 days (continue for 48h after lesions disappear)	For mild infection	Not available in the UK
Azole group (imidazoles)	Miconazole[a]	***Oral gel*** 20mg/g; 5–10mL oral gel q.d.s. for 7–14 days (continue for 48h after lesions disappear)	For mild infection. Useful in management of denture stomatitis and angular cheilitis (has anti-staphylococcal action). Smaller volumes of gel (i.e. 2.5mL) may suffice in localized lesions	£7.50
Azole group (triazoles)	Fluconazole	***Capsules*** 50mg, 150mg, 200mg *or* ***Oral suspension***[a] 50mg/5mL, 200mg/5mL; 100–200mg once daily for 7–14 days; use as a mouthwash and swallow	For moderate–severe infection. Immunosuppressed[b] patients and those with oesophageal infection require higher doses (e.g. 200–400mg once daily) for longer (e.g. 14–21 days)	£1.25 (capsules) £35 (oral suspension)
	Itraconazole	***Capsules*** 100mg; 100mg once daily for 7–14 days	For moderate–severe infection resistant to fluconazole. In immunosuppressed[b] patients, use 200mg once daily for 14–21 days	£2 (capsules)
		Oral solution[a,c] 10mg/mL; 200mg (20mL) once daily for 7–14 days; use as a mouthwash and swallow	Authorized for immunosuppressed[b] patients; when fluconazole-resistant infection, use 200mg (20mL) b.d. for 2–4 weeks	£55 (oral solution)

a. treatments with a topical action should be taken after food and drink (avoid for 1h after use) with dentures removed and held near the oral lesions for as long as possible (≥1min) before swallowing; for denture-related candidiasis, dentures should also be disinfected (see Management strategy, Correct the correctable above)

b. e.g. patients with neutropenia or HIV/AIDS

c. because of the difference in bio-availability, the oral solution is *not* interchangeable with the capsules on a mg for mg basis (see Management strategy, Drug treatment above).

Undesirable effects

Common (<10%, >1%): headache (azole antifungals); dizziness (**fluconazole** and **itraconazole**); GI symptoms, e.g. dyspepsia, nausea and vomiting, abdominal pain, diarrhoea (**fluconazole** and **itraconazole**); rashes; pruritus; hypokalaemia (**fluconazole** and **itraconazole**).
Uncommon, rare or very rare (<1%): anaphylaxis, hepatitis, cholestasis, hepatic failure, adrenal suppression (**itraconazole**), reduced libido, gynaecomastia, impotence, menstrual disturbances.

Dose, use and supply

See Table 1. With topical treatment, dentures should be removed temporarily before each dose is given. With topical treatment and **itraconazole** *oral solution*, food and drink should be avoided for 1h after each dose. Note:

- because **chlorhexidine** binds to **nystatin** and leads to inactivation of both drugs, **chlorhexidine** mouthwash should *not* be used at the same time as **nystatin** oral suspension.[19] The problem can be avoided if **chlorhexidine** is used ≥30min before **nystatin**
- the absorption of **itraconazole** capsules is improved if taken with an acidic drink, e.g. cola.

1 Finlay I and Davies A (2005) Fungal Infections. In: Davies A and Finlay I (eds), *Oral Care in Advanced Disease*. Oxford: Oxford University Press. pp. 55–71.
2 Davies AN *et al.* (2006) Oral candidosis in patients with advanced cancer. *Oral Oncology*. **42**: 698–702.
3 Davies AN *et al.* (2008) Oral candidosis in community-based patients with advanced cancer. *Journal of Pain and Symptom Management*. **35**: 508–514.
4 Astvad K *et al.* (2015) Oropharyngeal Candidiasis in Palliative Care Patients in Denmark. *Journal of Palliative Medicine*. **18**: 940–944.
5 Samonis G *et al.* (1998) Oropharyngeal candidiasis as a marker for esophageal candidiasis in patients with cancer. *Clinical Infectious Diseases*. **27**: 283–286.
6 Samaranayake L (1990) Host factors and oral candidosis. In: Samaranayake L and MacFarlane T (eds), *Oral Candidosis*. London: Wright. pp. 66–103.
7 Bagg J *et al.* (2003) High prevalence of non-albicans yeasts and detection of anti-fungal resistance in the oral flora of patients with advanced cancer. *Palliative Medicine*. **17**: 477–481.
8 Sweeney P and Davies A (2010) Oral hygiene. In: Davies A and Epstein J (eds), *Oral Complications of Cancer and its Management*. Oxford: Oxford University Press. pp. 43–51.
9 Worthington HV *et al.* (2010) Interventions for treating oral candidiasis for patients with cancer receiving treatment. *Cochrane Database of Systematic Reviews*. **7**: CD001972. www.thecochranelibrary.com.
10 Lyu X *et al.* (2016) Efficacy of nystatin for the treatment of oral candidiasis: a systematic review and meta-analysis. *Drug design, development and therapy*. **10**: 1161–1171.
11 Pappas PG *et al.* (2016) Clinical practice guideline for the management of candidiasis: 2016 update by the Infectious Diseases Society of America. *Clinical Infectious Diseases*. **62**: e1–50.
12 Zhang LW *et al.* (2016) Efficacy and safety of miconazole for oral candidiasis: a systematic review and meta-analysis. *Oral Diseases*. **22**: 185–195.
13 Davies A *et al.* (2006) Antifungal drug resistance amongst yeasts isolated from patients with advanced cancer. *Supportive Care in Cancer*. **14**: 645.
14 Nyst MJ *et al.* (1992) Gentian violet, ketoconazole and nystatin in oropharyngeal and esophageal candidiasis in Zairian AIDS patients. *Annales de la Societe Belge de Medecine Tropicale*. **72**: 45–52.
15 Vazquez J (1999) Options for the management of mucosal candidiasis in patients with AIDS and HIV infection. *Pharmacotherapy*. **19**: 76–87.
16 MHRA (2012) All medical devices and medicinal products containing chlorhexidine. Risk of anaphylactic reaction due to chlorhexidine allergy. *Medical Devices Alert*. MDA/2012/2075. www.gov.uk/drug-device-alerts.
17 Baxter K and Preston CL *Stockley's Drug Interactions*. London: Pharmaceutical Press. www.medicinescomplete.com (accessed December 2017).
18 MHRA (2016) Topical miconazole, including oral gel: reminder of potential for serious interactions with warfarin. *Drug Safety Update*. www.gov.uk/drug-safety-update.
19 Barkvoll P and Attramadal A (1989) Effect of nystatin and chlorhexidine digluconate on Candida albicans. *Oral Surgery Oral Medicine and Oral Pathology*. **67**: 279–281.
20 Davies A (2015) Oral Care. In: Cherny NI et al. (eds), *Oxford Textbook of Palliative Medicine*, 5th edn. Eds Cherny NI *et al.* Oxford University Press, Oxford, UK.

Updated (minor change) November 2021

METRONIDAZOLE

Class: Antibacterial and antiprotozoal.

Indications: Anaerobic and protozoal infections, *Helicobacter pylori* eradication (as part of combination treatment), malodour caused by fungating cancers (topical gel), †pseudomembranous colitis.

Pharmacology

Metronidazole is highly active against anaerobic or microaerophilic bacteria and protozoa. It is a prodrug, with low intracellular oxygen concentrations favouring conversion into the active form. Metronidazole does not require a specific transport mechanism to enter cells and reacts with multiple cellular targets; consequently, compared with other antibacterials, resistance to metronidazole is uncommon.

Metronidazole, either systemically (PO or IV) or topically, is used to reduce malodour from fungating cancers and decubitus ulcers.[1] The malodour is caused by dimethyl trisulfide and volatile fatty acids produced by bacteria colonizing moist necrotic tissue.[2]

Metronidazole is metabolized in the liver; the main hydroxy metabolite has antibacterial activity. Accumulation may occur in severe hepatic impairment and can exacerbate hepatic encephalopathy (see Chapter 18, p.753). In renal impairment, there is no accumulation of metronidazole, and no dose adjustment is necessary. The hydroxy metabolite does accumulate; this is of uncertain clinical significance. Note. **Tinidazole** (not UK) is similar to metronidazole, with a longer duration of action (it is given either b.d. or once daily).[3] It causes less GI disturbance than metronidazole.

Bio-availability 80–100% PO; 60–80% PR; 60% gel PV, 25% pessary PV.

Onset of action 20–60min PO; 5–12h PR.

Time to peak plasma concentration 1–2h PO; 3h PR.

Plasma halflife 6–11h.

Duration of action 8–12h.

Cautions

Hepatic impairment (see Dose and use). Monitoring of FBC and LFTs advised with systemic use >10 days (see Undesirable effects). Concurrent use of alcohol (see Drug interactions). May exacerbate existing neurological disease. Photosensitivity (topical gel).

Drug interactions

Metronidazole can increase the INR in patients taking **warfarin** or coumarins; there are case reports of increased plasma concentrations of **ciclosporin, fluorouracil, lithium** and **phenytoin**.

The metabolism of metronidazole is increased by **phenobarbital** and possibly **phenytoin**; consider a 2–3 times increase in the dose of metronidazole if not achieving the desired clinical effect.[4]

Metronidazole has been linked to a **disulfiram**-like reaction with alcohol.[5] Like **disulfiram**, metabolites of metronidazole can inhibit alcohol dehydrogenase, xanthine oxidase and aldehyde dehydrogenase. This could lead to acidosis, noradrenaline (norepinephrine) excess, and accumulation of acetaldehyde,[6] the latter being responsible for symptoms such as flushing, headaches, epigastric discomfort, nausea and vomiting. However, there is *no* hard evidence of a clinically important reaction between alcohol and metronidazole, rather the reverse.[4,5]

Even so, because of warnings in the PIL and SPC, patients should be advised that they may experience mild anorexia, and sometimes vomiting, if they drink alcohol when taking metronidazole. Any risk with topical or PV metronidazole is presumably lower because of smaller doses and lower systemic absorption.[7] In the USA (but not the UK), patients are advised to avoid liquid medicines containing alcohol during metronidazole treatment.

Undesirable effects

Very common (>10%): abdominal pain, nausea and vomiting, diarrhoea.

Common (<10%, >1%): skin irritation (topical use).

Very rare (<0.01%): epilepsy, encephalopathy, aseptic meningitis, optic neuropathy, peripheral neuropathy (dose-related, generally reversible on discontinuation), blood dyscrasias (neutropenia, thrombocytopenia, pancytopenia), cholestatic hepatitis, pancreatitis (generally reversible on discontinuation), darkening of urine (due to metabolite).

Dose and use

Limit dose to a maximum of 400mg PO b.d. in elderly, frail patients and 400mg PO once daily if significant hepatic impairment, e.g. patients with incipient or actual hepatic encephalopathy.

Anaerobic infections

- metronidazole 400mg PO t.d.s. for 1 week; administration with food may reduce the risk of nausea and vomiting.

Oral suspensions are available for those with swallowing difficulties, but are significantly more expensive and best taken on an empty stomach (also see Chapter 28, Table 2, p.863).

If PO is not possible, metronidazole can be given IV or PR. Standard practice is 500mg IVI q8h for 1 week, or 1g PR t.d.s for 3 days then 1g b.d. for a further 4 days.

Malodour caused by a fungating cancer

Topical

High-quality evidence of topical use is limited,[8,9] but most patients appear to benefit.[10-13] About half report complete resolution of the odour. Improvement generally occurs within 2 days but can take up to 1 month.[12] Topical application to a fungating cancer can be considered when:

- the cancer is relatively small (and thus easily accessible for topical application)
- the cancer is very sloughy and poorly vascularized (which will reduce systemic access by metronidazole)
- systemic treatment is impractical, e.g. because of dysphagia
- systemic treatment causes unacceptable effects.

The metronidazole is applied as a 0.75% gel:[1,11,14]

- after cleansing the wound, apply the gel liberally, about 1g/cm^2
- pack large cavities with paraffin gauze smeared in the gel
- cover with a non-adherent and then an absorbent dressing
- repeat once daily–b.d. as long as beneficial.

Traditionally, some centres have used a crushed 200mg tablet in lubricating gel; others crush a 500mg tablet and sprinkle the powder directly onto the wound once or twice daily.[15,16] These approaches are off-label, but cheaper (see Supply).

Note. Supporting data for topical use relate mostly to patients in richer countries. The situation in poorer countries is generally different, with, typically, late referrals and deeper inaccessible infection. In these circumstances, PO treatment is better.

Systemic

After the initial treatment, a maintenance dose of metronidazole is continued indefinitely (Box A).[17]

Preliminary data from one centre in India suggests that maintenance metronidazole to reduce malodour from locally recurrent/residual carcinoma of the cervix also reduces the risk of vesicovaginal and rectovaginal fistula formation.[18]

Box A Metronidazole for malodourous fungating cancer[17]

Odour classification

SNIFFF: Smell Nil (absent), Faint (not offensive), Foul (offensive but tolerable) or Forbidding (offensive and intolerable).

Malodour regimen

Regardless of severity, start with metronidazole 400mg PO t.d.s.

Review after 1 week and continue treatment based on SNIFFF test:

- *Nil or Faint*: 200mg once daily indefinitely
- *Foul*: continue 400mg t.d.s. for 1 more week; then 200mg once daily indefinitely
- *Forbidding*: continue 400mg t.d.s. for 2 more weeks; then 200mg twice daily indefinitely.

If there is concern that the patient may not attend for review, give information about continuing treatment at the initial appointment.

General care

Teach low-cost home-based wound care, and environmental hygiene.

6

Supply

Metronidazole (generic)

Tablets 200mg, 400mg, 7 days @ 400mg t.d.s. = £4.
Tablets 500mg, 7 days @ 500mg t.d.s. = £39.
Oral suspension (as benzoate) 200mg/5mL, 7 days @ 400mg t.d.s. = £70.
IV infusion 5mg/mL, 100mL = £3.25.

Flagyl® (Sanofi)
Suppositories 500mg, 1g, 3 days @ 1g t.d.s. and 4 days @ 1g b.d. = £39.

Topical products
Anabact® (CHS)
Gel 0.75%, 15g = £5.75, 30g = £8, 40g = £16.

Metrogel® (Galderma)
Gel 0.75%, 40g = £23.

Note. Other topical metronidazole creams and gels are available; they are authorized for exacerbation of rosacea and are generally more expensive.
Crushing 200mg tablets in lubricating gel or crushing 500mg tablets directly into the wound cost about £0.70 or £2 respectively per topical application compared with £5.75 for proprietary gel.

Zydoval® (Mylan)
Vaginal gel 0.75%, 40g pack with 5 applicators = £4.25. *One applicator delivers a 5g dose of metronidazole 0.75%.*

1 Finlay IG *et al.* (1996) The effect of topical 0.75% metronidazole gel on malodorous cutaneous ulcers. *Journal of Pain and Symptom Management.* **11**: 158–162.
2 Shirasu M *et al.* (2009) Dimethyl trisulfide as a characteristic odor associated with fungating cancer wounds. *Bioscience, Biotechnology and Biochemistry.* **73**: 2117–2120.
3 Carmine AA *et al.* (1982) Tinidazole in anaerobic infections: a review of its antibacterial activity, pharmacological properties and therapeutic efficacy. *Drugs.* **24**: 85–117.
4 Preston CL. *Stockley's Drug Interactions.* London: Pharmaceutical Press www.medicinescomplete.com (accessed September 2021).
5 Williams CS and Woodcock KR (2000) Do ethanol and metronidazole interact to produce a disulfiram-like reaction? *Annals of Pharmacotherapy.* **34**: 255–257.
6 Harries D *et al.* (1990) Metronidazole and alcohol: potential problems. *Scottish Medical Journal.* **35**: 179–180.
7 Plosker G (1987) Possible interaction between ethanol and vaginally administered metronidazole. *Clinical Pharmacy.* **6**: 189–193.
8 Adderley U and Holt IG (2014) Topical agents and dressings for fungating wounds. *Cochrane Database of Systematic Reviews.* CD003948. www.cochranelibrary.com.
9 da Costa Santos CM *et al.* (2010) A systematic review of topical treatments to control the odor of malignant fungating wounds. *Journal of Pain and Symptom Management.* **39**: 1065–1076.
10 Gethin G *et al.* (2014) Current practice in the management of wound odour: an international survey. *International Journal of Nursing Studies.* **51**: 865–874.
11 Watanabe K *et al.* (2016) Safe and effective deodorization of malodorous fungating tumors using topical metronidazole 0.75 % gel (GK567): a multicenter, open-label, phase III study (RDT.07.SRE.27013). *Supportive Care in Cancer.* **24**: 2583–2590.
12 Kalinski C *et al.* (2005) Effectiveness of a topical formulation containing metronidazole for wound odor and exudate control. *Wounds.* **17**: 84–90.
13 Villela-Castro D *et al.* (2018) Polyhexanide versus metronidazole for odor management in malignant (fungating) wounds. A double-blinded randomized, clinical trial. *Journal of Wound, Ostomy & Continence Nursing.* **45**: 413–418.
14 Thomas S and Hay N (1991) The antimicrobial properties of two metronidazole medicated dressings used to treat malodorous wounds. *Pharmaceutical Journal.* **246**: 264–266.
15 Al-Arjeh G *et al.* (2020) Crushed metronidazole in managing chronic nonsurgical wound malodor in patients with cancer: preliminary findings. *Journal of Palliative Medicine.* **23**: 308–309.
16 Hu J *et al.* (2020) Successful management of malodor from fungating tumors using crushed metronidazole tablets. *JAAD Case Reports.* **6**: 26–29.
17 George R *et al.* (2017) Improving malodour management in advanced cancer: a 10-year retrospective study of topical, oral and maintenance metronidazole. *BMJ Supportive and Palliative Care.* **7**: 286–291.
18 George R *et al.* (2019) Regular low-dose oral metronidazole is associated with fewer vesicovaginal and rectovaginal fistulae in recurrent cervical cancer: results from a 10-year retrospective cohort. *Journal of Global Oncology.* **5**: 1–10.

Updated (minor change) September 2021

RIFAMPICIN

Class: Rifamycin antibacterial.

Indications: Infection (in combination with other antibacterials to treat tuberculosis, leprosy and serious staphylococcal infections; meningococcal prophylaxis), †cholestatic pruritus.[1,2]

Pharmacology

The bactericidal activity of rifampicin is due to inhibition of bacterial RNA polymerase. The antipruritic effect in cholestasis is mediated through agonist activity at the pregnane X receptor (PXR), which increases bile acid elimination and inhibits synthesis of the enzyme autotaxin.[1,3]

Previously, cholestatic pruritus was thought to be caused by bile acid accumulation, but plasma concentrations do not correlate with the severity of pruritus, nor with response to antipruritic treatments.[3] In contrast, autotaxin activity does correlate with the intensity of pruritus in cholestasis.[3] Autotaxin catalyses the conversion of cell membrane phospholipids to the lipid signalling molecule lysophosphatidic acid (LPA). The plasma concentration of LPA also correlates with the severity of cholestatic pruritus, and falls when there is benefit from rifampicin, bile acid sequestrants or biliary drainage.[4] How LPA causes pruritus in cholestasis is uncertain, but mechanisms may include nerve activation and altered immune function. In nerve cells, binding of LPA to the LPA_5 receptor can activate transient receptor potential ankyrin 1 (TRPA1) and vanilloid 1 (TRPV1) ion channels, both of which are associated with pruritus.[3] However, LPA levels can be increased in diseases not associated with pruritus, suggesting that additional cofactors may be involved.

Pooled RCT data (n=71) support the efficacy of rifampicin in cholestatic pruritus due to chronic liver disease, mostly primary biliary cholangitis (80%). In two of the trials (n=42), pruritus reduced by 25mm (95% CI −18 to −31mm) on a 100mm visual analogue scale.[5] The RCTs were short-term (≤2 weeks), but successful treatment for ≤2 years has been reported.[6] Thus, in this setting, rifampicin is recommended when bile acid sequestrants (e.g. **cholestyramine**) have not provided adequate symptom control.[1,2] **Sertraline** may also benefit cholestatic pruritus, but because of comparatively less RCT experience, specialty guidelines generally position it below rifampicin.[1,2] However, in a small RCT (n=36), **sertraline** (100mg once daily) and rifampicin (300mg once daily) provided similar benefit when first assessed after 4 weeks of use.[7] For the management of pruritus in complete biliary obstruction, see p.825.

The absorption of rifampicin is halved by food. Metabolites also have antibacterial effects and are excreted in bile (70%). Up to 30% of a dose is excreted in the urine, about half as unchanged drug. Halflife doubles in cirrhosis and acute or chronic hepatitis.[8,9]

Bio-availability ≥95%.[9]
Onset of action ≥2 days (for pruritus).[10]
Peak plasma concentration 2–4h.
Plasma halflife 3–5h initially; 2–3h after repeat dosing (due to auto-induction).
Duration of action no data for pruritus.

Cautions

Renal impairment (for doses >600mg/24h), hepatic impairment (see Dose and use). Jaundice is listed as a contra-indication by the UK manufacturer and a warning by the US manufacturer, but rifampicin was well tolerated in eight patients with jaundice and pruritus associated with hepatic metastases.[10] The risk of hepatotoxicity is increased with pre-existing hepatic impairment; monitor carefully when used for cholestatic pruritus (see Chapter 18, p.755).

Uncorrected vitamin K deficiency, see Undesirable effects.[11]

Drug interactions

Concurrent use with **isoniazid** and some antiretrovirals increases the risk of serious hepatotoxicity; concurrent use of **saquinavir/ritonavir** is contra-indicated.

Concurrent use of **atazanavir**, **darunavir**, **fosamprenavir**, **saquinavir** and **tipranavir** is contra-indicated, due to substantially decreased plasma concentrations which may lead to loss of antiviral efficacy and/or development of viral resistance.

Avoid concurrent use with **apixaban**, **dabigatran**, **edoxaban**, **rivaroxaban**, azole antifungals, hormonal contraceptives, because these are likely to be rendered ineffective.

Rifampicin induces various enzymes involved in drug metabolism, including in oxidation (a potent inducer of CYP2B6, CYP2C19, and CYP3A4), glucuronidation (UGT1A1) and glutathione conjugation (GSTA1). Thus, caution is required with concurrent use of drugs which are metabolized by these enzymes, as rifampicin may reduce their effect and conversely cause toxicity when it is discontinued, e.g. **fentanyl** (see p.785). Note. For pro-drugs, rifampicin can increase exposure to active metabolites, e.g. rifampicin can increase the antiplatelet effect of **clopidogrel.**

Reports of interactions where close monitoring ± dose adjustment are required are listed in Table 1. Onset and offset of enzyme induction is gradual (see p.785), thus clinical effects may not become fully evident for 2–3 weeks after rifampicin is started or discontinued.

Conversely, some drugs may reduce the effect of rifampicin:

- antacids (reduced absorption); generally avoided by separating the administration time by ≥2h
- **phenobarbital** (may increase clearance).

6

Table 1 Clinically important cytochrome P450 interactions with rifampicin[a,12]

Drug effect ↓ by rifampicin	*Specific drugs within a class*
Anti-androgens	Abiraterone, darolutamide, enzalutamide
Antiarrhythmics	Dronedarone
Anticoagulants	Apixaban[b], dabigatran[b], edoxaban[b], rivaroxaban[b], warfarin (and other coumarins)[c]
Antidiabetics	Canagliflozin, glibenclamide, gliclazide, repaglinide, linagliptin, pioglitazone, rosiglitazone (not UK), tolbutamide
Antipsychotics	Aripiprazole, clozapine, haloperidol, lurasidone[b], risperidone
Azole antifungals	Fluconazole[d], itraconazole[b], ketoconazole[b], voriconazole[b]
Benzodiazepines	Alprazolam, diazepam, lorazepam (IV only), midazolam[e], nitrazepam, triazolam[b] (not UK)
Bronchodilators	Aminophylline, theophylline
Calcium channel blockers	Diltiazem, nifedipine (PO only, not IV), verapamil
Cannabinoids	Cannabis extract (Sativex®)
Corticosteroids	Dexamethasone, prednisolone
Digoxin	
Doxycycline	
Fesoterodine[b]	
Fexofenadine	
Hormonal contraceptives[b]	All, including emergency hormonal contraceptives
Lamotrigine	
Macrolides	Clarithromycin, telithromycin[b]
Neurokinin-1 antagonists	Aprepitant, fosaprepitant
NSAIDs	Celecoxib, diclofenac, etoricoxib
Opioids	Alfentanil, buprenorphine, codeine, fentanyl (all routes), methadone, morphine, oxycodone
Opioid antagonists	Naldemedine, naloxegol
Phenytoin/fosphenytoin	
Ramelteon (not UK)	
Statins[f]	All
Terbinafine	
Tolvaptan	
Z-drug hypnotics	Zaleplon, zolpidem, zopiclone

a. *not* an exhaustive list; limited to drugs most likely to be encountered in palliative care and *excludes* anticancer, antiviral, HIV and immunosuppressive drugs (seek specialist advice)
b. likely to be ineffective PO (and IV, where available); avoid concurrent use
c. onset within 1 week of starting rifampicin and persists for about ≤5 weeks after its withdrawal
d. generally with IV but not PO fluconazole; however, reports of therapeutic failure with PO fluconazole in patients with severe fungal infection
e. likely to be ineffective PO, avoid concurrent use; up to 60% reduction in AUC for IV
f. effect may increase or decrease depending on timing of administration and duration of concurrent use.

Undesirable effects

Nausea and anorexia (3% of patients with cholestatic pruritus[13]), diarrhoea (check for *Clostridium difficile* toxin; pseudomembranous colitis reported), orange discolouration of sweat, saliva, urine, faeces and tears (may stain contact lenses), flushing or rash (generally mild and transient; discontinue if purpuric or urticarial).

Adrenal insufficiency due to increased catabolism of adrenal steroids.

Hepatotoxicity occurs in 5% of patients with primary biliary cholangitis or primary sclerosing cholangitis, 1–5 months after starting rifampicin, occasionally longer; stopping rifampicin leads to a full recovery.[14]

Hypersensitivity reactions (flu-like symptoms, urticaria, thrombocytopenia, haemolysis, renal failure) are more common with intermittent therapy used for some infections, but occurred in <2% of patients using rifampicin continuously for cholestatic pruritus.[13] Generally resolve if rifampicin is stopped.

Rarely, severe prolongation of the prothrombin time (via altered production/metabolism of vitamin K); correct by giving vitamin K (p.632) and stopping rifampicin.[11]

Dose and use

Monitoring

Check LFTs, U+E and FBC before starting treatment and if symptoms suggestive of hepatotoxicity occur (e.g. nausea, vomiting, abdominal pain, worsening LFTs, pruritus). Although repeating these tests routinely is also suggested, the intervals vary, e.g. the SPC suggests every 2 weeks, others after 6 and 12 weeks of starting, or after any dose increase.[1,2,15] Monitoring of prothrombin time is recommended for patients at risk of bleeding.

With tuberculosis, it is recommended that rifampicin is stopped if ALT increases three times the upper limit of normal (when jaundice and/or symptoms of hepatitis present) or five times (when asymptomatic).[15] In cancer patients with progressive biliary obstruction, LFTs will deteriorate, but rifampicin-induced hepatotoxicity should be considered as a potential reversible cause.

†Cholestatic pruritus

Compared with rifampicin, there are less RCT data for **sertraline**, but efficacy appears similar; given its tolerability, familiarity and fewer drug interactions, *PCF* recommends that **sertraline** is generally tried before **rifampicin** (see Chapter 26, Table 1, p.829).

- start with rifampicin 150mg PO at bedtime
- if necessary, increase to 300mg at bedtime after 1 week (sooner if pruritus is severe and prognosis short)
- usual maximum dose 300mg b.d. (in hepatic impairment the SPC advises a maximum of 8mg/kg/24h).

Although generally advised to take rifampicin on an empty stomach to optimize absorption, when used for pruritus, strict adherence to this is probably unnecessary.

When PO administration is not possible, the same dose of rifampicin may be given by intravenous infusion (see Supply for further details).

Supply

Rifampicin (generic)
Capsules 150mg, 300mg, 28 days @ 150mg b.d. = £12.

Rifadin (Sanofi-Aventis)
Capsules 150mg, 300mg, 28 days @ 150mg b.d. = £10.
Oral syrup 100mg/5mL, 28 days @ 150mg b.d. = £15.
Intravenous infusion (powder for reconstitution) 600mg vial, supplied with 10mL solvent = £9. *Reconstitute with solvent provided; the displacement value of the powder may be significant, e.g. 0.48mL; consult local reconstitution guidelines. Further dilute the required dose with glucose 5% or sodium chloride 0.9% to a final concentration of 1.2mg/mL and infuse over 2–3h.*

1 Hirschfield GM *et al.* (2018) The British Society of Gastroenterology/UK-PBC primary biliary cholangitis treatment and management guidelines. *Gut.* **67**: 1568-1594.

2 Lindor KD *et al.* (2019) Primary biliary cholangitis: 2018 practice guidance from the American Association for the Study of Liver Diseases. *Hepatology.* **69**: 394-419.

3 Sanjel B and Shim W-S (2020) Recent advances in understanding the molecular mechanisms of cholestatic pruritus: A review. *BBA – Molecular Basis of Disease.* **1866**: 165958.

4 Sun Y *et al.* (2016) Autotaxin, pruritus and primary biliary cholangitis (PBC). *Autoimmunity Reviews.* **15**: 795–800.

5 Siemens W *et al.* (2016) Pharmacological interventions for pruritus in adult palliative care patients. *Cochrane Database of Systematic Reviews.* **11**: CD008320. www.thecochranelibrary.com.

6 Bachs L *et al.* (1992) Effects of long-term rifampicin administration in primary biliary cirrhosis. *Gastroenterology.* **102**: 2077–2080.

7 Ataei S *et al.* (2019) Comparison of Sertraline with Rifampin in the treatment of Cholestatic Pruritus: A Randomized Clinical Trial. *Rev Recent Clin Trials.* **14**: 217-223.

8 Acocella G (1978) Clinical pharmacokinetics of rifampicin. *Clinical Pharmacokinetics.* **3**: 108–127.

9 Riess W (1969) Pharmacokinetic studies in the field of rifamycins. Proceedings of the 6th International Congress of Chemotherapy. *University of Tokyo Press.* **2**: 905–913.

10 Price TJ *et al.* (1998) Rifampicin as treatment for pruritus in malignant cholestasis. *Supportive Care in Cancer.* **6**: 533–535.

11 Sampaziotis F and Griffiths WJH (2011) Severe coagulopathy caused by rifampicin in patients with primary sclerosing cholangitis and refractory pruritus. *British Journal of Clinical Pharmacology.* **73**: 826–827.

12 Baxter K and Preston CL. *Stockley's Drug Interactions.* London: Pharmaceutical Press, www.medicinescomplete.com (accessed February 2021).

13 Khurana S and Singh P (2006) Rifampin is safe for treatment of pruritus due to chronic cholestasis: a meta-analysis of prospective randomized-controlled trials. *Liver International.* **26**: 943-948.

14 Webb GJ *et al.* (2018) Low risk of hepatotoxicity from rifampicin when used for cholestatic pruritus: a cross-disease cohort study. *Alimentary Pharmacology and Therapeutics.* **47**: 1213–1219.

15 ATS (2006) An official ATS statement: hepatotoxicity of antituberculosis therapy. *American Journal of Respiratory and Critical Care Medicine.* **174**: 935–952

Updated (minor change) April 2021

6

URINARY TRACT INFECTIONS

Escherichia coli (*E. coli*) and other Gram-negative enterobacteria, particularly those producing extended-spectrum beta-lactamases or carbepenamase, are becoming resistant to several antibacterials, including **trimethoprim**, **gentamicin**, quinolones and cephalosporins.[1] This possibility should be considered in patients with recurrent urinary infection. Appropriate specimens for culture should be taken, and any previous microbiology reviewed.

If a multiresistant isolate has been identified previously, e.g. a **gentamicin**-resistant coliform in urine, treatment should be discussed with a medical microbiologist, because the usual first-line treatment may not be appropriate.

E. coli is the commonest cause of urinary tract infection (UTI).[2,3] UTIs are more common in women. They are categorized as lower (cystitis) or upper (pyelonephritis), and uncomplicated or complicated. Lower UTIs generally present with typical symptoms of cystitis; even when these are present, an upper UTI should be suspected in the presence of fever >38°C, loin pain and/or costovertebral angle tenderness.

UTIs are considered uncomplicated when they occur in otherwise healthy premenopausal women with normal urinary tracts; this includes upper UTIs *without* urosepsis. UTIs are considered complicated when they occur in men, children, pregnant women, women with abnormal urinary tracts and the elderly (particularly if immunocompromised or with co-morbidities that make diagnosis challenging, e.g. dementia).[4] UTIs *with* urosepsis (i.e. severe systemic response to infection with persistent hypotension despite fluid resuscitation, causing end-organ damage and tissue anoxia) are always complicated. Complicated UTIs are caused by a broader range of bacteria that are more likely to be resistant to antibacterials.[5]

Diagnosis

Uncomplicated lower UTI

Diagnosis can be made based on history if a woman has typical or severe symptoms and signs of a UTI without vaginal irritation or discharge suggestive of an alternative diagnosis; *dipstick testing (see below) and urine culture are irrelevant.*

In the community, in non-catheterized women three symptoms independently predict UTI: cloudy urine, dysuria and recent-onset nocturia:

- presence of all three symptoms has a positive predictive value of 82%
- absence of all three symptoms had a negative predictive value of 67%.[6]

Thus, using a symptom score alone will lead to a missed diagnosis in about one third of UTIs.

With dipsticks, nitrites are most predictive, followed by leucocytes (leucocyte esterase+ or greater) and blood (haemolysed trace or greater). For dipstick tests in combination:

- nitrite+ and *either* blood+ *or* leucocyte esterase+: positive predictive value 92%
- nitrite+ or leucocyte esterase and blood *both*+: positive predictive value about 80%
- nitrite, leucocyte esterase and blood *all* –: negative predictive value 76% (Box A).[6]

Thus, the use of a dipstick alone will lead to a missed diagnosis in about one quarter of UTIs.

Box A Urine dipsticks and the diagnosis of UTI in non-catheterized women ≤65 years with few or mild symptoms

Urine dipstick testing is generally *not* advised in patients >65 years because of the prevalence of asymptomatic bacteriuria (see Box B).[7]

Use a urine dipstick that measures urinary pH and specific gravity, and the presence and amount of:

- glucose
- ketone
- blood
- protein
- nitrite, a bacterial metabolite
- leucocyte esterase (produced by inflammation/infection).

When to do the test

- if patient has few or mild symptoms of UTI
- if typical or severe symptoms of UTI, prescribe an antibacterial in accord with local policy, without using a dipstick.

How to do the test

- clean external genitalia with sterile water
- take a mid-stream specimen of urine (or in-and-out catheter sample under aseptic conditions)
- dip the whole strip into the urine container and remove immediately
- drag the edge of the strip against the container rim to remove excess urine and start timing
- compare each test pad on the strip to the corresponding row of colour blocks on the bottle label
- read each test pad at the time shown on the bottle, starting with the shortest time first.

Late readings are of no value.

Significance of the results

Nitrite positive or leucocyte and blood positive or all three positive: make a working diagnosis of UTI; prescribe an antibacterial in accord with local policy. Urine specimen for culture *not* required unless risk factors present, e.g. recent hospital admission, recurrent UTIs.

Nitrite, leucocyte and blood all negative: tentatively exclude UTI; do *not* send urine specimen for culture unless definite urinary tract symptoms.

A negative culture may suggest an alternative diagnosis, e.g. urethritis caused by sexually transmitted infections (STIs) (e.g. *Chlamydia*, *Neisseria*, *Trichomonas*) or interstitial cystitis. Although the traditional criterion for a positive urine culture is $\geq 10^5$ colony-forming units (cfu)/mL, some studies have demonstrated that this is insensitive in 30–50% of women who have lower UTI confirmed by bladder aspirate but have only 10^2–10^4 cfu/mL in voided urine. Thus, in a woman with symptoms of uncomplicated UTI, a culture report of 'no growth' should be treated with caution, and a colony count of $\geq 10^3$ cfu/mL is microbiologically diagnostic.[3]

A small proportion of UTIs are caused by a mixed infection. Thus, when a patient with typical symptoms of a UTI has a 'mixed growth' culture, consider repeating the MSU and treating for UTI.[7]

Note. High cfu counts in MSU or catheter samples in patients *without* symptoms of UTI (asymptomatic bacteriuria) do *not* require antibacterial treatment (Box B).

Box B Asymptomatic bacteriuria (ABU)

ABU increases with age, occurring in ≤50% of women and ≤40% of men in long-term elderly care facilities. It is defined as bacteriuria $\geq 10^5$ cfu/mL of same-species bacteria in two consecutive MSU samples in women or one sample in men, *or* $\geq 10^2$ cfu/mL of same-species bacteria in one catheterized sample in men or women *without* symptoms of UTI.

ABU is important to recognize, because antibacterial treatment of ABU does *not* prevent development of symptomatic UTI or reduce the risk of severe UTI, urosepsis or death, but does expose the patient to the undesirable effects of antibacterials and contributes towards antimicrobial resistance.

Differentiation between ABU and symptomatic UTI in some patients can be challenging, e.g. those with impaired cognitive function. Careful history-taking from those who know the patient, with details of the impact of previous antibacterial treatment, will help prevent unnecessary treatment.[8,9]

6

Complicated UTI

Diagnosis is based on history and examination; *dipsticks are less reliable in these circumstances and their use discouraged.*[7] A complicated UTI is likely if there is new onset dysuria *or* ≥2 of:

- new urinary frequency/urgency
- new urinary incontinence
- new or worsening delirium or debility
- new suprapubic pain
- visible haematuria
- change in temperature: ≥38°C *or* ≤36°C *or* >1.5°C above baseline twice in the last 12h.

However, in frail, elderly or hospitalized patients, a complicated UTI may present with atypical clinical symptoms (e.g. features of systemic infection but no localizing features such as dysuria, frequency, urgency or loin pain) or just be suspected because of the onset of delirium. When there are *no* urinary symptoms and *no* signs of systemic infection, delay starting an antibacterial until the results of urine culture are available.

Pyelonephritis should be suspected if there is new loin pain, flu-like illness or myalgia, nausea or vomiting, or changes in temperature (≥38°C or ≤36°C). A diagnosis of sepsis should be considered using a local or national screening tool, e.g. NEWS2.[10]

To confirm the presence of bacteria and identify antibacterial sensitivity, MSU should be collected before starting antibacterial therapy in patients at risk of a complicated UTI and those associated with:

- recurrent UTI
- haematuria (macroscopic or on dipstick testing)
- impaired immunity, e.g. from immunosuppressive treatment or poorly controlled diabetes mellitus
- moderate–severe renal impairment
- a hospital admission (>7 days in last 6 months)
- a care home resident.

Management

Remember: before prescribing an antibacterial, always ask about drug allergies and check previous urine culture and sensitivity results. Prescribe antibacterials according to local guidelines.

The dose and frequency of many antibacterials are reduced in renal impairment.

Lower UTI

In women presenting to their GP, one approach is to prescribe paracetamol or NSAID to relieve painful cystitis, with an antibacterial to start only if symptoms worsen or persist for >48h.[11]

However, this is not appropriate in patients receiving palliative care. Prompt, empirical antibacterial therapy is indicated for symptoms that are moderate–severe or if symptoms are mild but urine dipstick test is positive. Start antibacterial according to local guidelines or treat according to NICE guidelines (Table 1).

In frail women struggling with tablet burden, consider **fosfomycin**, because it is a single-dose treatment. For those unable to swallow tablets or with an EFT, consider **trimethoprim** oral suspension or soluble **fosfomycin** granules, because **nitrofurantoin** suspension is expensive. In men, if the first-line antibacterial is not suitable or symptoms persist for >48h, treat as for pyelonephritis (see below), but consider the possibility of an alternative diagnosis, e.g. acute prostatitis.

Complicated UTI and pyelonephritis

Prompt antibacterial therapy is indicated, guided by severity of symptoms and risk of developing complications, which is higher in immunocompromised patients, those with poorly controlled diabetes mellitus and those with abnormal urinary tracts. Start antibacterial according to local guidelines or Table 1.[15]

If IV antibacterials are indicated, review after 48h and switch to PO if possible. Second-line antibacterials vary from region to region; if necessary, consult a medical microbiologist.[5]

Where IV access is unwanted or difficult to maintain, the following regimens are as effective as parenteral dosing until afebrile for >48h:[16-18]

- IM **ceftriaxone** 1g, repeated once 18–36h later, followed by PO **cefalexin** for 10 days
- IM **ceftriaxone** 1g single dose, followed by PO **cefixime** for 10 days (or other antibacterial according to sensitivities).

Some centres give **ceftriaxone** SC. To reduce discomfort from IM/SC **ceftriaxone**, it can be reconstituted using **lidocaine** 1%. For full details, see p.509.

Recurrent UTI

Defined as ≥2 UTIs within 6 months or ≥3 UTIs within 12 months. It may be caused by the same or different strains of bacteria. Antibacterial prophylaxis in a single dose can be considered when there is an identifiable trigger, e.g. sexual intercourse. When there is no identifiable trigger, consider daily antibacterial prophylaxis, following local guidance and after discussion with a medical microbiologist (Table 1).

Topical (but *not* PO) oestrogen is an option for post-menopausal women with recurrent UTI.[19,20] Vaginal oestrogen applied as a cream or ring (but not as a pessary) reduces the incidence of recurrent UTI by 30–45%. Undesirable effects include breast tenderness and vaginal bleeding.

Although **cranberry** supplementation has generated much interest, it should no longer be encouraged as a means of preventing recurrent UTI (Box C). Similarly, there is insufficient evidence of benefit from PO/intravaginal probiotics or D-mannose to recommend their widespread use.[21-24] Thus, in a palliative care population, prophylactic antibacterials are more effective and cheaper.[20]

Catheter-associated UTI (CA-UTI)

In catheterized patients, bacterial colonization is common, occurring in up to 30% of patients catheterized for >7 days and almost universally in those catheterized for >28 days. It should not be investigated or treated unless symptomatic, because generally bacteriuria does not progress to UTI.

CA-UTI is defined as $\geq 10^3$ cfu/mL of one or more bacterial species in one catheter sample or one MSU in patients who have had a catheter removed within the previous 48h. Patients who develop CA-UTI may not present with fever or symptoms referable to the urinary tract. Non-specific symptoms such as rigors, malaise and new-onset delirium are more common, so thorough evaluation for alternative sources of infection should also be conducted.[12]

If CA-UTI is clinically suspected, do *not* perform a urine dipstick test, because it is unreliable, but send urine for culture and then start empirical treatment according to local guidance;[25] alternatively, see Table 1.

Consider removing the catheter. If this is not possible and the catheter has been in place for >7 days, change it as soon as possible to improve clinical and bacteriological cure rates.[12,26]

For second line antibacterials, consult a medical microbiologist.

Table 1 Selected summary of NICE guidance for treatment of UTI: PO unless stated otherwise[5,9,12]

Situation	*First-line antibacterials*	*Second-line antibacterials (when first-line unsuitable or persistent symptoms >48h)*
Lower UTI in non-pregnant women	Nitrofurantoin[a] 100mg m/r b.d. for 3 days *or* Trimethoprim[b] 200mg b.d. for 3 days	Nitrofurantoin[a] if not already tried *or* Pivmecillinam 400mg stat, followed by 200mg t.d.s. for 3 days *or* Fosfomycin 3g single dose
Lower UTI in men	Trimethoprim[b] 200mg b.d. for 7 days *or* Nitrofurantoin[a] 100mg m/r b.d. for 7 days	Consult medical microbiologist
Complicated UTI and pyelonephritis	Cefalexin 500mg b.d.–t.d.s. (1–1.5g t.d.s.–q.d.s. for severe infections) for 7–10 days **When culture results available and bacteria sensitive** Co-amoxiclav 500/125mg t.d.s. for 7–10 days *or* Trimethoprim[b] 200mg b.d. for 14 days *or* Ciprofloxacin[c] 500mg b.d. for 7 days **Parenteral route if vomiting, severely unwell or sepsis[d]** Ceftriaxone 1–2g IV once daily *or* Cefuroxime 750mg–1.5g IV t.d.s.– q.d.s. *or* Ciprofloxacin[c] 400mg IV b.d.–t.d.s.	Consult medical microbiologist
Prophylaxis for recurrent UTI	Long-term trimethoprim[b] 100mg at night *or* Nitrofurantoin[a] 50–100mg at night	Consult medical microbiologist
CA-UTI	**No upper UTI symptoms** Trimethoprim[b] 200mg b.d. for 7 days *or* Nitrofurantoin[a] 100mg m/r b.d. for 7 days *or* Amoxicillin 500mg t.d.s. for 7 days (when culture results available and bacteria sensitive) If upper UTI symptoms, or if vomiting, severely unwell or sepsis, treat as for complicated UTI and pyelonephritis above	Pivmecillinam 400mg stat, followed by 200mg t.d.s. for 7 days

a. avoid when eGFR <45mL/min/1.73m^2 (unless no alternatives and eGFR >30mL/min/1.73m^2; see SPC)[13]
b. if renal impairment and/or low risk of resistance, e.g. not used ≤3 months, young patient, not in residential care facility
c. because ciprofloxacin can rarely cause disabling and potentially irreversible undesirable effects, e.g. tendinitis, tendon rupture, muscle or joint pain, it is recommended to: limit its use to severe infections; use with caution in patients >60 years; avoid in patients receiving corticosteroids; stop immediately if musculoskeletal symptoms develop[14]
d. for sepsis, also give a stat dose of IV gentamicin 5–7mg/kg; monitor plasma levels if regular once daily use becomes necessary.

Prophylactic antibacterials for CA-UTI

Long-term catheterization

Because of the risk of increasing antibacterial resistance, continuous prophylaxis against CA-UTI in long-term catheterized patients is not recommended, even though there is some evidence to suggest it reduces the risk of symptomatic UTI.[27,28] Prophylactic antibacterials for routine catheter changes are *not* recommended unless the patient:

- has a history of UTI associated with catheter changes *or*
- is significantly immunosuppressed (e.g. neutropenic from recent chemotherapy) *or*
- experiences trauma during catheter change, i.e. frank haematuria or ≥2 attempts at catheterization.

In such cases, single-dose treatment according to local guidelines is sufficient.[29]

Short-term catheterization

Routine antibiotic prophylaxis before, during or at time of removal of a short-term catheter is not recommended, particularly because of increasing antibacterial resistance.[12] The only group of patients consistently demonstrated to benefit are post-surgical patients with a urinary catheter >5 days or following prostate surgery, where antibacterial prophylaxis given at the time of catheter removal halves the risk of symptomatic UTI (11% to 5%, NNT 18).[30-32]

Alternative approaches

In catheterized patients, consider a urinary antiseptic to help prevent recurrent CA-UTIs (but *not* for treatment), e.g. **methenamine hippurate** (p.616). There is no evidence to support use of **cranberry** supplementation to prevent CA-UTI (Box C).[33]

Box C Cranberry supplementation for prevention of recurrent UTI

Cranberry juice inhibits bacterial adherence to the urinary tract mucosa by disrupting the binding of bacterial macromolecules to receptors on mucosal epithelial cells.[34] This effect has been shown *in vitro* with *Escherichia coli*, and is produced by pro-anthocyanidins (PAC) present in cranberries (and blueberries).[34]

Cranberry juice does not cure established infection but its use has generated popular and scientific interest as a means of preventing UTIs.[24,35,36] The evidence is mixed and interpretation made difficult by the use of different formulations (with widely differing PAC content, e.g. juice or powder), doses, outcomes and patient populations.

Almost all of the recent large RCTs have been negative, and the overwhelming evidence is for little or no effect.[20,37-43]

Thus, the use of cranberry supplementation should *not* be encouraged as a means of preventing recurrent UTIs.[44] Prophylactic antibacterials are more effective and cheaper, and should be considered with advice from a microbiologist.[45,46]

Patients who do take cranberry juice should be made aware of the potential for this to inhibit cytochrome P450 activity (see Chapter 19, p.781).[47] Regular use of cranberry juice has been linked to an increase in or fluctuation of INR values in patients taking warfarin (predominantly metabolized by CYP2C9).[48] This prompted the recommendation in the UK that the concurrent use of cranberry products and warfarin should be avoided.[49,50] If a patient taking warfarin consumes variable amounts of cranberry juice or other cranberry supplements, the INR should be monitored more closely.

A possible interaction between cranberry juice extracts and tacrolimus, resulting in subtherapeutic levels of the latter, has also been reported.[51]

Supply

Amoxicillin (generic)

Capsules 250mg, 500mg, 7 days @ 250mg t.d.s. = £0.50; two doses of 3g = £0.50.

Oral suspension 125mg/5mL, 250mg/5mL, 7 days @ 250mg t.d.s. = £1.50.

Oral suspension (sachet of powder to mix with water) 3g, two doses = £10.

Cefalexin (generic)
Tablets 250mg, 500mg, 7 days @ 500mg t.d.s. = £2.25.
Capsules 250mg, 500mg, 7 days @ 500mg t.d.s. = £1.50.
Oral suspension 125mg/5mL, 250mg/5mL, 7 days @ 500mg t.d.s. = £3.50.

Ceftriaxone (generic)
Injection (powder for reconstitution) 1g and 2g vial = £3.50 and £12.

Cefuroxime (generic)
Injection (powder for reconstitution) 750mg and 1.5g vial = £2.25 and £4.75.

Co-amoxiclav (generic)
Tablets 250/125 (amoxicillin 250mg, clavulanic acid 125mg), 7 days @ 375mg t.d.s. = £1.50.
Tablets 500/125 (amoxicillin 500mg, clavulanic acid 125mg), 7 days @ 625mg t.d.s. = £1.75.
Oral suspension 250/62 (amoxicillin 250mg as trihydrate, clavulanic acid 62.5mg as potassium salt)/5mL, 7 days @ 10mL t.d.s = £5.

Ciprofloxacin (generic)
Tablets 100mg, 250mg, 500mg, 750mg, 7 days @ 500mg b.d. = £1.25.
Oral suspension 250mg/5mL, 7 days @ 500mg b.d. = £45.
Infusion 2mg/mL, 400mg (200mL) bottle or bag = £15 or £12 respectively.

Fosfomycin (generic)
Granules 3g sachet = £4.75.

Gentamicin sulfate (generic)
Injection 40mg/mL, 1mL amp and 2mL vial = £1.50, 2mL amp = £1.

Nitrofurantoin (generic)
Tablets 50mg, 100mg, 7 days @ 50mg q.d.s. = £8.50.
Capsules 50mg, 100mg, 7 days @ 50mg q.d.s. = £11.
Oral suspension 25mg/5mL, 7 days @ 50mg q.d.s. = £416.

Macrobid® (Goldshield)
Capsules m/r 100mg, 7 days @ 100mg b.d. = £9.50.

Pivmecillinam (generic)
Tablet 200mg, 3 days @ 200mg t.d.s. = £5.50.

Trimethoprim (generic)
Tablets 100mg, 200mg, 7 days @ 200mg b.d. = £1.25.
Oral suspension 50mg/5mL, 7 days @ 200mg b.d. = £19.

1 UK Health Security Agency (2021) English surveillance programme for antimicrobial utilisation and resistance (ESPAUR) report 2020–2021. www.gov.uk.
2 Vitetta L *et al.* (2000) Bacterial infections in terminally ill hospice patients. *Journal of Pain and Symptom Management.* **20**: 326–334.
3 Hooton TM (2012) Clinical practice. Uncomplicated urinary tract infection. *New England Journal of Medicine.* **366**: 1028–1037.
4 Johansen TE *et al.* (2011) Critical review of current definitions of urinary tract infections and proposal of an EAU/ESIU classification system. *International Journal of Antimicrobial Agents.* **38 Suppl**: 64–70.
5 NICE (2018) Pyelonephritis (acute): antimicrobial prescribing. Guideline 111. www.nice.org.uk.
6 Little P *et al.* (2009) Dipsticks and diagnostic algorithms in urinary tract infection: development and validation, randomised trial, economic analysis, observational cohort and qualitative study. *Health Technology Assessment.* **13**: 1–73.
7 Public Health England (2020) Diagnosis of urinary tract infections. Quick reference tool for primary care for consultation and local adaptation. www.gov.uk/phe.
8 Zalmanovici Trestioreanu A *et al.* (2015) Antibiotics for asymptomatic bacteriuria. *Cochrane Database of Systematic Reviews.* CD009534. www.cochranelibrary.com.
9 NICE (2018) Urinary tract infection (lower): antimicrobial prescribing. Guideline 109. www.nice.org.uk.
10 Royal College of Physicians (2017) National Early Warning Score (NEWS) 2. Standardising the assessment of acute-illness severity in the NHS. Updated report of a working party. www.rcplondon.ac.uk.
11 Little P (2017). Antibiotics or NSAIDs for uncomplicated urinary tract infection? *British Medical Journal.* **359**: j5037.
12 NICE (2018) Urinary tract infection (catheter-associated): antimicrobial prescribing. Guideline 113. www.nice.org.uk.
13 MHRA (2014) Nitrofurantoin now contraindicated in most patients with an estimated glomerular filtration rate (eGFR) of less than 45 ml/min/1.73m². Drug Safety Update. **8**. www.gov.uk/drug-safety-update.

14 MHRA (2019) Fluoroquinolone antibiotics: new restrictions and precautions for use due to very rare reports of disabling and potentially long-lasting or irreversible side effects. *Drug Safety Update*. **12**. www.gov.uk/drug-safety-update.
15 Lutters M and Vogt-Ferrier MB (2008) Antibiotic duration for treating uncomplicated, symptomatic lower urinary tract infections in elderly women. *Cochrane Database of Systematic Reviews*. **3**: CD001535. www.cochranelibrary.com.
16 Pohl A (2007) Modes of administration of antibiotics for symptomatic severe urinary tract infections. *Cochrane Database of Systematic Reviews*. CD003237. www.cochranelibrary.com.
17 Millar LK *et al.* (1995) Outpatient treatment of pyelonephritis in pregnancy: a randomized controlled trial. *Obstetrics and Gynaecology*. **86**: 560–564.
18 Sanchez M *et al.* (2002) Short-term effectiveness of ceftriaxone single dose in the initial treatment of acute uncomplicated pyelonephritis in women. A randomised controlled trial. *Emergency Medicine Journal*. **19**: 19–22.
19 Perrotta C *et al.* (2008) Oestrogens for preventing recurrent urinary tract infection in postmenopausal women. *Cochrane Database of Systematic Reviews*. CD005131. www.cochranelibrary.com.
20 NICE (2018) Urinary tract infection (recurrent): antimicrobial prescribing. Guideline 112. www.nice.org.uk.
21 Grin PM *et al.* (2013) Lactobacillus for preventing recurrent urinary tract infections in women: meta-analysis. *Canadian Journal of Urology*. **20**: 6607–6014.
22 Schwenger EM *et al.* (2015) Probiotics for preventing urinary tract infections in adults and children. *Cochrane Database of Systematic Reviews*. CD008772. www.cochranelibrary.com.
23 Kranjcec B *et al.* (2013) D-mannose powder for prophylaxis of recurrent urinary tract infections in women: a randomized controlled trial. *World Journal of Urology*. **173**: 1281–1287.
24 Wawrysiuk S *et al.* (2019) Prevention and treatment of uncomplicated lower urinary tract infections in the era of increasing antimicrobial resistance-non-antibiotic approaches: a systemic review. *Archives of Gynecology and Obstetrics*. **300**: 821–828.
25 Schwartz DS and Barone JE (2006) Correlation of urinalysis and dipstick results with catheter-associated urinary tract infections in surgical ICU patients. *Intensive Care Medicine*. **32**: 1797–1801.
26 Raz R *et al.* (2000) Chronic indwelling catheter replacement before antimicrobial therapy for symptomatic urinary tract infection. *Journal of Urology*. **164**: 1254–1258.
27 Niël-Weise BS *et al.* (2012) Urinary catheter policies for long-term bladder drainage (review). *Cochrane Database of Systematic Reviews*. CD004201. www.cochranelibrary.com.
28 Fisher H *et al.* (2018) Continuous low-dose antibiotic prophylaxis for adults with repeated urinary tract infections (AnTIC): a randomised, open-label trial. *Lancet Infectious Diseases*. **18**: 957–968.
29 NICE (2017) Healthcare-associated infections: prevention and control in primary and community care. *Clinical Guideline*. CG139. www.nice.org.uk.
30 Lusardi G *et al.* (2013) Antibiotic prophylaxis for short-term catheter bladder drainage in adults. *Cochrane Database of Systematic Reviews*. CD005428. www.cochranelibrary.com.
31 Dieter AA *et al.* (2014) Oral antibiotics to prevent postoperative urinary tract infection: a randomized controlled trial. *Obstetrics and Gynecology*. **123**: 96–103.
32 Marschall J *et al.* (2013) Antibiotic prophylaxis for urinary tract infections after removal of urinary catheter: meta-analysis. *British Medical Journal*. **346**: F3147.
33 Gunnarsson A-K *et al.* (2017) Cranberry juice concentrate does not significantly decrease the incidence of acquired bacteriuria in female hip fracture patients receiving urine catheter: a double-blind randomized trial. *Clinical Interventions in Aging*. **12**: 137–143.
34 Micali S *et al.* (2014) Cranberry and recurrent cystitis: more than marketing? *Critical Reviews in Food Science and Nutrition*. **54**: 1063–1075.
35 Natural Medicines Comprehensive Database (2008) Cranberry. www.naturaldatabase.com (accessed 2008).
36 Tong H *et al.* (2006) Effect of ingesting cranberry juice on bacterial growth in urine. *American Journal of Health-System Pharmacy*. **63**: 1417–1419.
37 Jepson RG *et al.* (2012) Cranberries for preventing urinary tract infections. *Cochrane Database of Systematic Reviews*. **10**: CD001321. www.cochranelibrary.com.
38 Caljouw MA *et al.* (2014) Effectiveness of cranberry capsules to prevent urinary tract infections in vulnerable older persons: a double-blind randomized placebo-controlled trial in long-term care facilities. *Journal of the American Geriatrics Society*. **62**: 103–110.
39 Gallien P *et al.* (2014) Cranberry versus placebo in the prevention of urinary infections in multiple sclerosis: a multicenter, randomized, placebo-controlled, double-blind trial. *Multiple Sclerosis Journal*. **20**: 1252–1259.
40 Juthani-Mehta M *et al.* (2016) Effect of cranberry capsules on bacteriuria plus pyuria among older women in nursing homes: a randomized clinical trial. *Journal of the American Medical Association*. **316**: 1879–1887.
41 Letouzey V *et al.* (2017) Cranberry capsules to prevent nosocomial urinary tract bacteriuria after pelvic surgery: a randomised controlled trial. *British Journal of Obstetrics and Gynaecology*. **124**: 912–917.
42 Wang CH *et al.* (2012) Cranberry-containing products for prevention of urinary tract infections in susceptible populations: a systematic review and meta-analysis of randomized controlled trials. *Archives of Internal Medicine*. **172**: 988–996.
43 Fu Z *et al.* (2017) Cranberry reduces the risk of urinary tract infection recurrence in otherwise healthy women: a systematic review and meta-analysis. *Journal of Nutrition*. **147**: 2282–2288.
44 Nicolle LE (2016) Cranberry for prevention of urinary tract infection? Time to move on. *Journal of the American Medical Association*. **316**: 1873–1874.
45 Bosmans JE *et al.* (2014) Cost-effectiveness of cranberries vs antibiotics to prevent urinary tract infections in premenopausal women: a randomized clinical trial. *PLoS One*. **9**: e91939.
46 van den Hout WB *et al.* (2014) Cost-effectiveness of cranberry capsules to prevent urinary tract infection in long-term care facilities: economic evaluation with a randomized controlled trial. *Journal of the American Geriatrics Society*. **62**: 111–116.
47 Hodek P *et al.* (2002) Flavonoids-potent and versatile biologically active compounds interacting with cytochromes P450. *Chemico-Biological Interactions*. **139**: 1–21.
48 Rettie AE *et al.* (1992) Hydroxylation of warfarin by human cDNA-expressed cytochrome P-450: a role for P-4502C9 in the etiology of (S)-warfarin-drug interactions. *Chemical Research in Toxicology*. **5**: 54–59.
49 CSM (Committee on Safety of Medicines) (2004) Interaction between warfarin and cranberry juice: new advice. *Current Problems in Pharmacovigilance*. **30**: 10.
50 MHRA (2009) Warfarin: changes to product safety information Public assessment report. December.
51 Dave AA and Samuel J (2016) Suspected interaction of cranberry juice extracts and tacrolimus serum levels: a case report. *Cureus*. **8**: e610.

Updated December 2021

CELLULITIS IN A LYMPHOEDEMATOUS LIMB

The following should be read together with *Consensus Document on the Management of Cellulitis in Lymphoedema* produced by the British Lymphology Society.[1]
Note. The risk of infection is increased in an oedematous limb of any cause. Lymphatic failure is a common feature, due to injury (e.g. cancer, surgery) or being overwhelmed by excess capillary filtration (e.g. chronic heart failure).[2]

Cellulitis is an acute spreading inflammation of the skin and subcutaneous tissues characterized by erythema, warmth, swelling and pain. Generally, it occurs unilaterally rather than bilaterally. In lymphoedema, presentation may be more variable than 'classical' cellulitis, e.g. blotchy vs. well-demarcated erythema. The accompanying systemic upset may be minimal or severe with high fever and rigors; sepsis can occur.[2]

Generally, the diagnosis of cellulitis is based on the history and examination. CRP and WBC are raised in ≥80% and ≤50% of patients respectively and may help diagnosis and monitoring of response to treatment.[3] Blood cultures should be taken when there is sepsis or significant systemic upset and swabs when there are wounds ± pus.

In most episodes, the bacteria responsible are not isolated; when they are, both streptococci and *Staphylococcus aureus* are common.[3] However, overall, streptococci are considered responsible for most episodes of cellulitis (≥70%, based on serology studies).[1,3]

Management strategy

Preventive measures

Patients should be educated about:

- why they are susceptible to cellulitis, e.g. skin crevices harbour bacteria, reduced local immunity[3]
- the importance of daily skin care to improve and maintain skin integrity. Risk factors for cellulitis include cracked or macerated interdigital skin, dermatitis, wounds (including leg ulcers) and weeping lymphangiectasia (leaking lymph blisters on the skin surface)
- the primary importance of achieving optimal control of lymphoedema to reduce the risk of cellulitis[4]
- reducing other risks, e.g. protecting hands when gardening, cleaning cuts, treating fungal infections (e.g. **terbinafine** 1% cream once daily for 2 weeks) and ingrowing toenails
- the consequences of cellulitis, e.g. increased swelling, worsening fibrosis, reduced response to compression treatment
- the importance of seeking prompt medical attention and treatment if they suspect they may be developing cellulitis.

Patients who have had cellulitis in the past and who are travelling away from home should be supplied with an emergency 2-week supply of antibacterials (see QCG: Cellulitis in lymphoedema, p.532).

Non-drug treatment

- although compression garments should be avoided during the acute episode, they should be reapplied as soon as it is comfortable to do so
- daily skin hygiene measures should be continued: washing and gentle drying
- emollients should not be used where the skin is broken
- *if severe, bed rest is essential*, with the affected limb elevated in a comfortable position and supported on pillows.[5]

Drug treatment

The dose and frequency of many antibacterials are reduced in renal impairment.

Cellulitis should be treated promptly with antibacterials to prevent sepsis and increased morbidity from worsening swelling and accelerated fibrosis (Table 1, and QCG: Cellulitis in lymphoedema, p.532). Streptococci are believed to be the most common causal pathogens.[1,3,6] Although either **amoxicillin** or **flucloxacillin** are considered acceptable first-line PO antibacterials in this setting, the British Lymphology Society favours **amoxicillin** because of its lower minimum inhibitory concentration and possibly better tissue penetration.[1,6] However, when *Staphylococcus aureus* is suspected, **flucloxacillin** should be used.

Folliculitis, pus formation and crusting are indicative of *Staphylococcus aureus* infection, and **flucloxacillin** should definitely be used.

Table 1 Antibacterials for cellulitis[a] (PO unless stated otherwise)

Situation	*First-line antibacterials*	*If allergic to penicillin*	*Second-line antibacterials*	*Comments*
Acute cellulitis (home care) or emergency back-up supply of antibacterials	Amoxicillin 500mg t.d.s. *or* flucloxacillin 500mg q.d.s.	Erythromycin[b] 500mg q.d.s. *or* clarithromycin[b] 500mg b.d.	Clindamycin 300mg q.d.s. If fails to resolve, convert to first-line IV regimen below	Antibacterials are given for a minimum of 2 weeks from when a clinical response is first seen and continued until the acute inflammation has completely resolved; this may take 1–2 months.
Acute cellulitis + septicaemia (inpatient admission)	Flucloxacillin 2g IV q6h[10]	Clindamycin 600mg IV q6h[11]	Clindamycin 600mg IV q6h (if poor or no response by 48h)	Switch to flucloxacillin 500mg PO q.d.s. *or* clindamycin 300mg PO q.d.s. when: • no fever for 48h *and* • inflammation much resolved *and* • falling CRP. Then continue as above.
Prophylaxis if ≥2 episodes of cellulitis in a year	Phenoxymethylpenicillin 250mg b.d. (500mg b.d. if BMI ≥33)[12,13]	Erythromycin[b] 250mg b.d. *or* clarithromycin[b] 250mg once daily	Clindamycin 150mg once daily *or* cefalexin 125mg once daily *or* doxycycline 50mg once daily[c]	Consider stopping after 2 years if preventive measures are optimal. Consider *life-long* prophylaxis when there are ongoing risk factors or a relapse occurs off treatment.

a. but take note of local guidelines, particularly for IV antibacterials; seek advice of a medical microbiologist for cellulitis affecting the anogenital region, developing after an animal lick or bite, or not responding to recommended antibacterials

b. has a known risk of prolonged QT interval, and *torsade de pointes* and important drug interactions; if use is contra-indicated (see SPC, and QCG: Cellulitis in lymphoedema, p.532), use cefalexin (but not in patients with a history of serious penicillin allergy, i.e. anaphylaxis) or doxycycline as an alternative

c. in these circumstances, review by local specialist lymphoedema service and advice from a microbiologist are recommended. There is a need to balance the use of certain antibiotics (e.g. clindamycin, cefalexin) as prophylaxis against the risk of predisposing to *Clostridium difficile* infection.

The need for hospital admission and IV antibacterials is based on the degree of systemic upset.[7] They are needed when there is:

- sepsis (signs include pyrexia >38.3°C, delirium, tachycardia, hypotension)
- continuing or deteriorating systemic upset (± deteriorating local signs) despite 48h of PO antibacterial
- continuing or deteriorating local signs (± systemic upset) despite first- and second-line PO antibacterials.

The advice of a medical microbiologist should be obtained in unusual circumstances, e.g.:

- in anogenital cellulitis
- cellulitis developing shortly after an animal lick or bite
- failure to respond to the recommended antibacterials.

6

Remember: cellulitis is painful, and analgesics should be prescribed regularly and p.r.n. Because of a possible relationship between skin infections, NSAIDs and necrotizing fasciitis,[8] **paracetamol** and opioids are the preferred analgesics.[9]

Supply

Amoxicillin (generic)
Capsules 250mg, 500mg, 14 days @ 500mg t.d.s. = £2.50.
Oral suspension 125mg/5mL, 250mg/5mL, 14 days @ 500mg t.d.s. = £5.50.

Clarithromycin (generic)
Tablets 250mg, 500mg, 14 days @ 500mg b.d. = £5.
Oral suspension 125mg/5mL, 250mg/5mL, 14 days @ 500mg b.d. = £20.

Clindamycin (generic)
Capsules 75mg, 150mg, 300mg, 14 days @ 300mg q.d.s. = £16. *Price based on 150mg capsules; the 300mg capsules cost £71.*
Injection 150mg/mL, 2mL, 4mL amp, 600mg dose = £12.

Erythromycin (generic)
Tablets e/c 250mg, 14 days @ 500mg q.d.s. = £7.
Oral suspension (as ethyl succinate) 125mg/5mL, 250mg/5mL, 500mg/5mL, 14 days @ 500mg q.d.s. = £42.

Flucloxacillin (generic)
Capsules 250mg, 500mg, 14 days @ 500mg q.d.s. = £5.
Oral solution 125mg/5mL, 250mg/5mL, 14 days @ 500mg q.d.s. = £140.
Injection (powder for reconstitution) 250mg, 500mg, 1g vial, 2g vial, 2g dose = £6.

Phenoxymethylpenicillin (generic)
Tablets 250mg, 14 days @ 250mg b.d. = £1.50.
Oral solution 125mg/5mL, 250mg/5mL, 14 days @ 250mg b.d. = £12.

1 British Lymphology Society (2016) Consensus document on the management of cellulitis in lymphodema. www.thebls.com.
2 The Lymphoedema Support Network. (2018) Oedema in advanced ill health. Information for healthcare professionals. www.lymphoedema.org.
3 Cranendonk DR *et al.* (2017) Cellulitis: current insights into pathophysiology and clinical management. *The Netherlands Journal of Medicine*. **75**: 366–378.
4 Raff AB and Kroshinsky D (2016) Cellulitis: a review. *JAMA*. **316**: 325–337.
5 Twycross R and Wilcock A (2016) *Introducing Palliative Care*, 5th edn. Nottingham: palliativedrugs.com.
6 British Lymphology Society (2010) Consensus document on the management of cellulitis in lymphoedema: flucloxacillin versus amoxicillin. www.thebls.com.
7 Eron LJ *et al.* (2003) Managing skin and soft tissue infections: expert panel recommendations on key decision points. *Journal of Antimicrobial Chemotherapy*. **52 (Suppl 1)**: i3–17.
8 Sultan HY *et al.* (2012) Necrotising fasciitis. *British Medical Journal* **345**: e4274.
9 Anonymous (2007) Necrotising fasciitis, dermal infections and NSAIDs: caution. *Prescrire International*. **16**: 17.
10 Leman P and Mukherjee D (2005) Flucloxacillin alone or combined with benzylpenicillin to treat lower limb cellulitis: a randomised controlled trial. *Emergency Medical Journal*. **22**: 342–346.
11 Bisno AL and Stevens DL (1996) Streptococcal infections of skin and soft tissues. *New England Journal of Medicine*. **334**: 240–245.
12 Team UKDCTNs PT *et al.* (2012) Prophylactic antibiotics for the prevention of cellulitis (erysipelas) of the leg: results of the UK Dermatology Clinical Trials Network's PATCH II trial. *British Journal of Dermatology*. **166**: 169–178.
13 Thomas KS *et al.* (2013) Dermatology Clinical Trials Network's PATCH I Trial Team. Penicillin to prevent recurrent leg cellulitis. *New England Journal of Medicine*. **368**: 1695–1703.

Updated October 2019

Quick Clinical Guide: Cellulitis in lymphoedema

Cellulitis is a common complication of lymphoedema. It is associated with significant morbidity and may lead to sepsis. It may be difficult to identify the pathogen, but group A streptococci are considered the most common cause.

Evaluation

1 Clinical features can be more variable than 'classical' cellulitis and range *from*:
- mild symptoms of diffuse erythema (well defined or blotchy), warmth and increased swelling, *to*
- severe episodes of inflammation with pain, systemic upset and even sepsis.

2 Diagnosis is based on pattern recognition and clinical judgement. Elicit:
- history of current episode: date of onset, any precipitating factor (e.g. insect bite or trauma), treatment received to date
- past history: details of past cellulitis, precipitating factors, antibacterials taken
- examination: for erythema, warmth, swelling, tenderness, lymphangitis, local lymph node involvement. It is uncommon to have bilateral cellulitis.

3 Establish a baseline
- extent and severity of rash: if well demarcated, outline with pen and date
- level of systemic upset: temperature, pulse, blood pressure, CRP, WBC
- swab cuts or breaks in skin for microbiology before starting antibacterials; take blood cultures when hospital admission needed.

4 Arrange admission to hospital for IV antibiotics for patients with:
- sepsis (features include pyrexia >38.3°C, delirium, tachycardia, hypotension)
- significant systemic upset, e.g. feeling unwell, rigors, vomiting
- a lack of response to PO antibacterials.

Antibacterials

5 Cellulitis should be treated promptly with antibacterials to prevent sepsis and injury to the lymphatics. Antibacterials should be given for a minimum of 2 weeks from the time a definite clinical response is seen and continued until the acute inflammation has completely resolved; this may take 1–2 months.

6 The advice of a microbiologist should be obtained in unusual circumstances, e.g. anogenital cellulitis, cellulitis after an animal lick or bite, when there is a failure to respond to the recommended antibacterials.

7 Standard treatment at home (PO)

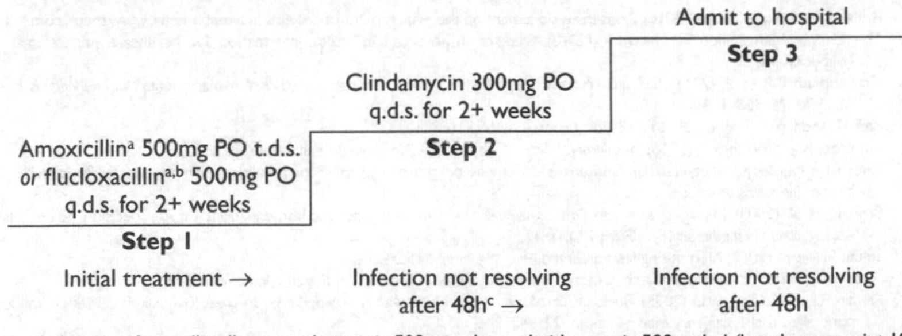

a. if a history of penicillin allergy, erythromycin 500mg q.d.s. or clarithromycin 500mg b.d. (but also see point 10)

b. if features suggest *Staphylococcus aureus* infection (e.g. folliculitis, pus, crusted dermatitis), flucloxacillin should definitely be used

c. if despite 48h of a step 1 antibacterial there are continuing or deteriorating systemic signs (± deteriorating local signs), admit to hospital; otherwise change to step 2 antibacterial.

8 Standard treatment in hospital (IV): follow local guidelines. The following reflect the recommendations of the British Lymphology Society and Lymphoedema Support Network. Switch to PO amoxicillin, flucloxacillin or clindamycin when no fever for 48h, inflammation settling and CRP falling (see point 7).

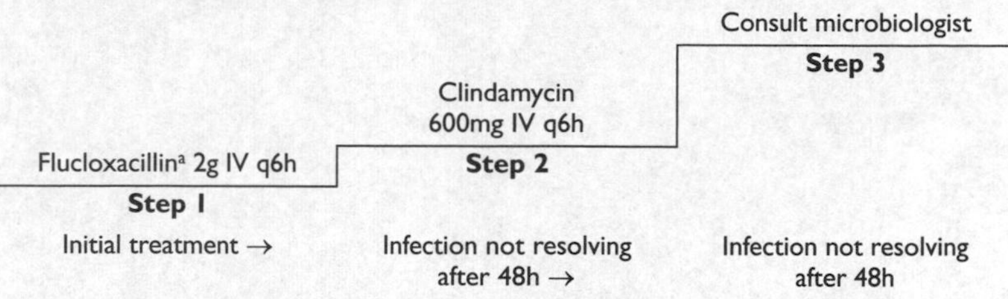

a. if a history of penicillin allergy, start on step 2.

9 If ≥2 episodes of cellulitis/year, review skin condition and skin care regimen and consider further steps to reduce limb swelling. Start PO antibacterial prophylaxis with:
- phenoxymethylpenicillin 250mg b.d. (500mg b.d. if BMI ≥33) for 2 years
- if allergic to penicillins, prescribe erythromycin 250mg b.d.; if not tolerated, use clarithromycin 250mg once daily (but see point 10)
- if cellulitis develops despite the above antibacterials, consider other once daily alternatives, e.g. clindamycin 150mg, cefalexin 125mg, or doxycycline 50mg; seek advice from a microbiologist and local specialist lymphoedema service
- if cellulitis develops after discontinuation of antibacterials after 2 years, treat the acute episode and then commence life-long prophylaxis
- if recurrent anogenital cellulitis, prescribe trimethoprim 100mg at bedtime.

10 Clarithromycin and erythromycin have a risk of prolonged QT interval and *torsade de pointes* and important drug interactions; certain concurrent drug combinations are contra-indicated (e.g. domperidone, statins) or need close monitoring ± dose adjustment. Alternative PO antibacterials: cefalexin 500mg t.d.s. (but not if a history of severe penicillin allergy), or doxycycline 200mg once daily stat then 100mg once daily. For prophylaxis, prescribe cefalexin 125mg or doxycycline 50mg once daily. Some antibacterials also interact with coumarins e.g. warfarin.

General

11 Remember:
- if severe, bed rest and elevation of the affected limb on pillows are essential
- cellulitis is painful; analgesics should be prescribed regularly and p.r.n. Avoid NSAIDs, because there is an increased risk of necrotizing fasciitis
- although compression garments should be avoided during the acute episode, they should be reapplied as soon as it is comfortable to do so
- daily skin hygiene measures should be continued: washing and gentle drying
- emollients should not be used in the affected area if the skin is broken.

12 Patients should be educated about cellulitis:
- why susceptible (skin crevices harbour bacteria, reduced immunity)
- that it causes increased swelling, more fibrosis, decreased response to compression
- daily skin care to improve and maintain skin integrity
- how to reduce risk by achieving optimal control of lymphoedema; also protect hands when gardening, clean cuts, treat fungal infections (terbinafine cream once daily for 2 weeks) and ingrowing toenails
- the need to obtain prompt medical attention if cellulitis occurs.

13 When away from home, patients should take a 2-week supply of PO amoxicillin 500mg t.d.s. *or* flucloxacillin 500mg q.d.s. for emergency use. If allergic to penicillins, erythromycin 500mg q.d.s. or clarithromycin 500mg b.d. (also see point 10).

Updated October 2019

7: ENDOCRINE SYSTEM AND IMMUNOMODULATION

7

BISPHOSPHONATES

Indications: Authorized indications vary among products and among countries; consult SPCs for details. They include tumour-induced hypercalcaemia; prevention of skeletal-related events (SRE) and pain in adults with advanced malignancies involving bone; †adjuvant analgesic in moderate–severe bone pain; †treatment of bone loss in patients at high risk of fracture receiving hormone deprivation therapy for early prostate or breast cancer; †prevention of bone metastases in post-menopausal women with early breast cancer; osteoporosis in post-menopausal women and men; prevention of corticosteroid-induced osteoporosis; Paget's disease.

Contra-indications: Hypocalcaemia. ***PO:*** Oesophageal abnormality (e.g. stricture or achalasia), inability to sit upright for 60min.

Pharmacology

The bisphosphonates are stable analogues of pyrophosphate, a naturally occurring regulator of bone metabolism. They have a high affinity for calcium ions and bind rapidly to hydroxyapatite crystals in mineralized bone. Subsequently, when the bone is resorbed, the bisphosphonate is released and taken up by osteoclasts, inhibiting their function and/or inducing their apoptosis (programmed cell death). Nitrogen-containing bisphosphonates (e.g. **alendronate, ibandronic acid, pamidronate disodium, zoledronic acid**) inhibit the mevalonate pathway vital for normal cellular function (e.g. vesicular trafficking, cell signalling, cytoskeleton function), and non-nitrogen-containing bisphosphonates (e.g. **sodium clodronate, disodium etidronate**) form cytotoxic ATP analogues. Nitrogen-containing bisphosphonates are more potent.[1] Thus, bisphosphonates interfere with the cancer-related increase in the number and osteolytic activity of osteoclasts which contributes to bone pain by the:

- production of an increasingly acidic environment (stimulating acid-sensing receptors on sensory nerves)
- destruction of sensory nerves (producing neuropathic pain)
- loss of bone mineral leading to mechanical instability (stimulating mechanoreceptors on sensory nerves in the periosteum).[2]

In vitro and in animals, bisphosphonates also have a direct anticancer effect by inhibiting cell migration, invasion and metastasis. Clinical studies suggest that bisphosphonates can reduce the risk of bone metastases developing (see p.540). Bisphosphonates have no impact on the effect of parathyroid hormone-related protein (PTHrP) or on renal tubular resorption of calcium.

Bisphosphonates are poorly absorbed PO, and this is reduced further by food. They are rapidly taken up by the skeleton, particularly at sites of bone resorption and where the mineral is more exposed, and they remain there for weeks–years.[3] Most of the remainder is bound to plasma

Table 1 Summary of selected indications for bisphosphonates and/or denosumab; see text for full details

Indication	*Bisphosphonates*	*Denosumab (see p.549)*
Tumour-induced hypercalcaemia (TIH)	IV bisphosphonate is the treatment of choice	SC denosumab: TIH refractory to bisphosphonate
Prevention of skeletal-related events in patients with advanced malignancies involving bone		
Breast cancer: with bone metastases	Zoledronic acid: give every 4 weeks for a minimum of 3–6 months, then every 3 months for 1–2 years	More effective but less cost-effective than zoledronic acid
Prostate cancer: hormone-relapsed with bone metastases	UK guidance recommends zoledronic acid. Although denosumab is more effective, it is less cost-effective and has a higher risk of osteonecrosis of the jaw	
Multiple myeloma: newly diagnosed (± radiologically evident bone disease) or relapsed or refractory disease	Zoledronic acid preferred unless renal impairment: give every 4 weeks for a minimum of 1 year	An alternative for patients with radiologically evident bone disease, particularly when renal impairment is present
Treatment of bone loss in patients at high risk of fracture receiving hormone deprivation therapy for early prostate or breast cancer		
Early prostate cancer: treated with androgen deprivation therapy	Zoledronic acid: give every 6–12 months	An alternative given every 6 months (generally when bisphosphonates are not tolerated, or when CrCl <30mL/min)
Early breast cancer: treated with an aromatase inhibitor or ovarian suppression (including premenopausal women rendered prematurely post-menopausal, e.g. by chemotherapy)	Either risedronate PO once a week or zoledronic acid IV every 6 months	An alternative, particularly in patients with hormone-receptor positive breast cancer receiving an aromatase inhibitor at low risk of disease recurrence
Prevention of bone metastases in post-menopausal women with early invasive breast cancer at high risk of recurrence		
Post-menopausal women (including those prematurely post-menopausal because of treatment) regardless of fracture risk	Either zoledronic acid IV every 3–6 months or ibandronic acid PO once daily; serves dual purpose of preventing bone metastases and treatment-induced bone loss	Not an alternative: ineffective
Prevention and relief of bone pain (see p.539)		
Prevention of corticosteroid-induced osteoporosis (see Box A, p.540)		

proteins. Non-nitrogen-containing bisphosphonates are metabolized to cytotoxic ATP analogues; other bisphosphonates are not metabolized and are excreted unchanged via the kidneys. The plasma proportion of the drug is eliminated generally within 24h. Thereafter, elimination is much slower as the remainder gradually seeps out of bone over many years. Comparison of the halflives of different bisphosphonates is complicated by this multiphasic elimination.

Bisphosphonates and the monoclonal antibody **denosumab** (p.549) have several indications, particularly in patients with cancer (Table 1).

Tumour-induced hypercalcaemia

Bisphosphonates given IV are the treatment of choice for hypercalcaemia of malignancy (Table 2).[4]

Table 2 Bisphosphonates and the initial treatment of tumour-induced hypercalcaemia[5,6]

	Zoledronic acid	*Pamidronate disodium*	*Ibandronic acid*
IV dose	4mg	30–90mg	2–6mg
Onset of effect	<4 days	<3 days	<4 days
Maximum effect	4–7 days	5–7 days	7 days
Duration of effect	4 weeks	2.5 weeks	2.5 weeks (4mg) 4 weeks (6mg)
Restores normocalcaemia	90%	70–75%	75%

For hypercalcaemia refractory to a bisphosphonate, **denosumab** (p.549) can be considered. This supersedes the previous occasional use of **zoledronic acid** *8mg* in those patients failing to respond to 4mg or relapsing within a few days of treatment. With the higher dose of **zoledronic acid**, normocalcaemia is achieved in 50% of the previous non-responders.[5] However, the median duration of response is only 2 weeks. Further, the incidence of renal impairment doubles with 8mg, so its use was abandoned in clinical trials and it is unauthorized.[7]

Prevention of skeletal-related events (SRE) in patients with advanced malignancies involving bone

IV **pamidronate disodium**, IV **zoledronic acid** and PO/IV **ibandronic acid** are given long-term to patients with bone metastases to decrease the incidence of SRE. Onset of benefit is 2–3 months. SRE can include pathological fracture, radiotherapy to bone, spinal cord compression, surgery to bone and pain. However, the SRE used as outcomes in studies vary (e.g. radiological vs. clinical pathological fracture) and can limit direct comparison of study findings. Thus, more recent trials use symptomatic skeletal events as outcomes, defined as radiation to bone, symptomatic pathological fracture, surgery to bone or symptomatic spinal cord compression.[8] Only studies ≥6 months in duration have shown a reduction in fractures, hypercalcaemia and the need for radiotherapy. Studies ≥1 year in duration have also shown a reduced need for orthopaedic surgery. There is no impact on the occurrence of spinal cord compression.[9,10]

Various national guidelines recommend with provisos the routine use of bisphosphonates for the treatment and prevention of SRE in patients with:[11]

- symptomatic myeloma, whether or not bone lesions are evident[12,13]
- breast cancer with bone metastases[14,15]
- hormone-relapsed prostate cancer with bone metastases.[16,17]

Specialty guidelines generally recommend the preventive use of either **zoledronic acid** or **denosumab** for all patients with bone metastases arising from breast or hormone-relapsed prostate cancer, and for selected patients with other solid tumours, i.e. those considered at high risk of an SRE with a likely prognosis ≥3 months and multiple bone metastases, although there is limited evidence from clinical trials in the latter group of patients.[11,18,19]

The optimal dosing schedule or duration of treatment for solid tumours has not been established. However, in patients with bone metastases from breast or prostate cancer, a typical regimen is **zoledronic acid** given every 4 weeks for a minimum of 3–6 months, followed by every 12 weeks for 1–2 years.[20-22] Bisphosphonates are generally continued for as long as they are tolerated or until there is a substantial decline in the patient's performance status. However, a pause in treatment can be considered for those patients with a durable response to systemic treatment, few bone metastases and low risk of fracture.

Multiple myeloma

In patients with myeloma, bisphosphonates reduce SRE, including vertebral fracture, and are recommended for all patients newly diagnosed with multiple myeloma (even in the absence of myeloma bone disease on imaging) or with relapsed or refractory myeloma.[12] They may also reduce pain, both through prevention of painful SRE and through a possible direct anti-tumour effect. Meta-analyses are not wholly consistent, but **zoledronic acid** is probably the most effective bisphosphonate and may prolong overall survival, and is thus recommended in guidelines.[23] There is no consensus on duration of treatment, but a typical regimen is **zoledronic acid** every 4 weeks for a minimum of 1 year. For patients whose myeloma has completely responded, **zoledronic acid** can then be paused; for those with a very good partial response, the frequency is reduced to every 3–6 months, and for those with poorer responses, **zoledronic acid** is continued unchanged for as long as tolerated or until there is a substantial decline in the patient's performance status.[13,24]

Denosumab (p.549) is an alternative for patients with *myeloma bone disease seen on imaging*, particularly in patients with renal impairment.[12] However, it is no more effective than **zoledronic acid** in reducing SRE and does not improve overall survival. Thus, because of its lower cost and dosing frequency, guidelines generally favour **zoledronic acid** over **denosumab**. Nonetheless, there are certain subgroups of patients for whom **denosumab** is favoured, i.e. those with newly diagnosed myeloma for whom autologous stem cell transplantation is intended (see p.550).

Breast cancer

In patients with breast cancer and bone metastases, bisphosphonates given with chemotherapy or hormonal therapy delay time to developing SRE, reduce the risk and rate of developing SRE by <30%, and improve quality of life. Compared with placebo, **zoledronic acid** 4mg IV given every 4 weeks for 1 year reduces the proportion of patients experiencing ≥1 SRE from 50% to 30%.[25] Treatment every 2 weeks provides no greater benefit.[26] After 1 year, a 12-weekly regimen has been shown to maintain benefit, and may be satisfactory after 3–6 months of 4-weekly treatment.[20,21,27]

Zoledronic acid is more effective than PO **ibandronic acid**; it may also be more effective than **pamidronate disodium** and IV **ibandronic acid**.[10,28,29] Conversely, **denosumab** (p.549) is more effective than **zoledronic acid**. However, some have questioned the cost-effectiveness of the modest health gains at substantial additional cost.[30] Guidelines suggest that either IV **zoledronic acid** or SC **denosumab** should be started in all patients with breast cancer and bone metastases, whether or not they are symptomatic.[11,31]

Prostate cancer

In early and metastatic prostate cancer controlled by androgen ablation, there is little or no benefit from bisphosphonates in relation to SRE, quality of life or survival.[17,32–35]

In patients with hormone-relapsed prostate cancer with bone metastases, both **zoledronic acid** and **denosumab** (p.549) reduce total number of SREs.[36] **Zoledronic acid** given for >15 months reduces the risk (by <40%) and rate of developing SRE.[37,38] Although **denosumab** appears more effective than **zoledronic acid** in reducing SRE risk and increasing time to first SRE (21 months vs. 17 months),[39] this is offset by a 10% higher incidence of osteonecrosis of the jaw.[16,40]

However, the pivotal trials of both **zoledronic acid** and **denosumab** pre-date approval of newer treatment options for hormone-relapsed prostate cancer, e.g. **abiraterone**, **enzalutamide**, all of which reduce SRE. Neither **zoledronic acid** nor **denosumab** improve survival,[36] and the question of cost-effectiveness remains.[41]

Thus, the place of **denosumab** and **zoledronic acid** in conjunction with these newer treatments is still to be determined.[16,28,42] As a result, bisphosphonates and **denosumab** are used more frequently in some regions (e.g. USA)[8] than others (e.g. Europe) and in the UK where guidelines recommend **zoledronic acid** but not **denosumab**.[17]

Radium-223 is an alternative in men with hormone-relapsed prostate cancer and symptomatic bone metastases. Compared with placebo it delays time to first symptomatic skeletal event (15 vs. 10 months) and reduces risk of spinal cord compression by half, with a small increase in overall survival (15 vs. 11 months).[43] These results were independent of bisphosphonate use, although in patients on regular bisphosphonates, the results were better, suggesting a synergistic effect.

Bisphosphonates as analgesics

Bisphosphonates are used in two ways:

Prophylactic use

IV/PO bisphosphonates given over months–years are recommended in myeloma, breast cancer and metastatic hormone-relapsed prostate cancer, to reduce the risk and rate of developing potentially painful SRE. This could lead to a delay in the development and/or worsening of bone pain. However, evidence in support of this is mixed. For example, in a systematic review, *no* analgesic benefit of bisphosphonates was seen in 22 of 28 RCTs, mostly involving patients with breast cancer, prostate cancer or myeloma.[44] Generally, bone pain was not the focus of these studies; few used it as a primary end point, and others did not require it as an inclusion criterion. Further, even when assessed, the use of differing and often non-validated measures of pain and analgesic use make comparisons difficult.

Of the studies showing benefit, most were in patients with breast cancer or myeloma and mild–moderate pain, with moderate relief obtained from an IV bisphosphonate given over several months.[10,23] A direct anti-cancer effect of bisphosphonates, seen particularly in breast cancer and myeloma, may be relevant. Thus, in the prophylactic use setting, the analgesic effect is limited to preventing the development of more painful SRE.

†Adjuvant analgesics for moderate–severe bone pain

The role of bisphosphonates as adjuvant analgesics for bone pain is unclear. IV bisphosphonates are given as adjuvant analgesics for moderate–severe bone pain not responding to usual analgesic and anticancer approaches, with the expectation of a more rapid analgesic effect, potentially from their anti-inflammatory effect (see Pharmacology). Onset of pain relief is about 2 weeks and is most likely in patients with moderate pain receiving IV bisphosphonates.[25,45–49] **Denosumab** (p.549) is an alternative and has similar modest benefit.[31] However, supporting data are limited/low quality. Thus, for patients with painful bone metastases despite optimized analgesia and systemic anticancer therapy, *PCF* advises:

- if localized, consider palliative radiotherapy;[50] reserve the use of a bisphosphonate (see Dose and use) for when this is ineffective or inappropriate
- if more widespread, consider:
  - ▷ a radionuclide, e.g. radium-223, in patients with metastatic hormone-relapsed prostate cancer[16,51]
  - ▷ IV **zoledronic acid** or, if unavailable, IV **pamidronate** (see Dose and use) in patients with a prognosis of ≥2 weeks and not already receiving prophylactic bisphosphonates or SC **denosumab**.

†Treatment of bone loss in patients at high risk of fracture receiving hormone deprivation therapy for early prostate or breast cancer

Androgen and oestrogen deprivation therapy accelerates bone turnover, leading to a reduction in bone mineral density (BMD) and increase in fracture incidence (by 40–50% in women; comparable data for men unavailable). Thus, specialty guidelines generally suggest that in early stage prostate or breast cancer, men treated with androgen deprivation therapy or women treated with an aromatase inhibitor or ovarian suppression (including premenopausal women rendered prematurely post-menopausal, e.g. by chemotherapy) should have their bone health monitored every 1–2 years for fracture risk.[11,52,53]

An overall fracture risk is determined, based on BMD and the presence of additional risk factors, e.g. age >65 years, current or past smoker, personal or family history of fragility fracture, long-term corticosteroid use. Correctable risk factors should be addressed and all advised to consume a calcium-enriched diet, to exercise moderately, and take **vitamin D** supplements, with bisphosphonate or **denosumab** therapy reserved for those at greatest risk. Oral calcium supplements are recommended for all patients taking **denosumab** unless hypercalcaemia is present.

In early prostate cancer, in patients with a high fracture risk, **zoledronic acid** every 6–12 months is an accepted treatment.[11,16,54] Although **denosumab** every 6 months (p.551) is authorized for this indication, generally it is used when bisphosphonates are poorly tolerated, or in renal impairment (CrCl <30mL/min).[11,16,17]

In early breast cancer, in patients with a high fracture risk, both PO and IV bisphosphonates can be used, e.g.:[52,55,56]

- **risedronate** 35mg PO once a week
- **zoledronic acid** 4mg IV every 6 months.

Denosumab (p.549) may be an alternative, particularly in patients with hormone receptor-positive breast cancer receiving an aromatase inhibitor.[52,57] Note. Certain groups of women may already be receiving **zoledronic acid** to reduce the risk of bone metastases (see below).

†Prevention of bone metastases in post-menopausal women with early invasive breast cancer at high risk of recurrence

Bisphosphonates (but *not* **denosumab**) reduce the incidence of bone metastases and lead to a small improvement in survival in women with early invasive breast cancer at high risk of recurrence (e.g. node-positive), *without* bone metastases, who are either post-menopausal or premenopausal but rendered prematurely post-menopausal by gonadotrophin-releasing hormone (GnRH) analogues.[10,57–60] Consequently, guidelines recommend bisphosphonates (e.g. **zoledronic acid** 4mg IV every 3–6 months or **ibandronic acid** 50mg PO once daily[61]) as an adjuvant therapy regardless of their fracture risk.[53,62] In this setting, bisphosphonates serve the dual purpose of preventing bone metastases and treatment-induced bone loss.

Bisphosphonates are *not* recommended for the prevention of bone metastases in other solid tumours.

Prevention of osteoporosis in patients receiving long-term corticosteroids (Box A)

Box A Prevention of corticosteroid-induced osteoporosis[63,64]

Concurrent bone-protection therapy is recommended for patients taking corticosteroids equivalent to prednisolone ≥7.5mg/day for ≥3 months at high risk of osteoporotic fracture, i.e.:

- men or women ≥70 years, *or*
- women of any age with previous osteoporotic fracture.

For patients outside these categories, some guidelines suggest treatment only for those at high risk of osteoporotic fracture, identified by a validated risk tool (e.g. FRAX or QFracture) ± BMD measurement. However, recent guidance recommends bone-protection therapy for *all* men and women receiving such doses of corticosteroids, irrespective of age and risk of osteoporotic fracture.[65]

Management

Correctable risk factors should be addressed, e.g. stop smoking and reduce alcohol intake, and all advised to consume a calcium-enriched diet, to exercise moderately and take vitamin D supplements.

When treatment is based on 10-year fracture risk:

- >1%: oral bisphosphonate, e.g. †alendronic acid 70mg once weekly
- >10%: IV bisphosphonate, e.g. zoledronic acid 5mg once a year.

Denosumab 60mg SC every 6 months is an alternative in post-menopausal women >65 years unable to tolerate oral bisphosphonates. Teriparatide is another alternative; *seek endocrinology advice*.

For palliative care patients receiving long-term corticosteroids, an annual IV bisphosphonate may represent the most convenient approach; use of an IV bisphosphonate or denosumab for another reason (e.g. hypercalcaemia of malignancy) removes the need for additional bone-protection therapy.

Cautions

Renal impairment (see Dose and use, and Chapter 17, p.746). Vitamin D deficiency (increased risk of hypocalcaemia).[66] Invasive dental procedures (risk of osteonecrosis of the jaw).

Drug interactions

Concurrent use increases the risk of:

- prolonged hypocalcaemia and hypomagnesaemia with an aminoglycoside[67]
- hypocalcaemia and dehydration with loop diuretics
- renal impairment with other nephrotoxic drugs
- renal impairment with **thalidomide** in multiple myeloma.

For PO bisphosphonates, avoid taking PO products containing **calcium** and antacids (and other products containing **aluminium**, **magnesium** or **iron**) for 1–2h after each dose (see Antacids and antiflatulents, Box A, p.2).

Undesirable effects

Very common (>10%): transient pyrexia and flu-like symptoms (see below), fatigue, headache, anxiety, hypertension, anaemia, thrombocytopenia, cough, arthralgia, myalgia, bone pain, *asymptomatic* hypocalcaemia, hypomagnesaemia, hypophosphataemia.

Oral products in particular may cause anorexia, dyspepsia, nausea, vomiting, abdominal pain, diarrhoea or constipation.

Common (<10%, >1%): sleep disturbance, psychosis, tachycardia, atrial fibrillation or flutter,[68] hypertension, syncope, breathlessness, leucopenia, infusion site reactions, renal impairment (see below), hypokalaemia, osteonecrosis of the jaw (see below).

Rare (<0.1%, >0.01%): ocular inflammation (see below), angioedema, acute renal failure, nephrotic syndrome (**pamidronate disodium**), *symptomatic* hypocalcaemia (e.g. tetany), atypical femoral fractures (see below).

Very rare (<0.01%): osteonecrosis of the external auditory canal (see below), Stevens–Johnson syndrome (**ibandronic acid**).

Acute systemic inflammatory reactions after IV bisphosphonates

Bone pain sometimes occurs <12h after IV bisphosphonates. Systemic reactions, more common with IV nitrogen-containing bisphosphonates, manifest as mild fever (occasionally rigors), myalgia, arthralgia, nausea and vomiting in 25–50% of patients, generally <2 days after IV infusion and lasting 1–2 days. Can be treated with **paracetamol** or NSAIDs. Generally lessen with repeat doses or with prophylactic **paracetamol** or NSAID.[69]

Renal toxicity

Renal impairment is common (about 10%) with both **zoledronic acid** and **pamidronate disodium** (when given as 90mg over 2h).[5] It is uncommon (<1%) with **alendronate**, **clodronate**, **ibandronic acid** or **risedronate**.[70–72]

With **zoledronic acid** 4mg, increases in plasma creatinine lead to treatment delay or discontinuation in about 1% and 3% of patients respectively.[73] Increases in creatinine levels >3 times the upper limit of normal were seen in 0.4% of patients.[71] There have been reports of life-threatening renal failure caused by toxic acute tubular necrosis in patients treated with **zoledronic acid**, e.g. 72 cases among >430,000 patients (<0.02%).[74,75] Other risk factors were often present, including dehydration, pre-existing renal impairment and concurrent use of other nephrotoxic drugs.

Renal impairment often manifests <2 months after starting treatment. Mild impairment tends to recover a few days–several months after discontinuing **zoledronic acid**, but, in those with renal failure, the damage is generally permanent.[10]

The risk of renal toxicity is reduced by adhering to the recommended dose and infusion rate, ensuring adequate hydration, monitoring renal function, and adjusting the dose of bisphosphonate as appropriate or discontinuing treatment if there is deterioration, and avoiding the concurrent use of other nephrotoxic drugs.

Osteonecrosis of the jaw and external auditory canal

All bisphosphonates PO and IV (and **denosumab**) have been implicated as a risk factor for osteonecrosis of the jaw (ONJ).[76,77] The true incidence of ONJ is difficult to identify, but ranges for patients receiving long-term **zoledronic acid** or **pamidronate disodium** for metastatic bone disease are 0.3–8% and 3–5% respectively.[78,79] Although osteonecrosis has been reported after 4 months, generally patients have been receiving bisphosphonates for years (median duration 2–3 years). Additional risk factors for ONJ include invasive dental procedures (reported in about 60% of patients), poor dental health, blood clotting disorders, anaemia, and possibly chemotherapy, angiogenesis inhibitors and corticosteroids.

The jaw bones may be particularly susceptible to osteonecrosis because of the combination of repeated low-level local trauma (e.g. from chewing, dentures) and ease of infection from microbes. Trauma and infection increase the demand for bone repair, which the bisphosphonate-inhibited bone cannot meet, resulting in localized bone necrosis; the anti-angiogenic effect of bisphosphonates may also contribute.

ONJ can present as an asymptomatic bony exposure in one or more sites in the mandible or maxilla, or with orofacial pain, trismus, offensive discharge from a cutaneous fistula, chronic sinusitis because of an oro-antral fistula, and numbness in the mandible or maxilla.[69] If probed, the necrotic bone is generally non-tender and may not bleed. There may be osteomyelitis with oral-cavity flora or *Actinomyces* species. ONJ may show as mottled bone on a plain radiograph and be confused with bone metastases on a bone scan. Pathological fracture can occur.

There is no effective treatment for ONJ.[80,81] Options include antiseptic mouthwashes and antimicrobials to treat infection, or dental surgery. Long-term outcomes are generally poor, with persistent symptoms and unresolved ONJ common, e.g. in patients with multiple myeloma and ONJ, it remains unresolved in up to one-quarter).[78,82–84] Thus, prevention is an important part of the recommended approach (Box B).

Box B Prevention and management of ONJ[69,78,85,86]

For PO bisphosphonates, advise patients to maintain good oral hygiene, attend routine dental check-ups and immediately report any oral symptoms, e.g. dental mobility, pain, swelling, to a doctor and dentist.

For IV bisphosphonates:

- explain the risk of ONJ and give the patient a reminder card (supplied by manufacturers)
- undertake preventive dental treatment before commencing long-term bisphosphonates, e.g. treat infection, extract teeth
- delay bisphosphonate treatment (unless a medical emergency) if there are unhealed oral lesions
- monitor with regular dental examinations, e.g. every 3 months; encourage good dental hygiene, including regular dental cleaning by a dental hygienist
- avoid invasive dental procedures during treatment, and advise patients to inform their dentist of bisphosphonate treatment; if treatment is required, consider a 'bisphosphonate holiday' for 3 months pre- and post-procedure
- minimize trauma, e.g. patients with loose dentures may require a soft reline or replacement
- advise patients to inform their doctor or dentist immediately if oral symptoms develop, e.g. loose teeth, pain, swelling, discharge or non-healing sores.

If urgent treatment precludes dental examination before starting a bisphosphonate, a dental referral and any treatment should be undertaken within 1–2 months for patients expected to receive long-term bisphosphonates.

If ONJ occurs:

- seek specialist advice from a dentist or oral surgeon with expertise in ONJ regarding temporary/permanent discontinuation; however, new lesions may continue to appear even after discontinuation
- treat infection, e.g. antimicrobials, chlorhexidine mouthwash, periodic minor debridement and wound irrigation
- avoid major debridement because it may exacerbate the situation
- avoid major surgery unless there is no alternative, e.g. due to sequestered bone, pathological fracture, oro-antral fistula.

Bisphosphonates PO or IV (and **denosumab**) can also very rarely cause osteonecrosis of the external auditory canal. Reports are for both cancer-related and osteoporosis indications, although generally in patients treated for >2 years. Possible risk factors include corticosteroid use and chemotherapy ± local infection or trauma. Patients should be counselled to report ear pain, discharge or infection during treatment.[87]

Hypocalcaemia

Hypocalcaemia is a risk with all bisphosphonates, although less than with **denosumab** (p.549). Patients who have undergone thyroid surgery may be at increased risk. Although asymptomatic hypocalcaemia is classified as very common, symptomatic hypocalcaemia is rare. However, life-threatening cases have been reported with **zoledronic acid**. For all indications other than tumour-induced hypercalcaemia:

- pre-existing hypocalcaemia must be corrected before the initial dose of **zoledronic acid**
- patients should receive daily oral supplementation with **calcium** and **vitamin D** (see Dose and use).

For the treatment of hypocalcaemia, see p.553.

Ocular toxicity

A rare undesirable effect is ocular inflammation, causing eye pain, redness, swelling, abnormal vision or impaired eye movement (due to rectus muscle oedema).[88] Typically, the onset is <2 days after the first or second infusion and affects both eyes. There may be other symptoms of an acute systemic reaction (see above). An urgent ophthalmology assessment is required, followed by appropriate treatment.

Patients with mild reactions, e.g. those that settle quickly without treatment, can generally continue to receive the same bisphosphonate. Those with more severe reactions, e.g. uveitis or scleritis, should not receive the same bisphosphonate again. Some tolerate a switch to a non-nitrogen-containing bisphosphonate, but specialist advice should be sought from the ophthalmologist ± endocrinologist.[69]

Other toxicities

Atypical femoral fractures: reported rarely and generally in patients treated for >5 years for osteoporosis. The absolute number of atypical fractures reported is far lower than the number of osteoporotic fractures prevented. They are often bilateral and can occur with no/minimal trauma. Patients should be advised to report new or unusual thigh, hip or groin pain.[89–91]

Musculoskeletal pain: severe (sometimes incapacitating) musculoskeletal pain has been reported after days, months or years of bisphosphonate treatment. It is particularly associated with PO bisphosphonates used for osteoporosis and Paget's disease. The pain is distinct from the arthralgia/myalgia associated with an acute systemic reaction (see above), and may respond to temporary or permanent discontinuation of the bisphosphonate.[92]

Dose and use

Because **zoledronic acid** is more effective, *PCF* favours it over **pamidronate disodium** as the bisphosphonate of first choice for tumour-induced hypercalcaemia and prevention of SRE in patients with advanced malignancies involving bone.

Generally, either a single bisphosphonate or **denosumab** (p.549) is used, but not both concurrently.

Tumour-induced hypercalcaemia

Stop and think! Tumour-induced hypercalcaemia can occur as a terminal event in a patient expected to die soon from progressive cancer. Are you justified in correcting a potentially fatal complication in a moribund patient?

All plasma calcium values should be albumin-corrected (see Box C).

Box C Correcting plasma calcium concentrations[a]

If the mean normal albumin for the local laboratory is 40g/L

Corrected calcium (mmol/L) = measured calcium + (0.022 x (40 – albumin g/L))

e.g. measured calcium = 2.45; albumin = 32

corrected calcium = 2.45 + (0.022 x 8) = 2.63mmol/L

(*normal range* = 2.12–2.65mmol/L)

a. most UK pathology laboratories automatically report an albumin-corrected plasma calcium concentration based on locally validated data.

7

For **zoledronic acid**, the SPC recommends treatment for an albumin-corrected plasma calcium ≥3mmol/L (Box C):

- patients should be well hydrated, using sodium chloride 0.9% IV if necessary
- give 4mg IVI in 100mL diluent (see Supply) over 15min
- if plasma calcium does not normalize, repeat after 1 week[4]
- in refractory hypercalcaemia, 8mg has been used, but this dose is unauthorized because of concerns about renal impairment (see Pharmacology)
- for patients with renal impairment:
  - ▷ CrCl ≥30mL/min: no dose adjustment is required
  - ▷ CrCl <30mL/min: avoid use (see Renal or hepatic impairment below).

For **pamidronate disodium**, the SPC recommends a dose dependent on the initial albumin-corrected plasma calcium concentration (Box C and Table 3). However, it has been suggested that 90mg should be given irrespective of the initial calcium level, to increase the probability of a response and to prolong its duration:[4]

- patients should be well hydrated, using sodium chloride 0.9% IV if necessary
- standard and maximum recommended dose is 90mg IVI in 500mL sodium chloride 0.9% over 4h
- repeat after 1 week if initial response inadequate
- repeat every 3–4 weeks according to plasma calcium concentration
- for patients with renal impairment:
  - ▷ CrCl ≥30mL/min: no dose adjustment is required
  - ▷ CrCl <30mL/min: avoid use (see Renal or hepatic impairment below).

Table 3 IV pamidronate disodium for tumour-induced hypercalcaemia[a]

Corrected plasma calcium concentration (mmol/L)	*Dose (mg)*
<3	15 or 30
3–3.5	30 or 60
3.5–4	60 or 90
>4	90

a. UK manufacturer's recommendations. Irrespective of the initial calcium level, many centres use 90mg to increase the probability of a response and to prolong its duration.[4]

Prevention of skeletal-related events (SRE) in patients with advanced malignancies involving bone

Onset of benefit is 2–3 months. Pre-existing hypocalcaemia must be corrected before starting bisphosphonate therapy. Daily oral supplements of elemental **calcium** 500mg and **vitamin D** 400 units are recommended, e.g. Calcichew® D3 Forte.

Baseline assessment and monitoring

Patients should be well hydrated, using sodium chloride 0.9% IV if necessary. Plasma creatinine should be measured before each dose of **zoledronic acid** or **pamidronate disodium**. Withhold treatment if:

- creatinine increases by ≥44micromol/L in patients with a *normal* baseline creatinine concentration (i.e. ≤124micromol/L), *or*
- creatinine increases by ≥88micromol/L in patients with a *raised* baseline creatinine concentration (i.e. >124micromol/L).

Treatment may be resumed at the same dose as before when plasma creatinine returns to within 10% of the baseline value. Discontinue treatment permanently if plasma creatinine fails to improve after 4–8 weeks.

Plasma calcium should be within the normal range before starting treatment with the initial dose of **zoledronic acid**.

To reduce the risk of ONJ, follow the guidelines in Box B.

For **zoledronic acid**:
- patients should be well hydrated, using sodium chloride 0.9% IV if necessary
- give 4mg IVI in 100mL diluent (see Supply) over 15min every 3–4 weeks (see Table 1 for duration of use); with appropriate support, this can be given at home[15]
- for use in patients with renal impairment, see Table 4; avoid use with CrCl <30mL/min (see Renal or hepatic impairment below).

Table 4 Dose reduction for zoledronic acid in cancer patients with renal impairment[a,b,c]

Baseline creatinine clearance (mL/min)	*Recommended dose (mg)*
>60	4 (no reduction)
50–60	3.5
40–49	3.3
30–39	3

a. manufacturer's recommendations for patients with multiple myeloma or bone metastases
b. no data exist for creatinine clearance <30mL/min because these patients were excluded from the studies
c. reduced doses must still be given in 100mL diluent IVI over 15min; see SPCs for preparation details, particularly if using the pre-diluted infusion products.

For **pamidronate disodium**:
- patients should be well hydrated, using sodium chloride 0.9% IV if necessary
- in *breast cancer with bone metastases*, give 90mg IVI in 250mL sodium chloride 0.9% over 1.5–2h every 3–4 weeks (review after 6 months)
- in *multiple myeloma*, give 90mg IVI in 500mL sodium chloride 0.9% *over 4h* every 4 weeks, because of greater risk of renal toxicity
- for patients with renal impairment:
  - ▷ CrCl ≥30mL/min: no dose adjustment is required but the infusion rate should not exceed 90mg/4h
  - ▷ CrCl <30mL/min: avoid use (see Renal or hepatic impairment section below).

†Adjuvant analgesics for moderate–severe bone pain

High-quality data are lacking, and such use is unauthorized (see Pharmacology). Consider when analgesics and radiotherapy are unsatisfactory and the patient is not already receiving prophylactic bisphosphonates or **denusomab** (p.549). **Zoledronic acid** is the drug of choice (see Prevention of SRE above). If not available:
- give **pamidronate disodium** 90mg IVI in 250mL sodium chloride 0.9% over 2h (50% of patients respond, generally within 1–2 weeks); if helpful, repeat 60–90mg every 3–4 weeks for as long as benefit is maintained.

Renal or hepatic impairment

For use in patients with renal impairment (CrCl ≥30mL/min), see details under specific indications above.

The use of bisphosphonates in patients with severe renal impairment or ESRF (CrCl <30mL/min) can be complicated, and specialist renal/endocrinology advice should be sought (also see Chapter 17, p.746). Reasons include the need for caution with fluid administration, the presence of other potentially contributing factors, e.g. tertiary hyperparathyroidism, use of vitamin D analogues or calcium-based phosphate binders, and the risk of further renal toxicity (see Undesirable effects). Renally safer options include **denosumab** (p.549) or reduced doses of **ibandronic acid** (Box D). Both are authorized in the UK for the prevention of SRE in patients with bone metastases from breast cancer/solid tumours and with severe renal impairment.

No dose adjustment is needed for **pamidronate disodium** in mild–moderate hepatic impairment; there are no data in severe hepatic impairment or for **zoledronic acid**; caution is advised by the manufacturer (also see Chapter 18, p.776). No dose adjustment is necessary for **ibandronic acid** in patients with hepatic impairment (Box D).

Box D Ibandronic acid

Ibandronic acid is a third-generation bisphosphonate which is available PO and IV and authorized in the UK for the indications below.

PO ibandronic acid may be as effective as IV zoledronic acid in preventing bone metastases and leads to a small improvement in survival in women with early breast cancer *without* bone metastases, who are either post-menopausal or premenopausal but rendered prematurely post-menopausal by gonadotrophin-releasing hormone (GnRH) analogues.[11,61]

IV ibandronic acid may be as effective as zoledronic acid in reducing SRE in patients with myeloma or metastatic bone disease (but *not* breast cancer).[29,95] It can be used PO for patients wanting to avoid IV treatment or at risk of renal impairment, but is less effective than IV.[74,75,96] The PO tablet is smaller and more easily swallowed than sodium clodronate tablets.

The incidence of undesirable events is low (see main text).[4,45] Renal impairment is no more frequent than with placebo, and ibandronic acid is the only bisphosphonate authorized for use in reduced doses in severe renal impairment (CrCl <30mL/min). Dose adjustment is not needed in hepatic impairment.

Dose and use

For full details, see SPC.

Tumour-induced hypercalcaemia

- patients should be well hydrated, using sodium chloride 0.9% IV if necessary
- if the albumin-corrected plasma calcium:
  - ▷ is ≥3mmol/L give 4mg IVI
  - ▷ is <3mmol/L give 2mg IVI
- for both, give the dose in 500mL sodium chloride 0.9% *or* glucose 5% over 2h.

Prevention of skeletal-related events (SRE) in patients with bone metastases from breast cancer (PO/IV) or †moderate–severe bone pain (IV)

Plasma calcium should be within the normal range before starting treatment; daily supplementation with calcium and vitamin D and steps to reduce the risk of ONJ are recommended, as for other bisphosphonates (see above).

For oral use:

- give 50mg PO once daily; adjust the dose in renal impairment:
  - ▷ CrCl 30–49mL/min: give 50mg PO on *alternate days*
  - ▷ CrCl <30mL/min: give 50mg PO *once a week.*

To maximize absorption and to minimize undesirable gastro-oesophageal effects, patients should take ibandronic acid tablets whole after an overnight fast with a glass of *plain tap water*, followed by a further fast while sitting upright for 1h.

For parenteral use:

- give 6mg IVI in 100mL sodium chloride 0.9% *or* glucose 5% over 15min every 3–4 weeks; adjust the dose in renal impairment:
  - ▷ CrCl 30–49mL/min: give 4mg in 500mL *over 1h* every 3–4 weeks
  - ▷ CrCl <30mL/min: give 2mg in 500mL *over 1h* every 3–4 weeks.

†Subcutaneous administration

If the IV route is inaccessible, the following bisphosphonates can be administered by CSCI, together with SC hydration.[93,94]

- **pamidronate disodium** 90mg in 1L sodium chloride 0.9% over 12–24h
- **sodium clodronate** (not UK or USA) 1,500mg in 50–250mL sodium chloride 0.9% or glucose 5% over 2–3h.

Denosumab (p.549), an SC injection, is an alternative.

Supply

Pamidronate disodium (generic)

Injection (concentrate for dilution and use as an infusion) 3mg/mL, 5mL, 10mL, 20mL and 30mL vial = £28, £55, £110 and £165 respectively; 9mg/mL, 10mL vial = £170; 15mg/mL, 1mL, 2mL, 4mL and 6mL amp = £30, £60, £119 and £170 respectively.

Zoledronic acid (generic)
Injection (concentrate for dilution and use as an infusion) 4mg/5mL, 5mL vial = £30–£175. *Further dilute in 100mL sodium chloride 0.9% or glucose 5%.*
Infusion 4mg/100mL, 100mL bag, vial or bottle = £85–£175.

Note. Zoledronic acid 5mg/100mL is available but only authorized for the treatment of Paget's disease, as an annual dose for osteoporosis in post-menopausal women or in men, and osteoporosis associated with long-term systemic glucocorticoid therapy.

Ibandronic acid (generic)
Tablets 50mg, 28 days @ 50mg once daily = £27.
Injection (concentrate for dilution) 1mg/mL, 2mL vial = £43; 6mL vial = £130.

Note. Ibandronic acid 150mg tablets and 1mg/mL prefilled 3mL syringe are available but only authorized for the treatment of post-menopausal osteoporosis.

1 Kuznik A *et al.* (2020) Bisphosphonates – much more than only drugs for bone diseases. *European Journal of Pharmacology.* **866**: 172773.
2 Falk S and Dickenson AH (2014) Pain and nociception: mechanisms of cancer-induced bone pain. *Journal of Clinical Oncology.* **32**: 1647–1654.
3 Cremers S *et al.* (2019) Pharmacology of bisphosphonates. *British Journal of Clinical Pharmacology.* **85**: 1052–1062.
4 Saunders Y *et al.* (2004) Systematic review of bisphosphonates for hypercalcaemia of malignancy. *Palliative Medicine.* **18**: 418–431.
5 Major P *et al.* (2001) Zoledronic acid is superior to pamidronate in the treatment of hypercalcaemia of malignancy: a pooled analysis of two randomized, controlled clinical trials. *Journal of Clinical Oncology.* **19**: 558–567.
6 Ralston SH *et al.* (1997) Dose-response study of ibandronate in the treatment of cancer-associated hypercalcaemia. *British Journal of Cancer.* **75**: 295–300.
7 Rosen LS *et al.* (2001) Zoledronic acid versus pamidronate in the treatment of skeletal metastases in patients with breast cancer or osteolytic lesions of multiple myeloma: a phase III, double-blind, comparative trial. *Cancer Journal.* **7**: 377–387.
8 Saad F *et al.* (2018) The role of bisphosphonates or denosumab in light of the availability of new therapies for prostate cancer. *Cancer Treatment Reviews.* **68**: 25–37.
9 Henk H *et al.* (2012) Evaluation of the clinical benefit of long-term (beyond 2 years) treatment of skeletal-related events in advanced cancers with zoledronic acid. *Current Medical Research and Opinion.* **28**: 1119–1127.
10 O'Carrigan B *et al.* (2017) Bisphosphonates and other bone agents for breast cancer. *Cochrane Database of Systematic Reviews.* **10**: CD003474. www.cochranelibrary.com.
11 Coleman R *et al.* (2020) Bone health in cancer: ESMO Clinical Practice Guidelines. *Annals of Oncology.* **31**: 1650–1663.
12 Terpos E *et al.* (2021) Treatment of multiple myeloma-related bone disease: recommendations from the Bone Working Group of the International Myeloma Working Group. *Lancet Oncology.* **22**: e119–e130.
13 Snowden JA *et al.* (2017) Guidelines for screening and management of late and long-term consequences of myeloma and its treatment. *British Journal of Haematology.* **176**: 888–907.
14 NICE (2014) Advanced breast cancer: diagnosis and treatment. *Clinical Guideline.* CG81. www.nice.org.uk.
15 SIGN (2013) Treatment of primary breast cancer. *Clinical Guideline* **134**. www.sign.ac.uk.
16 Mottet N *et al.* (2021) *European Association of Urology Prostate Cancer Guidelines.* www.uroweb.org (accessed May 2021).
17 NICE (2019) Prostate cancer: diagnosis and management. *Clinical Guideline* NG131. www.nice.org.uk.
18 Lopez-Olivo MA *et al.* (2012) Bisphosphonates in the treatment of patients with lung cancer and metastatic bone disease: a systematic review and meta-analysis. *Supportive Care in Cancer.* **20**: 2985–2998.
19 Escudier B *et al.* (2019) Renal cell carcinoma: ESMO Clinical Practice Guidelines for diagnosis, treatment and follow-up. *Annals of Oncology.* **30**: 706–720.
20 Himelstein AL *et al.* (2017) Effect of longer-interval vs standard dosing of zoledronic acid on skeletal events in patients with bone metastases: a randomized clinical trial. *JAMA.* **317**: 48–58.
21 Hortobagyi GN *et al.* (2017) Continued treatment effect of zoledronic acid dosing every 12 vs 4 weeks in women with breast cancer metastatic to bone: the OPTIMIZE-2 randomized clinical trial. *JAMA Oncology.* **3**: 906–912.
22 Ng T *et al.* (2021) Long-term impact of bone-modifying agents for the treatment of bone metastases: a systematic review. *Support Care Cancer.* **29**: 925–943.
23 Mhaskar R *et al.* (2017) Bisphosphonates in multiple myeloma: an updated network meta–analysis. *Cochrane Database of Systematic Reviews.* **12**: CD003188. www.cochranelibrary.com.
24 Morgan GJ *et al.* (2013) Long-term follow-up of MRC myeloma IX trial: survival outcomes with bisphosphonate and thalidomide treatment. *Clinical Cancer Research.* **19**: 6030–6038.
25 Kohno N *et al.* (2005) Zoledronic acid significantly reduces skeletal complications compared with placebo in Japanese women with bone metastases from breast cancer: a randomized, placebo-controlled trial. *Journal of Clinical Oncology.* **23**: 3314–3321.
26 Mystakidou K *et al.* (2006) A prospective randomized controlled clinical trial of zoledronic acid for bone metastases. *American Journal of Hospice and Palliative Medicine.* **23**: 41–50.
27 Amadori D *et al.* (2013) Efficacy and safety of 12-weekly versus 4-weekly zoledronic acid for prolonged treatment of patients with bone metastases from breast cancer (ZOOM): a phase 3, open-label, randomised, non-inferiority trial. *Lancet Oncology.* **14**: 663–670.
28 Palmieri C *et al.* (2013) Comparative efficacy of bisphosphonates in metastatic breast and prostate cancer and multiple myeloma: a mixed-treatment meta-analysis. *Clinical Cancer Research.* **19**: 6863–6872.
29 Barrett-Lee P *et al.* (2014) Oral ibandronic acid versus intravenous zoledronic acid in treatment of bone metastases from breast cancer: a randomised, open label, non-inferiority phase 3 trial. *Lancet Oncology.* **15**: 114–122.
30 Andronis L *et al.* (2018) Cost-effectiveness of treatments for the management of bone metastases: a systematic literature review. *Pharmacoeconomics.* **36**: 301–322.
31 Van Poznak C *et al.* (2017) Role of bone-modifying agents in metastatic breast cancer: an American Society of Clinical Oncology-Cancer Care Ontario focused guideline update. *Journal of Clinical Oncology.* **35**: 3978–3986.

32 Yuen KK *et al.* (2006) Bisphosphonates for advanced prostate cancer. *Cochrane Database Systematic Reviews*. **4**: CD006250. www.cochranelibrary.com.

33 Denham JW *et al.* (2014) Short-term androgen suppression and radiotherapy versus intermediate-term androgen suppression and radiotherapy, with or without zoledronic acid, in men with locally advanced prostate cancer (TROG 03.04 RADAR): an open-label, randomised, phase 3 factorial trial. *Lancet Oncology*. **15**: 1076–1089.

34 Smith MR *et al.* (2014) Randomized controlled trial of early zoledronic acid in men with castration-sensitive prostate cancer and bone metastases: results of CALGB 90202 (alliance). *Journal of Clinical Oncology*. **32**: 1143–1150.

35 James ND *et al.* (2016) Addition of docetaxel, zoledronic acid, or both to first-line long-term hormone therapy in prostate cancer (STAMPEDE): survival results from an adaptive, multiarm, multistage, platform randomised controlled trial. *Lancet*. **387**: 1163–1177.

36 Jakob T *et al.* (2020) Bisphosphonates or RANK-ligand-inhibitors for men with prostate cancer and bone metastases: a network meta-analysis. *Cochrane Database Systematic Reviews*. **12**: CD013020. www.cochranelibrary.com.

37 Saad F *et al.* (2002) A randomized, placebo-controlled trial of zoledronic acid in patients with hormone-refractory metastatic prostate carcinoma. *Journal of the National Cancer Institute*. **94**: 1458–1468.

38 James ND *et al.* (2016) Clinical outcomes and survival following treatment of metastatic castrate-refractory prostate cancer with docetaxel alone or with strontium-89, zoledronic acid, or both: the TRAPEZE randomized clinical trial. *JAMA Oncology*. **2**: 493–499.

39 Fizazi K *et al.* (2011) Denosumab versus zoledronic acid for treatment of bone metastases in men with castration-resistant prostate cancer: a randomised, double-blind study. *Lancet*. **377**: 813–822.

40 Beaver JA *et al.* (2018) Metastasis-free survival – a new end point in prostate cancer trials. *New England Journal of Medicine*. **378**: 2458–2460.

41 Tombal B (2015) Assessing the benefit of bone-targeted therapies in prostate cancer, is the devil in the end point's definition? *Annals of Oncology*. **26**: 257–258.

42 Attard G *et al.* (2016) Prostate cancer. *Lancet*. **387**: 70–82.

43 Parker C *et al.* (2013) Alpha emitter radium-223 and survival in metastatic prostate cancer. *New England Journal of Medicine*. **369**: 213–223.

44 Porta-Sales J *et al.* (2017) Evidence on the analgesic role of bisphosphonates and denosumab in the treatment of pain due to bone metastases: a systematic review within the European Association for Palliative Care guidelines project. *Palliative Medicine*. **31**: 5–25.

45 Wong R and Wiffen PJ (2002) Bisphosphonates for the relief of pain secondary to bone metastases. *Cochrane Database Systematic Reviews*. **2**: CD002068. www.cochranelibrary.com.

46 Groff L *et al.* (2001) The role of disodium pamidronate in the management of bone pain due to malignancy. *Palliative Medicine*. **15**: 297–307.

47 Kretzschmar A *et al.* (2007) Rapid and sustained influence of intravenous zoledronic acid on course of pain and analgesics consumption in patients with cancer with bone metastases: a multicenter open-label study over 1 year. *Supportive Cancer Therapy*. **4**: 203–210.

48 Hoskin P *et al.* (2015) A multicenter randomized trial of ibandronate compared with single-dose radiotherapy for localized metastatic bone pain in prostate cancer. *Journal of National Cancer Institute*. **107**: djv197.

49 WHO (2018) Guidelines for the pharmacological and radiotherapeutic management of cancer pain in adults and adolescents. World Health Organization, Geneva, Switzerland. www.who.int.

50 Fallon M *et al.* (2018) Management of cancer pain in adult patients: ESMO Clinical Practice Guidelines. *Annals of Oncology*. **29** (Suppl 4): iv166–191.

51 Sartor O *et al.* (2014) Effect of radium-223 dichloride on symptomatic skeletal events in patients with castration-resistant prostate cancer and bone metastases: results from a phase 3, doubleblind, randomised trial. *Lancet Oncology*. **15**: 738–746.

52 National Comprehensive Cancer Network Guidelines (2018) Breast cancer. www.nccn.org.

53 NICE (2018) Early and locally advanced breast cancer: diagnosis and management. *Clinical Guideline* NG101. www.nice.org.uk.

54 Droz JP *et al.* (2014) Management of prostate cancer in older patients: updated recommendations of a working group of the international society of geriatric oncology. *Lancet Oncology*. **15**: e404–e414.

55 Shapiro CL *et al.* (2019) Management of osteoporosis in survivors of adult cancers with nonmetastatic disease: ASCO Clinical Practice Guideline. *Journal of Clinical Oncology*. **37**: 2916–2946.

56 Kyvernitakis I *et al.* (2018) Prevention of breast cancer treatment-induced bone loss in premenopausal women treated with zoledronic acid: Final 5-year results from the randomized, double-blind, placebo-controlled ProBONE II trial. *Bone*. **114**: 109–115.

57 Gnant M *et al.* (2019) Adjuvant denosumab in postmenopausal patients with hormone receptor-positive breast cancer (ABCSG-18): disease-free survival results from a randomised, double-blind, placebo-controlled, phase 3 trial. *Lancet Oncology*. **20**: 339–351.

58 Early Breast Cancer Trialists' Collaborative Group (2015) Adjuvant biphosphonate treatment in early breast cancer: meta-analyses of individual patient data from randomised trials. *Lancet*. **386**: 1353–1361.

59 Coleman R *et al.* (2014) Adjuvant zoledronic acid in patients with early breast cancer: Final efficacy analysis of the AZURE (BIG 01/04) randomised open-label phase 3 trial. *Lancet Oncology*. **15**: 997–1006.

60 Coleman R *et al.* (2020) Adjuvant denosumab in early breast cancer (D-CARE): an international, multicentre, randomised, controlled, phase 3 trial. *Lancet Oncology*. **21**: 60–72.

61 Gralow JR *et al.* (2020) Phase III randomized trial of bisphosphonates as adjuvant therapy in breast cancer: S0307. *Journal of the National Cancer Institute*. **112**: 698–707.

62 Dhesy-Thind S *et al.* (2017) Use of adjuvant bisphosphonates and other bone-modifying agents in breast cancer: a Cancer Care Ontario and American Society of Clinical Oncology Clinical Practice Guideline. *Journal of Clinical Oncology*. **35**: 2062–2081.

63 NICE (2017) Technology appraisal guidance [TA464]: Bisphosphonates for treating osteoporosis (updated 2019). www.nice.org.uk.

64 NICE (2010) Technology appraisal guidance [TA204]: Denosumab for the prevention of osteoporotic fractures in postmenopausal women. www.nice.org.uk.

65 SIGN (2021) Management of osteoporosis and the prevention of fragility fractures. SIGN 142. www.sign.ac.uk.

66 Broadbent A *et al.* (2005) Bisphosphonate-induced hypocalcemia associated with vitamin D deficiency in a patient with advanced cancer. *American Journal of Hospice and Palliative Care*. **22**: 382–384.

67 Johnson M and Fallon M (1998) Symptomatic hypocalcaemia with oral clodronate. *Journal of Pain and Symptom Management*. **15**: 140–142.

68 MHRA (2008) Biphosphonates atrial fibrillation. *Drug Safety Update*. www.gov.uk/drug-safety-update.

69 Tanvetyanon T and Stiff PJ (2006) Management of the adverse effects associated with intravenous bisphosphonates. *Annals of Oncology*. **17**: 897–907.

70 Chang JT *et al.* (2003) Renal failure with the use of zoledronic acid. *New England Journal of Medicine*. **349**: 1676–1679.

71 Rosen LS *et al.* (2003) Long-term efficacy and safety of zoledronic acid compared with pamidronate disodium in the treatment of skeletal complications in patients with advanced multiple myeloma or breast carcinoma: a randomized, double-blind, multicenter, comparative trial. *Cancer*. **98**: 1735–1744.

72 De Roij van Zuiddewijn C *et al.* (2021) Bisphosphonate nephropathy: A case series and review of the literature. *British Journal of Clinical Pharmacology*. **87**: 3485–3491.
73 Vogel CL *et al.* (2004) Safety and pain palliation of zoledronic acid in patients with breast cancer, prostate cancer, or multiple myeloma who previously received bisphosphonate therapy. *Oncologist*. **9**: 687–695.
74 Body JJ *et al.* (2004) Oral ibandronate improves bone pain and preserves quality of life in patients with skeletal metastases due to breast cancer. *Pain*. **111**: 306–312.
75 Body JJ *et al.* (2004) Oral ibandronate reduces the risk of skeletal complications in breast cancer patients with metastatic bone disease: results from two randomised, placebo-controlled phase iii studies. *British Journal of Cancer*. **90**: 1133–1137.
76 West H (2011) Denosumab for prevention of skeletal-related events in patients with bone metastases from solid tumors: incremental benefit, debatable value. *Journal of Clinical Oncology*. **29**: 1095–1098.
77 Ruggiero SL *et al.* (2004) Osteonecrosis of the jaws associated with the use of bisphosphonates: a review of 63 cases. *Journal of Oral and Maxillofacial Surgery*. **62**: 527–534.
78 Beth-Tasdogan NH *et al.* (2017) Interventions for managing medication-related osteonecrosis of the jaw. *Cochrane Database of Systematic Reviews*. **10**: CD012432. www.cochranelibrary.com.
79 Yarom N *et al.* (2019) Medication-related osteonecrosis of the jaw: MASCC/ISOO/ASCO clinical practice guideline. *Journal of Clinical Oncology*. **37**: 2270–2290.
80 El-Rabbany M *et al.* (2017) Effectiveness of treatments for medication-related osteonecrosis of the jaw: a systematic review and meta-analysis. *The Journal of the American Dental Association*. **148**: 584–594.e2.
81 Zebic L and Patel V (2019) Preventing medication-related osteonecrosis of the jaw. *BMJ*. **365**: 1733.
82 Badros A *et al.* (2008) Natural history of osteonecrosis of the jaw in patients with multiple myeloma. *Journal of Clinical Oncology*. **26**: 5904–5909.
83 Hinson AM *et al.* (2015) Temporal correlation between bisphosphonate termination and symptom resolution in osteonecrosis of the jaw: a pooled case report analysis. *Journal of Oral and Maxillofacial Surgery*. **73**: 53–62.
84 Rollason V *et al.* (2016) Interventions for treating bisphosphonate-related osteonecrosis of the jaw (BRONJ). *Cochrane Database of Systematic Reviews* **2**: CD008455. www.cochranelibrary.com.
85 MHRA (2015) Denosumab (xgeva, prolia); intravenous biphosphonates: osteonecrosis of the jaw – further measures to minimise risk. *Drug Safety Update*. www.gov.uk/drug-safety-update.
86 MHRA (2009) Bisphosphonates: osteonecrosis of the jaw. www.gov.uk/drug-safety-update.
87 MHRA (2015) Bisphosphonates: Very rare reports of osteonecrosis of the external auditory canal. *Drug Safety Update*. www.gov.uk/drug-safety-update.
88 Fraunfelder FW and Fraunfelder FT (2003) Bisphosphonates and ocular inflammation. *New England Journal of Medicine*. **348**: 1187–1188.
89 MHRA (2011) Biphosphonates: atypical femoral fractures. *Drug Safety Update*. www.gov.uk/drug-safety-update.
90 FDA (2010) Drug safety communication: safety update for osteoporosis drugs, bisphosphonates, and atypical fractures. *FDA Drug Safety Communication*. www.fda.gov/drugs/drugsafety.
91 Black DM *et al.* (2019) Atypical femur fractures: review of epidemiology, relationship to bisphosphonates, prevention, and clinical management. *Endocrine Reviews*. **40**: 333–368.
92 FDA (2008) Bisphosphonates (marketed as actonel, actonel+ca, aredia, boniva, didronel, fosamax, fosamax+d, reclast, skelid, and zometa). Information for healthcare professionals. www.fda.gov/drugs.
93 Roemer-Becuwe C *et al.* (2003) Safety of subcutaneous clodronate and efficacy in hypercalcemia of malignancy: a novel route of administration. *Journal of Pain and Symptom Management*. **26**: 843–848.
94 Duncan AR (2003) The use of subcutaneous pamidronate. *Journal of Pain and Symptom Management*. **26**: 592–593.
95 Geng CJ *et al.* (2015) Ibandronate to treat skeletal-related events and bone pain in metastatic bone disease or multiple myeloma: a meta-analysis of randomised clinical trials. *British Medical Journal Open*. **5**: 1–10.
96 Costa L (2014) Which bisphosphonate to treat bone metastases? *Lancet Oncology*. **15**: 15–16.

Updated November 2021

DENOSUMAB

Class: Monoclonal antibody.

Indications: Authorized indications vary among products and among countries; consult SPCs for details. Prevention of skeletal-related events (SRE) in adults with advanced malignancies involving bone; †refractory tumour-induced hypercalcaemia (authorized in USA);[1] giant cell tumour of bone; treatment of bone loss in patients at high risk of fracture receiving hormone deprivation therapy for early prostate or †breast cancer, or long-term systemic corticosteroid therapy; osteoporosis in post-menopausal women and men.

Contra-indications: Hypocalcaemia, unhealed lesions from dental or oral surgery (also see Undesirable effects).

Pharmacology

Denosumab is a human monoclonal antibody that binds receptor activator of nuclear factor kappa β ligand (RANKL), a cytokine and member of the tumour necrosis factor superfamily. This prevents interaction between RANKL and the RANK receptor on osteoclasts, inhibiting their maturation, function and survival, and thereby bone resorption. Bisphosphonates also inhibit osteoclast function (via a different mechanism) and share similar indications and undesirable effects with denosumab but are significantly cheaper.

Denosumab is administered by SC injection. Pharmacokinetics in adults are unaffected by changes in age or renal function, although the risk of hypocalcaemia is increased in renal impairment (see Undesirable effects). Pharmacokinetics in hepatic impairment have not been studied, but are not expected to be altered.

Denosumab is used in a range of clinical settings, sometimes as a preferred alternative to a bisphosphonate, e.g. severe renal impairment, or when a bisphosphonate is ineffective (see Bisphosphonates, Table 1, p.536).

Prevention of skeletal-related events (SRE) in adults with advanced malignancies involving bone

SRE include pathological fracture, spinal cord compression, pain, and need for radiation or surgery to bone. Those used as outcomes vary among studies, as does their definition, e.g. radiological vs. clinical pathological fracture; this variation can limit direct comparison of study findings.

Denosumab is superior to **zoledronic acid** (p.535) in reducing the risk and rate of SRE in patients with bone metastases from solid tumours, particularly breast cancer.[2] Further, denosumab is more effective in delaying the development of painful SRE and the onset of moderate–severe pain in these patients.[3,4] However, any analgesic effect of denosumab is modest, and patients with *existing* bone pain should be managed with usual analgesic approaches.[5,6]

Although **zoledronic acid** is considered cost-effective in this setting, this has been questioned for denosumab, where the modest health gains are at substantial additional cost.[7] Except for cost, other factors influencing choice between **zoledronic acid** and denosumab include route of administration (IV vs. SC), along with the risks of renal toxicity or an acute phase response (both lower with denosumab), and of hypocalcaemia or osteonecrosis of the jaw (lower with **zoledronic acid**).

Breast cancer with bone metastases

Denosumab is superior to **zoledronic acid** (p.535) in delaying time to first and subsequent SRE, with a 20% reduction in skeletal morbidity rate (i.e. number of SRE/time at risk: 0.45 vs. 0.58 events per patient year). However, this was not associated with improvements in survival.[6,8,9]

Prostate cancer with bone metastases

In hormone-relapsed metastatic prostate cancer, compared with **zoledronic acid** (p.535), denosumab is more effective in reducing SRE risk and increasing the time to first SRE (21 vs. 17 months respectively).[10] Neither improve survival.[11] However, denosumab is less cost-effective and associated with a 10% higher incidence of osteonecrosis of the jaw. Consequently, UK guidelines recommend **zoledronic acid**.[12] Nonetheless, some non-UK guidelines recommend either **zoledronic acid** or denosumab.[13,14]

Of note, the pivotal trials of both **zoledronic acid** and denosumab pre-date approval of newer treatment options for hormone-relapsed prostate cancer, e.g. **abiraterone, enzalutamide**, all of which reduce SRE. Thus, the degree of added benefit of **zoledronic acid** and denosumab in this setting has not been determined.[15]

Other solid tumours

Despite limited evidence from clinical trials, specialty guidelines generally recommend either **zoledronic acid** (p.535) or denosumab for selected patients with other solid tumours, i.e. those considered at high risk of an SRE with a likely prognosis ≥3 months and multiple bone metastases.[6,9]

Overall, the preventive benefits of **zoledronic acid** or denosumab do *not* translate into improved survival.[4] Although a *post hoc* analysis of subgroups found that, compared with **zoledronic acid**, denosumab was associated with a small increase in median survival in NSCLC (9.5 vs. 8 months; HR 0.8; 95% CI 0.7–0.9; p=0.01),[16] no survival advantage was found when specifically examined in a subsequent RCT.[17]

Multiple myeloma

In multiple myeloma, denosumab is non-inferior to **zoledronic acid** in delaying the time to first SRE. It is associated with a lower incidence of renal toxicity (12% vs. 17%) but is less cost-effective.[18] Guidelines generally favour IV bisphosphonates, based on their lower cost and more flexible dosing intervals, e.g. **zoledronic acid** (see p.535).

Guidelines recommend denosumab as an option for patients with *myeloma bone disease seen on imaging*, particularly in those with renal impairment.[19] Further, for those patients with newly diagnosed myeloma for whom autologous stem cell transplantation is intended, denosumab prolongs progression-free survival by <11 months, but not overall survival. Thus, more recent guidelines recommend denosumab for this patient group, given every 4 weeks for a minimum of 2 years then every 3–6 months or paused in patients with at least a very good partial response. A single dose of **zoledronic acid** is recommended ≥6 months after discontinuation of denosumab to prevent rebound fragility fractures.[20]

Treatment of bone loss in patients at high risk of fracture receiving hormone deprivation therapy for early prostate or †breast cancer, or long-term systemic corticosteroid therapy

Androgen and oestrogen deprivation therapy accelerates bone turnover, leading to a reduction in bone mineral density and, in women, a 40–50% increase in fracture incidence. For information on assessment and management, see Bisphosphonates, p.535.[21]

In prostate cancer, only denosumab 60mg SC every 6 months is specifically authorized for this indication, reducing the incidence of vertebral fracture from 4% to 1.5% in a 3-year RCT.[22] However, **zoledronic acid** 4mg IVI every 6–12 months is an accepted alternative.[9,12]

In breast cancer, the use of a bisphosphonate PO/IV or denosumab 60mg SC appears sufficient to prevent treatment-related bone loss.[9] Because denosumab improves progression-free survival by 2–3% vs. placebo in post-menopausal women with early hormone-receptor positive breast cancer receiving an aromatase inhibitor and at low risk of disease recurrence, some guidelines recommend denosumab as the treatment of choice to prevent fractures in this group of patients.[9,23,24]

†Prevention of bone metastases

In women with stage 2/3 breast cancer at high risk of bone progression, denosumab does *not* improve bone metastasis-free, disease-free or overall survival.[25] Thus, bisphosphonates (p.535) but not denosumab are recommended for post-menopausal women (or pre-menopausal women treated with GnRH analogues) with early breast cancer at significant risk of recurrence.[9]

Denosumab is not generally recommended for prevention of bone metastases in patients with solid tumours (see Bisphosphonates, p.535).

†Tumour-induced hypercalcaemia

Denosumab is of benefit in hypercalcaemia (albumin-corrected plasma calcium ≥3.0mmol/L) that has failed to respond to bisphosphonate therapy. Initial dosing is at 1–2 week intervals (see Dose and use). In a large case series, by day 10, calcium levels were ≤2.9mmol/L in two-thirds of patients, with normocalcaemia achieved in one-third. Overall, some reduction was seen in 70% of patients, with normocalcaemia achieved in 64%, with a median duration of response of 15 weeks. However, some patients were also receiving anticancer treatment, e.g. chemotherapy.[1] Such use is authorized in the USA.

Giant cell tumour of bone

Denosumab is used to impede the growth of giant cell tumours of the bone in skeletally mature adolescents and adults, improving local control and/or facilitating less invasive surgical treatments.[26]

Bio-availability 60–80% SC (partly due to pre-systemic catabolism).
Onset of action 3 days (80% reduction in bone resorption markers ≤1 week).
Time to peak plasma concentration 10 days.
Plasma halflife 28 days.
Duration of action weeks–months.

Cautions

Renal impairment or ESRF (increased risk of hypocalcaemia). Patients with risk factors for osteonecrosis of the jaw or of the external auditory canal (see Undesirable effects, and p.541).

Drug interactions

Clinically significant pharmacokinetic interactions have not been reported and are unlikely.

Undesirable effects

Very common (>10%): breathlessness, diarrhoea, hypocalcaemia (see below), musculoskeletal pain.
Common (<10%, >1%): hypophosphataemia, hyperhidrosis, osteonecrosis of jaw (see below), need for tooth extraction, rash. New primary cancers (see below).

Rare (<0.1%, >0.01%): atypical femoral fracture.
Not known: osteonecrosis of external auditory canal.

Hypocalcaemia

In patients with bone metastases from solid tumours, hypocalcaemia is twice as common with denosumab 120mg (10%) than **zoledronic acid** (5%).[27] In multiple myeloma, the incidence is 17% vs. 12% respectively.[18] It mostly occurs ≤2 weeks after starting treatment and can be severe and life-threatening.[28] Those with renal impairment or ESRF are at increased risk.

Severe hypocalcaemia is rare with denosumab 60mg, and generally occurs in those with additional risk factors for hypocalcaemia, e.g. electrolyte imbalance, severe renal impairment/dialysis.[27,29]

Pre-existing hypocalcaemia must be corrected before starting denosumab. Except when used for tumour-induced hypercalcaemia, daily oral supplementation with calcium and vitamin D is recommended. Calcium levels should be monitored regularly, particularly in those at increased risk, e.g. with severe renal impairment/dialysis (see Dose and use).[28]

Osteonecrosis of the jaw and external auditory canal

The incidence of osteonecrosis of the jaw (ONJ) with denosumab 120mg is similar to that with **zoledronic acid** in multiple myeloma (around 4%). Some studies report an incidence of ≤4% in patients with bone metastases from solid tumours receiving denosumab.[30] However, a recent meta-analysis reported the incidence as 0.5–2.1% after 1 year of treatment with denosumab, slightly higher than 0.4–1.6% after 1 year of treatment with **zoledronic acid.**[18,27,31] Duration of exposure, history of tooth extraction, poor oral hygiene, use of a dental appliance and concurrent or previous chemotherapy affect the risk of ONJ. It can also occur ≤5 months after stopping treatment (see p.541). Patients should be counselled and issued with cards to remind them of the precautions to follow before and during treatment, including the need for dental check-ups (also see p.541). Unhealed lesions from dental or other oral surgery is a contra-indication to the use of denosumab 120mg (see Dose and use).[32]

As with bisphosphonates, osteonecrosis of the external auditory canal can also occur. The incidence is unknown. Possible risk factors include corticosteroid use, chemotherapy ± local infection or trauma. Patients should be counselled to report ear pain, discharge or infection during treatment.[33]

The risk of ONJ and osteonecrosis of the external auditory canal is related to cumulative dose and is thus less with denosumab 60mg.[27,32]

Other toxicities

Atypical femoral fractures: As with bisphosphonates, rare cases of atypical femoral fracture have been reported affecting the subtrochanteric and diaphyseal regions, often bilateral, associated with minimal or no trauma. Patients should be advised to report new or unusual thigh, hip or groin pain.[34] Denosumab should be discontinued and an orthopaedic opinion obtained.

Discontinuation fractures: Unlike bisphosphonates, denosumab is not taken up into bone. In osteoporosis, after discontinuation of denosumab, bone turnover increases within 3 months, bone mineral density falls to baseline levels within 12 months and there is an increased risk of multiple vertebral fractures, probably due to a rebound increase in osteoclast activity.[35] Thus, when used for osteoporosis, denosumab should be administered regularly, and if discontinued, a bisphosphonate used instead to preserve at least some of the bone mineral density gained during denosumab treatment.[36,37] In cancer, by extrapolation, such considerations are probably even more relevant given the stimulating effect of cancer on osteoclasts; thus, denosumab is generally given indefinitely until the patient is in the last weeks of life (or it is substituted for **zoledronic acid**; see Box B).[9,38]

Discontinuation hypercalcaemia in patients with giant cell tumour of bone and in patients with growing skeletons: Clinically significant hypercalcaemia has occurred in patients with giant cell tumour of bone within weeks–months of stopping denosumab. This is probably due to a rebound increase in osteoclast activity. Such patients should be regularly monitored for signs and symptoms of hypercalcaemia (± plasma calcium) along with their need for calcium and vitamin D supplementation. Similarly, hypercalcaemia has also occurred after denosumab is stopped in patients with growing skeletons. (Note. The manufacturer does *not* recommend its use in this setting.)[39]

Infection: RANK receptors are also expressed on immune cells, e.g. lymphocytes, macrophages. Although denosumab potentially could impede immune activation, a meta-analysis of RCTs in osteoporosis suggests no significantly increased risk of severe infection.[40] Nonetheless, in one large RCT, more participants receiving denosumab than placebo experienced severe skin infections, mostly erysipelas/

cellulitis of the lower limb, although numbers affected were small (15 vs. 3).[41] It is suggested that inhibition of RANKL in keratinocytes could reduce the number of regulatory T cells, increasing the inflammatory response to a skin infection and thereby resulting in a more severe appearance.[42] Studies in other settings, including advanced cancer, have found no increased risk of infection.[42]

New primary cancers: In a pooled analysis of four studies of patients with advanced cancer involving bone and receiving treatment to reduce SRE (median duration around 1 year), the incidence of a new primary cancer was twice as common with denosumab 120mg (1.1%) vs. **zoledronic acid** 4mg (0.6%). A more recent meta-analysis of 25 RCTs has found a similar risk between denosumab 60mg SC every 6 months up to 48 months and any comparator.[43] The full implications of this recent observation and relation to higher dose of denosumab are currently uncertain.[44]

Dose and use

Generally, either denosumab or a bisphosphonate (p.535) is used, but not both concurrently.

Pre-existing hypocalcaemia must be corrected before starting denosumab, along with any underlying cause, e.g. vitamin D deficiency. During treatment with denosumab (unless given for hypercalcaemia), daily oral supplements of elemental **calcium** ≥500mg and **vitamin D** 400 units should be given, e.g. Calcichew® D3 Forte.

Denosumab is administered as an SC injection into the thigh, abdomen or upper arm. To reduce discomfort at the site of injection, allow the vial to reach room temperature before use (also see Supply).

Baseline assessment and monitoring

All plasma calcium values are albumin-corrected (see Bisphosphonates, Box C, p.543).

Unless hypercalcaemia is present, plasma calcium should be within the normal range before the initial dose of denosumab is given. Thereafter, it should be monitored as a minimum:[28]
- within 2 weeks of an initial 120mg dose; consider ongoing monitoring, e.g. before each dose, in patients with risk factors for hypocalcaemia, e.g. severe renal impairment/dialysis
- within 2 weeks of an initial 60mg dose in patients with risk factors for hypocalcaemia
- before each 6-monthly 60mg dose
- if symptoms of hypocalcaemia occur; counsel patients to report muscle spasms, twitches, cramps, and numbness or tingling in the fingers, toes or around the mouth.

If hypocalcaemia occurs, when mild (plasma calcium ≥1.9–2.2mmol/L and asymptomatic), an increase in PO calcium supplementation to 2–4g/24h may suffice. However, severe (plasma calcium <1.9mmol/L) or symptomatic hypocalcaemia is a *medical emergency* and requires IV calcium gluconate (Box A).[45]

Box A Emergency treatment of hypocalcaemia

Hypocalcaemia increases the risk of cardiac arrhythmia. IV calcium administration can cause hypotension, cardiac arrhythmia and precipitate digoxin toxicity. *Continuous heart rate monitoring* is required in patients at higher risk of cardiotoxicity, e.g. those with ECG changes, cardiac disease or taking digoxin. Recommendations on the need for *continuous ECG monitoring* vary, ranging from the ideal of its routine use to, as a minimum, in the high-risk group above.[45,46]

Stop or slow the infusion if bradycardia or hypotension occurs. For patients with raised plasma phosphate levels, consult specialist renal and/or endocrinology guidance.

Initial treatment
- give 10–20mL calcium gluconate 10% (2.2–4.4mmol) IV diluted in 50–100mL sodium chloride 0.9% or glucose 5% over 10min
- use a central or large peripheral vein because of the risk of irritation
- repeat the dose until the patient is asymptomatic.

Follow-up infusion
- give 100mL calcium gluconate 10% (22mmol) IVI diluted in 1L sodium chloride 0.9% or glucose 5% at a rate of 50–100mL/h; titrate to achieve normocalcaemia
- check calcium levels 2h after the infusion.

The following precautions should be taken to reduce the risk of ONJ (also see Undesirable effects, and p.541):[28]

- denosumab 120mg; a dental examination and appropriate preventive dentistry is recommended before treatment. Denosumab should not be started if patients require dental or jaw surgery, or if they have not recovered from oral surgery
- denosumab 60mg; check for ONJ risk factors before treatment and, if present, a dental examination and appropriate preventive dentistry are recommended.

Patients should be counselled on the risks and to report symptoms associated with hypocalcaemia, ONJ, osteonecrosis of the ear and atypical fracture.

Prevention of skeletal-related events (SRE) in adults with advanced malignancies involving bone

For all patients with breast or hormone-relapsed prostate cancer with bone metastases, whether symptomatic or not. For selected patients with other solid tumours (i.e. those considered at high risk of an SRE with a likely prognosis >3 months) or multiple myeloma:

- give 120mg SC every 4 weeks
- continue indefinitely, until patient is in last weeks of life (also see Box B).

Box B Prevention of SRE in patients with a limited prognosis

PCF notes that:

- the cost-effectiveness of the additional benefit of denosumab over zoledronic acid for the prevention of SRE is questionable
- the risk of discontinuation fractures is greater with denosumab than zoledronic acid
- speciality guidelines generally recommend the use of either.

Thus, for patients with cancer referred to a specialist palliative care service who have progressive metastatic bone disease despite monthly denosumab, unless there is severe renal impairment, *PCF* recommends considering replacing denosumab with zoledronic acid. For patients with a limited prognosis, zoledronic acid would need to be given only once, 4 weeks after the last dose of denosumab. However, if necessary, the zoledronic acid can be repeated every 3 months (see p.535).[9]

Treatment of bone loss in patients at high risk of fracture receiving hormone deprivation therapy for early prostate or †breast cancer, or long-term systemic corticosteroid therapy

In addition to general measures (see Pharmacology), in those considered high risk:

- give 60mg SC every 6 months.

Bisphosphonates (p.535) are suitable alternatives.

†Tumour-induced hypercalcaemia

XGEVA® is authorized for this indication in the USA. Generally, used for hypercalcaemia refractory to bisphosphonate therapy (see Pharmacology):

- give 120mg SC every 4 weeks; *give additional 120mg SC doses on days 8 and 15 of the first month of therapy*
- monitor at regular intervals for ongoing benefit.

Giant cell tumour of bone

Denosumab is authorized as an alternative to surgery. Dose schedule as per tumour-induced hypercalcaemia above.

Supply

XGEVA® (Amgen)

Injection 70mg/mL, 120mg vial = £310.

Prolia® (Amgen)

Injection (prefilled syringe) 60mg/mL, 1mL = £183.

XGEVA® and Prolia® should be stored long-term in a refrigerator (2–8°C); do not freeze. They may be removed and stored at room temperature, in the original cartons, to protect from light, for up to 30 days (see SPCs). Do not shake the vial or syringe.

1 Hu MI *et al.* (2014) Denosumab for treatment of hypercalcemia of malignancy. *Journal of Endocrinology and Metabolism*. **99**: 3144–3152.

2 O'Carrigan B *et al.* (2017) Bisphosphonates and other bone agents for breast cancer. *Cochrane Database of Systematic Reviews*. **10**: CD003474. www.cochranelibrary.com.

3 von Moos R *et al.* (2013) Pain and health-related quality of life in patients with advanced solid tumours and bone metastases: integrated results from three randomized, double-blind studies of denosumab and zoledronic acid. *Supportive Care in Cancer*. **21**: 3497–3507.

4 Sun L and Yu S (2013) Efficacy and safety of denosumab versus zoledronic acid in patients with bone metastases: a systematic review and meta-analysis. *American Journal of Clinical Oncology*. **36**: 399–403.

5 Porta-Sales J *et al.* (2017) Evidence on the analgesic role of bisphosphonates and denosumab in the treatment of pain due to bone metastases: a systematic review within the European Association for Palliative Care guidelines project. *Palliative Medicine*. **31**: 5–25.

6 Van Poznak C *et al.* (2017) Role of bone-modifying agents in metastatic breast cancer: an American Society of Clinical Oncology-Cancer Care Ontario focused guideline update. *Journal of Clinical Oncology*. **35**: 3978–3986.

7 Andronis L *et al.* (2018) Cost-effectiveness of treatments for the management of bone metastases: a systematic literature review. *PharmacoEconomics*. **36**: 301–322.

8 von Moos R *et al.* (2019) Management of bone health in solid tumours: from bisphosphonates to a monoclonal antibody. *Cancer Treatment Reviews*. **76**: 57–67.

9 Coleman R *et al.* (2020) Bone health in cancer: ESMO Clinical Practice Guidelines. *Annals of Oncology*. **31**: 1650–1663.

10 Fizazi K *et al.* (2011) Denosumab versus zoledronic acid for treatment of bone metastases in men with castration-resistant prostate cancer: a randomised, double-blind study. *Lancet*. **377**: 813–822.

11 Jakob T *et al.* (2020) Bisphosphonates or RANK-ligand-inhibitors for men with prostate cancer and bone metastases: a network meta-analysis. *Cochrane Database of Systematic Reviews*. **12**: CD013020. www.cochranelibrary.com.

12 NICE (2019) Prostate cancer: diagnosis and management. *Clinical Guideline* NG131. www.nice.org.uk.

13 Beaver JA *et al.* (2018) Metastasis-free survival – a new end point in prostate cancer trials. *New England Journal of Medicine*. **378**: 2458–2460.

14 Mottet N *et al.* (2021) Prostate Cancer Guidelines. Arnhem: European Association of Urology. https://uroweb.org/guideline/prostate-cancer/ (accessed May 2021).

15 Saad F *et al.* (2018) The role of bisphosphonates or denosumab in light of the availability of new therapies for prostate cancer. *Cancer Treatment Reviews*. **68**: 25–37.

16 Scagliotti GV *et al.* (2012) Overall survival improvement in patients with lung cancer and bone metastases treated with denosumab versus zoledronic acid: subgroup analysis from a randomized phase 3 study. *Journal of Thoracic Oncology*. **7**: 1823–1829.

17 Peters S *et al.* (2020) A randomized open-label phase III trial evaluating the addition of denosumab to standard first-line treatment in advanced NSCLC: the European Thoracic Oncology Platform (ETOP) and European Organisation for Research and Treatment of Cancer (EORTC) SPLENDOUR trial. *Journal of Thoracic Oncology*. **10**: 1647–1656.

18 Raje N *et al.* (2018) Denosumab versus zoledronic acid in bone disease treatment of newly diagnosed multiple myeloma: an international, double-blind, double-dummy, randomised, controlled, phase 3 study. *Lancet Oncology*. **19**: 370–381.

19 Anderson K *et al.* (2018) Role of bone-modifying agents in multiple myeloma: American Society of Clinical Oncology Clinical Practice guideline update. *Journal of Clinical Oncology*. **36**: 812–818.

20 Terpos E *et al.* (2021) Treatment of multiple myeloma-related bone disease: recommendations from the Bone Working Group of the International Myeloma Working Group. *Lancet Oncology*. **22**: e119–e130.

21 Sawamura M (2017) Effects of denosumab on bone metabolic markers and bone mineral density in patients treated with glucocorticoids. *Internal Medicine*. **56**: 631–636.

22 Smith MR *et al.* (2009) Denosumab in men receiving androgen-deprivation therapy for prostate cancer. *New England Journal of Medicine*. **361**: 745–755.

23 Gnant M *et al.* (2019) Adjuvant denosumab in postmenopausal patients with hormone receptor-positive breast cancer (ABCSG-18): disease-free survival results from a randomised, double-blind, placebo-controlled, phase 3 trial. *Lancet Oncology*. **20**: 339–351.

24 Shapiro CL *et al.* (2019) Management of osteoporosis in survivors of adult cancers with nonmetastatic disease: ASCO Clinical Practice Guideline. *Journal of Clinical Oncology*. **37**: 2916–2946.

25 Coleman R *et al.* (2020) Adjuvant denosumab in early breast cancer (D-CARE): an international, multicentre, randomised, controlled, phase 3 trial. *Lancet Oncology*. **21**: 60–72.

26 Van der Heijden L *et al.* (2020) Current concepts in the treatment of giant cell tumour of bone. *Current Opinion in Oncology*. **32**: 332–333.

27 Lipton A *et al.* (2012) Superiority of denosumab to zoledronic acid for prevention of skeletal-related events: a combined analysis of 3 pivotal, randomised, phase 3 trials. *European Journal of Cancer*. **48**: 3082–3092.

28 MHRA (2014) Denosumab: updated recommendations. *Drug Safety Update*. www.gov.uk/drug-safety-update.

29 Body JJ *et al.* (2018) Hypocalcaemia in patients with prostate cancer treated with a bisphosphonate or denosumab: prevention supports treatment completion. *BMC Urology*. **18**: 81.

30 Smith MR *et al.* (2012) Denosumab and bone-metastasis free survival in men with castration-resistant prostate cancer: results of a phase 3, randomised, placebo-controlled trial. *Lancet*. **379**: 39–46.

31 Limones A *et al.* (2020) Medication-related osteonecrosis of the jaws (MRONJ) in cancer patients treated with denosumab VS. zoledronic acid: A systematic review and meta-analysis. *Medicina Oral Patologia Oral y Cirugia Bucal*. **25**: e326–e336.

32 MHRA (2015) Denosumab (Xgeva, Prolia); intravenous biphosphonates: osteonecrosis of the jaw – further measures to minimise risk. *Drug Safety Update*. www.gov.uk/drug-safety-update.

33 MHRA (2017) Denosumab (Prolia, Xgeva): reports of osteonecrosis of the external auditory canal. *Drug Safety Update*. www.gov.uk/drug-safety-update.

34 MHRA (2013) Denosumab 60mg (Prolia). Rare cases of atypical femoral fracture with long-term use. *Drug Safety Update*. www.gov.uk/drug-safety-update.
35 Cummings SR *et al.* (2018) Vertebral fractures after discontinuation of denosumab: A post hoc analysis of the randomized placebo-controlled FREEDOM Trial and its extension. *Journal of Bone and Mineral Research*. **33**: 190–198.
36 Reid IR *et al.* (2017) Bone loss after denosumab: only partial protection with zoledronate. *Calcified Tissue International.* **101**: 371–374.
37 Tsourdi E *et al.* (2021) Fracture risk and management of discontinuation of denosumab therapy: a systematic review and position statement by ECTS. *The Journal of Clinical Endocrinology & Metabolism*. **106**: 264–281.
38 MHRA (2020) Denosumab 60mg (Prolia): increased risk of multiple vertebral fractures after stopping or delaying ongoing treatment. *Drug Safety Update*. www.gov.uk/drug-safety-update.
39 MHRA (2018) Denosumab (Xgeva®) for giant cell tumour of bone: risk of clinically significant hypercalcaemia following discontinuation. *Drug Safety Update*. www.gov.uk/drug-safety-update.
40 von Keyserlingk C *et al.* (2011) Clinical efficacy and safety of denosumab in postmenopausal women with low bone mineral density and osteoporosis: a meta-analysis. *Seminars in Arthritis and Rheumatism*. **41**: 178–186.
41 Cummings SR *et al.* (2009) Denosumab for prevention of fractures in postmenopausal women with osteoporosis. *New England Journal of Medicine*. **361**: 756–765.
42 Watts NB *et al.* (2012) Infections in postmenopausal women with osteoporosis treated with denosumab or placebo: coincidence or causal association? *Osteoporosis International*. **23**: 327–337.
43 Rosenberg D (2021) Denosumab is not associated with risk of malignancy: systematic review and meta-analysis of randomized controlled trials. *Osteoporosis International*. **3**: 413–424.
44 MHRA (2018) Denosumab (Xgeva®) for advanced malignancies involving bone: study data show new primary malignancies reported more frequently compared to zoledronate. *Drug Safety Update*. www.gov.uk/drug-safety-update.
45 Turner J *et al.* (2016) Society for Endocrinology Endocrine Emergency Guidance: emergency management of acute hypocalcaemia in adult patients. *Endocrine Connections*. **5**: G7–G8.
46 UKMI (2017) How is acute hypocalcaemia treated in adults? *Medicines Q&A*. www.sps.nhs.uk.

Updated November 2021

SYSTEMIC CORTICOSTEROIDS

Indications: Suppression of inflammatory and allergic disorders, cerebral oedema, nausea and vomiting with chemotherapy; †see Box A.

Box A Off-label indications for systemic corticosteroids in advanced cancer[1]

This list of off-label uses is not totally comprehensive. Inclusion does not mean that a systemic corticosteroid is necessarily the treatment of choice. Further, the evidence base for some indications is only expert opinion.[2]

Specific
Appetite stimulant
Spinal cord compression[3]
Nerve compression
Breathlessness caused by:
  pneumonitis (after radiation therapy)
  lymphangitic carcinomatosis
  tracheal compression/stridor
Superior vena caval obstruction[4]
Obstruction of hollow viscus:
  bronchus[5]
  ureter
  GI[6,7]
Discharge from rectal tumour (can give either PO or PR)
Paraneoplastic fever
Nausea and vomiting in cancer resistant to standard measures (see p.264)

Pain relief[a]
Pain associated with spinal cord or nerve compression
Pain caused by a tumour in a confined organ or body cavity, e.g. raised intracranial pressure
Radiation-induced inflammation[8]

Anticancer hormone therapy
Prostate cancer[9]
Haematological malignancies
Lymphoproliferative disorders

a. RCT evidence is mixed, but overall suggests that the use of corticosteroids for cancer pain per se outside of the above indications has little benefit.[10,11] In an adequately powered study of cancer patients with moderate pain of various causes, 1 week of methylprednisolone 32mg/24h PO significantly improved anorexia and fatigue, but not average daily pain or opioid use.[11]

Contra-indications: Systemic infection, unless considered to be life-saving and specific anti-infective therapy is employed.

Pharmacology

The adrenal cortex secretes **hydrocortisone** (cortisol), which has glucocorticoid activity and weak mineralocorticoid activity.[12] It also secretes aldosterone, which has mineralocorticoid activity. Thus, in deficiency states, physiological replacement is best achieved with a combination of **hydrocortisone** and **fludrocortisone**, a mineralocorticoid.

In many disease states, corticosteroids are used primarily as potent anti-inflammatory agents. The anti-inflammatory action is mediated via several interacting mechanisms,[12] in contrast to the more specific impact of NSAIDs on prostaglandin synthesis (see p.341). Thus, as anti-inflammatory agents, corticosteroids are potentially more effective than NSAIDs. However, certainly when used long-term, corticosteroids are likely to cause more numerous and more serious undesirable effects (see below).

When comparing the relative anti-inflammatory (glucocorticoid) potencies of corticosteroids, their water-retaining properties (mineralocorticoid effect) should also be borne in mind (Table 1). Thus, **hydrocortisone** is not used for long-term disease suppression because large doses would be required and these would cause troublesome fluid retention. On the other hand, the moderate anti-inflammatory effect of **hydrocortisone** makes it a useful corticosteroid for topical use in inflammatory skin conditions; both topical and systemic undesirable effects are minimal.

Prednisolone is the most frequently used corticosteroid for disease suppression. **Dexamethasone**, with high glucocorticoid activity but insignificant mineralocorticoid effect, is particularly suitable for high-dose anti-inflammatory therapy. It is 7 times more potent than **prednisolone**, i.e. 2mg of **dexamethasone** is approximately equivalent to 15mg of **prednisolone** (Box B, p560) and it has a long duration of action (Table 1). Some corticosteroid esters, e.g. of **betamethasone** and of **beclometasone**, exert a marked topical effect; use is made of this property with skin applications and bronchial inhalations (see Emollients, p.677 and Inhaled corticosteroids, p.140).

Appetite stimulant

Corticosteroids have traditionally been used in patients with advanced cancer as a 'tonic' to improve appetite ± wellbeing. Although most patients appear to benefit,[13,14] RCTs suggest a large placebo effect.[15,16]

A systematic review found overall evidence of a beneficial effect on appetite from corticosteroids, but variation in drug, dose and quality of the RCTs made it impossible to recommend a particular regimen.[17] Results are mixed, e.g. a recent RCT found no significant difference in the proportion of responders after 1 week of PO **dexamethasone** 4mg/day (65%), **megestrol acetate** 480mg/day (80%) or placebo (60%).[16]

In a real-world setting, mostly involving patients with advanced cancer, 1 week of **dexamethasone** (mean/median dose 4mg/day) improved anorexia in about 70% (30% completely). Although generally well tolerated, one third reported ≥1 harm, mostly mild–moderate in severity, the most common being mood disturbance (e.g. euphoria, agitation, depression or mania), insomnia and hyperglycaemia.[13]

Guidelines recommend that a short-term trial of a corticosteroid (or progestogen, see p.599) may be offered for appetite stimulation in patients with advanced cancer using **dexamethasone** 3–4mg/day PO or equivalent, with the duration of treatment dependent on treatment goals and assessment of risk vs. benefit.[18]

However, both corticosteroids and progestogens should *not* be regarded as 'anticachexia' agents (see p.600). Any weight gain relates to fluid retention ± increased fat, rather than to increased skeletal muscle mass. This could make mobilizing more difficult in an already debilitated patient. In addition, the catabolic effect of corticosteroids on skeletal muscle, exacerbated by reduced levels of physical activity, may well further weaken the patient, rendering corticosteroids suitable for short-term use only (e.g. ≤2 weeks).[2]

Nausea and vomiting

Dexamethasone is an integral part of standard management of chemotherapeutic nausea and vomiting.[19] Its anti-emetic effect may be mediated through a direct central action at the solitary tract nucleus, a direct anti-inflammatory effect on damaged tissue, or through reduced expression of serotonin receptors.[20]

In palliative care, **dexamethasone** is often used when all else fails as an add-on anti-emetic (see QCG: Nausea and vomiting, p.264). However, supporting data are limited, with some suggesting that **dexamethasone** does not add to the anti-emetic efficacy of **metoclopramide** or phenothiazines in patients with advanced cancer.[21]

Obstructive syndromes

In obstructive syndromes (Box A), corticosteroids may help by reducing inflammation at the site of the obstruction, thereby increasing the lumen of the obstructed hollow viscus. Corticosteroids (e.g. **dexamethasone** 8mg/24h SC) may improve bowel obstruction, but do not affect survival. The incidence of undesirable events is low.[6,22] High-dose corticosteroids (**dexamethasone** equivalent 20–40mg/24h PO) relieved stridor within 12h in three patients with upper airway obstruction from infiltrating tumour.[5]

Brain metastases

Dexamethasone is recommended for treatment of adults with symptomatic brain metastases; no benefit is seen in patients with asymptomatic brain metastases. **Dexamethasone** 4–8mg/24h PO provides temporary symptomatic relief for patients with mild symptoms related to raised intracranial pressure from cerebral oedema. If patients have severe symptoms or are at risk of herniation, doses of ≥16mg/24h PO are recommended. Symptom relief from **dexamethasone** reduces over time, and undesirable effects increase. Thus, ideally, the dose of **dexamethasone** should be reduced after 1 week and discontinued after 2–4 weeks.[23] However, unless patients receive additional treatment (e.g. palliative radiotherapy), they will experience a recurrence of their symptoms at some point as the dose of **dexamethasone** is decreased. Thus, it may be necessary to taper more slowly or continue maintenance **dexamethasone** indefinitely in some patients.

Whole-brain radiotherapy may cause nausea, vomiting, headache, fever and a transient worsening of neurological symptoms. **Dexamethasone** should be continued for 1 week after treatment and then tapered over 2–4 weeks.[24,25]

Spinal cord compression

Spinal cord compression must be treated as an emergency; patients with paraparesis do better than those who are totally paraplegic.[3,26,27] Because corticosteroids inhibit inflammation, stabilize vascular membranes and reduce spinal cord oedema, their use in spinal cord compression often results in a dramatic reduction in pain and an early improvement in the patient's physical status.

Traditionally, **dexamethasone** has been used as the corticosteroid of choice, sometimes initially given IV. However, given its high PO bio-availability (Table 1), IV administration seems unnecessary. A typical PO regimen would be:[3]

- a stat dose of **dexamethasone** 16mg PO
- continue with 16mg PO each morning until surgery completed or radiotherapy started
- maintain on 8mg PO each morning until radiotherapy completed
- taper (and discontinue) over 1–2 weeks after the completion of radiotherapy or surgery.

If there is neurological deterioration during the dose reduction, the dose should be increased again to the previous satisfactory dose and maintained at that level for a further 2 weeks before attempting to taper the dose again. About one quarter of patients require maintenance **dexamethasone** in order to preserve neural function.

Very high initial doses of **dexamethasone** (96–100mg stat and once daily for 3 days, then tapering to zero over 2 weeks) are not justified. They provide little or no more benefit than 16mg, but are associated with a definite risk of a major adverse event (>10%), particularly acute GI perforation (3%, at any level from the stomach to the sigmoid colon), GI haemorrhage, sepsis, and possibly even death.[28]

For pharmacokinetic details, see Table 1

Table 1 Selected pharmacokinetic details of commonly used corticosteroids[29,30]

Drug	*Anti-inflammatory potency*	*Approximate equivalent dose (mg)*	*Sodium-retaining potency*	*Oral bio-availability (%)*	*Onset of action*	*Peak plasma concentration*	*Plasma halflife (h)*	*Duration of action (h)*	*Relative affinity for lung tissue*	*Daily dose (mg) above which adrenal suppression possible*	
										Male	*Female*
Hydrocortisone	1	20	1	96	No data	1h PO	1.5	8–12	1	20–30	15–25
Prednisone[a] and prednisolone	4	5	0.25	75–85	No data	1h PO	3.5	12–36	1.6	7.5–10	7.5
Dexamethasone	25–50[b]	0.5–1	<0.01	78	8–24h IM[c]	1–2h PO	4.5	36–54	1	1–1.15	1
Betamethasone				98	No data	10–36min IV	6.5	24–48			

a. biologically inert prednisone is converted by the liver to prednisolone
b. thymic involution assay
c. acute allergic reactions.

Box B Approximate equivalent anti-inflammatory doses of corticosteroids

This list takes no account of either mineralocorticoid effects or variations in duration of action.

Corticosteroid	*Approximate equivalent anti-inflammatory dose*
Cortisone acetate	25mg
Hydrocortisone	20mg
Prednisone	5mg
Prednisolone	5mg
Methylprednisolone	4mg
Triamcinolone	4mg
Betamethasone	750microgram
Dexamethasone	750microgram

Cautions

Risk of life-threatening adrenal insufficiency at times of significant intercurrent illness, trauma or surgical procedure (see Dose and use).

Diabetes mellitus, psychotic illness.

There is a small overall increased risk of GI bleed or perforation from the use of corticosteroids alone compared with placebo (2.9% vs. 2%; OR 1.42, 95%CI 1.22–1.66).[31] This is mostly explained by their high occurrence in hospitalized patients (38 vs. 26 per 1,000 patients), probably because of the association between severe illness and stress ulceration. In ambulatory patients, their occurrence was low (1.8 vs. 0.7 per 1,000 patients), with no significant difference in risk. *However, there is a 15 times increase in risk when corticosteroids are given concurrently with NSAIDs* (p.346).[32-34]

Prolonged courses of corticosteroids increase susceptibility to infections and increase their severity. Clinical presentation may be atypical; the signs of infection (including peritonitis) may be masked. Serious infections (e.g. septicaemia, tuberculosis, pneumocystis pneumonia) may reach an advanced stage before diagnosis. Live vaccines should not be given; the antibody response to other vaccines may be diminished.[35]

Renal or hepatic impairment (because of the salt- and water-retaining properties of corticosteroids), also see Chapters 17 and Chapter 18, p.746 and p.776.

Drug interactions

Corticosteroids antagonize oral hypoglycaemics and **insulin** (glucocorticoid effect), antihypertensives and diuretics (mineralocorticoid effect). Increased risk of hypokalaemia if high doses of corticosteroids are prescribed with β_2 agonists (e.g. **salbutamol**, **terbutaline**).

CYP3A4 is important in the metabolism of most corticosteroids, and caution is required with the concurrent use of drugs that inhibit or induce this enzyme (see Chapter 19, Table 8, p.790). Reports of interactions include:

- **itraconazole** (potent CYP3A4 inhibitor) decreases the metabolism of corticosteroids; e.g. for **dexamethasone**, this increases the AUC and maximum plasma concentration by up to 3 times.
- **carbamazepine**, **phenobarbital**, **phenytoin**, **primidone**, **rifabutin** and **rifampicin** (potent CYP3A4 inducers) increase the metabolism of corticosteroids. This is more pronounced with long-acting glucocorticoids; thus **phenytoin** may reduce the bio-availability of **dexamethasone** to 25–50%, and larger doses (double or more) will be needed when prescribed concurrently.[36]
  Dexamethasone itself can affect plasma **phenytoin** concentrations (may either rise or fall).

Concurrent prescription of a corticosteroid increases the INR in patients already taking **warfarin**, necessitating a dose reduction in about 50% of patients.[37] Thus, the INR should be checked weekly for 2–3 weeks when a corticosteroid is started or dose altered.

Magnesium trisilicate can reduce the absorption of **dexamethasone** and possibly other corticosteroids by ≤75% (see Antacids and antiflatulents, p.1); separate the administration of each drug by ≥2h.

Undesirable effects

See Box C–Box F.

Box C Undesirable effects of corticosteroids[33]

Glucocorticoid effects
Adrenal suppression[a]
Avascular bone necrosis
Cataract (prednisolone 15mg/24h or equivalent for several years = 75% risk; also seen with long-term inhaled steroids)[38]
Central serous chorioretinopathy[39]
Diabetes mellitus or deterioration of glycaemic control in known diabetics (see p.585)
Infection (increased susceptibility):
- candidosis (debatable, see p.511)
- septicaemia (may delay recognition)
- tuberculosis (may delay recognition)
- PCP pneumonia
- chickenpox[b], measles[c] (increased severity)

Psychiatric disturbances (Box D)
Muscle wasting and weakness (Box E)
Osteoporosis → fracture[d]
Peptic ulceration (particularly if given with an NSAID)
Suppression of growth (in child)

Mineralocorticoid effects
Hypertension
Potassium loss
Sodium and water retention → oedema

Cushingoid features
Acne
Bruising
Hirsutism
Lipodystrophy after ≥8 weeks of treatment in 30–70% of patients (reversible on stopping treatment):
- moon face
- buffalo hump
- increased abdominal fat
- reduced subcutaneous fat in limbs

Striae

a. see Dose and use
b. if exposed to infection, non-immune patients should be given varicella-zoster immunoglobulin
c. if exposed to infection, consider use of IM pooled immunoglobulin (Ig) in non-immune patients[40]
d. consider prophylactic bisphosphonate therapy in patients receiving long-term corticosteroids (see p.535).

Box D Corticosteroid-induced psychiatric disturbances[13,41-43]

Incidence

Reports range from 13–62% of those prescribed a corticosteroid.
Prevalence is higher in women, and more likely with higher doses.

Clinical manifestations

Symptoms generally occur 4–6 days after starting a corticosteroid, but this is highly variable and they can occur even after cessation of treatment.

Manifestations are mostly mild or moderate, but can be severe, and include:
- depression (40%)
- mania (25%)
- paranoid ('steroid') psychosis (15%)
- delirium (10%)
- bipolar disorder (5%).

Insomnia, anxiety, agitation and euphoria are also common. Educating patients about the possible risk of undesirable psychiatric effects may improve the reporting of symptoms.

Management

Reduce or discontinue the causal corticosteroid if possible.[41]

Environmental conditions should be optimized to minimize agitation.[44] Symptoms may take 1–2 weeks to resolve.[42]

If the corticosteroid cannot be stopped or symptoms are intolerable, atypical antipsychotics should be prescribed for patients with psychosis, aggression or agitation.

Although antidepressants may exacerbate agitation and psychosis, they are generally helpful in depressed patients who require long-term corticosteroids.

All patients with corticosteroid-induced psychiatric disturbance should be evaluated for suicidal ideation.

Prognosis

A history of:
- psychiatric disease does not make a corticosteroid-induced psychiatric disturbance more likely
- previous corticosteroid-induced disturbance does not necessarily mean that a second disturbance will occur if corticosteroids are represcribed.[43]

Box E Systemic corticosteroid myopathy[45,46]

Glucocorticoids cause atrophy of limb and respiratory muscles. It is a dose-related effect which generally manifests only after ≥2 months of treatment with dexamethasone >4mg/24h or prednisolone >40mg/24h. Can occur earlier and with lower doses.

If the chronological sequence fits with corticosteroid myopathy, a presumptive diagnosis should be made and the following steps taken:

- explanation to patient and family
- discuss need to compromise between maximizing therapeutic benefit and minimizing undesirable effects
- halve corticosteroid dose (generally possible as a single step)
- consider changing from dexamethasone to prednisolone (non-fluorinated corticosteroids cause less myopathy)
- attempt further reductions in dose at intervals of 1–2 weeks
- arrange for physiotherapy (disuse exacerbates myopathy)
- emphasize that weakness should improve after 3–4 weeks (provided cancer-induced weakness does not supervene).

Box F Pseudorheumatism

Patients receiving corticosteroids for rheumatoid arthritis occasionally develop myalgia, arthralgia, malaise, rhinitis, conjunctivitis, painful itchy skin nodules, weight loss and pyrexia; so-called steroid pseudorheumatism.[47]

It is sometimes also seen in cancer patients receiving large doses of corticosteroids or when a very high dose is reduced rapidly to a lower dose. Most likely to be affected are those:

- receiving prednisolone 100mg/24h for several days in association with chemotherapy
- with spinal cord compression given dexamethasone 96mg IV/24h for 3 days[48] (followed by a rapidly reducing oral dose)[a]
- on high doses of dexamethasone to reduce raised intracranial pressure associated with brain metastases
- reducing to an ordinary maintenance dose after a prolonged course.

a. such a high dose is unnecessary; 10mg IV is as effective as 96mg.[28]

Dose and use

In patients who have taken **prednisolone** ≥5mg (or equivalent) daily for ≥4 weeks by *any* route, the occurrence of any significant intercurrent illness, trauma or surgical procedure necessitates a temporary increase in corticosteroid dose (or, if stopped within the past 3 months, a temporary re-introduction) to compensate for a reduced adrenocortical response caused by the corticosteroid treatment; see national guidance for full details on dose adjustments required to cover sick days, surgery or invasive treatment.[49]

For the emergency management of adrenal crisis see Box H.

Given the many and significant undesirable effects of corticosteroids, and the potentially deleterious effect of rapid withdrawal, corticosteroids should be prescribed cautiously:

- for defined symptoms potentially responsive to corticosteroid therapy
- always bearing in mind potential benefit vs. risk
- at a low–moderate dose, titrated to clinical effect (Note. Higher than usual doses may be necessary with concurrent use of an enzyme-inducing drug; see Drug interactions)
- for a time-limited trial, e.g. 1 week is generally sufficient to assess for benefit for anorexia[13]
- wean the patient to the lowest effective dose or discontinue if no clinical/symptomatic benefit seen.[50]

Further:

- monitor blood glucose before starting, and regularly during treatment (e.g. every 1–2 weeks), particularly in patients at risk of diabetes (also see Drugs for diabetes mellitus, Box C p.585)
- prescribe a PPI if patient is at high risk of peptic ulceration or bleeding, e.g. past history of either, acutely unwell, concurrent NSAID use (also see p.346)

- if expected to take PO corticosteroids for ≥3 weeks, give patients a steroid *treatment* card (Box G). Consider also for those taking:
  - ▷ frequent (>4/year) shorter courses of PO corticosteroids
  - ▷ inhaled corticosteroids (see p.141)
- patients who are corticosteroid dependent (includes those on long-term PO corticosteroids) should also receive a steroid *emergency* card (see Box H).

Box G Steroid treatment card information[a]

I am a patient on STEROID treatment which must not be stopped suddenly.

- If you have been taking this medicine for more than 3 weeks, the dose should be reduced gradually when you stop taking steroids unless your doctor says otherwise.
- Read the patient information leaflet given with the medicine.
- Always carry this card with you and show it to anyone who treats you (for example a doctor, nurse, pharmacist or dentist).
- For 1 year after you stop the treatment, you must mention that you have taken steroids.
- If you become ill or if you come into contact with anyone who has an infectious disease, consult your doctor promptly.
- If you have never had chickenpox, you should avoid close contact with people who have chickenpox or shingles. If you do come into contact with chickenpox, see your doctor urgently.
- Make sure that the information on the card about your current dose is kept up to date.

a. official steroid treatment card available from www.nhsforms.co.uk.

Box H Steroid emergency card information[a,49]

This should be given to patients dependent on corticosteroids, i.e. those:

- with primary adrenal insufficiency
- with adrenal insufficiency due to hypopituitarism
- taking prednisolone ≥5mg (or equivalent) daily for ≥4 weeks by *any* route of administration, i.e. oral, topical, inhaled, intranasal, or intra-articular
- taking prednisolone ≥40mg (or equivalent) daily for >1 week, or repeated short PO courses
- taking a course of PO corticosteroids ≤1 year of stopping long-term therapy.

The card highlights this dependency, and how omitting or stopping the corticosteroid, along with illness or surgery, can precipitate an adrenal crisis, that can present with vomiting, diarrhoea, dehydration and shock. The emergency treatment consists of:

- *immediate* hydrocortisone 100mg IV/IM, *followed by*:
  - ▷ hydrocortisone 200mg/24h CIVI in glucose 5%, *or*
  - ▷ hydrocortisone 50mg IV/IM q.d.s. (100mg if severely obese)
- rapid rehydration with sodium chloride 0.9%
- liaising with the endocrinology team.

Further information is available from https://www.endocrinology.org/adrenal-crisis

a. official steroid emergency card available from www.nhsforms.co.uk.

For corticosteroid replacement therapy (e.g. in hypo-adrenalism), a typical regimen is **hydrocortisone** 20mg each morning and 10mg each evening, with **fludrocortisone** 100–300microgram each morning.

Except for **hydrocortisone**, corticosteroids can be given in a single daily dose each morning. However, when tablet burden is an issue, higher doses of **dexamethasone** (i.e. >8mg) can be halved and administered as a morning and a lunchtime dose. Giving doses later in the day should be generally avoided, as this increases the risk of corticosteroid-induced adrenal suppression and insomnia. Nonetheless, even with morning doses, **temazepam** or **diazepam** at bedtime is sometimes needed to counter insomnia or agitation.

PO

In palliative care, **dexamethasone** is generally the systemic corticosteroid of choice for anti-emesis, anorexia, raised intracranial pressure, obstruction of a hollow viscus and spinal cord compression. The initial dose varies according to indication (Table 2). For more information about dose adjustment and duration of treatment, see the relevant sections in Pharmacology above.

Table 2 Typical PO and SC/IV starting doses for dexamethasone, expressed as dexamethasone base[a]; before use, read the relevant sections in Pharmacology

Indication	*PO dose*	*SC/IV dose (volume)*	
		3.3mg/mL formulation	*3.8mg/mL formulation*
Appetite stimulant[b]	2–4mg[18]	1.7–3.3mg (0.5–1mL)	1.9–3.8mg (0.5–1mL)
Anti-emetic[c]	8–16mg[19,51,52]	6.6–13.2mg (2–4mL)	7.6–15.2mg (2–4mL)
Obstruction of hollow viscus	8–16mg[6]	6.6–13.2mg (2–4mL)	7.6–15.2mg (2–4mL)
Raised intracranial pressure	8–16mg[53]	6.6–13.2mg (2–4mL)	7.6–15.2mg (2–4mL)
Spinal cord compression	16mg	13.2mg (4mL)	15.2mg (4mL)

a. generally given once daily in the morning (see text)
b. prednisolone 15–30mg PO each morning is an alternative
c. also see QCG: Nausea and vomiting, p.264.

SC/IV

In the UK, **dexamethasone** is available in injectable formulations as the *sodium phosphate* salt. However, all dosing advice, prescribing and labelling must now be expressed as **dexamethasone** *base*.[54,55]

There is further potential for confusion because different brands of injection vary in their strength, presentation, preservative/solvent content and storage requirements. For more details, see Table 3.[56]

All the injectable formulations are suitable for SC use.

In palliative care, **dexamethasone** is traditionally given SC rather than IM/IV, with the initial dose varying according to indication and strength of the injectable formulation (Table 2).

Traditionally, for ease of prescribing, conversion of PO to SC/IV **dexamethasone** was made on a 1:1 basis (e.g. 4mg PO = 4mg SC/IV). Following recent labelling and formulation changes, the injectable formulations contain either 3.3mg/mL or 3.8mg/mL **dexamethasone** *base* (Tables 2 and 3). Thus, continuing with an exact 1:1 conversion will lead to an unnecessarily complex and wasteful use of ampoules and vials. Because the conversion between PO and SC/IV **dexamethasone** only requires the selection of a reasonable starting dose, *PCF* recommends that:

- for pragmatic purposes, when converting between PO and SC/IV routes, both 3.3mg and 3.8mg **dexamethasone** *base* of the injectable formulations can be considered approximately equivalent to **dexamethasone** *base* 4mg PO
- the SC/IV dose prescribed should take into account which injectable formulation is being used so as to avoid wasteful use of vials/ampoules (Tables 2 and 3)
- the dose should be subsequently titrated according to response
- *for consistency and to avoid confusion between colleagues and departments, clinicians should observe local guidelines and use the locally available injection formulation.*

Betamethasone *base* 4mg/mL injection provides an alternative of similar potency to **dexamethasone**. However, there is no cost advantage and there is less experience of its use.

CSCI

CSCI compatibility of dexamethasone with other drugs: because it is an alkaline drug, therapeutic doses of **dexamethasone** often cause compatibility problems. To minimize the risk of precipitation, it should always be the last drug added to an already dilute combination of drugs. In addition, different injectable formulations may react differently when mixed (see Chapter 29, p.892).

Dexamethasone has a long duration of action; therapeutic doses can generally be given as a bolus SC injection once daily, which avoids the risk of precipitation (see p.887).

To reduce CSCI site reactions, **dexamethasone** 1mg is sometimes added to other drugs when compatibility data permit (see p.895).

Rectal use

Anecdotally, a corticosteroid enema may help reduce excessive discharge from a rectal cancer. However, current options are limited and the costs significantly higher (see Supply). A trial of **budesonide** foam enema 2mg PR every 1–2 days is one option, but a PO corticosteroid may be more practical.

Other uses

For use in the management of anaphylaxis, see p.920.
For inhaled corticosteroids, see p.140.
For depot corticosteroid injections, see p.649.
For topical corticosteroids, see p.679.

7

Stopping corticosteroids

If after 7–10 days the corticosteroid fails to achieve the desired effect, it should be stopped. It is often possible to stop corticosteroids abruptly (Box I). However, if there is uncertainty about disease or symptom resolution, withdrawal should be guided by monitoring disease activity or the symptom.

Particularly if it has been taken for >3 weeks, rapid withdrawal of a corticosteroid may result in a corticosteroid withdrawal syndrome. This may cause an array of symptoms and signs similar to those of pseudorheumatism (Box F). The syndrome is treated by restarting the corticosteroid or increasing the dose to that given before the onset of withdrawal symptoms.[57] Acute adrenal insufficiency may also occur, see Box H.

Box I Recommendations for withdrawing systemic corticosteroids[40]

Abrupt withdrawal

Systemic corticosteroids may be stopped abruptly in those whose disease is unlikely to relapse *and* who have received treatment for <3 weeks *and* are not in the groups below.

Gradual withdrawal

Gradual withdrawal of systemic corticosteroids is advisable in patients who:

- have received >3 weeks treatment
- have received prednisolone >40mg/24h or equivalent, e.g. dexamethasone 4–6mg for >1 week
- have had a second dose in the evening
- have received repeated treatments
- are taking a short course within 1 year of stopping long-term treatment
- have other possible causes of adrenal suppression.

During corticosteroid withdrawal, higher doses may initially be reduced rapidly (e.g. by 25–50% every 3–4 days) until near-physiological doses are reached (e.g. prednisolone 7.5–10mg/24h or equivalent, e.g. dexamethasone 1–2mg/24h). Thereafter, reductions should be made more slowly (e.g. at *weekly* intervals: prednisolone by 1–2mg; dexamethasone 2mg → 1mg → 0.5mg → stop) to allow the adrenals to recover and to prevent a hypo-adrenal crisis (malaise, profound weakness, hypotension, etc.). The patient should be monitored during withdrawal in case of deterioration; this will necessitate a return to a higher dose, and subsequent attempts at withdrawal to be at a slower rate.

If physiological stress, e.g. from infection, trauma or surgery, occurs within 1 week of stopping the corticosteroid, additional corticosteroid cover should be prescribed to compensate for adrenal suppression.

In patients who are moribund and no longer able to swallow tablets, it is generally acceptable to discontinue corticosteroids abruptly,[50] although sometimes a maintenance dose may be indicated to prevent distress from symptomatic hypo-adrenalism.

Occasionally, a patient with a brain tumour or multiple brain metastases requests that **dexamethasone** is stopped because, despite its continued use, there is progressive physical deterioration and/or cognitive impairment. In this circumstance, it is often best to reduce the **dexamethasone** step by step on a daily basis. This gives the patient time to reconsider. *Ensure appropriate analgesia is prescribed in case headache develops as the intracranial pressure increases.* If the patient becomes drowsy or swallowing becomes difficult, switch any PO anti-epileptic to one that can be given parenterally, e.g. **midazolam** (see p.174), **levetiracetam** (p.312), **valproate** (p.307), **phenobarbital** (p.315).

If the patient becomes semi-conscious and cannot communicate clearly, the presence of headache may manifest as grimacing or general restlessness. However, as in all moribund patients, it is important to exclude other common reasons for agitation, e.g. a full bladder or rectum, and discomfort and stiffness secondary to immobility.

Supply

Dexamethasone formulations in the UK

Conventional PO tablets are formulated as **dexamethasone** *base*; the soluble tablets, oral solution and injectable formulations are formulated as **dexamethasone** *sodium phosphate*. The *BNF*, SPCs and product labels now all use **dexamethasone** *base* for labelling and dosing advice.

In countries where soluble tablets or an oral solution of **dexamethasone** are not available, the contents of an ampoule for injection can be used PO (see Chapter 28, Table 2, p.863).

Dexamethasone (generic)
Tablets 500microgram, 2mg, 4mg, 28 days @ 2mg once daily = £3. *For higher doses, the 4mg are significantly more expensive than using the 2mg tablets.*
Oral solution (sugar-free) 2mg/5mL, 10mg/5mL, 20mg/5mL, 28 days @ 2mg (5mL) once daily = £34.
Soluble tablets (sugar-free) 2mg, 4mg, 8mg, 28 days @ 2mg once daily = £4.25.
Injection see Table 3.

Table 3 Dexamethasone injectable formulations (UK)[54,55]

	Aspen	*Hameln*	*Panpharma, Pfizer or Wockhardt*
Dexamethasone base	3.8mg/mL[a]	3.3mg/mL[b]	3.3mg/mL[b]
Presentation (all glass)	1mL vial	1mL, 2mL amp	1mL, 2mL amp, 2mL vial[c]
Storage	Refrigerate at 2–8°C	<25°C	<25°C
Other[d]		Contains propylene glycol 20mg/mL	2mL vial[c] contains sodium sulphite 0.07mg/mL
Cost	£2	1mL = £2.50 2mL = £2.50	1mL = £1.25–2.50 2mL = £2–£4.75[c]

a. dexamethasone base 3.8mg ≈ dexamethasone sodium phosphate 5mg
b. dexamethasone base 3.3mg ≈ dexamethasone sodium phosphate 4.3mg
c. 2mL vial available only from Pfizer
d. all formulations except the Panpharma/Wockhardt products and 1mL Pfizer ampoule contain disodium edetate.

Betamethasone (generic)
Tablets (soluble) 500microgram, 28 days @ 2mg once daily = £65.
***Injection* betamethasone** 4mg/mL (base) 1mL = £7.50.

Budesonide
Budenofalk® (Dr Falk Pharma)
Foam enema 2mg/metered application, 14-application canister with applicators = £57.

Entocort® (Tillotts Pharma)
Enema 2mg/100mL, 7 single enemas = £34.

Hydrocortisone (generic)
Tablets 10mg, 20mg 28days @ 20mg each morning and 10mg each evening = £10.

Fludrocortisone (generic)
Tablets 100microgram, 28 days @ 100microgram each morning = £3.25. *Some brands require storage in a fridge.*

Prednisolone (generic)
Tablets 1mg, 2.5mg, 5mg, 10mg, 20mg, 25mg, 30mg, 28 days @ 15mg once daily = £2.25.
Tablets e/c 1mg, 2.5mg, 5mg, 28 days @ 15mg once daily = £5.50.
Tablets soluble 5mg, 28 days @ 15mg once daily = £34.
Oral solution 1mg/mL, 10mg/mL, 28 days @ 15mg once daily = £78.
Retention enema **prednisolone** (as ***sodium phosphate***) 20mg in 100mL, 7 single enemas = £15.
Retention foam enema **prednisolone** (as ***metasulfobenzoate sodium***) 20mg/metered application, 14-application canister with applicators = £185.
Suppositories **prednisolone** (as ***sodium phosphate***) 5mg, 10 = £12.

1 Hardy J *et al.* (2001) A prospective survey of the use of dexamethasone on a palliative care unit. *Palliative Medicine*. **15**: 3–8.
2 Hardy J *et al.* (2021) Practice review: evidence-based quality use of corticosteroids in the palliative care of patients with advanced cancer. *Palliative Medicine*. **35**: 461–472.
3 NICE (2008) Metastatic spinal cord compression. *Clinical Guideline*. CG75. www.nice.org.uk.
4 Rowell NP and Gleeson FV (2002) Steroids, radiotherapy, chemotherapy and stents for superior vena caval obstruction in carcinoma of the bronchus: a systematic review. *Clinical Oncology (Royal College of Radiologists)*. **14**: 338–351.
5 Elsayem A and Bruera E (2007) High-dose corticosteroids for the management of dyspnea in patients with tumor obstruction of the upper airway. *Supportive Care in Cancer*. **15**: 1437–1439.
6 Feuer DJ and Broadley KE (2017) Corticosteroids for the resolution of malignant bowel obstruction in advanced gynaecological and gastrointestinal cancer. *Cochrane Database of Systematic Reviews*. CD001219. www.cochranelibrary.com.
7 Laval G *et al.* (2000) The use of steroids in the management of inoperable intestinal obstruction in terminal cancer patients: do they remove the obstruction? *Palliative Medicine*. **14**: 3–10.
8 Fabregat C *et al.* (2019) Pain flare-effect prophylaxis with corticosteroids on bone radiotherapy treatment: a systematic review. *Pain Practice*. **20**:101–109.
9 Ndibe C *et al.* (2015) Corticosteroids in the management of prostate cancer: a critical review. *Current Treatment Options in Oncology*. **16**: 6.
10 Haywood A *et al.* (2015) Corticosteroids for the management of cancer-related pain in adults. *Cochrane Database of Systematic Reviews*. **4**: CD010756. www.cochranelibrary.com.
11 Paulsen O *et al.* (2014) Efficacy of methylprednisolone on pain, fatigue, and appetite loss in patients with advanced cancer using opioids: a randomized, placebo-controlled, double-blind trial. *Journal of Clinical Oncology*. **32**: 3221–3228.
12 Rhen T and Cidlowski JA (2005) Antiinflammatory action of glucocorticoids--new mechanisms for old drugs. *New England Journal of Medicine*. **353**: 1711–1723.
13 Hatano Y *et al.* (2016) Pharmacovigilance in hospice/palliative care: the net immediate and short-term effects of dexamethasone for anorexia. *BMJ Supportive & Palliative Care*. **6**: 331–337.
14 Lundstrom S *et al.* (2009) The existential impact of starting corticosteroid treatment as symptom control in advanced metastatic cancer. *Palliative Medicine*. **23**: 165–170.
15 Willox JC *et al.* (1984) Prednisolone as an appetite stimulant in patients with cancer. *British Medical Journal*. **228**: 27.
16 Currow DC *et al.* (2021) A randomized, double-blind, placebo-controlled trial of megestrol acetate or dexamethasone in treating symptomatic anorexia in people with advanced cancer. *Scientific Reports*. **11**: 2421.
17 Miller S *et al.* (2014) Use of corticosteroids for anorexia in palliative medicine: a systematic review. *Journal of Palliative Medicine*. **17**: 4824–4825.
18 Roeland EJ *et al.* (2020) Management of cancer cachexia: ASCO guideline. *Journal of Clinical Oncology*. **38**: 2438–2453.
19 MASCC/ESMO (2019) Antiemetic guideline. Available from www.mascc.org.
20 Chu CC *et al.* (2014) The cellular mechanisms of the antiemetic action of dexamethasone and related glucocorticoids against vomiting. *European Journal of Pharmacology*. **722**: 48–54.
21 Vayne-Bossert P *et al.* (2017) Corticosteroids for adult patients with advanced cancer who have nausea and vomiting (not related to chemotherapy, radiotherapy, or surgery). *Cochrane Database of Systematic Reviews*. **7**: CD012002. www.cochranelibrary.com.
22 Minoura T *et al.* (2018) Practice patterns of medications for patients with malignant bowel obstruction using a nationwide claims database and the association between treatment outcomes and concomitant use of H2-blockers/proton pump inhibitors and corticosteroids with octreotide. *Journal of Pain and Symptom Management*. **55**: 413–419.
23 Vecht C *et al.* (1994) Dose-effect relationship of dexamethasone on Karnofsky performance in metastatic brain tumors. A randomized study of doses of 4, 8 and 16 mg per day. *Neurology*. **44**: 675–680.
24 Soffierri R *et al.* (2011) Brain Metastases. In: Gilhus NE *et al.* (eds). *European Handbook of Neurological Management*. Volume 1. (2e). Blackwell Publishing Ltd.
25 Tsao MN (2015) Brain metastases: advances over the decades. *Annals of Palliative Medicine*. **4**: 225–232.
26 Cowap J *et al.* (2000) Outcome of malignant spinal cord compression at a cancer center: implications for palliative care services. *Journal of Pain and Symptom Management*. **19**: 257–264.
27 da Silva GT *et al.* (2015) Prognostic factors in patients with metastatic spinal cord compression secondary to lung cancer: a systematic review of the literature. *European Spine Journal*. **24**: 2107–2113.
28 George R *et al.* (2015) Interventions for the treatment of metastatic extradural spinal cord compression in adults. *Cochrane Database of Systematic Reviews*. **9**: CD006716. www.cochranelibrary.com.

29 Swartz S and Dluhy R (1978) Corticosteroids: clinical pharmacology and therapeutic use. *Drugs*. **16**: 238–255.
30 Demoly P and Chung K (1998) Pharmacology of corticosteroids. *Respiratory Medicine*. **92**: 385–394.
31 Narum S *et al.* (2014) Corticosteroids and risk of gastrointestinal bleeding: a systematic review and meta-analysis. *BMJ Open*. **4**: e004587.
32 Ellershaw J and Kelly M (1994) Corticosteroids and peptic ulceration. *Palliative Medicine*. **8**: 313–319.
33 Fardet L *et al.* (2007) Corticosteroid-induced adverse events in adults: frequency, screening and prevention. *Drug Safety*. **30**: 861–881.
34 Piper JM *et al.* (1991) Corticosteroid use and peptic ulcer disease: role of nonsteroidal anti-inflammatory drugs. *Annals of Internal Medicine*. **114**: 735–740.
35 Yamaguchi T *et al.* (2014) Pneumocystis pneumonia in patients treated with long-term steroid therapy for symptom palliation: a neglected infection in palliative care. *American Journal of Hospice and Palliative Care*. **31**: 857–861.
36 Chalk J *et al.* (1984) Phenytoin impairs the bioavailability of dexamethasone in neurological and neurosurgical patients. *Journal of Neurology, Neurosurgery, and Psychiatry*. **47**: 1087–1090.
37 Hazlewood KA *et al.* (2006) Effect of oral corticosteroids on chronic warfarin therapy. *Annals of Pharmacotherapy*. **40**: 2101–2106.
38 Jick S *et al.* (2001) The risk of cataract among users of inhaled steroids. *Epidemiology*. **12**: 229–234.
39 MHRA (2017) Corticosteroids: rare risk of central serous chorioretinopathy with local as well as systemic administration. *Drug Safety Update*. www.gov.uk/drug-safety-update.
40 British National Formulary. Section 6: Corticosteroids (systemic). London: BMJ Group and Pharmaceutical Press. www.medicinescomplete.com (accessed September 2021).
41 Warrington TP and Bostwick JM (2006) Psychiatric adverse effects of corticosteroids. *Mayo Clinic Proceedings*. **81**: 1361–1367.
42 Brown ES and Suppes T (1998) Mood symptoms during corticosteroid therapy: a review. *Harvard Review of Psychiatry*. **5**: 239–246.
43 Stiefel FC *et al.* (1989) Corticosteroids in cancer: neuropsychiatric complications. *Cancer Investigation*. **7**: 479–491.
44 Twycross R *et al.* (2021) *Introducing Palliative Care* (6e). Pharmaceutical Press, London.
45 Eidelberg D. Steroid myopathy. In: Rottenberg DA, editor. *Neurological Complications of Cancer Treatment*. Boston: Butterworth-Heineman; 1991. p. 185–191.
46 Schakman O *et al.* (2008) Mechanisms of glucocorticoid-induced myopathy. *Journal of Endocrinology*. **197**: 1–10.
47 Rotstein J and Good R (1957) Steroid pseudorheumatism. *AMA Archives of Internal Medicine*. **99**: 545–555.
48 Greenberg H *et al.* (1979) Epidural spinal cord compression from metastatic tumour: results with a new treatment protocol. *Annals of Neurology*. **8**: 361–366.
49 Simpson H *et al.* (2020) Guidance for the prevention and emergency management of adult patients with adrenal insufficiency. *Clinical Medicine*. **20**: 371–378. www.rcpjournals.org.
50 Rousseau P (2004) Sudden withdrawal of corticosteroids: a commentary. *American Journal of Hospice and Palliative Care*. **21**: 169–171.
51 Gralla R *et al.* (1999) Recommendations for the use of antiemetics: evidence-based, clinical practice guidelines. *Journal of Clinical Oncology*. **17**: 2971–2994.
52 Editorial (1991) Ondansetron versus dexamethasone for chemotherapy-induced emesis. *Lancet*. **338**: 478.
53 Kirkham S (1988) The palliation of cerebral tumours with high-dose dexamethasone: a review. *Palliative Medicine*. **2**: 27–33.
54 MHRA (2014) Dexamethasone 4mg/mL injection (Organon Laboratories Limited) reformulation with changes in name, concentration, storage conditions, and presentation. *Drug Safety Update*. **3**: www.mhra.gov.uk/Safetyinformation.
55 UK Medicines Information (2014) Dexamethasone injection. *In use product safety assessment report*. www.ukmi.nhs.uk.
56 Palliativedrugs.com (2014) Use of dexamethasone formulations in palliative care: a palliativedrugs.com reponse to recent changes. *News (December)*. www.palliativedrugs.com.
57 Margolin L *et al.* (2007) The steroid withdrawal syndrome: a review of the implications, etiology, and treatments. *Journal of Pain and Symptom Management*. **33**: 224–228.

Updated October 2021

DEMECLOCYCLINE

Class: Tetracycline antibacterial and vasopressin receptor antagonist.

Indications: Symptomatic hyponatraemia caused by paraneoplastic syndrome of inappropriate antidiuretic hormone secretion (SIADH).

Contra-indications: Patients with hypovolaemic hyponatraemia, e.g. caused by severe diarrhoea, vomiting or adrenal insufficiency.

Pharmacology

Pathogenesis and clinical features of SIADH

There are many causes of SIADH, including a range of drugs (Box A). In paraneoplastic SIADH, there is ectopic secretion of arginine vasopressin (antidiuretic hormone, ADH) or vasopressin-like peptides by the cancer.[1] In small cell lung cancer (SCLC), an elevated arginine vasopressin can be detected in about 40% of patients, although in most it is asymptomatic. Risk factors for developing SIADH include poor diet (particularly low sodium intake compared to volume of water ingested), nausea and pain, along with other situations associated with a stress response, which increases ADH secretion. Additional risk factors in patients taking SSRIs include older age, female sex, low body weight and concurrent use of diuretics.[2-4]

Box A Causes of SIADH[a,3,5]

Cancer
Acute myeloid leukaemia
Carcinoid
Head and neck
Lymphoma
Pancreas
Prostate
Small cell lung

Treatment
Chemotherapy, e.g.
- cyclophosphamide
- vincristine

Drugs[a]
- carbamazepine
- haloperidol
- opioids
- oxcarbazepine
- PPIs
- phenothiazines
- SSRIs
- TCAs
- valproate

Post-neurosurgery

Miscellaneous
Central nervous system
- cerebral thrombosis
- encephalitis
- head injury
- meningitis
- multiple sclerosis
- subarachnoid haemorrhage

Psychiatric
- psychosis
- schizophrenia

Pulmonary
- lung abscess
- pneumonia
- positive pressure ventilation
- tuberculosis

Recreational drugs
- ethanol
- nicotine

a. many other drugs are associated with hyponatraemia via a different mechanism, including effects on sodium and water homeostasis (e.g. diuretics), increasing renal sensitivity to ADH (e.g. NSAIDs) and by resetting the osmostat (e.g. venlafaxine).

Clinical features of SIADH depend on both the level and rate of decline of the plasma sodium concentration (Box B). Even moderate levels of hyponatraemia (i.e. plasma sodium 125–129mmol/L) are associated with an increased risk of cognitive impairment and falls. Asymptomatic hyponatraemia indicates chronic rather than acute SIADH. Hyponatraemia is considered acute if it develops <48h.

Hyponatraemia (with consequential intracellular cerebral oedema), possibly caused by SIADH, should be considered in all patients who develop drowsiness, confusion or seizures while taking a TCA or SSRI.

Diagnosis of SIADH can only be made once hypo-adrenalism, hypothyroidism, hypopituitarism and severe renal impairment have been excluded. For accurate diagnosis of the cause of hyponatraemia, paired serum and urine sodium and osmolality should be requested. Diagnosis is based on the following criteria:

- hyponatraemia (<132mmol/L)
- low plasma osmolality (<275mOsmol/kg)
- urine osmolality >100mOsm/kg
- urine sodium concentration always >20mmol/L, and generally >40mmol/L (Note. An unreliable indicator when dietary sodium and water intake abnormal, or patient taking a diuretic)
- normal plasma volume.[6,7]

If plasma volume is altered, consider alternative causes of hyponatraemia: if hypervolaemic, e.g. heart failure or cirrhosis; if hypovolaemic, e.g. severe vomiting, diarrhoea or diuretic therapy. When concomitant causes of hyponatraemia are suspected, discuss with an endocrinologist.[8]

Box B Clinical features of hyponatraemia

Moderate	**Severe**
Anorexia	Vomiting
Nausea	Multifocal myoclonus
Headache	Drowsiness
Lassitude	Seizures
Confusion	Coma

The rate at which the hyponatraemia develops is more important than the absolute value, e.g. with rapid onset hyponatraemia, symptoms may occur at higher plasma sodium levels. Those with severe features require urgent treatment and close monitoring, ideally in an ICU.

Management of SIADH

Stop and think! Rarely, SIADH presents with severe symptoms in a patient expected to die soon from progressive cancer. Are you justified in attempting to correct a potentially fatal complication in a moribund patient?

Treatment is necessary only if the patient is symptomatic. When possible, stop the causal drug and/or treat the underlying cause of SIADH. Generally, the treatment of choice is restricting fluid intake to 500–1,000mL/24h (ideally 500mL below the 24h total urine volume).

However, fluid restriction is ineffective when urine osmolality is >500mOsm/kg,[3,9,10] and, in palliative care, fluid restriction is burdensome. In these circumstances, treatment with demeclocycline is generally preferable.

Most of the evidence for the effectiveness of demeclocycline in paraneoplastic SIADH comes from case series which report a rise in mean plasma sodium from about 120mmol/L to 135mmol/L.[11] The effect of demeclocycline is often apparent after 2–5 days and persists for several days after stopping treatment. *There is no need to restrict fluid during treatment.* Renal function should be monitored, particularly in patients with cirrhosis.

Because of the lack of RCT data and concerns about nephrotoxicity, European guidelines no longer recommend demeclocycline, favouring PO **urea** instead. However, there is also very limited evidence to support this approach.[3,12] American guidelines recommend demeclocycline if fluid restriction fails.[9]

Demeclocycline is a tetracycline derivative. It induces nephrogenic diabetes insipidus, i.e. inhibits the action of ADH on renal tubules, probably by antagonism of arginine vasopressin V_2-receptors.[3] There are at least three arginine vasopressin receptor subtypes. V_2-receptors are concentrated in renal collecting tubules, where antagonism leads to aquaresis, i.e. the excretion of water without significantly changing the total level of electrolyte excretion. V_2-receptors also occur in vascular endothelium, where antagonism results in vasodilation.

PO absorption of demeclocycline is incomplete and reduced by various metal ions (see Drug interactions). About 45% is excreted unchanged via the kidneys.

Bio-availability 60–80%.
Onset of action 2–5 days.
Time to peak plasma concentration 3–4h.
Plasma halflife 12h.
Duration of action several days.

Tolvaptan is an alternative arginine vasopressin V_2-receptor antagonist (VRA) (Box C).

Box C Tolvaptan (Samsca®)

Tolvaptan is an alternative VRA.[13,14] It decreases expression of aquaporin channels in the renal collecting ducts, resulting in increased free water clearance. Authorization differs in Europe and the USA (see country-specific SPCs/PIs).

European guidelines do not recommend tolvaptan for treatment of SIADH.[3] American guidelines recommend a limited role for tolvaptan in mild–moderate symptomatic SIADH.[9,15]

Tolvaptan is contra-indicated in anuria, in patients with hypovolaemic hyponatraemia, and in patients with severe cerebral symptoms of SIADH. Tolvaptan may attenuate the effects of vasopressin analogues, e.g. desmopressin, used to control bleeding.[16]

continued

Box C Continued

RCTs of tolvaptan for patients with SIADH have generally excluded patients with a plasma sodium of <120mmol/L. VRAs increase plasma sodium by an average of 4mmol/L compared to placebo, with a response seen in about 60% of patients vs. 25% receiving placebo.[12]

The effect of tolvaptan on morbidity and mortality in SIADH or hyponatraemia of any cause is unclear; few trials were designed to examine these outcomes.[12] Long-term data are limited, although one study demonstrated acceptable safety in patients with various causes of hyponatraemia after 4 years.[14,17] Tolvaptan has *not* been compared with fluid restriction and/or demeclocycline in SIADH.

Patients with paraneoplastic SIADH may be more sensitive to tolvaptan, necessitating a lower starting dose, e.g. 7.5mg daily.[18] With doses >60mg/24h, there is a risk of liver toxicity.[19] Patients receiving tolvaptan should *not* be fluid-restricted and should *not* receive IV normal or hypertonic saline (sodium chloride).[20]

Irreversible osmotic demyelination is a risk with any treatment which causes a too-rapid rise in plasma sodium (increase ≥12mmol/L in 24h).[16] Risk factors for osmotic demyelination include a baseline plasma sodium <120mmol/L, malnutrition, hypokalaemia, hypoxia, advanced liver disease and excessive alcohol use. Although VRAs increase the risk of a rapid increase in plasma sodium, there were no reports of osmotic demyelination in >1,800 patients in 10 studies.[12] When starting tolvaptan, plasma sodium levels should be checked at least every 6h for the first 48h.

Tolvaptan is expensive (see Supply), and the need to closely monitor plasma sodium will restrict the use of tolvaptan in palliative care. Further, it is subject to significant drug interactions via CYP3A4 inhibition and induction. However, it may have a role in recurrent severe hyponatraemia unresponsive to fluid restriction and demeclocycline.[21]

Cautions

Renal and hepatic impairment; lower doses (e.g. maximum dose <1g/24h) advised to avoid excessive systemic accumulation.[11] Risk of photosensitivity; warn patients not to expose skin to direct sunlight or sunlamps.

Drug interactions

The absorption of demeclocycline is reduced by the concurrent administration of **iron**, **calcium**, **magnesium**, **aluminium** or **zinc**, contained in the diet or some drugs, e.g. antacids, laxatives. Separate the administration of demeclocycline by ≥2h.

Demeclocycline depresses plasma prothrombin activity and, if used concurrently with **warfarin**, the dose of **warfarin** may need to be reduced. Risk of oral contraceptive failure (as with all antibacterials). Avoid concurrent **penicillin** use (tetracyclines possibly antagonize the effect of penicillins).

Undesirable effects

Nausea, vomiting, diarrhoea, renal impairment, photosensitivity (see Cautions), oesophagitis, discolouration of teeth during tooth development.
Rare (<0.1%, >0.01%): acute renal failure or nephritis.

Dose and use

Treat the patient and not the biochemical results.
If feasible, stop the causal drug and/or treat the underlying cause.

If symptomatic and cause of SIADH irreversible:

- start with 300mg PO t.d.s. on an empty stomach, e.g. 1h before food; take with plenty of water in an upright position to reduce the risk of oesophagitis; avoid milk, antacids, **iron** and **zinc** preparations at the same time
- if necessary, increase to 300mg q.d.s. after 2 weeks
- recommended maintenance dose = 300mg b.d.–t.d.s., but 150mg b.d.–t.d.s. is adequate in some patients.

Because of concerns around nephrotoxicity, renal function should be regularly monitored, e.g. at dose titration and every 4 weeks, and the lowest effective maintenance dose used. Stop demeclocycline if, despite dose titration, there is no benefit.

In patients unable to take drugs PO, demeclocycline can be given PR dispersed in 5mL of a methylcellulose carrier.[22] However, the powder may cause local irritation and inflammation.

Supply

Demeclocycline hydrochloride (generic)

Capsules 150mg, 28 days @ 300mg b.d. = £954.

Tolvaptan

Samsca® (Otsuka)

Tablets 7.5mg, 15mg, 30mg, 28 days @ 15mg or 30mg daily = £2,091.

Jinarc® (Otsuka)

Tablets 15mg, 30mg, 45mg, 60mg, 90mg, 28 days @ 15mg or 30mg daily = £1,208.

Jinarc® is authorized for use in autosomal dominant polycystic kidney disease. Combination packs of different strength tablets also available.

1 Sorensen J *et al.* (1995) Syndrome of inappropriate secretion of antidiuretic hormone (SIADH) in malignant disease. *Journal of Internal Medicine.* **238**: 97–110.
2 Jacob S and Spinler SA (2006) Hyponatremia associated with selective serotonin-reuptake inhibitors in older adults. *Annals of Pharmacotherapy.* **40**: 1618–1622.
3 Spasovski G *et al.* (2014) Clinical practice guideline on diagnosis and treatment of hyponatraemia. *European Journal of Endocrinology.* **170**: G1–47.
4 Renneboog B *et al.* (2006) Mild chronic hyponatremia is associated with falls, unsteadiness, and attention deficits. *American Journal of Medicine.* **119**: e1–8.
5 Liamis G *et al.* (2008) A review of drug-induced hyponatremia. *American Journal of Kidney Disease.* **52**: 144–153.
6 Smellie WS and Heald A (2007) Hyponatraemia and hypernatraemia: pitfalls in testing. *BMJ.* **334**: 473–476.
7 Ellison DH and Berl T (2007) Clinical practice. The syndrome of inappropriate antidiuresis. *New England Journal of Medicine.* **356**: 2064–2072.
8 Jacob P *et al.* (2019) Hyponatraemia in primary care. *BMJ.* **365**: l1774.
9 Verbalis JG *et al.* (2013) Diagnosis, evaluation, and treatment of hyponatremia: expert panel recommendations. *American Journal of Medicine.* **126 (Suppl 1)**: S1–42.
10 Grant P *et al.* (2015) The diagnosis and management of inpatient hyponatraemia and SIADH. *European Journal of Clinical Investigation.* **45**: 888–894.
11 Miell J *et al.* (2015) Evidence for the use of demeclocycline in the treatment of hyponatraemia secondary to SIADH: a systematic review. *International Journal of Clinical Practice.* **69**: 1396–1417.
12 Nagler EV *et al.* (2018) Interventions for chronic non-hypovolaemic hypotonic hyponatraemia. *Cochrane Database of Systematic Reviews.* **6**: CD010965. www.cochranelibrary.com
13 Schrier RW *et al.* (2006) Tolvaptan, a selective oral vasopressin V2-receptor antagonist, for hyponatremia. *New England Journal of Medicine.* **355**: 2099–2112.
14 Amin A and Meeran K (2010) New drugs for hyponatraemia. *BMJ.* **341**: c6219.
15 Berl T (2015) Vasopressin antagonists. *New England Journal Medicine.* **372**: 2207–2216.
16 MHRA (2012) Tolvaptan (Samsca): over-rapid increase in serum sodium risking serious neurological events. *Drug Safety Update.* www.gov.uk/drug-safety-update
17 Berl T *et al.* (2010) Oral tolvaptan is safe and effective in chronic hyponatremia. *Journal of the American Society of Nephrology.* **21**: 705–712.
18 Kenz S *et al.* (2011) High sensitivity to tolvaptan in paraneoplastic syndrome of inappropriate ADH secretion (SIADH). *Annals of Oncology.* **22**: 2696.
19 MHRA (2013) Tolvaptan (Samsca): risk of liver injury. *Drug Safety Update.* www.gov.uk/drug-safety-update
20 Peri A and Combe C (2012) Considerations regarding the management of hyponatraemia secondary to SIADH. *Best Practice and Research Clinical Endocrinology and Metabolism.* **26 (Suppl 1)**: S16–26.
21 Mumby C and Adam S (2012) Tolvaptan use in a patient with metastatic small cell lung cancer. *Lung Cancer.* **75**: S59–S60.
22 Hussain I *et al.* (1998) Rectal administration of demeclocycline in a patient with syndrome of inappropriate ADH secretion. *International Journal of Clinical Practice.* **52**: 59.

Updated (minor change) March 2022

DESMOPRESSIN

Class: Vasopressin analogue.

Indications: Authorized indications vary between formulations and products; consult SPCs for full details. Pituitary diabetes insipidus, primary nocturnal enuresis, idiopathic nocturnal polyuria, nocturia associated with multiple sclerosis, †nocturia or nocturnal polyuria associated with other urinary tract disorders; mild–moderate haemophilia and von Willebrand's disease; †last-resort treatment for severe bleeding associated with platelet dysfunction.

Contra-indications: Current or previous hyponatraemia (including SIADH), coronary insufficiency, unstable angina, hypertension, concurrent use with diuretics, psychogenic and alcohol abuse-related polydipsia, renal impairment (creatinine clearance <50mL/min), type 2B and platelet-type (pseudo) von Willebrand's disease, patients >65 years (for primary nocturnal enuresis and nocturia associated with multiple sclerosis only).

Pharmacology

Desmopressin is an analogue of the pituitary antidiuretic hormone, **vasopressin**. It stimulates arginine vasopressin V_2-receptors in the medullary collecting tubules, increasing water resorption by the renal tubules, thereby reducing urine volume. The antidiuretic effect of desmopressin is 3–10 times greater than that of **vasopressin**, and it has a longer duration of action. Unlike **vasopressin**, it has no vasoconstrictor effect. Desmopressin is ineffective in nephrogenic diabetes insipidus.[1]

Desmopressin also stimulates V_2-receptors on endothelial cells, leading to the release of stored von Willebrand factor and factor VIII. This augments platelet function and enhances haemostasis, hence its use as a last resort in certain bleeding states, including those associated with severe renal or hepatic impairment.[2]

Bio-availability 3–4% intranasal; 0.1–0.2% PO.

Onset of action 1h intranasal; 2h PO.

Plasma halflife 0.4–4h intranasal; 2–3h PO.

Duration of action 5–24h intranasal; 6–8h PO.

Cautions

CHF, raised intracranial pressure, cystic fibrosis. Take care to avoid fluid overload, because with excessive water intake there is an increased risk of hyponatraemia. The effect of desmopressin may be potentiated in the elderly, particularly women, and by drugs which cause fluid retention, e.g. NSAIDs and corticosteroids. In renal impairment, the antidiuretic effect is less. Avoid in moderate–severe renal impairment. Food may reduce the absorption of tablets.

Drug interactions

Loperamide triples the desmopressin plasma concentration after PO administration.[3] The concurrent use of drugs which increase the endogenous secretion of vasopressin, notably **carbamazepine, chlorpromazine, lamotrigine**, NSAIDs, opioids, SSRIs, and TCAs, increases the risk of symptomatic hyponatraemia.

Undesirable effects

Water retention and hyponatraemia is a risk particularly in patients treated with desmopressin for an indication other than pituitary diabetes insipidus. In extreme cases this may result in hyponatraemic seizures.

Common (<10%, >1%): tablets and high doses of nasal spray (≥40microgram/24h): headache, dizziness, dry mouth, abdominal pain, nausea. Nasal spray: nosebleeds, nasal congestion or rhinitis, sore throat. IV: facial flushing, tachycardia, mild transient systemic arterial hypotension.

Rare or very rare (<0.1%): IV: increase in thrombo-embolic events, e.g. myocardial infarction, aggression in children.

Dose and use

Desmopressin products for SL administration are known as oral lyophilisates. Although all desmopressin products contain desmopressin *acetate*, the SL products are labelled with the dose expressed as desmopressin *base*.

To minimize the risk of symptomatic hyponatraemia, keep to the recommended starting doses and avoid fluid overload by advising patients to:

- avoid drinking large amounts of fluid
- restrict fluid to the minimum which satisfies thirst:
  - ▷ from 1h before until 8h after the dose given for enuresis/nocturia
  - ▷ continually with repeated doses for bleeding.

The monitoring required to detect fluid retention (weight, blood pressure) ± hyponatraemia (plasma sodium) varies between indication; *see SPC and obtain advice from an endocrinologist.*

Treatment should be stopped if plasma sodium concentration <135mmol/L. In addition, fluid should be restricted if any of the following develop:

- unusually severe or prolonged headache, nausea or vomiting, confusion (symptoms associated with hyponatraemia); *advise patient to seek immediate medical help*
- progressive increase in blood pressure and/or body weight
- plasma sodium concentration <130mmol/L
- plasma osmolality <270mosmol/kg.

When a patient has fully recovered from an episode of fluid overload, desmopressin can be restarted at an appropriate dose, with strict fluid restriction enforced.

When given for enuresis/nocturia:

- review after 3 months and stop if symptoms have not improved
- *stop desmopressin during any acute intercurrent illness impacting on fluid/electrolyte balance, e.g. diarrhoea, vomiting.*

Pituitary diabetes insipidus

Tablets (PO or SL) should be used first-line. The nasal spray should be used only when tablets are not suitable:

- start with 100microgram PO t.d.s., 60microgram SL t.d.s. (or 10–20microgram intranasally at bedtime)
- if necessary, increase dose progressively every few days
- effective dose is generally 100–400microgram PO t.d.s., 120–240microgram SL t.d.s. (or 10–20microgram intranasally at bedtime–b.d.).

A parenteral formulation for SC/IM/IV use (1–4microgram daily) is available if necessary.

Primary nocturnal enuresis, idiopathic nocturnal polyuria and nocturia

Exclude other causes which require specific therapy, e.g. urinary tract infection, diabetes mellitus, CHF. A lower starting dose is advised in the elderly, particularly women, who are more sensitive to the effects of desmopressin, and when other risk factors for hyponatraemia are present.[4,5]

Primary nocturnal enuresis (children >5 years, adults <65 years)

Treat only with PO or SL tablets:

- start with 200microgram PO or 120microgram SL at bedtime
- if necessary, after 1–2 weeks, increase dose to 400microgram PO or 240microgram SL at bedtime.[1,6]

Idiopathic nocturnal polyuria in adults (including adults >65 years)[7]

This is defined as voiding overnight >20% (>33% in patients aged >65 years) of (normal) total 24h urine volume. It is the only type of nocturia authorized for treatment with desmopressin in patients aged >65 years (Noqdirna® SL):

- in women, 25microgram SL 1h before bedtime
- in men, 50microgram SL 1h before bedtime
- in those >65 years, check plasma sodium before treatment and after 3 days and 4 weeks
- dose increase is *not* recommended in patients aged >65 years.

Compared with placebo, time to first void is increased by 40–50min and the mean number of voids is reduced by 0.2–0.4, suggesting little or no benefit in some patients.

In men, doses ≥100microgram are generally necessary. If higher doses are considered for patients <65 years, switch to an alternative SL desmopressin product to aid adherence, because the largest tablet size of Noqdirna® is 50microgram.[5,8]

†Nocturia or nocturnal polyuria associated with other urinary tract disorders in adults

In women <65 years with nocturia or nocturnal polyuria associated with overactive bladder or urinary incontinence, give desmopressin only if insufficient response to a urinary antimuscarinic (p.611).[9-11]

In men with nocturia or nocturnal polyuria associated with benign prostatic obstruction (BPO) or overactive bladder, give desmopressin only if insufficient response to a selective α_1-antagonist (see p.609) or a urinary antimuscarinic (p.611), respectively.[10,11] The degree of benefit may be relatively small, e.g. the addition of desmopressin to an α-blocker in men with BPO reduces the mean number of nocturnal voids by only 0.5.[12]

For both men and women:

- start with 50–100microgram PO at bedtime
- check plasma sodium before treatment and after 3 days
- if necessary, after 1–2 weeks, increase dose to maximum 200microgram.

A late-afternoon loop diuretic is an alternative.[13,14]

Nocturia associated with multiple sclerosis

Give only in adults aged <65 years when other treatments have failed:

- do *not* give >1 dose/24h
- start with 10–20microgram intranasally at bedtime to reduce nocturia or in the morning to reduce daytime frequency
- a trial of 40microgram may occasionally be justified, but higher doses (e.g. 60microgram) are associated with a higher risk of hyponatraemia and generally do not provide additional benefit.[15,16]

†Severe surface bleeding associated with platelet dysfunction

Although the benefit is small, desmopressin is used as a last-resort treatment (i.e. when other measures are insufficient) for severe surface bleeding associated with platelet dysfunction caused by, e.g. hepatic impairment,[17] renal impairment, paraproteinaemia. Obtain advice from a haematologist before use:

- give a single dose of:
  - ▷ desmopressin 0.3–0.4microgram/kg IVI (in 50mL sodium chloride 0.9% over 20min) *or*
  - ▷ desmopressin 0.3–0.4microgram/kg SC (using Octim® to minimize injection volume) *or*
  - ▷ desmopressin 3microgram/kg intranasally
- if necessary, repeat once daily up to a total of 4 days.

Because of the mechanism of action of desmopressin (releasing stored von Willebrand factor and factor VIII from the vascular endothelium), the second and subsequent injections provide only about two-thirds of the benefit of the first injection.[18-20]

Supply

Table 1 Desmopressin formulations and use in palliative care

Indications	*PO*	*SL*	*Nasal*	*Parenteral*
Pituitary diabetes insipidus	Yes (DDAVP® or generic)	Yes (DDAVP® Melt)	Yes[a] (Desmospray® or generic)	Yes (DDAVP)
Primary nocturnal enuresis	Yes[b] (Desmotabs® or generic)	Yes[b] (DesmoMelt®)	No	
Idiopathic nocturnal polyuria		Yes (Noqdirna®)		
Nocturia associated with multiple sclerosis (where other treatments have failed)			Yes[b] (Desmospray® or generic)	
†Nocturia (other causes)	†Yes			
†Severe surface bleeding with platelet dysfunction			†Yes	†Yes

a. intranasal formulations should *not* be used first-line

b. contra-indicated in adults >65 years.

Desmopressin *acetate* (generic)
Tablets 100microgram, 200microgram, 28 days @ 200microgram t.d.s. = £73.

Desmotabs (Ferring)
Tablets 100microgram, 200microgram, 28 days @ 200microgram t.d.s. = £82.

DDAVP® (Ferring)
Tablets 100microgram, 200microgram, 28 days @ 200microgram t.d.s. = £82.

Oral lyophilisate products
DesmoMelt (Ferring)
Tablets SL 120microgram, 240microgram, 28 days @ 120microgram t.d.s. = £85.

DDAVP® Melt (Ferring)
Tablets SL 60microgram, 120microgram, 240microgram, 28 days @ 120microgram t.d.s. = £85.

Noqdirna® (Ferring)
Tablets SL 25microgram, 50microgram, 28 days@ 25microgram (women) or 50microgram (men) once daily = £15.

Nasal products
Desmopressin *acetate* (generic)
Nasal spray 10microgram/metered spray, 60 dose bottle = £25.
Desmospray (Ferring)
Nasal spray 10microgram/metered spray, 60 dose bottle = £25.

Octim® (Ferring)
Nasal spray 150microgram/metered spray, 25 dose bottle = £577.

Parenteral products
Desmopressin *acetate*
DDAVP (Ferring)
Injection 4microgram/mL, 1mL amp = £1.25; for SC/IM/IV injection or IVI.

Octim® (Ferring)
Injection 15microgram/mL, 1mL amp = £19; for SC injection or IVI; *store at room temperature and protect from light.*

1 Cvetkovic RS and Plosker GL (2005) Desmopressin: in adults with nocturia. *Drugs*. **65**: 99–107; discussion 108–109.
2 Van de Walle *et al.* (2007) Desmopressin 30 years in clinical use: a safety review. *Current Drug Safety*. **2**: 232–238.
3 Callreus T et *al.* (1999) Changes in gastrointestinal motility influence the absorption of desmopressin. *European Journal of Clinical Pharmacology*. **55**: 305–309.
4 Juul KV et *al.* (2011) Gender difference in antidiuretic response to desmopressin. *American Journal of Renal Physiology*. **300**: F1116–1122.
5 Weiss JP et *al.* (2012) Desmopressin orally disintegrating tablet effectively reduces nocturia: Results of a randomized, double-blind, placebo-controlled trial. *Neurourology Urodynamics*. **31**: 441–447.
6 NICE (2010) Bedwetting in under 19s. *Clinical guideline* **CG11**. www.nice.org.uk
7 Burkhard FC et *al.* (2017) European association of urology guideline: urinary incontinence. www.uroweb.org/guidelines (Accessed June 2018).
8 Drugs and Therapeutics Bulletin (2017) Desmopressin for nocturia in adults. **55**: 30–32.
9 NICE (2015) Urinary incontinence in women: management. *Clinical Guideline*. **CG171**: www.nice.org.uk
10 Ebell MH et *al.* (2014) A systematic review of the efficacy and safety of desmopressin for nocturia in adults. *Journal of Urology*. **192**: 829–835.
11 Friedman FM and Weiss JP (2013) Desmopressin in the treatment of nocturia: Clinical evidence and experience. *Therapeutic Advances in Urology*. **5**: 310–317.
12 Han J et *al.* (2017) Desmopressin for treating nocturia in men. *Cochrane Database of Systematic Reviews*.
13 NICE (2015) The management of lower urinary tract symptoms in men *Clinical Guideline* **CG97**: www.nice.org.uk
14 Gravas S et *al.* (2017) European association of urology guidelines: treatment of non-neurogenic male luts including benign prostatic obstruction. www.uroweb.org/guidelines (Accessed June 2018).
15 Panicker JN et *al.* (2015) Lower urinary tract dysfunction in the neurological patient: clinical assessment and management. *Lancet Neurology*. **14**: 720–732.
16 Bosma R et *al.* (2005) Efficacy of desmopressin in patients with multiple sclerosis suffering from bladder dysfunction: a meta-analysis. *Acta Neurologica Scandinavica*. **112**: 1–5.

17 Lisman T *et al.* (2010) Hemostasis and thrombosis in patients with liver disease: the ups and downs. *Journal of Hepatology*. **53**: 362–371.
18 Mannucci PM and Tripodi A (2012) Hemostatic defects in liver and renal dysfunction. *Hematology* **2012**: 168–173.
19 Caldwell SH (2014) Management of coagulopathy in liver disease. *Gastroenterology & hepatology*. **10**: 330–332.
20 Stanca CM *et al.* (2010) Intranasal desmopressin versus blood transfusion in cirrhotic patients with coagulopathy undergoing dental extraction: a randomized controlled trial. *Journal of Oral Maxillofacial Surgery*. **68**: 138–143.

Updated (minor change) September 2021

DRUGS FOR DIABETES MELLITUS

Diabetes UK has commissioned and published recommendations on the management of patients with diabetes at the end of life.[1] These should be read together with this monograph.

Indications: Diabetes mellitus not controlled by diet.

Contra-indications: Generally, antidiabetic drugs should not be given by the PO or SC route during sepsis or after major trauma; seek advice from the diabetes team. Also see the Pharmacology sections for specific contra-indications for individual drugs.

Background

Diabetes mellitus comprises a group of metabolic diseases characterized by hyperglycaemia resulting from defects in insulin secretion, insulin action or both. There are two main types of diabetes mellitus (Box A). Some patients exhibit features of both type 1 and type 2 diabetes, making a definite classification difficult.

Box A Classification of diabetes mellitus

Type 1 (<10% of all cases)
Typically develops in children, young people, and adults <30 years old, but can occur at any age. There is a lack of insulin because of immune-mediated destruction of the β-cells in the pancreas. Symptoms develop rapidly, and the diagnosis is based on the presence of characteristic symptoms plus a high blood glucose concentration. All patients require insulin.

Type 2
Typically develops in adults >40 years old, although it is increasingly manifesting in younger people because of obesity. The pancreas does not produce sufficient insulin for the body's needs, and generally there is also marked insulin resistance, i.e. cells are not able to respond to the insulin that is produced. Symptoms tend to develop gradually, with a long delay (possibly years) before diagnosis. Treatment is based on modification of diet and weight loss, together with various antidiabetic drugs; some patients require insulin.

In the UK, 7% of the general population and 25% of care home residents have diabetes mellitus.[1,2] Nearly 40% of cancer patients have impaired glucose tolerance demonstrated by an oral or IV glucose tolerance test.[3] In cancer, corticosteroids are the most common cause of drug-induced hyperglycaemia (p.585), but thiazides, **furosemide**, **levothyroxine**, **octreotide** and atypical antipsychotics (e.g. **olanzapine**, **risperidone**) are also potential precipitants.[4]

In patients with symptoms suggestive of diabetes mellitus (e.g. thirst, polydipsia and/or polyuria), a diagnosis can be made on the basis of the following criteria:

- fasting blood glucose concentrations of ≥7mmol/L (normal <5.6mmol/L) *or*
- random blood glucose concentrations of ≥11.1mmol/L *or*
- 2h post-load blood glucose ≥11.1mmol/L (normal <7.8mmol/L) during oral glucose tolerance test *or*
- glycated haemoglobin (HbA_{1c}) ≥48mmol/mol (≥6.5%).

In *asymptomatic* patients, ≥2 of the above must be present. Measurement of HbA_{1c} is the recommended and most convenient diagnostic test for diabetes mellitus. However, HbA_{1c} reflects glycaemia in the preceding 2–3 months. Thus, it is *not* suitable as the sole test for patients with recent onset hyperglycaemia, e.g. in those:

- at high risk of diabetes and acutely ill
- taking medications that may cause a rapid rise in blood glucose, e.g. corticosteroids, atypical antipsychotics (see list above)
- with short duration of symptoms suggestive of diabetes mellitus
- with symptoms suggestive of type 1 diabetes at any age
- with acute pancreatitis or recent pancreatic surgery
- with conditions affecting red cell turnover, e.g. anaemia, chronic kidney disease.[5]

Pharmacology

Drug treatment in type 1 diabetes mellitus

Insulin is an essential life-long treatment in type 1 diabetes and is sometimes needed in type 2 diabetes. Human sequence insulin is produced by bacteria, using recombinant DNA technology; this has effectively replaced enzymatic modification of animal insulin (mainly porcine, sometimes beef), which is now rarely used. Because insulin is classified as a biological medicine, it should be prescribed by brand.

Insulin products can be classified according to duration of action (Table 1). Because the plasma halflife for insulin is a few minutes, the time–activity profile is determined by factors that impact the absorption characteristics, e.g. dose, route, injection site, SC fat. Thus, there is significant intra- and inter-individual variation in the pharmacokinetics of any given dose. Further, sensitivity to insulin varies with, e.g. body weight, renal function. Individual dose titration is required to identify the appropriate dose.

Table 1 Pharmacokinetics of different types of insulin given by SC administration

Type	*Rapid-acting*	*Short-acting*	*Intermediate-acting*	*Long-acting*
Brand example	Novorapid®	Actrapid®	Insulatard®	Lantus®
Onset of action	10–20min	30min	1.5h	2h
Time to peak plasma concentration	40min[a]	1.5–2.5h	2–18h	Plateau <4h[b]
Duration of action	3–5h	7–8h	24h[c]	≥24h

a. 60–90min in type 2 diabetes mellitus
b. SC insulin glargine once daily takes 2–4 days to reach steady state[6]
c. maximum effect 4–12h.

Most patients with type 1 diabetes will be on a multiple **insulin** injection (basal–bolus) regimen, e.g. a long-acting or intermediate-acting insulin once or twice daily and rapid-acting insulin before meals. Some, particularly if they have difficulty with or prefer not to use multiple daily injections, may be using premixed insulin products, such as **biphasic insulin aspart** (e.g. NovoMix® 30) or **biphasic insulin lispro** (e.g. Humalog® Mix25®), which are mixtures of rapid- and intermediate-acting insulins. The ability of the patient to use the necessary equipment for insulin delivery also influences the type of insulin used and the regimen, e.g. those with poor eyesight may not be able to safely use an insulin pen injector. Increasingly, patients with type 1 diabetes mellitus are managed with insulin pump therapy and/or have continuous glucose sensing, e.g. Freestyle Libre®.[7]

Patients starting treatment with **insulin** for >3 months must inform the Driver and Vehicle Licensing Agency (DVLA) and their insurance company if they intend to drive. Drivers need to be particularly careful to avoid hypoglycaemia (see Driving and hypoglycaemia, p.587). Detailed guidance on eligibility to drive is available from the DVLA (www.gov.uk/diabetes-driving).

Drug treatment in type 2 diabetes mellitus

There are several different classes of antidiabetic drugs, with differing modes of action (Table 2). Guidelines recommend initial therapy with a single non-insulin antidiabetic drug (monotherapy).

Class	Examples	Mechanism of action	Risk of hypoglycaemia[a]	Comment
Biguanides	Metformin	Decrease hepatic gluconeogenesis, increase uptake of glucose by muscle	–	Tend to cause weight loss; may cause nausea and diarrhoea; low risk of lactic acidosis. GI undesirable effects may be reduced with m/r metformin. See Dose and use for use in renal impairment
Sulfonylureas	Gliclazide, tolbutamide, glibenclamide (not UK), chlorpropamide (not UK)	Increase insulin secretion	++ with longer-acting glibenclamide, chlorpropamide	Original class of oral antidiabetic drugs; relatively inexpensive. Used when metformin not tolerated or as part of dual or triple therapy
Gliptins (DPP-4/dipeptidyl peptidase-4 inhibitors)	Alogliptin, linagliptin, saxagliptin, sitagliptin, vildagliptin	Incretin mimetics: increase insulin secretion and lower glucagon secretion	±	Some authorized as monotherapy if metformin contra-indicated or not tolerated (see text). Second- or third-line drugs, for use particularly in patients at high risk of hypoglycaemia.[8] Some gliptins suitable for use in renal impairment/failure (seek advice). Can use with insulin. Stop if symptoms of pancreatitis develop
Meglitinides	Repaglinide, nateglinide	Increase insulin secretion	–	Relatively fast onset and short duration of action; permits flexible regimen
Glitazones (thiazolidinediones)	Pioglitazone	Reduce peripheral insulin resistance	±	Authorized as monotherapy if metformin contra-indicated or not tolerated; or as second- or third-line drug in combination therapy. Causes fluid retention, exacerbates CHF
GLP-1 (glucagon-like peptide-1) receptor agonists	Exenatide (SC b.d.), liraglutide (SC once daily), semaglutide (SC once weekly)	Incretin mimetics: increase insulin secretion and lower glucagon secretion; slow gastric emptying and increase satiety	–	Second- or third-line drugs, for use particularly in patients with a BMI ≥35kg/m^2.[8] Only to be given with insulin after specialist advice. Increased risk of diabetic ketoacidosis.[9] Stop if weight loss >1.5kg weekly or if symptoms of pancreatitis develop.[b] Initial nausea and vomiting common
SGLT2 (sodium-glucose co-transporter 2) inhibitors	Canagliflozin, dapagliflozin, empagliflozin, ertugliflozin	Inhibits renal resorption of glucose, causing glycosuria	±	Authorized as monotherapy if metformin inappropriate. Can use as dual therapy with other antidiabetic drugs, including insulin, or as triple therapy with metformin and a sulfonylurea. May promote weight loss. Stop if eGFR <45mL/min/1.73m^2, dehydration, peripheral vascular disease or foot ulceration.[10–12] Increased risk of diabetic ketoacidosis even with near normal blood glucose levels; test for ketones in acute illness.[13] Increased risk of necrotizing fasciitis.[14] Dapagliflozin may be used with insulin in patients with type 1 diabetes and BMI>27kg/m^2.[15]

a. – = rare; ± = average; ++ = high

b. the risk of pancreatitis is about 1 extra case per 10,000 patients.[16,17] Concern about pancreatic cancer is *not* supported by latest evidence.[18]

Treatment intensification to dual therapy (two non-insulin antidiabetic drugs) then to triple therapy (three non-insulin antidiabetic drugs or two non-insulin antidiabetic drugs with insulin) may be necessary.[8] However, choice of drugs in patients with advanced cancer requires additional consideration (see below). The risk of hypoglycaemia is greatest with **insulin** and sulfonylureas. Table 3 lists the pharmacokinetics of selected oral antidiabetic drugs generally preferred in palliative care.

Table 3 Pharmacokinetics of selected oral antidiabetic drugs

	Gliclazide	*Linagliptin*
Bio-availability	78%	30%
Onset of action	3–4h	No data
Time to peak plasma concentration	2–4h	1.5h
Plasma halflife	10–12h	12h
Duration of action	12–24h	No data

Biguanides: Metformin

Contra-indications: Metformin should not be used in patients with severe renal impairment (eGFR <30mL/min/1.73m^2). Reduce the maximum total daily dose in patients with an eGFR <60mL/min/1.73m^2 (see Dose and use). It should be withheld during and for 48h after testing with IV iodinated contrast agents or until renal function is normal.

Metformin is contra-indicated in patients with acute heart failure but not in those with chronic heart failure controlled on treatment. Because of the risk of lactic acidosis, withhold in patients with acute conditions that could cause tissue hypoxia or sudden deterioration in renal function, e.g. dehydration, severe infection, sepsis, shock, acute heart failure, respiratory failure, hepatic impairment, excessive alcohol intake. However, recent evidence suggests the risk of this has been over estimated.[19]

Immediate-release **metformin** is generally recommended as first-line therapy for patients with type 2 diabetes.[8,20] However, starting **metformin** is generally inappropriate in patients with advanced cancer because it promotes weight loss and commonly causes GI undesirable effects, e.g. nausea, heartburn, diarrhoea. For those patients with advanced cancer already taking **metformin**, consider reducing and stopping it when there is anorexia or other undesirable GI effects. Monitor blood glucose twice daily for several days to determine if an alternative antidiabetic drug is necessary. **Metformin** is also best *not* used in elderly, frail patients, particularly those with hepatic impairment or COPD.[1] Hypoglycaemia is rare with **metformin**.

Modified-release **metformin** is used in patients with GI disease and in those who develop undesirable GI effects with immediate-release **metformin**; these can occur even when previously tolerant of **metformin**. When undesirable effects are severe or fail to improve with the modified-release product, stop the **metformin**.

Sulfonylureas: Gliclazide

Contra-indications: Gliclazide should not be used in severe renal impairment (eGFR <30mL/min/1.73m^2) or severe hepatic impairment. The concurrent use of systemic or oromucosal **miconazole** is contra-indicated with **gliclazide.**

The effect of sulfonylureas can be sufficient to produce hypoglycaemia, particularly if there is renal or hepatic impairment. Thus, when the risk of hypoglycaemia is high (e.g. elderly (>75 years), frail patient, eGFR <40mL/min/1.73m^2, poor oral intake), avoid long-acting sulfonylureas (e.g. **chlorpropamide**, **glibenclamide**; neither UK) and use intermediate-acting sulfonylureas, e.g. **gliclazide** with caution. Dose reduction of **gliclazide** may be necessary if liver function deteriorates, and it should be stopped if moderate–severe hepatic impairment develops. If episodes of hypoglycaemia occur, stop **gliclazide**. In these circumstances, **linagliptin**, a gliptin, may be a safer alternative (see below).

The plasma concentration of sulfonylureas may be increased (effect enhanced) by **fluconazole** and **miconazole** and decreased (effect reduced) by **rifampicin** and **rifabutin**.

Gliptins: Linagliptin

Contra-indications: Suspected pancreatitis.

Linagliptin, **saxagliptin**, **sitagliptin** and **vildagliptin** (but not **alogliptin**) are authorized as monotherapy if **metformin** is contra-indicated or not tolerated. **Linagliptin** once daily has several advantages over **metformin** or a sulfonylurea in elderly or frail patients with a poor oral intake. There is a low risk of hypoglycaemia, it does not affect body weight and no dose adjustment is required in renal or hepatic impairment or the elderly.

Meglitinides: Repaglinide

Contra-indications: Repaglinide should not be used in severe hepatic impairment or concurrently with **gemfibrozil** (see below).

Meglitinides, e.g. **repaglinide**, are insulin secretagogues; they are only occasionally used in the UK.[8] They provide similar glucose control to sulfonylureas but act more rapidly and for a shorter time. **Repaglinide** is authorized as monotherapy or in combination with **metformin** when **metformin** alone is inadequate. Because of its rapid onset (15–60min) and short duration (4–6h) of action, **repaglinide** is given by 'pulse dosing' before meals, which may be useful in patients with a variable appetite and oral intake.

Gemfibrozil (a plasma lipid-lowering drug) increases plasma concentrations of **repaglinide** and concurrent use is contra-indicated. However, in palliative care, the continued use of **gemfibrozil** is generally unnecessary. Concurrent use of **clopidogrel** (used in thromboembolic disorders) with **repaglinide** is contra-indicated in Canada and cautioned in the UK because of the increase in plasma concentration of **repaglinide** and risk of severe hypoglycaemia.

Glitazones: Pioglitazone

Contra-indications: Pioglitazone should not be used in patients with CHF or a history of CHF and all patients should be monitored for symptoms and signs of CHF.[8,21] **Pioglitazone** is also contra-indicated in hepatic impairment or in patients with (or at risk of) bladder cancer.[22]

Pioglitazone can be used as monotherapy if **metformin** is contra-indicated or not tolerated, or as second- or third-line combination therapy with **metformin** and/or a sulfonylurea or **insulin**. No dose adjustment is required in renal impairment.

Pioglitazone is cautioned in patients with a high risk of fracture because it increases the risk of distal fracture, particularly in women.[23,24] It may also cause or worsen diabetic macular oedema. Because of these concerns, it is unlikely to be appropriate for use in patients with advanced cancer and should generally be stopped in this group. Its antidiabetic effects can persist for <2 months after it is stopped.

Gemfibrozil (a plasma lipid-lowering drug) and **clopidogrel** (used in thromboembolic disorders) both increase plasma concentrations of **pioglitazone**. Because this may result in severe hypoglycaemia, avoid concurrent use of either drug with **pioglitazone**. However, in palliative care, the continued use of **gemfibrozil** is generally unnecessary.

Insulin in type 2 diabetes

Insulin is sometimes needed in patients with type 2 diabetes. When adding **insulin** to oral antidiabetics, a dose that is equivalent to 10% of body weight in units of intermediate-acting **insulin** or long-acting **insulin** at bedtime may suffice, i.e. for a patient weighing 50kg, start on 5 units of **insulin**. However, it may be easier and safer for patients with advanced cancer to switch to an insulin-only regimen rather than combining **insulin** with existing oral therapy.[1] All patients started on **insulin** should be provided with an insulin passport and information booklet.[25]

Management overview in the last few weeks of life

The following sections provide advice about the management of common clinical scenarios in *the last few weeks of life*. Guidance from a diabetes team should be sought if in doubt. For corticosteroid-induced diabetes mellitus, see p.585.

Because the patient's prognosis is short (days, weeks, a few months), it is *not* necessary to maintain rigid dietary control or target theoretically ideal blood glucose levels to avoid long-term complications.[26] Measuring HbA_{1c} to determine the overall level of glycaemic control over 6–8 weeks is also irrelevant for most palliative care patients.

The goal is to preserve quality of life. Thus, the aim of treatment is the prevention of symptoms from hyperglycaemia or hypoglycaemia, ketoacidosis and hyperosmolar non-ketotic states. Set a realistic safe target, e.g. a pre-meal capillary (fingerstick) blood glucose of 6–15mmol/L. Because the threshold for symptomatic hyperglycaemia varies, the upper limit may need to be reduced in some patients. For the management of spikes of hyperglycaemia, see Box B.

Resetting blood glucose targets necessitates careful discussion with both patient and family.[1,27] When stable, monitor with a fasting capillary blood glucose test twice a week. Although not as accurate, urine tests for glucose may suffice: aim for <1+ urine glucose before evening meal.

Box B Management of spikes of hyperglycaemia in the last few weeks of life[28]

When a patient is otherwise well, common causes of spikes of hyperglycaemia include extra dietary sugar, missed dose of insulin/antidiabetics and incorrect insulin injection technique. Spurious high readings also occur with incorrect monitoring technique, e.g. finger contaminated with sugar.

If the patient is drinking and *not* dehydrated, septic or acutely unwell, they should *not* be treated with stat doses of rapid-acting insulin. Instead, monitor with regular capillary blood glucose tests and adjust their usual antidiabetic drug regimen if a particular pattern emerges.

However, if the patient is vomiting, dehydrated, becoming severely unwell or is insulin-dependent with blood glucose >14mmol/L for >3h, a stat dose of rapid-acting insulin, e.g. NovoRapid®, may be necessary.

Type 1 diabetes or type 2 diabetes treated with insulin

Generally, 1 unit of rapid-acting insulin, e.g. NovoRapid®, reduces the blood glucose by about 3mmol/L. However, because this varies, check what the patients' usual experience is, then:

- calculate the dose of rapid-acting insulin required to bring the blood glucose to <14mmol/L
- recheck capillary blood glucose hourly
- if blood glucose >14mmol/L after 2h, repeat stat rapid-acting insulin but consider increasing the dose
- repeat each step until blood glucose <14mmol/L.

Test blood or urine for ketones. If raised, manage as per sick day rules (see text) and seek advice from diabetes team.

Type 2 diabetes not treated with insulin

Manage as per sick day rules (see text).

Management of existing type 1 diabetes mellitus in the last few weeks of life

Patients with **insulin** *pumps* will generally be able to adjust pump settings to manage moderate variations in diet. However, advice from the diabetes specialist pump team is essential when, e.g.:

- complicated situations arise that necessitate a change in pump settings, e.g. marked reductions in oral intake, enteral feeding, starting corticosteroids, last days of life
- the pump is no longer wanted or can no longer be managed by the patient, and an alternative **insulin** regimen is required
- frequent alarms distress the patient or carers (patients with impaired hypoglycaemic awareness may have sensor-augmented pumps that sound an alarm, e.g. in the low–normal glucose range).[1,29]

Injections of **insulin** are an essential life-long treatment, including in the last days of life. However, for most patients, the **insulin** requirement decreases because of weight loss, anorexia, nausea and vomiting, diarrhoea and renal and/or hepatic impairment.

In patients on a basal–bolus regimen, the rapid-acting **insulins** (given to cover mealtimes), which produce a more rapid peak and have a greater risk of hypoglycaemia, are reduced or discontinued first. Intermediate- or long-acting **insulins** (given once daily or b.d. to provide background control) may subsequently need to be reduced as well.

Likewise, patients receiving premixed **insulins** containing rapid- and intermediate-acting **insulins** may need to switch to a basal regimen of intermediate- or long-acting **insulin** once daily or b.d. If a patient has months or weeks to live, it would be prudent to liaise with the diabetes team before making major changes to an established **insulin** regimen.

Sick day management in type 1 diabetes mellitus

To avoid serious metabolic complications, e.g. diabetic ketoacidosis, apply sick day rules when the patient is feeling particularly unwell and unable to manage normal oral intake or levels of activity:[1]

- *do not stop the basal insulin regimen*
- encourage the patient to sip sugar-free fluids, aiming for 100mL/h
- offer frequent small meals, e.g. soup, ice cream, milky drinks
- if the patient has symptoms of hyperglycaemia and dehydration, check capillary blood for glucose and ketones (if capillary ketone meter unavailable, test urine for ketones)
- if ketones are present, test blood glucose and ketones every 2h:
  - ▷ if ketones >1.5mmol/L in blood (or ++ in urine), give additional 10% of the current typical total daily **insulin** dose (i.e. including rapid-acting and basal **insulins** in basal–bolus regimen) as rapid-acting **insulin**, e.g. **NovoRapid®**, every 3–4h until capillary blood glucose <15mmol/L
  - ▷ if ketone levels do not improve and the patient is vomiting, seek urgent advice from the diabetes team and consider transfer to hospital because the patient may require treatment with a variable rate IVI of short-acting **insulin** and rehydration.

Note. Carers must be educated about sick day rules. Sick day rules are generally *not* relevant for patients entering the last days or hours of life.

Stopping insulin in type 1 diabetes mellitus in the last days of life

A decision to stop **insulin** completely should generally be taken only after discussion with the patient (if still has capacity) and the family. It is generally appropriate to stop **insulin** injections completely when the patient has become irreversibly unconscious as part of the dying process (not because of hypoglycaemia or diabetic ketoacidosis) and when all other life-prolonging treatments have been stopped.

If it is felt strongly that the **insulin** should be continued, a simple regimen can be used, e.g. once daily long-acting **insulin glargine**, with the minimum of routine monitoring, e.g. capillary blood glucose test once daily at teatime:

- if blood glucose is <8mmol/L, reduce **insulin** dose by 10%
- if blood glucose >20mmol/L, increase **insulin** dose by 10%.[1,30]

Management of type 2 diabetes in the last few weeks of life

Newly diagnosed type 2 diabetes mellitus in advanced cancer

The relative advantages and disadvantages of **insulin** and oral antidiabetics need to be taken into account, together with factors such as the patient's prognosis, food intake and the presence of other co-morbidities. **Insulin** provides rapid, effective and more predictable control, is easier to titrate and has less risk of prolonged hypoglycaemia compared with some oral antidiabetics. It is a better choice in patients with:

- a short prognosis (<3 months)
- co-morbidity contributing to hyperglycaemia, e.g. infection
- poor or erratic food intake
- contra-indications to the use of oral antidiabetics
- severe symptoms from hyperglycaemia.

With oral antidiabetics, control may take several weeks and be less effective, less predictable and harder to titrate than **insulin**. However, if oral antidiabetics are preferred, **linagliptin** is a good choice (see p.581 and Dose and use); if unavailable, an alternative is **gliclazide.**

When deciding the starting dose of **insulin**, the patient's build, oral intake and blood glucose levels must be considered. The dose is titrated to achieve a fasting blood glucose of 6–15mmol/L.

Doses of 0.1 units/kg/24h of a long-acting **insulin**, e.g. **insulin glargine** (given once daily), or intermediate-acting **insulin**, i.e. **isophane insulin** (given once daily or in two divided doses), will provide only a basal insulin supply, and thus it does not matter if a patient on this amount is not eating.

However, in patients who are still eating and require larger doses than this, **insulin glargine** is a better choice than **isophane insulin** because there is less probability of interprandial hypoglycaemia. It is given once daily and need not be given at the same time each day, thus easing the burden of injections on the patient/carer.[8,31] Given these advantages, it may be beneficial for patients on oral antidiabetics troubled by hypoglycaemic episodes or a burdensome tablet load to be switched to once daily injections of long-acting **insulin glargine**. Blood glucose should be monitored before each dose until the **insulin** dose is stable. The frequency of testing can then be reduced and the time of testing varied to monitor control during different parts of the day.

Rationalizing therapy in existing type 2 diabetes mellitus

If patients have a prognosis of weeks–months and are becoming increasingly dependent on carers to administer treatment, consider simplifying existing therapy:

- stop glitazones, gliptins, GLP-1 (glucagon-like peptide-1) receptor agonists and SGLT2 (sodium-glucose co-transporter 2) inhibitors if part of dual or triple therapy
- switch from combination of oral antidiabetic and **insulin** to **insulin** alone
- switch from b.d. to once daily **insulin glargine** (start with 75% of total b.d. dose)
- if in doubt, consult the diabetes team.

Sick day management in type 2 diabetes mellitus

To avoid serious metabolic complications, apply sick day rules when the patient is feeling particularly unwell and unable to manage normal food intake or levels of activity:

- encourage the patient to sip sugar-free fluids, aiming for 100mL/h
- offer frequent small meals, e.g. soup, ice cream, milky drinks
- check blood glucose only if symptoms of hyperglycaemia and dehydration develop.

For patients on diet alone, or any of the following: **metformin**, gliptin, glitazone or SGLT2 inhibitor:

- aim to maintain blood glucose ≤15mmol/L
- if the patient develops vomiting or diarrhoea, stop **metformin**, SGLT2 inhibitor.

For patients on any of the following: sulfonylurea, meglitinide, GLP-1 receptor agonist or **insulin**:

- if blood glucose <6mmol/L, consider reducing dose of sulfonylurea or **insulin**
- if blood glucose >15mmol/L, consider increasing dose of sulfonylurea or **insulin**
- stop all antidiabetic medicines if the patient is not eating, has no symptoms of hyperglycaemia and blood glucose <15mmol/L.[1]

Note. Sick day rules are generally *not* relevant for patients entering the last days or hours of life.

Stopping treatment in patients with type 2 diabetes

In advanced cancer, patients with insulin-treated type 2 diabetes may be able to stop **insulin**, and those with tablet-treated type 2 diabetes may be able to stop tablets, because of weight loss, anorexia, nausea and vomiting, and renal and/or hepatic impairment.

As patients approach the last few days of life, they are unlikely to be able to swallow any remaining oral antidiabetic drugs. These should be stopped, as should GLP-1 receptor agonist injections. Consider stopping low-dose **insulin** (e.g. intermediate or long-acting **insulin** <15 units total daily dose) if capillary blood glucose <10mmol/L. In most cases it will be appropriate to stop blood glucose monitoring too. However, if it is felt necessary to continue monitoring, conduct daily capillary blood glucose or urinalysis:

- if urine glucose >2+, check capillary blood glucose
- if capillary blood glucose >20mmol/L, give 0.1 units/kg SC rapid-acting **insulin**, e.g. **Novorapid®**
- recheck capillary blood glucose after 2h
- if capillary blood glucose still >20mmol/L, repeat SC rapid-acting **insulin**, titrating dose to response
- if rapid-acting **insulin** is required more than twice, consider starting a once daily morning dose of intermediate-acting **isophane insulin** or long-acting **insulin glargine**; start with a dose 25% lower than the total previous daily rapid-acting **insulin** dose.

If a patient requires a total daily dose of >15 units of **insulin** or a decision is made to continue **insulin**, switch to an intermediate or long-acting **insulin** (if not switched already) at a dose 25% lower than the previous total daily **insulin** dose, and manage as for type 1 diabetes (see above).[1,32]

Corticosteroid-induced diabetes mellitus

Diabetes mellitus occurs in about 10% of patients treated with corticosteroids.[33] It can occur with any corticosteroid and any formulation (including inhaled and topical)[34] and is dose-related. The greatest rise in blood glucose is likely to occur 2–3h after taking a corticosteroid, returning to normal 12–16h later with **prednisolone** and 24h later with **dexamethasone**.[1] Thus, treatment with a longer acting antidiabetic product, either a sulfonylurea or long-acting **insulin**, may cause nocturnal hypoglycaemia in patients with **prednisolone**-induced hyperglycaemia, but is less likely when **dexamethasone**-induced.[35] This should be taken into account when planning treatment. Appropriate assessment and monitoring should be undertaken (Box C).

Box C Corticosteroids and diabetes: blood glucose assessment and monitoring[1,36]

Target capillary blood glucose levels

These vary with prognosis:

- *last few weeks of life*: 6–15mmol/L (or <1+ urine glucose)
- *longer prognoses*: ideally 6–10mmol/L, although 6–12mmol/L is acceptable.

Before starting corticosteroids in patients with no previous diagnosis of diabetes

Check random capillary blood glucose; if ≤8mmol/L no further checks are necessary unless risk factors for hyperglycaemia present (see below), but if >8mmol/L take random *venous* blood glucose:

- if >7.8mmol/L, the patient is at risk of developing diabetes with corticosteroid therapy; check capillary blood glucose every 1–2 weeks unless risk factors for hyperglycaemia present (see below)
- if ≥11.1mmol/L, check *fasting* venous blood glucose; ≥7mmol/L indicates pre-existing undiagnosed diabetes mellitus; manage accordingly (see p.577).

Alternatively, HbA_{1c} can be checked in patients at high risk of developing diabetes as long as they are not acutely unwell (see p.577).

Monitoring capillary blood glucose: patients without diabetes but with risk factors for hyperglycaemia

Check once daily (pre- or 1–2h post either lunch or evening meal) in those with risk factors for hyperglycaemia (e.g. obesity, family history, previous gestational diabetes). If:

- <10mmol/L consistently, stop checking
- 10–11.9mmol/L, continue checking
- ≥12mmol/L, increase frequency of testing to q.d.s.; if ≥12mmol/L on 2 occasions/24h, manage as for corticosteroid-induced diabetes (Box D).

Patients at home receiving long-term corticosteroids who are at risk of hyperglycaemia should be provided with a glucose meter and instructed how to use it.

Monitoring capillary blood glucose: patients with known diabetes

- check q.d.s.
- in patients with type 1 diabetes, if capillary blood glucose >12mmol/L check daily for ketones and if raised, seek advice from diabetes team.

If corticosteroids are given b.d., consider switching to a once daily morning dose. If tablet load is a concern, soluble **prednisolone** tablets are available and **dexamethasone** can be given as an oral solution (see Systemic corticosteroids, p.556). If the patient develops corticosteroid-induced diabetes with a once-daily corticosteroid, see Box D.

If it is not possible to switch to a corticosteroid once daily, consider prescribing **gliclazide** 40mg PO b.d. titrated up to a maximum of 160mg b.d.. Nonetheless, **insulin** is more likely to be effective in this context, e.g. intermediate-acting **isophane insulin** b.d. or a basal-bolus regimen. Early morning hypoglycaemia is a risk; if this occurs on several occasions, or the patient is struggling to manage **isophane insulin** b.d., consider **insulin glargine** once daily in the morning. Seek advice from the diabetes team.

Box D Corticosteroids and diabetes: management of patients taking dexamethasone once daily in the morning[1,36]

If possible, stop the causative corticosteroid; when unavoidable, reduce to the minimum effective dose.

Corticosteroid-induced diabetes (no pre-existing diabetes)
Start gliclazide only if symptomatic hyperglycaemia >target levels (Box C) and ongoing corticosteroid treatment is unavoidable, e.g. >3 days. If drug treatment is necessary:

- start gliclazide 40mg PO each morning
- if necessary, increase by 40mg up to a maximum of 240mg each morning
- some centres stop gliclazide and *switch* to insulin if 160mg each morning is ineffective; seek advice from the diabetes team.

An alternative is to start an intermediate-acting insulin (e.g. isophane insulin 0.1–0.15 units/kg/24h SC) instead of gliclazide, particularly in patients with difficulty in swallowing. If blood glucose remains >target before evening meal, increase insulin dose by 10% every 2–3 days.[1]

Note. Only insulin is recommended for corticosteroid-induced diabetes resulting from dexamethasone treatment for COVID-19.[37]

Corticosteroid-exacerbated pre-existing non-insulin-dependent diabetes
If glycaemic control deteriorates when corticosteroids are started for a course of >3 days, antidiabetic treatment will need to be modified.

Type 2 diabetes not on gliclazide or insulin
Check capillary blood glucose before evening meal. If two consecutive readings of blood glucose >target:

- for patients already taking metformin, first titrate this to 1g PO b.d.
- otherwise, start gliclazide 40mg PO each morning
- if necessary, increase gliclazide by 40mg up to a maximum of 240mg each morning until blood glucose within target
- if blood glucose remains >target:
  - ▷ add an evening meal dose of gliclazide 40mg, increasing to 80mg if necessary (maximum total daily dose 320mg; some centres limit maximum total daily dose to 240mg gliclazide), *or*
  - ▷ *switch* gliclazide to a morning dose of an intermediate-acting insulin (e.g. isophane insulin 0.1–0.15 units/kg/24h SC). If blood glucose remains >target before evening meal, increase morning insulin dose by 10%; a dose of 0.3–0.5 units/kg/24h may be required.[38]

Type 2 diabetes on gliclazide
Check capillary blood glucose before evening meal. If two consecutive readings of blood glucose >target:

- adjust dose of gliclazide up to a maximum of 240mg PO each morning and 80mg with evening meal (maximum total daily dose 320mg; some centres limit maximum total daily dose to 240mg gliclazide)
- if blood glucose still remains >target:
  - ▷ *switch* gliclazide to a morning dose of an intermediate-acting insulin (e.g. isophane insulin 0.1–0.15 units/kg/24h SC). If blood glucose remains >target before evening meal, increase morning insulin dose by 10%; a dose of 0.3–0.5 units/kg/24h may be required.[38]

Corticosteroid-exacerbated pre-existing insulin-controlled diabetes mellitus
Insulin-controlled diabetes on once daily night-time insulin
Transfer night-time insulin injection to morning.
Check capillary blood glucose before evening meal. If blood glucose >target:

- increase dose by 10–20%
- if target not achieved after several titrations, consider switching to b.d. or basal–bolus insulin.

Insulin-controlled diabetes on b.d. insulin
Check capillary blood glucose before evening meal:

- If blood glucose >target and low risk of hypoglycaemia, consider increasing morning insulin by 10–20%.

continued

Box D Continued

Insulin-controlled diabetes on basal–bolus insulin

Check capillary blood glucose before lunch and evening meals:

- if blood glucose >target, increase rapid-acting insulin doses by 10–20%
- consider transferring evening basal dose insulin to morning.

Reducing the corticosteroid dose

Generally, blood glucose levels decline in parallel, but there may be a 'lag' time of up to several days. Review antidiabetic therapy after each change in corticosteroid dose.

In corticosteroid-*induced* diabetes, continue monitoring capillary blood glucose until normoglycaemia returns or, if persistent hyperglycaemia, a definitive test for diabetes is undertaken (see Background, p.577).

In corticosteroid-*exacerbated* diabetes, aim to gradually revert to pre-corticosteroid regimen.

Hypoglycaemia

Hypoglycaemia is a lower than physiologically normal blood glucose concentration. It is the most common undesirable effect of **insulin** and sulfonylureas. Elderly patients or those with renal impairment are at particular risk.

Metformin, **pioglitazone**, gliptins, GLP-1 receptor agonists and SGLT2 inhibitors are unlikely to cause hypoglycaemia unless prescribed with either **insulin** or a sulfonylurea. Hypoglycaemia can be precipitated by several drugs, including **warfarin**, **quinine**, fibrates, NSAIDs and SSRIs.

Hypoglycaemia can be described as mild if self-treated and severe if assistance by another person is needed. Any blood glucose less than 5mmol/L should be treated (Box E). For patients at risk, it helps to have a 'hypo box' containing everything necessary for treating hypoglycaemia and keep it in a prominent place. Carers must also be educated in how to manage hypoglycaemia.[28]

The risk of hypoglycaemia with a sulfonylurea or long-acting **insulin** can persist for 24–36h after the last drug dose, particularly when there is concurrent renal impairment, and regular blood glucose monitoring must be continued for this time, e.g. about q4h, timed as pre-meal, bedtime and middle of the night.

Malnourished patients with reduced hepatic glycogen stores have a reduced capacity to counteract hypoglycaemia, and **glucagon** treatment in these patients is likely to be less effective.

Driving and hypoglycaemia

Because DVLA rules are complex, frequently reviewed and vary according to group of driving licence, patients should be advised to check the DVLA website. Patients taking **insulin** >3 months must inform the DVLA and apply for a restricted licence. Patients with diabetes and a Group 1 licence should stop driving and inform the DVLA if they:

- experience 2 episodes of severe hypoglycaemia while awake in a year
- experience 1 episode of severe hypoglycaemia when driving
- develop impaired awareness of hypoglycaemia.

Drivers need to be particularly careful to avoid hypoglycaemia. Drivers treated with **insulin** should be advised to check their blood glucose before driving and, on long journeys, every 2h as specified by the DVLA to ensure blood glucose is >5mmol/L (www.gov.uk/diabetes-driving).

These precautions may also be necessary for drivers taking oral antidiabetic drugs that carry a risk of hypoglycaemia (e.g. long-acting sulfonylureas, meglitinides). Drivers treated with **insulin** should ensure that a supply of sugar is always available in the vehicle, and they should avoid driving if a meal is delayed.

If warning signs of hypoglycaemia develop, the driver should:

- stop the vehicle in a safe place
- switch off the ignition and move out of the driver's seat
- eat or drink a suitable source of sugar (see Box E)
- not drive again until 45min after the blood glucose has returned to normal.

Box E Treatment of hypoglycaemia[28,39]

Stop IVI insulin (if running).

For patients with insulin pump therapy:

- if able to manage own pump, give quick-acting carbohydrate (long-acting carbohydrate usually *not* needed) and consult diabetes team about adjusting pump infusion rate
- if unconscious patient, manage as below; if persistent hypoglycaemia remove cannula and pump and urgently consult diabetes team.

Conscious patient

1 Give one of the following *quick-acting* carbohydrate 15–20g PO:
   - 200mL of pure fruit juice
   - 60–80mL glucose in solution (250mg/mL), e.g. Lift/GlucoJuice®
   - 4–5 glucose tablets (4g/tablet), e.g. Lift/Glucotabs®
   - 3–4 heaped teaspoons *or* 4–5 lumps of sugar dissolved in water
   - 5 large jelly babies.

2 If the patient is not able to take tablets or drink but can still swallow, give 2 tubes of GlucoGel® or Dextrogel® squeezed into the mouth between the teeth and gums.

3 If the patient has a PEG, stop the feed, flush feeding tube with 30mL water and administer down the tube 60–80mL Lift/GlucoJuice® (*or* sugar dissolved in water as in point 1); repeat flush with 30mL water.

4 Repeat capillary blood glucose test after 10–15min; if blood glucose <4mmol/L, *repeat above steps up to a maximum of 3 treatments in total.*

5 Then, if blood glucose still remains <4mmol/L:
   - *if well-nourished*, give glucagon 1mg IM (can be given SC but will act more slowly)
   - *if malnourished or cachectic or PEG-fed*, give 150–200mL glucose 10% IV over 15min.

6 When the blood glucose is >4mmol/L and the patient has recovered, give 20g of a *long-acting* carbohydrate of the patient's choice, e.g.:
   - two biscuits
   - one slice of bread/toast
   - 200–300mL glass of cow's milk
   - if PEG-fed, connect feed and give 20g carbohydrate (see feed label)
   - normal meal if due (must contain carbohydrate)/restart PEG feed.

   Note. Patients given glucagon require double the above amount of *long-acting* carbohydrate (i.e. 40g) to replenish glycogen stores.

7 If the patient is aggressive, give IV glucose (as below).

Unconscious patient ± seizures

- treat patient using the **A**irway, **B**reathing, **C**irculation, **D**isability, **E**xposure (**ABCDE**) approach: ensure airway is clear and give high-flow oxygen via a mask, check breathing and circulation, obtain IV access. Stop insulin infusion if in situ
- then:
   - ▷ give 150–200mL glucose 10% IV over 15min, particularly if *malnourished or cachectic or PEG-fed*
   - ▷ *if well-nourished*, and no IV access available, give glucagon 1mg IM (can be given SC, but acts more slowly)
- repeat capillary blood glucose test after 10min; repeat glucose infusion if blood glucose <4mmol/L
- when conscious, give *quick-acting* carbohydrate drink (see points 1–3) followed by a starchy snack (see point 6)
- consider glucose 10% IV 100mL/h until the antidiabetic drug has been metabolized and blood glucose levels are stable (or if patient 'nil by mouth' and unable to take carbohydrate drink or snack).

Further measures

Discuss with diabetes team and review diabetes management:

- consider reducing or stopping oral antidiabetics or insulin in patients with type 2 diabetes
- consider reducing *but not stopping* insulin in patients with type 1 diabetes.

Impaired awareness of hypoglycaemia

This is an acquired syndrome associated with long-standing insulin-dependent diabetes. It is a consequence of autonomic neuropathy, which removes both the warning symptoms (sweating, tremor, pounding heartbeat) and the counter-regulatory mechanism of an adrenaline (epinephrine)-induced increase in blood glucose. Such patients tend to present with pallor, mental detachment ± drowsiness ± clumsiness. Some become irritable and aggressive, and others slip rapidly into hypoglycaemic coma. Specialist advice from the diabetes team should be sought.

Dose and use

To maximize safety, all regular and bolus doses of **insulin** must be measured and administered using an **insulin** syringe or commercial **insulin** pen device. IV syringes must never be used because they are calibrated in mL and not in **insulin** units. *'Units' must always be written in full.* Abbreviations, e.g. U or IU, should not be used; e.g. 10U could be mistakenly read as 100.[40,41] **Insulin** should be prescribed by brand.

Local guidelines influence the choice of oral antidiabetic drugs and **insulin.**

Gliclazide

- start with **gliclazide** 40–80mg PO each morning with breakfast
- if necessary, increase every 3 days to a maximum of 160mg b.d. with meals.

For use in corticosteroid-induced diabetes mellitus, see Box D.

Metformin

- start with **metformin** 500mg immediate-release tablets PO each morning with breakfast
- if necessary, increase by 500mg at weekly intervals; split the total daily dose into b.d. or t.d.s with meals
- maximum dose 1g t.d.s.
- for patients with:
  - ▷ *mild* renal impairment (eGFR 45–59mL/min/1.73m^2), reduce the total maximum daily dose to 2g/24h given as divided doses
  - ▷ *moderate* renal impairment (eGFR 30–44mL/min/1.73m^2), reduce the total maximum daily dose to 1g/24h given as divided doses
- for m/r formulations, generally a once daily dose with the evening meal is recommended, with a maximum daily dose of 2g/24h (see SPC); reduce the dose as above in moderate renal impairment.

Linagliptin

- give **linagliptin** 5mg PO once daily; it does not need to be taken with meals.

Insulin

- if the patient is already taking the maximum dose of an oral antidiabetic, and the fasting blood glucose is >15mmol/L, prescribe **insulin glargine** 0.1–0.2 units/kg/24h SC (given once daily) or **isophane insulin** 0.1–0.2 units/kg/24h SC (given once daily or in two divided doses)
- adjust the dose to achieve a fasting blood glucose of 6–15mmol/L and seek advice from the diabetes team if needed
- continuously rotate the injection site.

Also see p.583.

Supply

This is not a complete list; see BNF for additional details, including combination products.

Gliclazide (generic)

Tablets 40mg, 80mg (scored), 28 days @ 80mg each morning = £1.

Oral suspension (sugar-free) 40mg/5mL, 80mg/5mL, 28 days @ 80mg each morning = £21 (unauthorized; available as a special order; see Chapter 24, p.817). *Price based on specials tariff in the community.*

Metformin (generic)
Tablets 500mg, 850mg, 28 days @ 500mg each morning = £1.
Tablets m/r 500mg, 750mg, 1,000mg, 28 days @ 500mg each morning = £1.50.
Oral solution (sugar-free) 500mg/5mL, 850mg/5mL, 1,000mg/5mL, 28 days @ 500mg each morning = £6.

Linagliptin
Trajenta® (Boehringer Ingelheim)
Tablets 5mg, 28 days @ 5mg once daily = £33.

Insulin

All insulin products should be prescribed by brand. Take great care to check the insulin concentration. Although all insulin products have traditionally been 100 units/mL, other strengths are now available, e.g. long-acting **insulin degludec** (100 units/mL and 200 units/mL) and long-acting **insulin glargine** (100 units/mL and 300 units/mL).

Table 4 Types of human insulins (not an exhaustive list; see BNF)

Type	*Rapid-acting*	*Short-acting*	*Intermediate-acting*	*Long-acting*
Examples	Insulin aspart, insulin glulisine, insulin lispro	Insulin (soluble insulin short-acting; neutral insulin)	Isophane insulin	Insulin degludec, insulin detemir, insulin glargine[b]
Concentrations available	100 units/mL	100 units/mL	100 units/mL	100 units/mL, 200 units/mL, 300 units/mL
Brand example[a]	Novorapid®	Actrapid®	Insulatard®	Lantus®
Cost (10mL multidose vial)	£14	£7.50	£7.50	£28

a. most insulin products are also available as cartridges for use with dedicated re-usable injection pen devices or as pre-filled disposable pen devices
b. in clinical practice, insulin glargine is preferred to insulin degludec because insulin glargine has a shorter duration of action (36h vs 42h).

Mixed formulations of rapid-acting or short-acting insulins with intermediate-acting insulins are available, e.g. biphasic insulin aspart (Novomix® 30), biphasic insulin lispro (e.g. Humalog® Mix25®) or biphasic isophane insulin (e.g. Humulin® M3).

1 Diabetes UK (2021) End of life diabetes care: full strategy document commissioned by Diabetes UK 4th ed. Available from: www.diabetes.org.uk.
2 Holman N *et al.* (2011) The Association of Public Health Observatories (APHO) diabetes prevalence model: estimates of total diabetes prevalence for England, 2010–2030. *Diabetic Medicine*. **28**: 575–582.
3 Giovannucci E *et al.* (2010) Diabetes and cancer: a consensus report. *CA: A Cancer Journal for Clinicians*. **60**: 207–221.
4 Fathallah N *et al.* (2015) Drug-induced hyperglycaemia and diabetes. *Drug Safety*. **38**: 1153–1168.
5 WHO (2011) Use of glycated haemoglobin (HbA1c) in the diagnosis of diabetes mellitus. *World Healh Organization*.
6 Heinemann L *et al.* (2000) Time-action profile of the long-acting insulin analog insulin glargine (HOE901) in comparison with those of NPH insulin and placebo. *Diabetes Care*. **23**: 644–649.
7 NICE (2016) Type 1 diabetes in adults: diagnosis and management. NG17. www.nice.org.uk.
8 NICE (2019) Type 2 diabetes in adults: management. NG28. www.nice.org.uk.
9 MHRA (2019) GLP-1 receptor agonists: reports of diabetic ketoacidosis when concomitant insulin was rapidly reduced or discontinued. *Drug Safety Update*. **12**: 11. https://www.gov.uk/drug-safety-update.
10 MHRA (2017) SGLT2 inhibitors: updated advice on increased risk of lower-limb amputation (mainly toes). *Drug Safety Update*. https://www.gov.uk/drug-safety-update.
11 NICE (2016) Dapagliflozin in triple therapy for treating type 2 diabetes. *Technology Appraisal*. TA418. www.nice.org.uk.
12 NICE (2016) Canaglifozin, dapagliflozin and empagliflozin as monotherapies for treating type 2 diabetes. *Technology Appraisal*. TA390. www.nice.org.uk.

13 MHRA (2016) SGLT2 inhibitors (canagliflozin, dapagliflozin, empagliflozin): risk of diabetic ketoacidosis. *Drug Safety Update*. **9**: 9. https://www.gov.uk/drug-safety-update.
14 MHRA (2019) SGLT2 inhibitors: reports of Fournier's gangrene (necrotising fasciitis of the genitalia or perineum). *Drug Safety Update*. **12**: 7. https://www.gov.uk/drug-safety-update.
15 NICE (2019) Dapagliflozin with insulin for treating type 1 diabetes. *Technology Appraisal*. TA597. www.nice.org.uk.
16 Li L *et al.* (2014) Incretin treatment and risk of pancreatitis in patients with type 2 diabetes mellitus: systematic review and meta-analysis of randomised and non-randomised studies. *British Medical Journal*. **348**: 2366.
17 Faillie JL *et al.* (2014) Incretin based drugs and risk of acute pancreatitis in patients with type 2 diabetes: cohort study. *British Medical Journal*. **348**: 2780.
18 Azoulay L *et al.* (2016) Incretin based drugs and the risk of pancreatic cancer: international multicentre cohort study. *British Medical Journal*. **352**: i581.
19 Salpeter S *et al.* (2003) Risk of fatal and nonfatal lactic acidosis with metformin use in type 2 diabetes mellitus. *Cochrane Database of Systematic Reviews*. CD002967.
20 ADA (American Diabetes Association) (2014) Diagnosis and classification of diabetes mellitus. *Diabetes Care*. **37 (Suppl 1)**: S81–S90.
21 MHRA (2011) Insulin combined with pioglitazone: risk of cardiac failure. *Drug Safety Update*. https://www.gov.uk/drug-safety-update.
22 MHRA (2011) Pioglitazone: risk of bladder cancer. *Drug Safety Update*. **5**: https://www.gov.uk/drug-safety-update.
23 Loke YK *et al.* (2009) Long-term use of thiazolidinediones and fractures in type 2 diabetes: a meta-analysis. *Canadian Medical Association Journal*. **180**: 32–39.
24 Habib ZA *et al.* (2010) Thiazolidinedione use and the longitudinal risk of fractures in patients with type 2 diabetes mellitus. *Journal of Clinical Endocrinology and Metabolism*. **95**: 592–600.
25 National Patient Safety Agency (2011) The adult patient's passport for safer use of insulin. *Patient Safety Alert*. NPSA/2011/PSA2003. www.nrls.npsa.nhs.uk.
26 Angelo M *et al.* (2011) An approach to diabetes mellitus in hospice and palliative medicine. *Journal of Palliative Medicine*. **14**: 83–87.
27 Dikkers MF *et al.* (2013) Information needs of family carers of people with diabetes at the end of life: a literature review. *Journal of Palliative Medicine*. **16**: 1617–1623.
28 Joint British Diabetes Societies Inpatient Care Group (2021) The hospital management of hypoglycaemia in adults with diabetes mellitus. Available from: www.abcd.care.
29 Anonymous (2012) Insulin pump therapy. *Drug and Therapeutics Bulletin*. **50**: 105–108.
30 McCann M-A *et al.* (2006) Practical management of diabetes mellitus. *European Journal of Palliative Care*. **13**: 226–229.
31 Ciardullo AV *et al.* (2006) Effectiveness and safety of insulin glargine in the therapy of complicated or secondary diabetes: clinical audit. *Acta Diabetologica*. **43**: 57–60.
32 King EJ *et al.* (2012) The management of diabetes in terminal illness related to cancer. *Quarterly Journal of Medicine*. **105**: 3–9.
33 Pilkey J *et al.* (2012) Corticosteroid-induced diabetes in palliative care. *Journal of Palliative Medicine*. **15**: 681–689.
34 van der Linden MW *et al.* (2009) Topical corticosteroids and the risk of diabetes mellitus: a nested case-control study in the Netherlands. *Drug Safety*. **32**: 527–537.
35 Perez A *et al.* (2014) Glucocorticoid-induced hyperglycemia. *Journal of Diabetes*. **6**: 9–20.
36 Joint British Diabetes Societies Inpatient Care Group (2021) Management of hyperglycaemia and steroid (glucocorticoid) therapy. Available from: www.diabetes.org.uk.
37 Diabetes UK (2020) COncise adVice on Inpatient Diabetes (COVID:Diabetes): Dexamethasone therapy in COVID-19 patients: implications and guidance for the management of blood glucose in people with and without diabetes. Available from: www.diabetes.org.uk.
38 Bonaventura A and Montecucco F (2018) Steroid-induced hyperglycemia: an underdiagnosed problem or clinical inertia? A narrative review. *Diabetes Research and Clinical Practice*. **139**: 203–220.
39 Trend-UK (2020) Hypoglycaemia in adults in the community: recognition, management and prevention. https://trenddiabetes.online.
40 NICE (2019) Safer insulin prescribing. Key therapeutic topic ktt20. www.nice.org.uk.
41 National Patient Safety Agency (2010) Safer administration of insulin. *Patient Safety Alert*. NPSA/2010/RRR2013. www.nrls.npsa.nhs.uk.

Updated (minor change) February 2022

*OCTREOTIDE

Class: Somatostatin analogue.

Indications: Symptoms associated with unresectable hormone-secreting tumours, e.g. carcinoid, VIPomas, glucagonomas, acromegaly; prevention of complications after elective pancreatic surgery;[1] bleeding oesophageal varices in cirrhosis; †salivary, buccal and enterocutaneous fistulas;[2-4] †intractable diarrhoea;[5-12] †inoperable bowel obstruction in patients with cancer;[13,14] †hypertrophic pulmonary osteoarthropathy;[15] †ascites in cirrhosis and cancer;[16-18] †death rattle (noisy rattling breathing); †bronchorrhoea;[19,20] †reduction of tumour-related secretions.[18]

Pharmacology

Octreotide (like **lanreotide**) is a synthetic analogue of somatostatin with a longer duration of action.[21] Somatostatin is an inhibitory hormone found throughout the body. In the hypothalamus it inhibits the release of growth hormone, TSH, prolactin and ACTH. It inhibits the secretion of insulin, glucagon, gastrin and other peptides of the gastro-enteropancreatic system (i.e. peptide YY, neurotensin, VIP and substance P), reducing splanchnic blood flow, portal blood flow, GI motility, and gastric, pancreatic and small bowel secretion, and increasing water and electrolyte absorption.[22]

In type 1 diabetes mellitus, octreotide decreases insulin requirements. However, in type 2 diabetes, octreotide suppresses both insulin and glucagon release, leaving blood glucose concentrations either unchanged or slightly elevated.[23,24] Thus, octreotide (with dextrose) has been suggested as treatment for refractory sulfonylurea-induced hypoglycaemia.[25]

Somatostatin acts as an inhibitory neurotransmitter in the CNS, has anti-inflammatory and analgesic effects, and also inhibits cell proliferation.[26-29] Somatostatin analogues have a direct anticancer effect and improve time to progression ± prognosis in patients with neuroendocrine or solid tumours of the GI tract.[29-34] The combination of somatostatin analogues and targeted anticancer therapies (e.g. tyrosine kinase inhibitors) are now used in the treatment of some neuroendocrine tumours.

There are five somatostatin receptors (SST_{1-5}), each mediating a different biological action of somatostatin. Neuroendocrine tumours express various receptor profiles, but generally SST_2 or SST_5 predominate.[35] Octreotide and **lanreotide** bind with high affinity to SST_2 and with moderate affinity to SST_3 and SST_5. **Pasireotide**, developed more recently, has a broader receptor affinity profile ($SST_5 > SST_2 > SST_3 > SST_1$), and in acromegaly provides higher rates of biochemical control than octreotide (30% vs. 20%). Further, of patients failing to respond to octreotide, ≤20% respond to **pasireotide**.[35] This suggests **pasireotide** has a potential role in patients who are or have become refractory to octreotide (tolerance can occur after 12–18 months).[33] However, compared with octreotide, the incidence of hyperglycaemia and diabetes mellitus and potential for drug interactions are greater with **pasireotide**;[35] it is also more expensive (>£2,000 for the monthly depot injection).

Various radionuclides have been linked to somatostatin analogues for either diagnostic or therapeutic purposes. The latter are still in development and require the tumour to demonstrate high uptake on a somatostatin receptor radionuclide scan. Best results are seen in fitter patients without significant liver involvement.[33]

The inhibitory, antisecretory and absorptive effects of octreotide are utilized in a wide range of clinical settings.

Hormone-secreting tumours

Octreotide improves symptoms by inhibiting hormone secretion, e.g.:

- 5HT in carcinoid (improving flushing and diarrhoea)
- VIP in VIPomas (improving diarrhoea)
- glucagon in glucagonomas (improving rash and diarrhoea)
- TSH in pituitary adenomas.

Inoperable bowel obstruction in patients with cancer

For a suggested management approach, see QCG: Inoperable bowel obstruction (p.266).

Octreotide can provide rapid improvements in nausea and vomiting in this setting, although the evidence for benefit is generally low level and limited to short-term use.[36–38]

The optimal dose has not been formally identified, but reports suggest <50% of patients respond to the typical CSCI starting dose of 300microgram/24h,[39] and 75–90% respond to 600–800microgram/24h.[14,40] Although doses of up to 1,500microgram/24h have been used,[41] a dose of 600–800microgram/24h is generally sufficient to identify those likely to respond.[40,42] Benefit is less likely in obstruction of the gastric outlet or proximal small bowel.[39,43]

In a well-conducted RCT over 72h, there was no difference between octreotide 600microgram/24h CSCI and placebo in relation to the *complete* control of vomiting when given alongside a standardized regimen of bowel rest (IV hydration, PO clear fluids only ± NG tube) + SC/IV **dexamethasone** + SC/IV **ranitidine** (also chosen for its antisecretory effects; see p.27) and p.r.n. SC **hyoscine *butylbromide*.**[44] No differences were seen in the number of patients free of vomiting for all 3 days (about 30%), mean number of days free of vomiting (about 2 days), nausea, patients' global impression of change or quality of life scores.[45] Although mean pain was the same in both groups, those receiving octreotide required more **hyoscine *butylbromide***. Nonetheless, octreotide about halved the overall number of vomiting episodes. These findings suggest that, in this setting, octreotide can be reserved for instances when such a regimen fails to reduce the frequency of vomiting to an acceptable level.

In comparisons with **hyoscine *butylbromide*** (60–80mg/24h CSCI; p.15), octreotide (300–800microgram/24h CSCI) provided more effective and rapid improvements in nausea and vomiting and reduction in NG tube output.[40,46] However, in those patients responding to either drug, after 3–6 days overall symptom relief is similar, and NG tube removal possible with both.[40,46] A large database study (n=1,595) suggested that the addition of a corticosteroid to octreotide (± H_2 antagonist or PPI) increases the likelihood of NG tube removal at 4 and 7 days.[47]

Depot (long-acting) preparations of octreotide and **lanreotide** have also been explored in RCTs in this setting.[48,49] Although there was suggestion of some benefit, both studies had methodological limitations.[36]

Ascites

Octreotide 300microgram SC b.d. can suppress diuretic-induced activation of the renin–angiotensin–aldosterone system. Its use has improved renal function and Na^+ and water excretion in patients with cirrhosis and ascites receiving **furosemide** and **spironolactone** (p.73).[17,50]

Octreotide is also reported to reduce the rate of formation of malignant ascites.[16,18] In a pilot RCT of depot octreotide 30mg IM monthly for malignant ascites, the median time to next paracentesis was doubled (28 days vs. 14 days), although this did not reach statistical significance. Nonetheless, patients receiving octreotide had significantly less abdominal bloating, abdominal discomfort and shortness of breath.[51]

Octreotide may interfere with ascitic fluid formation in various ways, including by a reduction in splanchnic blood flow or by inhibiting vascular endothelial growth factor, which increases vascular permeability and also promotes angiogenesis and tumour growth.

Octreotide could be considered in patients with rapidly accumulating ascites requiring frequent paracentesis despite diuretic therapy (if indicated; see **Spironolactone**, p.73) and/or when an indwelling catheter is inappropriate or declined. Octreotide may also help resolve chylous ascites and/or pleural effusion from various causes.[52–61]

Other antisecretory effects

Octreotide reduces salivary production and may be of use in salivary or buccal fistulas.[2,4] Experience of its use in death rattle is limited.[62] The use of octreotide has led to rapid and sometimes complete control of bronchorrhoea (>1L/24h) in patients with diffuse adenocarcinoma of the lung.[19,20]

When given in conjunction with pancreatic surgery *for cancer* (but not for other conditions), octreotide reduces the risk of complications, e.g. fistulas.[1] If enterocutaneous fistulas complicate abdominal surgery, somatostatin analogues reduce the time to closure and length of hospital stay.[3] However, in a review limited to pancreatic fistula, evidence of benefit was lacking.[63]

Octreotide has been used for intractable diarrhoea from various causes, e.g. high-output ileostomies, AIDS, Crohn's disease, and following coeliac plexus block, radiation therapy, chemotherapy or bone marrow transplant.[6-12] In severe and/or complicated diarrhoea caused by chemotherapy or radiotherapy, octreotide is combined with **loperamide** (p.36). For those who have experienced severe chemotherapy-induced diarrhoea, prophylactic depot octreotide is recommended for subsequent cycles. In an RCT, octreotide failed to improve diarrhoea in patients with ileal pouch anastomosis (± pouchitis) following total colectomy for ulcerative colitis.[64]

Octreotide has also been used for the treatment of enterovesical fistula,[65] to improve mucous discharge from rectal cancers,[18] and, together with fasting ± TPN, for chylothorax of various aetiologies, including cancer.[61]

Pain

Octreotide is reported to have an analgesic effect in patients with cancer, e.g. in bone pain from metastatic carcinoid, in hypertrophic pulmonary osteoarthropathy, pain arising from GI cancer, or when given IT.[15,66–68] However, a small RCT found octreotide to be no better than placebo.[69]

Although octreotide slows GI transit time, mostly via inhibitory effects on the small bowel,[70] there is no evidence of an antispasmodic effect. Indeed, patients receiving octreotide for bowel obstruction required 3 times more doses of **hyoscine *butylbromide*** than those receiving placebo.[44] This has implications for the management of patients with bowel obstruction associated with colic (see QCG: Inoperable bowel obstruction, p.266).

The development of somatostatin analogues with a greater affinity for the receptors predominantly responsible for an anti-inflammatory effect (SST_1, SST_4) may prove more effective.[26] Octreotide may also be of value in chronic pancreatitic pain caused by hypertension in scarred ducts.[71,72] Benefit may be secondary to its antisecretory action.[73] (Suppressing exocrine function by administering **pancreatin** supplements (p.63) can also reduce pain in patients with chronic pancreatitis.[74])

Miscellaneous

At doses far below those necessary for an antisecretory effect (e.g. 1microgram SC t.d.s.), octreotide protects the stomach from NSAID-related injury, probably via its ability to reduce NSAID-induced neutrophil adhesion to the microvasculature.[75] Uncontrolled data suggest somatostatin analogues may reduce transfusion requirements in patients with angiodysplasia of the GI tract.[76] Benefit is also reported in the control of bleeding from peristomal varices.[77] However, a systematic review casts doubt on the value of octreotide in the acute management of bleeding oesophageal varices.[78]

Octreotide improves tolerance to being upright, in part by reducing splanchnic blood flow. Potentially this could benefit patients with postural hypotension caused by loss of the ability to vasoconstrict splanchnic blood vessels in response to standing.[79] Octreotide is used as an adjunct to IV dextrose in the treatment of hypoglycaemia caused by sulfonylurea overdose.[80]

Octreotide is generally given as an SC bolus or by CSCI,[81] but can be given IV (after dilution) when a rapid effect is required. Octreotide has also been administered IT as an analgesic.[66] A long-acting IM depot formulation is also available, but evaluation has been generally limited to hormone-secreting tumours.[82] Benefit from depot octreotide has been reported in an RCT for the prevention of chemotherapy-related diarrhoea[5] and in cancer patients with bowel obstruction.[83,84] **Lanreotide** is available in depot formulations only.

Onset of action 30min.
Time to peak plasma concentration 30min SC.
Plasma halflife 1.5h SC.
Duration of action 8h.

Cautions

In type 1 diabetes mellitus, **insulin** requirements may be reduced by up to 50%; monitor blood glucose concentrations to guide dose reductions with both **insulin** and oral hypoglycaemic agents. Insulinoma: may exacerbate hypoglycaemia.

Cirrhosis, renal failure requiring dialysis (both lead to reduced elimination, which may necessitate a dose reduction). May cause gallstones (although the manufacturer advises ultrasound examination of the gallbladder before treatment and then every 6–12 months, this is generally not necessary in palliative care). Avoid abrupt withdrawal of short-acting octreotide after long-term treatment (may precipitate biliary colic caused by gallstones/biliary sludge).

May cause bradycardia,[85] conduction defects or arrhythmias; use with caution in at-risk patients. Monitor thyroid function during long-term treatment (may cause hypothyroidism).

In patients with carcinoid, possibly by increasing catecholamine levels, anaesthesia and operations can provoke a sudden release of carcinoid hormones and cause a 'carcinoid crisis'. In addition to typical carcinoid symptoms (e.g. flushing, diarrhoea), life-threatening haemodynamic instability can occur. It is treated with IV octreotide and supportive measures, e.g. IV fluids. Traditionally, in an attempt to reduce the risk of a crisis, prophylactic octreotide is given peri-operatively, although the value of this has been questioned.[86]

Drug interactions

Octreotide increases the bio-availability of **bromocriptine** by about 40% (consider when using the combination in acromegaly).[87]

Octreotide markedly reduces plasma **ciclosporin** concentrations, and inadequate immunosuppression may result. Increase the **ciclosporin** dose by 50% before starting octreotide, and monitor the plasma concentration daily to guide further adjustments.[87]

Undesirable effects

Dry mouth, flatulence (lowers oesophageal sphincter tone), nausea, abdominal pain, diarrhoea, steatorrhoea (GI undesirable effects may be reduced by administering octreotide between meals or at bedtime), impaired glucose tolerance, hypoglycaemia (shortly after starting treatment), persistent hyperglycaemia (during long-term treatment), gallstones (10–20% of patients on long-term treatment), pancreatitis (associated with gallstones), vitamin B12 deficiency.

Dose and use

Octreotide is painful if given as an SC bolus injection. Warming the ampoule or vial to body temperature before injection by holding it in the hand reduces the pain. With CSCI, to reduce the likelihood of inflammatory reactions at the skin injection site, dilute to the largest volume possible, preferably in sodium chloride 0.9% (see Chapter 29, p.889).

7

The dose varies according to the indication (Table 1). To maximize the benefit (convenience and cost-effectiveness) of the multidose vials, the starting doses have been given in convenient fractions of 1mg (e.g. 250–500microgram rather than 300–600microgram). If necessary, the dose should be titrated upwards; higher doses are generally well tolerated.[88] However, after the desired response has been achieved, it may be possible to reduce to a lower maintenance dose.

Table 1 Dose recommendations for SC/CSCI octreotide

Indication	*Starting dose*[a]	*Maximum dose*[b]
Hormone-secreting tumours		
Acromegaly	100–200microgram t.d.s.	600microgram/24h[22]
Carcinoid, VIPomas, glucagonomas	50microgram once daily or b.d.	1,500microgram/24h; rarely 6,000microgram/24h[89]
†Intractable diarrhoea (including that caused by chemotherapy and radiotherapy)	250–500microgram/24h	1,500microgram/24h,[12,90] occasionally higher
†Inoperable bowel obstruction	250–500microgram/24h	750microgram/24h, occasionally higher
†Tumour-antisecretory effect	50–100microgram b.d.	600microgram/24h[18]
†Ascites	250–500microgram/24h	600microgram/24h[16]
†Bronchorrhoea	250–500microgram/24h[19,20]	
†Hypertrophic pulmonary osteoarthropathy	100microgram b.d.[15]	

a. doses rounded to maximize benefit from multidose vials
b. unrounded doses from the literature.

CSCI compatibility with other drugs: there are 2-drug compatibility data for octreotide in sodium chloride 0.9% with **diamorphine**, **haloperidol**, **hyoscine *butylbromide***, **hyoscine *hydrobromide***, **midazolam**, **morphine sulfate**, **ondansetron** and **oxycodone**.

Incompatibility may occur with **dexamethasone** or **levomepromazine**. More details and 3-drug compatibility data can be found on the www.palliativedrugs.com Syringe Driver Survey Database.

For compatibility charts for mixing drugs in WFI, see Appendix 3 (p.933).

Depot formulations

Depot formulations of octreotide 10–30mg, given IM every 4 weeks, are available (e.g. Sandostatin LAR®, Olatuton®). Higher (40–60mg) or more frequently administered (every 3 weeks) doses are sometimes required.[88] This has a relative bio-availability of about 60% compared with SC octreotide. Generally, the depot formulation is used only after symptoms have been controlled with SC octreotide.

Patients who have not previously received SC octreotide should have a test dose of 50–100microgram SC and, provided there are no unacceptable undesirable effects, then switch to the depot injection. The starting dose for those patients with acromegaly or gastro-enteropancreatic tumours who are adequately controlled is 20mg every 4 weeks. The depot formulation requires deep IM injection into the gluteal muscle; use alternate sides for subsequent injections.

In acromegaly, stop SC octreotide when the first depot injection is given; for other neuroendocrine tumours, continue the SC dose for 2 weeks.

In a survey, 40% of respondents reported the use of depot formulations in cancer-related bowel obstruction.[91] There is limited published long-term experience of their use in this setting, although benefit in a small number of patients with ovarian cancer for up to 15 months has been reported.[83] A reduction in NG tube output and symptomatic benefit is evident within 24h.[84]

Lanreotide

Patients can be started directly on either of the long-acting formulations. However, for palliative care, use of Somatuline Autogel® may be preferable, because it is given by deep SC injection into the superior external quadrant of the buttock:

- start with 60mg every 4 weeks for the first 3 months
- if necessary, increase to 120mg every 4 weeks.

If a switch between Sandostatin LAR® and Somatuline Autogel® is considered necessary, experience in patients with acromegaly suggests that Sandostatin LAR® 20mg is approximately equivalent to Somatuline Autogel® 90mg.[92]

Supply

For full details of storage and reconstitution details, see manufacturer's SPC.

For prolonged storage, keep all *unopened* ampoules, vials and pre-filled syringes in a refrigerator. Once opened, a multidose vial can be kept for up to 2 weeks at room temperature for day-to-day use (for a maximum of 10 punctures of the vial).

Octreotide

Octreotide (generic)

Injection (as acetate) 50microgram/mL, 1mL amp = £2.50; 100microgram/mL, 1mL amp = £5.50; 500microgram/mL, 1mL amp = £23.

Injection (as acetate) 50microgram/mL, 1mL prefilled syringe = £3.75; 100microgram/mL, 1mL prefilled syringe = £6; 500microgram/mL, 1mL prefilled syringe = £31.

Injection (as acetate) 200microgram/mL multidose vial, 1mg in 5mL = £65.

Sandostatin LAR® (Novartis)

Depot injection (microsphere powder for aqueous suspension), octreotide (as acetate) 10mg vial = £550; 20mg vial = £800; 30mg vial = £998; all supplied with diluent-filled syringe for deep IM injection every 28 days.

Olatuton® (Teva)

Depot injection (microsphere powder for aqueous suspension), octreotide (as acetate) 10mg vial = £495; 20mg vial = £719; 30mg vial = £899; all supplied with diluent-filled syringe for deep IM injection every 28 days.

Lanreotide

Somatuline LA® (Ipsen)

Long-acting injection (copolymer microparticles for aqueous suspension), lanreotide (as acetate) 30mg vial (with vehicle) = £323 for IM injection every 14 days.

Somatuline Autogel® (Ipsen)

Depot injection (prefilled syringe), lanreotide (as acetate) 60mg = £551; 90mg = £736; 120mg = £937; for deep SC injection into the superior external quadrant of the buttock every 28 days.

1 Gurusamy KS *et al.* (2012) Somatostatin analogues for pancreatic surgery. *Cochrane Database of Systematic Reviews.* **6**: CD008370. www.cochranelibrary.com.
2 Spinell C *et al.* (1995) Postoperative salivary fistula: therapeutic action of octreotide. *Surgery.* **117**: 117–118.
3 Coughlin S *et al.* (2012) Somatostatin analogues for the treatment of enterocutaneous fistulas: a systematic review and meta-analysis. *World Journal of Surgery.* **36**: 1016–1029.
4 Lam C and Wong S (1996) Use of somatostatin analog in the management of traumatic parotid fistula. *Surgery.* **119**: 481–482.
5 Rosenoff SH *et al.* (2006) A multicenter, randomized trial of long-acting octreotide for the optimum prevention of chemotherapy-induced diarrhea: results of the STOP trial. *Journal of Supportive Oncology.* **4**: 289–294.
6 Crouch M *et al.* (1996) Octreotide acetate in refractory bone marrow transplant-associated diarrhea. *Annals of Pharmacotherapy.* **30**: 331–336.
7 Harris A (1992) Octreotide in the treatment of disorders of the gastrointestinal tract. *Drug Investigation.* **4**: 1–54.
8 Dorta G (1999) Role of octreotide and somatostatin in the treatment of intestinal fistulae. *Digestion.* **60 (Suppl 2)**: 53–56.
9 Martelli L *et al.* (2017) Evaluation of the efficacy of octreotide LAR in the treatment of Crohn's disease associated refractory diarrhea. *Scandinavian Journal of Gastroenterology.* **52**: 564–569.
10 Yang A *et al.* (2016) Persistent diarrhea after celiac plexus block in a pancreatic cancer patient: case report and literature review. *Journal of Palliative Medicine.* **19**: 83–86.
11 Farthing MJ (1994) Octreotide in the treatment of refractory diarrhoea and intestinal fistulae. *Gut.* **35 (Suppl 3)**: s5–s10.
12 Bossi P *et al.* (2018) Diarrhoea in adult cancer patients: ESMO Clinical Practice Guidelines. *Annals of Oncology.* **29**: 126–142.
13 Mercadante S and Porzio G (2012) Octreotide for malignant bowel obstruction: twenty years after. *Critical Reviews in Oncology/Hematology.* **83**: 388–392.
14 Ripamonti C and Mercadante S (2004) How to use octreotide for malignant bowel obstruction. *Journal of Supportive Oncology.* **2**: 357–364.
15 Birch E *et al.* (2011) Treatment of painful hypertrophic osteoarthropathy associated with non-small cell lung cancer with octreotide: a case report and review of the literature. *BMJ Supportive and Palliative Care.* **1**: 189–192.
16 Cairns W and Malone R (1999) Octreotide as an agent for the relief of malignant ascites in palliative care patients. *Palliative Medicine.* **13**: 429–430.
17 Kalambokis G *et al.* (2005) Renal effects of treatment with diuretics, octreotide or both, in non-azotemic cirrhotic patients with ascites. *Nephrology, Dialysis, Transplantation.* **20**: 1623–1629.
18 Harvey M and Dunlop R (1996) Octreotide and the secretory effects of advanced cancer. *Palliative Medicine.* **10**: 346–347.
19 Hudson E *et al.* (2006) Successful treatment of bronchorrhea with octreotide in a patient with adenocarcinoma of the lung. *Journal of Pain and Symptom Management.* **32**: 200–202.
20 Pahuja M *et al.* (2014) The use of octreotide to manage symptoms of bronchorrhea: a case report. *Journal of Pain and Symptom Management.* **47**: 814–818.
21 Lamberts SWJ *et al.* (1996) Octreotide. *New England Journal of Medicine.* **334**: 246–254.
22 Gyr K and Meier R (1993) Pharmacodynamic effects of sandostatin in the gastrointestinal tract. *Digestion.* **54**: 14–19.
23 Davies R *et al.* (1989) Somatostatin analogues in diabetes mellitus. *Diabetic Medicine.* **6**: 103–111.
24 Lunetta M *et al.* (1997) Effects of octreotide on glycaemic control, glucose disposal, hepatic glucose production and counterregulatory hormone secretion in type 1 and type 2 insulin treated diabetic patients. *Diabetes Research and Clinical Practice.* **38**: 81–89.
25 Dougherty PP and Klein-Schwartz W (2010) Octreotide's role in the management of sulfonylurea-induced hypoglycemia. *Journal of Medical Toxicology.* **6**: 199–206.
26 Heyles Z *et al.* (2006) Effects of the somatostatin receptor subtype 4 selective agonist j-2156 on sensory neuropeptide and inflammatory reactions in rodents. *British Journal of Pharmacology.* **149**: 405–415.
27 Pinter E *et al.* (2006) Inhibitory effect of somatostatin on inflammation and nociception. *Pharmacology and Therapeutics.* **112**: 440–456.
28 Gadelha MR *et al.* (2017) Somatostatin receptor ligands in the treatment of acromegaly. *Pituitary.* **20**: 100–108.
29 Rinke A *et al.* (2017) Placebo-controlled, double-blind, prospective, randomized study on the effect of octreotide LAR in the control of tumor growth in patients with metastatic neuroendocrine midgut tumors (PROMID): results of long-term survival. *Neuroendocrinology.* **104**: 26–32.
30 Deming DA *et al.* (2005) A dramatic response to long-acting octreotide in metastatic hepatocellular carcinoma. *Clinical Advances in Hematology and Oncology.* **3**: 468–472; discussion 472–464.
31 Kouroumalis E *et al.* (1998) Treatment of hepatocellular carcinoma with octreotide: a randomised controlled study. *Gut.* **42**: 442–447.
32 Cascinu S *et al.* (1995) A randomised trial of octreotide vs best supportive care only in advanced gastrointestinal cancer patients refractory to chemotherapy. *British Journal of Cancer.* **71**: 97–101.
33 Walter T *et al.* (2012) New treatment strategies in advanced neuroendocrine tumours. *Digestive and Liver Disease.* **44**: 95–105.
34 Miljkovic MD *et al.* (2012) Novel medical therapies of recurrent and metastatic gastroenteropancreatic neuroendocrine tumors. *Digestive Diseases and Sciences.* **57**: 9–18.
35 Cuevas-Ramos D and Fleseriu M (2016) Pasireotide: a novel treatment for patients with acromegaly. *Drug design, development and therapy.* **10**: 227–239.
36 Obita GP *et al.* (2016) Somatostatin analogues compared with placebo and other pharmacologic agents in the management of symptoms of inoperable malignant bowel obstruction: a systematic review. *Journal of Pain and Symptom Management.* **52**: 901–919.
37 Walsh D *et al.* (2017) 2016 updated MASCC/ESMO consensus recommendations: Management of nausea and vomiting in advanced cancer. *Supportive Care in Cancer.* **25**: 333–340.
38 Davis M *et al.* (2021) Medical management of malignant bowel obstruction in patients with advanced cancer: 2021 MASCC guideline update. *Support Care Cancer.* **29**: 8089–8096.
39 Shima Y *et al.* (2008) Clinical efficacy and safety of octreotide (SMS201-995) in terminally ill Japanese cancer patients with malignant bowel obstruction. *Japanese Journal of Clinical Oncology.* **38**: 354–359.
40 Mystakidou K *et al.* (2002) Comparison of octreotide administration vs conservative treatment in the management of inoperable bowel obstruction in patients with far advanced cancer: a randomized, double-blind, controlled clinical trial. *Anticancer Research.* **22**: 1187–1192.
41 Weber C and Zulian GB (2009) Malignant irreversible intestinal obstruction: the powerful association of octreotide to corticosteroids, antiemetics, and analgesics. *American Journal of Hospice and Palliative Care.* **26**: 84–88.
42 Riley J and Fallon M (1994) Octreotide in terminal malignant obstruction of the gastrointestinal tract. *European Journal of Palliative Care.* **1**: 23–25.
43 Hisanaga T *et al.* (2010) Multicenter prospective study on efficacy and safety of octreotide for inoperable malignant bowel obstruction. *Japanese Journal of Clinical Oncology.* **40**: 739–745.

44 Currow DC *et al.* (2015) Double-blind, placebo-controlled, randomized trial of octreotide in malignant bowel obstruction. *Journal of Pain and Symptom Management.* **49**: 814–821.
45 McCaffrey N *et al.* (2020) Health-related quality of life in patients with inoperable malignant bowel obstruction: secondary outcome from a double-blind, parallel, placebo-controlled randomised trial of octreotide. *BMC Cancer.* **20**: 1050.
46 Peng X *et al.* (2015) Randomized clinical trial comparing octreotide and scopolamine butylbromide in symptom control of patients with inoperable bowel obstruction due to advanced ovarian cancer. *World Journal of Surgical Oncology.* **13**: 50.
47 Minoura T *et al.* (2018) Practice patterns of medications for patients with malignant bowel obstruction using a nationwide claims database and the association between treatment outcomes and concomitant use of H2-blockers/proton pump inhibitors and corticosteroids with octreotide. *Journal of Pain and Symptom Management.* **55**: 413–419.
48 Mariani P *et al.* (2012) Symptomatic treatment with lanreotide microparticles in inoperable bowel obstruction resulting from peritoneal carcinomatosis: A randomized, double-blind, placebo-controlled phase III study. *Journal of Clinical Oncology.* **30**: 4337–4343.
49 Laval G *et al.* (2012) SALTO: a randomized, multicenter study assessing octreotide LAR in inoperable bowel obstruction. *Bulletin Cancer.* **99**: E1–E9.
50 Kalambokis G *et al.* (2006) The effects of treatment with octreotide, diuretics, or both on portal hemodynamics in nonazotemic cirrhotic patients with ascites. *Journal of Clinical Gastroenterology.* **40**: 342–346.
51 Jatoi A *et al.* (2012) A pilot study of long-acting octreotide for symptomatic malignant ascites. *Oncology.* **82**: 315–320.
52 Yildirim AE *et al.* (2011) Idiopathic chylous ascites treated with total parenteral nutrition and octreotide. A case report and review of the literature. *European Journal of Gastroenterology and Hepatology.* **23**: 961–963.
53 Widjaja A *et al.* (1999) Octreotide for therapy of chylous ascites in yellow nail syndrome. *Gastroenterology.* **116**: 1017–1018.
54 Ferrandiere M *et al.* (2000) Chylous ascites following radical nephrectomy: efficacy of octreotide as treatment of ruptured thoracic duct. *Intensive Care and Medicine.* **26**: 484–485.
55 Sharkey AJ and Rao JN (2012) The successful use of octreotide in the treatment of traumatic chylothorax. *Texas Heart Institute Journal.* **39**: 428–430.
56 Zhou DX *et al.* (2009) The effectiveness of the treatment of octreotide on chylous ascites after liver cirrhosis. *Digestive Diseases and Sciences.* **54**: 1783–1788.
57 Pfammatter R *et al.* (2001) Treatment of hepatic hydrothorax and reduction of chest tube output with octreotide. *European Journal of Gastroenterology and Hepatology.* **13**: 977–980.
58 Dumortier J *et al.* (2000) Successful treatment of hepatic hydrothorax with octreotide. *European Journal of Gastroenterology and Hepatology.* **12**: 817–820.
59 Lee PH *et al.* (2005) Octreotide therapy for chylous ascites in a chronic dialysis patient. *Nephrology (Carlton).* **10**: 344–347.
60 Mincher L *et al.* (2005) The successful treatment of chylous effusions in malignant disease with octreotide. *Clinical Oncology.* **17**: 118–121.
61 Gupta A and Singh T (2016) Octreotide in malignant chylothorax: a case report. *BMJ Supportive & Palliative Care.* **6**: 122–124.
62 Clark K *et al.* (2008) A pilot phase II randomized, cross-over, double-blinded, controlled efficacy study of octreotide versus hyoscine hydrobromide for control of noisy breathing at the end-of-life. *Journal of Pain and Palliative Care Pharmacotherapy.* **22**: 131–138.
63 Gans SL *et al.* (2012) Systematic review and meta-analysis of somatostatin analogues for the treatment of pancreatic fistula. *British Journal of Surgery.* **99**: 754–760.
64 Van Assche G *et al.* (2012) Octreotide for the treatment of diarrhoea in patients with ileal pouch anal anastomosis: a placebo-controlled crossover study. *Colorectal Disease.* **14**: e181–e186.
65 Shinjo T *et al.* (2009) Treatment of malignant enterovesical fistula with octreotide. *Journal of Palliative Medicine.* **12**: 965–967.
66 Penn RD *et al.* (1992) Octreotide: A potent new nonopiate analgesic for intrathecal infusion. *Pain.* **49**: 13–19.
67 Befon S *et al.* (2000) Continuous subcutaneous octreotide in gastrointestinal cancer patients: pain control and beta-endorphin levels. *Anticancer Research.* **20**: 4039–4046.
68 Katai M *et al.* (2005) Octreotide as a rapid and effective painkiller for metastatic carcinoid tumor. *Endocrine Journal.* **52**: 277–2780.
69 De-Conno F *et al.* (1994) Subcutaneous octreotide in the treatment of pain in advanced cancer patients. *Journal of Pain and Symptom Management.* **9**: 34–38.
70 von der Ohe MR *et al.* (1995) Differential regional effects of octreotide on human gastrointestinal motor function. *Gut.* **36**: 743–748.
71 Donnelly PK *et al.* (1991) Somatostatin for chronic pancreatic pain. *Journal of Pain and Symptom Management.* **6**: 349–350.
72 Okazaki K *et al.* (1988) Pressure of papillary zone and pancreatic main duct in patients with chronic pancreatitis in the early state. *Scandinavian Journal of Gastroenterology.* **23**: 501–506.
73 Lembcke B *et al.* (1987) Effect of the somatostatin analogue sandostatin on gastrointestinal, pancreatic and biliary function and hormone release in man. *Digestion.* **36**: 108–124.
74 Draganov P and Toskes PP (2004) Chronic pancreatitis: controversies in etiology, diagnosis and treatment. *Revista Espanola de Enfermedades Digestivas.* **96**: 649–659.
75 Scheiman J *et al.* (1997) Reduction of NSAID induced gastric injury and leucocyte endothelial adhesion by octreotide. *Gut.* **40**: 720–725.
76 Sami SS *et al.* (2014) Review article: gastrointestinal angiodysplasia - pathogenesis, diagnosis and management. *Alimentary Pharmacology and Therapeutics.* **39**: 15–34.
77 Selby D and Jackson LD (2015) Octreotide for control of bleeding peristomal varices in palliative care. *Journal of Pain and Symptom Management.* **49**: e2–e4.
78 Gotzsche PC and Hrobjartsson A (2008) Somatostatin analogues for acute bleeding oesophageal varices. *Cochrane Database of Systematic Reviews.* **3**: CD000193. www.cochranelibrary.com.
79 Jarvis SS *et al.* (2012) A somatostatin analog improves tilt table tolerance by decreasing splanchnic vascular conductance. *Journal of Applied Physiology.* **112**: 1504–1511.
80 Glatstein M *et al.* (2012) Octreotide for the treatment of sulfonylurea poisoning. *Clinical Toxicology.* **50**: 795–804.
81 Mercadante S (1995) Tolerability of continuous subcutaneous octreotide used in combination with other drugs. *Journal of Palliative Care.* **11 (4)**: 14–16.
82 Scherubl H *et al.* (1994) Treatment of the carcinoid syndrome with a depot formulation of the somatostatin analogue lanreotide. *European Journal of Cancer.* **30A**: 1590–1591.
83 Matulonis UA *et al.* (2005) Long-acting octreotide for the treatment and symptomatic relief of bowel obstruction in advanced ovarian cancer. *Journal of Pain and Symptom Management.* **30**: 563–569.
84 Massacesi C and Galeazzi G (2006) Sustained release octreotide may have a role in the treatment of malignant bowel obstruction. *Palliative Medicine.* **20**: 715–716.
85 Kubota K *et al.* (2013) Octreotide acetate administration for malignant bowel obstruction induces severe bradycardia in patients with terminal stage cancer: two case reports. *Journal of Palliative Medicine.* **16**: 596–597.
86 Condron ME *et al.* (2016) Continuous infusion of octreotide combined with perioperative octreotide bolus does not prevent intraoperative carcinoid crisis. *Surgery.* **159**: 358–365.

87 Baxter K (ed) (2008) Stockley's Drug Interactions. In: Stockley I, (ed) (8e) Pharmaceutical Press, London.
88 Ludlam WH and Anthony L (2011) Safety review: dose optimization of somatostatin analogs in patients with acromegaly and neuroendocrine tumors. *Advances in Therapy*. **28**: 825–841.
89 Harris A and Redfern J (1995) Octreotide treatment of carcinoid syndrome: analysis of published dose-titration data. *Alimentary Pharmacology and Therapeutics*. **9**: 387–394.
90 Cello J *et al.* (1991) Effect of octreotide on refractory AIDS-associated diarrhea. A prospective, multicenter clinical trial. *Annals of Internal Medicine*. **115**: 705–710.
91 Palliativedrugs.com (2010) Octreotide - What is your experience? ; www.palliativedrugs.com.
92 Ashwell SG *et al.* (2004) The efficacy and safety of lanreotide Autogel in patients with acromegaly previously treated with octreotide LAR. *European Journal of Endocrinology*. **150**: 473–480.

Updated (minor change) January 2022

PROGESTOGENS

Class: Sex hormones.

Indications: Authorized indications vary between products; consult SPCs for details. Hormone therapy in advanced/recurrent endometrial cancer (use in breast, prostate and renal cancer has diminished);[1] anovulatory uterine bleeding; secondary amenorrhoea; mild–moderate endometriosis; †anorexia and cachexia in cancer and AIDS; †post-castration hot flushes in both women and men.

Contra-indications: *medroxyprogesterone acetate (MPA):* oestrogen-/progestogen-dependent cancer, cardiac disease (e.g. angina, atrial fibrillation, CHF), hepatic impairment, history of (or high risk of developing) thrombo-embolism, active thrombophlebitis, undiagnosed abnormal vaginal bleeding, pregnancy (known or suspected).

Pharmacology

In addition to natural **progesterone**, there are several classes of synthetic progestogens, e.g. derivatives of retroprogesterone, progesterone and 17α-hydroxyprogesterone (**cyproterone**, **MPA**, **megestrol acetate**).[2] Whereas all derivatives have a progestogenic effect on the uterus, there are differences in other biological effects (Table 1).

Table 1 Comparison of the biological effects of natural progesterone and selected synthetic progestogens[2]

Progestogen	*Effect*[a]		
	Androgenic	*Anti-androgenic*	*Anti-mineralocorticoid*
Progesterone	–	+	+
Cyproterone acetate	–	++	–
Megestrol acetate	+	+	–
MPA	+	–	–

++ effect present, + weak effect, – no effect

a. all the above possess similar progestogenic, anti-gonadotrophic, anti-oestrogenic and glucocorticoid effects.

In palliative care, **MPA** or **megestrol acetate** are used mostly in selected patients with cachexia–anorexia, although their efficacy in cachexia is debatable (see below). Progestogens may improve appetite by increasing levels of orexigenic neurotransmitters in the hypothalamus (e.g. neuropeptide Y), counteracting the anorexic effects of cytokines on the hypothalamus, or by interfering with the production of cytokines via their glucocorticoid anti-inflammatory effect.[3,4] *In vitro*, cytokine release from peripheral blood mononucleocytes is inhibited by both **MPA** and **megestrol acetate** in concentrations that would be achieved by daily doses of 1,500–2,000mg and 320–960mg respectively.[3] The release of serotonin is also inhibited and is considered one possible mechanism by which progestogens have an anti-emetic effect.[3]

Bio-availability of **MPA** and **megestrol acetate** is low (Table 2). Both **MPA** and **megestrol acetate** are highly protein-bound, mainly to albumin. **MPA** is metabolized extensively in the liver, by CYP3A4, and excreted mainly as glucuronides, whereas **megestrol acetate** is excreted mainly unchanged in the urine.

Table 2 Selected pharmacokinetic data[5,6]

	MPA	*Megestrol acetate*
Bio-availability	1–10%	No absolute data; reduced by 25% in fasting state
Time to peak plasma concentration	2–7h	1–3h
Plasma halflife	15–30h (PO)	15–20h

Cachexia and anorexia

Cachexia is common in cancer and other chronic diseases, impairing quality of life and increasing morbidity and mortality.[7] Cachexia is characterized by the loss of skeletal muscle ± body fat that cannot be fully reversed by conventional nutritional support. Loss of skeletal muscle is associated with impaired physical function and quality of life, whereas loss of fat (the body's main energy store) is associated with reduced survival. Recommended diagnostic criteria for cancer cachexia are:

- involuntary weight loss >5% in the past 6 months, or
- weight loss >2% in patients with either a BMI of <20kg/m^2 or skeletal muscle sarcopenia (absolute muscularity <5th centile of sex-specific norm).[8]

In cancer, a negative protein and energy balance is driven by the combination of reduced food intake (anorexia) and abnormal host metabolism resulting from factors produced by the cancer, e.g. proteolysis-inducing factor, or by the host in response to the cancer, e.g. cytokines. One outcome of this is a chronic inflammatory state, as evidenced by a raised serum CRP, the level of which relates to the degree and rate of weight loss.[9] Cytokines such as interleukin-1 and tumour necrosis factor-α act on the hypothalamus, muscle and fat tissues leading to anorexia, inefficient energy expenditure, wasting of skeletal and cardiac muscle, and loss of body fat. Management needs to address both the reduced nutritional intake and the abnormal host metabolism; increasing nutritional intake alone is generally ineffective.[10] Thus, a multimodal approach is generally recommended.[10,11] An RCT evaluating the combination of dietary counselling, nutritional support, anti-inflammatory drugs (NSAIDs, eicosapentanoic acid) and exercise is ongoing.[12]

Consensus recommendations emphasize the importance of early identification and intervention, and recognize that once cancer cachexia is advanced (patient has severe muscle wasting, ongoing catabolism, WHO performance status 3–4, metastatic disease refractory to therapy, and a prognosis of <3 months), a response to treatment is unlikely, and that the focus in these circumstances should be on symptom relief and psychosocial support.[8]

Megestrol acetate is used to stimulate appetite and weight gain. A large systematic review of 35 RCTs, totalling about 4,000 patients, mostly with cancer, AIDS (n=475) or other conditions (n=270), concluded that the quality of the evidence was very low.[13] Nonetheless, when compared with placebo, **megestrol acetate** increased appetite in about a quarter and weight (about 2kg) in about 1 in 12, but not overall quality of life. There was little difference in efficacy when compared with other drugs, e.g. **prednisolone**, except in patients with cancer, where **megestrol acetate** resulted in greater weight gain. For appetite stimulation, 160mg/day PO is probably the optimum dose; for weight gain, higher doses (≥400mg/day) appear more effective.[13,14] However, the RCTs used body weight as a primary outcome measure; none accurately evaluated changes in body composition (see below). Data from individual RCTs indicate that impotence occurred in 10–25% of men.[4,15-21] Further, compared with placebo, undesirable effects (e.g. oedema, thrombo-embolism) and sometimes deaths are more frequent in the patients treated with **megestrol acetate.**[13,22] Similar findings were reported in a study in frail elderly patients,[23] and, in consequence, enthusiasm for its use in this setting has declined. A subsequent systematic review limited to non-cancer conditions (18 trials, n=916) did not support the use of progestogens for cachexia, although there was evidence (albeit low quality) to support an appetite-stimulant effect.[24]

In studies that evaluated body composition, both **megestrol acetate** and **MPA** appear to increase fat mass but not fat-free mass, the part that includes skeletal muscle.[4,15,16,25] Thus it is likely that the gain in weight with progestogens (and corticosteroids), rather than representing the ideal increase in skeletal muscle *and* fat, is a less helpful retention of fluid or increase in fat only. This could make mobilizing more difficult in an already debilitated patient. In addition, the catabolic effect of progestogens on skeletal muscle could further weaken the patient. Catabolism may result from the glucocorticoid effect of progestogens, but they also suppress the amount and function of testosterone, which is anabolic.

Progestogens generally cost more than the equivalent dose of **dexamethasone** or **prednisolone**, which are also used as appetite stimulants (see Systemic corticosteroids, p.557). **Megestrol acetate** 800mg/day and **dexamethasone** 3mg/day are comparable with regard to appetite stimulation and non-fluid weight gain, although the latter was not accurately evaluated.[26] In this study, a high proportion of patients discontinued **dexamethasone** (36%) or **megestrol acetate** (25%) because of undesirable effects. **Dexamethasone** was more likely to cause cushingoid changes, myopathy, heartburn and peptic ulcers; **megestrol acetate** was associated with increased thrombo-embolism.[26] **Dexamethasone** is a fluorinated corticosteroid, a class which is more prone to cause muscle catabolism.[27] Thus, ideally, **dexamethasone** should be limited to short-term use (≤2 weeks).[28]

If long-term use of a corticosteroid is contemplated, a switch to the non-fluorinated **prednisolone** 10–20mg/day should be considered.[4] However, for patients expected to live months rather than weeks, progestogens may be more appropriate.[29] Caution is still required, as long-term progestogens can also cause cushingoid changes (25% of patients after 3 months in one study),[30] muscle catabolism and suppression of the hypothalamic–pituitary–adrenal axis.[31] The latter may present with non-specific symptoms, and a high level of clinical suspicion is required.[32] Additional corticosteroid replacement therapy would be a reasonable precaution in patients with serious infections or undergoing surgery.[4,33,34] Adrenal suppression is secondary to a central glucocorticoid effect on the hypothalamus and is dose-related; maximal suppression is seen with daily doses of **megestrol acetate** 200mg and **MPA** 1,000mg.[30]

In an attempt to improve outcomes, progestogens have been combined with other drugs.[29] The best evidence available is for NSAIDs, with some studies showing additional benefit, potentially via a reduction in the chronic inflammatory response.[35] However, other studies are negative and the overall evidence is insufficient to recommend such use.[29]

In conclusion, progestogens and systemic corticosteroids (p.556) can stimulate appetite and increase calorie intake, and as such can be considered for use in selected patients for anorexia. Progestogens may be better for long-term use than corticosteroids, but significant undesirable effects can occur. Starting doses should be low and titrated to the lowest effective dose. Both progestogens and corticosteroids are best *not* regarded as 'anticachexia' agents; any weight gain is likely to be because of an increase in fat and fluid retention, and the catabolism of skeletal muscle is *increased*, particularly in inactive people.

Cautions

Conditions that may be aggravated by potential fluid retention (e.g. CHF, renal impairment, hypertension); asthma, epilepsy, migraine, depression, diabetes (monitor).

MPA: hyperlipidaemia.

Megestrol acetate: history of/susceptibility to thrombo-embolism (particular caution with high dose), severe hepatic impairment.

Undesirable effects

May suppress the hypothalamic–pituitary–adrenal axis.[31] Possibility of glucocorticoid effects. May cause or worsen diabetes mellitus. Thrombo-embolism (5%).

Frequency not stated: hyperglycaemia, depression, insomnia, fatigue, hypertension, oedema/fluid retention, nausea, vomiting, constipation, cushingoid changes, bone mineral density loss, reduced libido, impotence, altered menstruation, breast tenderness, urticaria, acne.

Rare (<0.1%): jaundice, alopecia, hirsutism.

MPA: discontinue if any of the following develop: jaundice, hepatic impairment, significant increase in blood pressure, thrombo-embolic event, new onset migraine, severe visual disturbances.

Dose and use

Long-term progestogens can cause suppression of the hypothalamic–pituitary–adrenal axis (see Cachexia and anorexia). Maximal suppression is seen with daily doses of **megestrol acetate** 200mg and **MPA** 1,000mg. Additional corticosteroid replacement therapy would be a reasonable precaution in patients with serious infections or undergoing surgery (see p.562).

†Appetite stimulation

Given the relatively poor benefit:risk ratio (see above), the use of progestogens requires careful consideration, particularly in patients with conditions other than cancer or AIDS:

- start with **megestrol acetate** 80–160mg PO each morning
- if initial response poor, consider doubling the dose after 2 weeks[36,37]
- maximum dose generally 800mg PO/24h.

MPA 400mg PO each morning–b.d. is an alternative in countries where higher-strength tablets are available (e.g. 100mg, 200mg, 400mg).

†Hot flushes after surgical or chemical castration

- **MPA** 5–20mg PO b.d.–q.d.s. *or*
- **megestrol acetate** 80mg PO each morning; 40mg is used in countries where the 40mg tablet or oral suspension is readily available. The effect manifests after 2–4 weeks.[38]

Note. Better-tolerated alternatives are now generally used, e.g. SSRIs, **venlafaxine** (see Antidepressants, p.223).

Supply

Megestrol acetate

Tablets 40mg, 100 tablets = price unavailable (not UK, obtainable via import; see Chapter 24, p.817).

Oral suspension 40mg/mL; 240mL or 480mL = price unavailable (not UK, obtainable via import; see Chapter 24, p.817).

Megace® (Bausch & Lomb)

Tablets (scored) 160mg, 28 days @ 160mg each morning = £18.

Medroxyprogesterone acetate

Provera® (Pfizer)

Tablets (scored) 2.5mg, 5mg, 10mg, 100mg, 200mg, 400mg (unscored), 28 days @ 5mg b.d. = £7, 28 days @ 400mg each morning = £55.

Climanor® (ReSource Medical)

Tablets 5mg, 28 days @ 5mg b.d. = £6.50.

1 Colombo N *et al.* (2016) ESMO-ESGO-ESTRO consensus conference on endometrial cancer: diagnosis, treatment and follow-up. *Annals of Oncology.* **27**: 16–41.
2 Schindler AE *et al.* (2003) Classification and pharmacology of progestins. *Maturitas.* **46 (suppl 1)**: s7–s16.
3 Mantovani G *et al.* (1998) Cytokine involvement in cancer anorexia/cachexia: role of megestrol acetate and medroxyprogesterone acetate on cytokine downregulation and improvement of clinical symptoms. *Critical Reviews in Oncogenesis.* **9**: 99–106.
4 MacDonald N (2005) Anorexia-cachexia syndrome. *European Journal of Palliative Care.* **12 (suppl)**: 8s–14s.
5 Par Pharmaceuticals. Data on file.
6 Deschamps B *et al.* (2009) Food effect on the bioavailability of two distinct formulations of megestrol acetate oral suspension. *International Journal of Nanomedicine.* **4**: 185–192.
7 Laviano A *et al.* (2003) Cancer anorexia: clinical implications, pathogenesis, and therapeutic strategies. *Lancet Oncology.* **4**: 686–694.
8 Fearon K *et al.* (2011) Definition and classification of cancer cachexia: an international consensus framework. *Lancet Oncology.* **12**: 489-495.
9 Scott HR *et al.* (2002) The systemic inflammatory response, weight loss, performance status and survival in patients with inoperable non-small cell lung cancer. *British Journal of Cancer.* **87**: 264–267.
10 Peixoto da Silva S *et al.* (2020) Cancer cachexia and its pathophysiology: links with sarcopenia, anorexia and asthenia. *Journal of Cachexia, Sarcopenia and Muscle.* **11**: 619–635.
11 Maddocks M *et al.* (2016) Practical multimodal care for cancer cachexia. *Current Opinion in Supportive and Palliative Care.* **10**: 298–305.
12 Solheim TS *et al.* (2018) Cancer cachexia: rationale for the MENAC (multimodal –exercise, nutrition and anti-inflammatory medication for cachexia) trial. *BMJ Supportive & Palliative Care.* **8**: 258–265.
13 Ruiz Garcia V *et al.* (2013) Megestrol acetate for treatment of anorexia-cachexia syndrome. *Cochrane Database of Systemic Reviews.* **3**: CD004310. www.thecochranelibrary.com.
14 Saeteaw M *et al.* (2021) Efficacy and safety of pharmacological cachexia interventions: systematic review and network meta-analysis. *BMJ Supportive & Palliative Care.* **11**: 75–85.
15 Loprinzi CL *et al.* (1993) Phase III evaluation of four doses of megestrol acetate as therapy for patients with cancer anorexia and/or cachexia. *Journal of Clinical Oncology.* **11**: 762–767.
16 Simons JP *et al.* (1998) Effects of medroxyprogesterone acetate on food intake, body composition, and resting energy expenditure in patients with advanced, nonhormone-sensitive cancer: a randomized, placebo-controlled trial. *Cancer.* **82**: 553–560.
17 Jatoi A *et al.* (2002) Dronabinol versus megestrol acetate versus combination therapy for cancer-associated anorexia: a north central cancer treatment group study. *Journal of Clinical Oncology.* **20**: 567–573.

18 Jatoi A *et al.* (2003) On appetite and its loss. *Journal of Clinical Oncology*. **21 (suppl 9)**: 79–81.
19 Jatoi A *et al.* (2004) An eicosapentaenoic acid supplement versus megestrol acetate versus both for patients with cancer-associated wasting: a north central cancer treatment group and national cancer institute of canada collaborative effort. *Journal of Clinical Oncology*. **22**: 2469–2476.
20 Kropsky B *et al.* (2003) Incidence of deep-venous thrombosis in nursing home residents using megestrol acetate. *Journal of the American Medical Directors Association*. **4**: 255–256.
21 Garcia VR and Juan O (2005) Megestrol acetate-probably less effective than has been reported! *Journal of Pain and Symptom Management*. **30**: 4; author reply 5–6.
22 Ruiz-Garcia V *et al.* (2018)Megestrol acetate for cachexia-anorexia syndrome. A systematic review. *Journal of Cachexia, Sarcopenia and Muscle*. **9**: 444–452.
23 Bodenner D *et al.* (2007) A retrospective study of the association between megestrol acetate administration and mortality among nursing home residents with clinically significant weight loss. *American Journal Geriatric Pharmacotherapy*. **5**: 137–146.
24 Taylor JK and Pendleton N (2016) Progesterone therapy for the treatment of non-cancer cachexia: A systematic review. *BMJ Supportive & Palliative Care*. **6**: 276–286.
25 Loprinzi C *et al.* (1993) Body-composition changes in patients who gain weight while receiving megestrol acetate. *Journal of Clinical Oncology*. **11**: 152–154.
26 Loprinzi CL *et al.* (1999) Randomized comparison of megestrol acetate versus dexamethasone versus fluoxymesterone for the treatment of cancer anorexia/cachexia. *Journal of Clinical Oncology*. **17**: 3299–3306.
27 Faludi G *et al.* (1966) Factors influencing the development of steroid-induced myopathies. *Annals of the New York Academy of Sciences*. **138**: 62–72.
28 Hardy J *et al.* (2021) Practice review: evidence-based quality use of corticosteroids in the palliative care of patients with advanced cancer. *Palliative Medicine*. **35**: 461–472.
29 Roeland EJ *et al.* (2020) Management of cancer cachexia: ASCO guideline. *Journal of Clinical Oncology*. **38**: 2438–2453.
30 Willemse PH *et al.* (1990) A randomized comparison of megestrol acetate (ma) and medroxyprogesterone acetate (mpa) in patients with advanced breast cancer. *European Journal of Cancer*. **26**: 337–343.
31 Villarroel *et al.* (2008) Megestrol acetate-induced adrenal insufficiency. *Clinical Translational Oncology*. **10**: 235–237.
32 Dev R *et al.* (2007) Association between megestrol acetate treatment and symptomatic adrenal insufficiency with hypogonadism in male patients with cancer. *Cancer*. **110**: 1173–1177.
33 Naing KK *et al.* (1999) Megestrol acetate therapy and secondary adrenal suppression. *Cancer*. **86**: 1044–1049.
34 Lambert C *et al.* (2002) Effects of testosterone replacement and/or resistance exercise on the composition of megestrol acetate stimulated weight gain in elderly men: a randomized controlled trial. *Journal of Clinical Endocrinology and Metabolism*. **87**: 2100–2106.
35 Solheim TS *et al.* (2013) Non-steroidal anti-inflammatory treatment in cancer cachexia: A systematic literature review. *Acta Oncologica*. **52**: 6–17.
36 Donnelly S and Walsh TD (1995) Low-dose megestrol acetate for appetite stimulation in advanced cancer. *Journal of Pain and Symptom Management*. **10**: 182–183.
37 Vadell C *et al.* (1998) Anticachectic efficacy of megestrol acetate at different doses and versus placebo in patients with neoplastic cachexia. *American Journal of Clinical Oncology*. **21**: 347–351.
38 Loprinzi CL *et al.* (1996) Megestrol acetate for the prevention of hot flashes. *New England Journal of Medicine*. **331**: 347–352.

Updated (minor change) March 2022

*THALIDOMIDE

Class: Biologic response modifier.

Indications: Multiple myeloma, †lepromatous leprosy (erythema nodosum leprosum), †graft versus host disease (GVHD), †prevention of graft rejection, †recurrent aphthous stomatitis (e.g. HIV-related, connective tissue disease (Behcet's syndrome)), †paraneoplastic sweating, †paraneoplastic pruritus, †cachexia in HIV and cancer, †intractable GI bleeding, †intractable **irinotecan**-induced diarrhoea, †discoid lupus erythematosus.[1–3]

Contra-indications: Because it causes severe congenital abnormalities (absent or shortened limbs), thalidomide is contra-indicated in pregnant women and in women with childbearing potential unless strict contraception is implemented (see Dose and use).[4]

Pharmacology

Thalidomide is an immunomodulator with anticytokine, anti-integrin and anti-angiogenic properties.[3,5,6] It was withdrawn from use as a non-barbiturate hypnotic with anti-emetic properties in the early 1960s after it emerged that it was teratogenic (via binding cereblon, an E3 ligase protein).[3] Subsequently, it has been found to have immunomodulatory properties with potential for the treatment of various conditions.[7] However, its use is closely monitored, and it is prohibitively expensive (see Supply).

Thalidomide inhibits the synthesis of the pro-inflammatory cytokine tumour necrosis factor α (TNF-α) by monocytes,[8] and stimulates interleukin-2 and interferon-γ production (thereby stimulating human T lymphocytes).[9] It also inhibits chemotaxis of neutrophils and monocytes. Thalidomide antagonizes PGE_2, PGF_2, histamine, serotonin and acetylcholine.[10] It also affects several other mechanisms associated with inflammation and immunomodulation.[11] These properties probably account for the prevention of **irinotecan**-induced diarrhoea[12] and the amelioration of paraneoplastic sweating,[13] paraneoplastic pruritus (also see Chapter 26, p.825),[14–16] and cough in idiopathic pulmonary fibrosis.[17] This could also explain the beneficial effect of thalidomide in Crohn's disease and ulcerative colitis.[18]

An anti-inflammatory effect is also likely to explain benefit in the cachexia–anorexia syndrome in patients with cancer or HIV,[19–21] although high-quality evidence is limited.[22] Two small RCTs of thalidomide 100–200mg in patients with cancer found no overall benefit on body composition.[23,24] About half the patients experienced undesirable effects with the 200mg dose, particularly rash and drowsiness,[24] suggesting that a lower starting dose is advisable, e.g. 50–100mg at bedtime.

Despite promising case reports suggesting that thalidomide and its analogues (see below) may have an analgesic effect, a large RCT in complex regional pain syndrome (n=184) failed to show any benefit.[25–27]

The main antiproliferative and pro-apoptotic effects of thalidomide (and its analogues) in cancer cells are downstream consequences of binding cereblon.[3] Consistent benefit has been shown in several haematological cancers, but not solid tumours. It also inhibits angiogenesis by suppressing vascular endothelial growth factor, a potent angiogenic factor secreted by cancer cells in response to hypoxia. This property also provides the rationale underlying the use of thalidomide in refractory GI bleeding and epistaxis associated with underlying angiodysplasia.[28–32]

Analogues of thalidomide with similar anti-angiogenic, immunomodulatory and anti-inflammatory properties have been developed, e.g. **lenalidomide**, **pomalidomide**.[3] **Lenalidomide** is authorized in the treatment of multiple myeloma, and certain myelodysplastic syndromes that cause transfusion-dependent anaemia and mantle cell lymphoma (see SPC). It is also used in relapsed/refractory chronic lymphocytic leukaemia.[33] However, the analogues are also likely to carry serious teratogenic risk, are restricted in their availability, and are very expensive. Further, there is a dearth of experience with the analogues in symptom management and palliative care, and no obvious advantage over thalidomide.

The metabolism of thalidomide is almost completely by non-enzymatic hydrolysis in the plasma. Elimination is primarily via the kidneys, with <3% of the dose as unchanged thalidomide. Hepatic and renal impairment appear to have minimal effect on the metabolism and pharmacokinetics of thalidomide. However, because active metabolites are eliminated via the urine, patients with severe renal impairment should be carefully monitored for undesirable effects.

Bio-availability 67–93% PO in animals, no data in humans.

Onset of action varies from 2 days for lepromatous leprosy and paraneoplastic sweating to 1–2 months for GVHD and 2–3 months for rheumatoid arthritis.

Time to peak plasma concentration 2–6h, delayed by food.

Plasma half-life 6h (200mg/24h) to 18h (800mg/24h).[11]

Duration of action 24h.

Cautions

Treat as a 'cytotoxic' when handling. Thalidomide potentiates the sedative properties of barbiturates and alcohol, and increases the likelihood of extrapyramidal effects with **chlorpromazine** and **reserpine**.[10] Thalidomide should be used cautiously with other drugs that cause drowsiness, neuropathy or reduce the effectiveness of oral contraception (e.g. HIV protease inhibitors, **rifampicin**, **rifabutin**, **phenytoin**, **carbamazepine**).[10,34]

Undesirable effects

Neuropathy

Low-grade peripheral neuropathy occurs in >80% of patients receiving thalidomide, and severe neuropathy in 3–5%, generally after treatment lasting >6 months.[35,36] The incidence is higher in elderly patients, women, and in patients with pre-existing neuropathy or who are treated with neurotoxic chemotherapy, e.g. **vincristine**, **cisplatin**, **paclitaxel**.[36] Generally, the peripheral neuropathy presents as distal paraesthesia or dysaesthesia with or without sensory loss. Physical examination may be normal or show mildly decreased sensation in the distal limbs. Strength is usually preserved, but reflexes, particularly ankle jerks, may be depressed or absent. These symptoms, which are progressive, typically begin in the distal lower limbs and extend proximally and into the upper limbs.[37]

Although some studies have found a relationship between the cumulative dose and the occurrence of neuropathy,[38] others have not.[39] Nerve conduction studies typically show results consistent with a sensory axonal neuropathy. If a patient develops neuropathy, dose reduction or cessation may be required to decrease the likelihood of chronic painful neuropathy (see Dose and use).[40,41]

Some 80% of patients experience a mild decrease in bowel motility; this may reflect autonomic dysfunction, and can exacerbate constipation.[42]

Cardiovascular

Thalidomide and **lenalidomide** increase the risk of venous thrombo-embolism in patients with multiple myeloma, particularly when used in combination with high-dose corticosteroids and/or chemotherapy, and thromboprophylaxis is recommended.[43] Both thalidomide and **lenalidomide** increase the risk of arterial thrombosis, e.g. myocardial infarction, stroke.[44] The MHRA recommends thromboprophylaxis for patients at increased thrombotic risk for the first 5 months of treatment.[44] Generally this is with **LMWH** or **warfarin**. Although **aspirin** has been used, UK guidelines advocate this only in patients with no other risk factors for venous thrombo-embolism.[45,46]

7

Thalidomide is associated with arrhythmia, hypotension and oedema. Sinus bradycardia, generally mild, has been reported in ≤25% of patients.[47] Severe sinus bradycardia occurs in only 1–3% of patients.[47] Mild peripheral oedema has been reported in 15%. Orthostatic hypotension and dizziness also have been reported with thalidomide.[48] A dose-dependent decrease in supine systolic and diastolic pressures is seen up to 2h after dosing.[49] However, symptom-control doses should not affect blood pressure.

Skin

A pruritic and maculopapular rash may occur 10–14 days after starting treatment, starting on the trunk and extending to the back and proximal limbs. This is generally mild and resolves with the use of an emollient and dose reduction.[50] Severe skin reactions, such as Stevens–Johnson syndrome and toxic epidermal necrolysis, may also occur.[51] Skin complications seem more likely when thalidomide is combined with corticosteroids.

Other

These include drowsiness, seizures,[48] altered temperature sensitivity, pulmonary hypertension,[52] irregular menstrual cycles and hypothyroidism. Thalidomide can increase HIV viral load. Reactivation of varicella zoster (resulting in disseminated herpes zoster) and hepatitis B virus (resulting in acute hepatic failure) have occurred.[52,53] Myelosuppression is rare.

Tumour flare (a temporary increase in size of a cancerous lesion) may occur. When thalidomide is used to treat chronic lymphocytic leukaemia, some patients have experienced increased lymphadenopathy, enlargement of the spleen, and an increased lymphocyte count.[54]

Abnormal LFTs are common with **lenalidomide**. Serious (including fatal) instances of drug-related hepatitis have been reported in <1%, resulting in the recommendation for routine monitoring of LFTs (weekly for the first 8 weeks and monthly thereafter).[55] Patients with multiple myeloma treated with thalidomide or **lenalidomide** have a small increased risk of a second primary malignancy.[56,57]

Dose and use

Thalidomide is prohibitively expensive, and cost alone severely limits its use. In palliative care, thalidomide should *never* be considered as a first-line treatment. Its use should be considered only when more conventional treatments have failed and a full review of the potential benefits and harms has been undertaken with specialist colleagues.

There are several potential uses for thalidomide in palliative care (Table 1).[58] Female patients prescribed thalidomide must be counselled about the need for contraception, and male patients must use a condom. Written consent should be obtained.[59] Contraception should be used for ≥4 weeks before starting, during, and for 4 weeks after stopping treatment. Regular pregnancy testing is advised throughout treatment. Because thalidomide is present in the semen of men treated with the drug, even after vasectomy a latex condom must be used during sexual intercourse with women of childbearing potential.[60]

Table 1 Potential uses of PO thalidomide in palliative care[a]

Indication	*Dose*
†Aphthous ulcers in HIV+ disease	100–200mg at bedtime for 10 days[61]
†Paraneoplastic sweating	100–200mg at bedtime[62,63]
†Paraneoplastic pruritus[b]	100–200mg at bedtime[14–16]
†Cachexia–anorexia in HIV+ disease and cancer	50–200mg at bedtime[19–21]
†GI bleeding (associated with angiodysplasia/ radiation proctitis/cancer)	100–300mg at bedtime[31]
†Intractable irinotecan-induced diarrhoea	400mg at bedtime[12,64]

a. thalidomide is *not* the first-line treatment for any of these indications

b. also see Chapter 26, p.825.

For dose modifications if peripheral neuropathy occurs (i.e. paraesthesia, weakness and/or loss of reflexes), see Table 2.[4]

Table 2 Dose changes in thalidomide-related neuropathy[a]

Grade	*Impact of neuropathy*	*Dose modification*[b]
1	No loss of function	Consider reducing dose if symptoms worsen
2	Interferes with function but not with activities of daily living	Reduce dose or interrupt treatment. If no improvement or further deterioration, stop treatment. If improves to grade 1 or better, restart treatment (if the benefit:risk ratio remains favourable)
3	Interferes with activities of daily living	Stop treatment
4	Disabling	Stop treatment

a. based on first-line use in multiple myeloma

b. monitor the patient regularly during treatment, e.g. monthly in women of childbearing potential, otherwise every 3 months.

Supply

In the UK, thalidomide and **lenalidomide** are available through a strictly monitored pregnancy-prevention programme. Upon ordering through their distributor, pharmacies are contacted by the Celgene risk management department, registered, and sent full details of the pregnancy-prevention programme. Prescribers must complete a treatment initiation form and, subsequently, a prescription authorization form for each new supply. Further details can be obtained from rmp.uk.ire@celgene.com (0808 156 3059).

Thalidomide Celgene® (Celgene)
Capsules 50mg, 28 days @ 50mg at bedtime = £299.

Lenalidomide

Revlimid® (Celgene)
Capsules 2.5mg, 5mg, 7.5mg, 10mg, 15mg, 20mg, 25mg, 28 days @ 5mg at bedtime = £4,760.

1 Chen M *et al.* (2010) Innovative uses of thalidomide. *Dermatologic Clinics*. **28**: 577–586.
2 Hello M *et al.* (2010) Use of thalidomide for severe recurrent aphthous stomatitis: a multicenter cohort analysis. *Medicine (Baltimore)*. **89**: 176–182.
3 Millrine D and Kishimoto T (2017) A brighter side to thalidomide: its potential use in immunological disorders. *Trends in Molecular Medicine*. **23**: 348–361.
4 Celgene (2017) Thalidomide Celgene 50mg Hard Capsules. *SPC*. www.medicines.org.uk
5 Jacobson J (2000) Thalidomide: a remarkable comeback. *Expert Opinion in Pharmacotherapy*. **1**: 849–863.
6 De Sanctis JB *et al.* (2010) Pharmacological properties of thalidomide and its analogues. *Recent Patents on Inflammation and Allergy Drug Discovery*. **4**: 144–148.
7 Peuckmann V *et al.* (2000) Potential novel uses of thalidomide: focus on palliative care. *Drugs*. **60**: 273–292.
8 Sampaio E *et al.* (1991) Thalidomide selectively inhibits tumour necrosis factor alpha production by stimulated human monocytes. *Journal of Experimental Medicine*. **173**: 699–703.
9 Corral LG and Kaplan G (1999) Immunomodulation by thalidomide and thalidomide analogues. *Annals of the Rheumatic Diseases*. **58 (Suppl 1)**: I107–113.
10 Radomsky C and Levine N (2001) Thalidomide. *Dermatologic Clinics*. **19**: 87–103.
11 Bousvaros A and Mueller B (2001) Thalidomide in gastrointestinal disorders. *Drugs*. **61**: 777–787.
12 Govindarajan R *et al.* (2000) Effect of thalidomide on gastrointestinal toxic effects of irinotecan. *Lancet*. **356**: 566–567.
13 Deaner P (2000) The use of thalidomide in the management of severe sweating in patients with advanced malignancy: trial report. *Palliative Medicine*. **14**: 429–431.
14 Smith J *et al.* (2002) Use of thalidomide in the treatment of intractable itch. Poster abstract 21. In: *Palliative Care Congress*; Sheffield, UK.
15 Lowney AC *et al.* (2014) Thalidomide therapy for pruritus in the palliative setting –a distinct subset of patients in whom the benefit may outweigh the risk. *Journal of Pain and Symptom Management*. **48**: e3–5.
16 Goncalves F (2010) Thalidomide for the control of severe paraneoplastic pruritus associated with Hodgkin's disease. *American Journal of Hospice and Palliative Care*. **27**: 486–487.
17 Horton MR *et al.* (2012) Thalidomide for the treatment of cough in idiopathic pulmonary fibrosis: a randomized trial. *Annals of Internal Medicine*. **157**: 398–406.
18 Bramuzzo M *et al.* (2016) Thalidomide for inflammatory bowel disease: Systematic review. *Medicine*. **95**: e4239.
19 Gordon JN *et al.* (2005) Thalidomide in the treatment of cancer cachexia: a randomised placebo controlled trial. *Gut*. **54**: 540–545.
20 Davis M *et al.* (2012) A Phase II dose titration study of thalidomide for cancer-associated anorexia. *Journal of Pain and Symptom Management*. **43**: 78–86.
21 Reyes-Teran G *et al.* (1996) Effects of thalidomide on HIV-associated wasting syndrome: a randomized, double-blind, placebo-controlled clinical trial. *AIDS*. **10**: 1501–1507.
22 Reid J *et al.* (2012) Thalidomide for managing cancer cachexia. *Cochrane Database of Systematic Reviews*. **4**: CD008664. www.thecochranelibrary.com
23 Yennurajalingam S *et al.* (2012) The role of thalidomide and placebo for the treatment of cancer-related anorexia-cachexia symptoms: results of a double-blind placebo-controlled randomized study. *Journal of Palliative Medicine*. **15**: 1059–1064.
24 Wilkes EA *et al.* (2011) Poor tolerability of thalidomide in end-stage oesophageal cancer. *European Journal of Cancer Care (Engl)*. **20**: 593–600.
25 Song T *et al.* (2015) Involvement of peripheral TRPV1 channels in the analgesic effects of thalidomide. *Neurochemistry International*. **85-86**: 40–45.
26 Asher C and Furnish T (2013) Lenalidomide and thalidomide in the treatment of chronic pain. *Expert Opinion in Drug Safety*. **12**: 367–374.
27 Manning DC *et al.* (2014) Lenalidomide for complex regional pain syndrome type 1: lack of efficacy in a phase II randomized study. *Journal of Pain*. **15**: 1366–1376.
28 Engelen ET *et al.* (2015) Thalidomide for treatment of gastrointestinal bleedings due to angiodysplasia: a case report in acquired von Willebrand syndrome and review of the literature. *Haemophilia*. **21**: 419–429.
29 Craanen ME *et al.* (2006) Thalidomide in refractory haemorrhagic radiation induced proctitis. *Gut*. **55**: 1371–1372.
30 Karajeh MA *et al.* (2006) Refractory bleeding from portal hypertensive gastropathy: a further novel role for thalidomide therapy? *European Journal of Gastroenterology and Hepatology*. **18**: 545–548.
31 Lambert K and Ward J (2009) The use of thalidomide in the management of bleeding from a gastric cancer. *Palliative Medicine*. **23**: 473–475.
32 Franchini M *et al.* (2012) Novel treatments for epistaxis in hereditary hemorrhagic telangiectasia: a systematic review of the clinical experience with thalidomide. *Journal of Thrombosis and Thrombolysis*. **36**: 355–357.
33 Liang L *et al.* (2016) Efficacy of lenalidomide in relapsed/refractory chronic lymphocytic leukemia patient: a systematic review and meta-analysis. *Annals of Hematology*. **95**: 1473–1482.
34 Thomas D and Kantarjian H (2000) Current role of thalidomide in cancer treatment. *Current Opinion in Oncology*. **12**: 564–573.
35 Dimopoulos MA and Eleutherakis-Papaiakovou V (2004) Adverse effects of thalidomide administration in patients with neoplastic diseases. *American Journal of Medicine*. **117**: 508–515.
36 Mileshkin L *et al.* (2006) Development of neuropathy in patients with myeloma treated with thalidomide: patterns of occurrence and the role of electrophysiologic monitoring. *Journal of Clinical Oncology*. **24**: 4507–4514.
37 Wulff CH *et al.* (1985) Development of polyneuropathy during thalidomide therapy. *British Journal of Dermatology*. **112**: 475–480.
38 Fullerton P and O'Sullivan D (1968) Thalidomide neuropathy: a clinical, electrophysiological, and histological follow up study. *Journal of Neurology, Neurosurgery and Psychiatry*. **31**: 543–551.
39 Chapon F *et al.* (1985) [Neuropathies caused by thalidomide]. *Revue Neurologique (Paris)*. **141**: 719–728.
40 Gardner-Medwin J *et al.* (1994) Clinical experience with thalidomide in the management of severe oral and genital ulceration in conditions such as Behcet's disease. *Annals of Rheumatic Diseases*. **128**: 443–450.
41 Ochonisky S *et al.* (1994) Thalidomide neuropathy incidence and clinico-electrophysiologic findings in 42 patients. *Archives of Dermatology*. **130**: 66–69.
42 Grover JK *et al.* (2002) The adverse effects of thalidomide in relapsed and refractory patients of multiple myeloma. *Annals of Oncology*. **13**: 1636–1640.
43 Carrier M *et al.* (2011) Rates of venous thromboembolism in multiple myeloma patients undergoing immunomodulatory therapy with thalidomide or lenalidomide: a systematic review and meta-analysis. *Journal of Thrombosis and Haemostasis*. **9**: 653–663.
44 MHRA (2011) Thalidomide: risk of arterial and venous thromboembolism. *Drug safety update*. **(4) 12**: www.mhra.gov.uk/Safetyinformation

45 Palumbo A *et al.* (2011) Aspirin, warfarin, or enoxaparin thromboprophylaxis in patients with multiple myeloma treated with thalidomide: a phase III, open-label, randomized trial. *Journal of Clinical Oncology*. **29**: 986–993.
46 Bird JM *et al.* (2011) Guidelines for the diagnosis and management of multiple myeloma *British Journal of Haematology*. **154**: 32-75 www.bcshguidelines.com
47 Kaur A *et al.* (2003) Thalidomide-induced sinus bradycardia. *Annals of Pharmacotherapy*. **37**: 1040–1043.
48 Clark T *et al.* (2001) Thalidomid (Thalidomide) capsules: a review of the first 18 months of spontaneous postmarketing adverse event surveillance, including off-label prescribing. *Drug Safety*. **24**: 87–117.
49 Noormohamed F *et al.* (1999) Pharmacokinetics and hemodynamic effects of single oral doses of thalidomide in asymptomatic human immunodeficiency virus-infected subjects. *AIDS Research and Human Retroviruses*. **15**: 1047–1052.
50 Ng SS *et al.* (2002) Thalidomide, an antiangiogenic agent with clinical activity in cancer. *Biomedical and Pharmacology Journal*. **56**: 194–199.
51 Rajkumar SV *et al.* (2000) Life-threatening toxic epidermal necrolysis with thalidomide therapy for myeloma. *New England Journal of Medicine*. **343**: 972–973.
52 MHRA (2016) Thalidomide celgene: new important advice regarding viral reactivation and pulmonary hypertension. *Direct Healthcare Professional Communication*. www.gov.uk/drug-safety-update
53 Marriott J *et al.* (1997) A double-blind placebo-controlled phase II trial of thalidomide in asymptomatic HIV-positive patients: clinical tolerance and effect on activation markers and cytokines. *AIDS Research and Human Retroviruses*. **13**: 1625–1631.
54 Chanan-Khan A *et al.* (2005) Results of a phase 1 clinical trial of thalidomide in combination with fludarabine as initial therapy for patients with treatment-requiring chronic lymphocytic leukemia (CLL). *Blood*. **106**: 3348–3352.
55 MHRA (2013) Lenolidomide (Revlimid): risk of serious hepatic adverse drug reactions - routine monitoring of liver function now recommended. *Drug Safety Update*. **6**. www.mhra.gov.uk/Safetyinformation
56 MHRA (2011) Lenolidomide (Revlimid): risk of a second primary malignancy – update. *Drug Safety Update*. **5**. www.mhra.gov.uk/Safetyinformation
57 MHRA (2013) Thalidomide: risk of second primary malignancies. *Drug Safety Update*. **6**. www.mhra.gov.uk/Safetyinformation
58 Davis M and Dickerson E (2001) Thalidomide: dual benefits in palliative medicine and oncology. *American Journal of Hospice and Palliative Care*. **18**: 347–351.
59 Powell R and Gardner-Medwin J (1994) Guideline for the clinical use and dispensing of thalidomide. *Postgraduate Medical Journal*. **70**: 901–904.
60 Teo SK *et al.* (2001) Thalidomide is distributed into human semen after oral dosing. *Drug Metabolism and Disposition*. **29**: 1355–1357.
61 Jacobson J *et al.* (1997) Thalidomide for the treatment of oral aphthous ulcers in patients with human immunodeficiency virus infection. *New England Journal of Medicine*. **336**: 1487–1493.
62 Deaner P (1998) Thalidomide for distressing night sweats in advanced malignant disease. *Palliative Medicine*. **12**: 208–209.
63 Calder K and Bruera E (2000) Thalidomide for night sweats in patients with advanced cancer. *Palliative Medicine*. **14**: 77–78.
64 Govindarajan R (2000) Irinotecan and thalidomide in metastatic colorectal cancer. *Oncology (Williston Park)*. **14 (Suppl 13)**: 29–32.

Updated (minor change) January 2020

8: URINARY TRACT DISORDERS

8

TAMSULOSIN

Class: Uroselective α_1-adrenergic receptor antagonist (α_1 antagonist).

Indications: Symptoms associated with benign prostatic obstruction (BPO), †radiation-induced urethritis, †before trial without catheter inserted for acute urinary retention in men,[1] †medical management of urinary stones (5–10mm).[2]

Contra-indications: Symptomatic postural hypotension, severe hepatic impairment.

Pharmacology

Tamsulosin is a selective competitive antagonist at post-synaptic α_{1A}- and α_{1D}-adrenergic receptors, causing smooth muscle relaxation in the prostate gland, bladder neck, and possibly the detrusor (i.e. the bladder itself).[3,4]

In BPO, smooth muscle hyperplasia is estimated to be responsible for nearly half of the obstructive component. Tamsulosin is prescribed for men with moderate–severe voiding lower urinary tract symptoms (LUTS) (e.g. urinary hesitancy, poor urinary stream, incomplete bladder emptying, terminal dribble) and a moderately enlarged prostate gland (<30g). Tamsulosin reduces functional prostatic obstruction and increases maximum urinary flow rate. RCTs show that tamsulosin improves voiding LUTS by 30–45% compared to 10–30% for placebo. Symptoms generally improve within a few days, with a full response by 6 weeks. However, α_1 antagonists do not prevent acute urinary retention or the need for prostate surgery.[5]

Other selective α_{1A} antagonists, e.g. **alfuzosin**, **silodosin**, have similar symptomatic and urodynamic efficacy to tamsulosin. The use of non-selective α_1 antagonists, e.g. **doxazosin**, should generally be avoided because they have a higher risk of vascular-related undesirable effects, e.g. postural hypotension, when given alone or with antihypertensive drugs.[6,7] However, even with tamsulosin there is a small risk of postural hypotension, which may explain the association with an increased risk of falls and fractures in men >65 years.[8,9] Although the risk of postural hypotension is lower with **silodosin** compared with tamsulosin, there is an increased risk of sexual dysfunction, e.g. reduced/absent ejaculation.[10]

For men with moderate–severe voiding LUTS, a greater degree of prostatic enlargement (>30g) or a PSA >1.4nanogram/mL (surrogate marker for a prostate gland >30g)[11] and at risk of progressive obstruction, a 5α-reductase inhibitor, e.g. **dutasteride** or **finasteride**, should be considered. However, symptoms generally take 3–6 months to improve.[11] Combined treatment with α_1 antagonist and a 5α-reductase inhibitor is more effective than either agent alone, but has higher incidence of undesirable effects than monotherapy, and generally is neither necessary nor appropriate in patients with a prognosis of only 2–3 months.[12]

Of men with voiding LUTS associated with BPO, 15% also have significant storage LUTS (e.g. frequency, urgency, incontinence). Because tamsulosin may relax bladder smooth muscle, it may reduce detrusor instability and storage LUTS. Thus, in men with both voiding and storage LUTS, tamsulosin should be prescribed first. However, if storage LUTS persist, consider adding a urinary antimuscarinic (p.611). This has not been demonstrated to increase the risk of acute urinary retention, particularly in men with a post-voiding residual volume of <250mL.[13,14]

Tamsulosin 400–800microgram/24h reduces external beam radiotherapy-induced LUTS (voiding, storage and mixed types) in patients with prostate cancer. When started at least 5 days before prostate radiation brachytherapy, tamsulosin also reduces short-term LUTS.[15]

Tamsulosin is metabolized in the liver, primarily by CYP2D6 and CYP3A4; <10% is excreted unchanged in the urine. Bio-availability varies with food (take at the same time each day with respect to meals) and with formulation (only m/r available in the UK).

Bio-availability 55–100%.

Onset of action 4–8h; maximum benefit 4–8 weeks.

Time to peak plasma concentration 4–6h.

Plasma halflife 9–15h.

Duration of action <24h.

Cautions

Severe renal impairment (not studied).

Drug interactions

Concurrent use with epidural **morphine**, **sildenafil** or other α_1 antagonist increases the risk of postural hypotension.

Tamsulosin is metabolized mainly by CYP2D6 and CYP3A4. Caution should be taken with concurrent use of drugs that inhibit or induce these enzymes, e.g. **erythromycin**, particularly in those who are poor CYP2D6 metabolizers (see Chapter 19, Table 8, p.790).

Undesirable effects

Very common (>10%): dizziness, orthostatic hypotension, ejaculatory impairment.

Common (<10%, >1%): headache, asthenia, drowsiness or insomnia, amblyopia, chest pain, rhinitis, sinusitis, pharyngitis, cough, bitter taste, nausea, abdominal discomfort, diarrhoea, back pain, reduced libido, impotence or erectile dysfunction.

Uncommon (<1%, >0.1%): syncope, palpitations, vomiting, constipation, rash, pruritus, gynaecomastia.

Very rare (<0.01%, >0.001%): priapism.

Dose and use

Hesitancy of micturition

- tamsulosin 400microgram m/r PO once daily (because absorption is significantly affected by food, take at the same time each day with respect to meals)
- if necessary, increase to 800microgram m/r once daily after 2–4 weeks.[3]

†Before trial without catheter in men with acute retention

- tamsulosin 400microgram m/r PO once daily for 1–3 days before catheter removal.

Supply

Tamsulosin (generic)

Capsules m/r 400microgram, 28 days @ 400microgram once daily = £1.25.

Tablets m/r 400microgram, 28 days @ 400microgram once daily = £8.25.

Note. Tamsulosin 400microgram m/r capsules are available OTC for the treatment of functional symptoms of benign prostatic hyperplasia in men aged 45–75 years, to be taken for <6 weeks.

1 Fisher E *et al.* (2014) The role of alpha blockers prior to removal of urethral catheter for acute urinary retention in men. *Cochrane Database of Systematic Reviews*. **6**: CD006744. www.thecochranelibrary.com

2 Campschroer T *et al.* (2018) Alpha-blockers as medical expulsive therapy for ureteral stones. *Cochrane Database of Systematic Reviews*. **4**: CD008509. www.thecochranelibrary.com

3 Lyseng-Williamson KA *et al.* (2002) Tamsulosin: an update of its role in the management of lower urinary tract symptoms. *Drugs*. **62**: 135–167.

4 Yamada S *et al.* (2011) Alpha1-adrenoceptors and muscarinic receptors in voiding function - binding characteristics of therapeutic agents in relation to the pharmacokinetics. *British Journal of Clinical Pharmacology*. **72**: 205–217.

5 Djavan B *et al.* (2004) State of the art on the efficacy and tolerability of alpha1-adrenoceptor antagonists in patients with lower urinary tract symptoms suggestive of benign prostatic hyperplasia. *Urology*. **64**: 1081–1088.

6 Nickel JC *et al.* (2008) A meta-analysis of the vascular-related safety profile and efficacy of alpha-adrenergic blockers for symptoms related to benign prostatic hyperplasia. *International Journal of Clinical Practice*. **62**: 1547–1559.
7 Lowe FC (1997) Coadministration of tamsulosin and three antihypertensive agents in patients with benign prostatic hyperplasia: pharmacodynamic effect. *Clinical Therapeutics*. **19**: 730–742.
8 Welk B *et al.* (2015) The risk of fall and fracture with the initiation of a prostate-selective α antagonist: a population based cohort study. *British Medical Journal*. **351**: h5398.
9 Bird ST *et al.* (2013) Tamsulosin treatment for benign prostatic hyperplasia and risk of severe hypotension in men aged 40-85 years in the united states: risk window analyses using between and within patient methodology. *British Medical Journal*. **347**: f6320.
10 Jung JH *et al.* (2017) Silodosin for the treatment of lower urinary tract symptoms in men with benign prostatic hyperplasia. *Cochrane Database of Systematic Reviews*. **11**: CD012615. www.thecochranelibrary.com
11 NICE (2010) Lower urinary tract symptoms. The managment of lower urinary tract symptoms in men. *Clinical Guideline* **CG97**. www.nice.org.uk
12 Roehrborn CG *et al.* (2010) The effects of combination therapy with dutasteride and tamsulosin on clinical outcomes in men with symptomatic benign prostatic hyperplasia: 4-year results from the combat study. *European Urology*. **57**: 123–131.
13 Sarma AV and Wei JT (2012) Clinical practice. Benign prostatic hyperplasia and lower urinary tract symptoms. *New England Journal of Medicine*. **367**: 248–257.
14 Gravas S *et al.* (2017) European association of urology guideline: management of non-neurogenic male LUTS. www.uroweb.org/guidelines (Accessed September 2018).
15 Crawford ED and Kavanagh BD (2006) The role of alpha-blockers in the management of lower urinary tract symptoms in prostate cancer patients treated with radiation therapy. *American Journal of Clinical Oncology*. **29**: 517–523.

Updated (minor change) September 2021

URINARY ANTIMUSCARINICS

Class: Antimuscarinic (anticholinergic).

Indications: Symptoms of an overactive bladder: urgency (with or without urge incontinence), frequency (>8 times/day) and/or nocturia (waking more than once at night to void);[1] †bladder spasm.

Contra-indications: Bladder outflow obstruction, GI obstruction including paralytic ileus, severe ulcerative colitis, predisposition to narrow-angle glaucoma, myasthenia gravis. ***Darifenacin:*** severe hepatic impairment, *potent* inhibitors of CYP3A4 (see Drug interactions).

Pharmacology

Bladder muscle (detrusor) contains all subtypes of muscarinic receptor. M_2 and M_3 predominate, with M_2 outnumbering M_3 3:1. M_3 receptors are particularly important in relation to detrusor contraction; the function of M_2 receptors is less clear.

Oxybutynin hydrochloride has an antimuscarinic effect on bladder innervation. It is relatively selective for M_1 and M_3 receptor subtypes (see Antimuscarinics, p.4). It also has a direct papaverine-like antispasmodic effect on the detrusor.[2] It inhibits bladder contraction, relieves spasm induced by various stimuli, increases bladder capacity, and delays the desire to void in patients with a neurogenic bladder. **Oxybutynin** also has a topical anaesthetic effect on the bladder mucosa.[3] Newer antimuscarinics, e.g. **darifenacin**, **fesoterodine**, **solifenacin**, **trospium**, have higher M_3 receptor selectivity than older ones, e.g. **oxybutynin**, **tolterodine**.[4]

Oxybutynin (a tertiary amine) enters the CNS relatively easily, whereas **trospium** (a quaternary ammonium compound) does not. The M_1 receptor plays a significant role in modulating cognitive function, and centrally acting antimuscarinics with significant affinity for the M_1 receptor (e.g. **oxybutynin**) may cause cognitive impairment, delirium. The rate of cognitive decline increases with duration of antimuscarinic use.[5] Thus, it is recommended that cognitive function is monitored particularly in frail, elderly patients receiving such antimuscarinics. In theory, **trospium** and newer antimuscarinics that are more M_3-selective (e.g. **darifenacin**, **solifenacin**) should have fewer undesirable CNS effects.[6,7] However, in the RCTs that have specifically examined this, although **darifenacin** and **solifenacin** cause less cognitive dysfunction than **oxybutynin**, the difference is small.[8,9] Thus, when cognitive impairment or antimuscarinic burden are of particular concern, consider prescribing **trospium**[10] or **mirabegron**, a β_3 agonist, instead (Box A).[11]

Urinary antimuscarinics reduce frequency by 15–20% (vs. 10% with placebo), leakage episodes by 45–75% (vs. 20–45%) and urgency by 40% (vs. 35%), and have subjective improvement rates of 40–70% (vs. 20–50%).[12] The absolute probability of continence after 4 weeks of treatment is

15–30%. However, because of undesirable effects ± lack of benefit, ≤75% of patients discontinue treatment within 12 weeks.[11,13,14] For alternative drugs for the treatment of overactive bladder, nocturia or painful bladder spasm, see Box B and Box C.

Although there is some evidence suggesting that m/r formulations and higher doses of some newer drugs (e.g. **fesoterodine**, **solifenacin**) have greater efficacy than **oxybutynin**,[1] this is not reflected in recent systematic reviews and guidelines. Once daily m/r and TD formulations are better tolerated than immediate-release formulations, with immediate-release **oxybutynin** least well tolerated.[11,14]

Darifenacin, **oxybutynin**, **tolterodine** and **trospium** are all highly protein-bound and, except for **trospium**, are extensively hepatically metabolized via CYP450 enzyme pathways (Table 1). Active metabolites are produced for **tolterodine** (5-hydroxymethyl derivative; equipotent with **tolterodine**) and **oxybutynin** (N-desethyloxybutyin; uncertain clinical significance). Dose adjustment in renal and/or hepatic impairment may be necessary (see Dose and use).

Table 1 Pharmacokinetics of selected urinary antimuscarinics[15]

Drug	*Bio-availability PO (%)*	*T_{max} (h)*	*Plasma halflife (h)*	*Metabolism*
Darifenacin	15–20 (m/r)	7h (m/r)	13–19	CYP2D6 and CYP3A4
Oxybutynin	2–11[a]	0.5–1; 4–6h (m/r) 24–48h (TD)	2–3[b] 12–14 (m/r)	CYP3A4
Tolterodine	17[c]	1–3	2–3[c]	CYP2D6[d]
Trospium	10[e]	4–6	10–20 39 (m/r)	Renal excretion, largely unchanged[f]

a. immediate-release; increased by 50% with m/r tablets (with a corresponding reduction in the amount of active metabolite)
b. 4–5h in the elderly; lower doses can be given
c. bio-availability 65% and halflife 10h in poor metabolizers; however, this is *not* clinically significant because of the differences in protein-binding characteristics of tolterodine and the 5-hydroxymethyl active metabolite
d. active metabolite 5-hydroxymethyl derivative (equipotent with tolterodine); in poor metabolizers, the major metabolic pathway for tolterodine is via CYP3A4, to an inactive metabolite
e. immediate-release; reduced by ≤33% with m/r capsules; food further reduces bio-availability by ≤85%
f. in severe renal impairment, halflife and C_{max} can increase 2-fold and exposure (AUC) can increase 4-fold.

Cautions

See Antimuscarinics, p.4. Renal and hepatic impairment (see Dose and use), Parkinson's disease. ***Tolterodine:*** patients with risk factors for QT prolongation (see Chapter 20, p.797).

Drug interactions

Concurrent treatment with ≥2 antimuscarinic drugs (including antihistamines, phenothiazines and TCAs; see Antimuscarinics, Box B, p.4) will increase the likelihood of undesirable effects, and (when centrally acting) of central toxicity, e.g. restlessness, agitation, delirium (see Antimuscarinics, Box C, p.5). Children, the elderly, and patients with renal or hepatic impairment are more susceptible to the central effects of antimuscarinics.

For a full list of the relevant moderate/potent CYP450 inhibitors and inducers, also see Chapter 19, Table 8, p.790.

Oxybutynin

Concurrent use of drugs that are potent/moderate inhibitors of CYP3A4 (e.g. **clarithromycin**, **erythromycin**, **fluconazole**, **itraconazole**) could potentially cause toxicity, and necessitate a reduction in the dose of **oxybutynin**.

Darifenacin

Although the concurrent use of a potent CYP3A4 inhibitor (e.g. **clarithromycin**, **itraconazole**) is contra-indicated in the UK, it is permitted in the USA if the maximum **darifenacin** daily dose is limited to 7.5mg. Moderate CYP3A4 inhibitors (e.g. **erythromycin**, **fluconazole**) and potent inhibitors of CYP2D6 (e.g. **fluoxetine**, **paroxetine**) can also increase the overall exposure to **darifenacin**.

Darifenacin is a moderate inhibitor of CYP2D6 and may cause toxicity of drugs metabolized by CYP2D6 that have narrow therapeutic windows (e.g. **flecainide**, TCAs).

Tolterodine

Although **tolterodine** is metabolized by CYP2D6, potent inhibitors (e.g. **fluoxetine**, **paroxetine**) do *not* result in clinically significant interactions, as the active metabolite is equipotent with the parent drug. However, in CYP2D6 poor metabolizers, the main metabolic pathway is via CYP3A4, and potent CYP3A4 inhibitors increase the overall exposure to **tolterodine** (2-fold increase in exposure).[16] Because metabolizer status is rarely known, the concurrent use of a potent CYP3A4 inhibitor (e.g. **clarithromycin**, **itraconazole**) is not recommended in the UK; it is permitted in the USA if the dose of **tolterodine** is limited to 1mg b.d. or 2mg once daily for m/r formulations.

8

Trospium

Clinically significant pharmacokinetic interactions are unlikely. However, caution is advised with concurrent use of bile acid sequestrants (e.g. **colestipol**, **colestyramine**).

Undesirable effects

Antimuscarinic effects are common, including dry mouth, cognitive impairment and delirium, particularly in the frail and elderly (see Antimuscarinics, Box C, p.5); nausea and abdominal discomfort. Skin reactions are common with TD **oxybutynin**.

Dose and use

For the treatment of overactive bladder, recommended first-line drugs are:

- immediate-release **oxybutynin** because of the low cost of generic drug (but *not* in the frail elderly) *or*
- immediate-release **tolterodine** *or*
- **darifenacin** (a once daily m/r product).[14,17]

It may take 4 weeks to see the full response to treatment, thus the antimuscarinic should be reviewed after that and then every 6 months to determine whether it is still needed.[18] If ineffective, consider an alternative first-line treatment above, **fesoterodine** or **solifenacin**.

In patients with cognitive impairment, consider **trospium** or **mirabegron** (Box A). For alternative drugs for the treatment of overactive bladder, nocturia or painful bladder spasm, see Box B and Box C.

Note. In men, lower urinary tract symptoms (LUTS) most commonly relate to voiding difficulties associated with benign prostatic obstruction (BPO), and this requires a different approach (see **Tamsulosin**, p.609). **Tamsulosin** should also be used in men with both voiding and storage LUTS (e.g. frequency, urgency, incontinence). An antimuscarinic should only be used first-line for men with moderate–severe LUTS who have mainly overactive bladder/storage symptoms. However, an antimuscarinic should *not* be used in men with a post-void residual volume >150mL.[19,20]

Oxybutynin

- start with immediate-release **oxybutynin** 5mg PO b.d.
- if necessary, increase progressively to 5mg q.d.s.
- in patients >60 years or with renal or hepatic impairment, these doses should be halved
- if not tolerated, consider m/r or TD **oxybutynin** (more-expensive options; see Supply).

Do *not* use in patients >60 years at risk of a rapid deterioration in physical or mental health; consider m/r or TD **oxybutynin** or an alternative urinary antimuscarinic.[14]

Tolterodine

- usual dose is immediate-release **tolterodine** 2mg PO b.d.
- for patients with hepatic impairment, severe renal impairment or receiving concurrent treatment with a potent CYP3A4 inhibitor (see Drug interactions), the maximum dose is 1mg b.d.

If not tolerated, consider m/r (more expensive; see Supply).

Darifenacin

- start with **darifenacin** 7.5mg m/r PO once daily; this is the maximum dose in patients with moderate hepatic impairment (contra-indicated in severe hepatic impairment)
- if necessary, increase after 2 weeks to 15mg once daily; monitor closely for toxicity in patients receiving concurrent treatment with potent CYP2D6 and moderate CYP3A4 inhibitors (see Drug interactions).

Trospium

- immediate-release **trospium** 20mg PO b.d., on an empty stomach
- if not tolerated, consider m/r 60mg PO once daily, on an empty stomach (more expensive; see Supply)
- for patients with severe renal impairment or ESRF, use the immediate-release tablets and reduce the dose to 20mg once daily or on alternate days.

Box A Mirabegron

Indications: Overactive bladder and/or nocturia when an antimuscarinic is contra-indicated, poorly tolerated or ineffective.[21]

Contra-indications: Severe uncontrolled hypertension (systolic BP≥180mmHg and/or diastolic BP≥110mmHg).

Pharmacology

Mirabegron is a potent selective β_3 agonist. It increases bladder relaxation, increasing urinary storage, and reduces bladder contractions compared with placebo. It is probably as effective as an antimuscarinic but causes less dry mouth, is better tolerated, and may be safer in the frail elderly.[22] However, further studies lasting >3 months and with direct comparison to antimuscarinics are awaited.[10,11,21,23]
Bio-availability 29–35% (dose dependent).
Time to peak plasma concentration 3–4h.
Plasma halflife 50h.
Duration of action No data.

Cautions

Renal or hepatic impairment (see Dose and use). Hypertension (monitor blood pressure); use of uroselective antimuscarinics in patients with bladder outlet obstruction (risk of urinary retention). Patients with risk factors for QT prolongation (see Chapter 20, p.797).

Drug interactions

Mirabegron is metabolized and transported through multiple pathways. However, dose adjustment of mirabegron is *not* needed unless the patient is concomitantly receiving a potent CYP3A inhibitor in the presence of renal or hepatic impairment (see Dose and use).

Mirabegron is a moderate inhibitor of CYP2D6; caution should be taken with concurrent drugs that are metabolized by this enzyme and have a narrow therapeutic index, e.g. flecainide.

Undesirable effects (for full list see SPC)

Common (<10%, >1%) headache, dizziness, tachycardia, nausea, constipation, diarrhoea.
Uncommon (<1%, >0.1%) palpitations, atrial fibrillation, dyspepsia, gastritis, joint swelling.
Rare (<0.1%, >0.01%) urinary retention.

Dose and use

- mirabegron 50mg m/r PO once daily; adjust the dose in renal and hepatic impairment.

Renal impairment

- mild or moderate renal impairment *and* also taking concurrent potent CYP3A inhibitors (e.g. clarithromycin, itraconazole, ketoconazole): give 25mg m/r once daily
- severe renal impairment or ESRF: give 25mg m/r once daily; avoid in patients taking potent CYP3A inhibitors.

continued

Box A Continued

Hepatic impairment

- mild hepatic impairment *and* also taking concurrent potent CYP3A inhibitors: give 25 mg m/r once daily
- moderate hepatic impairment: give 25mg m/r once daily; avoid in patients taking potent CYP3A inhibitors
- severe hepatic impairment: not recommended (no information).

Although more expensive than urinary antimuscarinics, mirabegron is still considered cost-effective.[24,25] Combining mirabegron with a urinary antimuscarinic improves symptoms further without additional undesirable effects.[26]

Box B Alternative drugs for overactive bladder and/or nocturia

When a less-selective antimuscarinic is necessary for concurrent symptoms, consider:

- amitriptyline 10mg PO at night (see p.228)
- hyoscine *hydrobromide* 300microgram SL b.d.–q.d.s. (e.g. Kwells®).

For persistent nocturia (once other medical causes excluded), consider:

- a loop diuretic, e.g. furosemide 40mg PO once daily around 1700–1800h
- a vasopressin analogue, e.g. desmopressin (p.572), although hyponatraemia is a possible complication.[14,17]

For postmenopausal women with urinary incontinence and vulvovaginal atrophy, consider short-term topical intravaginal oestrogen.[27]

Box C Alternative drugs for painful bladder spasm

For painful bladder spasm despite an optimal dose of a uroselective antimuscarinic, consider switching to:

- amitriptyline 10mg PO at night (see p.228)
- hyoscine *hydrobromide* 300microgram SL b.d.–q.d.s. (e.g. Kwells®)
- hyoscine *butylbromide* 60–120mg/24h CSCI and 20mg SC p.r.n. (see p.15).

If the above are inadequate, consider intravesical treatments:

- morphine (10–20mg t.d.s. or diamorphine 10mg t.d.s. diluted in sodium chloride 0.9% to 20mL); instil through an indwelling catheter and clamp for 30min[28]
- bupivacaine t.d.s. (0.5% bupivacaine 10mL diluted in sodium chloride 0.9% to 20mL) used alone or with intravesical morphine.[29,30]

Supply

Oxybutynin (generic)

Tablets 2.5mg, 3mg, 5mg, 28 days @ 5mg b.d. = £2.
Oral solution 2.5mg/5mL, 5mg/5mL, 28 days @ 5mg b.d. = £372.

Modified-release products
Lyrinel® XL (Janssen-Cilag)
Tablets m/r 5mg, 10mg, 28 days @ 10mg once daily = £28.

Transdermal products
Kentera® (Orion)
TD patches 36mg (releasing 3.9mg/24h), 28 days @ 1 patch twice weekly = £27.

Tolterodine (generic)
Tablets 1mg, 2mg, 28 days @ 2mg b.d. = £1.75.
Capsules m/r 4mg, 28 days @ 4mg once daily = £7.

Darifenacin
Emselex® (Aspire Pharma)
Tablets m/r 7.5mg, 15mg, 28 days @ 7.5mg once daily = £25.

Trospium (generic)
Tablets 20mg, 28 days @ 20mg b.d. = £4.

Regurin® XL (Mylan)
Capsules m/r 60mg, 28 days @ 60mg once daily = £23.

Mirabegron
Betmiga® (Astellas)
Tablets m/r 25mg, 50mg, 28 days @ 50mg once daily = £27.

1 Madhuvrata P *et al.* (2012) Which anticholinergic drug for overactive bladder symptoms in adults. *Cochrane Database of Systematic Reviews.* **1**: CD005429. www.cochranelibrary.com.
2 Andersson KE (2011) Antimuscarinic mechanisms and the overactive detrusor: an update. *European Urology.* **59**: 377–386.
3 Robinson T and Castleden C (1994) Drugs in focus: 11. Oxybutynin hydrochloride. *Prescribers' Journal.* **34**: 27–30.
4 Abrams P *et al.* (2006) Muscarinic receptors: their distribution and function in body systems, and the implications for treating overactive bladder. *British Journal of Pharmacology.* **148**: 565–578.
5 Risacher SL *et al.* (2016) Association between anticholinergic medication use and cognition, brain metabolism, and brain atrophy in cognitively normal older adults. *JAMA Neurology.* **73**: 721–732.
6 Callegari E *et al.* (2011) A comprehensive non-clinical evaluation of the CNS penetration potential of antimuscarinic agents for the treatment of overactive bladder. *British Journal of Clinical Pharmacology.* **72**: 235–246.
7 Pagoria D *et al.* (2011) Antimuscarinic drugs: review of the cognitive impact when used to treat overactive bladder in elderly patients. *Current Urology Reports.* **12**: 351–357.
8 Wagg A *et al.* (2013) Randomised, multicentre, placebo-controlled, double-blind crossover study investigating the effect of solifenacin and oxybutynin in elderly people with mild cognitive impairment: the SENIOR study. *European Urology.* **64**: 74–81.
9 Kay G *et al.* (2006) Differential effects of the antimuscarinic agents darifenacin and oxybutynin ER on memory in older subjects. *European Urology.* **50**: 317–326.
10 Araklitis G *et al.* (2020) Cognitive effects of anticholinergic load in women with overactive bladder. *Clinical interventions in aging.* **15**: 1493–1503.
11 Harding CK *et al.* (2021) EAU guidelines on management of non-neurogenic female lower urinary tract symptoms (LUTS). www.uroweb.org/guidelines (accessed October 2021).
12 Novara G *et al.* (2008) A systematic review and meta-analysis of randomized controlled trials with antimuscarinic drugs for overactive bladder. *European Urology.* **54**: 740–763.
13 Buser N *et al.* (2012) Efficacy and adverse events of antimuscarinics for treating overactive bladder: network meta-analyses. *European Urology.* **62**: 1040–1060.
14 NICE (2019) Urinary incontinence and pelvic organ prolapse in women: management. **NG123**. www.nice.org.uk.
15 Gupta SK and Sathyan G (1999) Pharmacokinetics of an oral once-a-day controlled-release oxybutynin formulation compared with immediate-release oxybutynin. *Journal of Clinical Pharmacology.* **39**: 289–296.
16 Brynne N *et al.* (1999) Ketoconazole inhibits the metabolism of tolterodine in subjects with deficient CYP2D6 activity. *British Journal of Clinical Pharmacology.* **48**: 564–572.
17 NICE (2015) The management of lower urinary tract symptoms in men. *Clinical Guideline.* **CG97**. www.nice.org.uk.
18 Marinkovic SP *et al.* (2012) The management of overactive bladder syndrome. *British Medical Journal.* **344**: e2365.
19 Kaplan SA *et al.* (2010) Solifenacin treatment in men with overactive bladder: effects on symptoms and patient-reported outcomes. *Aging Male.* **13**: 100–107.
20 Gravas S *et al.* (2017) EAU guidelines on management of non-neurogenic male lower urinary tract symptoms (LUTS), incl. benign prostatic obstruction (BPO). www.uroweb.org/guidelines (accessed October 2021).
21 NICE (2013) Mirabegron for treating symptoms of overactive bladder. *Technology Appraisal* 290. www.nice.org.uk.
22 Chapple CR *et al.* (2013) Randomized double-blind, active-controlled phase 3 study to assess 12-month safety and efficacy of mirabegron, a beta(3)-adrenoceptor agonist, in overactive bladder. *European Urology.* **63**: 296–305.
23 Deeks E (2018) Mirabegron: A Review in Overactive Bladder Syndrome. *Drugs.* **78**: 833–844.
24 Aballéa S *et al.* (2015) Cost effectiveness of mirabegron compared with tolterodine extended release for the treatment of adults with overactive bladder in the United Kingdom. *Clinical Drug Investigation.* **35**: 83–93.
25 Nazir J *et al.* (2015) Cost-effectiveness of mirabegron compared with antimuscarinic agents for the treatment of adults with overactive bladder in the United Kingdom. *Value in Health.* **18**: 783–790.
26 Beder D *et al.* (2021) Overactive bladder in women. *British Medical Journal.* **375**: e063526.
27 Cody JD *et al.* (2012) Oestrogen therapy for urinary incontinence in post-menopausal women. *Cochrane Database of Systematic Reviews.* **10**: CD001405. www.cochranelibrary.com.
28 McCoubrie R and Jeffrey D (2003) Intravesical diamorphine for bladder spasm. *Journal of Pain and Symptom Management.* **25**: 1–3.
29 Chiang D *et al.* (2005) Management of post-operative bladder spasm. *Journal of Paediatrics and Child Health.* **41**: 56–58.
30 Hanno PM *et al.* (2014) Diagnosis and treatment of interstitial cystitis/bladder pain syndrome: American Urological Association Guideline. www.auanet.org (Accessed March 2018).

Updated January 2022

METHENAMINE HIPPURATE

Class: Urinary antiseptic.

Indications: Prophylaxis and long-term treatment of chronic or recurrent uncomplicated lower UTI in patients with or without catheters.

Contra-indications: Severe renal impairment (creatinine clearance <10mL/min; eGFR <10mL/min/1.73m^2), infection of the *upper* urinary tract (pyelonephritis), metabolic acidosis, hepatic impairment, severe dehydration, or gout; concurrent administration with sulfonamides or alkalizing agents (see Drug interactions).

Pharmacology

Unlike most antibacterials, methenamine hippurate does *not* act by impairing bacterial protein synthesis. In an acid environment (pH <5.5), methenamine hippurate dissociates into methenamine and hippuric acid. Methenamine is converted to formaldehyde, which is responsible for the bactericidal effect.[1] Most bacteria are sensitive to formaldehyde at concentrations of ≥20microgram/mL, and acquired resistance does not appear to develop.

Urea-splitting bacteria, e.g. *Pseudomonas aeruginosa*, produce ammonia, which increases the alkalinity of urine. This could inhibit the formation of formaldehyde, and thereby reduce the effect of methenamine. However, hippuric acid helps maintain an acidic environment.

8

Prophylaxis against UTI

Oral antibacterials are more effective than methenamine hippurate for prophylaxis. However, concern about acquired resistance with antibacterials has led to renewed interest in methenamine hippurate.[2] Nonetheless, current national guidelines do not recommend its use for prophylaxis against UTIs.[3]

In patients with a normal renal tract (e.g. patients without bladder stones or neuropathic bladder), methenamine hippurate may provide a small benefit with short- (<1 week) and long-term (>12 months) use.[4] In a retrospective study of 150 elderly patients with recurrent UTI and normal renal tracts (17% with catheters), methenamine taken for >1 year delayed time to first UTI from 3 to 11 months.[5]

However, trials have been conducted in disparate patient populations using variable doses and follow-up, making results difficult to generalize. As such, efficacy, indications, dose and length of treatment are unclear, and methenamine is not routinely recommended.[3]

Prophylaxis against catheter-associated UTI (CAUTI)

Bacterial colonization of indwelling catheters is common, occurring in ≤30% of patients catheterized for >7 days and almost 100% of those catheterized for >28 days. An intrinsic limitation of using urinary antiseptics to prevent CAUTI is that some urine-colonizing bacteria produce secretions that eventually thicken enough to form a protective biofilm attached to the catheter surface. This can embed both the bacteria and phosphate crystals in a matrix that is impervious to urinary antiseptics or acidifying catheter patency solutions.

In catheterized patients, methenamine hippurate may not remain in the bladder for sufficient time to be converted to formaldehyde and/or for any formaldehyde produced to be effective. Thus, intermittent clamping may increase the effectiveness of methenamine hippurate, although this has not been tested in an RCT. (Note. Catheter clamping should be avoided in patients with spinal cord compression above spinal cord level T7, because of the risk of autonomic dysreflexia.)

Long-term indwelling or intermittent self-catheterization

An RCT in people after spinal cord injury (some with indwelling urethral or suprapubic catheters, some using intermittent self-catheterization, and some reflex voiding) compared prophylactic methenamine hippurate with **cranberry juice** and placebo for 6 months or until first symptomatic UTI, and found that the incidence of symptomatic UTI was the same in all three groups.[6] Thus, routine use of urinary antiseptics in patients with long-term urethral catheters or who undergo regular intermittent catheterization is not recommended.[7,8]

Short-term catheterization following surgery

In an adequately powered RCT, methenamine hippurate given to patients following gynaecological surgery and catheterized for ≤3 days, and continued for 4 days after catheter removal, reduced the rate of CAUTI compared with placebo (3% vs. 14%).[9]

In a randomized blind non-inferiority trial following urogynaecological surgery, two doses of either methenamine hippurate (1g) or **ciprofloxacin** (500mg), starting at the time of catheter removal, resulted in similar rates of CAUTI (11% and 22% respectively required antibacterials;

p=0.16).[10] Thus, methenamine hippurate can be used to reduce the risk of CAUTI in patients catheterized for ≤7 days following surgery or instrumentation of the urinary tract.[11]

Bio-availability readily absorbed.
Onset of action >2h.
Plasma halflife 4h.
Duration of action no data.

Drug interactions

Methenamine hippurate should *not* be administered concurrently with:
- sulfonamides, because of the risk of crystalluria
- alkalizing agents, e.g. **acetazolamide, potassium** or **sodium citrate, sodium bicarbonate** (also present in some antacids), because of the need for an acidic urinary environment.

Undesirable effects

Uncommon (<1%, >0.1%): dyspepsia, nausea and vomiting, rash, pruritus. With chronic use, the formaldehyde produced from methenamine may irritate and inflame the bladder mucosa and lead to painful and frequent voiding, haematuria and proteinuria.

Dose and use

The optimum dose for a urinary antiseptic in patients with an indwelling catheter has not been determined. The recommended dose at some centres is methenamine hippurate 1g PO b.d.–t.d.s. The tablets may be crushed and taken with milk or fruit juice (see Chapter 28, Table 2, p.863). Some centres recommend urinary acidification with ascorbic acid or ammonium chloride.

Supply

Hiprex® (Meda)
Tablets 1g, 28 days @ 1g b.d. = £19.

1 Strom JJ and Jun H (1993) Effect of urine pH and ascorbic acid on the rate of conversion of methenamine to formaldehyde. *Biopharmaceutics and Drug Disposition.* **14**: 61–69.
2 Sihra N *et al.* (2018) Nonantibiotic prevention and management of recurrent urinary tract infection. *Nature Reviews Urology.* **15**: 750–776.
3 NICE (2018) Urinary Tract infection (recurrent): antimicrobial prescribing. *NICE Guideline* ***NG112***. www.nice.org.uk.
4 Lee BS *et al.* (2012) Methenamine hippurate for preventing urinary tract infections. *Cochrane Database of Systematic Reviews.* **10**: CD003265. www.thecochranelibrary.com.
5 Snellings M *et al.* (2020) Effectiveness of methenamine for UTI prevention in older adults. *Annals of Pharmacotherapy.* **54**: 359–363.
6 Lee BB *et al.* (2007) Spinal-injured neuropathic bladder antisepsis (SINBA) trial. *Spinal Cord.* **45**: 542–550.
7 Blok B *et al.* (2020) Neuro-urology. *European Association of Urology Guidelines*. www.uroweb.org. (Accessed March 2021).
8 NICE (2018) Urinary tract infection (catheter-associated): antimicrobial prescribing. *NICE guideline* ***NG113***. www.nice.org.uk.
9 Schiotz HA and Guttu K (2002) Value of urinary prophylaxis with methenamine in gynecologic surgery. *Acta Obstetricia Gynecologica Scandinavica.* **81**: 743–746.
10 Chu CM (2016) Methenamine hippurate versus ciprofloxacin to prevent postoperative urinary tract infection: results of a randomized controlled trial. *Female Pelvic Medicine and Reconstructive Surgery.* **22 (Suppl 1)**: S2–S3.
11 Chwa A *et al.* (2019) Evaluation of methenamine for urinary tract infection prevention in older adults: a review of the evidence. *Therapeutic Advances in Drug Safety.* **10**: 1–9.

Updated June 2021

CATHETER PATENCY SOLUTIONS

Indications: Catheter blockage.

General considerations

Catheters can block because of blood clots, bladder mucosal debris, small calculi and/or phosphate encrustations on the surface of an indwelling catheter. Encrustations are associated with colonization of the urine by urease-producing bacteria, e.g. *Proteus mirabilis*, *Pseudomonas aeruginosa* and *Klebsiella*. Urease breaks down urea to form ammonia, increasing the alkalinity of the urine and leading to the deposition of mainly phosphate crystals on the surface of the catheter.

Some bacteria produce secretions which eventually thicken enough to form a protective biofilm attached to the catheter surface. This can embed both bacteria and phosphate crystals in a matrix which is impervious to acidifying solutions or urinary antiseptics. Thus, repeated blockage with encrustation generally means that the catheter needs to be changed.[1,2]

The main purpose of a catheter patency solution is to reduce the frequency of catheter blockage. Although a Cochrane review found insufficient evidence to make firm recommendations,[3] the *BNF* states that **sodium chloride** 0.9% is generally adequate as a mechanical flush for removing mucosal debris or small blood clots, and that solutions containing **citric acid** 3% (e.g. **solution G**) may be helpful in dissolving retained blood clots.

In a palliativedrugs.com survey, **sodium chloride** 0.9% was most commonly used for both flushing out cell debris or blood clots (75% of respondents) and treating or preventing encrustation (>50%). **Solution G** was next most popular for these indications (<10% and 20–25% respectively). Few respondents used other solutions.[4]

Irrigation does *not* cure catheter-associated urinary tract infection (CAUTI).[5,6] Although the *BNF* states that **chlorhexidine** 0.02% irrigation can be used in the management of common bladder infections, it is ineffective against most *Pseudomonas* species, and may irritate the bladder mucosa and cause a burning sensation or haematuria.

Use of irrigations or prophylactic antibacterials to prevent CAUTI is *not* recommended by NICE or current European nursing guidelines.[7,8] Consideration can be given to the use of a PO urinary antiseptic to acidify the urine and to reduce the risk of CAUTI in patients catheterized for ≤7 days following surgery or instrumentation of the urinary tract (see **Methenamine hippurate**, p.616).

8

Dose and use

To reduce the likelihood of encrustations causing a blockage, latex catheters should be changed:
- uncoated: every 2 weeks
- Teflon-coated: every 4 weeks
- silicone-coated or hydrogel-coated: ≤6 weeks, depending on manufacturer's instructions.[8]

If the catheter is to be left for longer periods, a silicone catheter should be used with a catheter patency solution. These catheters are designed to remain in place for ≤3 months.[8]

Some patients are more prone to recurrent encrustation than others. If encrustations regularly cause blockage, keep a diary over ≥3 recatheterizations, calculate the average time for which a catheter remains patent, then schedule a catheter change before a blockage is likely.[2,7]

For flushing out blockages caused by mucosal debris or small blood clots:
- start with **sodium chloride** 0.9% p.r.n.
- if necessary, use routinely every few days or even every day[4]
- if this is inadequate for dissolving retained clots, change to **solution G**.

For prevention of phosphate encrustations or calculi:[1,4]
- start with **sodium chloride** 0.9% p.r.n. or **solution G** once or twice a week
- if necessary, increase frequency.

Commercially available sachets are preferable to using a bladder syringe, because they are less likely to force encrusted material (which contains bacteria) higher up the urinary tract.

Supply

Sodium chloride 0.9%

Sachet 50mL, 100mL = £3.50.

Brands include OptiFlo S®, Uro-Tainer sodium chloride®, Uriflex S®.

Solution G containing **citric acid** 3.23% with magnesium oxide, sodium bicarbonate and disodium edetate

Sachet 50mL, 100mL = £3.50 for both sizes.

Brands include OptiFlo G®, Uriflex G®, Uro-Tainer Suby G®.

1 Williams C and Tonkin S (2003) Blocked urinary catheters: solutions are not the only solution. *British Journal of Community Nursing*. **8**: 321–326.
2 Getliffe K (2002) Managing recurrent urinary catheter encrustation. *British Journal of Community Nursing*. **7**: 574, 576, 578–580.
3 Shepherd AJ *et al.* (2017) Washout policies in long-term indwelling urinary catheterisation in adults (review). *Cochrane Database Systematic Reviews*. **3**: CD004012. www.thecochranelibrary.com

4 Palliativedrugs.com Ltd. Urinary catheter patency solutions – do you use them? *Latest additions: Survey results (December 2010)*. www.palliativedrugs.com
5 Getliffe K (1996) Bladder instillations and bladder washouts in the management of catheterized patients. *Journal of Advanced Nursing*. **23**: 548–554.
6 Pomfret I *et al.* (2004) Using bladder instillations to manage indwelling catheters. *British journal of Nursing*. **13**: 261–267.
7 NICE (2017) Infection control. Prevention of healthcare-associated infections in primary and community care. *Clinical Guideline*. CG139. www.nice.org.uk
8 Geng A (2012) Evidence-based guidelines for best practice in urological health care. Catheterisation. Indwelling catheters in adults, urethral and suprapubic. *European Association of Urology Nurses*. http://nurses.uroweb.org

Updated January 2019

DISCOLOURED URINE

Patients need to be warned about drugs and other substances which can discolour urine (Box A). If the urine is red, it may be assumed to be blood and cause alarm.

The colour-banding in Box A is approximate, e.g. a drug listed under 'brown/orange/yellow' will most likely cause discolouration at some point in that range. Sometimes the colour is pH dependent.

Note. Urine colour will vary according to the concentration or dilution of the urine. Colouring agents in processed food can also affect urine colour.

Box A Selected causes of discoloured urine[a]

Black/dark brown
Iron (ferrous salts)

Brown/orange/yellow
Aloe
Carrots
Dantrolene
Heparin
Nitrofurantoin
Paprika
Quinine
Retinol (vitamin A)
Riboflavin (vitamin B2)
Rifampicin
Senna (pH dependent)
Sulfasalazine
Sulfonamides
Warfarin

Brown/red/pink
Beetroot (alkaline urine)
Blackberries (acid urine)
Dantron
Ibuprofen
Levodopa-containing medicines, e.g. co-beneldopa (levodopa + benserazide) and co-careldopa (levodopa + carbidopa)
Metronidazole (acid urine)
Naphthalene-based dyes in foods and medicines, e.g. Ponceau 4R
Nefopam
Phenothiazines
Phenytoin
Rhubarb (pH dependent)
Senna (alkaline urine)

Purple
Degradation of tryptophan by urinary bacteria (see text)

Blue/green
Amitriptyline[1]
Chlorophyll breath mints
FD & C Dye No. 1 (used in foods and medicines)
Promethazine (injection)
Propofol[2]
Pseudomonas aeruginosa (pyocyanin; alkaline urine)
Triamterene

Milky colour
Diffuse glomerular nephritis
Lipids
Neutrophils
Phosphates
Radiographic dyes
Urates

a. excludes discolouration that occurs only when urine is left 'on standing' and causes unlikely to be encountered in palliative care.

Purple urine bag syndrome is caused by the breakdown of dietary tryptophan metabolites by bacteria in urine, ultimately producing indigo (blue) and indirubin (red) in alkaline urine.[3–5] Chronic urinary tract infection, long-term catheterization, constipation and immobility are the main risk factors. Although harmless, purple urine bag syndrome causes the urine to develop a strong, unpleasant odour, which becomes more noticeable over time and in warm conditions. This distresses patients more than the discolouration. Changing the drainage bag more frequently, e.g. every 3 days rather than every 5–7 days, helps to avoid the build-up of the odour. Indwelling long-term catheters may also need changing more often than normal.[5]

1 Beeley L (1986) What drugs turn urine green? *British Medical Journal*. **293**: 750.
2 Leclercq P *et al.* (2009) Green urine. *Lancet*. **373**: 1462.
3 Al-Jubouri MA and Vardhan MS (2001) A case of purple urine bag syndrome associated with Providencia rettgeri. *Journal of Clinical Pathology*. **54**: 412.
4 Ribeiro JP *et al.* (2004) Case report: purple urine bag syndrome. *Critical Care (London, England)*. **8**: R137.
5 Robinson J (2003) Purple urinary bag syndrome: a harmless but alarming problem. *British Journal of Community Nursing*. **8**: 263–266.

Updated July 2018

9: NUTRITION AND BLOOD

9

ANAEMIA

In adults, anaemia is defined as a haemoglobin (Hb) concentration:

- <130g/L in men
- <120g/L in non-pregnant women.[1]

Alternatively, the lower limit of the normal range for the laboratory performing the test can be used.

Anaemia is common in chronic disease. Associated symptoms include fatigue, breathlessness and weakness. In patients with cancer, 30–60% are anaemic at diagnosis, with its prevalence and severity increasing with more advanced disease.[2] The main causes are:

- anaemia of chronic disease (ACD) / anaemia of inflammation
- iron deficiency anaemia (IDA)
- chemotherapy-induced anaemia
- vitamin B_{12} deficiency
- folate deficiency
- malignant infiltration of the marrow
- haemolytic anaemia
- renal failure.

The most common form in cancer and in other diseases associated with inflammation is ACD, a cytokine-mediated disorder of iron homeostasis (Box A).

Box A Anaemia of chronic disease / anaemia of inflammation[3-5]

Present in >60% of anaemic patients with advanced cancer.

The hormone hepcidin, produced by hepatocytes, plays a key role in iron homeostasis. It binds to and inhibits ferroportin, the only known iron export protein.

Systemic inflammation increases the production of hepcidin and thereby inhibition of ferroportin. There is a decrease in both the absorption of dietary iron and in the release of iron from body stores, and consequently serum iron levels fall. Evolutionary advantages for this may include reduction of iron available for bacterial growth and conservation of iron for other tissues, e.g. muscle.

Thus, anaemia of inflammation is associated with a *functional* iron deficiency, i.e. insufficient iron is available for erythropoiesis, despite generally normal or increased iron stores. In contrast, iron deficiency anaemia is caused by low iron stores, an *absolute* iron deficiency.

Further, systemic inflammation also leads to reductions in:

- renal production of, and bone marrow response to, erythropoietin
- erythrocyte production
- erythrocyte lifespan.

Conversely, the production of white blood cells increases.

Novel treatments for anaemia of inflammation are in development, e.g. monoclonal anti-hepcidin antibodies.

It is important to distinguish between the various types of anaemia because treatment differs. There is no simple test to diagnose ACD. When clinically suspected, several parameters can be taken into account (Table 1).[6] Further, it is difficult to diagnose IDA in the presence of ACD because red cell indices are less reliable when there is systemic inflammation, indicated by a raised CRP. When patients have both ACD and IDA, the anaemia may be more severe and microcytic. Alternative methods of diagnosing IDA in the presence of ACD, such as hepcidin assays and serum transferrin receptor assays, remain experimental.[7-9]

Table 1 Anaemia of chronic disease (ACD) vs. iron deficiency anaemia (IDA)

	ACD	*IDA*	*ACD and IDA*
Red cell appearance	Normochromic, normocytic[a]	Hypochromic, microcytic	Hypochromic, microcytic
Plasma ferritin (microgram/L) Normal values: Men 40–300 Women 20–200	High/high–normal (>100)	Low[b] (<30)	Intermediate–normal (<100)
Transferrin saturation (%)[c] Normal values: Men 15–55 Women 12–55	Low–normal	Low/very low	Low–normal
Reticulocyte count	Low	Low	Low
Plasma iron	Low	Low	Low

a. anaemia may become microcytic if long-standing

b. ferritin reflects iron stores but rises during an acute phase response, e.g. to trauma, infection and some cancers; thus, ferritin may be normal or elevated in patients with IDA and cancer or inflammatory illness

c. reflects availability of iron to erythropoietic cells; calculated by dividing plasma iron by total iron-binding capacity (TIBC).

Treatment

In addition to trying to correct the underlying cause(s), there are three potential treatment options for anaemia due to IDA and/or ACD:

- **iron** (oral or IV)
- blood transfusion
- erythropoiesis-stimulating agent, e.g. SC **erythropoietin**.

The most appropriate choice is influenced by the severity of symptoms, likelihood of benefit, specific circumstances and patient preference. Although IM **iron** is available (iron dextran), its use is discouraged; the injections are painful, may cause permanent skin staining and are no safer than IV **iron**.

Iron deficiency anaemia (IDA)

Where IDA alone is diagnosed, **ferrous sulfate** PO is generally prescribed (p.626). There is no inherent advantage to using the IV route, providing PO **iron** is tolerated and absorbed sufficiently to exceed any ongoing loss. The Hb concentration should rise by about 20g/L over 3–4 weeks, and thus full benefit can take weeks–months.

IV **iron** is indicated when PO **iron** is poorly tolerated or ineffective or a more reliable response is required in specific circumstances, e.g. patients with renal failure receiving haemodialysis, after an acute GI bleed, and those undergoing surgery or myelosuppressive chemotherapy.[10-14] In some palliative care centres, IV **iron** is used because replacement can be given in 1–2 infusions, thereby reducing tablet burden. Compared with older IV **iron** products, the newer products are safer. Some have expressed concerns about the potential for IV **iron** to increase the growth of bacteria and cancer cells.[15,16] Thus, some centres avoid IV **iron** in patients who have active infection (also see Ferrous sulfate, Box A, p.628).[17,18]

Blood transfusion is the treatment of choice in severe IDA causing cardiovascular symptoms, e.g. angina or CHF, because it provides almost immediate benefit.

Anaemia of chronic disease (ACD)

In the palliative care setting, blood transfusion remains the treatment of choice for patients with symptomatic ACD.

Blood transfusion

There are limited data on effectiveness, duration of response and which patients are most likely to benefit.[19-21] In a prospective study of >100 transfusions in palliative care patients, 80% improved at least one anaemia symptom (fatigue, breathlessness or weakness); in 50% this was their primary anaemia symptom. Benefit was greatest in those requiring considerable assistance and frequent medical care, or in bed >50% of the time (i.e. AKPS 40–50%), but was not assessed beyond 7 days.[22] A systematic review found 30–70% of patients reported subjective benefit, although most returned to baseline ≤14 days after transfusion.[23] Because 1/4–1/3 had died by day 14, a high proportion of patients would have been in their last days of life.

Blood transfusion can cause transfusion reactions and anaphylaxis, and may increase the risk of stroke, myocardial infarction, acute renal failure and cancer recurrence.[18]

Systematic reviews have examined restrictive (trigger Hb 70–80g/dL) vs. liberal (trigger Hb 90–100g/dL) transfusion strategies and found no overall difference in mortality or hospital stay.[24,25] However, in the restrictive transfusion group, there was a trend towards higher mortality in patients with acute coronary syndrome. Thus, in haemodynamically stable patients, NICE guidance suggests a transfusion-trigger threshold of 70g/L and a target Hb sufficient to reduce symptoms of severe anaemia, i.e. 80–90g/L. For patients with symptomatic cardiovascular disease, the recommended values are a trigger threshold of 80g/L and a target of 90–100g/L.[10] Thus, for patients in the palliative care setting, a restrictive transfusion strategy should generally be followed; any deviation requires evidence of definite symptomatic benefit determined on an individual patient basis.[10,24,26]

9

Erythropoietin

Erythropoietin can be considered in patients with cancer-related anaemia but *only when receiving chemotherapy.*[18] This is because in the initial studies, **erythropoietin** increased cancer progression and reduced survival in patients not receiving chemotherapy. Some of the excess deaths related to CVS complications and VTE associated with high target Hb concentrations (>120g/L).[27,28] Subsequently, the MHRA changed the marketing authorization to stipulate that **erythropoietin** should only be given to patients receiving chemotherapy with a Hb concentration ≤100g/L, using a target Hb of ≤120g/L; further, it should be used with caution in patients receiving potentially curative treatment.[29,30] In the USA, **erythropoietin** is generally restricted to those receiving palliative chemotherapy.[17,31]

In more recent studies adhering to these parameters, the addition of IV **iron** to **erythropoietin** was more effective than PO **iron** (mean increases in Hb 8g/L vs. 5g/L respectively) and resulted in a moderate reduction in the need for transfusion.[32] No differences in survival during erythropoietin treatment, or overall, were seen. However, an increased risk of VTE remained (about 1.5 times increased risk).[33]

IV iron

Studies are currently examining the role of IV **iron** alone for ACD as a way to overcome the functional iron deficiency.[17,18] The use of IV **iron** as a means to reduce blood transfusion requirements can be considered on an individual patient basis.[17,18]

Anaemia of chronic disease (ACD) and iron deficiency anaemia (IDA)

Generally, in patients with ACD and suspected IDA, a therapeutic trial of PO **iron** can be considered *in low dose*, e.g. **ferrous sulfate** 200mg once daily for 4 weeks. Higher doses of PO **iron** increase hepcidin release, further reducing GI iron absorption (see Box A). If PO **iron** is poorly tolerated or ineffective, IV **iron** can be used (see Ferrous sulfate, Box A, p.628).[34-37]

However, in patients with cancer, IV **iron** is more effective than PO **iron** peri-operatively or when given to those receiving chemotherapy ± **erythropoietin**.[18,32] Although formal data are lacking, anecdotally, IV **iron** may also be more effective in cancer patients with ACD and IDA in the palliative care setting and is increasingly used.

For patients who have very symptomatic ACD and IDA, blood transfusion provides the most rapid improvement.[9,10]

1 WHO (2015) The global prevalence of anaemia in 2011. Geneva: World Health Organisation.

2 Maccio A *et al.* (2015) The role of inflammation, iron, and nutritional status in cancer-related anemia: results of a large, prospective, observational study. *Haematologica*. **100**: 124–132.

3 Neoh K *et al.* (2017) Estimating prevalence of functional iron deficiency anaemia in advanced cancer. *Supportive Care in Cancer*. **25**: 1209–1214.

4 Fraenkel PG (2015) Understanding anemia of chronic disease. *Hematology*. **2015**: 14–18.

5 Ganz T (2019) Anemia of inflammation. *The New England Journal of Medicine*. **381**: 1148–1157.

6 Thomas DW *et al.* (2013) Guideline for the laboratory diagnosis of functional iron deficiency. *British Journal of Haematology*. **161**: 639–648.

7 Camaschella C (2015) Iron-deficiency anemia. *New England Journal of Medicine*. **372**: 1832–1843.

8 Kelly AU *et al.* (2017) Interpreting iron studies. *British Medical Journal*. **357**: j2513.

9 Cullis JO (2011) Diagnosis and management of anaemia of chronic disease: current status. *British Journal of Haematology*. **154**: 289–300.

10 NICE (2015) Blood transfusion. *National Guideline* NG24. www.nice.org.uk.

11 Lopez A *et al.* (2016) Iron deficiency anaemia. *Lancet*. **387**: 907–916.

12 Gurusamy KS *et al.* (2014) Iron therapy in anaemic adults without chronic kidney disease. *Cochrane Database of Systematic Reviews*. **12**: CD010640. wwwthecochranelibrary.com.

13 Tang GH *et al.* (2019) Intravenous iron versus oral iron or observation for gastrointestinal malignancies: a systematic review. *European Journal of Gastroenterology & Hepatology*. **31**: 799–808.

14 Ferrer-Barceló L *et al.* (2019) Randomised clinical trial: intravenous vs oral iron for the treatment of anaemia after acute gastrointestinal bleeding. *Alimentary Pharmacology & Therapeutics*. **50**: 258–268.

15 Beguin Y *et al.* (2014) Epidemiological and nonclinical studies investigating effects of iron in carcinogenesis — a critical review. *Critical Reviews in Oncology/Hematology*. **89**: 1–15.

16 Litton E *et al.* (2013) Safety and efficacy of intravenous iron therapy in reducing requirement for allogeneic blood transfusion: systematic review and meta-analysis of randomised clinical trials. *British Medical Journal*. **347**: f4822.

17 National Comprehensive Cancer Network Practice Guidelines in Oncology (2016) Management of cancer- and chemotherapy-induced anemia. Version 1.2020. www.nccn.org (accessed January 2020).

18 Aapro M *et al.* (2018) Management of anaemia and iron deficiency in patients with cancer: ESMO Clinical Practice Guidelines. *Annals of Oncology*. **29**: iv96–iv110.

19 Uceda Torres ME *et al.* (2014) Transfusion in palliative cancer patients: a review of the literature. *Journal of Palliative Medicine*. **17**: 88–104.

20 To TH *et al.* (2016) Can we detect transfusion benefits in palliative care patients? *Journal of Palliative Medicine*. **19**: 1110–1113.

21 Chin-Yee N *et al.* (2018) Red blood cell transfusion in adult palliative care: a systematic review. *Transfusion*. **58**: 233–241.

22 To THM *et al.* (2017) The prospective evaluation of the net effect of red blood cell transfusions in routine provision of palliative care. *Journal of Palliative Medicine*. **20**: 1152–1157.

23 Preston NJ *et al.* (2012) Blood transfusions for anaemia in patients with advanced cancer. *Cochrane Database of Systematic Reviews*. **2**: CD009007. www.thecochranelibrary.com.

24 Carson JL *et al.* (2016) Transfusion thresholds and other strategies for guiding allogeneic red blood cell transfusion. *Cochrane Database of Systematic Reviews*. **10**: CD002042. www.thecochranelibrary.com.

25 Estcourt LJ *et al.* (2017) Restrictive versus liberal red blood cell transfusion strategies for people with haematological malignancies treated with intensive chemotherapy or radiotherapy, or both, with or without haematopoietic stem cell support. *Cochrane Database of Systematic Reviews*. **1**: CD011305. www.thecochranelibrary.com.

26 Brown E (2019) Blood transfusions: time for a change in practice? *British Medical Journal Supportive & Palliative Care*. **9**: 367–369.

27 Steensma DP (2007) Erythropoiesis stimulating agents. *British Medical Journal*. **334**: 648–649.

28 Bohlius J (2009) Recombinant human erythropoiesis-stimulating agents and mortality in patients with cancer: a meta-analysis of randomized trials. *Lancet*. **373**: 1532–1542.

29 MHRA (2007) Epoetins for the management of anaemia associated with cancer: risk of tumour progression and mortality. *Public assessment report*. www.gov.uk.

30 MHRA (2008) Recombinant human erythropoietins: treating anaemia in cancer. www.gov.uk/drug-safety-update.

31 NICE (2014) Erythropoiesis-stimulating agents (epoetin and darbepoetin) for treating anaemia in people with cancer having chemotherapy. *Technology Appraisal Guideline* TA323. www.nice.org.uk.

32 Mhaskar R *et al.* (2016) The role of iron in the management of chemotherapy-induced anemia in cancer patients receiving erythropoiesis-stimulating agents. *Cochrane Database of Systematic Reviews*. **2**: CD009624. www.thecochranelibrary.com.

33 Tonla T *et al.* (2012) Erythropoietin or darbepoetin for patients with cancer. *Cochrane Database of Systematic Reviews*. **12**: CD003407. www.thecochranelibrary.com.

34 Lindgren S *et al.* (2009) Intravenous iron sucrose is superior to oral iron sulphate for correcting anaemia and restoring iron stores in IBD patients: A randomized, controlled, evaluator-blind, multicentre study. *Scandinavian Journal of Gastroenterology*. **44**: 838–845.

35 O'Lone E *et al.* (2019) Parenteral versus oral iron therapy for adults and children with chronic kidney disease. *Cochrane Database of Systematic Reviews*. **2**: CD007857. www.thecochranelibrary.com.

36 Onken JE *et al.* (2014) A multicenter, randomized, active-controlled study to investigate the efficacy and safety of intravenous ferric carboxymaltose in patients with iron deficiency anemia. *Transfusion*. **54**: 306–315.

37 Bregman DB *et al.* (2013) Hepcidin levels predict nonresponsiveness to oral iron therapy in patients with iron deficiency anemia. *American Journal of Hematology*. **88**: 97–101.

Updated January 2021

FERROUS SULFATE

Class: Elemental salts.

Indications: Prevention and treatment of iron deficiency anaemia.

Contra-indications: Anaemia not caused by iron deficiency; haemosiderosis, haemochromatosis.

Pharmacology

Ferrous salts are better absorbed than ferric salts. Because there are only marginal differences in terms of efficiency of iron absorption, the choice of ferrous salt is based mainly on the incidence of undesirable effects and cost. Some undesirable effects relate directly to the amount of elemental iron, and improved tolerance after switching to another salt may be because the elemental iron content is less (Table 1). Modified-release formulations are designed to reduce undesirable effects by releasing iron gradually as the tablet or capsule passes down the GI tract.[1] However, these products are likely to carry most of the iron past the first part of the duodenum into parts of the intestine where iron absorption is poor. Such products have little therapeutic advantage and should not be used.[2]

Absorption of dietary (non-haem) iron may be increased by a high intake of red meat, poultry, fish or **ascorbic acid** (e.g. from fruits), but reduced by a high intake of phytates (e.g. in whole grain cereals), polyphenols (e.g. in tea, coffee), and **calcium** (e.g. in dairy products).[3]

Table 1 Elemental ferrous iron content of different iron salts

Iron salt	*Amount (mg)*	*Ferrous content (mg)*
Ferrous fumarate	200	65
Ferrous sulfate, dried (anhydrous)	200	65
Ferrous sulfate	300	60
Ferrous gluconate	300	35

Some oral formulations contain **ascorbic acid** or chelated iron. These modifications have been shown experimentally to produce a modest increase in the absorption of iron. However, the therapeutic advantage is minimal and the cost may be increased.[2] Further, **ascorbic acid** may increase GI irritation. There is no clinical justification for the inclusion of other therapeutically active ingredients such as the B group of vitamins (except **folic acid** for pregnant women).

Increasingly, relatively low doses of PO iron supplementation given once daily or on alternate days are recommended (see Dose and use).[4] This is because as the dose of PO iron increases, there is a corresponding increase in hepcidin levels, which inhibits iron absorption.[5-7] Although data are lacking for iron deficiency anaemia occurring concurrently with anaemia of chronic disease, where hepcidin levels are already increased, a low-dose approach is probably the most effective (also see Anaemia, p.623).

When treating iron deficiency, Hb should rise by about 20g/L over 3–4 weeks. Epithelial tissue changes such as atrophic glossitis and koilonychia also improve, but generally more slowly.

Cautions

Patients at increased risk from irritant GI effects, e.g. current or previous peptic ulcer, inflammatory bowel disease, intestinal strictures. In the upper GI tract, the risk of erosions appears highest with tablet formulations (direct contact of concentrated iron with mucosa) and lowest with liquid iron formulations.[8]

Drug interactions

Because of decreased PO absorption of iron, the other drug or both, ferrous sulfate should not be administered concurrently with antacids, bisphosphonates, **calcium** salts, **colestyramine**, **demeclocycline**, **levodopa**, **levothyroxine**, **penicillamine**, quinolone antibacterials, tetracyclines or **zinc**. Administration of iron products should be separated from the administration of these drugs by at least 2h.

Undesirable effects

Dyspepsia, nausea, epigastric pain, constipation and diarrhoea. Nausea and epigastric pain are dose-related, but the relationship between dose and altered bowel habit is not so clear.[2] Elderly patients are more likely to develop constipation, occasionally leading to faecal impaction; m/r products are more likely to cause diarrhoea, particularly in patients with inflammatory bowel disease.

Note. Liquid formulations may stain teeth. Urine and stools are discoloured (black), and this may result in a false-positive faecal occult blood test.

Dose and use

The diagnosis of iron deficiency should be confirmed before iron supplements are prescribed (see Anaemia, p.623).

Oral

Lower dose regimens providing 60–80mg/24h PO of *elemental iron* are as effective and better tolerated than higher doses (see Pharmacology), e.g.:

- ferrous *sulfate* (dried) 200mg PO once daily (65mg *elemental iron*/24h) *or* on alternate days.

After the Hb has risen to a normal concentration, treatment should be continued for a further 3 months to replenish the iron stores.[9]

This is also an appropriate prophylactic dose for patients at high risk of iron deficiency, e.g. those with a poor diet, malabsorption, and after total or subtotal gastrectomy.

For optimal absorption, iron products should be taken on an empty stomach with plenty of water. However, this may cause undesirable GI effects because of direct irritant action on the GI tract. If undesirable GI effects occur, options include:

- reduce the dose, e.g. once daily → alternate days
- take with food (but may reduce absorption by up to 50%; avoid taking at the same time as cereal, tea, coffee, eggs and dairy products; see Pharmacology)
- switch to a liquid formulation (may be less damaging to GI mucosa)[8]
- dilute liquid formulations and swallow through a straw to prevent discolouration of the teeth
- if problems persist, give IV iron (see below).

IV iron

Generally, IV iron (Box A) is reserved for when PO iron is not tolerated or is ineffective. However, it is the preferred option in several specific circumstances (also see Anaemia, p.623). Although IM iron is available (iron dextran), its use is discouraged; the injections are painful, may cause permanent skin staining, and are no safer than IV iron.

Box A IV iron

For an overview of the role of IV iron in iron deficiency anaemia, anaemia of chronic disease, or when both co-exist, see Anaemia (p.623).

There are four IV iron complexes available in the UK: ferric carboxymaltose, iron dextran, ferric derisomaltose (iron isomaltoside 1000) and iron sucrose. They appear to be equally effective.[10]

Indications: Authorized indications vary among products; see SPCs for details. Iron deficiency anaemia in inflammatory bowel disease, chronic kidney disease, otherwise when PO iron is ineffective, not tolerated, or there is a need to deliver iron rapidly; †cancer-related anaemia in patients receiving chemotherapy and erythropoietin; †patients with NYHA stage III–IV heart failure.[11]

Contra-indications: Risk factors for hypersensitivity reactions to IV iron, including asthma, eczema, history of allergic disorders, active rheumatoid arthritis. Use in hepatic or renal impairment varies among products; see SPCs for details.

Cautions

Active infection (may aid bacterial growth).

Undesirable effects

Common (<10%, >1%): nausea, injection site reactions.
Uncommon (<1%, ≥0.1%): severe hypersensitivity reactions, seizures, malaise, dizziness, tremor, chest pain, tachycardia, arrhythmias, myalgia, arthralgia, sweating.
Rare (<0.1%, ≥0.01%): anaphylaxis.

continued

Box A Continued

The newer IV iron products are less likely to cause hypersensitivity reactions than the older high molecular weight iron dextran, now withdrawn from use. Nonetheless, rarely, severe hypersensitivity reactions, including anaphylaxis, occur, even after previous IV doses have been tolerated. Thus, *IV iron should only be given where resuscitation facilities are immediately available*, and patients should be monitored during and for at least 30min after the infusion.[12,13]

Dose and use

Iron deficiency anaemia

Dose regimens vary for each product, with the required dose traditionally calculated using the Ganzoni formula (see individual SPCs). A simplified dose calculation is available for Ferinject® and Monofer®; these products are also popular because the required dose can generally be administered over 1–2 infusions.

For example, the dose for ferric derisomaltose (Monofer®):

Haemoglobin (g/dL)	*Body weight*		
	<50kg	*50–<70kg*	*≥70kg*
≥10	500mg	1,000mg	1,500mg
<10	500mg	1,500mg	2,000mg

The maximum dose that can be administered in a single IVI is 20mg/kg iron; thus, where necessary, the remainder of the dose is given in a second IVI, 7–10 days later. The iron can be given undiluted or diluted, e.g. in 100mL sodium chloride 0.9%. Doses >1,000mg are infused over ≥30min and lower doses over ≥15min. Hypotensive episodes can occur if administered too rapidly.

Bolus IV doses are used in some circumstances (see SPC).

In iron deficiency anaemia, check Hb after 4 weeks; when severe, consider checking ferritin to monitor iron stores. If anaemia has not corrected, confirm diagnosis of iron deficiency anaemia and repeat IV iron.

Concurrent iron deficiency anaemia and anaemia of chronic disease

There is no established dose regimen. Consider giving half the dose calculated for iron deficiency anaemia (see above). To monitor treatment, seek haematology advice.[14]

Supply

See below.

Supply

Oral products

Ferrous sulfate, dried (generic)

Tablets 200mg (65mg iron), 28 days @ 200mg once daily = £1.

Ferrous sulfate

Ironorm® (Wallace)

Oral drops 125mg (25mg iron)/mL, 28 days @ 375mg (3mL) once daily (75mg elemental iron/24h) = £168.

Ferrous *fumarate* (generic)

Tablets 210mg (68mg iron), 28 days @ 210mg once daily = £0.75.
Tablets 322mg (104mg iron), 28 days @ 322mg once daily = £0.75.
Capsules 305mg (99mg iron), 28 days @ 305mg once daily = £0.50.
Oral solution 140mg (45mg iron)/5mL, 28 days @ 280mg (10mL) once daily (90mg elemental iron/24h) = £5.50.

Ferrous *gluconate* (generic)
Tablets 300mg (35mg iron), 28 days @ 600mg once daily (70mg elemental iron/24h) = £2.

Parenteral products
Ferric carboxymaltose
Ferinject® (Vifor)
Injection 50mg/mL; 2mL, 10mL and 20mL vial = £20, £96 and £154; *contains sodium 0.24mmol/mL.*

Iron dextran
Cosmofer® (Pharmacosmos)
Injection 50mg/mL; 2mL and 10mL amp = £8 and £40.

Ferric derisomaltose (iron isomaltoside 1000)
Diafer® (Pharmacosmos)
Injection 50mg/mL, 2mL amp = £17. *Authorized for iron deficiency in patients with ESRF on dialysis.*

Monofer® (Pharmacosmos)
Injection 100mg/mL; 1mL, 5mL, 10mL vial = £11, £84, £170.

Iron sucrose
Venofer® (Vifor)
Injection 20mg/mL, 5mL vial = £10.

1 Cancelo-Hidalgo MJ *et al.* (2013) Tolerability of different oral iron supplements: a systematic review. *Current Medical Research and Opinion*. **29**: 291–303.
2 British National Formulary Section 9.1.1.2 Oral Iron. London: BMJ Group and Pharmaceutical Press. www.medicinescomplete.com (accessed January 2020).
3 Heath AL and Fairweather-Tait SJ (2002) Clinical implications of changes in the modern diet: iron intake, absorption and status. *Best Practice and Research Clinical Haematology*. **15**: 225–241.
4 Rimon E *et al.* (2005) Are we giving too much iron? Low-dose iron therapy is effective in octogenarians. *The American Journal of Medicine*. **118**: 1142–1147.
5 Stoffel NU *et al.* (2017) Iron absorption from oral iron supplements given on consecutive versus alternate days and as single morning doses versus twice-daily split dosing in iron-depleted women: two open-label, randomised controlled trials. *Lancet Haematology*. **4**: e524–e533.
6 Stoffel NU *et al.* (2020) Iron absorption from supplements is greater with alternate day than with consecutive day dosing in iron-deficient anemic women. *Haematologica*. **105**: 1232–1239.
7 Muñoz M *et al.* (2018) The safety of available treatment options for iron-deficiency anemia. *Expert Opinion Drug Safety*. **17**: 149–159.
8 Sunkara T *et al.* (2017) Iron pill gastritis: an under diagnosed condition with potentially serious outcomes. *Gastroenterology Research*. **10**: 138–140.
9 Lopez A *et al.* (2016) Iron deficiency anaemia. *Lancet*. **387**: 907–916.
10 Mhaskar R *et al.* (2016) The role of iron in the management of chemotherapy-induced anemia in cancer patients receiving erythropoiesis-stimulating agents. *Cochrane Database of Systematic Reviews*. **2**: CD009624. www.cochranelibrary.com.
11 Drozd M *et al.* (2017) Iron therapy in patients with heart failure and iron deficiency: review of iron preparations for practitioners. *American Journal of Cardiovascular Drugs*. **17**: 183–201.
12 MHRA (2013) Intravenous iron and serious hypersensitivity reactions: stengthened recommendations. *Drug Safety Update*. www.gov.uk/drug-safety-update.
13 Rampton D *et al.* (2014) Hypersensitivity reactions to intravenous iron: guidance for risk minimization and management. *Haematologica*. **99**: 1671–1676.
14 Ganz T (2019) Anemia of inflammation. *The New England Journal of Medicine*. **381**: 1148–1157.

Updated (minor change) September 2021

ASCORBIC ACID (VITAMIN C)

Class: Vitamin.

Indications: Scurvy, †enhancement of wound healing, †recurrent urinary infections.

Pharmacology

Ascorbic acid (vitamin C) is a powerful reducing agent. It is obtained from dietary sources of fresh fruit and vegetables, e.g. blackcurrants, kiwifruit, broccoli, red pepper and oranges. It cannot be synthesized by the body. It is involved in the hydroxylation of proline to hydroxyproline, which is necessary for the formation of collagen. The failure of this accounts for most of the clinical effects found in deficiency (scurvy), e.g. keratosis of hair follicles with 'corkscrew hair', perifollicular haemorrhages, swollen spongy infected and bleeding gums, loose teeth, spontaneous bruising and haemorrhage, anaemia and failure of wound healing. Repeated infections are also common. In healthy adults, a dietary intake of about 30–60mg/24h is necessary; in scurvy, a rapid clinical response is seen with ≥250mg/24h in divided doses.

A beneficial effect of megadose ascorbic acid therapy has been claimed for many conditions,[1] including the common cold, asthma, atherosclerosis, cancer, psychiatric disorders, increased susceptibility to infections related to abnormal leucocyte function, infertility and osteogenesis imperfecta. Ascorbic acid has also been tried in the treatment of wound healing, pain in Paget's disease and opioid withdrawal. There are few RCTs to substantiate these claims.

Systematic reviews of ascorbic acid for the prevention and treatment of cancer have found no conclusive evidence of benefit.[2-4] However, ascorbic acid deficiency is common in cancer patients, and low plasma concentrations have been associated with shorter survival.[5] Further, dietary ascorbic acid intake and supplement use following a diagnosis of breast cancer are associated with a reduced mortality risk for cancer and other causes.[6]

Ascorbic acid alone or with β-carotene and vitamin E does not prevent the development of colorectal adenoma.[7] Ascorbic acid does reduce the severity of a cold, but not its incidence.[8] Enthusiasm for high-dose ascorbic acid for HIV+ people waned after many died from disease progression.[9] Although it has been postulated that ascorbic acid might help prevent ischaemic heart disease, in contrast to other antioxidant vitamins, little benefit is seen in RCTs.[10,11] Of more concern are data which indicate that a total daily dose as small as 500mg has a pro-oxidant effect which could result in genetic mutation.[12]

Absorption occurs mainly from the proximal small intestine by a saturable process. In health, body stores of ascorbic acid are about 1.5g, although larger stores may occur with intakes higher than 200mg/24h. It is renally excreted as oxalic acid, unchanged ascorbic acid and small amounts of dehydro-ascorbic acid. Ascorbic acid is used to acidify urine in patients with alkaline urine and recurrent urinary infections.

Drug interactions

In patients with renal impairment, because of an increased risk of aluminium toxicity, avoid concurrent use of ascorbic acid and **aluminium**-containing products.

Aspirin reduces the absorption of ascorbic acid by up to a third.

Undesirable effects

GI symptoms may occur at doses of >1g/24h.[13] Doses of >3g/24h may result in diarrhoea, acidosis, glycosuria, oxaluria and renal stones. Tolerance may occur with prolonged use of large doses, resulting in symptoms of deficiency if intake is reduced.

In the past, some centres used undissolved effervescent ascorbic acid tablets (available OTC) for debriding the tongue. However, such use has fallen out of favour because the acidity may:

- exacerbate a sore or inflamed mouth
- contribute to the demineralization of teeth
- predispose to oral infections (see p.665).

Further, if not completely dissolved or swallowed when lying down, the tablets could cause localized oesophagitis.

Dose and use

Vitamin C deficiency

- for florid scurvy, give 100mg PO t.d.s. for 4 weeks
- otherwise, give 100mg PO once daily; continue indefinitely in undernourished patients, particularly the elderly.

†Enhancement of wound healing

- give 100mg PO b.d. for 4 weeks.

†Acidification of urine

- give 100–200mg PO b.d.; test urine with litmus paper until a constant acid result is obtained.

Supply

Ascorbic acid (generic)

Tablets 50mg, 100mg, 200mg, 500mg, 28 days @ 100mg once daily = £14.

Tablets (chewable) 100mg, 500mg, 1000mg, 28 days @ 100mg once daily = £4.

1 Ovesen L (1984) Vitamin therapy in the absence of obvious deficiency. What is the evidence? *Drugs*. **27**: 148–170.
2 Coulter ID *et al.* (2006) Antioxidants vitamin C and vitamin E for the prevention and treatment of cancer. *Journal of General Internal Medicine*. **21**: 735–744.
3 Jacobs C *et al.* (2015) Is there a role for oral or intravenous ascorbate (vitamin C) in treating patients with cancer? A systematic review. *Oncologist*. **20**: 210–223.
4 van Gorkom GNY *et al.* (2019) The effect of vitamin C (ascorbic acid) in the treatment of patients with cancer: a systematic review. *Nutrients*. **11**: 977.
5 Mayland CR *et al.* (2005) Vitamin C deficiency in cancer patients. *Palliative Medicine*. **19**: 17–20.
6 Harris HR *et al.* (2014) Vitamin C and survival among women with breast cancer: a meta-analysis. *European Journal of Cancer*. **50**: 1223–1231.
7 Greenberg E *et al.* (1994) A clinical trial of antioxidant vitamins to prevent colorectal adenoma. Polyp Prevention Study Group. *New England Journal of Medicine*. **331**: 141–147.
8 Hemila H (1994) Does vitamin C alleviate the symptoms of the common cold? a review of current evidence. *Scandinavian Journal of Infectious Diseases*. **26**: 1–6.
9 Abrams D (1990) Alternative therapies in HIV infection. *AIDS*. **4**: 1179–1187.
10 Rimm E (1993) Vitamin E consumption and the risk of coronary heart disease in men. *New England Journal of Medicine*. **328**: 1450–1456.
11 Stampfer M (1993) Vitamin E consumption and the risk of coronary disease in women. *New England Journal of Medicine*. **328**: 1444–1449.
12 Podmore I *et al.* (1998) Vitamin C exhibits pro-oxidant properties. *Nature*. **392**: 559.
13 Beveridge C (2002) Basic Nutrition. In: Repchinsky C, LeBlanc C (eds), *Patient Self Care* (1st edn). Canadian Pharmacists Association, Ottawa. pp. 339–358.

Updated August 2019

VITAMIN K

Class: Vitamin.

Indications: Reversal of anticoagulant effects of **warfarin** and other coumarins (**phytomenadione**); bleeding (actual or threatened) associated with a low plasma level of factor II (prothrombin) or factor VII, due to, e.g. hepatic impairment (particularly obstructive jaundice), dietary deficiency (**menadiol sodium phosphate**).

Pharmacology

Vitamin K is a fat-soluble vitamin. Phytomenadione (vitamin K_1) is the active form, and is present in green vegetables, dairy products and soya bean oil. In addition, vitamin K is synthesized by bacteria in the terminal ileum and colon. **Phytomenadione** is available for parenteral use. **Menadiol sodium phosphate** is a water-soluble synthetic vitamin K analogue. It can be given PO to prevent vitamin K deficiency in patients with fat malabsorption or to correct dietary deficiency.

Phytomenadione is necessary for the synthesis of coagulation factors II, VII, IX and X, and of proteins involved in bone calcification. Oral coumarins block the recycling of vitamin K metabolites in the liver, and thus block the synthesis of the coagulation factors. This block is circumvented by exogenous vitamin K; adequate factor VII levels are restored within 6h (IV) and 12h (PO) of vitamin K administration.

Hepatic stores of vitamin K are depleted in <3 days of dietary restriction. In patients with advanced cancer, >20% are vitamin K deficient.[1] Patients who are malnourished, have fat malabsorption (e.g. in biliary obstruction or liver disease) or are having prolonged courses of antibacterials which sterilize the GI tract are at risk of deficiency and a rapid rise in prothrombin time (PT) and activated partial thromboplastin time (APTT).

Phytomenadione and vitamin K analogues do *not* reverse heparin-induced anticoagulation (see p.102) or bleeding associated with direct oral anticoagulants (see p.95).

Bleeding tendency in hepatic impairment

Vitamin K is *not* indicated routinely in chronic hepatic impairment, because blood coagulation is 'rebalanced' by a reduction of both procoagulant and anticoagulant factors.[2] If a patient with severe hepatic impairment or failure develops surface bleeding (e.g. petechiae, purpura, multiple bruising, epistaxis, gum bleeding, bleeding from GI tract), PT should be checked and, if prolonged, vitamin K replacement is indicated. However, its use should be limited to conscious patients with a reasonable performance status for whom other supportive measures are deemed appropriate (e.g. blood transfusion). Vitamin K should not be used in moribund patients in an attempt to prevent an imminent inevitable death.

Because vitamin K deficiency is rarely the primary cause of coagulopathy in severe hepatic impairment or failure, replacement may only partially correct the PT. A persistently prolonged PT following administration of vitamin K may indicate the existence of a clotting factor deficiency caused by impaired hepatic synthesis. Other underlying conditions may also contribute to the bleeding tendency, e.g. renal failure, sepsis.[2]

Onset of action ≤6h (to normalize the INR).[3]

Plasma halflife 1.5–3h.

Cautions

Unless there is major bleeding, **phytomenadione** should generally not be given to patients with a prosthetic heart valve; obtain advice from a haematologist and consider using **human prothrombin complex** or fresh frozen plasma instead.

Severe hepatic impairment (Konakion® MM); contains glycocholic acid, which can displace bilirubin.

Oral absorption of **menadiol sodium phosphate** is reduced by concurrent administration with **colestyramine** or **liquid paraffin (mineral oil)**.

Undesirable effects

Rarely, anaphylactoid reaction after IV use.

Dose and use

Phytomenadione (Konakion® MM) is given by slow IV injection over at least 30sec, generally 3–5min, or by IVI diluted in 50mL of glucose 5% over 20–30min (protect from light).
Konakion® MM formulation must not be given IM.

Reversal of excessive warfarin anticoagulation

Obtain advice from a haematologist and use the British Society for Haematology guidelines.[3–5]

Major bleeding

- stop **warfarin** *and*
- give **human prothrombin complex** IVI (Box A) *and*
- give **phytomenadione** 5mg slow IV; check INR after 3h:
  - ▷ repeat the dose if necessary; each time check INR after 3h
  - ▷ maximum dose = 40mg/24h.

Note. Fresh frozen plasma produces suboptimal anticoagulation reversal and should be used only if **human prothrombin complex** is not available. Recombinant factor VIIa is *not* recommended for emergency reversal of anticoagulation.

Minor bleeding INR >5

- stop **warfarin** *and*
- give **phytomenadione** 1–3mg slow IV and recheck INR after 24h; repeat the dose if INR still >8
- restart **warfarin** when INR <5.

No bleeding but prolonged INR

- INR >5: withhold 1–2 doses of **warfarin** and reduce maintenance dose
- INR ≥8: stop **warfarin,** give **phytomenadione** 1–5 mg *by mouth* using the injection formulation, and recheck INR after 24h; repeat the dose if INR still >8
- restart **warfarin** when INR <5.

Box A Human prothrombin complex

Human prothrombin complex contains coagulation factors II, VII, IX, X with proteins C and S. Several human prothrombin complexes (also known as dried prothrombin complex or prothrombinase complex concentrate) are commercially available, but dosing regimens vary according to the product, patient's weight and INR; e.g. for Beriplex®:

- INR 2–3.9 → 25 units/kg (maximum dose 2,500 units)
- INR 4–6 → 35 units/kg (maximum dose 3,500 units)
- INR >6 → 50 units/kg (maximum dose 5,000 units)

The reconstituted Beriplex® product should be given IVI at a maximum rate of 8mL/min.

See individual SPCs for full details.

Supply

Beriplex P/N® (CSL Behring UK)

Injection (powder and solvent for reconstitution) factors II, VII, IX and X, 250 units, 500 units and 1,000 units = £128, £255 and £510 respectively.

For reversal of warfarin anticoagulation for emergency or planned surgery, obtain advice from a haematologist.

Reversal of bleeding (actual or threatened) associated with a low plasma level of factor II (prothrombin) or factor VII, e.g. from hepatic impairment or dietary deficiency

- give **menadiol phosphate** 10mg PO once daily
- check PT after 3 days and, if still raised, increase the dose progressively up to 40mg once daily (rarely necessary) until maximal PT correction is achieved
- once maximal PT correction is achieved:
  - ▷ *in malabsorption:* give a maintenance dose of **menadiol phosphate** 5–10mg PO once daily and monitor PT regularly[6]
  - ▷ *in hepatic impairment:* stop **menadiol phosphate** and recheck PT if signs of surface bleeding return
- in hepatic impairment, if **menadiol phosphate** is unavailable, consider giving phytomenadione 2.5–10mg *by mouth* using the injection formulation.

If serious bleeding:

- give **phytomenadione** injection (Konakion® MM) 10mg slow IV (see above)
- if IV access difficult, consider using the Konakion® MM Paediatric *formulation* 10mg, which can be administered IM
- **human prothrombin complex** may also be necessary.

In patients with hepatic impairment, the risk of venous thrombosis is often paradoxically increased. Thus, in this situation, **human prothrombin complex** should be used only in emergency situations after specialist advice and with regular coagulation monitoring.

Note. **Desmopressin** (p.572) may improve haemostasis in patients with hepatic platelet dysfunction.

Supply

Phytomenadione

Konakion® MM (Roche)

Injection (colloidal) phytomenadione 10mg/mL in a mixed micelles vehicle, 1mL (10mg) amp = £0.50. *For IV or IVI use only, do not use IM.* PO use is off-label.

Konakion® MM Paediatric (Roche)

Injection (colloidal) phytomenadione 10mg/mL in a mixed micelles vehicle, 0.2mL (2mg) amp = £1. *Konakion® MM Paediatric may be administered PO, IM, IV.*

Menadiol phosphate (generic)
Tablets menadiol sodium phosphate equivalent to 10mg of menadiol phosphate, 7 days @ 10mg once daily = £14.
Oral suspension 5mg/5mL, 30mL = £60 (unauthorized product, available as a special order; see Chapter 24, p.817). *Price based on Specials tariff in community.*

1 Harrington DJ *et al.* (2008) A study of the prevalence of vitamin K deficiency in patients with cancer referred to a hospital palliative care team and its association with abnormal haemostasis. *Journal of Clinical Pathology*. **61**: 537–540.
2 Tripodi A and Mannucci PM (2011) The coagulopathy of chronic liver disease. *New England Journal of Medicine*. **365**: 147–156.
3 Hunt BJ and Levi M (2018) Urgent reversal of vitamin K antagonists. *British Medical Journal*. **360**: 78–80.
4 Makris M *et al.* (2012) Guideline on the management of bleeding in patients on antithrombotic agents. *British Journal of Haematology*. **160**: 35–46.
5 British National Formulary Section 3.2 Oral anticoagulants. London: BMJ Group and Pharmaceutical Press. www.medicinescomplete.com (accessed January 2018).
6 Jagannath VA *et al.* (2017) Vitamin K supplementation for cystic fibrosis. *Cochrane Database of Systematic Reviews*. **8**: CD008482. www.thecochranelibrary.com

Updated May 2018

POTASSIUM

Class: Element.

Indications: Hypokalaemia (<3.5mmol/L).

Pharmacology

In palliative care, hypokalaemia is most common in patients receiving non-potassium-sparing diuretics, particularly if also taking a corticosteroid. Hypokalaemia is also associated with chronic diarrhoea and persistent vomiting. Correction of hypokalaemia is important in patients taking **digoxin** or other anti-arrhythmic drugs because of the risk of an arrhythmia. Potassium supplements are seldom required, with small doses of diuretics given to treat hypertension.

When larger doses of thiazide or loop diuretics are given to eliminate oedema, potassium-sparing diuretics (e.g. **amiloride**, **spironolactone**) rather than potassium supplements are preferable. Dietary supplements also help to maintain plasma potassium; 10mmol of potassium is contained in a large banana and in 250mL of orange juice.

When treating hypokalaemia, potassium *chloride* is generally the salt of choice because of associated hypochloraemia. However, occasionally, hypokalaemia is associated with a hyperchloraemic metabolic acidosis, and an alkalinizing salt will be preferable, e.g. potassium *bicarbonate* or potassium *citrate* (not UK). Co-existing hypomagnesaemia should always be corrected (see p.638).

Drugs are a common cause of hyperkalaemia in hospitalized patients (see Drug interactions), particularly in association with pre-existing or new renal impairment. When *mild–moderate* (i.e. 5.5–6.5mmol/L, with no ECG changes or symptoms), dose reduction or stopping the causal drug may be all that needs to be done. However, other causes may need to be considered, e.g. hypoaldosteronism, tumour lysis syndrome, **digoxin** toxicity. Spurious results can also occur, e.g. as a result of haemolysis, marked leukocytosis or thrombocytosis. Repeating the sample and/or obtaining advice from the clinical chemistry laboratory may be necessary. For the treatment of *severe* hyperkalaemia, see below.

Cautions

Use smaller doses of potassium when there is renal impairment.

Drug interactions

Hyperkalaemia may result if used concurrently with drugs that increase the plasma potassium concentration, e.g. by impairing renal potassium excretion via interference with the renin–angiotensin–aldosterone system (e.g. ACE inhibitors, angiotensin II receptor antagonists, LMWH/**heparin**, potassium-sparing diuretics, NSAIDs, **ciclosporin**, **tacrolimus**, **trimethoprim**), promoting shifts in cellular potassium (e.g. β-blockers, particularly non-selective), or containing potassium (e.g. laxatives such as Movicol®).

Undesirable effects

Oesophageal or GI ulceration, nausea and vomiting. Liquid or effervescent formulations are distasteful.

Dose and use

The normal adult daily requirement and the typical dietary intake of potassium is 40–80mmol. Whenever possible, orange juice and bananas should be used as a palatable source of potassium (see Pharmacology above).

To minimize nausea and vomiting, potassium supplements are best taken during or after a meal. Effervescent or liquid products are preferable; m/r formulations, e.g. Slow-K®, are not recommended, because of a greater risk of gastric irritation.

Prevention of hypokalaemia

- potassium *chloride*, e.g. Sando-K® 1–2 tablets b.d. (24–48mmol/24h K^+) *or*
- prescribe a potassium-sparing diuretic, e.g. **amiloride** 5–10mg once daily (maximum 20mg once daily) or **spironolactone** 25–200mg/24h.

Treatment of hypokalaemia

- potassium *chloride*, e.g. Sando-K® 2 tablets t.d.s. (72mmol/24h K^+)
- if the patient is hyperchloraemic, prescribe potassium *bicarbonate* effervescent tablets instead
- if hypokalaemia persists, investigate for possible magnesium deficiency (see p.638).

Emergency treatment of hyperkalaemia

Stop and think! Are you justified in correcting a potentially fatal complication in a moribund patient?

Urgent treatment is required when hyperkalaemia is severe (≥6.5mmol/L) or with any level ≥5.5mmol/L accompanied by ECG changes (e.g. reduced or absent P waves, PR prolongation, QRS widening) and/or symptoms (e.g. muscle weakness, paraesthesia, palpitation). An approach is summarized in Box A. However, this is only part of the management of hyperkalaemia, and specialist advice should be obtained as necessary.

Box A Emergency treatment of severe hyperkalaemia[1,2]

Stop potentially contributory or antagonistic drugs

These include ACE inhibitors, angiotensin II receptor antagonists, potassium-sparing diuretics, potassium-containing laxatives (e.g. Movicol®), NSAIDs and trimethoprim.

β-blockers and digoxin should also be stopped, as they antagonize the effect of insulin and β_2 agonists (see below).

Reduce the risk of cardiac arrhythmia

This is always the first step.

Give calcium gluconate 10mL of 10% solution IV over 2min; any improvement in ECG abnormalities will be seen in <3min; stop if bradycardia develops.

If necessary, repeat the same dose every 5–10min until improvement is obtained; some patients require up to 50mL.

Duration of action is 30–60min, and further doses may be required.

Note. Calcium gluconate can precipitate digoxin toxicity; give in 100mL of glucose 5% IV over 20min in patients using digoxin (seek specialist advice).

continued

Box A Continued

Shift potassium into cells

When hyperkalaemia is severe (≥6.5mmol/L), insulin is generally given.

β_2 agonists (e.g. salbutamol) can be as effective.

Both reduce the plasma potassium concentration by about 0.5–1mmol/L.

Some guidelines do not recommend β_2 agonists as a sole treatment because some patients, e.g. those who are dialysis-dependent or using β-blockers or digoxin, are less likely to respond.

The combination of insulin with nebulized salbutamol is more effective than either alone, with the latter helping to reduce the hypoglycaemic effect of the insulin.

These interventions do not remove potassium from the body, but buy time for more definitive treatment to be carried out.

Insulin

- add 10 units soluble insulin (e.g. Actrapid®) to 50mL glucose 50% and give IV into a large vein over 5min
- onset of effect 15min, duration of action at least 1h and commonly 4–6h
- if it becomes necessary to repeat the dose of insulin, additional glucose is not required if plasma glucose is ≥15mmol/L.

β_2 agonist

- give salbutamol 10–20mg nebulized over 10–30min (10mg in patients with ischaemic heart disease)
- when a nebulizer is not available, use salbutamol 1,200microgram (12 puffs) inhaled over 2min via a spacer device
- onset of effect 15–30min, duration of action 2h or more.

Monitoring treatment

- recheck urea and electrolytes after 30min, 1h and then q2h for 6h
- when insulin used, check blood glucose after 15min, 30min and then q1h for 6h, as delayed hypoglycaemia can occur.

Other measures

If the combined approach above fails to work, emergency dialysis may be necessary to remove potassium from the body (if appropriate to the patient's overall circumstances).

Calcium polystyrene sulfonate resin (Calcium Resonium®) 15g PO q.d.s. is also used together with regular lactulose to increase potassium loss from the GI tract. However, it is not an emergency treatment because it has a slow onset of action (4–24h). It is contra-indicated in hypercalcaemia. It is unpalatable and can be poorly tolerated; it can also cause constipation.

Supply

Potassium *chloride*

Sando-K® (HK Pharma)

Tablets effervescent potassium bicarbonate 400mg and potassium chloride 600mg equivalent to potassium 470mg (12mmol K^+) and chloride 285mg (8mmol Cl^-), 7 days @ 2 t.d.s. (72mmol/24h K^+ and 48mmol/24h Cl^-) = £4.25.

Kay-Cee-L® (Geistlich)

Oral syrup potassium chloride 7.5% (1mmol/mL K^+ and 1mmol/mL Cl^-), 7 days @ 20mL t.d.s. (60mmol/24h K^+) = £7.50.

Potassium *bicarbonate*

Tablets effervescent potassium bicarbonate 500mg, potassium acid tartrate 300mg (6.5mmol K^+), 7 days @ 2 q.d.s. (52mmol/24h K^+) = £92; *dose depends on acid–base balance as well as plasma potassium concentration.*

1 GAIN (Guidelines and Audit Implementation Network) (2014) Guidelines for the treatment of hyperkalaemia in adults. Available from: www.rqia.org.uk
2 Batterink J *et al.* (2015) Pharmacological interventions for the acute management of hyperkalaemia in adults. *Cochrane Database of Systematic Reviews*. Issue 10: CD01034. www.cochranelibrary.com

Updated August 2019

MAGNESIUM

Class: Metal element.

Indications: Hypomagnesaemia, constipation (see p.57), †arrhythmia, †eclampsia, †asthma (nebulized), †myocardial infarction.

Pharmacology

Magnesium is the second most abundant intracellular ion after potassium. It is involved in >600 enzymatic reactions and is a co-factor for many biological processes, most of which use ATP. It is important for bone mineralization, cell growth and proliferation, glycolysis, muscular relaxation, protein synthesis (including DNA synthesis, stability and repair) and neurotransmission. About half of the total body magnesium is in soft tissue, and the other half in bone. Less than 1% is in blood; thus serum magnesium concentration is a poor predictor of overall body stores.[1-3] Intracellular magnesium is mostly bound to ribosomes, phospholipids and nucleotides.[3]

The recommended total daily intake is about 6–12mmol/24h. However, magnesium intake is falling as the use of processed and fast foods increases, and, increasingly, people are failing to meet this requirement.[2,4] Thus, the incidence of chronic magnesium deficiency is probably increasing, with possible health implications, but is unrecognized because of the diagnostic limitations of serum magnesium (see below).[2,4]

Magnesium competes with calcium for absorption in the small intestine, probably by active transport. The normal serum magnesium is 0.7–1.1mmol/L. However, some have argued that for optimal health, the lower limit for serum magnesium should be considered to be 0.85mmol/L.[2] This is based on a progressive increase in the frequency of magnesium deficiency seen with serum levels between 0.85mmol/L and 0.75mmol/L (from <10% to 90%), which is associated with an increased risk of morbidity, e.g. impaired glucose tolerance, type 2 diabetes mellitus, and mortality, e.g. sudden cardiac death.[2,4] Most of the serum magnesium is in the ionized active form, with about 30% bound to albumin and inactive. Hypo-albuminaemia may lead to artificially low serum magnesium levels.

Magnesium is excreted by the kidneys, 3–12mmol/24h. Magnesium and calcium share the same transport system in the renal tubules, and there is a reciprocal relationship between the amounts excreted.

Magnesium deficiency can result from:

- *reduced intake*, e.g. an inadequate dietary intake (common)
- *reduced absorption*, e.g. small bowel resection, cholestasis, pancreatic insufficiency, diarrhoea, stoma, fistula, PPIs (rare and generally with prolonged use, e.g. >1 year; see p.31)
- *increased excretion*, e.g. alcoholism, diabetes mellitus, interstitial nephritis, diuretic phase of acute tubular necrosis, hyperthyroidism, hyperparathyroidism, hyperaldosteronism, some drugs (e.g. aminoglycosides, **amphotericin**, anti-epidermal growth factor receptor monoclonal antibodies, **cisplatin, ciclosporin**, loop diuretics).

Cisplatin accumulates within renal tubular cells, resulting in cellular injury/death which manifests as hypomagnesaemia ± acute kidney injury. **Cisplatin** accumulation and kidney damage is enhanced by magnesium deficiency and reduced by magnesium replacement.[5,6] The risk of hypomagnesaemia with **cisplatin** is dose-dependent and increases with cumulative doses (40% cycle 1 → 100% cycle 6).[7] It can persist for 4–5 months, and sometimes years, after completing treatment.[8,9] Although generally mild and asymptomatic, it can be severe and symptomatic.

Hypomagnesaemia is an emerging toxicity of anti-epidermal growth factor receptor monoclonal antibodies, e.g. **cetuximab, panitumumab**.[10,11] The risk increases in the elderly, in those with a higher baseline serum magnesium, and with duration of treatment (e.g. 5% <3 months → 50% >6 months of **cetuximab**).[10] It is reversible, with magnesium levels returning to normal 4–6 weeks after discontinuation of treatment.[10]

When magnesium deficiency develops acutely, the symptoms may be obvious and severe, particularly muscle cramps, which aids diagnosis (Box A). In chronic deficiency, symptoms may be insidious in onset, less severe and non-specific.

In animal studies, magnesium deficiency results in an increased release of substance P and other mediators from nerve endings. These activate immune cells to release histamine and cytokines, producing a pro-inflammatory state and increased levels of oxygen-derived free radicals and nitric oxide. Manifestations include:[12-14]

- cutaneous vasodilatation → erythema and oedema
- leukocytosis
- inflammatory lesions in cardiac muscle
- atherogenesis
- increased levels of oxidative stress
- hyperalgesia.

In humans, the incidence of magnesium deficiency increases with age (due to poor diet, reduced intestinal absorption, increased urinary loss etc.) and obesity. Magnesium deficiency, ageing and obesity are all associated with low-grade inflammation and increased oxidative stress. This has led some to postulate that magnesium deficiency is a contributing factor to age- and obesity-related diseases such as diabetes mellitus, cardiac failure, some cancers (e.g. breast, colon), and hypertension.[13,15-18] In support of this, there is an inverse relationship between serum magnesium and CRP and also risk of metabolic syndrome.[19,20] Magnesium supplementation has attenuated the elevated CRP in some patient groups, e.g. cardiac failure and older adults, but not others, e.g. obese adults.[19] The underlying mechanisms remain to be clarified, but in part may relate to magnesium acting as a natural 'calcium antagonist'.[3] Thus, in magnesium deficiency, intracellular calcium levels increase, activating processes which contribute to inflammation.[17]

Serum magnesium is associated with muscle performance, e.g. in the elderly[21] and in patients with coronary artery disease.[22] In both of these groups, the use of magnesium supplements can improve exercise capacity.[22,23] However, results are mixed; e.g. in patients with diabetes, the use of magnesium supplements or the correction of mild magnesium deficiency is of inconsistent benefit.[1]

Hypomagnesaemia (and hypokalaemia) are risk factors for drug-induced *torsade de pointes* arrhythmia. Thus, when using a drug known to prolong the QT interval, e.g. **methadone**, monitoring of serum electrolytes is generally recommended in patients with cardiac disease or other risk factors for prolonged QT, and in those at risk of electrolyte imbalance, e.g. because of vomiting, diarrhoea or diuretics (see Chapter 20, p.797).[24]

Hypermagnesaemia is rare and is seen most often in patients with renal impairment who take OTC medicines containing magnesium. Serum concentrations >4mmol/L produce drowsiness, vasodilation, slowing of atrioventricular conduction and hypotension. Over 6mmol/L there is profound CNS depression and muscle weakness (Box A). Calcium gluconate IV is used to help reverse the effects of hypermagnesaemia.

Generally, the clinical history will indicate the most likely cause of hypomagnesaemia. When this is not the case, if necessary, the distinction between renal and non-renal causes can be made by measuring urinary magnesium excretion (Box B).

In deficiency states that develop more insidiously, the serum magnesium is an insensitive guide to total body stores and hypomagnesaemia is not always present.[25,26] In this situation, the finding of a low urinary excretion of magnesium (Box B) may help the diagnosis. Currently, the best method for detecting magnesium deficiency is the magnesium loading test (Box C).[25,27,28]

If it is not possible to perform a magnesium loading test, hypokalaemia (± hypocalcaemia) not responding to potassium (± calcium) supplementation should raise the possibility of magnesium deficiency, and a trial of magnesium replacement therapy should be considered.[1] Magnesium deficiency results in hypokalaemia via increased potassium loss in the urine, and hypocalcaemia by reducing the release of and tissue sensitivity to PTH.[3]

Magnesium blocks calcium channels, including the NMDA-receptor–channel, and this probably accounts for its analgesic effect (Box D).[29-33] However, despite the overall positive outcome from numerous RCTs, the role of magnesium as an analgesic in palliative care is yet to be determined, and ideally such use should be in the setting of a clinical trial.

Box A Symptoms and signs of magnesium deficiency and excess

Magnesium deficiency	Magnesium excess
Muscle	Muscle
weakness	weakness
tremor	hypotonia
twitching	loss of reflexes
cramps	Sensation of warmth (IV)
tetany (positive Chvostek's sign)	Flushing (IV)
Paraesthesia	Drowsiness
Apathy	Slurred speech
Depression	Double vision
Delirium	Delirium
Choreiform movements	Hypotension
Nystagmus	Cardiac arrhythmia
Seizures	Respiratory depression
Prolonged QT interval	Nausea and vomiting
Cardiac arrhythmia, including *torsade de pointes*	Thirst
Increased pain (?)	Hypermagnesaemia
Hypomagnesaemia (not always)	
Hypokalaemia	
Hypocalcaemia	
Hypophosphataemia	

Box B Distinguishing between renal and non-renal causes of hypomagnesaemia

In hypomagnesaemia caused by renal wasting, renal excretion of magnesium is increased. The converse is true in non-renal causes of deficiency, e.g. poor intake or increased GI loss, because the kidney conserves magnesium.

Either a 24h urine collection can be used to measure total magnesium excretion, or a random urine specimen used to calculate the fractional excretion of magnesium (FEMg):

$$\text{FEMg} = \left[\frac{\text{urine Mg (mmol/L)} \times \text{plasma Cr (micromol/L)}}{(0.7 \times \text{plasma Mg (mmol/L)}) \times \text{urinary Cr (micromol/L)}}\right] \times 100$$

In a patient with hypomagnesaemia and normal renal function:

- total excretion >4mmol/24h or FEMg >2% indicates renal wasting
- total excretion <4mmol/24h or FEMg <2% indicates a non-renal cause.

Urinary magnesium excretion is a less reliable indicator in the presence of diabetes, renal impairment and drugs that increase renal excretion of magnesium, e.g. diuretics.

Box C The magnesium loading test[27]

Collect pre-infusion urine sample for urinary magnesium (Mg):creatinine (Cr) ratio. Measure Mg and Cr in mmol/L; divide the Mg value by the Cr value to calculate the Mg:Cr ratio.

By IVI over 4h, give 0.1mmol/kg of elemental magnesium, using magnesium sulfate 50% (contains elemental magnesium 2mmol/mL; see Supply) diluted to 50mL with 5% glucose.

Simultaneously, start a 24h urine collection for magnesium and creatinine. Measure the total amounts of magnesium and creatinine excreted in mmol (*not* the concentrations in mmol/L).

Calculate % magnesium retention:

$$1 - \left[\frac{\text{24h urinary Mg (mmol)} - (\text{pre-infusion urinary Mg/Cr ratio (mmol/L)} \times \text{24h urinary Cr (mmol)})}{\text{dose of elemental magnesium infused (mmol)}}\right] \times 100$$

>50% retention implies definite deficiency.

Box D Magnesium as an analgesic

A number of studies have explored the effects of magnesium, mostly as an adjuvant analgesic for postoperative pain.

A meta-analysis of 27 RCTs concluded that peri-operative IV magnesium reduces postoperative pain and analgesic requirements in patients undergoing cardiovascular, orthopaedic and urogenital surgery.[32]

Further, 8 RCTs of spinal magnesium have all reported lower pain scores and decreased analgesic requirements.[34-41]

In an RCT of PO magnesium in patients with neuropathic pain, although the frequency of pain paroxysms and the emotional component of behaviour improved, there was no overall difference in pain intensity or quality of life.[42]

Cancer cells preferentially accumulate magnesium, which is used to activate or inhibit various metabolic and genetic pathways in order to promote cell survival and proliferation.[43] Animal studies suggest that magnesium deficiency inhibits the growth of the primary cancer but exacerbates metastatic disease, possibly by enhancing inflammation.[43] The relevance of these findings for patients is unknown.

9

Cautions

Generally, parenteral magnesium should not be given to patients with heart block or severe renal impairment. Risk of hypermagnesaemia in patients with renal impairment.

Undesirable effects

Flushing, sweating and sensation of warmth IV; diarrhoea PO. Also see features of magnesium excess in Box A.

Dose and use

Severe (serum magnesium <0.5mmol/L) and symptomatic hypomagnesaemia generally necessitates >1mmol/kg of magnesium; the route of choice is IV, given in divided doses over 3–5 days.[1,44]

Mild or asymptomatic hypomagnesaemia may be treated PO. If the cause of the magnesium deficiency persists, PO maintenance therapy will be needed.

In mild–moderate renal impairment, reduce IV replacement doses by 50% and monitor plasma magnesium daily. In severe renal impairment, avoid IV replacement if possible.

Prevention of deficiency

- magnesium-rich foods, e.g. meat, seafood, green leafy vegetables, cereals and nuts
- potassium-sparing diuretics, e.g. **amiloride**, also preserve magnesium.

IV correction of chronic deficiency

Because the degree of deficiency is difficult to determine from the plasma magnesium, replacement is empirical, guided by symptoms, plasma magnesium and renal function. Guidelines vary widely in their recommended doses, duration of infusion and need for monitoring, e.g. heart rate/rhythm, blood pressure and respiratory rate; as a minimum, these should be checked at baseline and if the patient feels unwell during an infusion. The infusion should be through a dedicated line into a central or peripheral vein. The following are examples.

Serum magnesium <0.5mmol/L with symptoms (life-threatening), e.g. arrhythmia, seizure

- give 8mmol IV over 10–15min
- give as 4mL of magnesium sulfate injection 50% (elemental magnesium 2mmol/mL) diluted to 10mL with sodium chloride 0.9% or dextrose 5%
- follow with IVI replacement as below.

Serum magnesium <0.5mmol/L with symptoms (not life-threatening)

- on the first day give about 0.5mmol/kg IVI, then 0.25mmol/kg IVI daily for 2–5 days until the deficiency is corrected
- give as an appropriate dose of magnesium sulfate injection 50% (elemental magnesium 2mmol/mL) added to 250mL sodium chloride 0.9% or dextrose 5% (maximum concentration 0.2mmol/mL)
- infuse over a convenient time interval, e.g. 1.5h; ensure the infusion rate is restricted to ≤0.6mmol/min to avoid exceeding the maximum renal tubular resorption capacity for magnesium
- if undesirable effects occur, e.g. hypotension, increase the infusion time, e.g. up to 4h
- check serum magnesium levels daily during replacement; there may be artificially high serum levels until equilibration occurs with the intracellular compartment.

IV is the parenteral route of choice. If PO and IV routes are not feasible, options include (in order of preference):

- IM magnesium sulfate: in severe deficiency, give 0.25–0.5mmol/kg/24h as above in divided doses, e.g. multiple injections q4–6h of magnesium sulfate injection 50% (elemental magnesium 2mmol/mL); can be painful. Although dilution to 0.8mmol/mL is recommended by some, this further reduces the practicality of this approach
- CSCI magnesium sulfate: data are limited, but use of an isotonic solution is recommended, i.e. 25mmol of magnesium sulfate in 100mL WFI.[45,46] Smaller maintenance doses may be more practical; 8mmol of magnesium sulfate diluted to 32mL with WFI was successfully given CSCI over 24h for about 2 months, replacing the need for frequent IV replacement.[47]

Serum magnesium >0.5mmol/L and <0.75mmol/L without symptoms

Begin with a trial of PO replacement. The main limiting factor is diarrhoea, as magnesium salts are generally poorly absorbed PO and have a laxative effect. It is uncommon with doses <40mmol/24h, and the risk is reduced by a gradual introduction and by taking magnesium with or after food.

Several magnesium PO products are now authorized for the treatment and prevention of magnesium deficiency, but are expensive:

- magnesium *aspartate* oral powder sachets (magnesium 10mmol/sachet):
  - ▷ give 1–2 sachets once daily dissolved in 50–200mL water, orange juice or tea (10–20mmol/24h)
- magnesium *glycerophosphate* chewable tablets or capsules (magnesium 4mmol):
  - ▷ give 1–2 tablets/capsules t.d.s. (12–24mmol/24h)
- magnesium *glycerophosphate* oral solution (magnesium 5mmol/5mL):
  - ▷ give 5mL q.d.s. (20mmol/24h).

Traditionally, other PO magnesium products, either unauthorized or authorized for other indications, e.g. laxatives, have been used.[48]

Although plasma magnesium levels may respond immediately to PO replacement, generally 6–12 months is required to *fully* correct a deficiency.[49] If poorly tolerated or ineffective, and in patients with a shorter prognosis, use IV replacement as above.

PO maintenance

To prevent recurrence of the deficit, prescribe magnesium ~24mmol/24h in divided doses with food. PO is used unless poorly tolerated or ineffective, e.g. malabsorption.

Supply

Magnesium *aspartate*

AsparMag® (Essential-Healthcare)

Oral powder elemental magnesium 10mmol sachets, 28 days @ 2 sachets once daily = £39.

Magnesium *glycerophosphate* (generic)

Tablets (chewable) elemental magnesium 4mmol tablets, 28 days @ 2 tablets t.d.s. (24mmol/24h) = £52. *Standard tablets are available (Mag-4®) but are significantly more expensive.*

Capsules elemental magnesium 1.6mmol, 2mmol, 4mmol, 28 days @ 8mmol t.d.s. = £127.

Oral solution elemental magnesium 4mmol/5mL, 5mmol/5mL 28 days @ 5mmol/5mL q.d.s. (20mmol/24h) = £90.

Magnesium *sulfate*

Injection 10% (100mg/mL), elemental magnesium 0.4mmol/mL, 10mL amp = £6.50.

Injection 50% (500mg/mL), elemental magnesium 2mmol/mL, 2mL, 5mL, 10mL amps = £1.75, £4.50 and £2.25 respectively; 20mL, 50mL and 100mL vials = £6.50, £9 and £8 respectively.

1 Martin KJ *et al.* (2009) Clinical consequences and management of hypomagnesemia. *Journal of the American Society of Nephrology*. **20**: 2291-2295.
2 Elin RJ (2010) Assessment of magnesium status for diagnosis and therapy. *Magnesium Research*. **23**: 1–5.
3 de Baaij JH *et al.* (2015) Magnesium in man: implications for health and disease. *Physiological Reviews*. **95**: 1–46.
4 Rosanoff A *et al.* (2012) Suboptimal magnesium status in the United States: are the health consequences underestimated? *Nutrition Reviews*. **70**: 153–164.
5 Yamamoto Y *et al.* (2016) Hydration with 15 mEq magnesium is effective at reducing the risk for cisplatin-induced nephrotoxicity in patients receiving cisplatin (>/=50 mg/m2) combination chemotherapy. *Anticancer Research*. **36**: 1873–1877.
6 Romani AM (2015) Cisplatin-induced renal toxicity magn...ified: role of magnesium deficiency in AKI onset. *American Journal of Physiology Renal Physiology*. **309**: F1005–1006.
7 Hodgkinson E *et al.* (2006) Magnesium depletion in patients receiving cisplatin-based chemotherapy. *Clinical Oncology*. **18**: 710–718.
8 Schilsky RL *et al.* (1982) Persistent hypomagnesemia following cisplatin chemotherapy for testicular cancer. *Cancer Treatment Reports*. **66**: 1767–1769.
9 Buckley JE *et al.* (1984) Hypomagnesemia after cisplatin combination chemotherapy. *Archives of Internal Medicine*. **144**: 2347–2348.
10 Costa A *et al.* (2011) Hypomagnesaemia and targeted anti-epidermal growth factor receptor (EGFR) agents. *Target Oncology*. **6**: 227–233.
11 Cao Y *et al.* (2010) Meta-analysis of incidence and risk of hypomagnesemia with cetuximab for advanced cancer. *Chemotherapy*. **56**: 459–465.
12 Mazur A *et al.* (2007) Magnesium and the inflammatory response: potential physiopathological implications. *Archives of Biochemistry and Biophysics*. **458**: 48–56.
13 Tejero-Taldo MI *et al.* (2006) The nerve-heart connection in the pro-oxidant response to Mg-deficiency. *Heart Failure Reviews*. **11**: 35–44.
14 Maier JA (2012) Endothelial cells and magnesium: implications in atherosclerosis. *Clinical Science*. **122**: 397–407.
15 Barbagallo M *et al.* (2009) Magnesium homeostasis and aging. *Magnesium Research*. **22**: 235–246.
16 Nielsen FH (2010) Magnesium, inflammation, and obesity in chronic disease. *Nutrition Reviews*. **68**: 333–340.
17 King DE (2009) Inflammation and elevation of C-reactive protein: does magnesium play a key role? *Magnesium Research*. **22**: 57–59.
18 Song Y *et al.* (2005) Magnesium intake, C-reactive protein, and the prevalence of metabolic syndrome in middle-aged and older U.S. women. *Diabetes Care*. **28**: 1438–1444.
19 Dibaba DT *et al.* (2014) Dietary magnesium intake is inversely associated with serum C-reactive protein levels: meta-analysis and systematic review. *European Journal of Clinical Nutrition*. **68**: 510–516.
20 Dibaba DT *et al.* (2014) Dietary magnesium intake and risk of metabolic syndrome: a meta-analysis. *Diabetic Medicine*. **31**: 1301–1309.
21 Dominguez LJ *et al.* (2006) Magnesium and muscle performance in older persons: the InCHIANTI study. *American Journal of Clinical Nutrition*. **84**: 419–426.
22 Pokan R *et al.* (2006) Oral magnesium therapy, exercise heart rate, exercise tolerance, and myocardial function in coronary artery disease patients. *British Journal of Sports Medicine*. **40**: 773–778.
23 Veronese N *et al.* (2014) Effect of oral magnesium supplementation on physical performance in healthy elderly women involved in a weekly exercise program: a randomized controlled trial. *American Journal of Clinical Nutrition*. **100**: 974–981.
24 Al-Khatib SM *et al.* (2003) What clinicians should know about the QT interval. *Journal of the American Medical Association*. **289**: 2120–2127.
25 Dyckner T and Wester P (1982) Magnesium deficiency – guidelines for diagnosis and substitution therapy. *Acta Medica Scandinavica*. **661**: 37–41.
26 Ismail Y and Ismail AA (2010) The underestimated problem of using serum magnesium measurements to exclude magnesium deficiency in adults; a health warning is needed for "normal" results. *Clinical Chemistry and Laboratory Medicine*. **48**: 323–327.
27 Ryzen E *et al.* (1985) Parenteral magnesium testing in the evaluation of magnesium deficiency. *Magnesium*. **4**: 137–147.
28 Crosby V *et al.* (2000) The importance of low magnesium in palliative care. *Palliative Medicine*. **14**: 544.
29 Zeng C *et al.* (2016) Analgesic effect and safety of single-dose intra-articular magnesium after arthroscopic surgery: a systematic review and meta-analysis. *Scientific Reports*. **6**: 38024.
30 Crosby V *et al.* (2000) The safety and efficacy of a single dose (500mg or 1g) of intravenous magnesium sulfate in neuropathic pain poorly responsive to strong opioid analgesics in patients with cancer. *Journal of Pain and Symptom Management*. **19**: 35–39.
31 Chiu HY *et al.* (2016) Effects of intravenous and oral magnesium on reducing migraine: a meta-analysis of randomized controlled trials. *Pain Physician*. **19**: E97–112.
32 Guo BL *et al.* (2015) Effects of systemic magnesium on post-operative analgesia: is the current evidence strong enough? *Pain Physician*. **18**: 405–418.
33 Bujalska-Zadrozny M *et al.* (2017) Magnesium enhances opioid-induced analgesia - What we have learnt in the past decades? *European Journal of Pharmaceutical Sciences*. **99**: 113–127.
34 Bilir A *et al.* (2007) Epidural magnesium reduces postoperative analgesic requirement. *British Journal of Anaesthesia*. **98**: 519–523.
35 Arcioni R *et al.* (2007) Combined intrathecal and epidural magnesium sulfate supplementation of spinal anesthesia to reduce post-operative analgesic requirements: a prospective, randomized, double-blind, controlled trial in patients undergoing major orthopedic surgery. *Acta Anaesthesiologica Scandinavica*. **51**: 482–489.
36 Farouk S (2008) Pre-incisional epidural magnesium provides pre-emptive and preventive analgesia in patients undergoing abdominal hysterectomy. *British Journal of Anaesthesia*. **101**: 694–699.
37 Ghatak T *et al.* (2010) Evaluation of the effect of magnesium sulphate vs. clonidine as adjunct to epidural bupivacaine. *Indian Journal of Anaesthesia*. **54**: 308–313.
38 Yousef AA and Amr YM (2010) The effect of adding magnesium sulphate to epidural bupivacaine and fentanyl in elective caesarean section using combined spinal-epidural anaesthesia: a prospective double blind randomised study. *International Journal of Obstetrics and Anesthesia*. **19**: 401–404.
39 Ouerghi S *et al.* (2011) The effect of adding intrathecal magnesium sulphate to morphine-fentanyl spinal analgesia after thoracic surgery. A prospective, double-blind, placebo-controlled research study. *Annales Francaises d'Anesthethesie et de Reanimation*. **30**: 25–30.
40 Khalili G *et al.* (2011) Effects of adjunct intrathecal magnesium sulfate to bupivacaine for spinal anesthesia: a randomized, double-blind trial in patients undergoing lower extremity surgery. *Journal of Anesthesia*. **25**: 892–897.
41 Khezri MB *et al.* (2012) Comparison of postoperative analgesic effect of intrathecal magnesium and fentanyl added to bupivacaine in patients undergoing lower limb orthopedic surgery. *Acta Anaesthesiol Taiwan*. **50**: 19–24.
42 Pickering G *et al.* (2011) Oral magnesium treatment in patients with neuropathic pain: a randomized clinical trial. *Magnesium Research*. **24**: 28–35.
43 Castiglioni S and Maier JA (2011) Magnesium and cancer: a dangerous liason. *Magnesium Research*. **24**: S92–100.

44 Miller S (1995) Drug-induced hypomagnesaemia. *Hospital Pharmacy*. **30**: 248–250.
45 UK Medicines Information (2017) How is acute hypomagnesaemia treated in adults. *Medicines Q&A*. www.evidence.nhs.uk.
46 UK Medicines Information (2019) Can magnesium sulfate be given subcutaneously? *Medicines Q&A*. www.evidence.nhs.uk.
47 Fenning SJ *et al.* (2018) Subcutaneous magnesium in the advanced cancer setting. *BMJ Supportive & Palliative Care*. **8**: 191–193.
48 UK Medicines Information (2015) What oral magnesium preparations are available in the UK and which preparation is preferred for the treatment and prevention of hypomagesaemia? *Medicines Q&A*. www.evidence.nhs.uk.
49 Zang X *et al.* (2016) The circulating concentration and 24-h urine excretion of magnesium dose- and time-dependently respond to oral magnesium supplementation in a meta-analysis of randomized controlled trials. *Journal of Nutrition*. **146**: 595–602.

Updated (minor change) December 2021

ZINC

Class: Metal element.

Indications: Zinc deficiency (zinc sulfate), Wilson's disease (zinc acetate), †anorexia due to taste changes, †wound healing.

Pharmacology

Zinc is an essential trace element with multiple functions. It is present in >300 enzymes, and has catalytic, structural and regulatory functions (Box A).[1-3] It occurs in all tissues, particularly muscle and bone, and to a lesser extent in skin and liver. Most is intracellular, and much is intranuclear. Plasma contains only 0.1% of the body's zinc, mostly bound to albumin.[4]

Box A Physiological functions of zinc

Gene expression and cellular stability
Zinc-dependent RNA and DNA polymerases and reverse transcriptase
Cell proliferation and differentiation
Regulation of apoptosis (cell-specific; either increases or decreases)
Zinc-finger transcription factors
Structural maintenance of biomembranes

Homeostasis and metabolism
Cellular signal and transmission
Hormone storage, synthesis and action, e.g. sex and thyroid hormones
Metabolism of proteins, carbohydrates and lipids
Tissue growth and repair
Neurosensory (cognition, behavioural response, taste, smell, appetite)

Antioxidant
Protects from free radical reactions
Component of super oxide dismutase (SOD)
Induces metal-binding protein production
Membrane stabilization

Anti-inflammatory
Inhibits expression of pro-inflammatory cytokines (IL-4, IL-6 and TNF-α)

Immune response
Thymulin activity
T-cell maturation and differentiation
Regulates cytokine production
Natural killer cell activity
T-lymphocyte activation
Direct effect on DNA for immune cell proliferation

Homeostasis is achieved primarily through regulation of intestinal absorption. When dietary zinc is high, intestinal metal-binding proteins increase, and these slow absorption.[3] With a very high intake, secondary homeostatic mechanisms operate, e.g. increased renal excretion and redistribution of tissue zinc.[4]

There are no significant stores of zinc in the body, and a constant dietary intake is essential. The UK reference nutrient intake (RNI) for daily dietary (elemental) zinc is 5.5–9.5mg in men and 4–7mg for women.[2,5] Sources include meat, seafood, dairy products, wholegrain cereals, legumes and nuts. Bio-availability of dietary zinc is about 20–30%, and is lower from plant sources because of phytate binding.[2]

Excessive intake is generally safe. However, acute and chronic poisoning has been reported.[3,6] Prolonged ingestion of high doses (50–300mg/24h elemental zinc) is associated with impaired immune function with leucopenia and neutropenia, sideroblastic anaemia and reduced ferritin levels. It can lead to secondary copper deficiency with increased low:high density lipoprotein cholesterol ratio and HbA_{1c}.[3,6] The safe upper levels for elemental zinc intake recommended in the UK are 25mg/day from supplements and 40mg/day in total (i.e. from supplements and diet combined).[6,7]

In the brain, zinc acts as a neurotransmitter, binding to a zinc-sensing G-coupled protein receptor, and also as a neuromodulator via interactions with multiple other channels and receptors, e.g. AMPA, $GABA_A$, NMDA, with an overall inhibitory effect.[8,9] However, as a consequence of various insults (e.g. trauma, ischaemia, hypoglycaemia), zinc may accumulate to toxic levels and cause neural damage and apoptosis. Further, altered zinc homeostasis is associated with the pathogenesis of depression, schizophrenia and various neurodegenerative diseases, e.g. Alzheimer's disease, MND/ALS, multiple sclerosis, Parkinson's disease.[8,10]

Zinc concentrations can be measured in the cellular components of blood (RBC, mononuclear cells and platelets), plasma, urine, faeces, skin, hair and saliva. Cellular zinc is sensitive, but measurement is complex.[11] Consequently, plasma concentration is widely used instead, with zinc deficiency defined as <15micromol/L.[12] However, plasma zinc may not reflect total body zinc, and is influenced by various factors, e.g. plasma protein, drugs (see Cautions), infection and inflammation.[2,6,11,13] Thus, when zinc deficiency is clinically suspected, even if the plasma zinc concentration is within the normal range, a therapeutic trial of replacement therapy should be considered.

Zinc deficiency can occur relatively rapidly as a result of inadequate dietary intake, poor intestinal absorption or increased loss due to conditions such as cancer, malabsorption, alcoholism, cirrhosis of the liver, renal disease, sickle cell anaemia and AIDS. Metal-binding proteins, in addition to binding zinc and other heavy metals such as copper, have a protective role scavenging toxic metals and free radicals, and improving immunity. However, in stressful states, e.g. inflammation and with increasing age, levels increase and bind more intracellular zinc. Consequently, the persistent sequestration of zinc leads to reduced bio-availability and a relative deficiency state.[3,14] The effects of zinc deficiency are numerous and reflect its multifunctional role and importance in gene expression, protein synthesis and enzyme function (Box B).[2,3,14]

Cellular zinc homeostasis is altered in many cancers and may contribute towards cell proliferation and metastasis. In most cancers, changes in zinc transporter expression and function result in reduced cell zinc levels; in some, levels are increased, e.g. breast cancer.[15]

Zinc may have a contributory role in cachexia. Systemic inflammation affects zinc transporters in cell membranes, leading to zinc accumulation in the liver and also skeletal muscle where, it is suggested, it could enhance protein catabolism and inhibit protein synthesis.[16] Further, this redistribution is also proposed to cause a deficiency of zinc elsewhere, resulting in systemic features of zinc deficiency, e.g. anorexia, hypogonadism and impaired immunity, which are common features of cachexia.[16] The beneficial effect on zinc-related anorexia is linked to an increase in leptin levels and by influencing the hypothalamic neuropeptides which regulate appetite.[17,18]

Treating zinc deficiency improves wound healing. Use of PO or topical zinc preparations in the absence of zinc deficiency has produced mixed results.[19-21]

Correction of zinc deficiency may improve dry mouth (xerostomia) and disturbances of taste and smell.[22-24] Improvement in taste acuity is also reported in idiopathic and radiotherapy-induced taste disorders,[24-27] but not in chronic renal failure or if drug-induced.[12,24] However, the evidence is of insufficient quality to make definite recommendations for this use of zinc.

Box B Consequences of zinc deficiency

Immunological
Increased risk of infections due to impaired cellular immunity
Reduced neutrophils, monocytes, natural killer cells
Reduced T-helper$_1$ cytokines (IL-2 and IFN-γ)
Reduced thymulin activity
Increased inflammation secondary to increased pro-inflammatory cytokines, NO, COX-2 and NF-κB

Other cellular effects
Increased apoptosis
Increased oxidative stress with lipid peroxidation of mitochondrial membranes

Haematological
Defective platelet aggregation
Iron-deficiency anaemia

Neuropsychological
Impaired smell, taste and vision
Impaired cognition
Behavioural disturbance
Depression

Gastro-intestinal
Anorexia
Diarrhoea
Gastric acid and pepsin secretion, causing mucosal damage

Hormonal
Thyroid hormone function
Hypogonadism and infertility

Dermatological
Dermatitis
Alopecia
Nail dystrophy
Delayed wound healing

Zinc deficiency is common in a wide range of oral mucosal diseases, present in up to one quarter of patients with, e.g., recurrent aphthous stomatitis, atrophic glossitis, burning mouth syndrome and idiopathic xerostomia.[28] In a small RCT, zinc supplementation reduced the severity of chemotherapy-related mucositis and xerostomia.[29]

Zinc acetate and zinc gluconate lozenges are of benefit in the common cold, shortening its duration by about one third (~3 days).[30,31] Benefit is seen with 80–90mg/24h elemental zinc, with higher doses no more effective. A lozenge is dissolved in the mouth every 2–3h while awake, starting within 24h of the onset of symptoms and continued for the duration of the cold. Prophylactic supplementation cannot be recommended, because of insufficient data. Note. Many OTC zinc products either contain an insufficient dose or include substances that bind zinc, e.g. citric acid.

There is inconclusive or insufficient evidence regarding zinc's effectiveness as a treatment for male infertility.[2] In combination with other antioxidant supplements, zinc may be of benefit in slowing the progression of age-related macular degeneration.[32]

Zinc *acetate* (± chelating agents **penicillamine, trientine**) is also used under specialist supervision to prevent the absorption of copper from the GI tract in Wilson's disease.[2]

Cautions

Acute renal impairment (zinc may accumulate). If taken for prolonged periods, monitor zinc and copper plasma concentrations, FBC and plasma cholesterol to detect incipient zinc toxicity and copper deficiency.

Drug interactions

PO zinc decreases GI absorption of PO bisphosphonates, chelating agents (**penicillamine, trientine**), **iron**, and quinolone and tetracycline antimicrobials. Absorption of PO zinc is decreased by **calcium** and **iron** supplements, chelating agents (**penicillamine, trientine**), phosphorus-containing products and tetracyclines. Separating administration times by 2–3h avoids these interactions.

Thiazides and loop diuretics increase the urinary excretion of zinc and, if used long-term, may lead to deficiency.

Undesirable effects

More common: gastric irritation, gastritis, dyspepsia, abdominal pain, nausea, vomiting, diarrhoea; these can be reduced by giving PO zinc with or after food.
Less common: headache, lethargy and irritability.

Dose and use

Zinc deficiency

- elemental zinc ≤50mg PO t.d.s., e.g. zinc sulfate (Solvazinc®) 1 tablet (elemental zinc 45mg) dissolved in water once daily–t.d.s. with or after food.

Supply

Solvazinc® (Galen)
Tablets effervescent zinc sulfate monohydrate 125mg (elemental zinc 45mg), 28 days @ 1 tablet t.d.s. = £12.

Many zinc products are available OTC (citrate, gluconate, glycinate, oxide and sulfate salts) as dietary supplements and as symptomatic treatment for the common cold.

1 Frassinetti S *et al.* (2006) The role of zinc in life: a review. *Journal of Environmental Pathology, Toxicology and Oncology*. **25**: 597–610.
2 Mason P (2006) Physiological and medicinal zinc. *Pharmaceutical Journal*. **276**: 271–274.
3 Stefanidou M *et al.* (2006) Zinc: a multipurpose trace element. *Archives of Toxicology*. **80**: 1–9.
4 King JC *et al.* (2000) Zinc homeostasis in humans. *Journal of Nutritrion*. **130**: 1360S–1366S.
5 COMA (1991) Committee on medical aspects of food and nutrition policy. Dietary reference values for food energy and nutrients for the United Kingdom. Report of the panel on dietary reference values. Hmso, london.
6 Expert Group on Vitamins and Minerals (EVM) (2003) Risk assessment: zinc: In: *Safe Upper Levels for Vitamins and Minerals*. pp.253–262. London: Food Standards Agency. Available from: www.food.gov.uk
7 Mason P (ed.) (2016) *Dietary Supplements*. London: Pharmaceutical Press. www.new.medicinescomplete.com (accessed July 2018).
8 Portbury SD and Adlard PA (2017) Zinc signal in brain diseases. *International Journal of Molecular Sciences*. **18**: 2506.
9 Sunuwar L *et al.* (2017) The zinc sensing receptor, znr/gpr39, in health and disease. *Frontiers Bioscience, Landmark*. **22**: 1469–1492.
10 Bredholt M and Frederiksen JL (2016) Zinc in multiple sclerosis: a systematic review and meta-analysis. *ASN Neuro*. **8**: 1–9.
11 Hambridge M (2003) Biomarkers of trace mineral intake and status. *Journal of Nutritrion*. **133**: 948S–955S.
12 Heyneman CA (1996) Zinc deficiency and taste disorders. *Annals of Pharmacotherapy*. **30**: 186–187.
13 Alpers DH (1994) Zinc and deficiencies of taste and smell. *Journal of the American Medical Association*. **272**: 1233–1234.
14 Wessels I *et al.* (2017) Zinc as a gatekeeper of immune function. *Nutrients*. **9**: 1286.
15 Bafaro E *et al.* (2017) The emerging role of zinc transporters in cellular homeostasis and cancer. *Signal Transduction and Targeted Therapy*. **2**: e17029.
16 Siren PM and Siren MJ (2010) Systemic zinc redistribution and dyshomeostasis in cancer cachexia. *Journal of Cachexia Sarcopenia Muscle*. **1**: 23–33.
17 Ezeoke CC and Morley JE (2015) Pathophysiology of anorexia in the cancer cachexia syndrome. *Journal of Cachexia, Sarcopenia and Muscle*. **6**: 287–302.
18 Suzuki H *et al.* (2011) Zinc as an appetite stimulator – the possible role of zinc in the progression of diseases such as cachexia and sarcopenia. *Recent Patents on Food, Nutrition and Agriculture*. **3**: 226–231.
19 Wilkinson EA (2014) Oral zinc for arterial and venous leg ulcers. *Cochrane Database of Systematic Reviews*. **9**: CD001273. www.thecochranelibrary.com
20 Momen-Heravi M *et al.* (2017) The effects of zinc supplementation on wound healing and metabolic status in patients with diabetic foot ulcer: a randomized, double-blind, placebo-controlled trial. *Wound Repair and Regeneration*. **25**: 512–520.
21 Lin PH *et al.* (2018) Zinc in wound healing modulation. *Nutrients*. **10**: 16 doi:10.3390.

22 Tanaka M (2002) Secretory function of the salivary gland in patients with taste disorders or xerostomia: correlation with zinc deficiency. *Acta Otolaryngolica Supplementum*. 134–141.

23 Henkin RI *et al.* (1999) Efficacy of exogenous oral zinc in treatment of patients with carbonic anhydrase vi deficiency. *American Journal of Medical Sciences*. **318**: 392–405.

24 Kumbargere Nagraj S *et al.* (2017) Interventions for managing taste disturbances. *Cochrane Database of Systematic Reviews*. **12**: CD010470. www.thecochranelibrary.com

25 Heckmann SM *et al.* (2005) Zinc gluconate in the treatment of dysgeusia – a randomized clinical trial. *Journal of Dental Research*. **84**: 35–38.

26 Ripamonti C *et al.* (1998) A randomized, controlled clinical trial to evaluate the effects of zinc sulfate on cancer patients with taste alterations caused by head and neck irradiation. *Cancer*. **82**: 1938–1945.

27 Najafizade N *et al.* (2013) Preventive effects of zinc sulfate on taste alterations in patients under irradiation for head and neck cancers: a randomized placebo-controlled trial. *Journal of Research in Medical Sciences*. **18**: 123–126.

28 Bao ZX *et al.* (2016) Serum zinc levels in 368 patients with oral mucosal diseases: A preliminary study. *Medicina Oral, Patologia Oral Y Cirufia Bucal*. **21**: e335–340.

29 Arbabi-kalati F *et al.* (2012) Evaluation of the efficacy of zinc sulfate in the prevention of chemotherapy-induced mucositis: a double-blind randomized clinical trial. *Archives of Iranian Medicine*. **15**: 413–417.

30 Hemila H *et al.* (2016) Zinc acetate lozenges for treating the common cold: an individual patient data meta-analysis. *British Journal of Clinical Pharmacology*. **82**: 1393–1398.

31 Hemila H (2017) Zinc lozenges and the common cold: a meta-analysis comparing zinc acetate and zinc gluconate, and the role of zinc dosage. *Journal of the Royal Society of Medicine Open*. **8**: 2054270417694291.

32 NICE (2018) Age related macular degeneration. *Clinical Guideline*. NG82 www.nice.org.uk

Updated January 2019

10: MUSCULOSKELETAL AND JOINT DISEASES

10

DEPOT CORTICOSTEROID INJECTIONS

Indications: Inflammation of joints and soft tissues, †pain in superficial bones (e.g. rib, scapula, iliac crest), †intractable pain caused by spinal metastases, †malignant (peritoneal) ascites.

Contra-indications: Untreated local or systemic infection. Must *not* be given IV or IT.

Pharmacology

Corticosteroids have an anti-inflammatory effect; they reduce the concentration of algesic substances present in inflammation which sensitize nerve endings.[1] Further, in animal studies, when injected locally around an injured nerve, corticosteroids have been shown to have a direct inhibitory effect on the spontaneous activity associated with nerve injury.[2]

For many years depot injections of corticosteroids have been given epidurally in selected patients with non-malignant radicular (nerve root) compression pain associated with spinal pathology, e.g. lumbar disc herniation, sciatica.[3] However, a systematic review found only weak RCT evidence for their efficacy.[4] Even so, in patients with spinal metastases and intractable radicular pain, clinical experience indicates that ED depot corticosteroids are sometimes helpful.

Cautions

Depot formulations may result in suppression of the hypothalamic–pituitary–adrenal axis for up to 4 weeks. National guidance recommends that patients taking the equivalent of **prednisolone** ≥5mg daily for ≥4 weeks by *any* route should be warned not to abruptly stop treatment, and should be given both a steroid *treatment* and a steroid *emergency* card (see Systemic corticosteroids, p.562, Box G, p.563, and Box H, p.563).[5] Also see national guidance for full details on dose adjustments required to cover sick days, surgery or invasive treatment.[5]

History of severe affective disorders (e.g. depression, bipolar disorder) or steroid-induced psychosis, epilepsy, glaucoma, myasthenia gravis, hypertension, CHF, predisposition to thrombophlebitis, peptic ulceration, diverticulitis, ulcerative colitis, severe hepatic impairment, renal impairment, hypothyroidism, osteoporosis.

Depot formulations may result in symptomatic hperglycaemia for several days in patients with diabetes mellitus. Injection under a rib may be complicated by a pneumothorax.

Corticosteroids may mask or alter the presentation of infection in immunocompromised patients; such patients should not receive live vaccines and, if exposed to chickenpox, should receive varicella-zoster immunoglobulin.

Drug interactions

Pharmacodynamic interactions include antagonism of antihypertensive, antidiabetic and diuretic drugs, and increased risk of hypokalaemia if used concurrently with β_2 agonists (e.g. **salbutamol**, **terbutaline**) or other potassium-wasting drugs.

Undesirable effects

Undesirable effects associated with systemic corticosteroids can also occur with depot injections (see Systemic corticosteroids, p.560), including adrenal suppression.

Occasionally, a patient develops lipodystrophy (local fat necrosis) which results in an indentation of the overlying skin.

ED injection of **methylprednisolone *acetate*** (unauthorized route) has been associated with wound dehiscence and with loss of sphincter control.

Dose and use

Patients who are corticosteroid-dependent should be given both a steroid *treatment* and a steroid *emergency* card (see Cautions).

Injection into and/or over painful bone secondary[6]

- infiltrate the skin and SC tissues overlying the point of maximal bone tenderness with local anaesthetic
- with the tip of the needle pressing against the tender bone, inject depot **methylprednisolone *acetate*** 80mg in 2mL
- if there are two painful bones, inject 40mg at each spot; generally, limit the total amount given at any one time to 80mg.

Also, for rib lesions, reposition the needle under the rib and inject 5mL of **bupivacaine** 0.5% to anaesthetize the intercostal nerve. Complete or good relief occurs in about 70% of patients. If of benefit, injections can be repeated if the pain returns, but not within 2 weeks.

†Epidural injection[3]

Depot **methylprednisolone *acetate*** 80mg in 2mL (unauthorized route). A single ED injection is given, followed if necessary by a further 1–2 injections at 3–4 week intervals. The effect of ED corticosteroids is unpredictable and may not peak until 1 week after an injection. Depot corticosteroids cannot be injected through an ED bacterial filter. In some countries, depot **triamcinolone** or a *non-depot* formulation of **dexamethasone *sodium phosphate*** is used for ED injection.

†Malignant (peritoneal) ascites

After a preliminary paracentesis, instil intra-abdominally via the drain:

- **triamcinolone *acetonide*** 8mg/kg, to a maximum of 520mg (13 vials of the 40mg/mL depot injection) *or*
- **methylprednisolone *acetate*** 10mg/kg, to a maximum of 640mg (8 vials of the 80mg/2mL depot injection).

In an open study, the mean interval between paracentesis doubled to 18 days.[7] When neither of the above are available, another alternative is **triamcinolone *hexacetonide*** 10mg/kg, to a maximum of 640mg (32 ampoules of the 20mg/mL depot injection); however, it is more expensive.

Supply

Methylprednisolone *acetate*
Depo-Medrone® (Pfizer)
Depot injection (aqueous suspension) 40mg/mL, 1mL vial = £3.50, 2mL vial = £6, 3mL vial = £9.

Triamcinolone *acetonide*
Adcortyl® Intra-articular/Intradermal (Bristol-Myers Squibb)
Depot injection (aqueous suspension) 10mg/mL, 5mL vial = £3.75. *Contains benzyl alcohol.*

Kenalog® Intra-articular/Intramuscular (Bristol-Myers Squibb)
Depot injection (aqueous suspension) 40mg/mL, 1mL vial = £1.50. *Contains benzyl alcohol.*

Triamcinolone *hexacetonide* (generic)
Depot injection (aqueous suspension) 20mg/mL, 1mL amp = £12. *Contains benzyl alcohol.*

1 Pybus P (1984) Osteoarthritis: a new neurological method of pain control. *Medical Hypothesis*. **14**: 413–422.
2 Devor M *et al.* (1985) Corticosteroids reduce neuroma hyperexcitability. In: HL Fields *et al.* (eds), *Advances in Pain Research and Therapy*, Vol 9. Raven Press, New York, pp. 451–455.
3 McLain RF *et al.* (2004) Epidural steroids for back and leg pain: mechanism of action and efficacy. *Cleveland Clinic Journal of Medicine*. **71**: 961–970.
4 Armon C *et al.* (2007) Assessment: use of epidural steroid injections to treat radicular lumbosacral pain: report of the Therapeutics and Technology Assessment Subcommittee of the American Academy of Neurology. *Neurology*. **68**: 723–729.
5 Simpson H *et al.* (2020) Guidance for the prevention and emergency management of adult patients with adrenal insufficiency. *Clinical Medicine*. **20**: 371–378.
6 Rowell NP (1988) Intralesional methylprednisolone for rib metastases: an alternative to radiotherapy? *Palliative Medicine*. **2**: 153–155.
7 Mackey J *et al.* (2000) A phase II trial of triamcinolone hexacetanide for symptomatic recurrent malignant ascites. *Journal of Pain and Symptom Management*. **19**: 193–199.

Updated (minor change) October 2021

RUBEFACIENTS AND OTHER TOPICAL PRODUCTS

Indications: Soft tissue pains (rubefacients, topical NSAIDs), pain relief in osteoarthritis of the hand or knee (**capsaicin** cream 0.025%, topical NSAIDs),[1] post-herpetic neuralgia (after lesions have healed), diabetic neuralgia (**capsaicin** cream 0.075%), peripheral neuropathic pain (**capsaicin** TD patch 8%), †notalgia paraesthetica.

Contra-indications: Inflamed or broken skin.
Capsaicin TD patch 8%: Do not apply to the face or head.
Topical NSAIDs: If nasal polyps or history of asthma, angioedema, urticaria or acute rhinitis precipitated by aspirin or another NSAID.

Pharmacology

Rubefacients act by counter-stimulation of the skin, closing the pain 'gate' in the dorsal horn of the spinal cord.[2,3] Further benefit is obtained by the inclusion of **levomenthol (menthol)**. This cools the skin for several hours by acting on heat-sensitive transient receptor potential (TRP) channels expressed on sensory nerve endings.[4,5] **Levomenthol**-containing rubefacients have been used as home remedies for tension headache, muscle spasm and joint pain. (**Levomenthol** is also an ingredient in several topical antipruritic products; see p.685.)

Capsaicin

Capsaicin, a naturally occurring alkaloid found in chilli peppers and related plants, is a TRPV1 (vanilloid type 1) agonist. TRPV1 is a cation channel found on nociceptors and activated by heat, acidity and inflammation. Thus, **capsaicin** initially causes a sensation of warmth or pain, depending on concentration. However, the resultant calcium influx inactivates the TRPV1 channel and adjacent N- and T-type voltage-gated calcium channels, reducing excitability of the nociceptor. A variety of 'upstream' effects have been observed, including substance P depletion.[6]

In an open study of topical **capsaicin** cream 0.025% in post-axillary dissection pain, 12 of 18 women reported benefit after 1 month, eight of whom had a good or excellent response; after 6 months, most still had good relief.[7] An RCT of **capsaicin** cream 0.075% for 6 weeks gave comparable results: 8 of 13 patients had ≥50% improvement, five of whom had a good or excellent result.[8] Benefit was mainly in relation to stabbing pain.

In an RCT in 99 patients with persistent neuropathic pain after cancer surgery, **capsaicin** cream 0.075% produced a mean reduction in pain scores of >50%, compared with <20% for placebo. Improvement was seen most often in women with post-mastectomy pain.[9]

However, a systematic review was unable to reach a firm conclusion about benefit from 0.075% **capsaicin** cream in neuropathic pain generally.[10]

A TD patch containing **capsaicin** 8% is available for diabetic and non-diabetic painful neuropathy, e.g. post-herpetic or HIV. This was developed to deliver high-concentration **capsaicin** to the cutaneous nociceptors in a single application, thereby achieving rapid 'knock-out' of their function, as opposed to the periods of enhanced sensitivity and slow desensitization seen after repeated application of 0.025% and 0.075% creams. A systematic review found that TD **capsaicin** provided long-term pain relief after a single application. There was moderate quality evidence for post-herpetic neuralgia, with NNTs of 8.8 and 7 for patients grading themselves as 'much or very much better' at 8 and 12 weeks respectively. NNT values for reductions in pain intensity of ≥30% and ≥50% at 8 and 12 weeks were between 10 and 12. The quality of evidence was very low in other conditions. In HIV-related neuropathy, the NNT for reduction in pain intensity of ≥30% at 12 weeks was 11. In diabetic neuropathy, compared to placebo, about 10% and 3% more patients obtained a reduction in pain intensity of ≥30% and ≥50% respectively, at 12 weeks.[11] TD **capsaicin** patches are generally restricted to specialist pain clinics, when more usual options are either ineffective or not tolerated.

Capsaicin cream is of benefit in histamine-related pruritus, aquagenic pruritus, and pruritus associated with uraemia, nodular prurigo, psoriasis and post-axillary dissection syndrome (see Topical antipruritics, p.685).[5,12] Benefit is also seen with pruritus caused by notalgia paraesthetica (nerve injury, often caused by entrapment, of the dorsal ramus of the T2–T6 thoracic nerves, which causes pruritus and/or altered sensation in the areas of skin between or below the shoulder blade on either side of the back).[13,14]

Topical NSAIDs

Topical NSAIDs are of value for the relief of pain associated with soft tissue trauma, e.g. strains and sprains, inflammation of superficial joints, early osteoarthritis of the hand or knee.[1,15] Topically applied salicylates and some other NSAIDs can achieve local high SC concentrations and therapeutically effective concentrations within synovial fluid and peri-articular tissues similar to those seen after PO administration.[16-19]

A Cochrane review compared topical NSAIDs with placebo in *acute* musculoskeletal pain over about 1 week and found using moderate- to high-quality evidence that the NNTs for a 50% reduction in pain were lowest for **diclofenac** Emulgel® (1.8) and **ketoprofen** gel (2.5).[15] In *chronic* musculoskeletal pain (mostly hand and knee osteoarthritis) assessed over 6–12 weeks, NNTs for the same outcome were higher: **diclofenac** gel (9.8) and **ketoprofen** gel (6.9).[15] The evidence for all other topical salicylate or NSAID therapies was considered low/very low.

Pharmacokinetic details for **capsaicin** products and topical NSAIDs are shown in Table 1.

Table 1 Pharmacokinetic details for capsaicin products and topical NSAIDs

	Capsaicin cream 0.025% and 0.075%	*Capsaicin TD patch 8%*	*Topical NSAIDs*
Onset of action	Counter-stimulation generally immediate. 1 week in osteoarthritis, but full effect may not be seen for ≤2 months. 2–4 weeks in neuralgia	1–14 days in peripheral neuropathy	Product- and drug-dependent
Duration of action	No data; manufacturers advise applying q4–6h	≥12 weeks in peripheral and HIV-related neuropathy; manufacturers advise a 3-month gap between applications	Product- and drug-dependent; manufacturers advise applying b.d.–q.d.s.

Cautions

General

Avoid contact with eyes, mucous membranes and inflamed or broken skin; discontinue if rash develops. Do not cover with occlusive dressings or tight bandages.

Capsaicin cream 0.025% and 0.075%

Avoid hot baths or showers immediately before application, because they can enhance the burning sensation. Avoid inhaling the vapour from the cream. Wash hands immediately after application (unless treating the hands, in which case wash them 30min after application).

*Capsaicin TD patch 8%

Unstable or poorly controlled blood pressure, heart disease (see Undesirable effects). The painful burning sensation may necessitate local cooling (e.g. with a cold compress) or systemic analgesia. Avoid inhaling the vapour from the patch. Special precautions are required for handling (see Dose and use).

Topical NSAIDs

History of peptic ulcer, renal disease or asthma. Wash hands immediately after application (unless treating the hands, in which case wash them 30min after application). May cause photosensitivity, particularly **ketoprofen**. Avoid exposing the treated area to sunlight when using topical **ketoprofen**, and for 2 weeks afterwards.

Provided very large amounts are not applied, undesirable effects and drug interactions are much less likely with topical NSAIDs, because plasma concentrations are much lower, than with systemic NSAIDs. Conversely, skin reactions (e.g. rash) occur more commonly with topical NSAIDS.[1]

Undesirable effects

The commonest undesirable effect of **capsaicin** cream is tingling, stinging or burning at the site of application. This effect is thought to be related to the initial release of substance P from C fibres. The stinging and burning generally decreases with continued applications, often clearing in a few days but sometimes persisting for >4 weeks. Some patients discontinue treatment because of this. Runny eyes and respiratory tract irritation, causing coughing and sneezing, may result from rubbing the eyes and/or inhaling **capsaicin** vapour when applying the cream. Breathlessness and exacerbation of asthma have occurred occasionally.

Almost all patients experience local erythema and a burning sensation with **capsaicin** TD patches, unless the area is pretreated with local anaesthetic (see Dose and use). Other common local effects (1–10% of patients) are itching, blistering, swelling and dryness. Uncommon symptoms (1–10 per 1,000 patients) include eye irritation, raised blood pressure, arrhythmia (including atrioventricular block), palpitations, cough, throat irritation, loss of taste sensation, muscle spasm, reduced sensation in limbs, local wheals, prickling sensation and bruising.

Large quantities of topical NSAIDs have been associated with systemic effects (e.g. hypersensitivity, rash, asthma, renal impairment[20]) and potentiation of **warfarin**, occasionally leading to bleeding.[21] Local reactions include drying, reddening, burning sensations and contact dermatitis. A Cochrane review found that, in short-term studies, topical NSAIDs and placebo produced a similar incidence of local reactions and systemic undesirable effects (about 6% and 3% respectively).[15]

Dose and use

Capsaicin cream 0.025–0.075%

- apply a pea-sized amount t.d.s.–q.d.s. (the manufacturers specify q.d.s. initially for the 0.025% cream), leaving at least 4h between applications.

The burning sensation associated with the application of **capsaicin** cream is intensified and/or prolonged when larger quantities are applied (particularly with the higher strength) or if initially applied less frequently than t.d.s.–q.d.s. If the burning is severe, topical **lidocaine** or another local anaesthetic can be applied before **capsaicin** in the first few weeks of treatment.

Because heat and humidity influence dysaesthesia, patients should avoid activities that cause excessive sweating, e.g. exercise, taking a hot bath, immediately before application. Occlusion and tight bandaging should also be avoided.

Patients should apply the cream using gentle massage, avoiding contact with eyes, mucous membranes and broken/inflamed skin. *Patients must wash their hands after applying the cream to avoid subsequent unintentional contact with the eyes (unless treating the hands, in which case wash them 30min after application).*

*Capsaicin TD patch 8%

Health professionals should wear nitrile gloves when handling the patches and cleansing solution; latex gloves do *not* provide adequate protection. Also consider using protective masks and safety glasses to avoid accidental contact of aerosolized **capsaicin** particles with the eyes and mucous membranes, particularly when removing the patch.

- mark out the most painful areas with ink
- depending on the size of the painful areas, up to 4 patches may be applied simultaneously, or a patch may be cut to fit
- wash the skin in the treatment area with soap and water and dry thoroughly; any hair may be clipped but not shaved
- because most patients experience a burning sensation when the patches are applied, pretreat the area with topical **lidocaine** or another local anaesthetic 1h before applying the patches; wash off the local anaesthetic cream/ointment and thoroughly dry the skin before applying the **capsaicin** patch
- leave patches in place for:
  - ▷ 30min if applied to the feet
  - ▷ 1h if applied elsewhere
- if necessary, disposable socks or an open-weave bandage can be used to keep the patch in place
- when removing patches, roll them inwards to enclose the remaining **capsaicin**
- use the cleansing gel supplied to remove any traces of **capsaicin** from the patient's skin, both after any accidental contact and after removing the patches; leave the gel on the skin for 1min then wipe off
- wash the skin with soap and water after using the cleansing gel
- treatment can be repeated after 3 months if necessary.

Used patches, gloves, wipes, socks and bandages should be placed in a plastic bag and disposed of safely.

Topical NSAIDs

- generally apply b.d.–q.d.s.

Supply

Capsaicin

Zacin® (Teva)
Cream 0.025%, 45g = £18.

Axsain® (Teva)
Cream 0.075%, 45g = £15.

Qutenza® (Astellas)
TD patch 8% (contains 179mg **capsaicin**), 1 patch (with cleansing gel) = £210.

Diclofenac

Voltarol Emulgel® (GlaxoSmithKline)
Gel 1.16%, 100g = £4.50; 2.32% 30g, 50g, 100g = £4.50, £6.50 and £11; *also available OTC.*

Ketoprofen (generic)

Gel 2.5%, 50g, 100g = £1.50 and £3.25.

For **levomenthol** products, see Topical antipruritics, p.685.

1 NICE (2013) Osteoarthritis. *Clinical Knowledge Summaries*. http://cks.nice.org.uk
2 Melzack R and Wall P (1965) Pain mechanisms: a new theory. *Science*. **150**: 971–979.
3 Melzack R. (1991) The gate control theory 25 years later: new perspectives on phantom limb pain. In: Bond M, Charlton J, Woolf C, editors. *Proceedings of the VIth World Congress on Pain* Amsterdam: Elsevier Science. pp. 9–21.
4 Peier AM *et al.* (2002) A TRP channel that senses cold stimuli and menthol. *Cell*. **108**: 705–715.
5 Patel T *et al.* (2007) Menthol: a refreshing look at this ancient compound. *Journal of the American Academy of Dermatology*. **57**: 873–878.
6 Fattori V *et al.* (2016) Capsaicin: current understanding of its mechanisms and therapy of pain and other pre-clinical and clinical uses. *Molecules*. **21**: 844.
7 Watson C *et al.* (1989) The postmastectomy pain syndrome and the effect of topical capsaicin. *Pain*. **38**: 177–186.
8 Watson CPN and Evans RJ (1992) Post-mastectomy pain syndrome and topical capsaicin: a randomized trial. *Pain*. **51**: 375–379.
9 Ellison N *et al.* (1997) Phase III placebo-controlled trial of capsaicin cream in the management of surgical neuropathic pain in cancer patients. *Journal of Clinical Oncology*. **15**: 2974–2980.
10 Derry S and Moore RA (2012) Topical capsaicin (low concentration) for chronic neuropathic pain in adults. *Cochrane Database of Systematic Reviews*. CD010111. www.thecochranelibrary.com

11 Derry S *et al.* (2017) Topical capsaicin (high concentration) for chronic neuropathic pain in adults. *Cochrane Database of Systematic Reviews*. **1**: CD007393. www.thecochranelibrary.com
12 Xander C *et al.* (2013) Pharmacological interventions for pruritus in adult palliative care patients. *Cochrane Database of Systematic Reviews*. **6**: CD008320. www.thecochranelibrary.com
13 Bernstein JE (1988) Capsaicin in dermatologic disease. *Seminars in Dermatology*. **7**: 304–309.
14 Breneman D *et al.* (1992) Topical capsaicin for treatment of hemodialysis-related pruritus. *Journal of the American Academy of Dermatology*. **26**: 91–94.
15 Derry S *et al.* (2017) Topical analgesics for acute and chronic pain in adults – an overview of Cochrane Reviews. *Cochrane Database of Systematic Reviews*. **5**: CD008609. www.thecochranelibrary.com
16 Mondino A *et al.* (1983) Kinetic studies of ibuprofen on humans. Comparative study for the determination of blood concentrations and metabolites following local and oral administration. *Medizinische Welt*. **34**: 1052–1054.
17 Chlud K and Wagener H (1987) Percutaneous nonsteroidal anti-inflammatory drug (NSAID) therapy with particular reference to pharmacokinetic factors. *EULAR Bulletin*. **2**: 40–43.
18 Peters H *et al.* (1987) Percutaneous kinetics of ibuprofen (German). *Aktuelle Rheumatologie*. **12**: 208–211.
19 Dominkus M *et al.* (1996) Comparison of tissue and plasma levels of ibuprofen after oral and topical administration. *Arzneimittelforschung*. **46**: 1138–1143.
20 O'Callaghan C *et al.* (1994) Renal disease and use of topical NSAIDs. *British Medical Journal*. **308**: 110–111.
21 Makris UE *et al.* (2010) Adverse effects of topical nonsteroidal antiinflammatory drugs in older adults with osteoarthritis: a systematic literature review. *Journal of Rheumatology*. **37**: 1236–1243.

Updated (minor change) December 2019

10

SKELETAL MUSCLE RELAXANTS

Skeletal muscle relaxants are used to relieve painful chronic muscle spasm and spasticity associated with neural injury, e.g. paraplegia, post-stroke, multiple sclerosis and, sometimes, motor neurone disease/amyotrophic lateral sclerosis (MND/ALS),[1] and also troublesome cramp. †**Baclofen** (p.658) is also used to relieve hiccup. Most skeletal muscle relaxants act centrally (Table 1).

Table 1 Skeletal muscle relaxants; see individual monographs for more detailed explanation and references

Site of action	*Mode of action*	*Examples*	*Comments*
Central nervous system	$GABA_A$ mimetic	Benzodiazepines (p.163)	Avoid prolonged use (≥4 weeks)
	$GABA_B$ agonist	Baclofen (p.658)	A common first-line choice
	α_2 agonist	Tizanidine (p.662)	
	N-type Ca_V blocker	Gabapentin (p.297)	
	CB_1 agonist	Cannabinoids (p.251)	Limited efficacy; reserved for spasticity refractory to conventional treatments
Skeletal muscle	Ryanodine Ca channel blocker[a]	Dantrolene (p.661)	Severe hepatotoxicity
		Quinine (Box C)	QT prolongation; thrombocytopenia

a. by blocking ryanodine calcium channels on the sarcoplasmic reticulum, dantrolene and quinine reduce the release of calcium responsible for muscle contraction.

Spasticity

All skeletal muscle relaxants may reduce voluntary muscle power. This can be a disadvantage in people with hemiplegia or paraplegia if increased spastic muscle tone is what enables them to walk or function more independently. Thus, generally, dose escalation should be spread out over 4–8 weeks to balance the benefits of reduced spasticity with possible loss of functional performance and independence.

In contrast, in patients unable to use their limbs because of severe spasticity or paralysis or motor weakness, the dose can be escalated more rapidly. For these patients, sedation is likely to be the dose-limiting factor.[2]

There is low-level evidence that spasticity in multiple sclerosis can be improved by exercise programmes, magnetic stimulation and electromagnetic therapies.[3]

Cramp

Cramp has many causes (Box A), including drugs (Box B). With diuretics, it relates to volume depletion ± electrolyte imbalance, i.e. loss of sodium and magnesium (p.638). Cramp with **cisplatin** possibly relates to both hypomagnesaemia and peripheral neuropathy. In many cases, the mechanism is not known.

As always, it is important to consider correcting the correctable. Cramp cannot be induced or sustained in a stretched muscle, and calf stretching movements (both active and passive) and exercise are useful non-drug measures, particularly before going to bed,[4] despite the lack of a strong evidence base.[5,6]

Drug treatment of lower limb muscle cramp is similar to that of spasticity.[7] The use of **quinine** to relieve nocturnal cramp is now discouraged (Box C).

Box A Causes of cramp[4]

Idiopathic
Exercise
Old age (nocturnal leg cramps)

Acute extracellular volume depletion
Diuretics
Excessive sweating ('heat cramps')
Haemodialysis
GI fluid loss (diarrhoea, vomiting)

Drugs (Box B)

Endocrine
Hypo-adrenalism
Hypothyroidism
Pregnancy

Lower motor neurone disorders
MND/ALS
Neuropathy
Radiculopathy

Metabolic
Cirrhosis
Hypomagnesaemia
Renal impairment

Miscellaneous
Autoimmune disease
(antibodies to voltage-gated potassium channels)
Hereditary disorders

Box B Drug-induced cramps[4]

ACE inhibitors
- enalapril
- ramipril

Amitriptyline
Amphotericin B
β_2-agonists
- salbutamol
- terbutaline

Bisphosphonates
- pamidronate
- zoledronic acid

Celecoxib

Chemotherapy
- cisplatin
- vincristine

Cimetidine
Clofibrate (not UK)
Diuretics
Lithium
Statins
Steroids
- beclometasone (by inhaler)
- medroxyprogesterone acetate
- prednisolone

Choice of drug

Baclofen, **dantrolene**, **tizanidine** and **diazepam** are all authorized for use in spasticity. **Baclofen**, **tizanidine** and **diazepam** act principally on spinal and supraspinal sites within the CNS; **dantrolene** (and **quinine**) acts on muscle; see Table 1. There is no clear evidence that any one drug is superior to the others.[15-17]

If there is no concurrent indication for a benzodiazepine, **baclofen** is generally a good first-line choice, particularly if long-term treatment is likely. For the use of **diazepam** as a muscle relaxant, see p.171.

Use in renal or hepatic impairment

Skeletal muscle relaxants differ in their potential to cause toxicity when renal or hepatic function is impaired. For information on their use in ESRF and severe hepatic impairment, see Chapter 17 (p.746) and Chapter 18 (p.776).

Box C Quinine and cramp

Quinine is more effective than placebo in reducing the frequency and intensity of cramp at doses of 200–500mg/24h, most commonly 300mg.[8]

Compared to placebo, undesirable effects were higher with quinine, the most common being GI (6%), headache (5%) and tinnitus (1%). These were mostly minor, with no difference seen in major undesirable effects or withdrawals.[8]

Even so, various regulatory agencies consider that, because alternatives are available, the collective risks associated with using quinine for cramp are too high to permit continued routine use:

- rare but serious undesirable effects:
  - ▷ thrombocytopenia → severe bleeding (several deaths have been reported)
  - ▷ haemolytic–uraemic syndrome → permanent renal damage
  - ▷ cardiac arrhythmias → via prolongation of the QT interval or worsening of underlying conduction defect
- toxicity in overdose → permanent blindness or death
- serious drug interactions with, e.g., digoxin, warfarin.[9-11]

Consequently, the MHRA advises that quinine should not be used for nocturnal cramp unless the following criteria are all met:

- treatable causes have been ruled out
- non-drug measures have failed
- cramps regularly cause loss of sleep
- they are very painful or frequent.[9]

Further, a case control study of patients with idiopathic cramp or restless legs found a small but significant increased risk of all-cause mortality in those receiving quinine ≥100mg/24h for at least 1 year compared with those not receiving quinine. There was a dose and age effect; mortality was greater in those *under* 50.[12]

Typical doses of quinine are:

- quinine *sulfate* 200mg at bedtime, increased if necessary to 300mg at bedtime
- quinine *bisulfate* (not UK) 300mg at bedtime (equivalent to *sulfate* 200mg).

During the early stages of treatment, patients should be monitored for signs of thrombocytopenia, e.g. unexplained petechiae, bruising or bleeding.

Treatment should be discontinued after 4 weeks if there is no benefit, and interrupted approximately every 3 months to re-evaluate benefit.[5,9]

In people with MND/ALS, there is limited evidence to support one treatment over another for cramp;[13] NICE guidelines recommend quinine first-line because (in 2016) it was cheaper than baclofen and other drugs.[14] However, the costs of quinine and baclofen PO are now similar.

Table 2 Anti-epileptics for treating cramp[a,4]

Drug	*Dose*
Gabapentin	300mg at bedtime;[18] up to 900mg t.d.s.[19,20]
Carbamazepine	100–200mg at bedtime[4]
Phenytoin	100–200mg once daily[4]

a. also see Anti-epileptics, p.280.

Other options

Anti-epileptics are used to treat cramp unresponsive to more conventional approaches (Table 2). Indeed, NICE guidelines specifically mention the use of **gabapentin** for the management of spasticity in MND/ALS.[14]

More invasive treatments for spasticity include IT **phenol**. This is neurotoxic and can cause urinary and faecal incontinence. The use of indwelling devices to deliver IT **baclofen** has generally superseded the use of **phenol**.[7,20]

Botulinum toxin (BTX) injections are largely reserved for treatment of contractures. The BTX-type A light chain acts as a zinc endopeptidase and interferes with acetylcholine release.[21] The toxin is injected into each spastic muscle separately and reduces spasticity in a dose-dependent manner.[22] Its use is rarely relevant in palliative care. It has been used in people with neurodegenerative disorders, e.g. MND/ALS, to manage drooling and, less commonly, in people with dysphagia secondary to upper oesophageal sphincter dysfunction.[23,24]

1 Zafonte R *et al.* (2004) Acute care management of post-TBI spasticity. *Journal of Head Trauma Rehabilitation*. **19**: 89–100.
2 Noth J and Fink GR. Spasticity. In: Voltz R, Bernat J, Borasio GD, Maddocks I, Oliver D, Portenoy RK, editors. *Palliative care in neurology*. Contemporary neurology series. Oxford: Oxford University Press; 2004. p. 154.
3 Amatya B *et al.* (2013) Non pharmacological interventions for spasticity in multiple sclerosis. *Cochrane Database of Systematic Reviews*. **2**: CD009974. www.thecochranelibrary.com.
4 Miller TM and Layzer RB (2005) Muscle cramps. *Muscle Nerve*. **32**: 431–442.
5 NHS (2018) Clinical knowledge summary. Leg cramps. www.cks.nice.org.uk.
6 Blyton F *et al.* (2012) Non-drug therapies for lower limb muscle cramps. *Cochrane Database of Systematic Reviews*. **1**: CD008496. www.thecochranelibrary.com.
7 Kita M and Goodkin D (2000) Drugs used to treat spasticity. *Drugs*. **59**: 487–495.
8 El Tawil S *et al.* (2015) Quinine for muscle cramps. *Cochrane Database of Systematic Reviews*. **4**: CD005044. www.thecochranelibrary.com.
9 MHRA (2010) Quinine: not to be used routinely for nocturnal leg cramps. *Drug Safety Update*. **3**: www.gov.uk/drug-safety-update.
10 FDA (2010) Qualaquin (quinine sulfate): new risk evaluation and mitigation strategy - risk of serious hematological reactions. www.fda.gov/Safety/MedWatch.
11 MHRA (2017) Quinine: reminder of dose-dependent QT-prolonging effects; updated medicine interactions. *Drug Safety Update*.
12 Fardet L *et al.* (2017) Association between long-term quinine exposure and all-cause mortality. *JAMA*. **317**: 1907–1909.
13 Ng L *et al.* (2017) Symptomatic treatments for amyotrophic lateral sclerosis/motor neuron disease. *Cochrane Database of Systematic Reviews*. **1**: CD011776. www.thecochranelibrary.com.
14 NICE (2016) Motor neurone disease: assessment and management. *Clinical Guideline*. NG42. www.nice.org.uk.
15 Shakespeare DT *et al.* (2003) Anti-spasticity agents for multiple sclerosis. *Cochrane Database of Systematic Reviews*. **4**: CD001332. www.thecochranelibrary.com.
16 Chou R *et al.* (2004) Comparative efficacy and safety of skeletal muscle relaxants for spasticity and musculoskeletal conditions: a systematic review. *Journal of Pain and Symptom Management*. **28**: 140–175.
17 Baldinger R *et al.* (2012) Treatment for cramps in amyotrophic lateral sclerosis/motor neuron disease. *Cochrane Database of Systematic Reviews*. **4**: CD004157. www.thecochranelibrary.com.
18 Serrao M *et al.* (2000) Gabapentin treatment for muscle cramps: an open-label trial. *Clinical Neuropharmacology*. **23**: 45–49.
19 Paisley S *et al.* (2002) Clinical effectiveness of oral treatments for spasticity in multiple sclerosis: a systematic review. *Multiple Sclerosis*. **8**: 319–329.
20 Royal College of Physicians (2004) Multiple Sclerosis: National clinical guidelines for diagnosis and management in primary and secondary care.
21 Brin M (1997) Dosing, administration and a treatment algorithm for use of botulinum toxin A for adult-onset of spasticity. *Muscle and Nerve*. **20 ((Suppl 6))**: 208–220.
22 Royal College of Physicians of London (2018) Spasticity in adults: management using botulinum toxin. National guidelines. www.rcplondon.ac.uk
23 Young CA *et al.* (2011) Treatment for sialorrhea (excessive saliva) in people with motor neuron disease/amyotrophic lateral sclerosis. *Cochrane Database of Systematic Reviews*. **5**: CD00698. www.thecochranelibrary.com.
24 Regan J *et al.* (2014) Botulinum toxin for upper oesophageal sphincter dysfunction in neurological swallowing disorders. *Cochrane Database of Systemstic Reviews*. **7**: CD009968. www.thecochranelibrary.com.

Updated July 2019

BACLOFEN

Class: Skeletal muscle relaxant.

Indications: Spasticity ± painful flexor muscle spasms of voluntary (skeletal) muscle, resulting from spinal or CNS lesions; †hiccup.

Contra-indications: PO: Active peptic ulcer (baclofen stimulates gastric acid secretion).
IT: treatment-resistant epilepsy.

Pharmacology

Baclofen is a chemical congener of the naturally occurring neurotransmitter GABA.[1] It acts upon the GABA-receptor, inhibiting the release of the excitatory amino acids glutamate and aspartate, principally at the spinal level and also at supraspinal sites, thereby decreasing spasm in skeletal muscle.[2,3] It is preferable to **diazepam** for long-term use (e.g. in patients with chronic neurological disease such as multiple sclerosis[4]), because it avoids the problem of **diazepam** dependence. Further, its use is not associated with tolerance; it retains its antispasmodic effects even after many years of continued use.[5] Baclofen relieves hiccup, possibly by a direct effect on the diaphragm.

In patients with severe chronic spasticity in whom PO treatment is ineffective or poorly tolerated, baclofen can be given IT. However, a neurologist must be consulted before using this route. An overdose can cause rostral progression of hypotonia, respiratory depression, coma and, occasionally, seizures.[6] Symptoms of underdosing are generally limited to a return of the patient's baseline spasticity and rigidity. A life-threatening withdrawal syndrome can occur if IT baclofen is abruptly discontinued (see Cautions).

Baclofen is predominantly excreted unchanged in the urine (70–80%); accumulation and toxicity can occur in renal impairment (see Dose and use).

Bio-availability >90% PO.

***Onset of action* PO:** for hiccup, 4–8h; for muscle spasm, 1–2 days; for spasticity, 3–4 days. **IT:** for spasticity: bolus, 30–60min; infusion, 6–8h.

Time to peak plasma concentration 0.5–3h.

Plasma halflife 3.5h; 4.5h in the elderly.

Duration of action 6–8h.[7]

10

Cautions

Withdrawal: abrupt withdrawal of PO baclofen may precipitate serious psychiatric reactions, e.g. agitation, confusion, hallucinations, paranoia, delusions, psychosis. Thus, discontinue by gradual dose reduction over 1–2 weeks, or longer if withdrawal symptoms occur.[8] Sudden withdrawal of IT baclofen or failure of the IT pump may lead to a potentially fatal withdrawal syndrome (Box A).

Box A IT baclofen withdrawal syndrome[6,9]

Cause

Sudden cessation of IT baclofen (e.g. delivery device failure).

Reported with a wide range of doses (50–1,500microgram/24h).

Clinical features

Symptoms evolve over 1–3 days:

- prodromal pruritus or paraesthesia, ± priapism
- seizures (early and/or late onset)
- tachycardia, hypotension or labile blood pressure
- fever (→ hyperthermia)
- dysphoria and malaise → decreased level of consciousness
- spasticity and rigidity greater than patient's baseline
- rhabdomyolysis → hepatic and renal failure, DIC
- coma (→ death).

Management

Restart the IT baclofen infusion as soon as possible.

Cardiopulmonary support as necessary.

High-dose baclofen PO or by enteral feeding tube (up to 120mg/24h); see Chapter 28, Table 2, p.863.

If necessary, give a benzodiazepine by CSCI/CIVI (e.g. midazolam) titrated to achieve muscle relaxation, normothermia, stabilization of blood pressure and cessation of seizures.

Use with caution in patients with severe psychiatric disorders, epilepsy, Parkinson's disease, respiratory impairment, stroke, history of peptic ulceration, renal impairment (see Dose and use, and Chapter 17, p.746), liver impairment (monitor LFTs) (see Chapter 18, p.776), diabetes mellitus, hesitancy of micturition (may precipitate urinary retention), patients who use spasticity to maintain posture or to aid function. Drowsiness may affect skilled tasks and driving; effects of alcohol enhanced.

Because PO baclofen can increase gastric acid secretion, use is cautioned against in patients with a previous peptic ulcer, and contra-indicated in those with an active peptic ulcer. However, data are limited and the clinical relevance of this is unknown, e.g. one study found an overall *increase* in gastric pH.[10]

Undesirable effects

Very common (>10%): sedation, drowsiness, nausea.

Common (<10%, >1%): dizziness; fatigue; muscle hypotonia, pain or weakness; ataxia; tremor; insomnia; headache; visual disturbances; nystagmus; psychiatric disturbances; hypotension; respiratory depression; dry mouth; vomiting; constipation or diarrhoea; urinary frequency or incontinence; dysuria; hyperhidrosis; rash.

Uncommon, rare or very rare (<1%, >0.001%): paradoxical increase in spasticity, seizures (particularly in known epileptics), joint pain, hypothermia, paraesthesia, taste disturbance, abdominal pain, hepatic impairment, urinary retention, impotence.

Dose and use

The starting dose intervals and titration steps given here are more cautious than those in the SPC.

Starting doses are the same for muscle spasm, spasticity and †hiccup:

- start with 5mg PO once daily–t.d.s.; the risk of GI irritation is less if taken after food
- if necessary, increase by 5mg b.d.–t.d.s. every 3 days, but more slowly if troublesome undesirable effects, particularly in the elderly
- effective doses for hiccup are often relatively low, e.g. 5–10mg t.d.s., but it may be necessary to increase to 20mg t.d.s. (see Prokinetics, Table 2, p.25)
- for spasticity, the typical effective dose is generally ≤20mg q.d.s. (maximum 100mg/24h)
- effective doses for muscle spasm fall somewhere in between.

With spasticity, if no improvement with maximum tolerated dose after 6 weeks, *withdraw gradually over 1–2 weeks.*

An undesirable degree of hypotonia may occur, but generally can be relieved by reducing the daytime dose and increasing the evening dose.

Parenteral administration

Baclofen CSCI has been used to prevent a withdrawal reaction when PO and enteral tube administration become impossible.[11] The solution for IT infusion was used for several days at a dose of 10mg/24h. However, this is expensive and, if used, should be short-term (e.g. 4–5 days) to prevent a potential withdrawal reaction.

IT administration is restricted to specialist use.

Renal impairment

In moderate–severe renal impairment, baclofen toxicity (particularly reduced level of consciousness) will occur[12] unless the total daily dose is reduced:

- for patients with creatinine clearance (Cl_{cr}) 10–20mL/min, start with 5mg PO once daily–b.d. and titrate to response
- for patients with Cl_{cr} <10mL/min, avoid if possible but, if unavoidable, start with 5mg PO once daily and titrate to response.[13]

Also see Chapter 17, p.746.

Supply

Baclofen (generic)

Tablets 10mg, 28 days @ 10mg t.d.s. = £1.50.

Oral solution (sugar-free) 5mg/5mL, 10mg/5mL, 28 days @ 10mg t.d.s. = £7 and £30 respectively.

****IT injection*** (for test dose) 50microgram/mL, 1mL amp = £2.50.

****IT solution for infusion*** (for use with implantable pump) 500microgram/mL, 20mL amp = £50; 2mg/mL, 5mL and 20mL amp = £50 and £250 respectively.

1 Zafonte R et al. (2004) Acute care management of post-TBI spasticity. *Journal of Head Trauma Rehabilitation*. **19**: 89–100.
2 Ramirez FC and Graham DY (1992) Treatment of intractable hiccup with baclofen: results of a double-blind randomized, controlled, crossover study. *American Journal of Gastroenterology*. **87**: 1789–1791.
3 Guelaud C *et al.* (1995) Baclofen therapy for chronic hiccup. *European Respiratory Journal*. **8**: 235–237.
4 NICE (2014) Multiple sclerosis in adults: management. *Clinical Guideline*. CG186. www.nice.org.uk
5 Gaillard JM (1977) Comparison of two muscle relaxant drugs on human sleep: diazepam and parachlorophenylgaba. *Acta Psychiatrica Belgica*. **77**: 410–425.
6 Coffey RJ *et al.* (2002) Abrupt withdrawal from intrathecal baclofen: recognition and management of a potentially life-threatening syndrome. *Archives of Physical Medicine and Rehabilitation*. **83**: 735–741.
7 Kochak GM *et al.* (1985) The pharmacokinetics of baclofen derived from intestinal infusion. *Clinical Pharmacology and Therapeutics*. **38**: 251–257.
8 CSM (Committee on Safety of Medicines and Medicines Control Agency) (1997) Reminder! Severe withdrawal reactions with baclofen can be prevented by gradual dose reduction. *Current Problems in Pharmacovigilance*. **23**: 6.
9 Mohammed I and Hussain A (2004) Intrathecal baclofen withdrawal syndrome – a life-threatening complication of baclofen pump: a case report. *BMC Clinical Pharmacology*. **4**: 6.
10 Ciccaglione AF and Marzio L (2003) Effect of acute and chronic administration of the GABA B agonist baclofen on 24 hour pH metry and symptoms in control subjects and in patients with gastro-oesophageal reflux disease. *Gut*. **52**: 464–470.
11 Remi C and Albrecht E (2014) Subcutaneous use of baclofen. *Journal of Pain and Symptom Management*. **48**: e1–3.
12 Su W *et al.* (2009) Reduced level of consciousness from baclofen in people with low kidney function. *British Medical Journal*. **339**: b4559.
13 Ashley C and Dunleavy A (2014). *The Renal Drug Database*. Abingdon: CRC Press. http//renaldrugdatabase.com (accessed March 2017).

Updated (minor change) September 2021

DANTROLENE SODIUM

Class: Skeletal muscle relaxant.

Indications: Chronic severe spasticity of skeletal muscle.

Contra-indications: Hepatic impairment, particularly active liver disease, e.g. hepatitis or cirrhosis (may cause severe liver damage); acute muscle spasm or where spasm is useful in maintaining posture, balance or walking.

Pharmacology

Unlike **baclofen** and **diazepam**, dantrolene acts directly on skeletal muscle by binding to ryanodine receptors, thereby reducing the amount of intracellular calcium available for contraction.[1] It produces fewer central undesirable effects than **baclofen** and **diazepam** and, if necessary, can be used concurrently with these drugs in an attempt to produce a better balance between muscle relaxation and undesirable effects, e.g. unacceptable drowsiness.[2]

Dantrolene is metabolized in the liver mainly to the active hydroxylated metabolite, which is nearly as potent as the parent drug, and the acetamide metabolite, which has weak muscle relaxant activity. It is excreted in the urine, mainly as metabolites with a small amount of unchanged dantrolene; some is excreted in the bile.

Bio-availability 35% PO.
Onset of action up to 1 week.
Time to peak plasma concentration up to 3h.
Plasma halflife 5–9h.
Duration of action no data.

Cautions

Compromised pulmonary function, particularly COPD; predisposition to or actual cardiovascular impairment. Avoid concurrent use with other hepatotoxic drugs (see Chapter 18, p.755).

Undesirable effects

Drowsiness, dizziness, muscle weakness, general malaise, fatigue and diarrhoea (all generally transient). However, diarrhoea may be severe and may necessitate stopping dantrolene temporarily or permanently.

Common (>1%): Seizure, visual disturbances, speech disturbances, headache, pericarditis, pleural effusion, respiratory depression, nausea, vomiting, abdominal pain, anorexia, fever, skin rash, elevation of LFTs.

Severe hepatotoxicity develops rarely, most often after 1–12 months, and is more likely in people over 30 years old, women (particularly those taking oral contraceptives), and with doses >400mg/24h.[3] Fatalities have occurred only with doses >200mg/24h.[4,5]

Dose and use

Because of the risk of hepatotoxicity with long-term use, discontinue if no benefit is observed after 6 weeks of treatment. Perform LFTs before starting treatment and then at regular intervals, e.g. monthly, throughout treatment.

The dose of dantrolene should be built up slowly:
- start with 25mg once daily
- initially increase by no more than 25mg/24h weekly
- above 100mg/24h, larger increments are permissible (see SPC)
- usual effective dose 75mg t.d.s.
- maximum recommended dose 100mg q.d.s.

Supply

Dantrium® (Forum Health Products)
Capsules 25mg, 100mg, 28 days @ 75mg t.d.s. = £43.

Dantrolene (generic)
Oral suspension 10mg/5mL, 25mg/5mL, 100mg/5mL, 28 days @ 75mg t.d.s. = £30 (unauthorized; available as a special order, see Chapter 24, p.817); *price based on specials tariff in the community.*

1 Zafonte R *et al.* (2004) Acute care management of post-TBI spasticity. *Journal of Head Trauma Rehabilitation.* **19**: 89–100.
2 Krause T *et al.* (2004) Dantrolene–a review of its pharmacology, therapeutic use and new developments. *Anaesthesia.* **59**: 364–373.
3 Kim JY *et al.* (2011) Safety of low-dose oral dantrolene sodium on hepatic function. *Archives of Physical Medicine and Rehabilitation.* **92**: 1359–1363.
4 Utili R *et al.* (1977) Dantrolene-associated hepatic injury. Incidence and character. *Gastroenterology.* **72**: 610–616.
5 Wilkinson S *et al.* (1979) Hepatitis from dantrolene sodium. *Gut.* **20**: 33–36.

Updated (minor change) September 2021

TIZANIDINE

Class: Skeletal muscle relaxant.

Indications: Spasticity in multiple sclerosis, spinal cord injury or disease.

Contra-indications: Severe hepatic impairment; patients for whom spasm is useful in maintaining posture, balance or walking; concurrent use with potent CYP1A2 inhibitors, e.g. **ciprofloxacin, fluvoxamine**.

Pharmacology

Tizanidine, like **clonidine**, is a central α_2 agonist within the CNS at supraspinal and spinal levels.[1] It inhibits spinal polysynaptic reflex activity. This reduces the sympathetic outflow, which in turn reduces muscle tone. Tizanidine has no direct effect on skeletal muscle, neuromuscular junctions or monosynaptic spinal reflexes. Tizanidine reduces pathologically increased muscle tone, including resistance to passive movements, and alleviates painful spasms and clonus.[2] In spasticity, tizanidine is comparable in efficacy to **diazepam** and **baclofen**,[3] and has superior tolerability.[4]

Tizanidine is well absorbed but undergoes extensive first-pass metabolism in the liver, mainly by CYP1A2, to inactive metabolites which are mostly excreted by the kidneys. Wide interindividual variability in the effective plasma concentration means that the optimal dose must be titrated slowly over 2–4 weeks. Maximum effects occur within 2h of administration.[5]

Bio-availability 40% PO.
Onset of action 1–2h; peak response 8 weeks.
Time to peak plasma concentration 1.5h.
Plasma halflife 2.5h; up to 14h ± 10h in renal failure.[6]
Duration of action 'relatively short' (SPC).

Cautions

Elderly, renal impairment (see Chapter 17, p.746), cardiovascular disorders. Drowsiness may affect performance of skilled tasks, e.g. driving.

If possible, avoid concurrent use in high doses with other drugs that can cause QT interval prolongation.

In patients taking ≥12mg/24h, LFTs should be monitored monthly for the first 4 months, because of a risk of hepatotoxicity (see Chapter 18, p.755); discontinue if LFTs remain persistently raised at >3 times the upper limit of normal.

Avoid abrupt withdrawal, particularly after long-term use or high doses (risk of rebound hypertension and tachycardia); monitor blood pressure during withdrawal.

Drug interactions

Tizanidine plasma concentrations are increased by CYP1A2 inhibitors, potentially leading to severe hypotension. Avoid concurrent use with potent CYP1A2 inhibitors, e.g. **ciprofloxacin** (and possibly **enoxacin** (not UK)), **fluvoxamine**. Use with caution with other CYP1A2 inhibitors, e.g. **cimetidine**, **norfloxacin**, **oestrogens**, **progestogens** (see Chapter 19, Table 8, p.790).

Concurrent administration with antihypertensive drugs may potentiate hypotension; with **digoxin** may potentiate bradycardia.

Undesirable effects

Drowsiness, weakness and dry mouth in more than two-thirds of those taking it;[7] drowsiness and weakness may be less than with **diazepam** and **baclofen**.[8]

Hypotension and dizziness, nausea and other GI disturbances. Less frequently insomnia, bradycardia, hallucinations and hepatotoxicity (rare if dose ≤12mg/24h).

Dose and use

Slow upward titration helps to reduce undesirable effects:

- start with 2mg PO once daily
- if necessary, increase by 2mg every 3–4 days; build up to 2mg q.d.s. before increasing individual doses
- effective dose generally ≤24mg/24h
- maximum recommended dose 36mg/24h.

In elderly patients and those with severe renal impairment (creatinine clearance <25mL/min), an even slower titration is recommended. Because of the prolonged plasma halflife in renal impairment, the manufacturer recommends slow titration with a *single* daily dose (also see Chapter 17, p.746).

Avoid abrupt withdrawal; if possible, taper higher doses over several weeks (see Cautions).

Supply

Tizanidine (generic)
Tablets 2mg, 4mg, 28 days @ 8mg t.d.s. = £11 or £42 respectively.
Oral solution or suspension 2mg/5mL, 28 days @ 8mg t.d.s. = £76 or £72 respectively (unauthorized; available as a special order, see Chapter 24, p.817); *price based on specials tariff in community*.

1 Zafonte R *et al.* (2004) Acute care management of post-TBI spasticity. *Journal of Head Trauma Rehabilitation*. **19**: 89–100.
2 Wallace J (1994) Summary of combined clinical analysis of controlled clinical trials with tizanidine. *Neurology*. **44 (11 Suppl 9)**: s60–s69.
3 Lataste X *et al.* (1994) Comparative profile of tizanidine in the management of spasticity. *Neurology*. **44 (11 Suppl 9)**: s53–s59.

4 Kamen L *et al.* (2008) A practical overview of tizanidine use for spasticity secondary to multiple sclerosis, stroke, and spinal cord injury. *Current Medical Research and Opinion*. **24**: 425–439.
5 Wagstaff A and Bryson H (1997) Tizanidine. A review of its pharmacology, clinical efficacy and tolerability in the management of spasticity associated with cerebral and spinal disorders. *Drugs*. **53**: 435–452.
6 Keyser E and Ohnhaus E (1986) *Data on file*. Pharmacokinetic study with Sirdalud (tizanidine, DS 103–282) in patients with renal insufficiency.
7 Nance P *et al.* (1997) Relationship of the antispasticity effect of tizanidine to plasma concentration in patients with multiple sclerosis. *Archives of Neurology*. **54**: 731–736.
8 Smith H and Barton A (2000) Tizanidine in the management of spasticity and musculoskeletal complaints in the palliative care population. *American Journal of Hospice and Palliative Care*. **17**: 50–58.

Updated (minor change) September 2021

11: EAR, NOSE AND OROPHARYNX

MOUTHWASHES

Cleaning and freshening the mouth

Lemon glycerine mouth swabs should not be used, because the lemon flavouring and the glycerine have a drying effect.[1]

For home use, one of the following rinses made with tepid water is generally satisfactory:

- mix 1/2 teaspoon of **sodium chloride** (table salt) in 1 cup (approximately 250mL)
- mix 1/4–1/2 teaspoon of **sodium bicarbonate** (baking soda) in 1 cup
- mix 1/4 teaspoon of **sodium chloride** and 1/4 tablespoon of **sodium bicarbonate** in 1 cup.[2]

Chlorhexidine mouthwashes are used to prevent/treat various oral infections (e.g. periodontal disease, oral candidosis)[3,4] and to sterilize dentures and other prostheses.[5] Although **chlorhexidine** inhibits the formation of plaque on teeth, it does not remove established plaque; this requires toothbrushing or, when calcified (tartar), professional dental cleaning.

Note. **Chlorhexidine** is inactivated by ingredients in some toothpastes. Thus, if a patient is using both, the use of the mouthwash should be delayed for ≥30min after using toothpaste. Further, because **chlorhexidine** binds to **nystatin** and leads to inactivation of both drugs, it is important to delay giving **nystatin** oral suspension for ≥30min after using **chlorhexidine** mouthwash.[6]

Most brands of **chlorhexidine** mouthwash contain alcohol, which may cause discomfort; diluting the mouthwash with an equal amount of water may reduce this;[5] however, an alcohol-free product is available. **Chlorhexidine** can stain the teeth and tongue, and this is exacerbated by drinking tea and coffee. The staining can be removed by professional dental cleaning.

Debridement

Generally, a coated ('furred') tongue is indicative of inadequate salivary gland function (most likely drug-induced). Debride the tongue by gentle brushing with a soft toothbrush (special care, baby) or use of a tongue scraper, and consider a saliva stimulant (see p.668); start frequent routine mouth care to help prevent a recurrence.

In the past, some centres used effervescent **ascorbic acid** tablets or pineapple for debriding. However, such use is now considered poor practice. Both agents are acidic and thus may exacerbate a sore or inflamed mouth, contribute to the demineralization of teeth, and predispose to oral infections (see p.666).

Cautions

The MHRA has issued an alert for products or medical devices containing **chlorhexidine** following reports of anaphylaxis, including one precipitated by the use of a **chlorhexidine** skin wipe.[7]

Use

Rinse the mouth with the recommended volume, generally 10–15mL, for about 30–60 seconds and then spit out:

- home-made **sodium chloride** or **sodium bicarbonate** mouthwashes can be used p.r.n.; see above for details
- **chlorhexidine** has a prolonged duration of action and generally needs to be used only b.d., either undiluted or diluted with an equal volume of warm water
- use **hydrogen peroxide** mouthwash undiluted after meals and at bedtime.

Note. Avoid using a mouthwash immediately after toothbrushing; mouthwash rinses away the protective fluoride contained in the toothpaste.

Supply

Chlorhexidine gluconate (generic)
Mouthwash 0.2% (2mg/mL), 300mL = £2; *original, aniseed or mint flavour.*
Mouthwash (alcohol-free) 0.2% (2mg/mL), 300mL = £3.

Hydrogen peroxide
Peroxyl® (Colgate Palmolive)
Mouthwash 1.5% (15mg/mL), 300mL = £3.

1 Poland JM *et al.* (1987) Comparing Moi-Stir to lemon-glycerin swabs. *American Journal of Nursing.* **87**: 422-424.
2 British Columbia Cancer. (2019) Symptom Management Guidelines: Oral mucositis. www.bccancer.bc.ca
3 Chow A. (2010) Oral bacterial infections. In: Davies AN, Epstein JB (eds). *Oral Complications of Cancer and its Management* Oxford: Oxford University Press. pp. 185-193.
4 Finlay I and Davies A. Fungal Infections. In: Davies A, Finlay I, editors. *Oral Care in Advanced Disease.* Oxford: Oxford University Press; 2005. p.55–71.
5 Sweeney P. (2005) Oral hygiene. In: Davies A, Finlay I (eds). *Oral Care in Advanced Disease.* Oxford: Oxford University Press. pp. 21–35.
6 Barkvoll P and Attramadal A (1989) Effect of nystatin and chlorhexidine digluconate on Candida albicans. *Oral Surgery Oral Medicine and Oral Pathology.* **67**: 279–281.
7 MHRA (2012) All medical devices and medicinal products containing chlorhexidine. Risk of anaphylactic reaction due to chlorhexidine allergy. *Medical Devices Alert.* MDA/2012/2075. www.gov.uk/drug-device-alerts

Updated November 2019

ARTIFICIAL SALIVA

Dry mouth (xerostomia) is managed by saliva stimulants or substitutes. Although 99% of saliva is water, the remaining 1% comprises a wide range of electrolytes and molecules which are important for saliva's many roles, e.g. lubrication, cleansing, antimicrobial action, taste, digestion, buffering, and remineralization of teeth.[1] The lack of lubricant (i.e. mucin) explains why sipping water gives only short-lived relief.

Artificial saliva is a poor substitute for natural saliva. Thus, a saliva stimulant should be used in preference (unless contra-indicated). Chewing gum acts as a saliva stimulant and is as effective as, and preferred to, mucin-based artificial saliva.[2] The gum should be sugar-free and, in patients with dentures, low-tack, e.g. Biotene®, Freedent®. Further, chewing sugar-free gum, particularly those containing xylitol, helps reduce the formation of dental caries.[3]

If dry mouth remains a problem, **pilocarpine** or **bethanechol** should be considered (see p.668). Acidic products should *not* be used as saliva stimulants, because they predispose to oral infection (e.g. dental caries, oral candidosis) and cause demineralization of the teeth (leading to dental erosion and dental pain). For patients who do not respond to, or cannot tolerate, saliva stimulants, artificial saliva is an option.

The ideal artificial saliva should be easy to use, pleasant, effective and well tolerated.[4] Further, it should have a neutral pH and contain fluoride (to enhance remineralization of the teeth).[5] Although a Cochrane review highlighted a lack of strong evidence,[6] RCTs indicate that mucin-based products are more effective and better tolerated than cellulose-based ones.[7-9]

The mucin comes from the stomach of pigs, and this may be an issue for some patients (e.g. Jews, Muslims, vegetarians). There is no good evidence that gels are more effective or last longer than sprays.

Undesirable effects

Unpleasant taste, irritation of the mouth, nausea and/or diarrhoea in ≤30% of patients (mucin-based artificial saliva).[2,10]

Dose and use

PCF regards sugar-free chewing gum as the saliva stimulant of choice for most patients. For patients with dentures, it should be low-tack, e.g. Biotene®, Freedent®.

Artificial salivas or saliva stimulants with an acidic pH should be avoided.

The duration of effect of artificial salivas is relatively short, due to a combination of swallowing and evaporation. Thus, artificial salivas may need to be taken every 10–30min, and also before (and sometimes during) meals. To optimize benefit, the gels should be massaged into the oral soft tissues. Proprietary artificial salivas with a neutral pH include:

- AS Saliva Orthana® (mucin-based sprays and lozenges); lozenges are ACBS classified (see Supply)
- Biotène Oralbalance® gel
- BioXtra® gel; ACBS classified (see Supply).

Supply

Some products, e.g. AS Saliva Orthana® lozenges and BioXtra® gel, are classified in the UK as borderline substances and have ACBS approval only for dry mouth associated with radiotherapy or sicca syndrome. The prescriber must endorse an NHS FP10 prescription for one of these products with 'ACBS', otherwise the Prescription Pricing Authority will investigate whether it has been issued for an approved indication.

Mucin-based (porcine)
AS Saliva Orthana® (CCMed Ltd)
Oral spray 50mL bottle = £5; 500mL refill = £34.
Lozenges 30 = £3.50 (ACBS).

Cellulose-based
Biotène Oralbalance® (GlaxoSmithKline Consumer Healthcare)
Saliva replacement gel 50g = £4.50.

BioXtra® (RIS Products)
Saliva replacement gel 40mL tube = £4, 50mL spray = £4 (ACBS).

1 Davies A (2005) Salivary gland dysfunction. In: Davies A, Finlay I (eds). *Oral Care in Advanced Disease*. Oxford: Oxford University Press. pp. 97–114.
2 Davies AN (2000) A comparison of artificial saliva and chewing gum in the management of xerostomia in patients with advanced cancer. *Palliative Medicine*. **14**: 197–203.
3 Newton JT *et al.* (2019) A systematic review and meta-analysis of the role of sugar-free chewing gum in dental caries. *JDR Clinical & Translational Research*. (Epub ahead of print).
4 Epstein JB and Stevenson-Moore P (1992) A clinical comparative trial of saliva substitutes in radiation-induced salivary gland hypofunction. *Special Care Dentistry*. **12**: 21-23.
5 Davies A (2010) Salivary gland dysfunction. In: Davies AN, Epstein JB (eds). *Oral Complications of Cancer and its Management.* Oxford: Oxford University Press. pp. 203-223.
6 Furness S *et al.* (2011) Interventions for the management of dry mouth: topical therapies. *Cochrane Database of Systematic Reviews*. CD008934. www.cochranelibrary.com
7 S'Gravenmade E *et al.* (1974) The effect of mucin-containing artificial saliva on severe exerostomia. *International Journal of Oral Surgery*. **3**: 435–439.
8 Vissink A *et al.* (1983) A clinical comparison between commercially available mucin- and CMC-containing saliva substitutes. *International Journal of Oral Surgery*. **12**: 232–238.
9 Visch L *et al.* (1986) A double-blind crossover trial of CMC- and mucin-containing saliva substitutes. *International Journal of Oral and Maxillofacial Surgery*. **15**: 395–400.
10 Davies A *et al.* (1998) A comparison of artificial saliva and pilocarpine in the management of xerostomia in patients with advanced cancer. *Palliative Medicine*. **12**: 105–111.

Updated November 2019

PILOCARPINE

Class: Parasympathomimetic.

Indications: Xerostomia (dry mouth) after radiotherapy for head and neck cancer, dry mouth (and dry eyes) in Sjögren's syndrome, †drug-induced dry mouth.

Contra-indications: Intestinal or urinary obstruction, or when increased intestinal or urinary tract motility could be harmful (e.g. after recent surgery); when miosis could be harmful (e.g. narrow-angle glaucoma, acute iritis); unstable asthma.

Pharmacology

Pilocarpine is a parasympathomimetic (predominantly muscarinic) drug with mild β-adrenergic activity which stimulates secretion from exocrine glands, including salivary glands. A systematic review suggests that about 40–50% of patients with radiotherapy-induced dry mouth respond to pilocarpine, with a time to response of up to 12 weeks.[1] However, undesirable effects are common, and were the main reason for withdrawal from studies (≤15% of patients taking 5mg t.d.s.).

About 90% of patients with drug-induced dry mouth respond to pilocarpine, with benefit seen in <24h.[2] In an RCT, half of the patients preferred pilocarpine because it was more effective, and half preferred the comparator **mucin**-based artificial saliva, mainly because it was a spray and not a tablet.[2] Undesirable effects were much more common in patients receiving pilocarpine (84% vs. 22%), which resulted in about a quarter of the patients withdrawing from the study.

Alternatives to pilocarpine are used at some centres, e.g. **bethanechol**.[3,4] Pharmacokinetic data for **bethanechol** are limited. Because of poor GI absorption, it is recommended to take **bethanechol** on an empty stomach. Although cheaper than pilocarpine, it has a slower onset of action (30–90min) and possibly a shorter duration of action;[5] however, in practice, t.d.s.–q.d.s. dosing appears satisfactory.

Bio-availability 96% PO.
Onset of action 20min (drug-induced dry mouth); up to 3 months (after radiation).
Time to peak plasma concentration 1h.
Plasma halflife 1h.
Duration of action 3–5h (single dose).

Cautions

Pilocarpine may antagonize the effects of antimuscarinic drugs, e.g. inhaled **ipratropium bromide**. Concurrent use with β antagonists (β-blockers) may cause cardiac conduction disturbances.

Cognitive or psychiatric disorder, epilepsy, parkinsonism. Miosis may affect vision and driving ability, particularly at night. Cardiovascular disease (changes in haemodynamics or heart rhythm), hyperthyroidism, COPD (increased bronchial smooth muscle tone, airway resistance and bronchial secretions). Peptic ulcer (increased acid secretion), gallstones or biliary tract disease (increased biliary smooth muscle contraction). Renal impairment (no reliable human data on metabolism and excretion), kidney stones (potential for renal colic).

Reduce dose in moderate–severe hepatic impairment.

Undesirable effects

Very common (>10%): headache, flu-like syndrome, nausea, urinary frequency, sweating.
Common (<10%, >1%): dizziness, asthenia, chills, blurred vision, eye pain, conjunctivitis, flushing, palpitations, hypertension (after initial hypotension), rhinitis, abdominal pain, dyspepsia, vomiting, diarrhoea or constipation, rash, pruritus.

Undesirable effects with **bethanechol** are similar to pilocarpine but generally less severe.

Dose and use

The manufacturer recommends t.d.s. during or directly after meals, but, given its duration of action (3–5h), there is scope for greater flexibility. Adding a dose at bedtime reduces the likelihood of the patient waking in the night with an excessively dry mouth.[6]

In drug-induced dry mouth, 5mg PO q.d.s. is generally effective, but after radiotherapy 10mg q.d.s. may be needed:

- start with 5mg PO t.d.s. and at bedtime
- if necessary and if tolerated, increase the dose to 10mg q.d.s. after 2 days if the dry mouth is drug-induced, and after 4 weeks if radiation-induced
- if no improvement with 10mg q.d.s., stop after 4 days if the dry mouth is drug-induced, and after 12 weeks if radiation-induced.

In patients with moderate–severe hepatic impairment, start on a lower total daily dose, e.g. 5mg b.d., and increase to 5mg q.d.s. if well tolerated.

Some centres use the eyedrop formulation PO: 3 drops of a 4% solution contain 6mg. It is cheaper than tablets (see Supply), but appears to be less effective and is not always acceptable to patients.[7]

Bethanechol is used when pilocarpine is ineffective or poorly tolerated; for drug-induced dry mouth:

- start with 25mg PO t.d.s. on an empty stomach, e.g. 30min before meals
- if necessary, frequency can be increased to q.d.s.
- reduce dose to 10mg if patients experience excessive salivation.

Supply

Pilocarpine (generic)

Eyedrops 4% (40mg/mL), 10mL, 28 days @ 3 drops (6mg) PO q.d.s. = £48. (10mL lasts approximately 15 days.)

Salagen® (Merus Labs)

Tablets 5mg, 28 days @ 5mg q.d.s. = £55.

Bethanechol

Myotonine® (Glenwood)

Tablets *(scored)* 10mg, 25mg, 28 days @ 25mg t.d.s. = £23.

1 Davies AN and Thompson J (2015) Parasympathomimetic drugs for the treatment of salivary gland dysfunction due to radiotherapy. *Cochrane Database of Systematic Reviews*. **10**: CD003782. www.thecochranelibrary.com

2 Davies A *et al.* (1998) A comparison of artificial saliva and pilocarpine in the management of xerostomia in patients with advanced cancer. *Palliative Medicine*. **12**: 105–111.

3 Epstein J *et al.* (1994) A clinical trial of bethanechol in patients with xerostomia after radiation therapy. A pilot study. *Oral Surgery, Oral Medicine and Oral Pathology*. **77**: 610–614.

4 Davies A (2005) Salivary gland dysfunction. In: Davies A and Finlay I (eds) *Oral Care in Advanced Disease*. Oxford University Press, Oxford. pp. 97–114.

5 McEvoy GK. *American Hospital Formulary Service*. Maryland, USA: American Society of Health-System Pharmacists. www.medicinescomplete.com (accessed April 2017).

6 Davies A (2014) *Personal communication*.

7 Nikles J *et al.* (2015) Testing pilocarpine drops for dry mouth in advanced cancer using n-of-1 trials: A feasibility study. *Palliative Medicine*. **29**: 967–974.

Updated November 2019

DRUGS FOR ORAL INFLAMMATION AND ULCERATION

'Oral stomatitis' refers to any inflammation ± ulceration of the mouth and lips, whereas 'oral mucositis' tends to be restricted to stomatitis caused by local radiotherapy, chemotherapy, haematopoietic stem cell transplantation, or other anti-cancer modalities.

The causes of oral ulceration include trauma (physical, chemical), recurrent aphthous ulceration, infection, cancer, skin conditions, nutritional deficiencies, GI conditions, haematopoietic disorders and drug treatment (Box A). It is important to determine the cause so that, if appropriate, specific treatment is given as well as symptomatic treatment. For example, ill-fitting dentures which cause traumatic ulceration (and/or mucosal hyperplasia) should be relined or, ideally, replaced.[1]

Box A Drug-related oral ulceration[a,b]

Alimentary
Pancreatin

Analgesics
NSAIDs

Antibiotics
Aztreonam
Clarithromycin
Proguanil
Vancomycin

Anticancer
Chemotherapy[c]
- Bleomycin
- Doxorubicin
- 5-Fluoro-uracil
- Melphalan
- Mercaptopurine
- Methotrexate

Immunotherapy
Targeted therapy

Anti-rheumatic
Allopurinol
Gold
Methotrexate
Penicillamine

Antivirals
Foscarnet
Protease inhibitors
Zalcitabine

Cardiac
ACE inhibitors
Isoprenaline (not UK)
Labetalol
Losartan
Nicorandil
Phenindione

Corticosteroids
Flunisolide (not UK)

Dental
Sodium lauryl sulfate

Diabetic
Dipeptidyl peptidase-4 inhibitors

Immunomodulators
Azathioprine
Interferons
Interleukin-2
Molgramostim
Sirolimus
Tacrolimus

Psychotropics
Carbamazepine
Fluoxetine
Lithium
Olanzapine
Phenytoin
Sertraline

Other
Alendronic acid
Emepronium (not UK)
Potassium chloride

a. not an exhaustive list

b. excipients, e.g. ethanol or propylene glycol, in oral formulations, e.g. Sativex® spray (see Cannabinoids, p.251), can also cause oral ulceration

c. can occur with any chemotherapy, but particularly those listed.

Management strategy

The symptomatic management of oral inflammation and ulceration involves measures which:

- maintain oral hygiene
- relieve pain
- protect ulcerated mucosa
- treat secondary infection
- reduce inflammation.

Advice should be sought from an oral medicine specialist if unexplained ulceration persists for >3 weeks.

Maintain oral hygiene

Simple mouthwashes, e.g. **sodium chloride ± sodium bicarbonate**, can be soothing, help to maintain oral hygiene, and prevent secondary infection (see p.665).[2] The temperature of the mouthwash appears to be important, with tepid ones being more soothing than cold or warm ones.

Pain relief

Topical analgesics

These include:

- local anaesthetics
- NSAIDs
- antihistamines
- opioids.

Local anaesthetics

The efficacy of topical local anaesthetics depends on the formulation, duration of application (at least 5min is required) and site of application. There are limited data to support their use in oral mucositis, and any effect is of short duration.[3] They are less effective in more keratinized areas of the mouth, e.g. the palate.[4]

Some systemic absorption of the local anaesthetic occurs, which is increased by mucosal inflammation. However, plasma concentrations are generally low, and toxicity has been reported only in exceptional circumstances (see p.77). With all topical local anaesthetics, care must be taken not to produce pharyngeal anaesthesia before meals, because this could lead to aspiration and choking:

- **lidocaine** ointment 5% (has a water-miscible base), rubbed gently onto the affected areas before food and p.r.n.
- **lidocaine** spray 10% (Xylocaine®), applied thinly to the ulcer using a cotton bud before food and p.r.n. (unauthorized use)
- **oxetacaine** in combination with **aluminium hydroxide–magnesium hydroxide** oral suspension (available as a special order), is used for post-radiation oesophagitis and candidosis which is causing painful swallowing (see p.1).

Various OTC products are also available.

NSAIDs

Benzydamine, an NSAID, also has local anaesthetic and antimicrobial effects.[5,6] It is available as a mouthwash or spray, and can ease the discomfort associated with oral stomatitis. It is recommended for the prevention of oral mucositis secondary to radiotherapy (± chemotherapy) for head and neck cancer:

- **benzydamine** 0.15% mouthwash: rinse or gargle 15mL for 20–30sec before spitting out; repeat q1.5–3h p.r.n. Dilute with an equal volume of water if stinging occurs.[7]

Excessive use of **choline salicylate** dental gel or confinement under a denture can result in oral irritation and/or ulceration. Remove any dentures before use and wait ≥30min before re-inserting:

- **choline salicylate** 8.7% oromucosal gel (e.g. Bonjela®): apply 1–2cm by gentle massage q3h p.r.n.; maximum recommended dose 6 applications/day.

Other options include **flurbiprofen** lozenges (can also result in oral ulceration).

Antihistamines

Diphenhydramine (not UK) is an antihistamine with a topical analgesic effect. It has been used for decades for oral mucositis, particularly in the USA. Generally, it is given as a locally prepared mouthwash, often in combination with other products; e.g. 5mL would contain equal parts (about 1.7mL) of **diphenhydramine** 12.5mg/5mL + **lidocaine** viscous 2% + antacid (containing **aluminium hydroxide**, **magnesium hydroxide** and **simeticone**). Similarly, **doxepin**, a TCA and a potent H_1- and H_2-receptor antagonist, has also been used as a mouthwash (not UK).[8]

However, oral mucositis guidelines consider the evidence insufficient to recommend the use of **diphenhydramine** or **doxepin**.[7,9] Further, in a recent RCT of radiation-induced mucositis, although both **diphenhydramine** (combined as above) and **doxepin** mouthwashes reduced pain scores statistically significantly more than placebo, the improvement was not considered clinically meaningful for either.[10]

Opioids

Opioids have a topical analgesic effect on inflamed tissue and can be used as a mouthwash. Some recommend that the mouthwash is subsequently swallowed in order to combine a systemic analgesic effect with the topical one:

- special order **morphine sulfate** 2mg/mL solution: take 10mg in 5mL q3–4h; hold in the mouth for 2min *and then spit out or swallow*; some patients need higher doses, occasionally 30mg q3–4h.[11,12] Note. The commercially available products contain alcohol and should *not* be used
- locally prepared **morphine sulfate** 1–5mg/mL gel: initially 3mL q4–8h; hold in mouth for 10min *and then spit out or swallow*.

Also see **morphine**, p.410.

Systemic analgesics

Systemic analgesics include non-opioids and opioids given as for other pains, balancing benefit against undesirable effects. For severe mucositis (patient unable to eat ± unable to drink) with

11

inadequate pain relief from topical measures, a parenteral opioid should be administered either by patient-controlled analgesia, continuous infusion with p.r.n. boluses as required, or transdermal administration (e.g. **fentanyl**).[7] Chemotherapy patients often have a permanent IV access which can be used.

Protect the ulcerated areas

Coating agents are of limited value, because they can be difficult to apply and they do not relieve persistent oral inflammatory pain. However, by adhering to and coating the denuded surface, they may help to reduce contact pain, e.g. from eating or drinking. Available agents include:

- **carmellose (carboxymethylcellulose) sodium** (Orabase® paste, Orahesive® powder): apply the paste to, or sprinkle the powder onto, the sore area after food
- **polyvinylpyrrolidone** and **sodium hyaluronate** oral gel (Gelclair®): t.d.s. p.r.n., ideally 30–60min before eating; mix contents of 1 sachet with 40mL water, rinse around mouth for at least 1min, gargle and then spit out; an expensive option
- **sucralfate** (unauthorized use): given as a rinse-and-swallow suspension is *not* of benefit in chemotherapy- or radiation-induced oral mucositis.[13] It may help in other types of oral stomatitis, but it is expensive and cheaper agents should be tried first (see Supply). Give as a suspension 1g/5mL q.d.s.; rinse around the mouth for 2–3min and then spit out or, when inflammation extends beyond the mouth, swallow.

Treat secondary infection

Antiseptic and antibacterial mouthwashes may help prevent or treat secondary infection, particularly with multiple ulcers not easily accessible to covering pastes:

- *prevention:* **chlorhexidine gluconate** mouthwash 0.2%, ideally alcohol-free (see p.665)
- *treatment:* **doxycycline** suspension 100mg in 10mL q.d.s. for 3 days (unauthorized use; prepared by mixing a dispersible tablet or the contents of a capsule with a small quantity of water); rinse around the mouth for 2–3min and then spit out.

Alternative mouthwashes, if available, include **tetracycline** 0.25% (2.5mg/mL)[14] *or* **minocycline** 0.5% (5mg/mL);[15] use 5mL q.d.s.

For oral candidosis, see p.511.

Reduce the inflammation

Topical corticosteroids are useful in the management of certain types of oral ulceration, e.g. recurrent aphthous ulceration (Box B). However, corticosteroids do *not* feature in the management of oral mucositis. Systemic corticosteroids are generally reserved for severe ulcerative conditions, e.g. pemphigus vulgaris.

Box B Treatment of aphthous ulcers[16]

Corticosteroids

Corticosteroids are the mainstay of treatment. Use as soon as symptoms/ulcers appear; avoid in oral infections. Options include:

- hydrocortisone oromucosal tablets 2.5mg q.d.s. for up to 5 days; tablets are placed at the site of the ulcers and left to dissolve
- beclometasone metered-dose aerosol inhaler 50microgram or 100microgram sprayed into the mouth b.d.; for difficult-to-reach sites such as the soft palate and oropharynx, or widespread inflammation (unauthorized use)
- betamethasone soluble tablets 500microgram, dispersed in 20mL water and rinsed around the mouth q.d.s.; for difficult-to-reach sites, or widespread inflammation (unauthorized use).

Supply

The following list is selective.

Topical analgesics
Lidocaine (generic)
Ointment 5% in a water-miscible base, 15g = £8.50.

Xylocaine® (Aspen Pharma Trading)
Spray 10%, 50mL = £6.50. Apply thinly to ulcer using cotton bud (unauthorized use).

For **oxetacaine** with **aluminium hydroxide–magnesium hydroxide** oral suspension see p.1.

Benzydamine (generic)
Oral rinse (mouthwash) 0.15%, 300mL = £6.50.
Oromucosal spray 0.15%, 30mL = £2.75.

Choline salicylate dental gel BP
Bonjela® (Reckitt Benckiser)
Oral gel 8.7%, 15g = £3; also available OTC.

Flurbiprofen
Strefen® (Reckitt Benckiser)
Lozenges 8.75mg, 16 = £3.50.

Also see **Morphine**, p.410.

Coating agents
Orabase® (ConvaTec)
Oral paste containing **carmellose sodium** 16.7%, **gelatin** 16.7% and **pectin** 16.7%, 30g = £2.25.

Orahesive® (ConvaTec)
Powder containing **carmellose sodium**, **gelatin** and **pectin**, equal parts, 25g = £2.50.

Gelclair® (Cambridge Laboratories)
Oral gel containing **polyvinylpyrrolidone** and **sodium hyaluronate**, 28 days @ one 15mL sachet t.d.s. = £137.

Sucralfate (generic)
Oral suspension (sugar-free) 1g/5mL, 28 days @ 5mL q.d.s. = £269.

Antiseptic and antibacterial mouthwashes
For **chlorhexidine gluconate** mouthwashes, see p.665.

Doxycycline (generic)
Capsules 50mg, 100mg (as hyclate), 3 days @ 100mg q.d.s. = £1.

Vibramycin-D® (Pfizer)
Dispersible tablets doxycycline 100mg, 3 days @ 100mg q.d.s. = £7.25.

Corticosteroids
Hydrocortisone (generic)
Oromucosal tablets 2.5mg (as sodium succinate), 5 days @ 2.5mg q.d.s. = £9.

Beclometasone (generic)
Aerosol inhalation 50microgram/metered dose, 200-dose inhaler = £2.75; 100microgram/metered dose, 200-dose inhaler = £5.00.

Betamethasone (generic)
Tablets soluble (sugar-free) 500microgram, 5 days @ 500microgram q.d.s. = £11.50.

1 Walls A (2005) Domiciliary dental care. In: Davies A, Finlay I (eds) *Oral Care in Advanced Disease*. Oxford: Oxford University Press. pp. 37–45.
2 Hong CHL *et al.* (2019) Systematic review of basic oral care for the management of oral mucositis in cancer patients and clinical practice guidelines. *Supportive Care in Cancer*. **27**: 3949–3967.
3 Saunders DP *et al.* (2013) Systematic review of antimicrobials, mucosal coating agents, anaesthetics, and analgesics for the management of oral mucositis in cancer patients. *Supportive Care in Cancer*. **21**: 3191–3207.
4 Meecham J (2005) Oral pain. In: Davies A, Finlay I (eds). *Oral Care in Advanced Disease*. Oxford: Oxford University Press. pp. 134–143.
5 Turnbull RS (1995) Benzydamine Hydrochloride (Tantum) in the management of oral inflammatory conditions. *Journal Canadian Dental Association*. **61**: 127–134.

6 Fanaki NH and el-Nakeeb MA (1992) Antimicrobial activity of benzydamine, a non-steroid anti-inflammatory agent. *Journal of Chemotherapy*. **4**: 347–352.
7 Ariyawardana A *et al.* (2019) Systematic review of anti-inflammatory agents for the management of oral mucositis in cancer patients and clinical practice guidelines. *Supportive Care in Cancer*. **27**: 3985–3995.
8 Epstein JB *et al.* (2007) Management of pain in cancer patients with oral mucositis: follow-up of multiple doses of doxepin oral rinse. *Journal of Pain and Symptom Management*. **33**: 111–114.
9 Nicolatou-Galitis O *et al.* (2013) Systematic review of anti-inflammatory agents for the management of oral mucositis in cancer patients. *Supportive Care in Cancer*. **21**: 3179–3189.
10 Sio TT *et al.* (2019) Effect of doxepin mouthwash or diphenhydramine-lidocaine-antacid mouthwash vs placebo on radiotherapy-related oral mucositis pain: the alliance A221304 randomized clinical trial. *JAMA*. **321**: 1481–1490.
11 Cerchietti LC *et al.* (2002) Effect of topical morphine for mucositis-associated pain following concomitant chemoradiotherapy for head and neck carcinoma. *Cancer*. **95**: 2230–2236.
12 Cerchietti L (2007) Morphine mouthwashes for painful mucositis. *Supportive Care in Cancer*. **15**: 115–116.
13 Elad S *et al.* (2020) MASCC/ISOO clinical practice guidelines for the management of mucositis secondary to cancer therapy. *Cancer*. **126:** 4423–4431.
14 Gorsky M *et al.* (2007) Topical minocycline and tetracycline rinses in treatment of recurrent aphthous stomatitis: a randomized cross-over study. *Dermatology Online Journal*. **13**: 1.
15 Yarom N *et al.* (2017) The efficacy of minocycline mouth rinses on the symptoms associated with recurrent aphthous stomatitis: a randomized, double-blind, crossover study assessing different doses of oral rinse. *Oral surgery, oral medicine, oral pathology and oral radiology*. **123**: 675–679.
16 NICE (2017) Aphthous ulcer. *Clinical Knowledge Summary*. www.nice.org.uk

Updated (minor change) November 2021

CERUMENOLYTICS

Indications: Impacted earwax (cerumen).

Contra-indications: perforated ear drum, presence of myringotomy tubes (grommets), recent ear surgery.

Pharmacology

Cerumen impaction is defined as an accumulation of earwax which causes symptoms, prevents adequate examination of the ear, or both; it does not necessarily imply complete obstruction.[1,2] Symptoms associated with impacted earwax include deafness, tinnitus, fullness, itching, otalgia, discharge and chronic cough. Asymptomatic earwax does *not* need to be removed.

Earwax is secreted to provide a protective film on the skin of the external ear canal. It is generally expelled naturally. The risk of impaction is increased in children, the elderly, people with learning disabilities, and when natural expulsion is obstructed, e.g. by anatomical abnormalities of the ear canal, hearing aids, or inappropriate use of cotton buds to clean the ears.[1,3]

Removal of impacted earwax generally requires ear syringing ± pretreatment with a cerumenolytic. Syringing without pretreatment is effective in about three-quarters of patients;[3,4] with pretreatment, success approaches 100%.[1] However, pretreatment with water 15–30min before syringing is as effective as applying drops b.d. for several days.[4,5] It works in nearly all cases and is more convenient for patients.[6] In those where syringing fails to remove the wax, common sense dictates that drops should be continued for several days before a further attempt.[3,6]

Syringing can cause undesirable effects, including pain, minor damage to the external ear canal, and otitis externa; less commonly, perforation of the tympanic membrane and vertigo (the latter generally if the water is too cold).[1]

Used alone, cerumenolytics are less effective, with 5 days of use completely clearing wax in only 20% of ears (vs. 5% with no treatment).[7] Cerumenolytics are classified as either water-based (e.g. water, sodium chloride 0.9%, **sodium bicarbonate** 5%), oil-based (e.g. **almond oil, olive oil**), or non-water-/non-oil-based (e.g. **urea–hydrogen peroxide**).[4] Water-based products are true cerumenolytics (i.e. break up keratin within earwax),[8] whereas oil-based products lubricate and soften the earwax. The mechanism of action of non-water-/non-oil-based products is unclear. Nonetheless, no one cerumenolytic appears to be any more effective than another, including water or sodium chloride 0.9%.[7]

Management strategy

PCF regards water (tap or sterile) or sodium chloride 0.9% as cerumenolytics of choice.

- use drops alone for at least 4 days (e.g. 3–4 drops b.d.)
- if this fails, proceed to syringing
- if this fails, use drops for 3–4 more days and syringe again
- if syringing fails on the second occasion, proceed to manual removal using curette, probe, forceps, suction or hook.

To minimize the risk of damaging the ear canal and tympanic membrane, manual removal after failed syringing is best undertaken by those with specialist training.[1,3]

Supply

Although OTC products are available, their relative effectiveness is unproven, and they appear to be no better than water or sodium chloride 0.9%. Thus, none is recommended. Some proprietary products contain potentially irritant constituents.[2]

Sodium chloride 0.9% (generic)
Injection (use as ear drops) 10mL = £0.50.
Nasal drops (use as ear drops) 10mL = £1; available OTC.

11

1 Wright T (2015) Ear wax. *BMJ Clincial Evidence*. http://clinicalevidence.bmj.com
2 Roland PS *et al.* (2008) Clinical practice guideline: cerumen impaction. *Otolaryngology – Head and Neck Surgery*. **139 (3 Suppl 2)**: S1–S21.
3 McCarter DF *et al.* (2007) Cerumen impaction. *American Family Physician*. **75**: 1523–1528.
4 Hand C and Harvey I (2004) The effectiveness of topical preparations for the treatment of earwax: a systematic review. *British Journal of General Practice*. **54**: 862–867.
5 Pavlidis C and Pickering JA (2005) Water as a fast acting wax softening agent before ear syringing. *Australian Family Physician*. **34**: 303–304.
6 Eekhof JA *et al.* (2001) A quasi-randomised controlled trial of water as a quick softening agent of persistent earwax in general practice. *British Journal of General Practice*. **51**: 635–637.
7 Aaron K *et al.* (2018) Ear drops for the removal of ear wax. *Cochrane Database of Systematic Reviews*. **7**: CD012171. www.thecochranelibrary.com
8 Chalishazar U and Williams H (2007) Back to basics: finding an optimal cerumenolytic (earwax solvent). *British Journal of Nursing*. **16**: 806–808.

Updated November 2019

12: SKIN

EMOLLIENTS

Indications: Dry or rough skin.

Introduction

Emollients soften and increase the hydration of the outermost layer of the epidermis (stratum corneum). This increases the integrity and resilience of the skin and so helps to protect the skin from irritants, allergens and microbes.[1] Emollients also hydrate skin by preventing loss of water. Older patients are particularly likely to develop dry skin (asteotic dermatitis). Other common causes include:

- varicose (stasis) dermatitis
- drying environments
- excessive washing
- diuretics
- drug reactions
- radiotherapy.

Types of emollients

Emollients vary in greasiness, depending on the amount of oil and water they contain (Table 1). Creams and ointments are most commonly used. However, other formulations may be used for specific indications. The choice of emollient depends on many factors.

Ointments are greasy because of their structure, even when their water content is high. Anhydrous ointments provide an occlusive film of oil over the surface of the skin. The water trapped under the ointment passes back into the stratum corneum, which then swells up, improving skin barrier function.

Some creams contain **propylene glycol**, which gives a smoother texture and facilitates application. The properties of oily lotions are comparable to those of creams but, because they are more liquid, they can be applied more easily to large areas and are easier to apply to hairy skin. Both creams and oily lotions have a cooling effect on the skin (heat lost by evaporation of the water content).

Humectants are substances which attract moisture to, and retain it in, the stratum corneum, e.g. **urea**, **glycerol**, **lactic acid**, **alpha-hydroxy acids**, **propylene glycol** and **sodium pidolate**.[2] Adequate hydration is generally obtained with creams containing **urea** 5–10%[3,4] and, for patients with only mild–moderate dryness, this may be more cosmetically acceptable than using an ointment. **Urea** at higher concentrations of 20–30% is antipruritic, breaks down keratin, decreases the thickness of the stratum corneum, and is used in scaling conditions such as ichthyosis.[3] However, humectants may be irritating, particularly on inflamed skin, when humectant-free creams or ointments may be preferable.

Cautions

Fabrics, e.g. clothing, dressings and bedding, in contact with paraffin-based emollients, e.g. **emulsifying ointment BP** or **liquid paraffin and white soft paraffin ointment NPF** (**liquid paraffin** in **white soft paraffin** 50:50), are easily ignited by a naked flame. The risk is

Table 1 Emollient formulations

	Description	*Features*	*Potential limitations*
Ointments	Grease-based	Increased absorption	Messy Difficult to apply to hairy areas May occlude hair follicles Perspiration can be trapped under the ointment, causing discomfort from excessive body heat and moisture Avoid applying to large areas
Creams	Emulsions of water and oil; vary between greasy (water in oil; 'rich creams') to aqueous (oil in water; 'light creams')	Cosmetically acceptable Suitable for face and flexures May be used for large areas	May contain fragrances or preservatives that may cause sensitization and burning/stinging ± erythema. Avoid use in those with atopic dermatitis (eczema), other than as a soap substitute
Lotions	Solutions, suspensions or emulsions from which water evaporates leaving a thin coating of powder or oil	Suitable for wet rashes and hairy areas Spread well Useful for soaks or wet dressings	Only emulsions containing oil have an emollient effect; other lotions are drying Often contain alcohol, which will sting broken skin
Sprays	Oil in volatile silicone	Spray on, so application is quick No touching the skin No contamination from the hands	Make skin and surfaces slippery
Soap substitutes	Available as creams, lotions or ointments	Unlike soaps, no detergent properties	
Bath additives	Oil; often contain an antimicrobial or antipruritic	Although used, scientific evidence suggests little benefit	Make skin and surfaces slippery; particular care needed when bathing Additives can cause contact dermatitis if used excessively

increased when the products are applied to large areas of the body and fabrics become soaked with them. Patients should keep away from fire or flames, and not smoke when using these products, particularly if applying large quantities. Washing the fabric, even at high temperatures, may not totally remove the emollient.[5]

Undesirable effects

Proprietary emollients often contain additives and fragrances (perfumes), which are potentially allergenic (Table 2). Concern about **lanolin** is largely misplaced; many emollients contain refined (hypoallergenic) **lanolin**, which is rarely responsible for contact dermatitis.[6]

Official advice states that emollients containing **arachis** (peanut) **oil** should not be used by patients with peanut or soya allergy.[7] However, unlike *crude* **arachis oil**, the *refined* oil used in pharmaceutical products is not allergenic, and thus is highly unlikely to cause allergic reactions in people with (whole) peanut allergy.[8,9]

Aqueous cream sometimes causes burning/stinging ± erythema when used as an emollient. This has been linked to sodium lauryl sulfate (SLS), an ingredient of the emulsifying wax BP used to prepare aqueous cream, but may be caused by other sensitizing ingredients. The reaction generally occurs within 20min of applying the cream, but is rarely severe.

Should sensitization occur, use a proprietary emollient which does not contain SLS or emulsifying wax BP, e.g. Diprobase® cream (also see Table 4).[10]

In patients with atopic dermatitis (eczema), particularly children, although **aqueous cream** can be used as a soap substitute, it should *not* be used as an emollient.[11]

Table 2 Potential skin allergens in topical emollient products

Allergen	*Comment*
Fragrances (perfumes)[a,3,12]	
Preservatives (particularly parabens and cresols)[a,3,12]	In many creams, lotions and some ointments
Emulsifying agents and ointment bases (particularly sodium lauryl sulfate and cetostearyl alcohols)[a,3,12]	In many creams, lotions and ointments
Wool fat derivatives (includes lanolin)[a,3,12]	In many creams and ointments
Topical local anaesthetics	
Neomycin	
Ethyl alcohol	In some products and skin wipes
Chlorhexidine[13]	In antimicrobial products
Rubber additives (plasticizers, preservatives)	Undersheets, elastic stockings, etc.
Paraphenylenediamine, chromates	In leather
Tea tree oil[14]	

a. the BNF lists potential sensitizers, which mainly fall into these categories.

Dose and use

In hairy patients prone to folliculitis, to reduce the risk of further episodes, creams and ointments should be applied using downward strokes in the direction of hair growth, particularly on the legs.[15]

Choice of emollient involves consideration of:

- patient preference
- area to be treated, e.g. ointments are generally acceptable for the legs and trunk but not the face, and ointment may be necessary for the thicker skin of the palms and soles
- ingredients; does it contain known or potential allergens?
- degree of dryness; very dry skin often requires an ointment initially
- packaging, e.g. patients with weak hands may find removing screw-top lids or squeezing tubes difficult

- patient's lifestyle
- season; ointments are less well tolerated in the summer
- cost-effectiveness.

Emollients should be applied as frequently as needed to keep the skin well hydrated. This is generally twice daily. Very dry skin may require more frequent applications. Enough emollient should be applied to make the skin glisten.[15] However, if the emollient is applied too thickly, it may make the patient uncomfortable, hot or itchy, and may stain clothing.

The emollient should be applied immediately after a bath or shower when the skin is most hydrated. The patient should shake off excess water or lightly dab dry with a soft towel, and then apply the emollient to the damp skin. Emollients are essential for maintaining skin condition and should continue to be used at least once daily even when the dryness has improved/resolved.

It is helpful to demonstrate the use of the recommended emollient (or one of comparable consistency) to the patient and the family or carers. This is particularly useful in patients with unsightly skin who may feel ostracized, and for whom physical contact (touch) generally provides real psychological benefit.

In practice, to optimise adherence to treatment, *the best emollient is the one which a patient is happy to use*. This implies that it is both cosmetically acceptable and effective, and preferably should not be expensive. For example, many patients like the silky feel of **colloidal oatmeal** (e.g. Aveeno®), particularly on their hands and face. Average quantities required for b.d. application for 1 week are shown in Table 3.

Table 3 Quantities required for b.d. application for 1 week

	Creams and ointments (g)	*Lotions (mL)*
Face	15–30	100
Groins and genitalia	15–25	100
Both hands	25–50	200
Scalp	50–100	200
Both arms or both legs	100–200	200
Trunk	400	500

A light cream (e.g. Cetraben®, Diprobase®, E45®) or emollient lotion b.d. generally suffices with mild–moderate degrees of dryness (Table 4). For severe dryness, an ointment will be needed (e.g. Epaderm®, Hydromol®).

Soap should *not* be used, because of its drying effect on the skin. It contributes to the breakdown of the skin barrier by raising the pH; this enhances protease activity, inhibits lipid synthesis, and promotes bacterial colonization. Use instead a soap substitute (e.g. **aqueous cream BP**, **emulsifying ointment BP**, Cetraben® cream, Dermol® cream or lotion). Also see Table 4.

If emollient-related contact dermatitis is suspected, patch testing with the standard set of potential allergens may identify an allergen. If allergy is confirmed, a product which does not contain the allergen (and, ideally, any other added preservatives or fragrances) should be prescribed. However, not all contact dermatitis is allergic; sometimes it is caused by direct chemical irritation.

When there is an active inflammatory skin condition causing redness and eroded or scaly skin, apply a topical corticosteroid, preferably in ointment form, once daily to the affected area for 3–7 days or until the inflammation settles. Apply the corticosteroid 30–60min before or after any emollient has been applied. In practice, topical corticosteroids are prescribed mostly for dermatoses of the face and hands. Mild topical corticosteroids, e.g. **hydrocortisone** 1%, are generally used for the face. For the trunk, hands, feet or limbs, choose a moderately potent topical corticosteroid, e.g. **clobetasone butyrate** 0.05% or **betamethasone valerate** 0.025% ointment.

If the inflamed skin is deeply cracked and secondary infection is suspected, a topical corticosteroid + a topical antifungal and/or antibacterial should be prescribed; various combination products are available. *To minimize the risk of developing resistance, products containing antimicrobials must not be used p.r.n. but as a full course for 7 days.*

Lymphoedema

Skin care is just one component of multimodal lymphoedema management.[16,17] The following advice must be applied within the broader management context (also see p.529 and QCG: Cellulitis in lymphoedema, p.532).

The choice depends on the state of the skin but also on current fashion and local contracts:[18]

- if not obviously dry and flaky, a light cream can be applied once daily–b.d. as a prophylactic measure (e.g. Cetraben®, Diprobase®, E45®) or an alternative (see Table 4)
- if the skin is dry ± cracked, apply Epaderm®, Hydromol® or **liquid and white soft paraffin ointment NPF** (**liquid paraffin** in **white soft paraffin** 50:50)
- if there is a build-up of scales, wash the affected area with a light cream (see Table 4) using a circular motion in order to soften and lift off the scales; then apply **liquid and white soft paraffin ointment NPF**, and cover with a hydrocolloid dressing (e.g. Granuflex®) and bandage; repeat every 1–3 days until the skin condition is good
- if there are toe web fissures, take scrapings to look for fungus and, if present, treat appropriately, e.g. **clotrimazole** 1% or **terbinafine** 1% cream b.d. for 2 weeks.

Antipruritic emollients

If pruritus is caused by dry skin, rehydration of the skin will correct it. Thus, all emollients are antipruritic in this sense. However, some products have a specific antipruritic agent added, and can provide extra benefit in some patients (see Topical antipruritics, p.685).

12

Supply

This is not a complete list; see BNF for additional options.

Pharmaco-economics

Before prescribing a relatively expensive proprietary product, check to see whether, content for content, there is a cheaper essentially equivalent product.

Mild topical corticosteroid
Hydrocortisone (generic)
Cream 1%, 15g = £1, 30g = £1.75, 50g = £5.
Ointment 1%, 15g = £1.50, 30g = £3, 50g = £5.

Moderately potent topical corticosteroids
Betamethasone valerate
Betnovate-RD® (GSK)
Cream 0.025%, 100g = £3.25; *this is a quarter of the strength of Betnovate® cream. Excipients include cetostearyl alcohol, chlorocresol.*
Ointment 0.025%, 100g = £3.25; *this is a quarter of the strength of Betnovate® ointment.*

Clobetasone butyrate
Eumovate® (GSK)
Cream 0.05%, 30g = £2, 100g = £5.50. *Excipients include beeswax substitute, cetostearyl alcohol, chlorocresol.*
Ointment 0.05%, 30g = £2, 100g = £5.50.

Antifungal creams
Clotrimazole (generic)
Cream 1%, 20g = £1.50, 50g = £3.50.

Terbinafine (generic)
Cream 1%, 15g = £1.50, 30g = £3.

For more antifungal products, see Barrier products (p.688) and the *BNF*.

Table 4 Emollient and additive content of selected topical products[a]

	Emollient base	*Additional ingredients*	*Sensitizing excipients[b]*	*Supply*
Ointments				
Emulsifying ointment BP[c]	White soft paraffin 50% Emulsifying wax 30% Liquid paraffin 20%		Cetostearyl alcohol Sodium lauryl sulfate	500g = £4.75
Epaderm® ointment	Emulsifying wax 30% Yellow soft paraffin 30%			125g = £4, 500g = £6.50, 1kg = £12
White *or* yellow soft paraffin BP	Petroleum jelly (white or yellow)			100g = £2, 500g = £4
Liquid paraffin and white soft paraffin ointment NPF	Liquid paraffin 50% White soft paraffin 50%			250g = £1.75, 500g = £3.25
Hydromol®	Liquid paraffin 40% Emulsifying wax 30% Yellow soft paraffin 30%		Cetostearyl alcohol Sodium lauryl sulfate	125g = £3, 500g = £5, 1kg = £8.50
Oils				
Coconut oil BP	Coconut oil			OTC
Water-in-oil (rich) creams				
Aquaderm® hydrous ointment	Wool alcohols ointment 50%	Magnesium sulfate 0.5% Phenoxyethanol 1%		500g = £4.25
Aquadrate®	White soft paraffin	Urea 10%		30g = £1.75, 100g = £4.50
Lipobase®	Light liquid paraffin White soft paraffin		Cetostearyl alcohol Hydroxybenzoates (parabens)	50g = £1.50
Unguentum M®	Saturated neutral oil Liquid paraffin White soft paraffin		Cetostearyl alcohol Polysorbate 40 Propylene glycol Sorbic acid	500g = £8.50

continued

Table 4 Continued

	Emollient base	*Additional ingredients*	*Sensitizing excipients*[b]	*Supply*
Oil-in-water (light) creams				
Aqueous cream BP[c]	Emulsifying ointment 30%	Phenoxyethanol[d] 1%	Cetostearyl alcohol Sodium lauryl sulfate	100g = £0.75 500g = £2.25
Aveeno® cream	Emollient basis	Colloidal oatmeal	Benzyl alcohol Cetyl alcohol Isopropyl palmitate	ACBS, 100mL = £4, 500mL = £6.50
Cetraben®,[c]	White soft paraffin 13.2% Light liquid paraffin 10.5%		Cetostearyl alcohol Hydroxybenzoates (parabens)	50g = £1.50, 150g = £4, 500g = £6, 1kg = £12
Dermol®,[c] cream	Liquid paraffin 10% Isopropyl myristate 10%	Benzalkonium chloride 0.1% Chlorhexidine hydrochloride 0.1%	Cetostearyl alcohol	100g = £3, 500g = £6.50
Diprobase® cream	White soft paraffin 15% Liquid paraffin 6% Cetomacrogol 2.25%		Cetostearyl alcohol Chlorocresol	50g = £1.25, 500g = £6.50
E45® cream	White soft paraffin 14.5% Liquid paraffin 12.6% Lanolin[e] 1%		Cetyl alcohol Hydroxybenzoates (parabens)	50g = £2, 125g = £3.25, 350g = £6, 500g = £6
E45® Itch relief	Lauromacrogols 3% Liquid paraffin Octyldodecanol Cetyl palmitate Dimeticone	Glycerol 85% Urea 5%	Benzyl alcohol Polysorbates	50g = £2.75, 100g = £4.25, 500g = £15
Hydromol® cream	Liquid paraffin 13.8%	Sodium pidolate 2.5%	Cetostearyl alcohol Hydroxybenzoates (parabens)	50g = £2.25, 100g = £4.25, 500g = £12
Zerobase®	Liquid paraffin 11%		Cetostearyl alcohol Chlorocresol	50g = £1, 500g = £5.50

continued

Table 4 Continued

	Emollient base	*Additional ingredients*	*Sensitizing excipients*[b]	*Supply*
Lotions				
Aveeno® lotion	Emollient basis	Colloidal oatmeal	Benzyl alcohol Cetyl alcohol Isopropyl palmitate	ACBS, 500mL = £7
Dermol® 500 lotion	Liquid paraffin 2.5% Isopropyl myristate 2.5%	Benzalkonium chloride 0.1% Chlorhexidine hydrochloride 0.1%	Cetostearyl alcohol	500mL = £6
E45® lotion	White soft paraffin 10% Light liquid paraffin 4% Lanolin[e] 1% Cetomacrogol Glyceryl monostearate		Isopropyl palmitate Hydroxybenzoates (parabens) Benzyl alcohol	200mL = £2.50, 500mL = £4.50

a. list is not exhaustive; see BNF for alternative products
b. excipients which are associated, rarely, with sensitization
c. can be used as a soap substitute
d. or other antimicrobial
e. hypoallergenic anhydrous wool fat (hypoallergenic lanolin).

1 Cork MJ and Danby S (2009) Skin barrier breakdown: a renaissance in emollient therapy. *British Journal of Nursing*. **18**: 872, 874, 876–877.
2 Kraft JN and Lynde CW (2005) Moisturizers: what they are and a practical approach to product selection. *Skin Therapy Letter*. **10**: 1–8.
3 Sibbald D (2002) Dermatitis. In: Repchinsky C (ed.) *Patient Self-care* (2nd edn). Ottawa: Canadian Pharmacists Association. pp. 479–505.
4 Fluhr JW *et al.* (2008) Emollients, moisturizers, and keratolytic agents in psoriasis. *Clinics in Dermatology*. **26**: 380–386.
5 MHRA (2018) Emollients: new information about risk of severe and fatal burns with paraffin-containing and paraffin-free emollients. *Drug Safety Update*. **3**. www.gov.uk/drug-safety-update
6 Hoppe U, (ed) (1999) The Lanolin Book. Beierdorf AG, Hamburg, pp.
7 MHRA (2003) Medicines containing peanut (arachis) oil. *Current Problems in Pharmacovigilance*. **29**: 5.
8 Hourihane JO *et al.* (1997) Randomised, double blind, crossover challenge study of allergenicity of peanut oils in subjects allergic to peanuts. *British Medical Journal*. **314**: 1084–1088.
9 Keating MU *et al.* (1990) Immunoassay of peanut allergens in food-processing materials and finished foods. *Journal of Allergy and Clinical Immunology*. **86**: 41–44.
10 MHRA (2013) Aqueous cream: may cause skin irritation, particularly in children with eczema, possibly due to sodium lauryl sulphate content. *Drug Safety Update*. **6**. www.gov.uk/drug-safety-update
11 Cork MJ *et al.* (2003) An audit of adverse drug reactions to aqueous cream in children with atopic eczema. *The Pharmaceutical Journal*. **271**: 747–748.
12 Voegeli D (2008) Care or harm: exploring essential components in skin care regimens. *British Journal of Nursing*. **17**: 24-30.
13 MHRA (2012) All medical devices and medicinal products containing chlorhexidine. Risk of anaphylactic reaction due to chlorhexidine allergy. *Medical Devices Alert*. MDA/2012/2075. www.gov.uk/drug-device-alerts
14 Rubel DM *et al.* (1998) Tea tree oil allergy: what is the offending agent? Report of three cases of tea tree oil allergy and review of the literature. *Australasian Journal of Dermatology*. **39**: 244–247.
15 Lawton S (2009) Practical issues for emollient therapy in dry and itchy skin. *British Journal of Nursing*. **18**: 978–984.
16 Twycross R and Wilcock A (eds) (2016) *Introducing Palliative Care*. (5e). palliativedrugs.com Ltd, Nottingham, pp. 131–135.
17 Twycross R *et al.* (2000) *Lymphoedema*. Radcliffe Medical Press, Oxford.
18 Linnitt N (2000) Skin management in lymphoedema. In: Twycross RG *et al.* (eds). *Lymphoedema* Oxford: Radcliffe Medical Press. pp. 118–129.

Updated (minor change) September 2021

12

TOPICAL ANTIPRURITICS

Indications: Pruritus which fails to respond to an emollient and/or specific treatment.

Background

Pruritus may be caused by systemic disease (such as drug hypersensitivity, obstructive jaundice, endocrine disease, malignant disease), skin disease (e.g. eczema, urticaria, psoriasis, scabies) or drugs (e.g. opioids).

Dryness of the skin (xerosis) is the commonest cause of pruritus without an accompanying rash, and an emollient is the first-line treatment (see p.677). Dryness is associated with normal ageing, inflammatory skin conditions (e.g. atopic dermatitis), systemic disease (e.g. hypothyroidism, renal failure), and cachexia and general debility in advanced cancer.

Whenever possible, the treatment of pruritus should be cause-specific.[1,2] For example, in skin disorders:

- scabies: treat patient and the whole family with topical **permethrin** (preferred) or **malathion**[3,4]
- atopic dermatitis: use topical corticosteroid (+ emollient)[5]
- contact dermatitis: use topical corticosteroid, identify causal substance and avoid further contact.

In systemic disorders or when caused by opioids, a range of options exist (see Chapter 26, p.825). A topical antipruritic should be considered only if a bland emollient and cause-specific treatment fail to relieve.

Although topical products are not convenient to apply regularly to the whole body, many patients with generalized pruritus have patches of more intense discomfort and may benefit from more limited application.

Pharmacology

Traditional topical antipruritics include **phenol**, **levomenthol** (**menthol**) and **camphor**. **Phenol** 0.5–3% acts by anaesthetizing cutaneous nerve endings. **Levomenthol** 0.5–2% and **camphor** 0.5–3% may relieve pruritus by cooling the skin by acting on heat-sensitive transient receptor potential (TRP) channels expressed on sensory nerve endings.[6,7] Cooling the skin is known to reduce the intensity of histamine-induced pruritus, and patients who suffer from chronic pruritic conditions such as atopic dermatitis, psoriasis and uraemic pruritus often find that cold showers reduce the pruritus.

Capsaicin is a naturally occurring alkaloid found in the fruits of various species of Solanaceae (the nightshade family) and in pepper plants of the genus *Capsicum* (chilli peppers).[8] It acts by depleting substance P at sensory nerve endings. **Capsaicin** products are useful in relieving neuropathic pain (see p.651). Benefit has also been reported in histamine-related pruritus, aquagenic pruritus, and pruritus associated with uraemia, nodular prurigo, psoriasis and post-axillary dissection syndrome.[6]

A Cochrane review of pruritus in adult palliative care patients also found benefit in uraemic pruritus, but the methodological quality of the studies was low, introducing a risk of bias and thus preventing meaningful interpretation of the results.[9] **Capsaicin** has also been used successfully in the treatment of intractable pruritus ani.[10]

In practice, **capsaicin** will be applied to relatively limited areas of the skin. It often initially causes localized burning and stinging. This irritation subsides with repeated use, but patients may have difficulty continuing treatment. Patients should initially use **capsaicin** cream t.d.s.–q.d.s. (leaving at least 4h between applications; the manufacturers specify q.d.s. for the 0.025% cream) to overcome the irritation, after which the frequency of applications can be reduced. The mixed topical anaesthetic cream EMLA® (eutectic mixture of local anaesthetics; **lidocaine** 2.5% and **prilocaine** 2.5%), used in conjunction with **capsaicin**, may reduce the initial irritation.[11] Excessive use of a topical anaesthetic cream may result in acute transient systemic local anaesthetic neurotoxicity.[12]

Polidocanol (macrogol lauryl ether) is an anionic detergent with local anaesthetic properties.[13] Benefit has been reported in patients with pruritus associated with atopic dermatitis, non-atopic dermatitis and psoriasis, with the regular application of a cream containing 5% **urea** and 3% **polidocanol** (E45® Itch Relief Cream).[14,15]

Crotamiton 10% lotion (Eurax®) has a mild antiscabetic effect, which is probably the reason for its reputation as an antipruritic. However, in an RCT in patients with chronic pruritic dermatoses, **crotamiton** lotion was no more effective than its vehicle.[16]

Topical H_1 antihistamines, e.g. **diphenhydramine**, are of benefit only when the pruritus is cutaneous in origin and related to histamine release.[1] Topical **diphenhydramine** can cause contact dermatitis and photosensitivity; if used, limit to 3 days. Oral sedating H_1 antihistamines, e.g. **alimemazine**, **chlorphenamine**, may be helpful if sedation is desirable in intractable pruritus, e.g. if itch is disturbing sleep (see Chapter 26, p.825).

A **coal tar**-based shampoo, e.g. Capasal® or Polytar®, has a long tradition of use with scalp pruritus; when caused by seborrheic dermatitis, **ketoconazole** shampoo can be used.

Calamine lotion has traditionally been used for pruritus, and generally also contains **phenol** 0.5%. However, proprietary formulations are very drying and, because it is unsightly, **calamine** is unlikely to be acceptable except on a short-term basis, e.g. in acute contact dermatitis; avoid in dry skin conditions.

Doxepin

Doxepin is a TCA which is a potent H_1- and H_2-receptor antagonist. Its affinity for H_2-receptors is six times that of **cimetidine**.[17] It is also antimuscarinic and may antagonize the pruritic effects of substance P at skin receptors.

Doxepin 5% cream is reported to be of benefit in some patients with atopic dermatitis,[17-19] but long-term independent studies are lacking.[20] It is not generally suitable for children. It is possible that the benefit is systemic rather than topical. About 15% of patients complain initially of localized stinging or burning, and a similar proportion complain of drowsiness secondary to systemic absorption.[18] The sedation may help the antipruritic effect.

Doxepin cream is less effective than systemic treatment[21] (see Chapter 26, p.825), and allergic contact dermatitis may occur.[18] However, PO capsules are expensive (see Supply). Patients with contact allergy should not take the drug by mouth.[22]

Cautions

Because of:

- the risk of contact dermatitis, *discourage* the use of topical H_1 antihistamines and of local anaesthetics
- their drying effect, *discourage* the use of products containing **calamine** unless they contain oil (e.g. **calamine oily lotion BP**).

Calamine oily lotion BP (only available as a special order product) contains *refined* **arachis** (peanut) **oil**; official advice states that emollients containing **arachis** (peanut) **oil** should not be used by patients with peanut or soya allergy.[23,24] However, unlike *crude* **arachis oil**, the *refined* oil is not allergenic, and is highly unlikely to cause allergic reactions in people with (whole) peanut allergy.[25,26]

Polytar® products also contain traces of **arachis** (peanut) **oil** from the **coal tar** extraction process, and thus might cause allergic reactions in people with peanut or soya allergy.

Patients prescribed **doxepin**, either systemically or topically, should avoid the concurrent use of drugs which inhibit cytochrome P450, e.g. **cimetidine**, imidazole antifungals, macrolide antibacterials (see Chapter 19, Table 8, p.790). As with other TCAs, MAOIs should be discontinued ≥2 weeks before starting treatment with **doxepin**. Monitor carefully in patients with glaucoma, severe heart disease, cardiac arrhythmias, urinary hesitancy, severe liver disease or a history of mania. Because of the possibility of undesirable systemic effects, e.g. dizziness, antimuscarinic effects, headache or GI disturbances, avoid applying the cream to large areas of skin. The manufacturer recommends a maximum of 3g per application, covering no more than 10% of the body area.

Use

Because pruritus is commonly associated with dry skin, an emollient (moisturizer) should be tried first (see p.677). A light cream (oil in water), e.g. Cetraben®, Diprobase® or E45®, or an emollient lotion often suffices with mild–moderate degrees of dryness. Products containing **colloidal oatmeal** (Aveeno®) are popular because of their silky feel (see Emollients, Table 4, p.682). Storing creams and lotions in a refrigerator may increase benefit.

Levomenthol 0.5–5% is available as a proprietary product authorized for pruritus, e.g. Dermacool®. When a proprietary product is unavailable or unsuitable, **levomenthol** 0.5–2% (or **camphor** 0.5–3%) in a bland emollient base can be obtained as a special order (see Chapter 24, p.817) and applied topically t.d.s.–q.d.s.

Supply

Several OTC products contain **levomenthol** and **camphor** (with contents as high as 11%). These are marketed for rheumatic aches and pains, sprains or minor sports injuries, e.g. Tiger Balm Red®. Others are mainly intended for use on insect bites, and the unit size is small. 12

Note. This list is not exhaustive.

Levomenthol
Dermacool® (Pern Consumer Products)
Cream 0.5%, 1%, 2%, 5%, 100g tube = £4, 500g pump pack = £17.

Polidocanol (macrogol lauryl ether)
E45 Itch Relief® (Crookes)
Cream (oil in water) containing **urea** 5%, **macrogol lauryl ether** 3%, 100g = £4.25; 500g pump-pack = £15.

Coal tar
Capasal® Therapeutic Shampoo (Dermal Laboratories)
Shampoo containing **distilled coal tar** 1%, **coconut oil** 1%, **salicylic acid** 5%, 250mL = £4.50.

Polytar® Scalp Shampoo (GlaxoSmithKline Consumer Healthcare)
Shampoo containing **coal tar** solution 40mg/mL (4%), 150mL = £3.50. *May contain **arachis** (peanut) oil.*

Ketoconazole (generic)
Shampoo 2%, 120mL = £3.50.

Doxepin
Doxepin (generic)
Capsules 25mg, 50mg, 28 days @ 25mg, 50mg, 75mg at bedtime = £97, £154 and £291 respectively.

Xepin® (Cambridge Healthcare Supplies)
Cream 5%, 30g = £13.50.

See p.651 for **capsaicin** products.

---

1 Zylicz Z *et al.* (2004) *Pruritus in Advanced Disease*. Oxford University Press, Oxford.
2 Twycross R and Wilcock A (eds) (2016) *Introducing Palliative Care* (5th edn). palliativedrugs.com Ltd, Nottingham. pp. 228–232.
3 British National Formulary 13.2. Parasiticidal preparations. London: BMJ Group and Pharmaceutical Press. www.medicinescomplete.com (accessed November 2019).
4 Strong M and Johnstone P (2007) Interventions for treating scabies. *Cochrane Database of Systematic Reviews*. 3: CD000320. www.thecochranelibrary.com
5 Cork MJ (1999) Taking the itch out of eczema: how careful use of emollients can break the itch-scratch cycle of atopic eczema. *Asthma Journal*. 4: 16–20.

6 Patel T *et al.* (2007) Menthol: a refreshing look at this ancient compound. *Journal of the American Academy of Dermatology.* **57**: 873–878.
7 Peier AM *et al.* (2002) A TRP channel that senses cold stimuli and menthol. *Cell.* **108**: 705–715.
8 Towlerton GR and Rice AS. Topical analgesics for chronic pain. In: Rice AS *et al.* (eds). *Clinical Pain Management: Chronic Pain.* London: Arnold; 2003. p. 213–226.
9 Xander C *et al.* (2013) Pharmacological interventions for pruritus in adult palliative care patients. *Cochrane Database of Systematic Reviews.* **6**: CD008320. www.thecochranelibrary.com
10 Lysy J *et al.* (2003) Topical capsaicin--a novel and effective treatment for idiopathic intractable pruritus ani: a randomised, placebo controlled, crossover study. *Gut.* **52**: 1323–1326.
11 Yosipovitch G and Hundley JL (2004) Practical guidelines for relief of itch. *Dermatology Nursing.* **16**: 325–328; quiz 329.
12 Brosh-Nissimov T *et al.* (2004) Central nervous system toxicity following topical skin application of lidocaine. *European Journal of Clinical Pharmacology.* **60**: 683–684.
13 Vieluf D *et al.* (1992) Dry and itching skin – therapy with a new preparation, containing urea and polidocanol. *Zeitschrift fur Hautkrankheiten.* **67**: 816–821.
14 Hauss H *et al.* (1993) Comparative study of a formulation containing urea and polidocanol and a greasy cream containing linoleic acid in the treatment of dry, pruritic skin lesions [in German]. *Dermatosen in Beruf und Umwelt Occupational and Environmental Dermatoses.* **41**: 184–188.
15 Freitag G and Hoppner T (1997) Results of a postmarketing drug monitoring survey with a polidocanol-urea preparation for dry, itching skin. *Current Medical Research and Opinion.* **13**: 529–537.
16 Smith E *et al.* (1984) Crotamiton lotion in pruritus. *International Journal of Dermatology.* **23**: 684–685.
17 Drake L *et al.* (1994) Relief of pruritus in patients with atopic dermatitis after treatment with topical doxepin cream. The Doxepin Study Group. *Journal of the American Academy of Dermatology.* **31**: 613–616.
18 DTB (2000) Doxepin cream for eczema? *Drug and Therapeutics Bulletin.* **38**: 31.
19 Breneman D *et al.* (1997) Doxepin cream relieves eczema-associated pruritus within 15 minutes and is not accompanied by a risk of rebound upon discontinuation. *Journal of Dermatological Treatment.* **8**: 161–168.
20 Hoare C *et al.* (2000) Systematic review of treatments for atopic eczema. *Health Technology Assessment.* **4**: 1–191.
21 Smith P and Corelli R (1997) Doxepin in the management of pruritus associated with allergic cutaneous reactions. *Annals of Pharmacotherapy.* **31**: 633–635.
22 Bonnel RA *et al.* (2003) Allergic contact dermatitis from topical doxepin: food and Drug Administration's postmarketing surveillance experience. *Journal of the American Academy of Dermatology.* **48**: 294–296.
23 MHRA (2003) Medicines containing peanut (arachis) oil. *Current Problems in Pharmacovigilance.* **29**: 5.
24 Anonymous (2003) Peanut allergy research is published. *Pharmaceutical Journal.* **270**: 391.
25 Keating MU *et al.* (1990) Immunoassay of peanut allergens in food-processing materials and finished foods. *Journal of Allergy and Clinical Immunology.* **86**: 41–44.
26 Hourihane JO *et al.* (1997) Randomised, double blind, crossover challenge study of allergenicity of peanut oils in subjects allergic to peanuts. *British Medical Journal.* **314**: 1084–1088.

Updated November 2019

BARRIER PRODUCTS

Indications: Skin protection, napkin rash.

Introduction

Barrier products contain water-repellent substances which help to protect the skin and prevent maceration and infection. They can be used around stomas and in the perineal and peri-anal areas in patients with urinary or faecal incontinence, as long as the skin is intact. Once skin damage is present, typical barrier preparations generally have a limited role. However, a barrier product such as Cavilon No-Sting Barrier Film® or Medi Derma-S® Non Sting Barrier Film coats damaged skin with a protective film for ≤72h and thereby protects it from urine, faeces and other body fluids, and reduces friction and adhesive trauma from dressings.

A cream is less greasy than an ointment and is easier to apply and wash off. Most barrier creams and ointments are **silicone-**, **titanium**- or **zinc oxide**-based.[1] Some products contain *refined* **arachis** (peanut) **oil**. However, unlike *crude* **arachis oil**, the *refined* oil is not allergenic, and thus is highly unlikely to cause allergic reactions in people with (whole) peanut allergy.[2,3]

Cautions

If the damaged skin is infected, because barrier products prevent topical antimicrobials from penetrating the skin, delay their use until the infection has been treated.

Use

Ensure that infection is treated promptly with topical antifungals (more common) and/or antibacterials (less common).

Intertrigo

Intertrigo is an inflammatory dermatosis of skin folds, primarily caused by skin on skin friction. Exacerbating factors cause skin maceration and inflammation, e.g. obesity, heat, moisture, lack of air. Secondary fungal or bacterial infection is common. The wet component is the most easily modified, and drying the involved skin is essential. Initial treatment may comprise:

- cleanse with a soap substitute (e.g. Cetraben®); see Emollients, Table 4, p.682)
- dry well; blow-drying with a hand-held hair dryer can be used if necessary
- avoid tight clothing and non-breathable fabrics; change dressings and incontinence pads before they become saturated
- if infection is likely, and because fungal infection is more common, a topical broad-spectrum antifungal should be prescribed, e.g. **clotrimazole**
- if inflammation or pruritus are problematic, add a mild topical corticosteroid for 7–14 days, e.g. **hydrocortisone** 1% cream (see p.677); combination products containing both an antifungal and **hydrocortisone** 1% are available
- intertrigo not responding to the above measures may benefit from a combination product containing an antifungal, corticosteroid and an antibacterial (e.g. Trimovate® cream)
- when infection is widespread, the patient is immunocompromised, or topical treatment ineffective, give PO antifungal treatment, e.g. **fluconazole** 50mg PO once daily for 14 days
- when the wetness and infection has settled, begin to use a barrier product.

Protection around a stoma

Many products designed to protect the skin around a stoma from liquid effluent are available; a stoma-care nurse can advise on product selection. Sprays or wipes which dry to form a protective film are commonly used. An alcohol-free formulation is preferable, because it is less likely to sting or irritate the skin.

A barrier cream (e.g. Comfeel®, Medi Derma-S®) should be used prophylactically if the stoma effluent is liquid or if the stoma bag is being changed more than once daily. It is gently rubbed in, and any excess wiped off. If the skin becomes red and sore, a barrier film is used instead (e.g. Cavilon No-Sting Barrier Film ®, Medi Derma-S® Non Sting Barrier Film).

A topical corticosteroid can be used short-term to treat moderate–severe inflammation. Foam products are well tolerated, e.g. Bettamousse® (off-label use). Topical application of **beclometasone** dry powder inhaler has been reported successfully (also off-label use), without compromising the adhesion of the stoma bag, which can occur with creams and lotions.[4]

Incontinence

After cleansing with a soap substitute and gently drying, apply a barrier product to the affected area whenever the dressing or padding is changed.[1] Avoid excessive amounts of cream that could coat the pad and thereby interfere with its ability to absorb fluids.

Painful malignant wounds

An unauthorized topical product containing **lidocaine** 2% in Lutrol gel has been used up to b.d. with dressing changes for patients with pain from malignant wounds, especially in areas where dressings are difficult to apply and keep in place or are exposed to body fluids such as urine.[5,6] Benefit is from the barrier properties of the Lutrol gel in addition to the **lidocaine** (also see **lidocaine** medicated plasters, p.77). A fact sheet with further information can be obtained from the Document library of palliativedrugs.com. When the barrier properties are not required, lidocaine 5% ointment is an alternative.

For the use of topical **morphine** in wounds, see p.410.

Supply

The following is only a selection of the available products.

Cavilon Durable Barrier Cream® (3M)
Cream 2g sachet, 20 = £6.50, 28g tube = £3.25, 92g tube = £6.50.

Cavilon No-Sting Barrier Film® (3M)
Foam applicator 5 × 1mL = £4; 5 × 3mL = £6.50.
Pump spray 28mL = £6.

Comfeel® Barrier Cream (Coloplast)
Cream 60g = £5.

Conotrane® (Karo Pharma)
Cream containing **dimeticone 350** 22% and **benzalkonium chloride** 0.1%, 100g = £1, 500g = £3.50.

Medi Derma-S® Barrier Cream (Medicareplus).
Cream 2g sachet, 20 = £6, 28g tube = £3, 90g tube = £6.

Medi Derma-S® Non Sting Medical Barrier Film (Medicareplus)
Foam applicator 5 x 1mL = £3.75, 5 x 3mL = £6.
Pump spray 30mL = £5.25.
Aerosol spray 50mL = £9.

Zinc and castor oil (generic)
Ointment containing **zinc oxide** 7.5% in a **castor oil, arachis** (peanut) **oil, white beeswax** and **cetostearyl alcohol** base, 100g = £1.50, 500g = £5.25.

Lidocaine (generic)
Ointment **lidocaine** 5%, 15g = £8.25.
Topical gel **lidocaine** 2% in Lutrol gel, 5mL (unauthorized product, available as a special order from Oxford Pharmacy Store, Oxford Health NHS Foundation Trust; see Chapter 24, p.817).
There is a lead time of several days from order and the product is quite expensive.

Antifungal products
Clotrimazole (generic)
Cream **clotrimazole** 1%, 20g = £1.25, 50g = £3.50.

Canesten® (Bayer Consumer Care)
Solution **clotrimazole** 1%, 20mL = £2.50.
Spray **clotrimazole** 1%, 40mL = £4.75; *contains isopropyl alcohol.*

Miconazole
Daktarin® (Janssen-Cilag)
Cream **miconazole** 2% 30g = £1.75.
Powder spray (Daktarin Aktiv®) **miconazole** 0.16%, 100g = £3.75.

Topical corticosteroids
For **hydrocortisone** 1%, see p.677.

Bettamousse® (RPH Pharmaceuticals AB)
Foam (scalp application) containing **betamethasone valerate** 0.1%, 100g = £10.

Combined antifungal and topical corticosteroid products
Canesten HC® (Bayer)
Cream containing **clotrimazole** 1% and **hydrocortisone** 1%, 30g = £2.50.

Daktacort® (Janssen-Cilag)
Cream containing **miconazole** 2% and **hydrocortisone** 1%, 30g = £2.50.

Combined antibacterial, antifungal and moderate-potency topical corticosteroid
Trimovate® (Ennogen)
Cream containing **clobetasone butyrate** 0.05%, **oxytetracycline calcium** 3%, **nystatin** 100,000 units/g, 30g = £12.50.

1 Nazarko L (2007) Managing a common dermatological problem: incontinence dermatitis. *British Journal of Community Nursing.* **12**: 358–363.
2 Hourihane JO *et al.* (1997) Randomised, double blind, crossover challenge study of allergenicity of peanut oils in subjects allergic to peanuts. *British Medical Journal.* **314**: 1084–1088.
3 Keating MU *et al.* (1990) Immunoassay of peanut allergens in food-processing materials and finished foods. *Journal of Allergy and Clinical Immunology.* **86**: 41–44.
4 Boland J and Brooks D (2012) Topical application of a beclometasone steroid inhaler for treatment of stoma inflammation. *Palliative Medicine.* **26**: 1055–1056.
5 MacGregor K *et al.* (1994) Symptomatic relief of excoriating skin conditions using a topical thermoreversible gel. *Palliative Medicine.* **8**: 76–77.
6 Beynon T *et al.* (2003) Lutrol gel: a potential role in wounds? *Journal of Pain and Symptom Management.* **26**: 776–780.

Updated (minor change) September 2021

13: ANAESTHESIA

*KETAMINE

The use of ketamine is associated with upper GI, hepatobiliary, urinary and neuropsychiatric toxicity. Although most reports involve long-term recreational abusers, toxicity has also arisen after only 1–2 weeks of therapeutic use (Box A). Accordingly, the use of ketamine should be restricted to specialists in pain or palliative care for patients who have failed to obtain relief from standard drug and non-drug treatments.

Class: General anaesthetic.

Indications: Induction and maintenance of anaesthesia; pain in emergency medicine (IM/IV **esketamine**); treatment-resistant major depression (intranasal **esketamine**); †neuropathic, inflammatory, ischaemic limb and procedure-related pain unresponsive to standard treatments.[1,2]

Contra-indications: Any situation in which an increase in blood pressure would constitute a hazard. Concurrent use of **aminophylline** or **theophylline** (possible reduced seizure threshold).

Pharmacology

Ketamine, a derivative of phencyclidine (PCP), is a dissociative anaesthetic which has analgesic properties in sub-anaesthetic doses.[2,3] Both ketamine (racemic mixture) and **esketamine** (*S*-enantiomer) are available for clinical use. Ketamine is the most potent NMDA-receptor–channel blocker available for clinical use, binding to the PCP site when the channels are in the open activated state (Figure 1).[3] It also binds to a second membrane-associated site, which decreases the frequency of channel opening.[3]

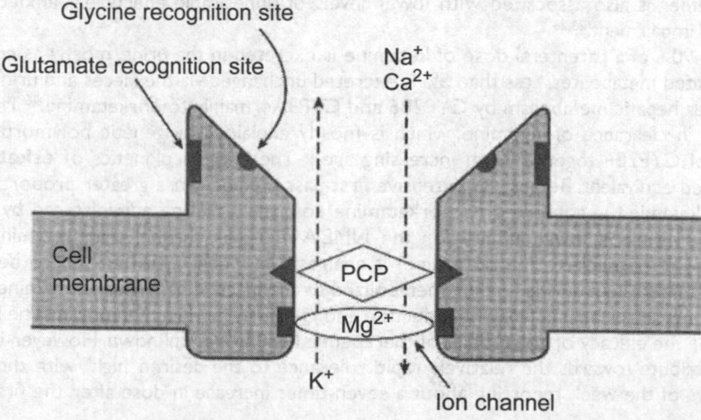

Figure 1 Diagram of the NMDA (excitatory) receptor–channel complex. The channel is blocked by magnesium (Mg^{2+}) when the membrane potential is at resting level (*voltage-dependent block*) and by drugs which act at the phencyclidine (PCP) binding site in the glutamate-activated channel, e.g. dextromethorphan, ketamine, methadone (*use-dependent block*).[4]

The NMDA-receptor–channel complex is composed of four subunits, generally two GluN1 in combination with two GluN2 (rarely GluN3) subunits, with binding of agonists (e.g. glutamate and glycine or serine) to all four units necessary for activation. There are several forms of the GluN2 (i.e. A–D) and GluN3 (i.e. A and B) subunits. This variation influences localization to synaptic or extra-synaptic sites and may partly explain the differences in clinical effects between NMDA-receptor–channel blocking drugs, e.g. ketamine and **memantine**.[5] Drugs are in development with greater selectivity for the various types of subunit.

The NMDA-receptor–channel complex is closely involved in the development of central sensitization of dorsal horn neurones which transmit pain signals.[4] At normal resting membrane potentials, the channel is blocked by magnesium and is inactive.[3] When the resting membrane potential is changed as a result of prolonged excitation, the channel unblocks and calcium moves into the cell. This leads to neuronal hyperexcitability and results in hyperalgesia and allodynia, and a reduction in opioid-responsiveness. These effects are probably mediated by the intracellular formation of nitric oxide and cyclic guanosine monophosphate.[3]

The reduction in opioid-responsiveness arises from cross-talk between opioid receptors and the NMDA-receptor channel. Opioid receptor activation results in phosphorylation and opening of the NMDA-receptor channel leading to a cascade of events which ultimately down-regulate the opioid receptor and its effects, thereby contributing towards tolerance and hyperalgesia.[3]

The NMDA-related sensitization is reflected in an increased temporal summation of pain (in response to a repeated brief painful stimulus), and its presence in patients with neuropathic pain helps predict benefit from ketamine.[6]

In addition to blocking the NMDA-receptor channel, ketamine has other actions, some of which may contribute to its analgesic effect.[2] These include opioid-like and anti-inflammatory effects,[7] and interactions with, e.g.:

- other calcium, potassium and sodium channels, e.g. hyperpolarization-activated cyclic nucleotide, AMPA
- cholinergic, dopaminergic and noradrenergic transmission
- descending inhibitory pathways.

Resultant changes in cellular processes, e.g. in gene expression and protein regulation, could explain ongoing benefit even after discontinuation of ketamine.[8]

Ketamine is generally administered PO or SC/CSCI.[9,10] It can also be administered IM, IV, SL, intranasally, PR and spinally (preservative-free formulation; not UK).[11-17] However, for spinal routes, concerns have been raised about the potential for neurotoxicity.[18] Ketamine has been given by CIVI in adults and children in combination with opioids (**fentanyl, morphine**) ± **midazolam** to control intractable pain and agitation.[19-21]

Because of its greater affinity and selectivity for the NMDA-receptor, the *S*-enantiomer (**esketamine**), as a parenteral analgesic, is about 4 times more potent than the *R*-enantiomer, and twice as potent as the racemic mixture.[22-24] When equi-analgesic doses are compared, the *S*-enantiomer is also associated with lower levels of undesirable effects, e.g. anxiety, tiredness, cognitive impairment.[23,25]

About 90% of a parenteral dose of ketamine is excreted in the urine, mostly as conjugates of hydroxylated metabolites. Less than 5% is excreted unchanged via the faeces and urine. Ketamine undergoes hepatic metabolism by CYP2B6 and CYP3A4, mainly to norketamine.[26] There is wide variation in clearance of ketamine, which is mostly explained by genetic polymorphism in the activity of CYP2B6 together with increasing age.[27] The pharmacokinetics of **esketamine** are considered equivalent. Because of extensive first-pass metabolism, a greater proportion of a PO dose of ketamine is converted to norketamine compared to one administered by injection.[28] Norketamine has a lower affinity for the NMDA-receptor channel than ketamine. Although norketamine (particularly *S*-norketamine) is analgesic in rodents, this remains to be clarified in humans.[29,30] Norketamine is further metabolized to the inactive dehydronorketamine.

Ketamine causes hepatic enzyme induction and enhances its own metabolism. The implications of this for the efficacy or tolerability of therapeutic ketamine is unknown. However, in abusers it may contribute towards the relatively rapid tolerance to the desired 'high', with those taking it most days of the week reporting about a seven-times increase in dose after the first 2 months of use.[31]

Ketamine increases sympathetic nervous system activity, and this is responsible for a number of effects, e.g. increases in heart rate, blood pressure, and salivary and tracheobronchial secretions, and bronchodilatation. When ketamine is used for procedural anaesthesia, a quarter of patients experience vivid dreams, misperceptions, hallucinations and alterations in body image and mood as emergent (psychotomimetic) phenomena, i.e. as the effects of a bolus dose wear off. The incidence is reduced to <10% by the concurrent use of **midazolam**.[32] Emergent phenomena occur to a lesser extent with the sub-anaesthetic analgesic doses given PO or CSCI, and generally can be controlled by concurrent administration of a benzodiazepine (e.g. **diazepam, midazolam**) or **haloperidol**.[15,33,34] Sub-anaesthetic doses of ketamine are associated with impaired attention, memory and judgement, and it is used as a pharmacological model for acute schizophrenia.[3]

Although ketamine is widely used as a short-term analgesic in various clinical settings (including peri-operatively, where it reduces pain and opioid requirements),[35,36] the potential for upper GI, hepatobiliary, urinary and neuropsychiatric toxicity (Box A) must be considered when contemplating its long-term use. In palliative care, ketamine should generally be reserved for pain that has failed to respond to standard analgesic drugs, including opioids and adjuvants (see Adjuvant analgesics, p.325).

Chronic non-cancer pain

A systematic review and meta-analysis of six RCTs in neuropathic or complex regional pain syndrome (CRPS) found moderate evidence of benefit from ketamine at 4 weeks after the beginning of treatment.[37] However, the authors concluded that further studies were required, in part because of methodological weaknesses in several of the RCTs and the meta-analysis being underpowered.[37] Separate systematic reviews in phantom limb pain and CRPS also found the evidence for ketamine limited and inconclusive.[38,39,40]

Nonetheless, ketamine is used in chronic non-cancer pain, generally when more usual treatments have failed, mostly by intermittent IVI. Caution is advised given the risk of undesirable effects (e.g. NNH=3 for psychotomimetic effects) and the lack of long-term safety data.[37,40,41]

Cancer pain

A systematic review of ketamine as an adjunct to opioids in cancer pain found only three studies of sufficient quality[15,42,43] and concluded that there is insufficient evidence to assess potential benefits and harms.[44] A subsequent large RCT of PO racemic ketamine in cancer-related neuropathic pain found no difference in duration of analgesic benefit between ketamine and placebo (median 0 days for both). However, most of the participants had cancer-treatment-related neuropathic pain (post chemotherapy/surgery) and were not taking opioids. Further, the bio-availability of the ketamine product used (encapsulated powder) is unknown, and it is only available as a special order (see Supply; p.698).[45]

Thus, in patients with cancer, evidence of ketamine's efficacy as an analgesic is mostly from case reports, retrospective surveys or uncontrolled studies in patients with refractory neuropathic or bone pain.[9,10,15,42,46-56] Nonetheless, it is considered a potentially useful treatment for cancer pain failing to respond to usual treatments, including opioids, non-opioids and adjuvant analgesics.[40]

Short-term 'burst' treatment with ketamine sometimes has a relatively long-lasting effect (i.e. several days to weeks and occasionally for months).[57,58] For example, ketamine 100mg/24h by CIVI for 2 days in a cancer patient, repeated a month later, reduced opioid requirements by 70%.[59] Similarly, in non-cancer patients taking regular strong opioids for ischaemic limb pain, a single 4h IV infusion of ketamine 600microgram/kg reduced opioid requirements during the next week.[60]

However, in a large case series, about a quarter of patients experienced severe undesirable effects from higher-dose 'burst' CSCI ketamine involving rapid dose escalation 100 → 300 → 500mg/24h over 3–5 days.[57] Further, in a 5-day RCT in cancer patients using the same regimen, there was no difference in the proportion responding in the ketamine and placebo arms (about 50% in each, based on average pain score).[43] There were fewer treatment failures at the maximum dose (25% vs. 50%), but more undesirable effects and withdrawals due to toxicity (19% vs. 2%).[43] *These results suggest that rapid titration involving such doses of CSCI ketamine is generally inadvisable.*[44]

Miscellaneous

Ketamine (generally IV/IM, alone or in combination with **morphine** or **midazolam**) can provide analgesia in severe acute pain due to trauma and other causes,[61,62] severe cancer treatment-related mucositis[63,64] and during painful procedures, e.g. change of dressings, reduction of fractures and dislocations.[65-67] There are reports of its successful use in children and adolescents with pain of various causes.[68]

Topical ketamine has been used as an oral rinse in cancer-treatment-related mucositis.[69,70] It has also been applied to the skin in various non-cancer pains,[71-73] although a recent large RCT where ketamine was one of several drugs applied as a gel was negative.[74]

Ketamine has a rapid antidepressant effect in patients with major depression and bipolar disorder, including a reduction in suicidal ideation, and is increasingly used when other treatments have failed.[75-77] Following a single IV dose (typically 500microgram/kg over 40–60min), up to 70% of patients respond, with improvements seen within hours. However, duration of benefit is generally ≤1 week.[75,77] Serial treatments (e.g. 6 doses given on alternate days) improve and maintain the response, but following completion most relapse within 1–6 weeks.[75] Ketamine 25mg b.d. PO also decreases the response time to an SSRI in newly diagnosed major depression.[78] The exact mechanism is unclear, but modulation of glutaminergic neurotransmission, AMPA receptor activation and the release of brain-derived neurotrophic factor appear important. The latter helps to restore neuroplasticity, e.g. through the formation of new synapses, more rapidly than seen with conventional antidepressants (see Antidepressants, p.210).[79] Although case reports of benefit are emerging from the palliative care setting,[80] the use of ketamine to treat major depression is best restricted to specialist mental health services.[81] Intranasal **esketamine** (Spravato®, see Supply) has recently been approved for use in treatment-resistant depression. Clinical trials of ketamine/ketamine-like drugs are ongoing.[79,82] There are preliminary reports of similar rapid but short-lasting benefit from ketamine in refractory anxiety.[83]

CIVI ketamine appears effective in refractory status epilepticus, but its place in clinical practice remains to be determined.[84]

Bio-availability 93% IM; 45% nasal; 30% SL; 30% PR; 20% PO.[85,86]

Onset of action 5min IM; 15–30min SC; 30min PO.

Time to peak plasma concentration no data SC; 30min PO; 1h norketamine.[87]

Plasma halflife 1–3h IM; 3h PO; 12h norketamine.[88]

Duration of action 30min–2h IM; 4–6h PO, sometimes longer.[89]

Cautions

History of psychiatric disorder; epilepsy, glaucoma, hypertension, heart failure, ischaemic heart disease, stroke, acute intermittent porphyria.[90] Hyperthyroidism (increased risk of hypertension and tachycardia). Conditions causing excessive upper airway secretions; ketamine both increases salivation and sensitizes the gag reflex, leading on rare occasions to laryngospasm. Severe hepatic impairment (consider dose reduction).

Because of reports of ketamine increasing CSF pressure, raised intracranial pressure (e.g. as a result of head injury, intracranial tumour, hydrocephalus) is a traditional caution. However, systematic reviews report no such concerns in ventilated patients with traumatic or non-traumatic brain injury.[91,92]

Drug interactions

Ketamine (and **esketamine**) is metabolized by CYP2B6 and CYP3A4 (see Pharmacology). Reports involving the CYP450 enzyme system are mostly limited to PO **esketamine**:

- **clarithromycin** and grapefruit juice (potent CYP3A4 inhibitors) increase the plasma concentration of **esketamine** and reduce that of norketamine[93,94]
- **ticlopidine** (potent CYP2C19 and weak CYP2B6 inhibitor) increases the AUC of **esketamine**[95]
- **rifampicin** and **St John's wort** (potent CYP3A4 inducers) decrease the plasma concentration of **esketamine**; **rifampicin** also following IV **esketamine**.[96,97]

Other potent inhibitors or inducers of these enzymes could have similar effects (see Chapter 19, Table 8, p.790). The clinical relevance of these interactions is unclear for both **ketamine** and **esketamine**.

Undesirable effects

Ketamine can be abused or diverted; careful monitoring is essential.

Dose-related psychotomimetic phenomena occur in about 40% of patients with CSCI ketamine; less with PO: euphoria, dysphasia, blunted affect, psychomotor retardation, vivid dreams, nightmares, impaired attention, memory and judgement, illusions, hallucinations, altered body image.

Delirium, drowsiness, dizziness, diplopia, blurred vision, nystagmus, altered hearing, hypertension, tachycardia, hypersalivation, nausea and vomiting. At higher anaesthetic doses, tonic–clonic movements are very common (>10%) but these have not been reported after PO use or with analgesic parenteral doses.

Erythema and pain at injection site. Upper GI, hepatobiliary, urinary and neuropsychiatric toxicity (Box A).

Box A Ketamine and upper GI, hepatobiliary, urinary and neuropsychiatric toxicity

Most data concern long-term frequent abusers of large doses of ketamine, generally by nasal insufflation (typically ~3.5g/24h for >3 years). Nonetheless, toxicity has been reported in patients, sometimes after only *days* of use.

The exact mechanism of the toxicity is unknown, but possible triggers include a direct irritant effect of ketamine or a metabolite, disruption of the epithelial barrier (e.g. in bladder, GI tract), and IgE-mediated hypersensitivity.[98]

Upper GI

Abdominal symptoms, e.g. epigastric pain or vomiting, are common in ketamine abusers, often preceding urinary tract toxicity. Presentation may be acute and severe, e.g. upper GI bleeding, perforated peptic ulcer.[99]

Investigations may reveal anaemia, oesophagitis, gastritis, gastro-duodenal erosions or ulceration.[99]

Management includes treatment of the acute complication and abstinence.[99]

Hepatobiliary

Abnormal LFTs have been associated with both ketamine abuse and therapeutic use, e.g. IV for maintenance anaesthesia (>10h) or infusions for pain relief (≥4 days).[100-103] In the latter, although abnormal LFTs were sometimes apparent after 4–5 days, in others it occurred only with a second infusion some 2 weeks later.[103]

In abusers, abdominal pain has been reported and, in some, dilatation or strictures of the common bile duct.[101,104,105]

The cause is unknown, but a contributing factor may be ketamine-related dysfunction of the sphincter of Oddi.[100,106]

With abstinence, the LFTs, abdominal pain and biliary duct dilatation generally improve. Some recommend regular monitoring of LFTs during the long-term therapeutic use of ketamine.[103]

Urinary tract

In three patients with chronic pain, urinary symptoms developed after receiving ketamine 650–800mg/24h PO for 5–18 months.[107] In another patient, severe damage necessitated cystectomy after 3 years of ketamine 240mg/24h PO for chronic back pain.[108] However, urinary symptoms developed after only 9 *days* in a 16 year-old receiving ketamine 8mg/kg/24h PO.[109]

Urinary tract problems are more widely documented in ketamine abusers. The risk appears related to both dose and frequency of use.[110]

Symptoms include frequency, urgency, urge incontinence, dysuria, haematuria and lower abdominal pain.[110-112]

Investigations (e.g. cystoscopy and biopsy, CT urogram) may show inflammation and ulceration of the mucosa, detrusor overactivity, decreased bladder capacity, vesico-ureteric reflux, perivesical inflammation, bladder and ureteric wall thickening, hydronephrosis, papillary necrosis and renal impairment. Irreversible damage leading to renal failure has occurred.

Most respond to abstinence (+ an NSAID ± a urinary antimuscarinic) with symptoms generally settling over several weeks.[113] However, despite abstinence, symptoms can persist, worsen or even develop. Additional analgesia (e.g. tramadol + gabapentin) is required by some, and for a few, intravesical instillations of hyaluronic acid.[113] Injections of botulinum toxin A into the bladder wall have also been used.[114] Rarely, surgery is required for patients with severely reduced bladder capacity ± upper urinary tract damage.[113,115]

Consequently, when patients receiving therapeutic ketamine experience urinary symptoms without evidence of bacterial infection, practitioners should consider stopping the ketamine and seeking the advice of a urologist.

continued

Box A Continued

Neuropsychiatric

There are no studies of neuropsychiatric effects in patients receiving therapeutic ketamine long-term.

A study of long-term ketamine abusers suggested a high incidence of moderate–severe depression (75%) and anxiety (50%), and only a low incidence of, at most, mild psychosis (<10%).[116] The relevance is uncertain; no definite link exists between ketamine abuse and mood disorder or psychosis.

Impairment of various cognitive functions has been described, e.g. in visual and verbal memory, selective attention and response inhibition, auditory attention.[117]

MRI changes were evident with *total estimated lifetime doses* of ≤3g.[118-120] Functional MRI showed dose-related alterations in the anterior cingulate cortex (decrease) and in the left precentral frontal gyrus (increase).[118]

These effects may be the consequence of long-term NMDA-receptor channel blockade. Dopamine depletion in the prefrontal cortex, a key area involved in working memory, is also reported in those abusing ≥200mg/week.[121] Ketamine is also directly neurotoxic, with dose-related MRI changes suggestive of disruption or damage to the white matter in the frontal and left temporoparietal regions.[119]

Memory impairments appear to improve with abstinence, but former abusers continue to score higher than controls on delusional symptoms.[122]

Dose and use

Because of the undesirable effects profile of ketamine, which includes upper GI, hepatobiliary, urinary and neuropsychiatric toxicity, prescription of ketamine as an analgesic should be restricted to specialists in pain or palliative care for patients who have failed to obtain adequate relief from standard non-drug and drug treatments, including the optimal use of opioids, non-opioids and adjuvant analgesics (p.325).[40] A toxicity monitoring form is available.[123]

In patients with a prognosis of more than a few weeks, once analgesia has been obtained, an attempt should be made to withdraw ketamine over 2–3 weeks. Benefit from a short course can last for weeks or even months, and the course can be repeated if necessary.[45] Thus, apart from patients with a prognosis of just days–weeks, long-term continuous ketamine should be used only as a last resort, i.e. in those patients with unsatisfactory analgesia from a short-course approach.

Note. Whole-body hyperalgesia and allodynia may occur if ketamine is abruptly stopped after ≥3 weeks of use.[124]

Ketamine is included in a law in England, Wales and Scotland relating to driving with certain drugs above specified plasma concentrations (see Chapter 22, p.809).

All doses in this section relate to racemic ketamine.

Dose recommendations vary widely, but ketamine is often started low dose PO (see below). In some centres, an initial test dose is given to assess tolerability and efficacy. The prophylactic concurrent administration of a benzodiazepine or an antipsychotic is also routine in some but not all centres, where it is reserved for more select circumstances (see below). Long-term success, i.e. both pain relief and tolerable undesirable effects, varies from <20% to about 50%.[12,13,51,125]

Some practitioners routinely reduce the background opioid dose by 25–50% when starting parenteral ketamine. If the patient becomes drowsy, the dose of opioid should be reduced. If a patient experiences dysphoria or hallucinations, the dose of ketamine should be reduced and a benzodiazepine prescribed, e.g. **diazepam** 5mg PO stat & at bedtime, **lorazepam** 1mg PO stat & b.d., **midazolam** 5mg SC stat and 5–10mg CSCI, or **haloperidol**, e.g. 2–5mg PO stat & at bedtime, or 2–5mg SC stat and 2–5mg CSCI.[34] In patients at greatest risk of dysphoria (those with high anxiety levels), these measures may be more effective if given before starting ketamine.

When switching from CSCI to PO after just a few days, a conversion ratio of 1:1 should be used.[52,126] However, after weeks–months of use, some have found that a *smaller* total daily dose (25–50% of the parenteral dose) can maintain a similar level of analgesia, e.g. 400mg/24h CSCI → 150mg/24h PO.[50] In both instances, the patient should be monitored closely and the dose titrated accordingly. When switching from PO to CSCI or CIVI, it is advisable to commence on a small dose and titrate as required.

By mouth[9,10,127-129]

In the UK, an oral solution can be obtained as a special order (see Supply). When this option is not available, use direct from a vial or dilute for convenience (immediately before administration) to 50mg/5mL; add a flavouring of the patient's choice, e.g. fruit cordial, to mask the bitter taste:

- start with 10–25mg t.d.s.–q.d.s. and p.r.n.
- if necessary, increase dose in steps of 10–25mg up to 100mg q.d.s.
- maximum reported dose 200mg q.d.s.[127,129]
- give a smaller dose more frequently if psychotomimetic phenomena or drowsiness occurs which does not respond to a reduction in opioid.

Unauthorized capsules can be obtained as a special order. However, these are expensive. Where the 100mg/mL vial is available (not UK), an oral solution can be prepared by a local pharmacy (Box B).

Subcutaneous injection[10]

- typically 10–25mg p.r.n.; some use 2.5–5mg
- if necessary, increase dose in steps of 25–33%.

CSCI[9,33,46,47,49,130]

Because ketamine is irritant, dilute to the largest volume possible, and consider the use of sodium chloride 0.9% as the diluent (see Chapter 29, p.889). Consider the use of prophylactic **diazepam**, **lorazepam**, **midazolam** or **haloperidol** (see above).

- start with 1–2.5mg/kg/24h
- if necessary, increase by 50–100mg/24h
- continue to titrate until adequate pain relief
- usual maximum 500mg/24h
- maximum reported dose 3.6g/24h.

CSCI compatibility with other drugs: there are 2-drug compatibility data for ketamine in WFI with **metoclopramide**, **midazolam** and **morphine sulfate**. For more details and 3-drug compatibility charts see Appendix 3.

There are 2-drug compatibility data for ketamine in sodium chloride 0.9% with **alfentanil**, **clonazepam**, **dexamethasone** (low-dose), **diamorphine**, **haloperidol**, **hydromorphone**, **levomepromazine**, **metoclopramide**, **midazolam**, **morphine sulfate** and **oxycodone**. For more details and 3-drug compatibility charts, see the extended Appendix 3 of the on-line *PCF* on *www.medicinescomplete.com*.

Intravenous injection[10,131,132]

For cancer pain:

- typically 2.5–5mg p.r.n.

To cover procedures that may cause severe pain:

- give 350microgram/kg (typically 25mg; some start with 5–10mg), over 1–2min preceded by, e.g. **midazolam** 100microgram/kg IV (typically 5–10mg; some start with 1–2mg) to reduce emergent phenomena
- use a maximum concentration of ketamine 50mg/mL; sodium chloride 0.9% or glucose 5% are suitable diluents.

The right dose should provide analgesia within 1–5min lasting for 10–20min.

There is a risk of marked sedation when ketamine and a benzodiazepine are given concurrently. Use only if competent in airway management and the patient can be adequately monitored.

Procedures of longer duration may require ketamine CIVI; obtain advice from an anaesthetist.

CIVI[21,133,134]

Dilute to a concentration of 1mg/mL with sodium chloride 0.9% or glucose 5%.

- give a single 'burst' of 600microgram/kg up to a maximum of 60mg over 4h (reduce dose by 1/3–1/2 in elderly/frail patients); monitor blood pressure at baseline and then hourly:
  - ▷ if necessary, repeat daily for up to 5 days
  - ▷ if *no* analgesic response to an infusion, increase the dose of the next one by 30%
  - ▷ further dose titrate according to response and/or undesirable effects
  - ▷ repeat the above if the pain subsequently recurs.[45]

Or:

- start with 50–150microgram/kg/h (typically 50–100mg/24h) and titrate as necessary (typical increments 25–50mg/24h)
- in one series of 46 patients with cancer:
  - ▷ 20% responded to ≤100mg/24h
  - ▷ typical dose 100–300mg/24h
  - ▷ no psychotomimetic effects were seen with doses <300mg/24h.

Supply

All products are Schedule 2 **CD**.

Ketamine (generic)

Capsules (Keticap®) 10mg, 40mg, 28 days @ 40mg q.d.s. = £223 (unauthorized products, available as a special order from the Specials Lab UK; see Chapter 24, p.817). *A 3–4 day order period is needed; the product has a 90-day shelf life.*

Oral solution or suspension (sugar-free) 50mg/5mL, 28 days @ 50mg q.d.s. = £59 or £46 (unauthorized products, available as a special order; see Chapter 24, p.817). *Price based on Specials tariff in community.*

Injection 50mg/mL, 10mL vial = £7.

Ketalar® (Pfizer)

Injection 10mg/mL, 20mL vial = £5; 50mg/mL, 10mL vial = £9.

Although use as an analgesic is unauthorized, ketamine injection can be prescribed both in hospitals and in the community. Community pharmacies can order ketamine injection through their usual Alliance Healthcare wholesale account. To initiate an account, contact head office (tel: 020 8391 2323).

Box B Preparation of ketamine 50mg/5mL oral solution: pharmacy guidelines

Note. An option when 100mg/mL vials are available (not UK).

Use ketamine 100mg/mL, 10mL vials, because this is the cheapest concentration. Raspberry syrup BP can be used for dilution, but this is too sweet for some patients. Alternatively, use purified water as the diluent and ask patients to add their own flavouring, e.g. fruit cordial, just before use to disguise the bitter taste.

To prepare 100mL of 50mg/5mL ketamine oral solution:

- mix 10mL vial of ketamine 100mg/mL for injection with 90mL purified water.

Store in a refrigerator, with an expiry date of 1 week from manufacture.

Esketamine

Esketamine (*S*-ketamine) is about *twice* as potent as the racemic mixture (see Pharmacology); thus, an equivalent dose of **esketamine** is about half that of the racemic mixture.

Spravato® (Janssen-Cilag)

Nasal spray 28mg/0.2mL, 0.2mL dose (1 spray/nostril) = £163.

Vesierra® (Pfizer)

Injection (preservative-free) 5mg/mL, 5mL amp = £2; 25mg/mL, 2mL amp = £2.75.

1 Persson J *et al.* (1998) The analgesic effect of racemic ketamine in patients with chronic ischemic pain due to lower extremity arteriosclerosis obliterans. *Acta Anaesthesiologica Scandinavica.* **42**: 750–758.
2 Iacobucci GJ *et al.* (2017) Ketamine: an update on cellular and subcellular mechanisms with implications for clinical practice. *Pain Physician.* **20**: e285–301.
3 Mion G and Villevieille T (2013) Ketamine pharmacology: an update (pharmacodynamics and molecular aspects, recent findings). *CNS Neuroscience and Therapeutics.* **19**: 370–380.
4 Richens A. The basis of the treatment of epilepsy: neuropharmacology. In: Dam M, editor. *A Practical Approach to Epilepsy.* Oxford: Pergamon Press; 1991. p. 75–85.
5 Johnson JW *et al.* (2015) Recent insights into the mode of action of memantine and ketamine. *Current Opinions in Pharmacology.* **20**: 54–63.
6 Bosma RL *et al.* (2018) Brain dynamics and temporal summation of pain predicts neuropathic pain relief from ketamine infusion. *Anesthesiology.* **129**: 1015–1024.
7 De Kock M *et al.* (2013) Ketamine and peripheral inflammation. *CNS Neuroscience and Therapeutics.* **19**: 403–410.
8 Sleigh J (2014) Ketamine- more mechanisms of action than just NMDA blockade. *Trends in Anaesthesia and Critical Care.* **4**: 76–81.
9 Luczak J *et al.* (1995) The role of ketamine, an NMDA receptor antagonist, in the management of pain. *Progress in Palliative Care.* **3**: 127–134.
10 Kotlinska-Lemieszek A and Luczak J (2004) Subanesthetic ketamine: an essential adjuvant for intractable cancer pain. *Journal of Pain andSymptom Management.* **28**: 100–102.
11 Lin T *et al.* (1998) Long-term epidural ketamine, morphine and bupivacaine attenuate reflex sympathetic dystrophy neuralgia. *Canadian Journal of Anaesthesia.* **45**: 175–177.
12 Haines D and Gaines S (1999) N of 1 randomised controlled trials of oral ketamine in patients with chronic pain. *Pain.* **83**: 283–287.
13 Batchelor G (1999) Ketamine in neuropathic pain. *The Pain Society Newsletter.* **1**: 19.
14 Beltrutti D *et al.* (1999) The epidural and intrathecal administration of ketamine. *Current Review of Pain.* **3**: 458–472.
15 Mercadante S *et al.* (2000) Analgesic effect of intravenous ketamine in cancer patients on morphine therapy: a randomized, controlled, double-blind, crossover, double-dose study. *Journal of Pain and Symptom Management.* **20**: 246–252.
16 Mercadante S *et al.* (2005) Alternative treatments of breakthrough pain in patients receiving spinal analgesics for cancer pain. *Journal of Pain and Symptom Management.* **30**: 485–491.
17 Singh V *et al.* (2018) Intranasal ketamine and its potential role in cancer-related pain. *Pharmacotherapy.* **38**: 390–401.
18 Vranken JH *et al.* (2005) Neuropathological findings after continuous intrathecal administration of S(+)-ketamine for the management of neuropathic cancer pain. *Pain.* **117**: 231–235.
19 Berger J *et al.* (2000) Ketamine-fentanyl-midazolam infusion for the control of symptoms in terminal life care. *American Journal of Hospice and Palliative Care.* **17**: 127–132.
20 Enck R (2000) A ketamine, fentanyl, and midazolam infusion for uncontrolled terminal pain and agitation. *American Journal of Hospice and Palliative Care.* **17**: 76–77.
21 Conway M *et al.* (2009) Use of continuous intravenous ketamine for end-stage cancer pain in children. *Journal of Pediatric Oncology Nursing.* **26**: 100–106.
22 Oye I *et al.* The chiral forms of ketamine as probes for NMDA receptor function in humans. In: Kameyama T, editor. *NMDA receptor Related Agents: biochemistry, pharmacology and behavior.* Ann Arbor, Michigan: NPP; 1991. p. 381–389.
23 White PF *et al.* (1980) Pharmacology of ketamine isomers in surgical patients. *Anesthesiology.* **52**: 231–239.
24 Mathisen L *et al.* (1995) Effect of ketamine, an NMDA receptor inhibitor, in acute and chronic orofacial pain. *Pain.* **61**: 215–220.
25 Pfenninger EG *et al.* (2002) Cognitive impairment after small-dose ketamine isomers in comparison to equianalgesic racemic ketamine in human volunteers. *Anesthesiology.* **96**: 357–366.
26 Hijazi Y *et al.* (2002) Contribution of CYP3A4, CYP2B6, and CYP2C9 isoforms to N-demethylation of ketamine in human liver microsomes. *Drug Metabolism & Disposition.* **30**: 853–858.
27 Li Y *et al.* (2015) CYP2B6*6 allele and age substantially reduce steady-state ketamine clearance in chronic pain patients: impact on adverse effects. *British Journal of Clinical Pharmacology.* **80**: 276–284.
28 Clements JA *et al.* (1982) Bio-availability, pharmacokinetics and analgesic activity of ketamine in humans. *Journal of Pharmaceutical Sciences.* **71**: 539–542.
29 Olofsen E *et al.* (2012) Estimation of the contribution of norketamine to ketamine-induced acute pain relief and neurocognitive impairment in healthy volunteers. *Anesthesiology.* **117**: 353–364.
30 Holtman JR, Jr. *et al.* (2008) Effects of norketamine enantiomers in rodent models of persistent pain. *Pharmacology, Biochemistry and Behavior.* **90**: 676–685.
31 Muetzelfeldt L *et al.* (2008) Journey through the K-hole: phenomenological aspects of ketamine use. *Drug Alcohol Dependence.* **95**: 219–229.
32 Sener S *et al.* (2011) Ketamine with and without midazolam for emergency department sedation in adults: a randomized controlled trial. *Annals of Emergency Medicine.* **57**: 109–114.
33 Hughes A *et al.* (1999) Ketamine. *CME Bulletin Palliative Medicine.* **1**: 53.
34 Giannini A *et al.* (2000) Acute ketamine intoxication treated by haloperidol: a preliminary study. *American Journal of Therapeutics.* **7**: 389–391.
35 Assouline B *et al.* (2016) Benefit and harm of adding ketamine to an opioid in a patient-controlled analgesia device for the control of postoperative pain: systematic review and meta-analyses of randomized controlled trials with trial sequential analyses. *Pain.* **157**: 2854–2864.
36 Bell RF *et al.* (2006) Perioperative ketamine for acute postoperative pain. *Cochrane Database of Systematic Reviews.* CD004603. www.cochranelibrary.com.
37 Michelet D *et al.* (2018) Ketamine for chronic non-cancer pain: A meta-analysis and trial sequential analysis of randomized controlled trials. *European Journal of Pain.* **22**: 632–646.
38 Alviar MJM (2016) Pharmacological interventions for treating phantom limb pain. *Cochrane Database of Systematic Reviews.* **10**: CD006380. www.cochranelibrary.com.
39 Connolly SB *et al.* (2015) A systematic review of ketamine for complex regional pain syndrome. *Pain Medicine.* **16**: 943–969.
40 Bell RF and Kalso EA (2018) Ketamine for pain management. *Pain reports.* **3**: e674.
41 Cohen SP *et al.* (2018) Consensus guidelines on the use of intravenous ketamine infusions for chronic pain from the American Society of Regional Anesthesia and Pain Medicine, the American Academy of Pain Medicine, and the American Society of Anesthesiologists. *Regional Anesthesia and Pain Medicine.* **43**: 521–546.
42 Yang CY *et al.* (1996) Intrathecal ketamine reduces morphine requirements in patients with terminal cancer pain. *Canadian Journal of Anaesthesia.* **43**: 379–383.

43 Hardy J *et al.* (2012) Randomized , double-blind, placebo-controlled study to assess the efficacy and toxicity of subcutaneous ketamine in the management of cancer pain. *Journal of Clinical Oncology.* **30**: 11–17.
44 Bell RF *et al.* (2017) Ketamine as an adjuvant to opioids for cancer pain. *Cochrane Database Systematic Reviews.* **6**: CD003351. www.cochranelibrary.com.
45 Fallon MT *et al.* (2018) Oral ketamine vs placebo in patients with cancer-related neuropathic pain: A randomized clinical trial. *JAMA Oncology.* **4**: 870–872.
46 Oshima E *et al.* (1990) Continuous subcutaneous injection of ketamine for cancer pain. *Canadian Journal of Anaesthetics.* **37**: 385–392.
47 Cherry DA *et al.* (1995) Ketamine as an adjunct to morphine in the treatment of pain. *Pain.* **62**: 119–121.
48 Mercadante S (1996) Ketamine in cancer pain: an update. *Palliative Medicine.* **10**: 225–230.
49 Bell R (1999) Low-dose subcutaneous ketamine infusion and morphine tolerance. *Pain.* **83**: 101–103.
50 Fitzgibbon EJ *et al.* (2002) Low dose ketamine as an analgesic adjuvant in difficult pain syndromes: a strategy for conversion from parenteral to oral ketamine. *Journal of Pain and Symptom Management.* **23**: 165–170.
51 Kannan TR *et al.* (2002) Oral ketamine as an adjuvant to oral morphine for neuropathic pain in cancer patients. *Journal of Pain and Symptom Management.* **23**: 60–65.
52 Benitez-Rosario M *et al.* (2003) A retrospective comparison of the dose ratio between subcutaneous and oral ketamine. *Journal of Pain and Symptom Management.* **25**: 400–402.
53 Fitzgibbon EJ and Viola R (2005) Parenteral ketamine as an analgesic adjuvant for severe pain: development and retrospective audit of a protocol for a palliative care unit. *Journal of Palliative Medicine.* **8**: 49–57.
54 Lauretti G *et al.* (1999) Oral ketamine and transdermal nitroglycerin as analgesic adjuvants to oral morphine therapy and amitriptyline for cancer pain management. *Anesthesiology.* **90**: 1528–1533.
55 Lossignol DA *et al.* (2005) Successful use of ketamine for intractable cancer pain. *Support Care Cancer.* **13**: 188–193.
56 Cheng HW *et al.* (2015) Successful analgesic use of ketamine infusion in malignant cord compression. *Pain Medicine.* **16**: 2045–2047.
57 Jackson K *et al.* (2010) The effectiveness and adverse effects profile of "burst" ketamine in refractory cancer pain. *Journal of Palliative Care.* **26**: 176–183.
58 Jackson K *et al.* (2001) 'Burst' ketamine for refractory cancer pain: an open-label audit of 39 patients. *Journal of Pain and Symptom Management.* **22**: 834–842.
59 Mercadante S *et al.* (2003) Burst ketamine to reverse opioid tolerance in cancer pain. *Journal of Pain and Symptom Management.* **25**: 302–305.
60 Mitchell AC and Fallon MT (2002) A single infusion of intravenous ketamine improves pain relief in patients with critical limb ischaemia: results of a double blind randomised controlled trial. *Pain.* **97**: 275–281.
61 Balzer N *et al.* (2021) Low-dose ketamine for acute pain control in the Emergency Department: a systematic review and meta-analysis. *Academic Emergency Medicine.* **28**: 444–454.
62 Andolfatto G *et al.* (2019) Prehospital analgesia with intranasal ketamine (PAIN-K): A randomized double-blind trial in adults. *Annals of Emergency Medicine.* **74**: 241–250.
63 White MC *et al.* (2011) Pain management in 100 episodes of severe mucositis in children. *Paediatric Anesthesia.* **21**: 411–416.
64 James PJ *et al.* (2010) The addition of ketamine to a morphine nurse- or patient-controlled analgesia infusion (PCA/NCA) increases analgesic efficacy in children with mucositis pain. *Paediatric Anaesthesia.* **20**: 805–811.
65 Arroyo-Novoa CM *et al.* (2011) Efficacy of small doses of ketamine with morphine to decrease procedural pain responses during open wound care. *Clinical Journal of Pain.* **27**: 561–566.
66 Kundra P *et al.* (2013) Oral ketamine and dexmedetomidine in adults' burns wound dressing--A randomized double blind cross over study. *Burns.* **39**: 1150–1156.
67 Norambuena C *et al.* (2013) Oral ketamine and midazolam for pediatric burn patients: a prospective, randomized, double-blind study. *Journal of Pediatric Surgery.* **48**: 629–634.
68 Sheehy KA *et al.* (2017) Subanesthetic ketamine for pain management in hospitalized children, adolescents, and young adults: a single-center cohort study. *Journal of Pain Research.* **10**: 787–795.
69 Slatkin NE and Rhiner M (2003) Topical ketamine in the treatment of mucositis pain. *Pain Medicine.* **4**: 298–303.
70 Shillingburg A *et al.* (2017) Treatment of severe mucositis pain with oral ketamine mouthwash. *Supportive Care in Cancer.* **25**: 2215–2219.
71 Finch PM *et al.* (2009) Reduction of allodynia in patients with complex regional pain syndrome: A double-blind placebo-controlled trial of topical ketamine. *Pain.* **146**: 18–25.
72 Gammaitoni A *et al.* (2000) Topical ketamine gel: possible role in treating neuropathic pain. *Pain Medicine.* **1**: 97–100.
73 Skavinski KA (2018) Opioid-sparing effects of topical ketamine in treating severe pain from decubitus ulcers. *Journal of Pain & Palliative Care Pharmacotherapy.* **32**: 170–174.
74 Brutcher RE *et al.* (2019) Compounded topical pain creams to treat localized chronic pain: A randomized controlled trial. *Annals of Internal Medicine.* **170**: 309–318.
75 Bobo WV *et al.* (2016) Ketamine for treatment-resistent unipolar and bipolar major depression: Critical review and implications for clinical practice. *Depression and Anxiety.* **33**: 698–710.
76 Bartoli F *et al.* (2017) Ketamine as a rapid-acting agent for suicidal ideation: A meta-analysis. *Neuroscience and Biobehavioral Reviews.* **77**: 232 –236.
77 Caddy C *et al.* (2015) Ketamine and other glutamate receptor modulators for depression in adults. *Cochrane Database of Systematic Reviews.* **9**: CD011612. www.cochranelibrary.com.
78 Arabzadeh S *et al.* (2018) Does oral administration of ketamine accelerate response to treatment in major depressive disorder? Results of a double-blind controlled trial. *Journal of Affective Disorders.* **235**: 236–241.
79 Palucha-Poniewiera A (2018) The role of glutamatergic modulation in the mechanism of action of ketamine, a prototype rapid-acting antidepressant drug. *Pharmacological reports.* **70**: 837–846.
80 Christensen A and Pruskowski J (2020) The role of ketamine in depression. *Journal of Palliative Medicine.* **23**: 136–138.
81 Royal College of Psychiatrists (2017) Position statement on ketamine to treat depression. www.rcpsych.ac.uk.
82 Dolgin E (2013) Rapid antidepressant effects of ketamine ignite drug discovery. *Nature Medicine.* **19**: 8.
83 Glue P *et al.* (2017) Ketamine's dose-related effects on anxiety symptoms in patients with treatment refractory anxiety disorders. *Journal of Psychopharmacology.* **31**: 1302–1305.
84 Fang Y and Wang X (2015) Ketamine for the treatment of refractory status epilepticus. *Seizure.* **30**: 14–20.
85 Chong CC *et al.* (2006) Bioavailability of ketamine after oral or sublingual administration. *Pain Medicine.* **7**: 469–469.
86 Yanagihara Y *et al.* (2003) Plasma concentration profiles of ketamine and norketamine after administration of various ketamine preparations to healthy Japanese volunteers. *Biopharmacentrics and Drug Disposition.* **24**: 37–43.
87 Grant IS *et al.* (1981) Pharmacokinetics and analgesic effects of IM and oral ketamine. *British Journal of Anaesthesia.* **53**: 805–810.

88 Domino E *et al.* (1984) Ketamine kinetics in unmedicated and diazepam premedicated subjects. *Clinical Pharmacology and Therapeutics.* **36**: 645–653.

89 Rabben T *et al.* (1999) Prolonged analgesic effect of ketamine, an N-methyl-D-aspartate receptor inhibitor, in patients with chronic pain. *Journal of Pharmacology and Experimental Therapeutics.* **289**: 1060–1066.

90 Ward J and Standage C (2003) Angina pain precipitated by a continuous subcutaneous infusion of ketamine. *Journal of Pain and Symptom Management.* **25**: 6–7.

91 Zeiler FA *et al.* (2014) The ketamine effect on ICP in traumatic brain injury. *Neurocritical Care.* **21**: 163–173.

92 Zeiler FA *et al.* (2014) The ketamine effect on intracranial pressure in nontraumatic neurological illness. *Journal of Critical Care.* **29**: 1096–1106.

93 Peltoniemi MA *et al.* (2012) S-ketamine concentrations are greatly increased by grapefruit juice. *European Journal of Clinical Pharmacology.* **68**: 979–986.

94 Hagelberg N *et al.* (2010) Clarythromycin, a potent inhibitor of CYP3A, greatly increases exposure to oral S-ketamine. *European Journal of Pain.* **14**: 625–629.

95 Peltoniemi MA *et al.* (2011) Exposure to oral S-ketamine is unaffected by itraconazole but greatly increased by ticlopidine. *Clinical Pharmacology and Therapeutics.* **90**: 296–302.

96 Peltoniemi MA *et al.* (2012) Rifampicin has a profound effect on the pharmacokinetics of oral S-Ketamine and less on intravenous S-ketamine. *Basic and Clinical Pharmacology and Toxicology.* **111**: 325–332.

97 Peltoniemi MA *et al.* (2012) St John's wort greatly decreases the plasma concentrations of oral S-ketamine. *Fundamental and Clinical Pharmacology.* **26**: 743 –750.

98 Jhang JF *et al.* (2015) Possible pathophysiology of ketamine-related cystitis and associated treatment strategies. *International Journal of Urology.* **22**: 816–825.

99 Liu SYW *et al.* (2017) Clinical pattern and prevalence of upper gastrointestinal toxicity in patients abusing ketamine. *Journal of Digestive Diseases.* **18**: 504–510.

100 Ng SH *et al.* (2010) Emergency department presentation of ketamine abusers in Hong Kong: a review of 233 cases. *Hong Kong Medical Journal.* **16**: 6–11.

101 Wong SW *et al.* (2009) Dilated common bile ducts mimicking choledochal cysts in ketamine abusers. *Hong Kong Medical Journal.* **15**: 53–56.

102 Dundee JW *et al.* (1980) Changes in serum enzyme levels following ketamine infusions. *Anaesthesia.* **35**: 12–16.

103 Noppers IM *et al.* (2011) Drug-induced liver injury following a repeated course of ketamine treatment for chronic pain in CRPS type I patients: a report of 3 cases. *Pain.* **152**: 2173–2178.

104 Wang JW *et al.* (2017) Ketamine abuse syndrome: Hepatobiliary and urinary pathology among adolescents in Flushing, NY. *Pediatric Emergency Care.* **33**: e24–e26.

105 Seto WK *et al.* (2011) Ketamine-induced cholangiopathy: a case report. *American Journal of Gastroenterology.* **106**: 1004–1005.

106 Lee ST *et al.* (2009) Apoptotic insults to human HepG2 cells induced by S-(+)-ketamine occurs through activation of a Bax-mitochondria-caspase protease pathway. *British Journal of Anaesthesia.* **102**: 80–89.

107 Storr TM and Quibell R (2009) Can ketamine prescribed for pain cause damage to the urinary tract? *Palliative Medicine.* **23**: 670–672.

108 Shahzad K *et al.* (2012) Analgesic ketamine use leading to cystectomy: a case report. *British Journal of Medical and Surgical Urology.* **5**: 188–191.

109 Gregoire MC *et al.* (2008) A pediatric case of ketamine-associated cystitis. *Urology.* **71**: 1232–1233.

110 Winstock AR *et al.* (2012) The prevalence and natural history of urinary symptoms among recreational ketamine users. *British Journal of Urology International.* **110**: 1762–1766.

111 Chu PS *et al.* (2008) The destruction of the lower urinary tract by ketamine abuse: a new syndrome? *British Journal of Urology International.* **102**: 1616–1622.

112 Shahani R *et al.* (2007) Ketamine-associated ulcerative cystitis: a new clinical entity. *Urology.* **69**: 810–812.

113 Yee CH *et al.* (2015) Clinical outcome of a prospective case series of patients with ketamine cystitis who underwent standardized treatment protocol. *Urology.* **86**: 236–243.

114 Zeng J *et al.* (2017) Effective treatment of ketamine-associated cystitis with botulinum toxin type a injection combined with bladder hydrodistention. *Journal of International Medical Research.* **45**: 792–797.

115 Jhang JF *et al.* (2017) Patient characteristics for different therapeutic strategies in the management ketamine cystitis. *Neurology and Urodynamics.* **36**: 687–691.

116 Fan N *et al.* (2016) Profiling the psychotic, depressive and anxiety symptoms in chronic ketamine users. *Psychiatry Research.* **237**: 311–315.

117 Ke X *et al.* (2018) The profile of cognitive impairments in chronic ketamine users. *Psychiatry Research.* **266**: 124–131.

118 Liao Y *et al.* (2012) Alterations in regional homogeneity of resting-state brain activity in ketamine addicts. *Neuroscience Letters.* **522**: 36–40.

119 Liao Y *et al.* (2010) Frontal white matter abnormalities following chronic ketamine use: a diffusion tensor imaging study. *Brain.* **133**: 2115–2122.

120 Liao Y *et al.* (2016) Decreased thalamocortical connectivity in chronic ketamine users. *PLoS ONE.* **11**: e0167381.

121 Narendran R *et al.* (2005) Altered prefrontal dopaminergic function in chronic recreational ketamine users. *American Journal of Psychiatry.* **162**: 2352–2359.

122 Morgan CJ and Curran HV (2012) Ketamine use: a review. *Addiction.* **107**: 27–38.

123 Palliativedrugs.com (2013) Ketamine monitoring chart. *Document Library.* Pain (neuropathic). www.palliativedrugs.com.

124 Mitchell AC (1999) Generalized hyperalgesia and allodynia following abrupt cessation of subcutaneous ketamine infusion. *Palliative Medicine.* **13**: 427–428.

125 Enarson M *et al.* (1999) Clinical experience with oral ketamine. *Journal of Pain and Symptom Management.* **17**: 384–386.

126 Benitez-Rosario MA *et al.* (2011) A strategy for conversion from subcutaneous to oral ketamine in cancer pain patients: efficacy of a 1:1 ratio. *Journal of Pain and Symptom Management.* **10**: 1098–1105.

127 Clark JL and Kalan GE (1995) Effective treatment of severe cancer pain of the head using low-dose ketamine in an opioid-tolerant patient. *Journal of Pain and Symptom Management.* **10**: 310–314.

128 Broadley K *et al.* (1996) Ketamine injection used orally. *Palliative Medicine.* **10**: 247–250.

129 Vielvoye-Kerkmeer A (2000) Clinical experience with ketamine. *Journal of Pain and Symptom Management.* **19**: 3.

130 Lloyd-Williams M (2000) Ketamine for cancer pain. *Journal of Pain and Symptom Management.* **19**: 79–80.

131 Mason KP *et al.* (2002) Evolution of a protocol for ketamine-induced sedation as an alternative to general anesthesia for interventional radiologic procedures in pediatric patients. *Radiology.* **225**: 457–465.

132 Schwenk ES *et al.* (2018) Consensus guidelines on the use of intravenous ketamine infusions for acute pain management from the American Society of Regional Anesthesia and Pain Medicine, the American Academy of Pain Medicine, and the American Society of Anesthesiologists. *Regional Anesthesia and Pain Medicine*. **43**: 456–466.
133 Hocking G *et al.* (2007) Ketamine: does life begin at 40? *Pain Clinical Updates IASP*. **XV**.
134 Okamoto Y *et al.* (2012) Can Gradual dose titration of ketamine for management of neuropathic pain prevent psychotomimetic effects in patients with advanced cancer? *American Journal of Hospice and Palliative Medicine*. **30**: 450–454.

Updated (minor change) July 2021

*PROPOFOL

Class: General anaesthetic.

Indications: Induction and maintenance of general anaesthesia, conscious sedation (diagnostic or therapeutic procedures, e.g. radiation therapy in children),[1] continuous sedation of intubated and mechanically ventilated patients ≥16 years on intensive care units, †refractory agitation or intolerable distress in the imminently dying, †intractable nausea and vomiting.[2]

Contra-indications: Continuous sedation in children ≤16 years; when used for sedation in children in intensive care, the death rate increased 2–3 times.[3] Propofol 0.5% is contra-indicated for maintenance of general anaesthesia or continuous sedation in intensive care in adults and children, and maintenance of conscious sedation in children (diagnostic or therapeutic procedures).

Allergy to eggs, soya or peanuts (the available products contain purified egg phosphatide, as an emulsifying agent, and soya bean oil).[4]

Pharmacology

Propofol is an ultrafast-acting IV anaesthetic agent. It is rapidly metabolized, mainly in the liver, to inactive compounds which are excreted in the urine. The incidence of untoward haemodynamic changes is low. Propofol reduces cerebral blood flow, cerebral metabolism and, less consistently, intracranial pressure.[5] The reduction in intracranial pressure is greater if the baseline pressure is raised. On discontinuation, patients rapidly regain consciousness (10–30min) without residual drowsiness.

In palliative care, propofol is occasionally used for refractory agitation or intolerable distress in the imminently dying.[6-9] Careful titration generally permits 'conscious sedation', i.e. patients open their eyes on verbal command, possess intact autonomic reflexes, and tolerate mild noxious stimuli.[2] Such use has also been described in children at the end of life, and algorithms to assist physicians considering initiation of palliative sedation therapy in children have been suggested.[10-12]

Propofol also has an anti-emetic effect, resulting in less postoperative vomiting compared with other anaesthetic agents.[13-15] Specific postoperative anti-emetic regimens have been designed.[16-18] Chemotherapy-related nausea and vomiting is also helped by adjunctive propofol.[19] In patients receiving non-platinum regimens who were refractory to a combination of **dexamethasone** and a $5HT_3$-receptor antagonist, propofol was of benefit in ≥80%.[20] Propofol has also been used to relieve refractory nausea and vomiting in other settings, including palliative care.[2,21] In the group of patients with bowel obstruction, propofol was more effective in relieving nausea than vomiting.

Animal studies suggest that the mechanism of action of propofol as an anti-emetic is by inhibition of serotonin release by enhancing GABA activity, possibly by direct GABA-mediated action on $5HT_3$-receptors in the area postrema/chemoreceptor trigger zone.[22]

Propofol also has antipruritic, anxiolytic, bronchodilator, muscle relaxant and anti-epileptic properties. A possible role in refractory status epilepticus requires further clarification.[23-25] Transient excitatory phenomena are seen occasionally (e.g. myoclonus, opisthotonus, tonic–clonic activity) during induction or recovery when blood levels are low, and presumably at a time when inhibitory centres but not excitatory centres have been depressed.[5,26,27]

Onset of action 30 seconds.

Time to peak effect 5min.

Plasma halflife 2–4min initial distribution phase; 30–60min slow distribution and initial elimination phase; 3–12h terminal elimination phase. The terminal elimination halflife may increase with prolonged use.

Duration of action 3–10min after single IV bolus.[28,29]

Cautions

Risk of cardiorespiratory depression. Propofol clearance will reduce if cardiac output falls. Involuntary movements and seizures have been reported, particularly in epileptics, during induction or recovery.[26,30] With prolonged use in intensive care, the following have been reported: ECG changes, including prolongation of the QT interval (see Chapter 20, p.797), cardiac arrhythmia, heart failure, hepatomegaly, renal failure, rhabdomyolysis, metabolic acidosis, hyperkalaemia and hyperlipidaemia; when these occur in combination, it is termed a propofol infusion syndrome.

Although in intensive care use it is good practice to check plasma lipid levels in patients receiving propofol for ≥3 days, it is unnecessary in patients whose expected prognosis is only days.

Diprivan® contains disodium edetate (EDTA), a chelating agent which can reduce circulating concentrations and increase urinary losses of trace metals, e.g. zinc. Supplements should be considered for patients who are not imminently dying and who are likely to receive prolonged propofol treatment, particularly those at particular risk of deficiency, e.g. from fluid loss, catabolic states or infection.

Undesirable effects

Very common (>10%): local pain at the injection site.
Common (<10%, >1%): headache, hypotension, bradycardia, transient apnoea.
Uncommon (<1%, >0.1%): thrombosis, phlebitis.
Rare: epileptiform movements, propofol infusion syndrome, euphoria during recovery, misuse resulting in addiction and/or death. Concerns over a growing incidence among medical staff with access to propofol, e.g. anaesthetists, has prompted moves to designate propofol a controlled drug, particularly in the USA.[31-33]

13

Dose and use

Propofol is an emulsion of oil-in-water. This gives it a white appearance and makes it a potential growth medium. Diprivan® contains EDTA, a chelating agent which binds to divalent metal ions and reduces their availability for bacterial growth, replication and cell wall integrity. However, the concentration (0.005%) is sufficient only to *retard* microbial growth for up to 12h in the event of accidental contamination.[34] Propofol-Lipuro® and some generic products do not contain preservatives. Thus, with all propofol products, strict aseptic technique must be employed to prevent microbial contamination, *and the container and IV line renewed every 6–12h, in accordance with the individual manufacturer's instructions.* The propofol products available in the UK must not be infused through a microbiological filter.

The use of propofol in palliative care should be restricted to units with access to the necessary expertise and equipment.

Undiluted propofol requires a computer-controlled volumetric infusion pump or IV syringe pump (see manufacturer's SPC for full details). It is given by CIVI as a 1% (10mg/mL) or 2% (20mg/mL) solution, using the antecubital vein (or a large vein in the forearm) to minimize the risk of pain.[35,36] Pain at the IV injection site appears rare with undiluted propofol CIVI as used in palliative care practice. If problematic, seek the advice of an anaesthetist; options include:

- injecting *preservative-free* **lidocaine** prior to the propofol infusion
- mixing *preservative-free* **lidocaine** with propofol 0.5% or 1% immediately before administration; see specific SPC for details. *Note. Propofol 2% injection should not be mixed with* ***lidocaine*** *or any other drug.*
- using propofol 0.5% (5mg/mL; Propofol-Lipuro®) for induction of anaesthesia or sedation for infusions in adults of a maximum duration of 1h.

Diluted propofol 1% injection can be administered through a less sensitive infusion control device, e.g. an in-line burette or drop counter, after dilution with glucose 5% (Diprivan®; see SPC for details). Dilution is advised with less sensitive infusion control devices, because the weaker concentration reduces the risk of severe overdose if the infusion runs fast. The concentration of propofol in the diluted solution must not be less than 2mg/mL, because this can disrupt the emulsion. Diluted propofol should be used within 6h. *Propofol 2% injection should not be diluted.*

Compatibility: see the specific SPC for full details; formulations of propofol differ between manufacturers, and compatibility data cannot be extrapolated from one product to another.

Propofol 1% injection is compatible with certain concentrations of **alfentanil** (Diprivan® only) and **lidocaine**, and can be diluted with glucose 5% before use. *Propofol 2% injection should not be diluted or mixed with any other drugs.*

Both propofol 1% and 2% can be added through a Y connector to a running infusion of glucose 5%, sodium chloride 0.9% or glucose 4% + sodium chloride 0.18%; the Y connector should be placed as close to the injection site as possible.

†Refractory agitation or intolerable distress in the imminently dying

Consider propofol only if standard treatments have failed, i.e. a sedative antipsychotic + a benzodiazepine (Figure 1).[2,6,37-39] However, generally, **phenobarbital** (p.315) should be used in preference to propofol, because it is less complicated for clinical staff to titrate and monitor.

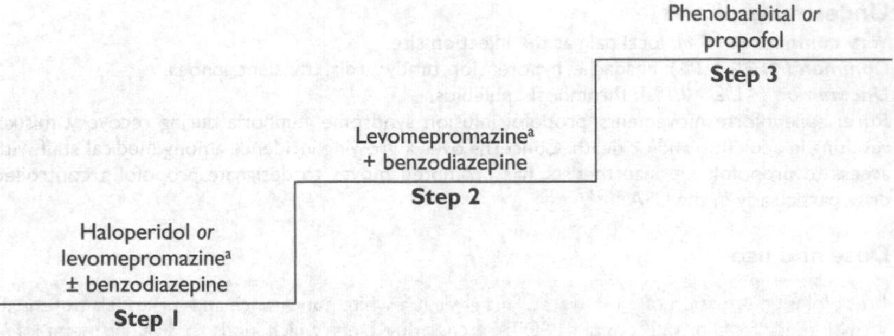

Figure 1 Drug treatment used at some centres for refractory agitation or intolerable distress in the imminently dying.

a. in countries where levomepromazine is not available, e.g. the USA, chlorpromazine is used instead.

Aim to titrate the dose until *conscious sedation* is achieved, i.e. patients open their eyes on verbal command but are not distressed by nursing interventions (e.g. mouth care, turning):

- remain with the patient throughout the initial titration process to ensure an effective and safe dose is found
- generally start with propofol 1mg/kg/h CIVI
- if necessary, increase by 0.5mg/kg/h every 5–10min until a satisfactory level of sedation is achieved; smaller dose steps can be used to fine-tune the treatment; most patients respond well to 1–2mg/kg/h
- to increase the level of sedation quickly, a bolus dose can be given by increasing the rate to 1mg/kg/*min* for a maximum of 1–2*min*
- monitor the patient closely during the first hour of treatment with respect to symptom relief and/or level of sedation, and then after 2h, 6h and 12h
- continue to monitor the effect of propofol and the level of sedation at least twice daily
- if the patient is too sedated (i.e. does not respond to a verbal command to open their eyes, shows no response to noxious stimuli) and/or there is evidence of drug-induced respiratory depression, the infusion should be turned off for 2–3min and restarted at a lower rate; occasionally this leads to a progressive reduction in dose because the patient has become unconscious as a result of their disease
- tolerance can develop, necessitating a dose increase, but generally not within 1 week
- long-term use of doses >4mg/kg/h is not recommended, because of increasing risk of undesirable effects
- if the patient does not respond to propofol 4mg/kg/h alone, supplement with **midazolam** by CSCI, starting with 10–30mg/24h
- it is important to replenish the infusion quickly when a container empties, because the effect of an infusion of propofol wears off after 10–30min
- *because propofol has no definite analgesic properties, analgesics should be continued.*

†*Intractable nausea and vomiting*

The use of propofol as an anti-emetic should be considered only if all other treatments have failed (see QCG: Nausea and vomiting, p.264).[2] Dose titration is generally slower for intractable nausea and vomiting than for refractory agitation or intolerable distress in the imminently dying:

- remain with the patient for at least 10min following any dose change to ensure that excessive sedation does not occur
- generally start with propofol 0.5mg/kg/h CIVI
- if necessary, increase by 0.25–0.5mg/kg/h every 30–60min until a satisfactory response is obtained; smaller dose steps can be used to fine-tune the treatment
- most patients respond well to 0.5–1mg/kg/h; doses >1mg/kg/h may result in sedation
- monitor the patient closely during the first hour of treatment with respect to symptom relief and/or level of sedation and then after 2h, 6h and 12h
- continue to monitor the effect of propofol and level of sedation at least twice daily
- if the patient is too sedated, the infusion should be turned off for 2–3min and then restarted at a lower rate
- if the patient responds well, reduce the infusion rate on a trial basis after 18–24h
- tolerance can develop, necessitating a dose increase, but generally not within 1 week
- it is important to replenish the infusion quickly when a container empties, because the effect of an infusion of propofol wears off after 10–30min
- when used solely for its anti-emetic effect in the last days of life, some centres reduce the dose of, or even discontinue, propofol when the patient becomes unconscious.

Supply

Propofol-Lipuro® (B. Braun)
Injection (emulsion) 5mg/mL (0.5%), 20mL amp = £3.50; *restricted to induction of general anaesthesia or induction of conscious sedation for diagnostic and therapeutic procedures in adults and children, and short-term sedation in adults (1h maximum duration of infusion).*

Propofol (generic)
Injection (emulsion) 10mg/mL (1%), 20mL vial or amp = £0.75 or £3 respectively.
Infusion (emulsion) 10mg/mL (1%) 50mL, 100mL vials = £5 and £19 respectively; 50mL prefilled syringe = £11.
Infusion (emulsion) 20mg/mL (2%), 50mL vial = £10; 50mL prefilled syringe = £15.

1 Harris EA (2010) Sedation and anesthesia options for pediatric patients in the radiation oncology suite. *International Journal of Pediatrics.* EPUB article ID 870921.

2 Lundstrom S *et al.* (2005) When nothing helps: propofol as sedative and antiemetic in palliative cancer care. *Journal of Pain and Symptom Management.* **30**: 570–577.

3 Anonymous (2001) Propofol (Diprivan) infusion: sedation in children aged 16 years or younger contraindicated. *Current Problems in Pharmacovigilance.* **27**: 10.

4 Hofer KN *et al.* (2003) Possible anaphylaxis after propofol in a child with food allergy. *Annals of Pharmacotherapy.* **37**: 398–401.

5 Mirenda J and Broyles G (1995) Propofol as used for sedation in the ICU. *Chest.* **108**: 539–548.

6 McWilliams K *et al.* (2010) Propofol for terminal sedation in palliative care: a systematic review. *Journal of Palliative Medicine.* **13**: 73–76.

7 Arantzamendi M *et al.* (2021) Clinical aspects of palliative sedation in prospective studies. A systematic review. *Journal of Pain and Symptom Management.* **61**: 831–844.

8 Fredheim OM *et al.* (2020) Clinical and ethical aspects of palliative sedation with propofol – a retrospective quantitative and qualitative study. *Acta Anaesthesiologica Scandinavica.* **64**: 1319–1326.

9 Bodnar J (2019) The use of propofol for continuous deep sedation at the end of life: A definitive guide. *Journal of Pain and Palliative Care Pharmacotherapy.* **33**: 63–81.

10 Hooke MC *et al.* (2007) Propofol use in pediatric patients with severe cancer pain at the end of life. *Journal of Pediatric Oncology Nursing.* **24**: 29–34.

11 Anghelescu DL *et al.* (2012) Pediatric palliative sedation therapy with propofol: recommendations based on experience in children with terminal cancer. *Journal of Palliative Medicine.* **15**: 1082–1090.

12 Miele E *et al.* (2019) Propofol-based palliative sedation in terminally ill children with solid tumours: a case series. *Medicine (Baltimore).* **98**: e15615.

13 Tramer M *et al.* (1997) Meta-analytic comparison of prophylactic antiemetic efficacy for postoperative nausea and vomiting: propofol anaesthesia vs omitting nitrous oxide vs total i.v. anaesthesia with propofol. *British Journal of Anaesthesia.* **78**: 256–259.

14 Sneyd JR *et al.* (1998) A meta-analysis of nausea and vomiting following maintenance of anaesthesia with propofol or inhalational agents. *European Journal of Anaesthesiology.* **15**: 433–445.

15 DeBalli P (2003) The use of propofol as an antiemetic. *International Anesthesiology Clinics.* **41**: 67–77.

16 Fujii Y *et al.* (2001) Small doses of propofol, droperidol, and metoclopramide for the prevention of postoperative nausea and vomiting after thyroidectomy. *Otolaryngology - Head and Neck Surgery.* **124**: 266–269.

17 Gan TJ *et al.* (1997) Determination of plasma concentrations of propofol associated with 50% reduction in postoperative nausea. *Anesthesiology*. **87**: 779–784.
18 Gan TJ *et al.* (1999) Patient-controlled antiemesis: a randomized, double-blind comparison of two doses of propofol versus placebo. *Anesthesiology*. **90**: 1564–1570.
19 Scher C *et al.* (1992) Use of propofol for the prevention of chemotherapy-induced nausea and emesis in oncology patients. *Canadian Journal of Anaesthesia*. **39**: 170–172.
20 Borgeat A *et al.* (1994) Adjuvant propofol enables better control of nausea and emesis secondary to chemotherapy for breast cancer. *Canadian Journal of Anaesthesia*. **41**: 1117–1119.
21 Hunter-Johnson L and Wheeler WL (2016) Use of propofol to manage nonmalignant intractable nausea and vomiting: a case study. *Journal of Palliative Medicine*. **19**: 252–253.
22 Cechetto DF *et al.* (2001) The effects of propofol in the area postrema of rats. *Anesthesia and Analgesia*. **92**: 934–942.
23 Rossetti AO (2007) Which anesthetic should be used in the treatment of refractory status epilepticus? *Epilepsia*. **48 (Suppl 8)**: 52–55.
24 Garcia Penas JJ *et al.* (2007) Status epilepticus: evidence and controversy. *Neurologist*. **13 (6 Suppl 1)**: S62–73.
25 Dulin JD *et al.* (2014) Management of refractory status epilepticus in an actively dying patient. *Journal of Pain and Palliative Care Pharmacotherapy*. **28**: 243–250.
26 Sneyd JR (1999) Propofol and epilepsy. *British Journal of Anaesthesia*. **82**: 168–169.
27 Meyer S *et al.* (2009) Propofol: pro- or anticonvulsant drug? *Anesthesia and Analgesia*. **108**: 1993–1994.
28 Jungheinrich C *et al.* (2002) Pharmacokinetics of the generic formulation Propofol 1 Fresenius in comparison with the original formulation (Disoprivan 1). *Clinical Drug Investigation*. **22**: 417–427.
29 Fechner J *et al.* (2004) Comparative pharmacokinetics and pharmacodynamics of the new propofol prodrug GPI 15715 and propofol emulsion. *Anesthesiology*. **101**: 626–639.
30 AstraZeneca (2006) *Data on file*.
31 Wilson C *et al.* (2010) The abuse potential of propofol. *Clinical Toxicology*. **48**: 165–170.
32 Charatan F (2009) Concerns mount over misuse of anaesthetic propofol among US health professionals. *British Medical Journal*. **339**: b3673.
33 Monroe T *et al.* (2011) The misuse and abuse of propofol. *Substance Use and Misuse*. **46**: 1199–1205.
34 AstraZeneca (2010) *Personal communication*.
35 Wijeysundera DN and Kavanagh BP (2011) Prevention of pain from propofol injection. *British Medical Journal*. **342**: d1102.
36 Jalota L *et al.* (2011) Prevention of pain on injection of propofol: systematic review and meta-analysis. *British Medical Journal*. **342**: d1110.
37 Cheng C *et al.* (2002) When midazolam fails. *Journal of Pain and Symptom Management*. **23**: 256–265.
38 Moyle J (1995) The use of propofol in palliative medicine. *Journal of Pain and Symptom Management*. **10**: 643–646.
39 Mercadante S *et al.* (1995) Propofol in terminal care. *Journal of Pain and Symptom Management*. **10**: 639–642.

Updated January 2022

14: PRESCRIBING IN PALLIATIVE CARE

In recent years, both national drug regulatory authorities and the general public have become increasingly concerned about the possibility of dangerous/life-threatening adverse drug reactions. Official documents and drug manufacturers' information often include a warning along the lines of:

> 'Use the lowest effective dose for the shortest possible time in order to reduce the risk of serious adverse events.'

This is, of course, one of the foundational principles of therapeutic drug use; it simply emphasises good practice. Official documents and drug manufacturers' information also highlight when caution is necessary in relation to, for example, hepatic and renal impairment.

In palliative care, many patients are elderly and debilitated, and many have impaired organ function. Accordingly, in *PCF*, it is assumed that prescribers will adopt an appropriately cautious approach in relation to both dose and duration of treatment (also see Getting the most out of PCF, p.xiv).

For information about prescribing for children or in patients with significant renal or hepatic impairment, see Chapter 16 (p.725), Chapter 17 (p.731) and Chapter 18 (p.753) respectively. For information about anticipatory prescribing in the community, see Chapter 15 (p.721).

GENERAL PRINCIPLES

Drugs should be used only within the context of a systematic approach, which is encapsulated in the acronym **EEMMA**:

- *Evaluation* of the impact of the illness on the patient and family, and of the causes of the patient's symptoms (often multifactorial)
- *Explanation* to the patient before starting treatment about what is going on, and what is the most appropriate course of action
- *Management:* correct the correctable, non-drug treatment, drug treatment
- *Monitoring*: frequent review of the impact of treatment; optimizing the doses of symptom-relief drugs to maximize benefit and minimize undesirable effects
- *Attention to detail:* do not make unwarranted assumptions; listen actively to the patient, respond to non-verbal and verbal cues.

In palliative care, the axiom *diagnosis before treatment* is still relevant. Even when cancer is responsible, a symptom may be caused by different mechanisms. For example, in lung cancer, vomiting may be caused by hypercalcaemia or by raised intracranial pressure (to name just two possible causes). Treatment often varies with the cause. Further, for many symptoms, the concurrent use of non-drug measures is equally important, and sometimes more important.

Attention to detail

Precision in taking a drug history

If a patient says, 'I take morphine every 4 hours', the doctor should ask, 'Tell me, when do you take your first dose?' 'And the second dose?' etc. It often turns out that the patient is taking morphine q.d.s. rather than q4h, and possibly p.r.n. rather than prophylactically.

A 90 year-old woman interpreted 'paracetamol four times a day' as meaning 0800h, 1200h, 1600h and 2000h. She was pain-free during the day but regularly woke between 0200h and 0300h in excruciating pain – so much so that she dreaded going to bed at night. Retiming her medication so that the doses were more equally spaced out around the clock (on waking, 1200h, 1800h, bedtime), resulted in a pain-free night.

'Think before you ink'

Consider non-drug options, but when prescribing any drug it is important for doctors to ask themselves:

'What is the treatment goal?'
'How can it be monitored?'
'What is the risk of undesirable effects?'
'What is the risk of drug interactions?'
'Can I stop any of the patient's other drugs?'

Safe prescribing

Safe prescribing is a skill and is crucial to success in symptom management. It extends to considering size, shape and taste of tablets and solutions, and avoiding doses which force patients to take more tablets, and/or open more containers, than would be the case if doses were 'rounded up' to a more convenient tablet size. For example, m/r **morphine** 100mg (one tablet, one container) is easier for the patient than 90mg (two tablets and two containers; 60mg + 30mg).

Safe prescribing requires good communication with patients, carers and other professionals. Poor communication contributes to about half of preventable drug errors.[1] A lack of information and involvement may leave patients dissatisfied.[2]

Good communication includes clear documentation (e.g. allergies, co-morbidities, prescription writing).[3-5] The use of a patient's 'logbook' is to be encouraged; this would include important contact names and telephone numbers.

Safe prescribing practice is particularly important in palliative care. Polypharmacy, debility, co-morbidities (e.g. renal and/or hepatic impairment), involvement of multiple professionals, and the use of higher-risk drugs are among the many factors which make patients particularly vulnerable to problems with adherence (compliance), medication errors, undesirable effects and drug interactions.

Keep it simple!

Polypharmacy in palliative care is the norm. In one study of patients receiving opioids, >25% were taking 10 or more different drugs concurrently.[6] Patients with diabetes and those with COPD or heart failure are likely to be among these. Drugs should be reviewed to see whether they are still necessary, e.g. long-term prophylactic medication such as statins, antihypertensives and oral hypoglycaemics, and stopped if possible.[7]

Clear written instructions

A home medicines chart is essential to prevent chaotic drug administration, e.g. one drug or other being taken in succession on the hour throughout the day with hardly any respite, and also to facilitate adherence.

Drug regimens should be written out in full for patients and/or families to work from. The recommendations published by the Royal Pharmaceutical Society[8] about the information to be recorded in writing when a patient transfers from one care provider to another also serve as a guide in relation to patients:

- name of drug (generic and, if appropriate, also brand)
- formulation and strength
- reason for use ('for pain', 'for bowels', etc.)
- dose (*x* mL, *y* tablets)
- frequency and times to be taken (Figure 1 and Figure 2).

Details about how to obtain further supplies should be included. An alternative system will be necessary if both the patient and the immediate family cannot read.

Hospice Home Care

Name *Linda Barton* **Age** *58* **Date** *7 July 2020*

Tablets/Medicines	2am	On waking	10am	2pm	6pm	Bed time	Purpose
MORPHINE (Oramorph 2mg in 1mL)		*10mL*	*10mL*	*10mL*	*10mL*	*20mL*	*pain relief*
HALOPERIDOL (1.5mg tablet)						*1*	*anti-sickness*
CELECOXIB (200mg capsule)			*1*			*1*	*pain relief*
SENNA (7.5mg/5mL liquid)			*10mL*			*10mL*	*for bowels*
ZOPICLONE (7.5mg tablet)						*1*	*for sleep*

If troublesome pain: take an extra 10mL of MORPHINE between regular doses.
If bowels remain constipated: increase SENNA to 15mL twice a day.

[Use this space for adding additional information, e.g. further advice about 'rescue' medication]

- Keep this chart with you so you can show your doctor or nurse this list of what you are taking.
- Ask for a fresh supply of your medication 2–3 days before you need it.
- Sometimes your medication may be supplied in different strengths or presentations. If you have any concerns about this, check with your pharmacist.
- In an emergency, phone ____________________ and ask to speak to ________________

Figure 1 Example of a patient's home medication chart (q4h).

Hospice Home Care

Name *Nicolas Crowthorne* **Age** *65* **Date** *7 July 2020*

Tablets/Medicines	*Breakfast*	*Midday meal*	*Evening meal*	*Bedtime*	Purpose
MORPHINE (MST 60mg tablet)	*1*			*1*	*pain relief*
CELECOXIB (200mg capsule)	*1*			*1*	*pain relief*
LANSOPRAZOLE (30mg capsule)	*1*				*to protect stomach*
SENNA (7.5mg/5mL liquid)	*10mL*			*10mL*	*for bowels*
HALOPERIDOL (1.5mg tablet)				*1*	*anti-sickness*

If troublesome pain: take MORPHINE SOLUTION (2mg in 1mL) 10mL, up to every 2 hours.

If bowels remain constipated: increase SENNA to 15mL twice a day.

[Use this space for adding additional information, e.g. further advice about 'rescue' medication]

- Keep this chart with you so you can show your doctor or nurse this list of what you are taking.
- Ask for a fresh supply of your medication 2–3 days before you need it.
- Sometimes your medication may be supplied in different strengths or presentations. If you have any concerns about this, check with your pharmacist.
- In an emergency, phone__________________ and ask to speak to ________________

Figure 2 Example of a patient's home medication chart (q.d.s.).

Generally, the drug that needs to be taken most frequently should act as the 'anchor' drug and, as far as possible, other drugs linked to its administration times. Although the SPC may indicate that an antibacterial should be given every 8 hours or every 6 hours, for PO administration there is generally no need to be so exact. Further, although patients with opioid-induced nausea are sometimes advised to take **metoclopramide** 30min before the opioid, in practice this is *rarely necessary*. However, certain drugs may need to have more precise timings, to ensure optimal symptom management, e.g.:

- drugs for diabetes mellitus
- anti-epileptics for seizure control
- desmopressin
- modified-release products, e.g. m/r opioids
- TD patches.

Antacids physically interact with many drugs, e.g. **azithromycin**, e/c products, quinolone antibacterials, **itraconazole** and tetracyclines, and reduce absorption. Accordingly, antacids should ideally be taken 2h before or after these drugs (see p.1, p.511 and p.568).

Drugs and food

Some SPCs and PILs indicate 'before food' (e.g. **lansoprazole**, p.31), or 'with/just after food' (e.g. NSAIDs, p.341), when this is not always necessary. Only when absolutely necessary should patients be asked to separate out drugs in relation to food. For example:

- when drug absorption is significantly affected by food. Box A lists drugs featured in *PCF* which, for maximal absorption, need to be taken either on an empty stomach or after food
- drugs which are known GI irritants. Box B lists those drugs featured in *PCF* for which food may reduce the risk or severity of undesirable GI effects.

In addition:

- drugs for diabetes and **pancreatin** should always be taken as recommended in relation to food/meal times
- in order to increase the contact time of the drug with the mucosa, food should *not* be taken immediately after drugs have been administered via the buccal mucosa (e.g. transmucosal **fentanyl**) or those used topically to treat oral ulceration or oral candidosis.

Box A Optimal absorption of drugs in relation to food[a,9,10]

Take on an *empty* stomach[b]	**Take *with* or *just after* food**
Antibacterials	Cefuroxime
demeclocycline[c]	Itraconazole *capsules*[d]
doxycycline[c]	Nitrofurantoin
flucloxacillin	Rivaroxaban
itraconazole *liquid*[d]	
phenoxymethylpenicillin	
tetracycline[c]	
rifampicin	
voriconazole	
Bisphosphonates[c]	
ibandronic acid[c]	
sodium clodronate[c]	
Propantheline	

a. these lists are limited to drugs featured in *PCF*

b. generally 30min before first food or drink of the day or 1h before and 2h after food at other times of the day

c. also avoid antacids, iron, zinc or milk for 2h before or after each dose to improve absorption

d. itraconazole liquid requires an empty stomach for full absorption, whereas food significantly improves the absorption of itraconazole capsules.

Box B Drugs for which food *may* reduce the risk of nausea/vomiting or GI irritation[a]

Baclofen	Iron
Corticosteroids	Potassium
Etamsylate (not UK)	Spironolactone
Metronidazole	Tinidazole
Misoprostol	Venlafaxine
NSAIDs[b]	Zinc

a. this list is limited to drugs that feature in the *PCF*
b. no substantial evidence.

Monitoring medication

It is often difficult to predict the optimum dose of a symptom-relief drug, particularly opioids, laxatives and psychotropics. Further, undesirable effects put drug adherence in jeopardy. Thus, arrangements must be made for monitoring the effects of medication. The responsibility for monitoring must be clearly stated; shared care is a definite risk factor for medication errors and problematic polypharmacy.[2,11]

Albumin binds acidic drugs, e.g. **phenytoin**, **warfarin**, **digoxin**, **naproxen** and **lorazepam**. When the albumin level is reduced by malnutrition, cirrhosis, nephrotic syndrome and/or end-stage renal disease, the proportion of unbound (active) drug increases. This increases the probability of toxicity with standard drug doses and normal total plasma drug concentrations, particularly with highly protein-bound drugs.

Most measured drug concentrations reflect the total drug concentration in the plasma (i.e. bound and unbound). Measuring free (unbound) levels of highly protein-bound drugs is not always possible, but formulas to 'correct' for low plasma protein concentrations are available for some drugs, e.g. **phenytoin** (see Anti-epileptics, Box A, p.288).

Compromise is sometimes necessary

It may be necessary to compromise on complete relief in order to avoid unacceptable undesirable effects. Antimuscarinic effects, e.g. dry mouth and visual disturbance, may limit dose escalation. Also, with inoperable bowel obstruction, it may be better to aim to reduce the incidence of vomiting to once or twice a day rather than to seek complete control.

Rescue ('as needed') medication

Patients need advice about what to do for intermittent symptoms, particularly break-through pain. Generally, it is good practice to err on the side of generosity in relation to the recommended frequency of p.r.n. medication. However, it does depend on the class and formulation of the drug in question, and whether the patient is an inpatient or at home.

In all circumstances, it is important that the dose and permitted frequency is stated clearly on the patient's medication chart (Figure 1 and Figure 2) and also verbally explained to the patient and the family.

Patients taking regular m/r strong opioid medication at home

The *corresponding* immediate-release opioid analgesic formulation should also be prescribed q1h p.r.n. in an appropriate dose (see p.323).

Patients taking regular immediate-release strong opioid medication at home

The *same* immediate-release opioid analgesic formulation should also be prescribed routinely q1h p.r.n. in an appropriate dose (see p.323).

With regular immediate-release strong opioids, if a patient needs an *occasional* rescue dose, say 40min or less before the next regular dose is due, it may suffice to give the next regular dose early. However, opinion is divided. Some specialists say that a p.r.n. dose should be given, followed in due course by the regular dose.

Patients taking regular analgesic medication other than a strong opioid

If a patient is receiving the maximum recommended dose of **paracetamol** or NSAID, a low dose of an immediate-release strong opioid/morphine can be prescribed *q2h p.r.n.* Recommendations for anti-emetics, laxatives and psychotropics are given in their respective sections.

Inpatients

Recommendations can be more generous because there are trained personnel to monitor the effect of any additional medication and thus prevent serious toxicity. For example, prescribing a range of permitted doses allows nurses to increase the amount given on their own initiative.

Example: Patient taking m/r **morphine** 100mg b.d.
Expected p.r.n. dose = 1/10–1/6 of total 24h dose, i.e. 20–30mg
Prescribe **morphine** immediate-release tablets/suspension 20–30mg q1h p.r.n.

In practice, nurses tend to start with the lower dose but increase to the top of the range if necessary. If two consecutive top-of-the-range doses at the maximum permitted frequency are insufficient, medical advice should be obtained and alternative measures considered, e.g. rapid titration with IV **morphine** (see p.404; and Morphine, Box B, p.411 and Box C, p.411), with a subsequent upward adjustment of the regular PO dose.

REVIEWING MEDICATION WHEN A PATIENT IS CLOSE TO DEATH

When a patient is clearly approaching death:

- *simplify medication:* stop long-term prophylactic medication if not already done, e.g. statins, antihypertensives, oral hypoglycaemics, **warfarin**
- *when the patient is moribund:* stop antidepressants and laxatives
- *anticipate and prescribe drugs p.r.n.* for common end-of-life problems, e.g. pain, breathlessness, vomiting, agitation, delirium, myoclonus, death rattle (see below)
- *prescribe all drugs both PO and SC/IV*
- *insulin-dependent diabetes:* reduce the dose of **insulin** as intake decreases (see p.582).
- *review need for IV hydration:* is it still appropriate? Can it be stopped?

For advice about stopping **dexamethasone** in patients with intracranial malignancy, see p.565.

In the last days, some nursing procedures normally regarded as essential may be discontinued. For example, standard care of pressure areas may cause a moribund patient to become distressed. If so, such care should be reduced or stopped.

'As needed' medication

Because patients close to death may well have increasing difficulty in swallowing, non-PO p.r.n. drugs should be prescribed (in addition to any existing PO p.r.n. drugs) in case of new distressing symptoms.

In some countries, SL, PR and TD products are preferred but, in the UK, SC injections are generally used. A typical pre-emptive regimen would include:

- **morphine** SC q1h p.r.n. (*dose depends on regular dose*) for pain, breathlessness, cough
- **haloperidol** 1–5mg SC q1h p.r.n. for nausea and vomiting, delirium
- **midazolam** 2.5–5mg SC q1h p.r.n. for anxiety, breathlessness; and, if seizures are likely, 10mg SC q1h p.r.n. (also see Anti-epileptics, Box B, p.291)
- **hyoscine *butylbromide*** 20mg SC q1h p.r.n. for bowel colic, death rattle.

Note. Charting all these drugs 'q1h p.r.n.' facilitates rapid dose titration. However, if after several q1h doses there is no benefit or any benefit is short-lived, it is important to consider if an alternative or an additional drug is needed (also see Chapter 15, p.721).

Other drugs may be necessary in various circumstances, e.g. renal failure (see Chapter 17, p.731), heart failure (see p.715) and Parkinson's disease (see p.717).

PRESCRIBING FOR THE ELDERLY

Elderly patients taking five or more drugs have a significantly increased risk of delirium and falls, the latter possibly related to postural hypotension.

The majority of patients receiving palliative care are elderly (≥65 years old). They are more likely to be receiving multiple drugs for existing co-morbid conditions. The addition of more drugs for symptom relief may adversely affect adherence and increases the risk of drug interactions (see Chapter 19, p.781) and adverse reactions.[6]

Presentation of adverse drug reactions in the elderly may be atypical and non-specific, and wrongly be attributed to a new medical problem. Drugs should be reviewed regularly and any of doubtful benefit should be stopped.[12,13] These include drugs for primary and secondary prevention which become irrelevant for a patient with a poor prognosis, e.g. statins, and drugs which do not treat symptoms caused by an underlying disease.[14,15]

Drug formulation and administration

Frail elderly patients may have difficulty swallowing tablets. They should be instructed to take tablets or capsules with fluid in an upright position to minimize the possibility of them remaining in the mouth or oesophagus and causing ulceration (e.g. NSAIDs, **temazepam**). Alternative formulations (e.g. liquid) or routes of administration (e.g. SC) may be preferable (see Chapter 28, p.853).

Pharmacokinetics

With increasing age, several changes occur which influence the pharmacokinetics of many drugs. The most important of these is the progressive decline in renal function. Drugs are excreted more slowly, and a lower dose may suffice, particularly for those with a narrow therapeutic ratio, e.g. **digoxin** (also see Chapter 17, p.731). Acute illness, particularly accompanied by dehydration, can lead to a rapid further reduction in renal clearance.

Reduction in liver size and blood flow may reduce hepatic metabolism (also see Chapter 18, p.753). Drugs with significant first-pass metabolism, e.g. **amitriptyline**, **glyceryl trinitrate**, **morphine**, may have higher bio-availability and a faster onset, necessitating starting with lower doses and/or at less frequent intervals.

Box C Examples of risks when prescribing for the elderly

Antidepressants
Postural hypotension, sedation, delirium, falls and femoral fracture.

Antimuscarinics
Falls, delirium, urinary retention, constipation.

Antihypertensives, digoxin, psychotropics
Undesirable effects more common; use smaller doses and monitor closely.

Hypoglycaemics
Chlorpropamide (not UK) and glibenclamide (not UK) are best avoided because of their long halflives and consequential risk of hypoglycaemia.

Night sedatives (hypnotics), including Z drugs
Cognitive impairment, delirium, falls, fractures; use a short course of a drug with a short halflife.

Nitrofurantoin
Lack of efficacy in patients with creatinine clearance <60mL/min because of inadequate urinary drug concentration.

NSAIDs
Serious GI bleeding is more common; may exacerbate fluid retention in patients with heart disease or renal impairment.

Reduction in lean body mass and increase in body fat will alter distribution of lipophilic drugs, e.g. benzodiazepines and **fentanyl**. When first given, these drugs will be stored in body fat, reducing their initial effect, but repeated administration may lead to prolonged release and significantly increased drug plasma concentrations.[14]

Pharmacodynamics

The ageing body has an increased sensitivity to drugs, notably centrally acting psychotropics and opioids (Box C).[16]

END-STAGE HEART FAILURE

In some *cancer patients*, chronic heart failure is a significant cause of breathlessness. It is important to recognize this and treat appropriately.

More detailed guidance about the care of patients with end-stage chronic heart failure is available from NICE[17] and elsewhere.[18,19] Resources include:

- *Supportive Care in Heart Failure*[20]
- *Heart Failure: From Advanced Disease to Bereavement*[21]
- *Heart Failure and Palliative Care: A Team Approach.*[22]

This section provides guidance about which drugs can be stopped to ease a patient's 'tablet burden' without adversely affecting the level of comfort.[23] In end-stage chronic heart failure, it is important *not* to stop 'disease control' medication which also has an important contribution in symptom relief. Unlike cancer, where disease-specific treatment tends to become increasingly burdensome and futile (and possibly counterproductive), the continued disease-specific treatment of chronic heart failure generally continues to be essential for symptom management even when end-stage (Figure 3). If in doubt, and for patients with chronic heart failure and preserved systolic ejection fraction, obtain advice from the patient's cardiologist or specialist heart failure nurse.

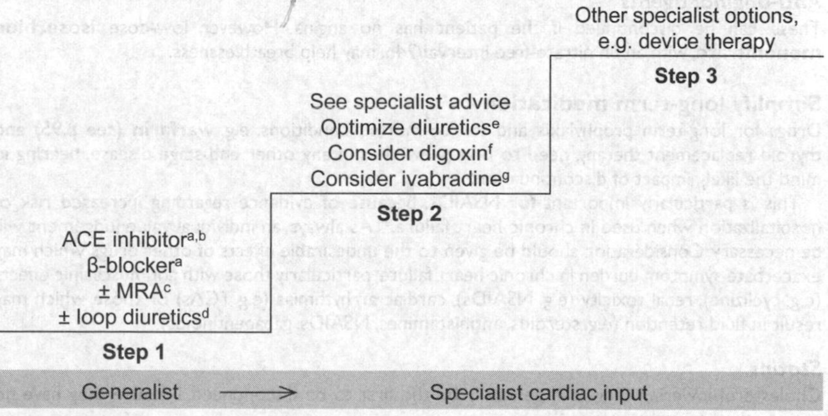

Figure 3 Synopsis of guidance for drug treatment of chronic heart failure with reduced systolic ejection fraction.

a. in all patients who are stable, i.e. minimal or no signs of fluid overload or depletion, even if asymptomatic
b. if an ACE inhibitor is not tolerated, substitute an adrenoreceptor blocker, e.g. losartan
c. mineralocorticoid antagonists (MRAs) include spironolactone and eplerenone
d. in patients with signs of fluid overload
e. thiazide diuretics and those affecting the renal distal tubule may be added, e.g. bendroflumethiazide, metolazone
f. digoxin can be considered irrespective of presence or absence of arrhythmias
g. ivabradine is used to slow heart rate to <75 beats per minute for those in sinus rhythm.

Drugs that improve survival and symptoms in patients with reduced ejection fraction

Aldosterone antagonists, angiotensin-converting enzyme (ACE) inhibitors; angiotensin receptor blockers; β-blockers

These should generally be continued, because there is good evidence that in chronic heart failure with a reduced systolic ejection fraction they slow progression, prolong survival, and improve symptom control.[24-30] Indications for considering a dose reduction or discontinuation on either a temporary or permanent basis are:

- symptomatic hypotension
- deteriorating renal function
- excessive tablet burden.

The patient's clinical condition, electrolytes and renal function should be monitored closely, and further dose adjustments made (up or down) as necessary (also see p.73).

Drugs that primarily improve symptoms in advanced disease

Loop diuretics

Furosemide (p.67) and **bumetanide** are widely used.[31] In very end-stage disease, the increasing dose necessary for symptom control may exacerbate renal dysfunction. However, unless the patient becomes anuric or clinically hypovolaemic, a loop diuretic should be continued for symptom management. **Furosemide** by CSCI may reduce the need for hospital admission (see p.70).[32,33]

Anti-arrhythmic drugs

Anti-arrhythmic drugs can generally be considered for discontinuation at a relatively early stage. Most anti-arrhythmics lower blood pressure and can contribute to fatigue. However, if *symptomatic* tachycardias are present, or rate control is also helping angina symptoms, it may be best to continue. **Amiodarone** has a very long halflife (6 months) and thus can generally be stopped in end-stage chronic heart failure.

Anti-anginal agents

These can be discontinued if the patient has no angina. However, low-dose **isosorbide mononitrate**, with an 8h nitrate-free interval/24h, may help breathlessness.

Simplify long-term medication

Drugs for long-term prophylaxis and for co-morbid conditions, e.g. **warfarin** (see p.95) and thyroid replacement therapy, need to be reviewed as in any other end-stage disease, bearing in mind the likely impact of discontinuation.

This is particularly important for NSAIDs, because of evidence regarding increased risk of hospitalization when used in chronic heart failure.[34] As always, an individual value judgement will be necessary. Consideration should be given to the undesirable effects of other drugs which may exacerbate symptom burden in chronic heart failure, particularly those with antimuscarinic effects (e.g. cyclizine), renal toxicity (e.g. NSAIDs), cardiac arrhythmias (e.g. TCAs) or those which may result in fluid retention (e.g. steroids, antihistamines, NSAIDs, gabapentinoids).

Statins

Cholesterol-lowering drugs can generally be the first to be discontinued, because they have no symptom-relieving properties.[35]

Antihypertensive drugs

These are generally inappropriate in end-stage disease.

Digoxin

In atrial fibrillation, **digoxin** may be important for rate control. Uncontrolled fast atrial fibrillation may be unpleasant for the patient and exacerbate symptoms. In patients in sinus rhythm, symptoms are less likely to worsen if digoxin is stopped.[36] If renal failure develops as the heart failure progresses, accumulation could lead to toxicity.

END-STAGE IDIOPATHIC PARKINSON'S DISEASE

Patients with idiopathic Parkinson's disease (IPD) can die directly from IPD or from a concurrent condition (e.g. cancer). Consequently, patients with IPD can be at differing stages as they approach death, and thus may have different degrees of dopamine responsiveness.

Even at the end of life, dopamine can be important for the control of rigidity, bradykinesia, tremor and pain in these patients. Thus, one of the key challenges is to assess and optimize dopamine treatment as patients deteriorate. A further challenge is trying to avoid centrally acting D_2 antagonists (e.g. antipsychotics, **metoclopramide**), because they exacerbate IPD, particularly rigidity and the associated pain.

Although predicting prognosis in idiopathic IPD is often difficult, a progressive decline in physical status, continuing weight loss, recurrent infections, cognitive impairment, swallowing problems, and episodes of aspiration pneumonia strongly suggest that the patient may be at the end stage. Given the unreliability of prognostication, frequent review is necessary. When deterioration is rapid, this may need to be daily (see p.713). Each patient requires careful individual evaluation, and, when possible, there should be ongoing liaison with an IPD specialist.

A rapid decline from diagnosis (within 3–5 years) with a poor response to **levodopa** could indicate a 'PD plus syndrome' (e.g. progressive supranuclear palsy, multiple system atrophy). Most of these patients die 6–10 years from the start of symptoms. The approach to palliative care in these conditions is the same as for IPD, namely determining dopamine responsiveness (often poorer in these groups) and avoiding drugs which may exacerbate symptoms (e.g. **haloperidol** and **metoclopramide**).

In the last few days of life, the patient with IPD is likely *not* to be able to swallow.[37] In patients with well-controlled IPD, dopaminergic drugs should generally be continued (see below). On the other hand, in patients dying with end-stage IPD, a *gradual* reduction of dopaminergic drugs is sometimes appropriate because of loss of efficacy and/or increased undesirable effects, e.g. agitation, delirium, hallucinations.[38] Note. Sudden withdrawal of dopaminergic drugs can lead to an acute dopamine depletion syndrome (neuroleptic/antipsychotic malignant syndrome); see Antipsychotics, Box A (p.192).

Rigidity

Rigidity is not always a major issue for patients with end-stage IPD, and many tolerate a reduction in their often complex IPD drug regimens. On the other hand, important causes of rigidity towards the end of life are:

- not getting dopaminergic drugs on time
- an inability to swallow medication
- worsening IPD which is less dopamine-responsive.

Thus, if the patient can still swallow, ensure that medication is given on time, and consider prescribing p.r.n. doses of dispersible Madopar®, e.g. 62.5mg (= **benserazide** 12.5mg + **levodopa** 50mg).

If the patient is not able swallow, consider giving previous dopaminergic medication via an existing PEG or an NG tube (see Chapter 28, Table 2, p.863). Alternatively, discuss the use of one of the following parenteral dopamine agonists with a PD specialist:

- TD **rotigotine** (most commonly used):
  - ▷ see www.pdmedcalc.co.uk for guidance on an appropriate starting dose based on existing dopaminergic drug use
  - ▷ replace the patch at about the same time each day, using a fresh site
  - ▷ if necessary, the dose can be increased every 3 days by 2mg/24h
  - ▷ maximum dose 8mg/24h in early-stage IPD, and 16mg/24h in end-stage IPD
- SC **apomorphine**; also prescribe prophylactic **domperidone** to prevent almost inevitable nausea.[39]

Relieving rigidity without causing delirium or hallucinations can be difficult. Both **rotigotine** and **apomorphine** can cause delirium ± agitation; generally use only with guidance from a PD specialist.

If dopaminergic medication is stopped, **midazolam** 5–10mg/24h by CSCI may help relieve rigidity. There is a risk of acute dopamine depletion syndrome (neuroleptic/antipsychotic malignant syndrome), and clinicians should be familiar with its features (see Antipsychotics, Box A, p.192). Optimal nursing care and gentle physiotherapy are also crucial.

Pain

Careful evaluation is needed to determine if pain is related to rigidity or to some other cause. Different pains often require different approaches to management:

- if related to rigidity, see above
- If not, consider:
  - ▷ non-drug treatment, e.g. positioning, nursing care, physiotherapy, massage, heat, TENS
  - ▷ drug treatment (see p.321).

Nausea and vomiting

Metoclopramide, **haloperidol** and **prochlorperazine** are D_2 antagonists (see p.258) and ideally should be avoided in IPD, because they will exacerbate rigidity and bradykinesia. Despite being D_2 antagonists, it may sometimes be necessary to prescribe small doses of **levomepromazine** (e.g. 3.125–6.25mg SC at bedtime; see p.201) or **olanzapine** (e.g. 1.25–2.5mg PO at bedtime; see p.203) if all else fails. A recent case report found **levomepromazine** 6.25mg SC p.r.n. effective and well tolerated in a patient receiving **rotigotine**.[40] Use of the latter may help protect against extra-pyramidal symptoms, with improvements reported in antipsychotic-induced parkinsonism.[41]

Anecdotal reports suggest that **cyclizine** may also exacerbate IPD. Anti-emetics *least* likely to exacerbate IPD are:

- **domperidone** (p.271)
- **ondansetron** (p.277). Note. Concurrent use with **apomorphine** contra-indicated
- **hyoscine *hydrobromide*** (p.18), but may exacerbate delirium.

Delirium and agitation

Remember: both **rotigotine** and **apomorphine** can cause delirium ± agitation.

There may be a need for a trade-off between increased rigidity (and the consequential pain) and the relief of a hyperactive delirium. However, there are many potential causes for delirium and agitation in end-stage IPD and, as always, a systematic approach is necessary:

- if feasible, treat any obvious underlying cause, e.g. constipation and/or urinary retention
- review dopaminergic drugs; discuss with the PD team the best order for stopping these
- this generally results in **levodopa** monotherapy, and perhaps reducing the dose of this as well
- if the patient can swallow, consider **quetiapine** (see p.189), an atypical antipsychotic available only as an oral product, but the one least likely to cause extrapyramidal movement disorders
- if the patient cannot swallow, consider a benzodiazepine (see p.163), *but be aware that this sometimes exacerbates delirium*, e.g.:
  - ▷ **midazolam** 2.5mg SC p.r.n.
  - ▷ **lorazepam** 0.5–1mg SL p.r.n.
- if the situation remains unsatisfactory, prescribe an injectable antipsychotic, e.g. **levomepromazine** 6.25mg SC p.r.n. (p.201).

The use of **levomepromazine** will generally result in a reduction in the patient's level of consciousness, but will exacerbate PD less than **haloperidol**.

Some patients with PD also have dementia, commonly Alzheimer's or dementia with Lewy bodies (DLB).[42,43] Extra care needs to be taken in DLB. About 50% of such patients are over-sensitive to antipsychotics and, if used, they will experience a marked exacerbation of the PD, reduced level of consciousness, increased delirium, and possibly acute dopamine depletion syndrome (neuroleptic/antipsychotic malignant syndrome) (see Antipsychotics, Box A, p.192).

1 Rothschild JM *et al.* (2002) Analysis of medication-related malpractice claims: causes, preventability, and costs. *Archives of Internal Medicine.* **162**: 2414–2420.

2 Spinewine A *et al.* (2005) Appropriateness of use of medicines in elderly inpatients: qualitative study. *British Medical Journal.* **331**: 935.

3 Kanjanarat P *et al.* (2003) Nature of preventable adverse drug events in hospitals: a literature review. *American Journal of Health System Pharmacy.* **60**: 1750–1759.

4 Jones TA and Como JA (2003) Assessment of medication errors that involved drug allergies at a university hospital. *Pharmacotherapy.* **23**: 855–860.

5 Neale G *et al.* (2001) Exploring the causes of adverse events in NHS hospital practice. *Journal of the Royal Society of Medicine.* **94**: 322–330.

6 Kotlinska-Lemieszek A *et al.* (2014) Polypharmacy in patients with advanced cancer and pain: a European cross-sectional study of 2282 patients. *Journal of Pain and Symptom Management.* **48**: 1145–1159.

7 Duerden M *et al.* (2013) Polypharmacy and medicines optimisation: making it safe and sound. Kings Fund, London. www.kingsfund.org.uk.

8 Royal Pharmaceutical Society (2012) Keeping patients safe when they transfer between care providers - getting the medicines right. www.rpharms.com.

9 BNF Appendix 3: Cautionary and advisory lables for dispensed medicines London: BMJ Group and Pharmaceutical Press. www.bnf.org (accessed April 2013).

10 Sweetman SC *Martindale: The Complete Drug Reference.* London: Pharmaceutical Press. www.medicinescomplete.com.

11 Dean B *et al.* (2002) Causes of prescribing errors in hospital inpatients: a prospective study. *Lancet.* **359**: 1373–1378.

12 Cruz-Jentoft AJ *et al.* (2012) Drug therapy optimization at the end of life. *Drugs & Aging.* **29**: 511-521.

13 Milton JC *et al.* (2008) Prescribing for older people. *British Medical Journal.* **336**: 606–609.

14 Hubbard RE *et al.* (2013) Medication prescribing in frail older people. *European Journal of Clinical Pharmacology.* **69**: 319–326.

15 Petrovic M *et al.* (2012) Adverse drug reactions in older people: detection and prevention. *Drugs & Aging.* **29**: 453–462.

16 O'Mahony D *et al.* (2015) STOPP/START criteria for potentially inappropriate prescribing in older people: version 2. *Age and Ageing.* **44**: 213–218.

17 NICE (2018) Chronic heart failure in adults: diagnosis and management. *Clinical Guideline.* NG106. www.nice.org.uk.

18 Ponikowski P *et al.* (2016) 2016 ESC Guidelines for the diagnosis and treatment of acute and chronic heart failure: the Task Force for the diagnosis and treatment of acute and chronic heart failure of the European Society of Cardiology (ESC). Developed with the special contribution of the Heart Failure Association (HFA) of the ESC. *European Journal of Heart Failure.* **18**: 891–975.

19 SIGN (2016) Management of chronic heart failure. *SIGN Guideline.* **147**: www.sign.ac.uk.

20 Beattie J and Goodlin S (2008) *Supportive Care in Heart Failure.* Supportive Care Series, Oxford University Press.

21 Johnson MJ (2012) *Heart Failure: From Advanced Disease to Bereavement.* End of Life Series. Oxford: Oxford University Press.

22 Johnson M *et al.* (2015) *Heart Failure And Palliative Care: A Team Approach* (2nd edn). CRC Press.

23 Cleland JG *et al.* (2000) Polypharmacy (or polytherapy) in the treatment of heart failure. *Heart Failure Monitor.* **1**: 8-13.

24 Jong P *et al.* (2002) Angiotensin receptor blockers in heart failure: meta-analysis of randomized controlled trials. *Journal of the American College of Cardiology.* **39**: 463–470.

25 Shibata MC *et al.* (2001) Systematic review of the impact of beta blockers on mortality and hospital admissions in heart failure. *European Journal of Heart Failure.* **3**: 351–357.

26 The SOLVD Investigators (1991) Effect of enalapril on survival in patients with reduced left ventricular ejection fractions and congestive heart failure. The SOLVD Investigators. *New England Journal of Medicine.* **325**: 293–302.

27 Consensus Trial Study Group (1987) Effects of enalapril on mortality in severe congestive heart failure. Results of the Cooperative North Scandinavian Enalapril Survival Study (CONSENSUS). *New England Journal of Medicine.* **316**: 1429–1435.

28 Pitt B *et al.* (2003) Eplerenone, a selective aldosterone blocker, in patients with left ventricular dysfunction after myocardial infarction. *New England Journal of Medicine.* **348**: 1309–1321.

29 Pitt B *et al.* (1999) The effect of spironolactone on morbidity and mortality in patients with severe heart failure. Randomized Aldactone Evaluation Study Investigators. *New England Journal of Medicine.* **341**: 709–717.

30 The RALES Investigators (1996) Effectiveness of spironolactone added to an angiotensin-converting enzyme inhibitor and a loop diuretic for severe chronic congestive heart failure (the Randomized Aldactone Evaluation Study [RALES]). *American Journal of Cardiology.* **78**: 902–907.

31 Faris R *et al.* (2012) Diuretics for heart failure. *Cochrane Database of Systematic Reviews.* CD003838. www.cochranelibrary.com.

32 Zacharias H *et al.* (2011) Is there a role for subcutaneous furosemide in the community and hospice management of end-stage heart failure? *Palliative Medicine.* **26**: 658–663.

33 Zatarain-Nicolas E *et al.* (2013) Subcutaneous infusion of furosemide administered by elastomeric pumps for decompensated heart failure treatment: initial experience. *Revista Espanola de Cardiologica (English Ed).* **66**: 1002–1004.

34 Arfe A *et al.* (2016) Non-steroidal anti-inflammatory drugs and risk of heart failure in four European countries: nested case-control study. *British Medical Journal.* **354**: i4857.

35 McGowan MP and Treating to New Target Study G (2004) There is no evidence for an increase in acute coronary syndromes after short-term abrupt discontinuation of statins in stable cardiac patients. *Circulation.* **110**: 2333–2335.

36 Digitalis Invesitgation Group (1997) The effect of digoxin on mortality and morbidity in patients with heart failure. *New England Journal of Medicine.* **336**: 525-533.

37 Goy ER *et al.* (2008) Neurologic disease at the end of life: caregiver descriptions of Parkinson disease and amyotrophic lateral sclerosis. *Journal of Palliative Medicine.* **11**: 548–554.

38 National Council of Palliative Care Neurological Conditions Group (2011) Consensus statement for the management of symptoms in idiopathic Parkinsons's Disease (PD) and related conditions in the last few days of life. www.ncpc.org.uk.

39 Dewhurst F *et al.* (2009) The pragmatic use of apomorphine at the end of life. *Palliative Medicine.* **23**: 777–779.

40 Hindmarsh J *et al.* (2019) The combination of levomepromazine (methotrimeprazine) and rotigotine enables the safe and effective management of refractory nausea and vomiting in a patient with idiopathic Parkinson's disease. *Palliative Medicine.* **33**: 109–113.

41 Di Fabio R *et al.* (2013) Low doses of rotigotine in patients with antipsychotic-induced parkinsonism. *Clinical Neuropharmacology.* **36**: 162–165.

42 McKeith IG *et al.* (2005) Diagnosis and management of dementia with Lewy bodies: third report of the DLB Consortium. *Neurology.* **65**: 1863–1872.

43 McKeith I (2002) Dementia with Lewy bodies. *British Journal of Psychiatry.* **180**: 144–147.

Updated (minor change) May 2021

15: ANTICIPATORY PRESCRIBING IN THE COMMUNITY

15

Anticipatory ('just in case') prescribing enables professional and informal carers to respond rapidly to an actual or potential symptom crisis in terminally ill patients at home. Drugs are prescribed to manage likely or foreseeable symptoms when treating reversible causes is no longer possible or desirable, including injections for when the PO route is no longer feasible.[1-4]

Drugs are kept with clear guidance about their intended use, administration authorization and record, and a stock balance sheet.[1-3,5]

Prescribing is only one component of planning for symptom crises.[6] Planning must integrate training, written guidance, along with rapid access to relevant patient information (e.g. an Advance Care Plan) and specialist palliative care advice, so that staff can respond confidently and effectively.[7,8] Good communication between daytime and out-of-hours services is essential.[7,9,10]

However, even when used optimally, anticipatory prescribing cannot cover every patient and every eventuality, e.g. unforeseen rapid deterioration ± crisis, when other approaches may be necessary, see Non-medical assessment and prescribing below.

CHOICE OF DRUGS

The choice of drugs should be sufficient to respond to the most common symptoms. Familiar drugs suitable for more than one indication are preferred (Table 1).

However, fixed lists of recommended drugs are unlikely to be suitable for all patients. Choice should be adapted to individual circumstances:

- co-morbid conditions:
  - ▷ Parkinson's disease: consider alternatives to antipsychotic anti-emetics (see p.718)
  - ▷ renal impairment: modify doses and perhaps choice of opioid (see p.743)
  - ▷ needle phobia: SL/buccal or PR alternatives
- present medication:
  - ▷ if taking PO **oxycodone**, parenteral **oxycodone** is generally preferable to morphine
- specific foreseeable problems:
  - ▷ seizures or major haemorrhage: modify dose of **midazolam** prescribed (see p.168)
  - ▷ mild–moderate haemorrhage: topical or SC tranexamic acid (p.114).

Table 1 Examples of drugs used for more than one symptom

Medication	*Indication*
Morphine sulfate	Pain Breathlessness Cough
Midazolam	Anxiety Seizures
Hyoscine *butylbromide*	Colic Respiratory secretions
Haloperidol or levomepromazine	Nausea Hyperactive delirium

ACCESSING ADDITIONAL DRUGS/SUPPORT

Because not all symptoms are foreseeable, anticipatory prescribing is generally combined with one or more of the approaches below to reduce delays in managing symptom crises.

Palliative care emergency kits

These contain a wider range of drugs and equipment (e.g. syringe driver), which can be kept at an out-of-hours (OOH) service provider's base or in a car. Local guidelines, contact numbers for specialist advice, and guidance on relevant local arrangements should be included with the kit or be easily accessible, remembering the wide range of care settings an OOH service provider may cover. To carry CDs, they must be able to demonstrate compliance with Home Office regulations.[11]

Extended community pharmacy schemes

These generally involve networks of community pharmacies able to offer extended opening hours, and carrying a locally agreed palliative care stock list. Some schemes reduce wastage by keeping less frequently used medicines in a smaller number of locations, typically close to OOH or community nursing teams (Table 2). Some also agree to provide palliative care information, advice and an emergency contacts list for patients, carers and clinicians. Examples of local practice are available in the Document library on www.palliativedrugs.com, filed under Medication issues (Out of hours issues).

Table 2 Isle of Wight community pharmacy palliative care stock list

Drug	*Form*	*Strength*	*Quantity stocked*
Commonly used medicines kept by all late-opening community pharmacies			
Cyclizine	Injection	50mg/mL	10
Dexamethasone	Injection	3.3mg/mL	10
Fentanyl	Injection	100microgram/2mL	10
Haloperidol	Injection	5mg/mL	10
Hyoscine *butylbromide*	Injection	20mg/mL	10
Levomepromazine	Injection	25mg/mL	10
Lorazepam	Tablets	1mg	28
Metoclopramide	Injection	10mg/2mL	2 × 12
Midazolam	Injection	10mg/2mL	2 × 10
Morphine sulfate	Injection	10mg/mL	10
Oxycodone hydrochloride	Injection	10mg/mL	10
Water	Injection	20mL	10
Infrequently used medicines kept by a single central pharmacy			
Clonidine	Injection	150microgram/mL	10
Levetiracetam	Injection	500mg/5mL	10
Methadone	Injection	10mg/mL	10
Morphine sulfate	Injection	30mg/mL	10
Octreotide	Injection	500microgram/mL	5
Ondansetron	Injection	4mg/2mL	10
Parecoxib	Injection	40mg	5
Phenobarbital	Injection	200mg/mL	10

Non-medical assessment and prescribing

Examples include:

- paramedics can give selected drugs without a prescription for a patient at the end of life, e.g. morphine sulfate for pain or breathlessness[12]
- non-medical prescribers, e.g. nurse specialists in an OOH community palliative care service
- Patient Group Directions enable suitably experienced clinical staff, e.g. paramedics, nurse specialists, to respond to selected symptom crises.

ANTICIPATORY CSCI (SYRINGE DRIVERS)

Recently, the risks inherent in anticipatory prescribing of drugs by CSCI have been highlighted, e.g. of unintentional under- or overdosing of a strong opioid.[13] However, some centres use anticipatory CSCI prescriptions for selected situations, when the following criteria are met:[14]

- the drug choice and dose is unlikely to change before next review
- all health professionals (including OOH) can:
  - ▷ recognise the situation for which the CSCI is intended *and*
  - ▷ have the expertise required to safely initiate the CSCI
- the initiation of the CSCI triggers a timely review by an appropriate clinician.

Examples include continuing drugs critical to symptom control when the PO route is lost (e.g. levetiracetam) or responding to recurrent symptom crises (e.g. anti-emetics). The situation must be reviewed frequently enough to ensure that the anticipatory CSCI prescription remains appropriate. Local service provision will influence whether or not the above criteria can be met.[14]

INTERMITTENT SC DRUG ADMINISTRATION BY INFORMAL CARERS

Injections are regularly given by relatives and other informal carers to children or adults with, for example, diabetes mellitus or cystic fibrosis. In palliative care, there are occasions when it is helpful to train a relative or other informal carer to give intermittent SC injections (including CDs):

- regular medication that cannot be taken by a less invasive route
- emergency medication for symptoms that may develop particularly during a patient's last days.

Multi-professional involvement is required to develop clear procedures to ensure the safety of the patient, provide support for the carer, minimise risks, and comply with legislative, regulatory and professional standards (see Box A). Examples of procedures and documentation are available on www.palliativedrugs.com.

Some emergency medication can be given by other routes (e.g. SL, buccal) rather than by injection. Similar procedures and safeguards are needed when delegating the administration of any medicinal product to a relative or other informal carer.[15]

Box A Procedures and safeguards for informal carers giving SC injections[15-19]

Careful evaluation of the situation by the healthcare team.

Informed consent obtained from the patient for administration by a named carer.

Informal carers, particularly if qualified nurses or doctors, must not feel pressured to give injections.

Both the patient and the carer should be able to opt out of the care arrangement at any time.

Carer's fears must be explored, including the possibility of the patient dying shortly after an injection.

Carers must:

- be trained and assessed as competent, and this should be documented in the patient's notes (together with the reason for using this approach)
- be provided with written information for each drug, including the name, dose, indication, common undesirable effects, interval before a repeat dose is permitted, maximum number of injections/24h
- keep a record of all injections given, including date, time, drug strength, formulation and dose, and name of person giving the injection
- be provided with contact telephone numbers for both in and out of hours.

Regular support and review of the situation must be carried out by a named health professional.

Close liaison with the primary health care team and all out-of-hours services ensuring that, e.g.:

- continuing the same formulation that the carer has been trained to use
- SC cannula are appropriately monitored and replaced when necessary.

1 NICE (2015) Care of dying adults in the last days of life. *Clinical Guideline NG31*. www.nice.org.uk.
2 Scottish Palliative Care Guidelines (2020) Anticipatory prescribing.: www.palliativecareguidelines.scot.nhs.uk (accessed May 2021).
3 Palliative Care Wales Anticipatory Prescribing. https://wales.pallcare.info/ (accessed May 2021).
4 Bowers B *et al.* (2019) Anticipatory prescribing of injectable medications for adults at the end of life in the community: A systematic literature review and narrative synthesis. *Palliative Medicine*. **33**: 160–177.
5 Gold Standards Framework (2006) Check list of contents for "Just in Case Boxes". www.goldstandardsframework.org.uk.
6 Health Service Ombudsman (2015) Dying without dignity. *Parliamentary and health service ombusman*. www.ombudsman.org.uk.
7 Williams H *et al.* (2019) Quality improvement priorities for safer out-of-hours palliative care: Lessons from a mixed-methods analysis of a national incident-reporting database. *Palliative Medicine*. **33**: 346–356.
8 Khalil H *et al. (2019) Challenges associated with anticipatory medications in rural and remote settings. Journal of Palliative Medicine*. **22**: 297–301.
9 Wilson E *et al.* (2020) An exploration of the experiences of professionals supporting patients approaching the end of life in medicines management at home. A qualitative study. *BMC Palliative Care*. **19**: 66.
10 Katz N *et al.* (2019) Pre-emptive prescription of medications for the management of potential, catastrophic events in patients with a terminal illness: A survey of palliative medicine doctors. *Palliative Medicine*. **33**: 178–186.
11 Care Quality Commission (2019) The safer management of controlled drugs.
12 JRCALC (2019) Clinical practice guidelines. Joint Royal Colleges Ambulance Liaison Committee. www.jrcalc.org.uk.
13 Bowers B *et al.* (2021) Anticipatory syringe pumps: benefits and risks. *BMJ Supportive & Palliative Care*. **0**: 1–2.
14 Howard P *et al.* (2019) Response to "Anticipatory syringe drivers: a step too far". *BMJ Support Palliative Care*. **8**.
15 Lau DT *et al.* (2012) Hospice providers' key approaches to support informal caregivers in managing medications for patients in private residences. *Journal of Pain and Symptom Management*. **43**: 1060–1071.
16 Bradford and Airedale NHS Trust (2006) Subcutaneous drug administration by carers (adult palliative care). www.palliativedrugs.com Document library.
17 NHS National Prescribing Centre (2009) A guide to good practice in the management of controlled drugs in primary care (England) 3rd Edition.
18 NHS Lothian (2009) Patients and or carers administration of subcutaneous drugs by intermittent injections: adult palliative care. Protocol, procedure and teaching guideline Version 2.
19 Lincolnshire Community Health Services NHS Trust (2015) The Lincolnshire policy for informal carer's administration of as required subcutaneous injections in community palliative care. (Version 8) St Barnabas Lincolnshire Hospice.

Updated August 2021

16: PRESCRIBING FOR CHILDREN

16

INTRODUCTION

Globally, there are about 21 million children who could benefit from palliative care each year.[1] In England, the prevalence rate is estimated to be 32 per 10,000 population aged 0–19.[2] There are about 50,000 children in the UK living with a life-limiting or life-threatening condition. About 2,500 children die from such a condition in England and Wales each year.[2]

Although cancer, after trauma, is the second most common condition causing death in children, most children needing palliative care have diagnoses other than cancer. The largest group have neurological or neuromuscular disorders, e.g. hypoxic brain injury or inherited progressive metabolic, muscle or degenerative disease.

The need for palliative care may extend over many years, sometimes from the time of diagnosis (including antenatally), and in parallel with ongoing treatment of the underlying condition and of any intercurrent illness. Evaluation in children is inherently more difficult than in most adults. Further, in children with life-limiting conditions, it is often difficult to identify the end stage, particularly with disorders other than cancer.

Common problems include cerebral irritability, intractable seizures, skeletal muscle spasm, dystonia, pain, swallowing and feeding difficulties, gastro-oesophageal reflux, breathlessness and troublesome secretions. Symptom evaluation is particularly difficult in children with cognitive impairment.[3-5]

When possible, use self-reporting tools appropriate to the child's age and ability.[6-9] A parent's report and observation by staff are important, particularly for evaluation of symptoms in children who are preverbal, nonverbal or cognitively impaired. Symptom scales and diaries may aid continuity among different carers and across different settings, e.g. home, school, hospital, palliative care unit, respite centre.

Ongoing care should be under the direction of a multiprofessional team,[5,10] including specialist paediatric palliative care,[5,11] ideally with advice from a paediatric pharmacist. Written individualized symptom management plans facilitate communication and consistency of care across different settings.[5]

GENERAL CONSIDERATIONS

The general comments in relation to prescribing for adults in palliative care (see Chapter 14, p.707) apply equally to children.

Extra care is needed when prescribing for children:

- prescribe only if there is a definite indication; always consider non-drug options
- become familiar with a limited range of drugs and their effects in children
- simplify regimens as much as possible
- try to avoid the need to administer drugs at school or when the child should be sleeping
- check dose calculations (often based on weight or surface area)
- round down to the nearest practical dose
- involve children in decisions about their medication (at a level appropriate to their age and understanding).

Children are at increased risk of medication errors because of:

- lack of evidence-based data
- the diversity and rarity of their conditions
- the need to calculate and adjust the dose for the age and/or weight of the child
- the lack of suitable dose formulations
- variations in recommended doses and administration regimens
- inconsistent presentation of recommended dose information (e.g. microgram/kg per dose, microgram/kg/h, mg per dose, total 24h dose).

Particular care is needed when prescribing in the neonatal period (<1 month), because of immature renal and liver function, immature reticular activating systems, and higher volumes of distribution.

Flexible personalized regimens make it easier for the child, increasing adherence and minimizing disruption to schooling and sleep. However, precise timing is important for some drugs, e.g. antidiabetics, anti-epileptics, **desmopressin** (also see p.707).

As far as possible, drugs should be prescribed within the terms of their marketing authorization. However, historically most drugs have been developed and tested in adults. Few are authorized for use in children or for indications for which they are regularly used. Many are not marketed in suitable dose form or strength, and there is little age-related information about adverse reactions.[12] As in adult palliative care, it is sometimes necessary to prescribe 'off-label', i.e. beyond a drug's authorized indications and/or routes of administration (see p.xix).[13]

Fortunately, there are several respected sources providing guidance about prescribing medication for children generally,[14-17] via enteral feeding tubes[18] (also see Chapter 28, p.853), for neonates[19] and in paediatric palliative care.[20-22] A Master Formulary is available from the Association for Paediatric Palliative Medicine.[23]

There is still a dearth of paediatric data for pharmacokinetics, pharmacodynamics and drug safety,[24] and practice has often evolved from personal experience and case series. To increase the body of knowledge, significant undesirable effects in children should be reported:

- in the UK:
  - ▷ through the Yellow Card website or app, https://yellowcard.mhra.gov.uk
  - ▷ through the PaedPalCare electronic forum, www.togetherforshortlives.org.uk/professionals/care_provision/care_forum
- in other countries which have similar national and specialist reporting schemes, e.g.:
  - ▷ FDA Medwatch, www.fda.gov/Safety/MedWatch (USA)
  - ▷ Medeffect, www.hc-sc.gc.ca/dhp-mps/medeff/index-eng.php (Canada)
  - ▷ Canadian Network of Palliative Care for Children, http://cnpcc.ca
- to www.palliativedrugs.com.

PHARMACOKINETICS AND PHARMACODYNAMICS

Children under 12 years tend to absorb and metabolize drugs differently from adults. Paediatric dosing based on weight alone may result in too small a dose in infants and children (because elimination does not change in direct proportion to weight) and too large a dose in neonates (who have immature drug-elimination pathways).[25]

Neonates (<1 month)

Relatively low renal and hepatic clearances and higher volumes of distribution result in a *longer halflife* for many drugs. This may necessitate lower doses at longer intervals. Neonates also have less fat and muscle and increased bio-availability. Drugs primarily metabolized by the liver should be administered with extreme care in those under 2 months.[26] There is a higher risk of respiratory depression with opioids (see Analgesics, below).[27]

Immaturity also affects pharmacodynamics; e.g. paradoxical reactions to benzodiazepines have been observed in neonates, particularly in premature infants, probably due to the delayed maturation of $GABA_A$ receptors.[28,29]

Infants and children (1 month–12 years)

Relatively high drug clearances and normal volumes of distribution result in a *shorter halflife* for many drugs. This may necessitate relatively higher doses at shorter intervals compared with adults. However, in infants, liver enzyme systems may still not be fully developed, and metabolic pathways may differ from those in older children. For example, **alfentanil, midazolam, morphine** all have *longer halflives* in infants (also in neonates).[26]

Monitoring drug concentrations

Monitoring plasma drug concentrations is distressing for children and generally of limited value, so should be considered only when dose adjustment on a clinical basis may be insufficient, e.g. **gentamicin, phenobarbital, phenytoin, teicoplanin**.

DECIDING THE DOSE

Appropriate paediatric dosing is guided by the physiological characteristics of the child and the pharmacokinetics of the drug.[16,26] Factors that need to be taken into account include the child's size, organ maturation, body composition, impact of disease at different stages, route of administration and interactions with other drugs.

Dosing by age may be particularly misleading in palliative care where, because of underlying disease, children are unlikely to be close to the mean weight for their age. Thus, generally, the dose is better determined by *body weight* than by age.

Body surface area tends to mirror physiological processes more closely, and this should be used to calculate doses for certain drugs, e.g. cytotoxics. Generally, doses in children should not exceed the maximum adult dose.

DRUG FORMULATION AND ADMINISTRATION

Most children are able to take medicines orally, and many continue to do so throughout their illness. An oral liquid may be easier to administer than tablets or capsules, particularly for young children who are very unwell and/or have dysphagia. An oral syringe should be used for accurate measurement of oral liquids. However, some oral liquids may not be suitable because of unacceptable amounts of sugar or excipients, e.g. ethanol, propylene glycol, sorbitol. The taste of unpleasant oral liquids/tablets can sometimes be masked by adding *small* quantities of food or fruit juice immediately before administration. However, medication should not be added to a feeding bottle or left mixed with food or fruit juice.

Tablets or capsules may be preferable to large volumes of unpleasant tasting oral liquids. Although generally off-label, many tablets or capsules can be modified to aid administration, e.g. opening capsules, dispersing tablets, splitting or crushing tablets. However, this is not a safe option for all formulations; e.g. do *not* split or crush m/r formulations (also see Chapter 28, Box A, p.857).

For advice on suitable alternative formulations, see Chapter 28 (p.853) and discuss with a clinical pharmacist. The use of alternative routes of administration (enteral feeding tube, buccal, intranasal, inhaled, PR, TD, SC, IV) is common in children.

Many seriously ill children are fed by nasogastric tube or gastrostomy, and these provide an alternative route of drug administration (see Chapter 28, p.853). However, close to death, GI absorption may be impaired. There is also the risk that drugs may continue to be administered via a feeding tube when no longer necessary or appropriate. Regular review is essential.

Buccal and intranasal administration are often used in children's palliative care because of ease of administration and rapid systemic absorption. Such routes avoid degradation by gastric acid, hepatic first-pass metabolism and the need for injections.[30] However, absorption can be affected by other factors, e.g. drug concentration or venous drainage of mucosal tissue, which results in significant interindividual variation in response. Some swallowing of the drug is also possible, with delayed absorption.[15,31]

Although not recommended by the manufacturers, some TD matrix (but *not* reservoir) patches can be cut.[23]

IM administration is particularly distressing for children and should generally be avoided. SC administration, e.g. via an indwelling SC cannula, may be appropriate and acceptable for children and is the route of choice for continuous infusions, particularly if there is no permanent central venous access.

SPECIFIC PRESCRIBING ADVICE

Analgesics

Paracetamol, NSAIDs, *strong* opioids and adjuvant analgesics are used to treat chronic pain in children associated with life-limited conditions and end-of-life care.[32] *Weak* opioids (p.376), such as **codeine** (p.378) and **tramadol** (p.383), are no longer recommended for use in children following safety concerns, including fatal respiratory depression. These are linked to genetic variations that can occur in metabolism (also see p.783).[33,34]

Strong opioids can generally be used safely in children for moderate or severe pain, although this may require careful explanation to parents and carers to allay fears. The transmucosal route (buccal, SL) is often used for p.r.n. doses of **morphine**, **diamorphine** or **fentanyl** to relieve break-through pain. As in adults, doses of transmucosal **fentanyl** products should be titrated against the child's pain. The dose needed may not correlate closely with background opioid requirements, although these should be taken into account.

When an appropriate strength is available, **fentanyl** and **buprenorphine** TD patches are often used as a convenient long-acting opioid formulation for children. Because of the risk of respiratory depression, TD medications should be used only after initial dose titration with an oral opioid. Extra care is necessary if a child becomes pyrexial, because this can accelerate the rate of diffusion from the patch (see Chapter 30, p.901).

Other than when used inappropriately, there is little evidence of TD opioids causing serious respiratory depression in children when the dose is individually titrated against the child's pain, *except in neonates* (<1 month). In the latter, late respiratory depression has been reported, >4h after immediate-release **morphine**.[35] Compared with children aged 2–12 years, the recommended doses per kg in those under 2 years are lower, and much lower in neonates.

Of the undesirable effects of opioids, pruritus and urinary retention are possibly more common, and nausea less common, than in adults.[36] Prophylactic anti-emetics are not provided routinely when opioids are prescribed for children.

Anti-emetics

Children probably have an age-related increased risk of dystonic reactions with D_2 antagonists, e.g. phenothiazines, **metoclopramide** (see Chapter 21, p.805). Such drugs should be used with caution in those <20 years.[37,38] **Metoclopramide** (p.268) has restricted indications and generally should not be used for >5 days and not at all in infants under 1 year.[39]

Domperidone (p.271) use in children is also under review because of concerns about undesirable cardiac effects and limited evidence of efficacy. It should be used only at the lowest dose and for the shortest time possible.[40]

Anti-epileptics

Many children with life-limiting or life-threatening conditions are on complicated anti-epileptic regimens. Interactions are common among anti-epileptics and are mostly caused by liver enzyme induction or inhibition. They are variable and unpredictable and may increase toxicity without a corresponding increase in anti-epileptic effect.

Anti-epileptics also have significant interactions with other drugs (see Anti-epileptics, p.280 and Chapter 19, p.781). Specialist paediatric neurology advice is recommended when titrating or reducing anti-epileptics in children.

Generally, anti-epileptics should *not* be stopped when a child is close to death. An alternative route of administration may be necessary. This could involve the addition or substitution of SC **midazolam** or **phenobarbital**.

Some anti-epileptics (**carbamazepine**, **clonazepam**, **diazepam**, **lorazepam**, **phenobarbital** and **valproate**) can be given PR but may need dose adjustment.[41] For example, the dose of **carbamazepine** should be increased by 25% when converting from PO to PR.[42] Rectal administration may also be possible for **lamotrigine**[43] and **vigabatrin**, but strong evidence is lacking.

Corticosteroids

In paediatric palliative care, the most common reason for prescribing a corticosteroid is headache and vomiting caused by raised intracranial pressure associated with an intracranial tumour. Compared with adults, children seem to experience a more rapid onset of relatively severe undesirable effects (particularly cushingoid facies, proximal myopathy, weight gain, changes in mood and behaviour); see p.560.

Accordingly, short courses of corticosteroids should be the norm, e.g. **dexamethasone** ≤500microgram/kg/day for 3–5 days for symptoms of raised intracranial pressure.[23] This approach often provides adequate symptom relief with less toxicity than continuous dosing. After a review of treatment goals, this can be repeated as necessary.[44]

Occasionally, continuous dosing may be needed. Because of increased undesirable effects and increased difficulty in weaning a child off corticosteroids, continuous dosing should be at the lowest effective dose and for the shortest time possible.[45,46]

1 World Health Organization (2018) Integrating palliative care and symptom relief into paediatrics: a WHO guide for health care planners, implementers and managers. *World Health Organization, Geneva*. www.who.int.

2 Fraser LK *et al.* (2012) Rising national prevalence of life-limiting conditions in children in England. *Pediatrics*. **129**: e923–e929.

3 Regnard C *et al.* (2007) Understanding distress in people with severe communication difficulties: developing and assessing the Disability Distress Assessment Tool (DisDAT). *Journal of Intellectual Disability Research*. **51**: 277–292.

4 Regnard C *et al.* (2003) Difficulties in identifying distress and its causes in people with severe communication problems. *International Journal of Palliative Nursing*. **9**: 173–176.

5 NICE (2016) End of life care for infants, children and young people with life-limiting conditions. *Clinical Guideline*. CG61. www.nice.org.uk.

6 Herr K *et al.* (2006) Pain assessment in the nonverbal patient: position statement with clinical practice recommendations. *Pain Management Nursing*. **7**: 44–52.

7 Wong D and Baker C (1988) Pain in children: comparison of assessment scales. *Pediatric Nursing*. **14**: 9–17.

8 von Baeyer CL and Spagrud LJ (2007) Systematic review of observational (behavioral) measures of pain for children and adolescents aged 3 to 18 years. *Pain*. **127**: 140–150.

9 von Baeyer CL (2009) Children's self-report of pain intensity: what we know, where we are headed. *Pain Research and Management*. **14**: 39–45.

10 EAPC Taskforce (2007) IMPaCCT: Standards for paediatric palliative care in Europe. *European Journal of Palliative Care*. **14**: 109–114.

11 Department of Health (2008) Better Care. Better Lives. http://www.dh.gov.uk/en/Publicationsandstatistics/Publications/PublicationsPolicyAndGuidance/DH_083106 (archived)

12 Jamieson L *et al.* (2016) Palliative medicines for children - a new frontier in paediatric research. *Journal of Pharmacy and Pharmacology*. **69**: 377–383.

13 AAP (American Academy of Pediatrics) (2014) Off-label use of drugs in children. *Pediatrics*. **133**: 563–567.

14 General Medical Council (GMC) (2007) 0-18. Guidance for all doctors. www.gmc-uk.org

15 Ballantine N and Bing Daglish E (2012) Chapter 17. Using Medications in Children. In: A Goldman et al. (eds) *Oxford Textbook of Palliative Care for Children 2e*. Oxford University Press, Oxford.

16 Paediatric Formulary Committee. BNF for Children (online) London: BMJ Group, Pharmaceutical Press, and RCPCH Publications. www.medicinescomplete.com.

17 Barker C *et al.* (2019) Prescribing Medicines for Children. London: Pharmaceutical Press www.medicinescomplete.com.

18 White R and Bradnam V. Handbook of Drug Administration via Enteral Feeding Tubes. London: Pharmaceutical Press www.medicinescomplete.com.

19 Ainsworth S (2014) Neonatal Formulary 7: drug use in pregnancy and the first year of life. *Wiley online library*. https://onlinelibrary.wiley.com.

20 International Children's Palliative Care Network (2008). www.icpcn.org.uk

21 Hain R and Jassal S (2016) Paediatric Palliative Medicine (2nd edition), Oxford Specialist Handbooks in Paediatrics. Oxford University Press, Oxford.

22 Jassal S (2016) Basic symptom control in paediatric palliative care: the Rainbows Children's Hospice Guidelines (edition 9.5). http://www.togetherforshortlives.org.uk

23 Association for Paediatric Medicine Master Formulary 2019 (5th edition). Available from: www.appm.org.uk.

24 Stephenson T (2005) How children's responses to drugs differ from adults. *British Journal of Clinical Pharmacology*. **59**: 670–673.

25 Anderson BJ and Holford NH (2013) Understanding dosing: children are small adults, neonates are immature children. *Archives of Disease in Childhood*. **98**: 737–744.

26 Bartelink IH *et al.* (2006) Guidelines on paediatric dosing on the basis of developmental physiology and pharmacokinetic considerations. *Clinical Pharmacokinetics*. **45**: 1077–1097.

27 Hartley C *et al.* (2018) Analgesic efficacy and safety of morphine in the Procedural Pain in Premature Infants (Poppi) study: randomised placebo-controlled trial. *Lancet*. **392**: 2595–2605.

28 Waisman D *et al.* (1999) Myoclonic movements in very low birth weight premature infants associated with midazolam intravenous bolus administration. *Pediatrics*. **104**: 579.
29 Ng E *et al.* (2002) Safety of benzodiazepines in newborns. *Annals of Pharmacotherapy*. **36**: 1150–1155.
30 Anderson BJ (2013) Goodbye to needles. *Archives of Disease in Childhood*. **98**: 718–719.
31 Lam JK *et al.* (2014) Oral transmucosal drug delivery for pediatric use. *Advanced Drug Delivery Reviews*. **73**: 50–62.
32 World Health Organization (2020) Guidelines on the management of chronic pain in children. *World Health Organization, Geneva*. www.who.int.
33 MHRA (2013) Codeine: restricted use as an analgesic in children and adolescents after European safety review. *Drug Safety Update*. www.gov.uk/drug-safety-update.
34 European Medicines Agency (2013) PRAC (Pharmacovigilance Risk Assessment Committee) recommends restricting the use of codeine when used for pain relief in children.
35 Zernikow B *et al.* (2006) Paediatric cancer pain management using the WHO analgesic ladder-results of a prospective analysis from 2265 treatment days during a quality improvement study. *European Journal of Pain*. **10**: 587–595.
36 Hain RDW (2006) Pharmacodynamics of morphine and M6G in children with cancer: analgesia and adverse effects. *International Conference in Paediatric Palliative Care*.
37 Grosset KA and Grosset DG (2004) Prescribed drugs and neurological complications. *Journal of Neurology, Neurosurgery, and Psychiatry*. **75 (Suppl 3)**: iii2–8.
38 van Harten PN *et al.* (1999) Acute dystonia induced by drug treatment. *British Medical Journal*. **319**: 623–626.
39 MHRA (2013) Metoclopramide: risk of neurological adverse effects - restricted dose and duration of use. *Drug Safety Update*. **7**: www.mhra.gov.uk/safetyinformation.
40 MHRA (2014) Domperidone: risk of cardiac side effects - indication restricted to nausea and vomiting, new contraindications, and reduced dose and duration of use. *Drug Safety Update*. **7**: www.mhra.gov.uk/safetyinformation.
41 Smith S *et al.* (2001) Guidelines for rectal administration of anticonvulsant medication in children. *Paediatric and Perinatal Drug Therapy*. **4**: 140–147.
42 Arvidsson J *et al.* (1995) Replacing carbamazepine slow-release tablets with carbamazepine suppositories: a pharmacokinetic and clinical study in children with epilepsy. *Journal of Child Neurology*. **10**: 114–117.
43 Birnbaum AK *et al.* (2000) Rectal absorption of lamotrigine compressed tablets. *Epilepsia*. **41**: 850–853.
44 Harrop E and Sen G (2010) The use of dexamethasone in children referred to a tertiary palliative care service who died from inoperable brain tumours over a 2 year period. What can we learn? Presented at Cardiff International Conference for Paediatric Palliative Care.
45 Waterson G (2006) Corticosteroids in the palliative phase of brain tumours. *Archives of Disease in Childhood*. **86 (Suppl 1)**: A76.
46 Glaser AW *et al.* (1997) Corticosteroids in the management of central nervous system tumours. Kids Neuro-Oncology Workshop (KNOWS). *Archives of Disease in Childhood*. **76**: 76–78.

Updated (minor change) September 2021

17: RENAL IMPAIRMENT

17

INTRODUCTION

Palliative care services are increasingly involved in the care of patients with chronic kidney disease, either alone or as a co-morbid condition. Because renal impairment often changes the pharmacokinetic and/or pharmacodynamic effects of a drug, this presents a challenge for prescribers.

Pharmacologically, the most important consequence of renal impairment is increased toxicity as a result of accumulation of a renally excreted drug ± active metabolites. Renal impairment also has many other consequences which may alter the effect of a drug, whether or not accumulation occurs, e.g. an enhanced sedative effect of a centrally acting drug (Box A).

Box A Drug-related consequences of renal impairment[1]

Pharmacokinetic

Absorption

↑ gastric pH, ↑ gut wall oedema → ↓ PO absorption
↓ hepatic enzyme function → ↓ first-pass metabolism → ↑ PO bio-availability

Distribution

↑ oedema/ascites → ↑ volume of distribution → ↓ effect of water-soluble drugs
↑ cachexia or dehydration → ↓ volume of distribution → ↑ effect of water-soluble drugs
↓ drug removal transporters in the blood–brain barrier, e.g. P-glycoprotein → ↑ CNS effects
↓ albumin levels and binding capacity → ↑ unbound (active) fraction of highly protein-bound drugs → ↑ effect (and metabolism)
↓ tissue binding → ↓ volume of distribution → ↑ effect

Metabolism

↓ hepatic enzyme function, particularly CYP450 → ↓ metabolism → variable effect depending on drug, e.g. pro-drug, active metabolite

Elimination

↓ GFR and ↓ tubular secretion → ↓ elimination of parent drug/active metabolite → ↑ effect, ↑ risk of toxicity
↓ drug removal transporters, e.g. P-glycoprotein → ↓ biliary and GIT elimination → ↓ elimination of parent drug/active metabolite → ↑ effect, ↑ risk of toxicity

Pharmacodynamic

Uraemia can alter the clinical response to certain drugs:
↑ sensitivity to drugs acting on the CNS
↑ risk of hyperkalaemia with potassium-sparing drugs
↑ risk of GI bleeding or oedema with NSAIDs
↓ efficacy or ↑ toxicity of drugs such as warfarin or statins (due to altered physiological or pathological processes involved in other conditions)
Electrolyte imbalance can increase the risk of cardiac arrhythmia with QT-prolonging drugs

Hypo-albuminaemia can lead to an increase in the proportion of free drug in highly protein-bound drugs, resulting in a greater therapeutic effect and, if the serum drug concentration is used to monitor treatment, difficulty in interpreting the results (see Chapter 14, p.712). In addition, there may be:

- reduced efficacy of some drugs acting on the kidneys, e.g. diuretics
- increased nephrotoxic effect of a drug, e.g. **allopurinol**, aminoglycosides, **ciclosporin**, **lithium**, NSAIDs; this may be particularly important for patients with mild–moderate renal impairment, which is made worse by such drugs.

Some of these problems can be overcome by:

- avoiding drugs which are nephrotoxic
- using alternative drugs which are not renally excreted
- reducing the total daily maintenance dose of a renally excreted drug, either by reducing the size of the individual doses or by increasing the interval between doses (see Dose adjustment in renal impairment, p.734)
- taking special care with drugs with a narrow therapeutic index, where undesirable effects are likely with accumulation of the drug or its metabolites.

ASSESSING RENAL FUNCTION

There are limitations to *all* the formula-based estimations of renal function, with none being suitable for all patients and all situations.

The glomerular filtration rate (GFR) is the best overall measure of renal function, but the most accurate ways of measuring GFR are impractical for routine use. Serum creatinine concentration has traditionally been used as a proxy, but is only a rough guide because a significant proportion of renal function may be lost before creatinine levels rise above the upper limit of normal, particularly in patients with a low body muscle mass or low protein intake. Thus, in practice, formula-based *estimations* of renal function using serum creatinine are used, typically:[2–4]

- estimated GFR (eGFR):
  - ▷ Chronic Kidney Disease Epidemiology Collaboration (CKD-EPI) formula
  - ▷ Modification of Diet in Renal Disease (MDRD) formula
- estimated creatinine clearance (CrCl):
  - ▷ Cockcroft–Gault formula.

Note. In acute kidney injury (AKI), changes in serum creatinine levels lag behind the development of the injury and the process of recovery. Thus, renal function will generally be overestimated during injury and underestimated during recovery.

Estimated GFR (eGFR)

eGFR are generally more accurate than estimated CrCl; they are reported by most clinical laboratories and used to classify *chronic* kidney disease (Table 1).[4]

The CKD-EPI eGFR is more accurate than the MDRD eGFR, particularly at higher levels of GFR, and is replacing the MDRD in many laboratories.[3–5] Changes in eGFR are more reliable than single estimates; e.g. for MDRD eGFR, a decrease of ≥15% is likely to represent a true change in renal function.[2]

eGFR are expressed as normalized values, i.e. what that individual's GFR would be if they had a body surface area of 1.73m^2. This can overestimate or underestimate renal function for patients with a body surface area less than or more than 1.73m^2 respectively.

eGFR may also be misleading in situations where creatinine production, volume of distribution or excretion rate are altered, and in patients with a clearance of <50mL/min.[6] Further, eGFR have not been validated for use (and are probably misleading) in a number of settings, including:

- children <18 years old
- elderly (≥75 years)
- AKI
- vegans
- malnourished patients
- muscle-wasting disease states
- amputees
- oedematous states
- pregnancy.

Table 1 eGFR classification of chronic kidney disease[a]

Category	*eGFR (mL/min/1.73m^2)*	*Description*[b]
G1	≥90	Normal renal function but renal disease based on urine findings or presence of structural abnormalities or genetic trait
G2	60–89	Mildly reduced renal function in the presence of renal disease (as above); in the absence of renal disease, an eGFR ≥60mL/min/1.73m^2 is considered normal
G3a	45–59	Mild to moderately reduced renal function
G3b	30–44	Moderate to severely reduced renal function
G4	15–29	Severely reduced renal function
G5	<15	End-stage renal failure (ESRF)

a. the albumin to creatinine ratio is used to further stratify the risk of adverse outcomes; for full details see NICE guidance[4]

b. evidence of damage or a reduced eGFR must be present for >3 months.

In palliative care patients who are elderly, malnourished, cachectic and/or oedematous, renal impairment may exist even when the *serum* creatinine or the eGFR are within normal limits, and it may be prudent to assume that there is at least some degree of renal impairment in such patients. Even when abnormal, the *serum* creatinine or the eGFR may both underestimate the actual degree of renal impairment.

Estimated creatinine clearance (CrCl)

The Cockcroft–Gault formula estimation of CrCl takes weight, rather than body surface area, into account (Box B). It is the preferred method for estimating renal function in patients who are:[7]

- elderly (≥75 years)
- at extremes of muscle mass (BMI <18kg/m^2 or >40kg/m^2)
- taking:
  - ▷ DOACs
  - ▷ nephrotoxic drugs
  - ▷ drugs with a narrow therapeutic index that are predominantly renally excreted.

Many palliative care patients are likely to be in one or more of the above categories. As with eGFR, estimated CrCl can be misleading in situations where creatinine production, volume of distribution or excretion rates are altered or are changing rapidly, e.g. in AKI.

Box B Estimation of renal function using Cockcroft–Gault formula[a,b]

$$\text{Creatinine clearance (mL/min)} = \frac{F \times [140 - \text{age (years)}] \times [\text{weight (kg)}]}{\text{serum creatinine (micromol/L)}}$$

F = 1.23 (male) or 1.04 (female)

Use *ideal* bodyweight where fat is likely to be the major contributor to weight:

Ideal body weight (kg) = Constant + 0.91 (Height (cm) – 152.4)

Constant = 50 (male) or 45.5 (female)

a. at extremes of muscle mass (BMI <18kg/m^2 or >40kg/m^2), it has also been suggested that *absolute* eGFR can be used to estimate renal function; see *BNF* for more details

b. an on-line calculation tool is available at www.mdcalc.com/creatinine-clearance-cockcroft-gault-equation.

DOSE ADJUSTMENT IN RENAL IMPAIRMENT

The need for dose reduction in renal impairment depends on the extent to which the drug and any active metabolite are renally excreted and how serious any undesirable effects of the drug may be:

- for drugs with minimal undesirable effects, a simple scheme for dose reduction is sufficient, i.e. start low and monitor for efficacy and toxicity
- for drugs with a small safety margin, dose adjustments should be based on an estimation of renal function (see below)
- for drugs where both efficacy and/or toxicity are closely related to serum concentration, ongoing treatment must be adjusted according to clinical response and serum concentration, e.g. **gentamicin**, **phenytoin** (see Monitoring drugs in renal impairment, below).

Dose adjustment may not always be needed, e.g. for a single dose, some loading doses, or drugs with a large safety margin where a critical serum concentration is needed (e.g. some antibacterials). For dose adjustment in patients on dialysis, see p.735.

Modifying drug dose based on renal function

In patients known to have *chronic* kidney disease or those at high risk of renal impairment, e.g. the elderly, and those with hypertension or diabetes, renal function should be assessed (see p.732) before prescribing a drug which may need dose modification.

Information on dose adjustments can then be made using the advice given in *PCF* or other resources such as the manufacturer's SPC, *The Renal Drug Handbook/Database*,[8] *Drug Prescribing in Renal Failure*[9] and the *BNF*. It should be noted that the advice will vary.[10] Further, some SPCs may include blanket contra-indications or cautions, or be unnecessarily restrictive because of lack of evidence/evaluation in renal impairment.[2] Knowledge of the pharmacokinetics and pharmacodynamics of a drug can help determine the level of risk for off-label use.

For historical reasons, dosing guidelines are generally based on CrCl values as an indication of renal function. This is also the case in *PCF*, particularly as for many palliative care patients, renal function is best estimated using CrCl (see p.733).

CrCl and eGFR are *not* interchangeable. Although the *BNF* states that for most drugs and most adult patients of average build and height eGFR can be used to determine dosage adjustment, this is inappropriate for the many palliative care patients with features that make eGFR unreliable (see p.732), or those taking DOACs, nephrotoxic drugs or renally excreted drugs with narrow therapeutic ranges. In these circumstances, the Cockcroft–Gault equation (Box B) must be used to calculate CrCl for drug dosing, irrespective of how the renal function is reported by the clinical laboratory.

Given the limitations of the estimates of creatinine clearance, any guidance should be regarded only as a useful approximation of a safe starting dose. Subsequent further adjustments are then based on response and undesirable effects, with monitoring of serum drug concentrations undertaken when appropriate.[11]

In AKI, appropriate caution needs to be applied when estimates of renal function are being used to inform dose adjustments (see p.732).

Monitoring drugs in renal impairment

When a drug dose modification has been necessary, or for drugs known to cause renal impairment, a clinical review and evaluation of renal function should be carried out within 2 weeks or at any time if drug-induced nephrotoxicity is suspected.[2]

For drugs with a narrow therapeutic range, e.g. **digoxin**, **gentamicin**, **phenytoin**, plasma levels must be measured and, where necessary, adjusted for hypo-albuminaemia using the formula modified for ESRF (see Chapter 14, p.712 and Anti-epileptics, Box A, p.288 for **phenytoin**).

PALLIATIVE CARE DRUGS FOR LONG-TERM USE IN END-STAGE RENAL FAILURE

Although ESRF is defined as an eGFR <15mL/min/1.73m^2, for *prescribing* purposes most sources of information use CrCl to guide drug dosing. Generally, CrCl <10mL/min is used to categorize patients with the greatest reduction in renal function, and this is used in *PCF* for dosing guidance for patients with ESRF.

Where necessary, the individual drug monographs contain specific information regarding dose adjustments for patients with renal impairment and CrCl >10mL/min.

This section provides guidance for prescribing drugs commonly used for palliative care symptom relief in patients with ESRF ± dialysis *with a prognosis of weeks–months or longer*. For patients in the last days of life, see the separate section below, p.750.

Tables 2–8 and the accompanying text were developed to provide user-friendly summaries to guide rational and safe prescribing in patients with ESRF (± dialysis), by raising awareness of:

- suitable drugs and their starting doses
- suitable alternatives when patients experience undesirable effects
- the potential risks of using a less 'renally safe' drug.

The tables cover the most common symptom-relief drug classes and highlight, when possible, the most, intermediate and least 'renally safe' drugs for *long-term* use. Because it is generally good practice to become experienced in using relatively few drugs well, the list is purposely limited.

The tables should be used in conjunction with the accompanying text, which highlights any general considerations for that class of drug and provides a commentary to help inform choice. As far as possible, specific prescribing advice is given. Even when a drug appears to be 'renally safe' from a metabolism/excretion point of view, other effects of renal impairment on drug action (Box A) mean that smaller starting doses and a slower titration than usual are generally advisable, particularly in the elderly and/or frail patient. Thus, the adage 'start low, go slow' will generally apply to the use of *any* drug, and particularly those with CNS effects.

In addition to the impact of ESRF and familiarity, the selection of the most appropriate symptom-relief drug in ESRF also requires the prescriber to consider any relevant additional factors such as the presence of concurrent symptoms, co-morbidities (e.g. cardiovascular disease, liver impairment), the need to avoid high-sodium and high-volume products, other drugs (e.g. in relation to risk of a drug–drug interaction, QT prolongation) and patient preference. Seek advice from a renal pharmacist.

Sometimes, the cautious use of a familiar drug may be preferable to an unfamiliar (albeit 'renally safer') one. Similarly, we do *not* advocate the automatic switching of patients to a 'renally safer' drug when an alternative is proving satisfactory. *This section aims to complement and not replace specialist renal unit guidance.*

Additional notes on the use of the tables:

- drugs are categorized as 'generally safe', 'use cautiously' and 'avoid if possible' from a *purely renal perspective*, according to their risk of accumulation with long-term use in ESRF
- consensus dosing guidelines are presented (for methodology behind their development, see Wilcock *et al.* 2017[12]). These include off-label use and, in some instances, despite an SPC contra-indication in this setting. However, it is impractical to highlight all cases of off-label use because this can vary according to country, brand, indication, formulation, dose, route of administration or patient population. Prescribers should be aware of the implications of off-label use; see p.xix.

Patients on dialysis

Generally, seek specialist renal advice. The dialysis columns in Tables 2–8 provide information on whether the effect of dialysis is sufficient to require a further change in the ESRF dosing regimen specified for that drug. Unless specified otherwise, the information is relevant for both peritoneal dialysis (PD; continuous ambulatory or automated) and thrice-weekly conventional haemodialysis (HD). However, because information is often limited and HD regimens are variable, some renal units adjust drug regimens for HD patients so that administration is timed to occur after the dialysis procedure, e.g. for **gabapentin, levetiracetam, pregabalin.**

Specialist renal advice should be sought for those patients on more frequent conventional HD, high flux dialysis or haemodiafiltration; drug removal is more likely, and closer monitoring is required.[8]

Table 2 Antidepressants and ESRF. Before use, see introductory and class-specific text

Antidepressant[a]	*Halflife in normal renal function (h)*	*Active metabolite(s)*[b]	*Accumulation in renal impairment*[c]	*Removed by dialysis*[d]	*Dose and comment*
Generally safe					
Sertraline[e]	26	No	No	No	Dose unchanged PO: start with 25mg each morning
Use cautiously					
Amitriptyline[e]	9–25	Yes	Possible	No	Lower doses may be sufficient PO: start with 10mg at bedtime *Not a first-line treatment for depression*
Citalopram[e]	36	Yes	Possible	No	Dose unchanged; lower doses may be sufficient PO: start with 10mg each morning
Nortriptyline[e]	15–39	Yes	Possible	No	Lower doses may be sufficient PO: start with 10mg at bedtime *Not a first-line treatment for depression*
Trazodone	5–13	Yes	Possible	No	Lower doses may be sufficient PO: start with 25–50mg at bedtime *Not a first-line treatment for depression*
Avoid if possible					
Duloxetine	8–17	No	Yes	No	If unavoidable, use lower doses PO: start with ≤30mg at bedtime
Mirtazapine[e]	20–40	Yes	Yes	No	If unavoidable PO: start with 15mg at bedtime
Venlafaxine	5 (11[f])	Yes	Yes	No	If unavoidable PO: start with 37.5mg daily, maximum 75–112.5mg/24h in divided doses *For HD patients* PO: dose after HD session to minimize undesirable effects

a. whichever antidepressant is used, because ESRF can have general effects on the pharmacokinetics and/or pharmacodynamics of a drug (see text), a slower than usual titration and close monitoring of the patient are required
b. of actual or potential clinical relevance in ESRF
c. of drug and/or active metabolite(s); 'possible' has been used when definitive data are lacking but accumulation is likely on clinical or theoretical grounds
d. sufficient to require a change in dosing regimen with PD or HD; for other forms of dialysis, seek specialist advice
e. because of a long halflife and time taken to reach steady state, undesirable effects with these antidepressants may only become apparent after several days or weeks of regular use
f. active metabolite.

Antidepressants (Table 2)[8,13–25]

Low starting doses and cautious titration are required for *all* antidepressants, regardless of whether they (± any active metabolites) are renally excreted. In ESRF there is increased sensitivity to drugs acting on the CNS, coupled with a risk of enhanced CNS-depressant effects from the variable pharmacokinetic changes (Box A), e.g.:

- all the featured antidepressants (apart from **venlafaxine**) are highly protein-bound
- all the featured antidepressants are dependent on one or more of CYP3A4, CYP2D6, CYP2C19 and CYP1A2
- metabolism will be further impaired in constitutionally poor metabolizers, e.g. of **amitriptyline**, **nortriptyline** (CYP2D6), **amitriptyline**, **citalopram** and **sertraline** (CYP2C19), and the risk of toxicity increased from a pharmacokinetic drug–drug interaction involving an inhibitor of the CYP450 enzyme(s).

Concurrent use of other drugs with CNS-depressant activity, e.g. opioids, increases the risk of toxicity.

Because of the time taken to accumulate, undesirable effects may become apparent only after days or weeks of regular use for those antidepressants with long halflives, e.g. **amitriptyline**, **citalopram**, **mirtazapine**, **nortriptyline**, **sertraline**.

Choice of antidepressant

From a renal perspective, the first-line antidepressant of choice for the treatment of depression in ESRF is **sertraline**. **Citalopram** can be used cautiously, but has a risk of prolongation of the QT interval (and increased risk of ventricular arrhythmia), e.g. as a result of possible accumulation, electrolyte imbalance, drug–drug interaction or concurrent use of other QT-prolonging drugs.

If an SSRI is not suitable, some renal units favour the cautious use of **mirtazapine** for depression, despite it being extensively excreted unchanged by the kidney and known to accumulate in ESRF.

Amitriptyline and **nortriptyline** may be used with caution for neuropathic pain, but starting doses in ESRF should be low. The presence of cardiac co-morbidity may limit their use.

For patients on PD or HD, none of the drugs in Table 2 require any additional changes to the ESRF dosing regimen.

Anti-emetics (Table 3)[8,13–15,22–28]

In addition to any specific advice, because of reduced elimination, for any individual anti-emetic, lower starting doses should be used and then cautiously titrated to response. This is because patients are at risk of an enhanced CNS-depressant effect as a result of reduced hepatic clearance (reduced CYP450 activity), reduced protein binding (increased unbound (active) fraction), and increased CNS levels and sensitivity (Box A). All of the featured anti-emetics are affected by one or more of these general consequences of renal impairment, albeit variably; e.g. **domperidone** does not cross the blood–brain barrier.

The risk of toxicity is also greater from a pharmacokinetic drug–drug interaction involving an inhibitor of the CYP450 enzyme. For example, CYP3A4 inhibitors will lead to reduced metabolism of **domperidone**.

The risk of prolongation of the QT interval (and the consequential increased risk of ventricular arrhythmia) is higher with **domperidone**, **haloperidol**, **levomepromazine** and **ondansetron**. The risk may be increased as a result of, e.g. drug accumulation, drug–drug interaction, or concurrent use of other drugs that either prolong the QT interval or cause electrolyte imbalance.

Because of the time taken to accumulate, undesirable effects may become apparent only after days or weeks of regular use for those anti-emetics with a long halflife, e.g. **cyclizine**, **haloperidol**, **levomepromazine**. Concurrent use of other drugs with CNS-depressant activity, e.g. opioids, increases the risk of toxicity of anti-emetics with central effects.

Choice of anti-emetic

Generally, all the anti-emetics used commonly in palliative care can be used in ESRF. Even those listed as 'use cautiously' are regularly used, in reduced doses, on renal units. Thus, choice should be primarily guided by the likely cause of the nausea and vomiting along with co-morbid conditions.

For patients on PD or HD, none of the drugs in Table 3 require any additional changes to the ESRF dosing regimen.

Table 3 Anti-emetics and ESRF. Before use, see introductory and class-specific text

Anti-emetics[a]	*Halflife in normal renal function (h)*	*Active metabolite(s)*[b]	*Accumulation in renal impairment*[c]	*Removed by dialysis*[d]	*Dose and comment*
Generally safe					
Cyclizine[e]	20	No	No	No	Dose unchanged; lower doses may be sufficient
Granisetron	4–11	No	No	No	Dose unchanged
Ondansetron	3–6	No	No	No	Dose unchanged
Prochlorperazine[e]	6–20	No	No	No	Lower doses may be sufficient
Use cautiously					
Domperidone[f]	7–9	No	Possible	No	PO: maximum 10mg daily–b.d.
Haloperidol[e]	12–38	Yes	Possible	No	For occasional use, dose unchanged For regular use, halve the usual dose *Also see Table 5 (Antipsychotics)*
Levomepromazine[e]	15–30	Yes	Possible	No	PO/SC: start with 6–6.25mg at bedtime and p.r.n. up to q8h; lower doses may be sufficient, e.g. 2.5mg–3mg
Metoclopramide[f]	4–6	No	Yes	No	PO/SC: start with 5mg t.d.s., maximum 10mg t.d.s.
Promethazine hydrochloride	5–14	No	No	No	PO: start with 10mg b.d., maximum 25mg t.d.s.

a. whichever anti-emetic is used, because ESRF can have general effects on the pharmacokinetics and/or pharmacodynamics of a drug (see text), a slower than usual titration and close monitoring of the patient are required
b. of actual or potential clinical relevance in ESRF
c. of drug and/or active metabolite(s); 'possible' has been used when definitive data are lacking but accumulation is likely on clinical or theoretical grounds
d. sufficient to require a change in dosing regimen with PD or HD; for other forms of dialysis, seek specialist advice
e. because of a long halflife and time taken to reach steady state, undesirable effects with these anti-emetics may only become apparent after several days or weeks of regular use
f. domperidone and metoclopramide should be used at the lowest effective dose for the shortest possible time because of concerns over prolonged QT interval or drug-induced movement disorders respectively.

Anti-epileptics (Table 4)[8,13–15,22–25,29–33]

In addition to any specific advice because of reduced elimination, for any anti-epileptic, lower starting doses should be used and then cautiously titrated to response. This is because patients are at risk of an enhanced CNS-depressant effect as a result of reduced hepatic clearance (reduced CYP450 activity), reduced protein binding (increased unbound (active) fraction) and increased

Table 4 Anti-epileptics and ESRF. Before use, see introductory and class-specific text

Anti-epileptic[a]	*Halflife in normal renal function (h)*	*Active metabolite(s)*[b]	*Accumulation in renal impairment*[c]	*Removed by dialysis*[d]	*Dose and comment*
Generally safe					
Carbamazepine[e]	16–36	Possible	Possible	No	Dose unchanged
Valproate	6–20	No	Possible	No	Dose unchanged; lower doses may be sufficient
Use cautiously					
Clonazepam[e]	20–60	Yes	Possible	No	Lower doses may be sufficient PO: start with 500microgram/24h *Also see Table 6 (Benzodiazepines and Z-drugs)*
Gabapentin	5–7	No	Yes	Yes	*For non-dialysis or PD patients* PO: start with 100mg on alternate nights and titrate slowly *For HD patients with a urine output >100mL/24h* PO: start with 100mg at bedtime; consider either a supplementary dose after each HD session or timing the daily dose post HD *For anuric HD patients* PO: start with 100mg stat and 100mg after every HD session; a regular maintenance dose is generally not required
Levetiracetam	6–8	No	Yes	Yes	*For non-dialysis patients* PO/IV: start with 250mg b.d., maximum dose 500mg b.d. If <50kg, dose on a mg/kg basis (see SPC) *For PD or HD patients* PO/IV: start with 750mg stat and give the maintenance dose (above) as a once daily dose, consider either a supplementary dose of 250–500mg after each HD session or timing the daily dose post HD
Oxcarbazepine	1–3 (9[f])	Yes	Yes	No data	PO: maximum starting dose 150mg b.d., lower doses may be sufficient, e.g. 75mg b.d., titrate by 75mg at weekly intervals

continued

Table 4 Continued

Anti-epileptic[a]	*Halflife in normal renal function (h)*	*Active metabolite(s)*[b]	*Accumulation in renal impairment*[c]	*Removed by dialysis*[d]	*Dose and comment*
Pregabalin	5–9	No	Yes	Yes	*For non-dialysis or PD patients* PO: start with 25mg once daily, maximum dose 75mg once daily *For HD patients* PO: consider either a supplementary dose of 25–100mg after each HD session or timing the daily dose post HD
Avoid if possible					
Phenobarbital[e]	75–120	No	Possible	No	If unavoidable, use only under specialist neurological advice
Phenytoin[e]	20–60	No	A clinically significant increase in the free (unbound fraction) can occur; high risk of toxicity due to the narrow therapeutic range	No	If unavoidable, dose as in normal renal function. Monitor plasma levels adjusted for hypo-albuminaemia in ESRF; see text and Anti-epileptics, Box A, p.288

a. whichever anti-epileptic is used, because ESRF can have general effects on the pharmacokinetics and/or pharmacodynamics of a drug (see text), a slower than usual titration and close monitoring of the patient are required

b. of actual or potential clinical relevance in ESRF

c. of drug and/or active metabolite(s); 'possible' has been used when definitive data are lacking but accumulation is likely on clinical or theoretical grounds

d. sufficient to require a change in dosing regimen with PD or HD; for other forms of dialysis, seek specialist advice

e. because of a long halflife and time taken to reach steady state, undesirable effects with these anti-epileptics may only become apparent after several days or weeks of regular use

f. active metabolite.

CNS levels and sensitivity (Box A). All the featured anti-epileptics are affected by one or more of these general consequences of renal impairment, albeit variably, e.g.:

- reduced protein binding affects the most highly protein-bound, e.g. **phenytoin** and **valproate** (for monitoring purposes or when toxicity is suspected, the free fraction plasma concentration should be measured)
- all but **levetiracetam**, **oxcarbazepine** and **gabapentin/pregabalin** are dependent on CYP450
- the risk of toxicity is also greater from a pharmacokinetic drug–drug interaction involving an inhibitor of CYP450 or other enzymes responsible for metabolism of the anti-epileptic. For example:
  - ▷ CYP3A4 inhibitors will lead to reduced metabolism of **carbamazepine**; CYP2C9 inhibitors, of **phenobarbital** and **phenytoin**; and CYP2C19 inhibitors, of **phenytoin**
  - ▷ **valproate**, by inhibiting epoxide hydrolase may reduce the metabolism of **carbamazepine**.

Concurrent use of other drugs with CNS-depressant activity, e.g. opioids, increases the risk of toxicity.[34,35] For example, the concurrent use of an opioid and a gabapentinoid increases the risk of respiratory depression and should generally be avoided;[34,35] an exception is when the combination is necessary for symptom relief in the last days of life (see p.750).

Because of the time taken to accumulate, undesirable effects may become apparent only after days or weeks of regular use for those anti-epileptics with a long halflife, e.g. **carbamazepine**, **clonazepam**, **phenobarbital**, **phenytoin**.

Choice of anti-epileptic

From a renal perspective, the first-line anti-epileptic of choice in ESRF is **valproate**. Although **carbamazepine** is also 'renally clean', it is disadvantaged by drug–drug interactions and is rarely used in palliative care. There does not appear to be any good evidence to support the commonly quoted advice to avoid modified-release formulations of anti-epileptics in ESRF.

Levetiracetam is increasingly used and the availability of a parenteral formulation is an advantage. It is primarily renally excreted, and thus accumulates in renal impairment. However, in reduced doses, it is authorized for use in ESRF (± dialysis), as are **gabapentin** and **pregabalin**. **Gabapentin** is used for pruritus and restless legs syndrome associated with ESRF,[36] and this may make its use for neuropathic pain a sensible multiple-purpose option. Nonetheless, in patients receiving haemodialysis, gabapentinoids have been associated with a higher risk of undesirable effects, e.g. altered mental status, falls and fractures.[37]

There is an increased risk of toxicity from **phenytoin**; further, it is disadvantaged by drug–drug interactions. If it cannot be avoided, monitor plasma levels corrected for hypo-albuminaemia using the formula modified for ESRF, see Anti-epileptics, Box A, p.288.

Phenobarbital is not generally used except in conjunction with specialist neurological advice.

For patients on PD or HD, specific changes to the dosing regimens are required for **gabapentin**, **levetiracetam** and **pregabalin**. The clinical effect should be monitored carefully for **valproate**, as the effect of dialysis may be variable.

Antipsychotics (Table 5)[8,13–15,22–26]

In addition to any specific advice because of reduced elimination, for any individual antipsychotic, lower starting doses should be used and then cautiously titrated to response. This is because patients are at risk of an enhanced CNS-depressant effect as a result of reduced hepatic clearance (reduced CYP450 activity), reduced protein binding (increased unbound (active) fraction) and increased CNS levels and sensitivity (Box A). All of the featured antipsychotics are affected by one or more of these general consequences of renal impairment, albeit variably, e.g.:

- all the featured antipsychotics are highly protein-bound
- all the featured antipsychotics are dependent on one or more of CYP3A4, CYP2D6, and CYP1A2; the risk of toxicity is greater from a pharmacokinetic drug–drug interaction with inhibitors of the relevant CYP450, e.g. **haloperidol**, **quetiapine**, **risperidone** (CYP3A4), **haloperidol** and **risperidone** (CYP2D6), and **olanzapine** (CYP1A2).

Undesirable effects may become apparent only after days or weeks of regular use for those antipsychotics with long halflives, e.g. **haloperidol**, **olanzapine**, **risperidone**. Concurrent use of other drugs with CNS-depressant activity, e.g. opioids, increases the risk of toxicity.

The risk of prolongation of the QT interval (and increased risk of ventricular arrhythmia) may be higher with **haloperidol** and lowest for **quetiapine**. The risk may be increased as a result of, e.g. drug accumulation, drug–drug interaction, concurrent use of other drugs that either prolong the QT interval or cause electrolyte imbalance.

Choice of antipsychotic

From a renal perspective, **olanzapine** is a good first-line choice in ESRF; it is also least dependent on CYP450 for its metabolism. **Haloperidol** can also be used cautiously, halving the dose for long-term use. For the use of **levomepromazine** as an anti-emetic, see Table 3.

For patients on PD or HD, **haloperidol**, **olanzapine** and **quetiapine** do not require any additional changes to the ESRF dosing regimen. **Risperidone** should be avoided due to unpredictable drug removal.

Benzodiazepines and Z-drugs (Table 6)[8,13–15,22–26,38–40]

In addition to any specific advice because of reduced elimination, for any individual benzodiazepine or Z-drug, lower starting doses should be used and then cautiously titrated to response. This is because patients are at risk of an enhanced CNS-depressant effect as a result of reduced hepatic clearance (reduced CYP450 activity), reduced protein binding (increased unbound (active) fraction) and increased CNS levels and sensitivity (Box A). All of the featured benzodiazepines and Z-drugs are affected by one or more of these general consequences of renal impairment, albeit variably; e.g. **lorazepam** elimination is not dependent on CYP450.

The risk of toxicity is also greater from a pharmacokinetic drug–drug interaction involving an inhibitor of the CYP450 enzyme mostly responsible for metabolism of the benzodiazepine or Z-drug, e.g. **diazepam** (CYP2C19, CYP3A4), and **midazolam**, **zolpidem**, **zopiclone** (CYP3A4).

The Z-drugs **zolpidem** and **zopiclone** have short halflives. All the featured benzodiazepines have a long halflife and thus take time to accumulate. In addition, **clonazepam** and **diazepam** have active metabolites that can accumulate. Undesirable effects may become apparent only after days or weeks of regular use.

Concurrent use of other drugs with CNS-depressant activity, e.g. opioids, increases the risk of toxicity.[34,35] For example, the concurrent use of an opioid and a benzodiazepine increases the risk of respiratory depression and should generally be avoided;[34,35] an exception is when the combination is necessary for symptom relief in the last days of life (see p.750).

Table 5 Antipsychotics and ESRF. Before use, see introductory and class-specific text

Antipsychotic[a]	*Halflife in normal renal function (h)*	*Active metabolite(s)*[b]	*Accumulation in renal impairment*[c]	*Removed by dialysis*[d]	*Dose and comment*
Generally safe					
Olanzapine[e]	34 (52 elderly)	No	No	No	Lower doses may be sufficient PO: maximum starting dose 5mg/24h
Use cautiously					
Haloperidol[e]	12–38	Yes	Possible	No	For occasional use, dose unchanged. For regular use, halve the usual dose *Also see Table 3 (Anti-emetics)*
Quetiapine	6–14	Yes	Possible	No	Lower doses may be sufficient PO: maximum starting dose 25mg/24h
Avoid if possible					
Risperidone[e]	20[f]	Yes	Yes	Yes	If unavoidable, use lower doses PO: maximum starting dose 500microgram b.d.; titrate in steps of 500microgram b.d. every 7 days *For PD or HD patients* Avoid due to unpredictable drug removal

a. whichever antipsychotic is used, because ESRF can have general effects on the pharmacokinetics and/or pharmacodynamics of a drug (see text), a slower than usual titration and close monitoring of the patient are required
b. of actual or potential clinical relevance in ESRF
c. of drug and/or active metabolite(s); 'possible' has been used when definitive data are lacking but accumulation is likely on clinical or theoretical grounds
d. sufficient to require a change in dosing regimen with PD or HD; for other forms of dialysis, seek specialist advice
e. because of a long halflife and time taken to reach steady state, undesirable effects with these antipsychotics may only become apparent after several days or weeks of regular use
f. total for the parent drug and active metabolite.

Choice of benzodiazepine or Z-drug

From a renal point of view, if a benzodiazepine is necessary, **lorazepam** is a good first-line choice. **Clonazepam** can also be used cautiously and is used by some renal units for restless legs syndrome associated with ESRF. **Diazepam** should be avoided if possible due to the risks of accumulation of an active metabolite with a very long halflife. Even so, some patients with ESRF tolerate it. **Zolpidem** or **zopiclone** is a good choice if a Z-drug is necessary for insomnia.

For patients on PD or HD, none of the drugs in Table 6 require any additional changes to the ESRF dosing regimen.

Table 6 Benzodiazepines and Z-drugs and ESRF. Before use, see introductory and class-specific text

Benzodiazepine or Z-drug[a]	*Halflife in normal renal function (h)*	*Active metabolite(s)*[b]	*Accumulation in renal impairment*[c]	*Removed by dialysis*[d]	*Dose and comment*
Generally safe					
Lorazepam[e]	10–20	No	Possible	No	Lower doses may be sufficient SL/PO: start with 500microgram/24h
Zolpidem	2.4	No	Possible	No	Lower doses may be sufficient PO: start with 5mg at bedtime
Zopiclone	5	No	No	No	Lower doses may be sufficient PO: start with 3.75mg at bedtime
Use cautiously					
Clonazepam[e]	20–60	Yes	Possible	No	Lower doses may be sufficient PO: start with 500microgram/24h *Also see Table 4 (Anti-epileptics)*
Avoid if possible					
Diazepam[e]	25–50 (≤200[f])	Yes	Yes	No	If unavoidable, use half the usual dose

a. whichever benzodiazepine or Z-drug is used, because ESRF can have general effects on the pharmacokinetics and/or pharmacodynamics of a drug (see text), a slower than usual titration and close monitoring of the patient are required

b. of actual or potential clinical relevance in ESRF

c. of drug and/or active metabolite(s); 'possible' has been used when definitive data are lacking but accumulation is likely on clinical or theoretical grounds

d. sufficient to require a change in dosing regimen with PD or HD; for other forms of dialysis, seek specialist advice

e. because of a long halflife and time taken to reach steady state, undesirable effects with these benzodiazepines may only become apparent after several days or weeks of regular use

f. active metabolite.

Opioids (Table 7)[8,13–15,22–24,26,34,41–47]

The guidance in this section is aimed at patients with ESRF ± dialysis and is also generally appropriate for use in patients with severe renal impairment. For dose adjustments in patients with lesser degrees of renal impairment, see the individual opioid drug monographs.

Chronic pain is common in patients with ESRF, and the cautious use of an opioid may be appropriate for certain pains when non-drug and non-opioid drug approaches are inadequate/inappropriate.

Because the use of strong opioids for chronic *non-cancer* pain is generally associated with lower benefits and higher risks,[48,49] specialist advice should be followed (e.g. Faculty of Pain Medicine)[50] and/or sought from chronic pain teams. For patients with ESRF taking an opioid, the higher risks are dose-dependent and include undesirable effects (e.g. altered mental status, falls and fractures), hospitalization and death.[34]

On the other hand, for pain in the last days of life that requires an opioid, this should be readily available and the dose appropriately titrated to ensure adequate pain relief (p.750).

In ESRF, opioids differ in their potential for toxicity. The evidence base is limited,[34,44] and recommendations need to be made partly on the basis of expert opinion.

In addition to specific advice because of reduced elimination, lower starting doses should be used for all opioids and cautiously titrated to response, not least because of the possibility of an enhanced CNS-depressant effect. This is because of the impact of renal impairment on hepatic function, e.g. reduced hepatic clearance (reduced CYP450 activity), reduced protein binding (increased unbound (active) fraction) and increased CNS levels and sensitivity (Box A). All opioids are affected variably by one or more of these general consequences of renal impairment, e.g.:

- **alfentanil, buprenorphine, fentanyl** and **methadone** are highly protein-bound
- **alfentanil, buprenorphine, codeine, dihydrocodeine, fentanyl, methadone, oxycodone** and **tramadol** are dependent on one or more of CYP3A4, CYP2D6 and CYP2B6; the risk of toxicity is greater from a pharmacokinetic drug–drug interaction with inhibitors of the relevant CYP450.

Undesirable effects may become apparent only after days or weeks of regular use for those opioids with long halflives, e.g. **methadone**. Concurrent use of other drugs with CNS-depressant activity increases the risk of toxicity.[34,35] For example, the concurrent use of an opioid and a benzodiazepine increases the risk of respiratory depression and should generally be avoided;[34,35] an exception is when the combination is necessary for symptom relief in the last days of life (see p.750).

Opioids with active metabolites include **codeine**, **diamorphine**, **dihydrocodeine**, **hydromorphone**, **morphine**, **oxycodone** and **tramadol**. All are significantly renally excreted and thus will accumulate with renal impairment, increasing the risk of toxicity.

Buprenorphine does have an active metabolite (norbuprenorphine) with similar opioid-receptor-binding affinities to **buprenorphine**, but norbuprenorphine does not normally cross the blood–brain barrier and thus has little, if any, central effect (see p.428).[51,52]

Choice of opioid

Although some opioids have advantages over other opioids in relation to prescribing in ESRF, a pragmatic approach is important. Thus, the cautious use of a more familiar opioid may be preferable to a less familiar (albeit 'renally safer') one. The ease of obtaining, administrating and titrating opioids are also important considerations, particularly in a community setting.

In ESRF, it is generally preferable to use a strong opioid that has no clinically relevant active metabolite, e.g. **alfentanil, buprenorphine, fentanyl, methadone.** However, there are practical limitations to their use (see below), including the lack of availability of PO products.

Clinical experience and limited objective data suggest that more familiar PO opioids (e.g. **oxycodone, hydromorphone**) are being used with caution in clinically stable patients in ESRF by, e.g.:

- starting with low doses
- reducing the frequency of administration
- titrating more cautiously/slowly.[34,42,45,53–55]

Increasingly, centres start with small doses of immediate-release **oxycodone** PO and then continue if tolerated (see Table 7). Immediate-release **hydromorphone** PO is an alternative, particularly in countries where low-dose (500microgram) products are available (not UK).

When the PO route is unavailable, **oxycodone** or **hydromorphone** can be given SC/CSCI if **alfentanil** or **fentanyl** SC/CSCI are impractical. TD **buprenorphine** or **fentanyl** patches are an alternative option when the pain is stable and opioid requirements are at least equivalent to the lowest-strength TD patch.

Interest in and clinical experience with **buprenorphine** (p.428) is growing, particularly TD.[43,56,57] For opioid-naïve patients, the lowest-strength **buprenorphine** TD patch (5microgram/h) should be used.

Although it has no active metabolites, **methadone** is for specialist use only, because of the unpredictable accumulation and risk of toxicity even in the absence of renal impairment (see p.469).

Fentanyl SC p.r.n. is a good choice when titration is required in *acute* pain. SL, buccal and nasal **fentanyl** products (see p.450) are suitable for p.r.n. use in sufficiently opioid-tolerant patients, e.g. for incident pain associated with dressing changes in patients with calciphylaxis (off-label use).[58]

At the end of life, consensus guidelines[41] favour **fentanyl** SC/CSCI (p.440) for analgesia. **Alfentanil** SC/CSCI (p.420) has also been used in this setting, particularly if the volume of **fentanyl** in a syringe driver becomes prohibitive. However, when used as a rescue analgesic, the short duration of action of **alfentanil** may necessitate frequent p.r.n. use (see p.420).

For patients on PD or HD, generally none of the drugs in Table 7 require any additional changes to the ESRF dosing regimen. However, caution is still necessary, particularly with **buprenorphine**, **fentanyl**, **hydromorphone** and **tramadol**. If loss of analgesia occurs before or soon after dialysis, give an additional dose of the opioid.

For anticipatory prescribing for patients in the last days of life, see Box C (p.750).

Table 7 Opioids and ESRF. Before use, see introductory and class-specific text

Opioid[a]	*Halflife in normal renal function (h)*	*Active metabolite(s)*[b]	*Accumulation in renal impairment*[c]	*Removed by dialysis*[d]	*Dose and comment*
Generally safe					
Alfentanil	1.5	No	No	No	Lower doses may be sufficient SC: start with 50–100microgram p.r.n. CSCI: start with 0.5–1mg/24h
Buprenorphine[e]	20–25 (IV) 24–69 (SL) 13–36 (TD)	No	Possible	Possible	SL/SC/CSCI: reduce initial dose by 25–50% TD: only use when pain is stable; start with 5microgram/h or a dose equivalent to previous opioid use
Fentanyl	4–16 (injection) 13–22 (TD)	No	Possible	No	Lower doses may be sufficient SC: start with 12.5–25microgram p.r.n. CSCI: start with 100–150microgram/24h TD: only use when pain is stable; use a dose equivalent to previous opioid use
*Methadone[e]	5–130	No	Possible	No	Use only under specialist palliative care advice Start with 50% of the usual dose; requires careful and *very slow* titration; accumulation occurs even without renal impairment (see p.469)
Use cautiously					
Hydromorphone	2.5	Yes	Yes	Possible (HD)	PO: start with 1.3mg q6h and p.r.n. SC: start with 0.25–0.5mg q6h and p.r.n. CSCI: start with 1mg/24h

continued

Table 7 Continued

Opioid[a]	*Halflife in normal renal function (h)*	*Active metabolite(s)*[b]	*Accumulation in renal impairment*[c]	*Removed by dialysis*[d]	*Dose and comment*
Oxycodone	2–4	Yes	Yes	No	PO: start with 1–2mg q6–8h and p.r.n. Once pain is controlled consider switching to equivalent dose of TD buprenorphine or fentanyl
Avoid if possible					
Codeine	3–4	Yes	Yes	No	If unavoidable PO: maximum 30mg q6h
Diamorphine	3min (IV); ≤5h[f]	Yes	Yes	No	If unavoidable SC: start with 2.5mg q8h
Dihydrocodeine	3.5–5	Yes	Yes	No	If unavoidable PO: start with 30mg q6h
Morphine	2–5	Yes	Yes	No	If unavoidable PO/SC: start with 1.25–2.5mg p.r.n. and once pain is controlled consider switching to an equivalent dose of TD buprenorphine or fentanyl
Tramadol	6	Yes	Yes	Possible (HD)	PO: start with 50mg q12h; maximum dose 200mg/24h

a. whichever opioid is used, because ESRF can have general effects on the pharmacokinetics and/or pharmacodynamics of a drug (see text), a slower than usual titration and close monitoring of the patient are required

b. of actual or potential clinical relevance in ESRF

c. of drug and/or active metabolite(s); 'possible' has been used when definitive data are lacking but accumulation is likely on clinical or theoretical grounds

d. sufficient to require a change in dosing regimen with PD or HD; for other forms of dialysis, seek specialist advice.

e. because of a long halflife and time taken to reach steady state, undesirable effects with these opioids may only become apparent after several days or weeks of regular use

f. active metabolite.

Miscellaneous (Table 8)[8,13–15,22–26,59,60]

The relative safety and dose adjustments for other common palliative care drugs in ESRF are shown in Table 8.

Full data have not been included for corticosteroids or laxatives. Corticosteroids, e.g. **dexamethasone**, **fludrocortisone**, **hydrocortisone**, **methylprednisolone**, **prednisolone**, can be used in normal doses. Similarly, commonly used laxatives, e.g. **bisacodyl**, **docusate**, **lactulose**, **macrogols** (polyethylene glycols), **senna**, are also generally safe in ESRF with doses unchanged. However, because of the amount of water required for their administration, **macrogols** should be used with caution, and bulking agents, e.g. **ispaghula** (psyllium) husk, avoided completely.

Loperamide is highly protein-bound, extensively metabolized by CYP3A4 and is a substrate for P-glycoprotein. In ESRF, lower doses may be sufficient, particularly in the presence of CYP3A4 and P-glycoprotein inhibitors, the latter potentially increasing the amount of loperamide within the CNS and the risk of central opioid effects.

Table 8 Miscellaneous drugs and ESRF. Before use, see introductory and class-specific text

Drug[a]	*Halflife in normal renal function (h)*	*Active metabolite(s)*[b]	*Accumulation in renal impairment*[c]	*Removed by dialysis*[d]	*Relative safety*	*Dose and comments*
Antidiarrhoeals						
Loperamide	9–14	No	No	No	**Use cautiously**	Dose unchanged; lower doses may be sufficient
Antimuscarinics						
Glycopyrronium	1–1.5	Yes	Yes	No data	**Avoid if possible**	If unavoidable SC: Start with 200microgram p.r.n.; lower doses may be sufficient
Hyoscine *butylbromide*	5–10	No	No	No	**Generally safe**	CSCI or PO: dose unchanged
Bisphosphonates and denosumab						
Denosumab	624	No	No	No	**Generally safe**	Dose unchanged, see text
Ibandronic acid	10–72	No	Yes	No	**Use cautiously**	For prevention of skeletal-related events in patients with bone metastases in breast cancer: PO: 50mg once weekly IVI: 2mg in 500mL sodium chloride 0.9% or glucose 5% over 1h every 3–4 weeks For tumour-induced hypercalcaemia, seek specialist renal unit advice
Pamidronate disodium	1–27	No	Yes	No	**Avoid if possible**	For tumour-induced hypercalcaemia, seek specialist renal unit advice
Zoledronic acid	146	No	Yes	No	**Avoid if possible**	See text
Corticosteroids					**Generally safe**	See text
Laxatives					**Generally safe**	See text

continued

Table 8 Continued

Drug[a]	*Halflife in normal renal function (h)*	*Active metabolite(s)*[b]	*Accumulation in renal impairment*[c]	*Removed by dialysis*[d]	*Relative safety*	*Dose and comments*
Non-opioids						
Paracetamol	1–4	Yes	Possible	No	**Use cautiously**	PO: start with 500mg q6–8h; maximum 3g/24h IV: see SPC; minimum interval 6h
Nefopam	4 (10–15)[e]	Yes	Possible	No	**Use cautiously**	PO: maximum 30mg t.d.s.
NSAIDs					**Avoid if possible**	See text
Skeletal muscle relaxants						
Baclofen	3–4	No	Yes	Yes	**Avoid if possible**	If unavoidable PO: maximum 5mg once daily *For HD patients* Dose after HD session
Tizanidine	3	No	Yes	No	**Use cautiously**	PO: start with 2mg once daily; if necessary, slowly titrate in 2mg steps. Only increase the frequency of administration if a single daily dose is inadequate

a. whichever drug is used, because ESRF can have general effects on the pharmacokinetics and/or pharmacodynamics of a drug (see text), a slower than usual titration and close monitoring of the patient are required

b. of actual or potential clinical relevance in ESRF

c. of drug and/or active metabolite(s); 'possible' has been used when definitive data are lacking but accumulation is likely on clinical or theoretical grounds

d. sufficient to require a change in dosing regimen with PD or HD; for other forms of dialysis, seek specialist advice

e. for active metabolite.

Hyoscine *butylbromide* is generally safe in ESRF. **Glycopyrronium** is significantly renally excreted, and the PO products (authorized for drooling in children) are contra-indicated in severe and ESRF. For both, there is potential for greater CNS penetration due to the changes to the blood–brain barrier.

Of the bisphosphonates, **pamidronate disodium** and **zoledronic acid** are both nephrotoxic, whereas the risk of renal toxicity with **ibandronic acid** is no greater than with placebo.[61] Thus, for the reduction of skeletal-related events in cancer, the risk–benefit balance favours the use of **ibandronic acid** over other bisphosphonates. An alternative in this setting is **denosumab**, which is authorized for use in renal impairment and does not require dose adjustment, although there is a high risk of hypocalcaemia (see p.552).

The management of tumour-induced hypercalcaemia can be complex in ESRF, because of the need for caution with fluid administration and presence of other potentially contributing factors, e.g. tertiary hyperparathyroidism, use of vitamin D analogues or calcium-based phosphate binders. **Denosumab** may be an option, but specialist renal unit advice should be sought.

For non-opioid analgesics, a reduced dose of **paracetamol** or **nefopam** is preferable to NSAIDs, which should be avoided due to their nephrotoxicity. However, in anuric patients on dialysis, NSAIDs can be used cautiously in normal doses, at the lowest effective dose and for as short a time as possible. Because of their low risk of systemic undesirable effects, topical NSAIDs can be used for acute musculoskeletal pain as long as the maximum approved dose is not exceeded.[34]

The choice of skeletal muscle relaxant in ESRF is not straightforward; for all, changes in the integrity of the blood–brain barrier may result in increased penetration into the CNS. **Baclofen** and **diazepam** (also see Table 6) are best avoided, because of the risks of accumulation. Even so, many renal units report that patients can tolerate low doses of **diazepam.** However, the better long-term option may be the cautious use of **tizanidine** in reduced doses. CYP1A2 inhibitors can significantly reduce the metabolism of **tizanidine**, and the concurrent use of **ciprofloxacin** and **fluvoxamine** is contra-indicated.

For patients on PD or HD, apart from baclofen for which dosing is recommended after HD, none of the featured drugs in Table 8 require any additional changes to the ESRF dosing regimen.

SIMPLIFYING LONG-TERM RENAL DRUGS

Patients with ESRF typically take numerous drugs to manage the various aspects of their kidney disease and co-morbidities. These drugs can be divided into categories according to function (see below). When to stop drugs as the end of life approaches will depend on:

- how close the patient is to death
- the purpose of the drug
- likely effects from stopping it
- the burden of taking tablets.

The guidance below should be used in conjunction with specialist renal advice.

Drugs for mineral and bone disease

Calcium and vitamin D preparations should be continued while the patient is swallowing or until they stop dialysis, because of the risk of hypocalcaemia. This is particularly important for the patient who has had a parathyroidectomy. However, for those who have not and are taking **cinacalcet**, a calcimimetic, this may generally be stopped earlier. Phosphate binders can be reduced or stopped as intake reduces, because their effect is on the food which is eaten.

Drugs for anaemia

For as long as it is desirable to maintain the haemoglobin for optimal symptom relief, **iron** (given as an infusion at dialysis) can be continued, as can **epoetins** until the final weeks.

Diuretics for fluid control

Patients may be taking high doses of diuretics; these should be continued if stopping them is likely to exacerbate symptoms.

Drugs for cardiovascular disease

ESRF patients may be taking **aspirin** and antihypertensives. These are often continued until dialysis is stopped, at which point BP targets can be relaxed for most patients to, e.g. <160/90.[62] Statins can also be discontinued in patients on conservative kidney management.

Drugs to maintain dialysis access

Warfarin should be continued until dialysis stops.

LAST DAYS OF LIFE

The two groups of patients for consideration in the last days of life are:
- those already on dialysis for whom a decision to stop dialysis has been made
- those with ESRF being treated with maximum conservative management (i.e. all renal care except dialysis) and who are now approaching death.

For the patient who stops dialysis, the mean survival is 8–10 days, whereas the duration of survival in the conservatively managed group is very variable, ranging from weeks to more than a year. Indicators that death may be approaching are similar to other non-malignant conditions:
- declining physical function
- increasing dependence
- increasing number of symptoms.[63]

Patients with ESRF experience more symptoms than patients with advanced cancer, with a mean of 20 symptoms in the last month of life.[64] Common symptoms in the last days include:
- breathlessness (may relate to fluid overload and acidosis)
- myoclonic jerks and seizures (relate to both increased drug toxicity and uraemia)
- delirium (also relates to both increased drug toxicity and uraemia).

Other symptoms particularly associated with ESRF may continue to be a major problem, e.g. pruritus (see Chapter 26, p.825) and restless legs. **Clonazepam** in low doses (Table 6) is often helpful in relieving restless legs, myoclonus and also neuropathic pain.

Occasionally, with severe fluid overload, if the patient still has a dialysis line in place, it may be appropriate to have a few hours of ultrafiltration to correct the overload.

Box C Anticipatory prescribing in patients with ESRF in the last days of life. Adapted from references[15,41]

Starting doses given below take into account the risk of accumulation and thus may be lower than used in other circumstances; see individual drug monographs and Chapter 14, p.712. All p.r.n. doses should be prescribed q1h.

Pain

Fentanyl or alfentanil SC are generally preferred; starting doses in opioid-naïve patients:
- fentanyl 12.5–25microgram SC p.r.n.
- alfentanil 50–100microgram SC p.r.n.

If ≥3 doses/24h, consider a CSCI.

If the above are unavailable, use oxycodone 1–2mg SC p.r.n.

Breathlessness

The prescribed strong opioid can be used for breathlessness as well as pain; when there is concurrent anxiety, combine with midazolam, e.g. 2.5mg SC p.r.n.

Noisy rattling breathing (pulmonary oedema excluded)

Hyoscine *butylbromide* 20mg SC p.r.n.; if ≥3 doses/24h, consider 40–120mg/24h CSCI.

Also see QCG: Death rattle (noisy rattling breathing), p.11.

Nausea and vomiting

Haloperidol 0.5–1mg SC p.r.n.; if ≥3 doses/24h, consider 1.5–3mg/24h CSCI.

Alternatively, levomepromazine 6.25mg SC p.r.n. or 6.25mg/24h CSCI.

Agitation, restlessness, myoclonus

Midazolam 2.5mg SC p.r.n.; if ≥3 doses/24h, consider 5–10mg/24h CSCI.

Delirium

Haloperidol or levomepromazine ± midazolam, starting with similar doses to above.

Pruritus

Topical emollient ± antipruritic, e.g. levomenthol 0.5–5%, applied q.d.s.

When refractory/contributing to agitation, add midazolam, e.g. 2.5mg SC p.r.n.

Anticipatory prescribing in patients with ESRF in the last days of life

The general principles for anticipatory prescribing in the last days of life apply; see Chapter 14, p.713. However, for patients with ESRF additional considerations apply, including anticipating symptoms associated with uraemia, e.g. encephalopathy (e.g. drowsiness, myoclonus, delirium), nausea, pruritus (Box C).

1 UK Medicines Information (2018) What factors need to be considered when dosing patients with renal impairment? *Medicines Q&A*. www.sps.nhs.uk.

2 Anonymous (2006) The patient, the drug and the kidney. *Drug and Therapeutics Bulletin*. **44**: 89–95.

3 Levey A *et al.* (2009) A new equation to estimate glomerular filtration rate. *Annals of internal medicine*. **150**: 604–612.

4 NICE (2021) Chronic kidney disease: assessment and management. *NICE guideline*. NG203. www.nice.org.uk.

5 UK Medicines Information (2018) Which estimate of renal function should be used when dosing patients with renal impairment? *Medicines Q&A*. www.sps.nhs.uk.

6 Holweger K *et al.* (2008) Novel algorithm for more accurate calculation of renal function in adults with cancer. *Annals of Pharmacotherapy*. **42**: 1749–1757.

7 MHRA (2019) Prescribing medicines in renal impairment: using the appropriate estimate of renal function to avoid the risk of adverse drug reactions. *Drug Safety Update*. www.gov.uk/drug-dafety-update.

8 Ashley C and Dunleavy A. *The Renal Drug Handbook*. Oxon: CRC Press, UK.

9 Brier M and Aronoff G (2007) *Drug Prescribing in Renal Failure (5e)*. ACP Press, Philadelphia.

10 Vidal L *et al.* (2005) Systematic comparison of four sources of drug information regarding adjustment of dose for renal function. *British Medical Journal*. **331**: 263.

11 Davison SN *et al.* (2010) Management of pain in renal failure. In: EJ Chambers *et al.* (eds) *Supportive Care for the Renal Patient* (2nd edn). Oxford: Oxford University Press. pp. 139–188.

12 Wilcock A *et al.* (2017) Therapeutic review: prescribing non-opioid drugs in end-stage kidney disease. *Journal of Pain and Symptom Management*. **54**: 776–787.

13 AHFS Drug Information. American Society of Health-System Pharmacists, Bethesda, Maryland, USA. www.medicinescomplete.com (accessed November 2021).

14 Buckingham R (ed) *Martindale: The Complete Drug Reference*. London: Pharmaceutical Press. www.medicinescomplete.com (accessed October 2021).

15 Brown *et al.* (2012) Kidney disease from advanced disease to bereavement. *Oxford Specialist Handbook* (2nd edn). Oxford: Oxford University Press.

16 Dawling S *et al.* (1982) Nortriptyline metabolism in chronic renal failure: metabolite elimination. *Clinical Pharmacology and Therapeutics*. **32**: 322–329.

17 Nagler EV *et al.* (2012) Antidepressants for depression in stage 3-5 chronic kidney disease: a systematic review of pharmacokinetics, efficacy and safety with recommendations by European Renal Best Practice (ERBP). *Nephrology Dialysis Transplant Perspectives*. **27**: 3736–3745.

18 Taylor D *et al.* (2021) Use of psychotropics in special patient groups: Renal Impairment. *The Maudsley Prescribing Guidelines* (14th edn). The South London and Maudsley NHS Foundation Trust, Oxleas NHS Foundation Trust. London: Informa Healthcare.

19 UK Medicines Information (2014) What is the first choice antidepressant for patients with renal impairment? *Medicines Q&A* 369.2. www.evidence.nhs.uk.

20 Bayer AJ *et al.* (1983) Pharmacokinetic and pharmacodynamic characteristics of trazodone in the elderly. *British Journal of Clinical Pharmacology*. **16**: 371–376.

21 Nilsen OG *et al.* (1993) Pharmacokinetics of trazodone during multiple dosing to psychiatric patients. *Pharmacology and Toxicology*. **72**: 286–289.

22 NHS Lothian (2011) Symptom control in patients with chronic kidney disease/renal impairment. *Palliative Care Guidelines*.

23 Royal Melbourne Hospital. *Nephrology Symptom Management Guidelines*. Australia. www.thermh.org.au (accessed November 2021).

24 Yorkshire Palliative Medicine Guidelines Group (2006) Clinical guidelines for the use of palliative care drugs in renal failure.

25 Micromedex Solution Truven Health Analytics, Inc. Ann Arbor, MI. www.micromedexsolutions.com (accessed January 2017).

26 Marie Curie Palliative Care Institute (2008) Guidelines for the LCP drug prescribing in advanced chronic kidney disease. *Liverpool Care Pathway for the dying patient*. Liverpool: National LCP Steering Group.

27 Dahl SG *et al.* (1982) Plasma and erythrocyte levels of methotrimeprazine and two of its nonpolar metabolites in psychiatric patients. *Therapeutic Drug Monitoring*. **4**: 81–87.28

28 Finn A *et al.* (2005) Bioavailability and metabolism of prochlorperazine administered via the buccal and oral delivery route. *Journal of Clinical Pharmacology*. **45**: 1383–1390.

29 Vulliemoz S *et al.* (2009) Levetiracetam accumulation in renal failure causing myoclonic encephalopathy with triphasic waves. *Seizure*. **18**: 376–378.

30 Tsanaclis LM *et al.* (1984) Effect of valproate on free plasma phenytoin concentrations. *British Journal of Clinical Pharmacology*. **18**: 17–20.

31 Sakkas GK *et al.* (2015) Current trends in the management of uremic restless legs syndrome: a systematic review on aspects related to quality of life, cardiovascular mortality and survival. *Sleep Medicine Reviews*. **21**: 39–49.

32 Asconape JJ (2014) Use of antiepileptic drugs in hepatic and renal disease. *Handbook of Clinical Neurology*. **119**: 417–432.

33 Gunal AI *et al.* (2004) Gabapentin therapy for pruritus in haemodialysis patients: a randomized, placebo-controlled, double-blind trial. *Nephrology, Dialysis, Transplantation*. **19**: 3137–3139.

34 Tobin DG *et al.* (2022) Opioids for chronic pain management in patients with dialysis-dependent kidney failure. *Nature Reviews: Nephrology*. **18**: 113–128.

35 MHRA (2020) Benzodiazepines and opioids: reminder of risk of potentially fatal respiratory depression. *Drug Safety Update*. www.gov.uk/drug-safety-update.

36 Cheikh Hassan HI *et al.* (2015) Efficacy and safety of gabapentin for uremic pruritus and restless legs syndrome in conservatively managed patients with chronic kidney disease. *Journal of Pain and Symptom Management*. **49**: 782–789.

37 Ishida JH *et al.* (2018) Gabapentin and pregabalin use and association with adverse outcomes among hemodialysis patients. *Journal of the American Society of Nephrology*. **29**: 1970–1978.

38 Kangas L *et al.* (1976) The protein binding of diazepam and N-demethyldiazepam in patients with poor renal function. *Clinical Nephrology*. **5**: 114–118.

39 Morrison G *et al.* (1984) Effect of renal impairment and hemodialysis on lorazepam kinetics. *Clinical Pharmacology and Therapeutics*. **35**: 646–652.

40 Verbeeck R *et al.* (1976) Biotransformation and excretion of lorazepam in patients with chronic renal failure. *British Journal of Clinical Pharmacology*. **3**: 1033–1039.

41 Douglas C *et al.* (2009) Symptom management for the adult patient dying with advanced chronic kidney disease: a review of the literature and development of evidence-based guidelines by a United Kingdom Expert Consensus Group. *Palliative Medicine*. **23**: 103–110.

42 UK Medicines Information (2016) Which opioids can be used in renal impairment? *Medicines Q&A* 402.3. www.evidence.nhs.uk.

43 Caraceni A *et al.* (2012) Use of opioid analgesics in the treatment of cancer pain: evidence-based recommendations from the EAPC. *Lancet Oncology*. **13**: e58–e68.

44 Sande TA *et al.* (2017) The use of opioids in cancer patients with renal impairment-a systematic review. *Supportive Care in Cancer*. **25**: 661–675.

45 King S *et al.* (2011) A systematic review of the use of opioid medication for those with moderate to severe cancer pain and renal impairment: a European palliative care research collaborative opioid guidelines project. *Palliative Medicine*. **25**: 525–552.

46 Dean M (2004) Opioids in renal failure and dialysis patients. *Journal of Pain and Symptom Management*. **28**: 497–504.

47 Davison SN (2019) Clinical pharmacology considerations in pain management in patients with advanced kidney failure. *Clinical Journal of the American Society of Nephrology*. **14**: 917–931.

48 Manchikanti L *et al.* (2017) Responsible, safe, and effective prescription of opioids for chronic non-cancer pain: American Society of Interventional Pain Physicians (ASIPP) guidelines. *Pain Physician*. **20**: s3–s92.

49 Els C *et al.* (2017) Adverse events associated with medium- and long-term use of opioids for chronic non-cancer pain: an overview of Cochrane Reviews. *Cochrane Database of Systematic Reviews*. **10**: CD012509. www.cochranelibrary.com.

50 Faculty of Pain Medicine (2017) Opioids aware: a resource for patients and healthcare professionals to support prescribing of opioid medicines for pain. Available from: www.fpm.ac.uk.

51 Hand CW *et al.* (1990) Buprenorphine disposition in patients with renal impairment: single and continuous dosing, with special reference to metabolites. *British Journal of Anaesthesia*. **64**: 276–282.

52 Elkader A and Sproule B (2005) Buprenorphine: clinical pharmacokinetics in the treatment of opioid dependence. *Clinical Pharmacokinetics*. **44**: 661–680.

53 Clemens KE and Klaschik E (2009) Morphine and hydromorphone in palliative care patients with renal impairment. *Anasthesiologie und Intensivmedizin*. **50**: 70–76.

54 Lee MA *et al.* (2001) Retrospective study of the use of hydromorphone in palliative care patients with normal and abnormal urea and creatinine. *Palliative Medicine*. **15**: 26–34.

55 Ferro CJ *et al.* (2004) Management of pain in renal failure. In: EJ Chambers *et al.* (eds) *Supportive Care for the Renal Patient*. Oxford: Oxford University Press., pp. 105–153.

56 Murtagh FE *et al.* (2007) The use of opioid analgesia in end-stage renal disease patients managed without dialysis: recommendations for practice. *Journal of Pain and Palliative Care Pharmacotherapy*. **21**: 5–16.

57 Boger RH (2006) Renal impairment: a challenge for opioid treatment? The role of buprenorphine. *Palliative Medicine*. **20 Suppl 1**: s17–s23.

58 Chinnadurai R *et al.* (2020) Pain management in patients with end-stage renal disease and calciphylaxis- a survey of clinical practices among physicians. *BMC Nephrology*. **21**: 403.

59 Cervelli MJ (2007). *The renal drug reference guide* (1st edn). Adelaide, South Australia Kidney Health.

60 Mimoz O *et al.* (2010) Nefopam pharmacokinetics in patients with end-stage renal disease. *Anaesthesia and Analgesia*. **111**: 1146–1153.

61 Geng CJ *et al.* (2015) Ibandronate to treat skeletal-related events and bone pain in metastatic bone disease or multiple myeloma: a meta-analysis of randomised clinical trials. *British Medical Journal Open*. **5**: 1–10.

62 Davison SN *et al.* (2019) Recommendations for the care of patients receiving conservative kidney management: Focus on management of CKD and symptoms. *Clinical Journal of the American Society of Nephrology*. **14**: 626–634.

63 Murtagh F and Sheerin N (2010) Conservative management of end-stage renal disease. In: Chambers EJ *et al.* (eds) *Supportive Care for the Renal Patient* (2nd edn). Oxford: Oxford University Press.

64 Murtagh FE *et al.* (2010) Symptoms in the month before death for stage 5 chronic kidney disease patients managed without dialysis. *Journal of Pain and Symptom Management*. **40**: 342–352.

Updated November 2021

18: HEPATIC IMPAIRMENT

The recommendations in this chapter are *not* comprehensive, more a direction of travel than a detailed road map. Specific recommendations are limited to common classes and types of drugs used in palliative care. For other drugs, see the relevant monograph and the manufacturer's SPC. However, some SPCs are unnecessarily restrictive.[1]

There will be occasions when hard evidence is not available and clinicians may have to *prescribe and proceed with caution*, e.g.:

- reduce polypharmacy as much as possible
- avoid hepatotoxic drugs if possible
- use a low starting dose
- reduce frequency of administration
- titrate upwards slowly
- monitor for both early and late onset toxicity (accumulation more likely if the plasma halflife is prolonged)
- ensure that the patient does not become constipated (may cause encephalopathy)
- beware of sedation (may cause, worsen or mask encephalopathy; Box A).

When deciding drug doses in hepatic impairment, it is important to also take the patient's overall clinical condition and rate of deterioration into account, and *not* rely solely on liver function tests (LFTs); of the latter, tests of synthetic liver function, i.e. albumin and clotting times, are considered more helpful and are included in the Child–Pugh score (see below).

INTRODUCTION

In palliative care, common liver problems encountered include cholestasis, liver metastases and chronic liver disease, e.g. secondary to alcohol or non-alcoholic fatty liver disease (NAFLD). Symptoms will vary with the underlying cause, but pain, fatigue, sleep disturbance, mood disturbance, pruritus, muscle cramps, anorexia and weight loss are common.

Cholestasis or liver metastases are characterized initially by abnormal LFTs, although synthetic liver function (i.e. albumin, clotting times) may be normal.

Chronic liver disease or progressive liver damage leads to fibrosis and subsequently cirrhosis. With severe cirrhosis, liver function is abnormal (decompensated) and the disorganized anatomy results in portal hypertension and complications such as oesophageal varices and the risk of major (sometimes fatal) haemorrhage, ascites, hepatic encephalopathy (Box A) and sepsis.

Patients with portal hypertension are at risk of hepatorenal syndrome. Portal hypertension leads to splanchnic vasodilation and a 'splanchnic steal syndrome', resulting in reduced arterial blood volume. Compensatory mechanisms initially maintain the systemic circulation but, when these fail, it can result in renal vasoconstriction, oliguria and functional renal insufficiency (hepatorenal syndrome).[2] This carries a prognosis of weeks to a few months (see Simplifying long-term hepatic drugs, p.777).

Box A Hepatic encephalopathy[3,4]

Hepatic encephalopathy is a neuropsychiatric disorder caused by effects on the CNS of toxins which accumulate in the blood because of inadequate hepatic detoxification.

It manifests as a spectrum of abnormalities affecting cognition, attention, functional ability, personality and intellect, and ranges from mild alteration of cognition ± drowsiness to coma. It is also characterized by neuromuscular symptoms such as flapping tremor (asterixis) and hyperreflexia.

The time course for hepatic encephalopathy can be episodic, recurrent (<6 months) or persistent (a pattern of behaviour changes that are always interspersed with relapses of overt hepatic encephalopathy). It can occur either spontaneously or be precipitated by constipation, sedatives, GI bleeding, dietary protein, uraemia, metabolic alkalosis and infections. Most of these result in an increase in blood levels of ammonia, the putative cause of the neuropsychiatric symptoms.

Grade 1
Minimal lack of awareness
Euphoria or anxiety
Shortened attention span
Impaired performance of addition

Grade 2
Lethargy or apathy
Minimal disorientation of time or place
Subtle personality changes
Inappropriate behaviour
Impaired performance of subtraction

Grade 3
Somnolence to stupor (but responsive to verbal stimuli)
Confusion
Gross disorientation

Grade 4
Coma (unresponsive to verbal or noxious stimuli)

When prescribing drugs in hepatic impairment, patients with decompensated liver function require the most caution. Unlike renal impairment, there is no one parameter which indicates the extent to which drug clearance will be affected by hepatic impairment. However, the Child–Pugh score, designed as a *prognostic aid in cirrhosis*, gives a general indication of the degree of hepatic impairment (Table 1).[5]

Table 1 Child–Pugh score; see footnote for interpretation

Factor	*Units*	*Score of 1*	*Score of 2*	*Score of 3*
Serum bilirubin	micromol/L mg/dL	<34 <2	34–51 2–3	>51 >3
Serum albumin	g/L g/dL	>35 >3.5	30–35 3–3.5	<30 <3
Prothrombin time (*or* INR)	%	>70 <1.7	40–70 1.7–2.3	<40 >2.3
Ascites		None	Easily controlled	Poorly controlled
Hepatic encephalopathy (see Box A)	grade	None	1–2 (subtle changes)	3–4 (drowsy–deep coma)

Child–Pugh A = score of 5–6 (well-compensated liver function); 1 year survival = 100%
Child–Pugh B = score of 7–9 (moderate functional impairment); 1 year survival = 80%
Child–Pugh C = score of 10–15 (severe impairment, hepatic decompensation); 1 year survival = 45%.

The drug literature generally refers to grades of hepatic impairment or to hepatic failure, and not to Child–Pugh scores. Pragmatically, one can regard Child–Pugh categories as roughly equivalent to mild, moderate and severe impairment. *However, it remains important to also take into account the patient's overall clinical condition, rate of deterioration and signs/symptoms of decompensated liver function.*

Drug-induced hepatotoxicity

Drug-induced hepatic impairment can be directly hepatocellular or secondary to biliary stasis (bile salts are hepatotoxic), or a combination of both. It is one of the main causes of *acute* liver failure (fulminant hepatic failure), characterized by jaundice, coagulopathy and encephalopathy, and is a medical emergency.

The underlying mechanism varies, but clinically it often resembles viral hepatitis: rapid onset malaise and jaundice with raised plasma aminotransferase concentrations.[6] Raised alkaline phosphatase and bilirubin concentrations predominate in hepatotoxicity secondary to cholestasis.

Hepatotoxic drug reactions can occur in any patient group, but the consequences can be particularly serious in those with pre-existing chronic liver disease. They can be divided into intrinsic (*predictable, dose-dependent*) and idiosyncratic (*unpredictable, dose-independent*). The intrinsic group is small because recommended doses are at levels known to be safe from early phase drug studies. Thus, predictable toxicity is associated with predisposing factors such as high doses (which may also occur from accumulation or drug interactions) and co-morbidity (alcoholism, malnutrition, genetic variation). Although not completely clear-cut, the following drugs used in palliative care are potential causes of predictable hepatotoxicity:

- **paracetamol**, generally with doses >4g/24h, *but toxicity has been reported with normal or lower doses in the presence of additional risk factors* (see p.331)
- **dantrolene**, particularly with doses ≥400mg/24h (see p.661)
- **fluconazole** and **itraconazole**, particularly if prolonged course and high dose
- **rifampicin**, used to treat cholestatic pruritus (see p.518)
- **tizanidine** ≥12mg/24h (see p.662)
- **valproate**; toxicity mostly limited to children <3 years (see p.307).[7]

LFTs, particularly synthetic liver function in patients with pre-existing hepatic impairment, should be monitored as per the individual SPCs.

On the other hand, most drugs at recommended doses can cause idiosyncratic (*dose-independent*) liver injury, with a frequency ranging from 1 in 1,000 to 1 in 100,000 patients, and with a female:male preponderance of 3:1.[6] Latency ranges from a few days to 6 months, occasionally longer.[8,9] Fatalities have been reported.[8]

Drug-induced mild elevation of liver enzymes is relatively common and, by itself, does *not* necessitate immediate discontinuation of the drug; the situation, including synthetic liver function tests, should be monitored. The enzymes often spontaneously revert to normal, but occasionally increasing concentrations will subsequently necessitate discontinuation.

Drugs used in palliative care most likely to cause idiosyncratic (*dose-independent*) drug-induced liver injury include:[10,11]

- NSAIDs, notably **diclofenac** (5/100,000 users/year)
- antimicrobials, notably **amoxicillin**, **co-amoxiclav**, fluoroquinolones, macrolides, **nitrofurantoin**
- **carbamazepine**, **valproate**
- PPIs.

In patients with hepatic impairment, drugs causing intrinsic (*predictable, dose-dependent*) toxicity do so at lower doses, but there is *not* a uniform increase in the risk of idiosyncratic (*unpredictable, dose-independent*) toxicity.[6]

The use of hepatotoxic drugs in a patient with cirrhosis increases the risk of hepatic encephalopathy (Box A).

PHARMACOLOGICAL IMPACT OF HEPATIC IMPAIRMENT

The liver is the main site for the metabolism of most drugs. However, hepatic reserve is large and, generally, unless drugs are metabolized mostly by a specific CYP450 pathway, e.g. **sertraline**, there must be severe hepatic impairment or decompensation for the overall intrinsic activity or capacity of the metabolizing enzymes to be altered to a clinically important extent.

However, hepatic impairment also has many other consequences which may alter the action or overall clearance of a drug (Box B). In addition, patient-related factors, e.g. disease type/severity and rate of change in LFTs/synthetic liver function, also contribute to the overall pharmacological impact.

Box B Summary of the impact of hepatic impairment on drug pharmacology[12,13]

Pharmacokinetic (see also main text below)

Absorption

↓ intestinal bile salts in cholestasis → ↓ absorption of lipid-soluble drugs

Ascites or oedematous bowel → ↓ absorption

↓ hepatic blood flow, e.g. cirrhosis, cardiac failure → ↓ first-pass metabolism → ↑ bioavailability

Distribution

Ascites → ↑ volume of distribution of water-soluble drugs

Hypo-albuminaemia or hyperbilirubinaemia → ↑ active unbound drug for highly protein-bound drugs

Metabolism

Accumulation of pro-drugs, drugs and/or metabolites

Active drugs: ↓ enzymatic function (e.g. CYP450) → ↑ effect/risk of toxicity, ↑ halflife

Pro-drugs: ↓ enzymatic function or capacity (e.g. CYP450) → ↓ effect

Elimination

Cholestasis → ↓ elimination of drugs excreted in bile → ↓ enterohepatic circulation

Pharmacodynamic

Altered receptor sensitivity to the effects of drugs

Anticoagulants → ↑ risk of bleeding

Antihypertensives → ↑ risk of hypotension

Benzodiazepines, psychotropics, opioids → ↑ sedation → ↑ encephalopathy

Diuretics → reduced response

Hypoglycaemics → ↑ risk of hypoglycaemia

NSAIDs → ↑ risk of GI bleeding; fluid retention; ↑ risk of hepatorenal syndrome

Secondary phenomena necessitating extra caution

Ascites: products with a high sodium content, and salt- and water-retaining drugs, e.g. NSAIDs, corticosteroids

Coagulopathy: anticoagulants, corticosteroids, NSAIDs, SSRIs

Disruption of the blood–brain barrier → higher CNS concentrations of some drugs, e.g. propranolol

Encephalopathy:

- increased sensitivity to hypnotics and other CNS depressants, including opioids
- diuretics, corticosteroids (if these cause hypokalaemia)
- drugs that constipate, e.g. antimuscarinics, opioids (slowed bowel transit time → increased ammonia absorption)

QT prolongation: ↑ risk of ventricular arrythmia with QT-prolonging drugs, e.g. citalopram

Renal impairment → ↓ elimination of renally excreted drugs, e.g. aminoglycosides

Spontaneous bacterial peritonitis: ↑ risk with PPIs.

Pharmacokinetic considerations

Also see Box B.

Absorption

Bile salts facilitate the absorption of lipid-soluble drugs. Thus, in cholestasis, absorption will be decreased, leading to reduced plasma concentrations and decreased efficacy, e.g. of **ibuprofen**.[12] Cholestasis will also decrease the absorption of lipid-soluble vitamins A, D, E and K, and may also affect enterohepatic circulation (see Elimination, below).

First-pass metabolism and systemic bio-availability

In cirrhosis, portosystemic shunts can lead to a decrease in blood flow through the liver. This can reduce first-pass metabolism of PO drugs, thereby *increasing* bio-availability. In severe hepatic impairment, the degree of caution required is related to the drug's usual PO bio-availability (Table 2).

Table 2 Effect of severe hepatic impairment on PO bio-availability[14]

Usual PO bio-availability	*Severe hepatic impairment*		*Examples*
	Effect on PO bio-availability	*Change to PO dosing regimen*	
High >70%	No change	Reduce maintenance dose[a]	Lorazepam, spironolactone
Moderate 40–70%	May increase	Initial doses should be in the low range of normal; reduce the maintenance dose	Amitriptyline, haloperidol, olanzapine
Low[b] <40%	May increase dramatically	Reduce both the initial dose and the maintenance dose	Domperidone, granisetron, morphine, ondansetron, propranolol, sertraline

a. to allow for associated decreased hepatic intrinsic metabolism, i.e. clearance; see below

b. low bio-availability does not necessarily mean high first-pass metabolism; low bio-availability can also relate to poor absorption from the GI tract.

Distribution and protein-binding

With highly protein-bound drugs (>80%), e.g. **phenytoin**, the proportion of free drug (free fraction) is greater in hypo-albuminaemia. Bilirubin binds to plasma proteins, and hyperbilirubinaemia can also increase the free fraction of highly protein-bound drugs. Depending on the characteristics of the drug, a greater free fraction means more drug is available for, e.g. distribution, action, elimination.

Water-soluble drugs, e.g. aminoglycoside antibiotics, will distribute into ascites and, in theory, could reduce systemic availability. Larger loading doses could be required but, in practice, this is unlikely to be a problem if the ascites is treated successfully or drained.

Metabolism

The liver typically converts active lipophilic drugs into inactive hydrophilic metabolites for excretion by the kidneys. However, pro-drugs such as **codeine**, **tramadol** and **oxcarbazepine** are metabolized by the liver into their active forms. Thus, severe hepatic impairment will reduce the efficacy of pro-drugs to a variable extent. Hepatic metabolism includes:

- *phase I (modification) reactions:* particularly oxidation catalysed by CYP450 enzymes in the endoplasmic reticulum (see Chapter 19, p.781)
- *phase II (conjugation) reactions:* particularly glucuronidation catalysed by glucuronyl transferases in the endoplasmic reticulum and cytosol.

In severe decompensated hepatic impairment, drugs predominantly metabolized in the liver will accumulate, with a greater likelihood of toxicity. Phase II enzymes are generally less affected than phase I enzymes, which are also affected to different degrees, e.g. CYP1A2, 2C19>2A6, 3A4>2C9, 2E1.[12] For drugs metabolized via CYP450, there is an increased risk of toxicity from a drug–drug interaction with the concurrent use of an inhibitor of the relevant CYP450 enzyme. The effect of concurrent use of an enzyme inducer is likely to be less predictable. In severe hepatic impairment, drug interactions may be unpredictable and fluctuate according to liver function. This requires the close monitoring of drugs with narrow therapeutic ranges, e.g. **warfarin**, direct-acting antivirals for hepatitis C.[15]

Impaired hepatic metabolic capacity may well go hand in hand with impaired hepatic synthetic functions, reflected in an elevated prothrombin time/INR and hypo-albuminaemia, and also by encephalopathy (Box A). These can be used as pointers to the need to reduce maintenance doses.

Elimination

In cholestasis, the clearance of drugs with predominant biliary elimination, e.g. **digoxin**, **fusidic acid**, **morphine**, **rifampicin** and many conjugated drug metabolites, will be impaired. Guidelines for dose reduction in cholestasis exist for many antineoplastic drugs, but are mostly lacking for other drugs with biliary elimination. Drugs that undergo enterohepatic circulation, e.g. **indometacin**, will be affected, but to an unpredictable extent.[12]

The dose of drugs with predominant renal elimination of unchanged drug ± active metabolite(s) may also have to be adjusted in patients with liver disease, because of associated hepatorenal syndrome. Note. Despite impaired renal function, the plasma creatinine concentration may be normal in patients with a reduced muscle mass. Thus, ideally, *creatinine clearance* should be used to determine the dose of drugs with predominant renal elimination in malnourished, cachectic or sarcopenic patients (see Chapter 17, p.731). Even so, the creatinine clearance tends to overestimate glomerular filtration in these circumstances, and the dose may still be too high.

Pharmacodynamic considerations

In severe cirrhosis, the pharmacodynamics of centrally acting drugs are also altered because of changes in the blood–brain barrier. Further, *moderate–severe hepatic impairment reduces renal clearance*, necessitating a reduction in the dose of renally excreted drugs (see Chapter 17, p.731). Thus, when hepatic and renal impairment occur concurrently, extra caution is necessary.

Also see Box B.

APPROACH TO PRESCRIBING IN LIVER DISEASE

Prescribing for a patient with liver disease should be individualized and pragmatic, balancing the risk vs. benefits in the context of overall goals of care. A cautious approach together with regular monitoring is required, particularly as the degree of impairment can fluctuate.

It is essential that prescribers are aware of the pharmacokinetics of the drug they are prescribing and the impact of hepatic impairment on drug pharmacology (Box B). Generally, the safer drugs are those with high PO bio-availability, minimal hepatic metabolism, low–moderate protein-binding, a short halflife, and no sedative, constipating or hepatotoxic effects.

Specific information on dose adjustment in patients with liver disease can be limited. SPCs often contain a blanket contra-indication (because of a lack of data) or provide nonspecific information.[16] Published guidance relies heavily on expert opinion and inevitably varies.[17]

PCF provides guidance for common palliative care drugs for long-term use in chronic severe hepatic impairment. Nonetheless, recommendations for dose adjustment can only be approximate and cannot replace careful clinical monitoring, including factors such as:

- underlying diagnosis/prognosis
- rate of disease progression
- changes in synthetic liver function/Child–Pugh score
- overall goals of care.

If in doubt, start with a low dose and titrate slowly to response (Box C).

Because patients with cirrhosis are prone to renal injury, *nephrotoxic* drugs, e.g. aminoglycosides, should be used with caution. However, this does not mean that essential drugs should be withheld, but that high-risk patients should be closely monitored.[7]

Box C 'Red flags' for considering dose reduction in severe hepatic impairment[12,18]

Consider dose reduction if prescribing a drug that normally:
- has low systemic PO bio-availability because of high first-pass hepatic extraction
- is highly protein-bound and the patient has hypo-albuminaemia (<30g/L) ± elevated plasma bilirubin
- is cleared mainly by phase I hepatic metabolism, e.g. CYP1A2, CYP2C19, CYP2D6 or CYP3A4 (see Chapter 19, Table 8, p.790), and has:
  - ▷ a narrow therapeutic range *or*
  - ▷ a long halflife.

Other factors indicative of severe hepatic impairment and possible need for dose reduction:
- prothrombin time >130% of normal
- platelets <150 x 10^9/L
- bilirubin >100micromol/L
- severe cirrhosis (i.e. Child–Pugh C)
- ascites
- hepatic encephalopathy
- hyponatraemia
- moderate renal impairment (eGFR <60mL/min/1.73m^2).

PALLIATIVE CARE DRUGS FOR LONG-TERM USE IN CHRONIC SEVERE HEPATIC IMPAIRMENT

Many drugs used in palliative care, e.g. antimuscarinics, benzodiazepines, opioids, cause CNS depression ± constipation and can either cause, worsen or mask hepatic encephalopathy (see Box A above, and individual sections below).

This section provides guidance for prescribing drugs commonly used for long-term palliative care symptom relief in patients with chronic severe hepatic impairment (roughly equivalent to Child–Pugh class C) *with a prognosis of weeks–months or longer*. For:
- acute hepatic impairment, seek specialist advice from a hepatologist
- mild–moderate hepatic impairment, see the individual drug monographs for any relevant information
- patients in the last days of life; see Last days of life, p.779.

Tables 3–10 and the accompanying text were developed to provide user-friendly summaries to guide rational and safe prescribing in patients with chronic severe hepatic impairment, by raising awareness of:
- suitable drugs and their starting doses
- suitable alternatives when patients experience undesirable effects
- the potential risks of using a less 'hepatically safe' drug.

The tables cover the most common symptom relief drug classes and highlight, when possible, the most, intermediate and least 'hepatically safe' drugs for long-term use. Because it is generally good practice to become experienced in using relatively few drugs well, the list is purposely limited.

The tables should be used in conjunction with the accompanying text which highlights any general considerations for that class of drug and provides a commentary to help inform choice.

As far as possible, specific prescribing advice is given. Even when a drug appears to be 'hepatically safe', because hepatic impairment can have general effects on pharmacokinetics and/or pharmacodynamics, *smaller starting doses, a slower than usual titration and close monitoring of the patient are advisable, particularly in elderly and/or frail patients.* Drugs with a long halflife may reach steady state only after 1–2 weeks or more of regular use, and undesirable effects may consequently be late onset. Thus, the adage 'start low, go slow' will generally apply to the use of any drug, and particularly those with CNS effects.

In addition to considering the impact of hepatic impairment and familiarity of use, the selection of the most appropriate drug also requires the prescriber to consider any relevant additional factors such as the presence of concurrent symptoms, co-morbidities (e.g. cardiovascular disease, renal impairment), use of other drugs (e.g. in relation to a drug–drug interaction, QT prolongation) and patient preference.

Sometimes the cautious use of a familiar drug may be preferable to an unfamiliar (albeit 'safer') one. Similarly, *PCF* does *not* advocate the automatic switching of patients to a 'safer' drug when an alternative is proving satisfactory. This section aims to complement and not replace specialist hepatology guidance.

Additional notes on the use of the tables:

- drugs are categorized as 'generally safer', 'use cautiously' and 'avoid if possible' from a *purely hepatic perspective*, according to the risk of accumulation and/or toxicity with long-term use in chronic severe hepatic impairment
- consensus dosing guidelines are presented. These include off-label use and, in some instances, despite an SPC contra-indication in this setting. However, it is impractical to highlight all cases of off-label or contra-indicated use, because this can vary according to country, brand, indication, formulations, dose, route of administration or patient population. Prescribers should be aware of the implications of off-label use, see p.xix.

Remember: recommendations can only be approximate and cannot replace clinical monitoring.

Analgesics: non-opioids (Table 3)

Pharmacokinetic changes

About 5–15% of a dose of **paracetamol** is hepatically metabolized to N-acetyl-p-benzoquinoneimine, a highly reactive hepatotoxic metabolite (see p.331). The halflife of **paracetamol** can be nearly doubled in hepatic impairment.[19] Despite this, PO **paracetamol** can still be used in severe hepatic impairment *at a reduced dose and provided there are no additional risk factors for toxicity* (see **Paracetamol**, Box B, p.334).[20] Although IV **paracetamol** is contra-indicated by the manufacturers in severe hepatic impairment, it is used by some liver units, at a maximum dose of 1g IV t.d.s.[21]

The use of NSAIDs in liver disease is associated with a higher risk of undesirable effects, e.g. renal impairment, bleeding from oesophageal varices (also see Box B).[22] Most NSAIDs are highly protein-bound and hepatically metabolized. Thus, most SPCs for NSAIDs include active liver disease or moderate–severe hepatic impairment as contra-indications. However, particularly in cancer, the potential analgesic benefit may well outweigh the risk.

The pharmacokinetics of **diclofenac** and **ibuprofen** appear not to be affected in hepatic impairment;[23] conversely, even mild hepatic impairment significantly affects the pharmacokinetics of **celecoxib**.[24]

Cholestasis may reduce the elimination of NSAIDs excreted in bile, e.g. **indometacin**, and may reduce or delay absorption of fat-soluble NSAIDs, e.g. **ibuprofen**.[12]

Hepatotoxicity is a rare unpredictable effect seen with most NSAIDs, including COX-2 inhibitors. **Diclofenac** may have the highest risk and **ibuprofen** the least.[1]

Choice of non-opioid analgesic

In severe hepatic impairment, the cautious use of reduced doses of PO **paracetamol** *provided there are no additional risk factors for toxicity* (see **Paracetamol**, Box B, p.334) is preferred to an NSAID, which generally should be avoided. Regular review to exclude other risk factors for toxicity, e.g. weight loss, is required.

If the use of an NSAID is unavoidable, **ibuprofen** is a reasonable choice in cholestatic and non-cholestatic liver disease. A PPI should be given concurrently (Table 10) due to the high GI risk, and renal function should be closely monitored.

For adjuvant analgesics, see Table 5, Table 7, Table 9 and Table 10.

18

Table 3 Non-opioid analgesics in severe hepatic impairment. Before use, see introductory and class-specific text

Drug	*PO bio-availability (%)*	*Protein-binding (%)*	*Halflife in normal liver function (h)*	*Significant hepatic metabolism*	*Significant biliary excretion of drug ± active metabolite(s)*	*Increase in halflife in severe hepatic impairment*	*Dose and comments*
Use cautiously							
Paracetamol[a]	<90	20–30	1–4	Yes; hepatotoxic metabolite (see p.331)	No	50–100%	PO/PR[b]: start with 500mg q8h; maximum 1g q8h
Avoid if possible							
NSAIDs							If unavoidable, use ibuprofen PO 200mg t.d.s. (see text)

a. use only when no additional risk factors for toxicity (see Paracetamol, Box B, p.334)

b. IV paracetamol is contra-indicated by the manufacturers, but is used by some liver units in reduced doses, e.g. 500mg–1g t.d.s. (also see text).

Analgesics: opioids (Table 4)

Regardless of the pharmacokinetic changes described below, in severe hepatic impairment there is an increased risk of toxicity with *all* opioids because of increased opioid receptor sensitivity and reduced integrity of the blood–brain barrier; further, their sedative ± constipating effects can cause, worsen or sometimes mask encephalopathy. A slower than usual titration and close monitoring of the patient are required.

The SPCs of most PO opioids include severe hepatic impairment as a contra-indication. M/r products should generally be avoided because of the prolonged duration of action if sedation becomes a problem. The exception may be for **morphine** in stable patients (see below).

Routine use of TD patches is not advised, because of the long duration of action and effects lasting for ≥20h after removal. In addition, pruritus may affect tolerability.

Pharmacokinetic changes

For most opioids, there is a risk of accumulation in severe hepatic impairment, because of either an increase in PO bio-availability (reduced first-pass metabolism) and/or decrease in hepatic metabolism. For opioids significantly metabolized via CYP450 (see Chapter 19, Table 1, p.783), there is an increased risk of toxicity from a drug–drug interaction with the concurrent use of an inhibitor of the relevant CYP450 enzyme (see, Chapter 19, Table 8, p.790).

For pro-drugs such as **codeine** and **tramadol** which are activated by hepatic metabolism, there is decreased production and metabolism of the active metabolite, leading to an unpredictable effect. There are a lack of data on the use of **dihydrocodeine**. Accordingly, weak opioids should be avoided in both moderate and severe hepatic impairment.

Morphine has a PO bio-availability of 35% (range 15–64%), which increases to almost 100% in patients with severe hepatic impairment with cirrhosis.[25] The plasma halflife is also increased, necessitating a decreased dose and frequency of administration of immediate-release products.[25,26] Generally, **morphine** should be avoided in patients with hepatorenal syndrome, because of the additional risk of toxicity from accumulation of morphine-6-glucuronide in severe renal impairment (see Chapter 17, p.743).[24] **Morphine** can cause spasm of the bile duct/sphincter of Oddi and is contra-indicated in biliary colic; this should be considered when the use of **morphine** is associated with abdominal pain.

Diamorphine (di-acetylmorphine) is, in effect, a pro-drug for **morphine** which is de-acetylated by digestive juices and body fluids (see p.417). Thus, *advice for* ***morphine*** *applies equally to* ***diamorphine***.

Buprenorphine (p.428) is only partly hepatically metabolized and, in theory, can be used cautiously in patients with cirrhosis. However, it is highly protein-bound and has a variable halflife, and a post-marketing study of IV use has shown higher plasma levels in patients with moderate–severe hepatic impairment. Two-thirds of **buprenorphine** is eliminated unchanged in the faeces, which could be relevant in patients with cholestatic disease. Further, although the active metabolite (norbuprenorphine) does not usually exert a central effect, this may change in situations where the blood–brain barrier becomes more permeable (see above). SL use is contra-indicated in severe hepatic impairment, and TD use is not recommended (see above).

Fentanyl pharmacokinetics are not altered in patients with cirrhosis after a single IV dose.[27] However, in severe hepatic impairment, **fentanyl** clearance is significantly reduced when administered CIVI.[28] With TD patches, the overall exposure to **fentanyl** is increased (AUC and C_{max} increased by 75% and 35% respectively), although the halflife following removal is unchanged.[24] **Fentanyl** is highly protein-bound and almost exclusively metabolized by the liver. It has a large volume of distribution, and only a relatively small fraction is available in the central compartment for hepatic uptake. Thus, clearance is mostly affected by changes in hepatic blood flow rather than reduced metabolism.

Alfentanil pharmacokinetics can be altered even in *mild* hepatic impairment.[24] **Alfentanil** is highly protein-bound, has a lower volume of distribution than **fentanyl**, and is metabolized almost exclusively by the liver.

Hydromorphone undergoes significant first-pass hepatic metabolism. In *moderate* hepatic impairment, because of increased bio-availability, both C_{max} and the AUC for PO **hydromorphone** are quadrupled, although surprisingly the halflife is unchanged. Thus, if **hydromorphone** is used, low starting doses at standard time intervals are advisable.[24,29] With severe hepatic impairment, the halflife will almost certainly increase, and the frequency of dosing should also be reduced. Parenterally, no data are available; based on pharmacokinetic parameters, parenteral **hydromorphone** may be safer than PO. **Hydromorphone** has low protein-binding, a short halflife and a relatively large volume of distribution, and the SPC suggests lower doses can be used with caution in hepatic impairment. However, the main metabolite, hydromorphone-3-glucuronide, has no analgesic activity but is a potent neuro-excitant and is renally excreted. Thus, **hydromorphone** should be avoided in hepatorenal syndrome.

For both PO and parenteral **oxycodone**, in severe hepatic impairment due to cirrhosis, the AUC and halflife are significantly increased, and the clearance decreased.[24,30] Thus, both PO and parenteral **oxycodone** are contra-indicated by the manufacturer in this setting; if use is unavoidable, both the dose and frequency of administration should be reduced.

The use of **methadone** requires specialist supervision because of the inherent risks of accumulation and toxicity even in patients without hepatic impairment (see p.469). In addicts receiving **methadone** maintenance, severe hepatic impairment increases halflife, but AUC and clearance are unchanged.[24] There are no data for the analgesic use of **methadone**. However, variability in bio-availability, high protein-binding and significant hepatic metabolism are likely to further complicate its use in severe hepatic impairment, and it is best avoided.

Choice of opioid analgesic

The use of all weak opioids is best avoided in severe hepatic impairment.

In some liver units, **fentanyl** SC/CSCI is the first-line choice in patients with severe hepatic impairment, particularly when there is concurrent renal impairment (see Chapter 17, p.743). Transmucosal **fentanyl** products may be an alternative option for break-through pain in those patients who have achieved the necessary degree of opioid tolerance (see p.457).

The cautious use of PO immediate-release **morphine** is a reasonable option, using lower starting doses and decreased dosing frequency. Generally, m/r products should be avoided. However, if continued regular use of immediate-release **morphine** is without problem, an m/r **morphine** product may be tried cautiously.

Antidepressants (Table 5)

Regardless of the pharmacokinetic changes described below, in severe hepatic impairment antidepressants with sedative ± constipating effects can cause, worsen or sometimes mask encephalopathy. A slower than usual titration and close monitoring of the patient are required.

Concurrent use of other drugs with sedative ± constipating effects, e.g. opioids, further increases the risk of toxicity.

Pharmacokinetic changes

Most antidepressants are highly protein-bound and hepatically metabolized by one or more CYP450 enzymes (see Antidepressants, Table 2, p.215). Metabolism will be further impaired in constitutionally poor metabolizers, e.g. of **amitriptyline**, **nortriptyline** (CYP2D6), **amitriptyline**, **citalopram** and **sertraline** (CYP2C19), and the risk of toxicity increased from a pharmacokinetic drug–drug interaction involving an inhibitor of the CYP450 enzyme(s).

Because of the time taken for drugs to accumulate, undesirable effects may become apparent only after days or weeks of regular use for those antidepressants with long halflives, e.g. **amitriptyline**, **citalopram**, **mirtazapine**, **nortriptyline**, **sertraline**.

TCAs are not a first-line treatment for depression. In palliative care, **amitriptyline** is used for neuropathic pain; its halflife does not appear to increase in severe hepatic impairment.

All SSRIs accumulate in severe hepatic impairment.[31] **Sertraline** has very high first-pass metabolism and protein-binding; **citalopram** less so, but is more dependent on biliary excretion for elimination.[14] Both have significantly increased halflives in severe hepatic impairment. **Citalopram** accumulation will increase the risk of prolongation of the QT interval (and thereby risk of ventricular arrhythmia; see p.797). The pharmacokinetic profiles of **fluoxetine**, **fluvoxamine** and **paroxetine** are no more favourable in severe hepatic impairment, and these drugs are also strong hepatic enzyme inhibitors (see p.232).

The clearance of **mirtazapine** is reduced in *mild* hepatic impairment and plasma concentration increases; accumulation also occurs in end-stage *renal* failure (see Chapter 17, p.737). Thus, **mirtazapine** is not a good choice in hepatorenal syndrome.

Table 4 Opioid analgesics in severe hepatic impairment. Before use, see introductory and class-specific text

Drug[a,b]	*PO bio-availability (%)*	*Protein-binding (%)*	*Halflife in normal liver function (h)*	*Significant hepatic metabolism*	*Significant biliary excretion of drug ± active metabolite(s)*	*Increase in halflife in severe hepatic impairment*	*Dose and comments*
Generally safer							
Fentanyl	N/A	80–85	4–16 (injection)	Yes; see text	No	No	Lower doses may be sufficient SC: start with 12.5–25microgram q1h p.r.n. CSCI: start with 100–150microgram/24h
Use cautiously							
Buprenorphine[c]	50 (SL)	96	20–25 (injection) 24–69 (SL)	No; but see text	Yes (66%)	Probably ↑	SL/SC: reduce initial dose by 25–50%
Diamorphine	No data	No data	3min (IV); ≤5h[d]	See morphine	See morphine	No	*Pro-drug*: see text; SC: start with 1.25–2.5mg q2–4h p.r.n CSCI: start with 5mg/24h
Morphine	15–64	20–35	2–5	Yes; active metabolite	Yes; see text	<100%	PO: start with 5mg q6–8h and q2–4h p.r.n. SC: start with 2.5mg q2–4h p.r.n. CSCI: start with 10mg/24h
Avoid if possible							
Alfentanil	N/A	92	1.5	Yes	No	Yes	If unavoidable SC: start with 50–100microgram q1h p.r.n. CSCI: start with 0.5–1mg/24h
Codeine	12–84	7	3–4	Yes; active metabolite	No	Yes	*Pro-drug*: reduced bio-transformation and thus reduced/unpredictable effect
Dihydrocodeine	20	No data	3.5–5	Yes; active metabolite	No data	Probably ↑	See text
Hydromorphone	32	<10	2.5	Yes; neurotoxic metabolite	No	Probably ↑	If unavoidable, decrease frequency of PO/SC immediate release products to q8h

Table 4 Continued

Drug[a,b]	*PO bio-availability (%)*	*Protein-binding (%)*	*Halflife in normal liver function (h)*	*Significant hepatic metabolism*	*Significant biliary excretion of drug ± active metabolite(s)*	*Increase in halflife in severe hepatic impairment*	*Dose and comments*
*Methadone[c]	40–100	60–90	5–130	Yes	Possible	Probably ↑	*Specialist use only* Requires careful and *slow* titration; accumulation occurs even without hepatic impairment (see p.469)
Oxycodone	60–87	45	2–4	Yes; active metabolite	No	<400%	If unavoidable PO: start with 2.5mg q8h and q2–4h p.r.n. SC: start with 1.5mg q2–4h p.r.n. CSCI: start with 5mg/24h
Tramadol	90 (multiple doses)	20	6	Yes; active metabolite	No	<300%	*Pro-drug*: reduced bio-transformation and thus reduced/unpredictable effect

a. whichever drug is used, because of the altered pharmacodynamic effects of opioids in severe hepatic impairment, a slower than usual titration and close monitoring of the patient are required

b. avoid m/r and TD products (see text)

c. because of the long halflife and time taken to reach steady state, undesirable effects with these opioids may only become apparent after several days or weeks of regular use

d. active metabolite.

Table 5 Antidepressants in severe hepatic impairment. Before use, see introductory and class-specific text

Drug[a]	*PO bio-availability (%)*	*Protein-binding (%)*	*Halflife in normal liver function (h)*	*Significant hepatic metabolism*	*Significant biliary excretion of drug ± active metabolite(s)*	*Increase in halflife in severe hepatic impairment*	*Dose and comments*
Use cautiously							
Amitriptyline[b]	45	96	9–25	Yes; active metabolite	No	No	PO: start with 5–10mg at bedtime *Not a first-line treatment for depression*
Citalopram[b]	80	<80	36	Yes; active metabolite	Yes (85%)	>200%	PO: start with 10mg once daily; maximum dose 16mg (oral solution) or 20mg (tablet) once daily
Mirtazapine[b]	50	85	20–40	Yes; active metabolite	No	Probably ↑	PO: start with 15mg at bedtime; maximum dose 30mg at bedtime
Avoid if possible							
Duloxetine	90	96	8–17	Yes	No	>200%	See text
Sertraline[b]	>44	98	26	Yes	No	>300%	Avoid unless for cholestatic pruritus: PO: start with 50mg once daily; maximum 100mg once daily (see text)
Trazodone	65	89–95	5–13 (doubles in elderly)	Yes; active metabolite	No	Probably ↑	*Not a first-line treatment for depression*
Venlafaxine[c]	13 (45 m/r)	27	5 (11)[d]	Yes; active metabolite	No	Yes	See text. If unavoidable PO: start with 37.5mg once daily

a. whichever drug is used, because of the altered pharmacodynamic effects of antidepressants in severe hepatic impairment, a slower than usual titration and close monitoring of the patient are required

b. because of the long halflife and time taken to reach steady state, undesirable effects with these antidepressants may only become apparent after several days or weeks of regular use

c. do not use m/r products

d. active metabolite.

Trazodone is not a first-line treatment for depression in palliative care. It undergoes extensive hepatic metabolism and has been associated with severe hepatotoxicity.

The halflife of **venlafaxine** is prolonged even in *mild* hepatic impairment, but with a large degree of inter-subject variation. The halflife of **duloxetine** more than doubles in *moderate* hepatic impairment, and the AUC almost quadruples. Thus, both are best avoided. Further, both **venlafaxine** and **duloxetine** accumulate in end-stage *renal* failure (see Chapter 17, p.737), making neither a good choice in hepatorenal syndrome.

Choice of antidepressant

Of the SSRIs generally used in palliative care (see p.232), the cautious use of **citalopram** is probably the best choice for patients with severe hepatic impairment, unless they have additional risk factors for QT prolongation or severe cholestasis. Because SSRIs decrease platelet aggregation and increase the risk of GI bleeding (see p.218), they are not a good choice in patients with coagulopathy or oesophageal varices. Although **sertraline** is generally best avoided, it is used for cholestatic pruritus (also see Chapter 26, p.825 and **Rifampicin**, p.518).

Cautious use of **mirtazapine** may also be an option and has a lower risk of bleeding than an SSRI. It should be avoided in patients with hepatorenal syndrome and discontinued if jaundice occurs. It is more sedating and associated with less nausea than SSRIs and is used in some liver units because of its beneficial effects on appetite and sleep.[31]

Amitriptyline may be used with caution for neuropathic pain. The presence of cardiac co-morbidity will limit its use.

Anti-emetics (Table 6)

Regardless of the pharmacokinetic changes described below, in severe hepatic impairment anti-emetics with sedative ± constipating effects can cause, worsen or sometimes mask hepatic encephalopathy. A slower than usual titration and close monitoring of the patient are required.

Concurrent use of other drugs with sedative ± constipating effects, e.g. opioids, further increases the risk of toxicity.

Pharmacokinetic changes

For anti-emetics metabolized via CYP450, e.g. **domperidone**, **haloperidol** and **ondansetron**, there is an increased risk of toxicity from a drug–drug interaction with the concurrent use of an inhibitor of the relevant CYP450 enzyme (see Chapter 19, Table 8, p.790).

The risk of prolongation of the QT interval (and thereby risk of ventricular arrhythmia) is higher with **domperidone**, **haloperidol**, **levomepromazine** and **ondansetron**. The risk may be increased as a result of, e.g. drug accumulation, drug–drug interaction, concurrent use of other drugs that either prolong the QT interval or cause electrolyte imbalance.

Because of the time taken for drugs to accumulate, undesirable effects may become apparent only after days or weeks of regular use for those anti-emetics with a long halflife, e.g. **cyclizine**, **haloperidol**, **levomepromazine**.

Domperidone has the advantage of not crossing the blood–brain barrier. However, in moderate hepatic impairment the AUC increases 3-times, the C_{max} and halflife increase 1.5-times and the unbound fraction by 25%. Thus, the SPC contra-indicates use in moderate–severe hepatic impairment.

In severe hepatic impairment, the halflife of **metoclopramide** increases by >100%, necessitating a dose reduction.[32,33] Similarly, clearance of **ondansetron** is reduced and the maximum dose limited.[34]

Although rare, **haloperidol**, **levomepromazine** and **prochlorperazine** (antipsychotic type anti-emetics) can cause hepatotoxicity (see Antipsychotics, p.771).

Choice of anti-emetic

Domperidone is the anti-emetic of choice in many liver units, despite the SPC contra-indication.[35] The starting dose should be halved and the risk/benefit assessed in patients with additional risk factors for QT prolongation. **Metoclopramide** and **ondansetron** are also commonly used in reduced doses. Note. **Ondansetron** is constipating, and an increased dose of laxatives may be required.

Table 6 Anti-emetics in severe hepatic impairment. Before use, see introductory and class-specific text

Drug[a]	*PO bio-availability (%)*	*Protein-binding (%)*	*Halflife in normal liver function (h)*	*Significant hepatic metabolism*	*Significant biliary excretion of drug ± active metabolite(s)*	*Increase in halflife in severe hepatic impairment*	*Dose and comments*
Use cautiously							
Domperidone[b]	12–18	>90	7–9	Yes	No	50%	PO: start with 5mg b.d.; maximum 10mg t.d.s.
Metoclopramide[b]	50–80	13–22	4–6	Yes	No	>100%	PO/SC: start with 5mg b.d.; maximum 10mg b.d.– t.d.s.
Ondansetron	56–71	70–76	3–6	Yes	No data	>300%	PO/SC: maximum 8mg/24h
Avoid if possible							
Cyclizine[c]	50%	No data	20	Yes	No data	No data	If unavoidable PO: start with 50mg b.d. SC: start with 25mg b.d.
Haloperidol[c]	45–75	92	12–38	Yes; active metabolite	Possible	No data	If unavoidable PO/SC: start with 500microgram at bedtime and q4h p.r.n. *Also see Table 8 (Antipsychotics)*
Levomepromazine[c]	20–40	No data	15–30	Yes; active metabolite	No data	No data	If unavoidable PO/SC: start with 2.5–3.125mg at bedtime and q4h p.r.n. *Also see Table 8 (Antipsychotics)*
Prochlorperazine[c]	6	96	15–20	Yes	No data	Probably ↑	If unavoidable Buccal: start with 3mg b.d. PO: start with 5mg t.d.s.

a. whichever drug is used, because of the altered pharmacodynamic effects of anti-emetics in severe hepatic impairment, a slower than usual titration and close monitoring of the patient are required

b. domperidone and metoclopramide should be used at the lowest effective dose for the shortest possible time because of concerns over prolonged QT interval or drug-induced movement disorders respectively

c. because of the long halflife and time taken to reach steady state, undesirable effects with these anti-emetics may only become apparent after several days or weeks of regular use.

Anti-epileptics (Table 7)

Regardless of the pharmacokinetic changes described below, in severe hepatic impairment anti-epileptics with sedative effects may cause, worsen or sometimes mask encephalopathy. A slower than usual titration and close monitoring of the patient are required.

Concurrent use of other drugs with sedative ± constipating effects, e.g. opioids, further increases the risk of toxicity.

Pharmacokinetic changes

Of the anti-epileptics generally used in palliative care (see p.280), the following should be considered in severe hepatic impairment:

- reduced protein-binding affects the most highly protein-bound, e.g. **phenytoin** and **valproate** (for monitoring purposes or when toxicity is suspected, the free fraction plasma concentration should be measured)
- all but **levetiracetam**, **oxcarbazepine** and **gabapentin/pregabalin** are dependent on CYP450
- the risk of toxicity is also greater from a pharmacokinetic drug–drug interaction involving an inhibitor of CYP450 or other enzymes responsible for metabolism of the anti-epileptic, e.g.:
  - ▷ CYP3A4 inhibitors will lead to reduced metabolism of **carbamazepine**; CYP2C9 inhibitors, of **phenobarbital** and **phenytoin**; and CYP2C19 inhibitors, of **phenytoin**
  - ▷ **valproate**, by inhibiting epoxide hydrolase, may reduce the metabolism of **carbamazepine**.

Because of the time taken for drugs to accumulate, undesirable effects may become apparent only after days or weeks of regular use for those anti-epileptics with a long halflife, e.g. **carbamazepine**, **clonazepam**, **phenobarbital**, **phenytoin**.

Oxcarbazepine is a pro-drug which is rapidly converted in the liver to an active metabolite (see p.304). The pharmacokinetics of **oxcarbazepine** and the metabolite are unchanged in mild–moderate hepatic impairment, but reduced biotransformation should be anticipated in severe impairment.

Because **phenytoin** is highly protein-bound, there is a danger of toxicity if the dose is not adjusted when a patient is hypo-albuminaemic (see Anti-epileptics, Box A, p.288) or is jaundiced. **Phenobarbital** is rarely used as an anti-epileptic in palliative care (see p.315). In a single-dose study, the halflife of **phenobarbital** increased from 86h to 130h in cirrhosis.[36] Because both **phenytoin** and **phenobarbital** should be avoided in patients with severe *renal* impairment (see Chapter 17, p.738), neither are a good choice in hepatorenal syndrome.

Levetiracetam (p.312), **gabapentin** and **pregabalin** (p.297) are not hepatically metabolized or excreted; in addition, they have low protein-binding and short halflives. Thus, they are a favourable choice in hepatic impairment. However, all require slow titration from low doses to minimize the sedative effects, and dose reduction if *renal* impairment is present.

Carbamazepine and **valproate** have been associated with hepatotoxicity and should be avoided if possible (see Drug-induced hepatotoxicity).

Choice of anti-epileptic

Levetiracetam is a good first-line choice for the long-term management of patients with a broad range of seizure types who also have severe hepatic impairment. It may also have a role in status epilepticus when benzodiazepines are insufficient (see p.312). However, it is renally excreted and a dose reduction is required when there is concurrent *renal* impairment (see p.312 and Chapter 17, p.738).

Gabapentin and **pregabalin** are also a good choice for long-term use as anti-epileptics or for neuropathic pain. Start with low doses and titrate slowly to reduce the risk of sedative effects; for patients with *renal* impairment, the dose may need to be further reduced (see p.297 and Chapter 17, p.738).

Table 7 Anti-epileptics in severe hepatic impairment. Before use, see introductory and class-specific text

Drug[a]	*PO bio-availability (%)*	*Protein-binding (%)*	*Halflife in normal liver function (h)*	*Significant hepatic metabolism*	*Significant biliary excretion of drug ± active metabolite(s)*	*Increase in halflife in severe hepatic impairment*	*Dose and comments*
Generally safer							
Gabapentin	30–75	<3	5–7	No	No	No data	Use low doses and titrate slowly PO: start with 100mg at bedtime, increase by 100mg/24h every 2–3 days; dose may need to be adjusted according to renal function (see text)
Levetiracetam	≥95	<10	6–8	No	No	No data	PO/IV: start with 250mg b.d.; dose may need to be adjusted according to renal function (see text)
Pregabalin	≥90	0	5–9	No	No	No data	Use low doses and titrate slowly PO: start with 25–50mg b.d.; dose may need to be adjusted according to renal function (see text)
Use cautiously							
Oxcarbazepine	≥95	40–60 metabolite	1–3 (metabolite = 9)	Yes; active metabolite	No	No data	*Pro-drug:* reduced bio-transformation and thus reduced/unpredictable effect; PO: start with 75mg b.d.
Avoid if possible							
Carbamazepine[b]	85–100	70–80	16–36	Yes; active metabolite	Possible	No data	If unavoidable, PO: start with 50mg b.d.
Clonazepam[b]	90	86	20–60	Yes; active metabolite	No	No data	*Not a first-line treatment for seizures* *Also see Table 9 (Benzodiazepines)*
Phenobarbital[b]	≥90	45–60	75–120	Yes	No data	<50%	If unavoidable, use only with specialist neurological supervision
Phenytoin[b]	90–95	90	20–60	Yes	Possible	No data	If unavoidable, monitor plasma levels adjusted for hypo-albuminaemia (see p.288)
Valproate	95	90–95	6–20	Yes	No	No data	If unavoidable, start with low dose and titrate slowly

a. whichever drug is used, because of the altered pharmacodynamic effects of anti-epileptics in severe hepatic impairment, a slower than usual titration and close monitoring of the patient are required

Antipsychotics (Table 8)

Regardless of the pharmacokinetic changes described below, in severe hepatic impairment antipsychotics with sedative ± constipating effects of can cause, worsen or sometimes mask encephalopathy. A slower than usual titration and close monitoring of the patient are required.

Concurrent use of other drugs with sedative ± constipating effects, e.g. opioids, further increases the risk of toxicity.

Pharmacokinetic changes

There are limited data on antipsychotics. The following should be borne in mind:

- *all* the featured antipsychotics are highly protein-bound
- *all* the featured antipsychotics are extensively metabolized in the liver and dependent on one or more of CYP3A4, CYP2D6 and CYP1A2; the risk of toxicity is greater from a pharmacokinetic drug–drug interaction with inhibitors of the relevant CYP450, e.g. **haloperidol**, **quetiapine**, **risperidone** (CYP3A4), **haloperidol** and **risperidone** (CYP2D6), **olanzapine** (CYP1A2).

Undesirable effects may become apparent only after days or weeks of regular use for those antipsychotics with long halflives, e.g. **haloperidol**, **olanzapine**, **risperidone**. Concurrent use of other drugs with CNS-depressant activity, e.g. opioids, increases the risk of toxicity.

The risk of prolongation of the QT interval (and thereby risk of ventricular arrhythmia) may be higher with **haloperidol** and lowest for **quetiapine**. The risk may be increased as a result of, e.g. drug accumulation, drug–drug interaction, concurrent use of other drugs that either prolong the QT interval or cause electrolyte imbalance.

Olanzapine has a long halflife and only moderate PO bio-availability. Based on this, a lower starting dose is recommended, only increasing with caution.

The halflife of **risperidone** is not significantly increased in patients with severe hepatic impairment. However, despite normal plasma levels, the free (unbound) fraction is increased by about 40%. Thus, lower doses are needed in severe hepatic impairment. The clearance of **risperidone** is reduced in *moderate renal* impairment (see Chapter 17, p.741). Thus, it is not a good choice in hepatorenal syndrome.

Quetiapine has a short halflife. Clearance is reduced by 25% in patients with stable alcoholic cirrhosis, thus lower doses are needed.

Antipsychotics can be associated with increased LFTs; rarely, significant hepatotoxicity can occur.[37]

Choice of antipsychotic

Generally, the long-term use of antipsychotics should be avoided in severe hepatic impairment.[31] If unavoidable, based on pharmacokinetic parameters, **quetiapine** is the best choice for the long-term treatment of psychosis, mania and bipolar disorder.

For the long-term use of antipsychotics as anti-emetics, see Anti-emetics, p.767 and Table 6. For the short-term use of antipsychotics in the last days of life, see Last days of life section, p.779.

Benzodiazepines and Z-drugs (Table 9)

Regardless of the pharmacokinetic changes described below, in severe hepatic impairment the sedative effects of benzodiazepines and Z-drugs can cause, worsen or sometimes mask encephalopathy.[38,39] A slower than usual titration and close monitoring of the patient are required.

Concurrent use of other drugs with CNS depressant ± constipating effects, e.g. opioids, further increases the risk of toxicity.

Pharmacokinetic changes

Of the featured benzodiazepines and Z-drugs generally used long-term in palliative care, all are significantly hepatically metabolized and contra-indicated in severe hepatic impairment. For those drugs metabolized by CYP450 enzymes, e.g. **diazepam**, **zopiclone** (see p.167), the risk of toxicity is greater from a pharmacokinetic drug–drug interaction involving an inhibitor of CYP450. Further, all the featured benzodiazepines (but not **zopiclone**) are highly protein-bound.

Table 8 Antipsychotics in severe hepatic impairment. Before use, see introductory and class-specific text

Drug[a]	*PO bio-availability (%)*	*Protein-binding (%)*	*Halflife in normal liver function (h)*	*Significant hepatic metabolism*	*Significant biliary excretion of drug ± active metabolite(s)*	*Increase in halflife in severe hepatic impairment (h)*	*Dose and comments*
Use cautiously							
Olanzapine[b]	60	93	34 (52 elderly)	Yes	Possible	No data	PO: start with 2.5–5mg at bedtime
Quetiapine[c]	100	83	6–14	Yes; active metabolite	No	Probably ↑	PO: start with 12.5mg b.d.; increase daily by 12.5mg
Risperidone[b]	99	90	20[d]	Yes; active metabolite	No	No	PO: start with 500microgram at bedtime; increase by 500microgram every 3–4 days
Avoid if possible							
Haloperidol[b]	45–75	92	12–38	Yes; active metabolite	Possible	No data	If unavoidable, PO/SC: start with 500microgram at bedtime and q4h p.r.n. *Also see Table 6 (Anti-emetics)*
Levomepromazine[b]	20–40	No data	15–30	Yes; active metabolite	No data	No data	*Not a first-line treatment for psychosis* *Also see Table 6 (Anti-emetics)*

a. whichever drug is used, because of the altered pharmacodynamic effects of antipsychotics in severe hepatic impairment, a slower than usual titration and close monitoring of the patient are required

b. because of the long halflife and time taken to reach steady state, undesirable effects with these antipsychotics may only become apparent after several days or weeks of regular use

c. avoid m/r products

d. total for the parent drug and active metabolite.

Table 9 Benzodiazepines and Z-drugs in severe hepatic impairment. Before use, see introductory and class-specific text

Drug[a]	*PO bio-availability (%)*	*Protein-binding (%)*	*Halflife in normal liver function (h)*	*Significant hepatic metabolism*	*Significant biliary excretion of drug ± active metabolite(s)*	*Increase in halflife in severe hepatic impairment (h)*	*Dose and comments*
Use cautiously							
Lorazepam[b]	90	85	10–20	Yes	No	See text	SL/PO: start with 500microgram/24h
Zopiclone	75	45–80	5	Yes; active metabolite	No	>100%	PO: start with 3.75mg at bedtime
Avoid if possible							
Clonazepam[b]	90	86	20–60	Yes; active metabolite	No	No data	See text; *also see Table 7 (Anti-epileptics)*
Diazepam[b]	90	95–99	25–50 (≤200[c])	Yes; active metabolites	No	>100%	See text
Temazepam	90	96	8–15	Yes	No	No	If unavoidable PO: start with 5mg at bedtime

a. whichever drug is used, because of the altered pharmacodynamic effects of benzodiazepines and Z-drugs in severe hepatic impairment, a slower than usual titration and close monitoring of the patient are required

b. because of the long halflife and time taken to reach steady state, undesirable effects with these benzodiazepines and Z-drugs may only become apparent after several days or weeks of regular use

c. active metabolite.

18

Table 10 Miscellaneous drugs in severe hepatic impairment. Before use, see introductory and class-specific text

Drug[a]	*PO bio-availability (%)*	*Protein-binding (%)*	*Halflife in normal liver function (h)*	*Significant hepatic metabolism*	*Significant biliary excretion of drug ± active metabolite(s)*	*Increase in halflife in severe hepatic impairment (h)*	*Relative safety*	*Dose and comments*
Acid suppressants								
Lansoprazole	80–90	97	1–2	Yes	No	<500%	**Use cautiously**	See text. PO: start with 15mg once daily; maximum dose 30mg once daily
Omeprazole	60	95	0.5–3	Yes	No	See text	**Use cautiously**	PO: start with 10mg once daily; maximum dose 20mg once daily
Ranitidine	50	15	2–3	No	No	No data	**Generally safer**	Dose unchanged; may need adjustment according to renal function
Antidiarrhoeals								
Loperamide	<1	80	9–14	Yes	No	No data	**Avoid**	If unavoidable PO: start with 2mg stat
Antimuscarinics								
Glycopyrronium	<5	No data	1–1.5	Possible	Possible	No data	**Use cautiously**	SC: start with 200microgram q2h p.r.n. CSCI: start with 600microgram/24h
Hyoscine *butylbromide*	<1	4	1–5	Possible	No data	No data	**Use cautiously**	SC: start with 20mg q1h p.r.n. CSCI: start with 60mg/24h
Bisphosphonates and denosumab								
Bisphosphonates	N/A	Variable	N/A	No	No	No data	**Generally safer**	Dose unchanged; may need adjustment according to renal function (see text)

continued

Table 10 Continued

Drug[a]	*PO bio-availability (%)*	*Protein-binding (%)*	*Halflife in normal liver function (h)*	*Significant hepatic metabolism*	*Significant biliary excretion of drug ± active metabolite(s)*	*Increase in halflife in severe hepatic impairment (h)*	*Relative safety*	*Dose and comments*
Denosumab	N/A	Variable	N/A	No	No	No data	**Generally safer**	Dose unchanged
Laxatives	N/A	N/A	N/A	N/A	N/A	N/A	**Generally safer**	Dose unchanged
Skeletal muscle relaxants								
Baclofen	>90	30	3–4	No	No	No data	**Use cautiously**	PO: start with 5mg once daily; dose may need adjustment according to renal function (see text)
Tizanidine	40	30	3	Yes	No	Probably ↑	**Avoid**	See text
Systemic corticosteroids								
Dexamethasone	78	77	4.5	Yes	No	Yes	**Use cautiously**	PO: start with 2–16mg once daily according to indication, see p.556
Other								
Octreotide	N/A	65	1.5	Yes	Possible	Yes	**Use cautiously**	SC: lower maintenance doses may be sufficient
Spironolactone	60–90	90	1.5 (14–17)[b]	Yes; active metabolites	Possible	<600%	**Use cautiously**	PO: once daily dose; monitor electrolytes closely, see p.73

a. whichever drug is used, because of the altered pharmacodynamic effects in severe hepatic impairment, a slower than usual titration and close monitoring of the patient are required
b. active metabolite.

Because of the time taken for drugs to accumulate, undesirable effects may become apparent only after days or weeks of regular use for those benzodiazepines with a long halflife, e.g. **clonazepam**, **diazepam**.

Although the halflife of **lorazepam** has been shown to double in cirrhosis, plasma clearance is *not* affected. The increased halflife is explained by an increased volume of distribution, caused by a reduction in plasma protein-binding.[39]

Temazepam is metabolized by direct conjugation and is not dependent on CYP450 metabolism, which may explain why the halflife is little changed in cirrhosis.[39,40]

The halflife of **diazepam** in healthy subjects is very long (≤5 days, with an active metabolite halflife of ≤8 days). In cirrhosis this more than doubles.[41]

Zopiclone is hepatically metabolized by CYP3A4. Although the halflife is relatively short in comparison to other sedatives, in patients with cirrhosis it more than doubles.[42] The SPC states that plasma clearance of **zopiclone** is delayed by 40%.

Choice of benzodiazepine or Z-drug

Generally, the use of benzodiazepines or Z-drugs as sedatives or anxiolytics should be avoided in severe hepatic impairment. If unavoidable, limit their use to the short-term, ideally <1 week. Based on pharmacokinetic parameters, **zopiclone** may be a reasonable choice as a night sedative, and **lorazepam** as an anxiolytic. **Lorazepam** is also used short-term to manage alcohol withdrawal symptoms; seek hepatology advice.[43]

For other indications, e.g. myoclonus, restless leg syndrome, muscle spasm and prophylaxis of seizures, longer-acting benzodiazepines (e.g. **clonazepam**, **diazepam**) should be generally avoided because they are not a first-line choice in these settings (see p.168) and have unfavourable pharmacokinetics in severe hepatic impairment.

For the emergency use of benzodiazepines for seizures, see p.290. For the use of **midazolam** in the last days of life, see Last days of life section, p.779.

Miscellaneous drugs (Table 10)

Regardless of the pharmacokinetic changes described below, in severe hepatic impairment drugs with sedative ± constipating effects can cause, worsen or sometimes mask encephalopathy. A slower than usual titration and close monitoring of the patient are required.

Concurrent use of other drugs with CNS depressant ± constipating effects, e.g. opioids, further increases the risk of toxicity.

The relative safety and dose adjustments for other common palliative care drugs for long-term use in severe hepatic impairment are shown in Table 10.

PPIs (p.31) are generally preferred to H_2-receptor antagonists (p.27). In patients with cirrhosis, it is recommended that PPI use be limited to specific indications, e.g. peptic ulcer disease, because of concerns of a possible association with poorer outcomes (e.g. increased risk of spontaneous bacterial peritonitis, hepatic encephalopathy and mortality).[44,45] In cirrhosis, there is a significant increase in overall exposure to **lansoprazole** and, to a lesser extent, **omeprazole**, leading some to recommend against their respective use in mild and severe hepatic impairment.[44] However, in practice, both have been used in severe hepatic impairment in lower PO doses.

When indicated, **ranitidine** (the *PCF* H_2 antagonist of choice; see p.27) has a favourable pharmacokinetic profile in severe hepatic impairment. It is not extensively hepatically metabolized, and has a short halflife and low protein-binding. However, dose reduction is needed with concurrent *renal* impairment.

Antidiarrhoeals, e.g. **loperamide**, should generally be avoided in severe hepatic impairment because of the risk of their constipating effect causing, worsening or masking encephalopathy. Further, **loperamide** is extensively hepatically metabolized, with most of the drug removed by first-pass metabolism. Thus, severe hepatic impairment may result in an increase in plasma levels of **loperamide**, increasing the risk of prolonged QT interval and CNS toxicity (see p.36).

There are a lack of pharmacokinetic data for antimuscarinic drugs in severe hepatic impairment. Unlike **hyoscine *hydrobromide*** (which should be avoided), **hyoscine *butylbromide*** and **glycopyrronium** do not generally cross the blood–brain barrier. However, because of the lack of data, potential for greater CNS penetration and their constipating effects, both **hyoscine *butylbromide*** and **glycopyrronium** should be used cautiously in severe hepatic impairment. For the use of antimuscarinics for noisy rattling breathing at the end of life, see Box D.

Despite the lack of data, based on their favourable pharmacokinetic profile, bisphosphonates can be used in severe hepatic impairment. They are not hepatically metabolized but are renally excreted. Reduced doses are required in patients with concurrent *renal* impairment, with **ibandronic acid** associated with less renal toxicity than other bisphosphonates (see Chapter 17, p.746). **Denosumab** (p.549) is an alternate osteoclast inhibitor that is generally safe in both hepatic and renal impairment.

Full data for laxatives have not been included. Generally, laxatives are not absorbed and can be used in usual doses. Laxatives should be routinely prescribed and carefully titrated against bowel movement for patients taking opioids, to minimize the risk of constipation (see QCG: Opioid-induced constipation, p.45). **Lactulose** and **macrogols** are used in the treatment of hepatic encephalopathy (see Simplifying long-term hepatic drugs, below).

Of the skeletal muscle relaxants used long-term, **baclofen** has a favourable pharmacokinetic profile in severe hepatic impairment. However, it should be used cautiously, with lower starting doses, because of its sedative properties. Further, toxicity can occur in moderate–severe *renal* impairment, see p.660. Because **tizanidine** is extensively hepatically metabolized and can cause hepatotoxicity in high doses (see Drug-induced hepatotoxicity, p.755), it should be avoided.

Systemic corticosteroids are generally mostly hepatically metabolized. Because of their salt- and water-retaining properties, they can cause or worsen ascites. They also have the potential to cause or worsen encephalopathy and to increase the risk of GI bleeding in patients with coagulopathy or oesophageal varices (Box B). Thus, **dexamethasone**, the most frequent systemic corticosteroid used in palliative care, should be used cautiously at the lowest effective dose.

The halflife of **octreotide** (p.591) may be increased in cirrhosis, and the SPC recommends adjusting the maintenance dose in these patients. **Octreotide** has an inhibitory effect on gallbladder motility and bile secretion; the clinical relevance of this in this setting is uncertain.

Spironolactone (p.73) is authorized in hepatic cirrhosis with ascites and oedema. The dose can generally be given once daily because of the significantly increased halflife in cirrhosis.[46] Because of the risk of electrolyte imbalance (particularly hyperkalaemia and hyponatraemia), close monitoring is required, see p.73.

SIMPLIFYING LONG-TERM HEPATIC DRUGS

Patients may be taking long-term drugs to manage the various aspects of their liver disease, e.g. ascites, encephalopathy, pruritus (see below). Generally, these should be continued in patients with a primary diagnosis of end-stage liver disease when a liver transplant is a possible option. However, their ongoing necessity can be reviewed as the end of life approaches, e.g. in those with a primary diagnosis of end-stage liver disease for whom a liver transplant is not appropriate, and in those with severe hepatic impairment caused by incurable cancer. The decision of when to stop these drugs is informed by considering the:

- prognosis of the patient
- purpose of the drug
- degree of hepatic impairment
- risk of undesirable effects from continuing the drug vs. the likely effects from stopping it
- burden of taking tablets.

Prognosis of patients with end-stage liver disease is variable. Although median survival is about 2 years, death can be relatively sudden and unexpected. Median survival is reduced in the presence of:

- severe or refractory encephalopathy (12 months)
- refractory ascites (6 months)
- hepatorenal syndrome; type 2 (3–6 months), type 1 (2–4 weeks).[47]

The guidance below should be used in conjunction with specialist hepatology advice.

Antibiotic prophylaxis for spontaneous bacterial peritonitis

Prophylactic antibiotics, e.g. **ciprofloxacin** 500mg once daily, are used to reduce the high risk of bacterial peritonitis from a long-term indwelling ascitic drain or peritoneal catheter. These can be discontinued in the last weeks of life.

Antihypertensives

These should generally be discontinued in the last weeks of life, because of the risk of hypotension/falls and subdural bleeds, unless being taken for prophylaxis of variceal bleeding (see below).

Antiretrovirals

Generally, these are continued as long as the patient is able to take them. Discussion with local HIV teams is advised.

Diuretics for management of ascites

Management of ascites should focus on maintaining comfort and symptom control. **Spironolactone ± furosemide** PO are the diuretics of choice (see p.73 and p.67) and should be continued if stopping is likely to exacerbate symptoms, and whilst the patient can tolerate PO tablets. They are generally discontinued in the last days of life. An ascitic drain can be considered for symptomatic relief.

Drugs for mineral and bone disease

Cirrhosis is a risk factor for osteoporosis, and many patients may be taking **calcium** and **vitamin D** supplements. These can be discontinued.

Drugs for management of hepatic encephalopathy

Oral drugs for the management of hepatic encephalopathy, e.g. **lactulose** (p.54), **macrogol** 3350 (off-label) and **rifaximin** 550mg b.d., should be continued as long as possible and/or tolerated, with the aim of inducing bowel movements twice a day. Where PO treatment is not possible and administration via naso-gastric tube is inappropriate, the use of **phosphate** enemas (p.59) may be considered.

Drugs for portal hypertension/prophylaxis of variceal bleeding

Where portal hypertension is being treated with beta-blockers, e.g. **carvedilol**, **propranolol**, these should be continued whilst the patient can tolerate PO tablets. ACE inhibitors should be stopped if renal function is poor or when ascites develops.

Drugs for pruritus

Pruritus can be a debilitating symptom of cholestasis of any cause, including cirrhosis, causing discomfort, poor sleep and anxiety. Identification of cause is important, and treatment for cholestatic-related pruritus should be continued if possible. Also see Chapter 26, p.825 and **Rifampicin**, p.518.

Immunosuppressants

Generally, these are continued as long as the patient is able to take them. Discussion with hepatology/liver transplant teams is advised for those taking immunosuppressants who have previously undergone transplantation.

Thiamine and vitamin supplements

Patients with alcohol-related liver disease may be taking **thiamine** and other vitamin supplements. These can be discontinued.

Vitamin K

Vitamin K replacement should be limited to conscious patients with a reasonable performance status for whom other supportive measures are deemed appropriate, e.g. blood transfusion. Vitamin K should not be used in moribund patients in an attempt to prevent an imminent inevitable death, see p.632.

LAST DAYS OF LIFE

Currently, there are no national guidelines for prescribing for patients with severe or end-stage hepatic impairment in the last days of life. Box D contains suggested starting doses for common symptoms based on consensus clinical experience. As the majority of drugs have CNS depressant effects ± cause constipation, one of the major challenges is to alleviate symptoms without precipitating or worsening encephalopathy. Thus, with all drugs, appropriate caution, close monitoring and individualized titration, initially with small doses, is required. Generally, SC p.r.n. injections are prescribed to facilitate this.

Box D Anticipatory prescribing in patients with severe or end-stage hepatic impairment in the last days of life

Starting doses given below are based on consensus clinical experience and take into account the risk of accumulation and toxicity; they may be lower than used in other circumstances; see individual drug monographs and Chapter 14, p.713. Generally, initial titration is with SC p.r.n. injections rather than CSCI.

Pain

In some liver units, fentanyl SC/CSCI is the first-line choice in patients with severe hepatic impairment, particularly when there is concurrent renal impairment (see Opioids section). However, it is uncertain if this outweighs the advantages of more cautious use of more familiar opioids in this setting. Starting dose in opioid-naïve patients:

- fentanyl 12.5–25microgram SC q1h p.r.n.
- morphine 2.5mg SC q1h p.r.n.

Breathlessness

Fentanyl can be used for breathlessness as well as pain; when there is concurrent anxiety, combine with midazolam 1–2.5mg SC q1h p.r.n.

Noisy rattling breathing

Hyoscine *butylbromide* 20mg SC q1h p.r.n.
Also see QCG: Death rattle (noisy rattling breathing), p.11.

Nausea and vomiting

Haloperidol 0.5–1mg SC q1h p.r.n.

Agitation, restlessness, myoclonus

Midazolam 1–2.5mg SC q1h p.r.n.

Delirium

Haloperidol ± midazolam, starting with similar doses and frequency to above.

1 Gupta NK and Lewis JH (2008) Review article: the use of potentially hepatotoxic drugs in patients with liver disease. *Alimentary Pharmacology and Therapeutics*. **28**: 1021–1041.

2 Low G *et al.* (2015) Hepatorenal syndrome: aetiology, diagnosis, and treatment. *Gastroenterology Research and Practice*. **15**: Article ID 207012.

3 Vilstrup H *et al.* (2014) Hepatic encephalopathy in chronic liver disease: 2014 practice guideline by the American association for the study of liver diseases and the European association for the study of the liver. *Hepatology*. **60**: 715–735.

4 Wijdicks EF (2016) Hepatic encephalopathy. *New England Journal of Medicine*. **375**: 1660–1670.

5 Albers I *et al.* (1989) Superiority of the Child-Pugh classification to quantitative liver function tests for assessing prognosis of liver cirrhosis. *Scandinavian Journal of Gastroenterology*. **24**: 269–276.

6 Lee WM (2003) Drug-induced hepatotoxicity. *New England Journal of Medicine*. **349**: 474–485.

7 Schenker S *et al.* (1999) Antecedent liver disease and drug toxicity. *Journal of Hepatology*. **31**: 1098–1105.

8 Banks AT *et al.* (1995) Diclofenac-associated hepatotoxicity: analysis of 180 cases reported to the food and drug administration as adverse reactions. *Hepatology*. **22**: 820–827.

9 Carrillo-Jimenez R and Nurnberger M (2000) Celecoxib-induced acute pancreatitis and hepatitis: a case report. *Archives of Internal Medicine*. **160**: 553–554.

10 Hernandez-Diaz S and Garcia-Rodriguez LA (2001) Epidemiologic assessment of the safety of conventional nonsteroidal anti-inflammatory drugs. *American Journal of Medicine*. **110 (Suppl 3A)**: 20s–27s.

11 Chalasani NP *et al.* (2014) American college of gastroenterology clinical guideline: The diagnosis and management of idiosyncratic drug-induced liver injury. *American Journal of Gastroenterology*. **109**: 950–966.

12 North-Lewis P (ed.) (2008) *Drugs and the liver* London: Pharmaceutical Press. pp. 103–126.

13 Weersink RA *et al.* (2020) Safe use of medication in patients with cirrhosis: pharmacokinetic and pharmacodynamic considerations. *Expert Opinion on Drug Metabolism & Toxicology*. **16**: 45–57.

14 Delco F *et al.* (2005) Dose adjustment in patients with liver disease. *Drug Safety*. **28**: 529–545.

15 MHRA (2017) Direct-acting antivirals to treat chronic hepatitis C: risk of interaction with vitamin K antagonists and changes in INR. *Drug Safety Update*. www.gov.uk/drug-safety-update.

16 Weersink RA *et al.* (2019) Evaluation of information in Summaries of Product Characteristics (SmPCs) on the use of a medicine in patients with hepatic impairment. *Frontiers in Pharmacology*. **10**: 1031.

17 Weersink RA *et al.* (2018) Evidence-based recommendations to improve the safe use of drugs in patients with liver cirrhosis. *Drug Safety*. **41**: 603–613.

18 UK Medicines Information (2014) What pharmacokinetic and pharmacodynamic factors need to be considered when prescribing drugs for patients with liver disease? *Medicines Q&A* 170.3. www.evidence.nhs.uk.

19 Forrest JA *et al.* (1979) Paracetamol metabolism in chronic liver disease. *European Journal of Clinical Pharmacology*. **15**: 427–431.

20 Hayward KL *et al.* (2016) Can paracetamol (acetaminophen) be administered to patients with liver impairment? *British Journal of Clinical Pharmacology*. **81**: 210–222.

21 King's College Hospital. (2018) Guidelines for the prescribing for symptom control in patients with hepatic impairment. London.

22 Lee YC *et al.* (2012) Non-steroidal anti-inflammatory drugs use and risk of upper gastrointestinal adverse events in cirrhotic patients. *Liver International*. **32**: 859–866.

23 Juhl RP *et al.* (1983) Ibuprofen and sulindac kinetics in alcoholic liver disease. *Clinical Pharmacology and Therapeutics*. **34**: 104–109.

24 Bosilkovska M *et al.* (2012) Analgesics in patients with hepatic impairment: Pharmacology and clinical implications. *Drugs*. **72**: 1645–1669.

25 Hasselstrom J *et al.* (1990) The metabolism and bioavailability of morphine in patients with severe liver cirrhosis. *British Journal of Clinical Pharmacology*. **29**: 289–297.

26 Tegeder I *et al.* (1999) Pharmacokinetics of opioids in liver disease. *Clinical Pharmacokinetics*. **37**: 17–40.

27 Haberer JP *et al.* (1982) Fentanyl pharmacokinetics in anaesthetized patients with cirrhosis. *British Journal of Anaesthesia*. **54**: 1267–1270.

28 Choi L *et al.* (2016) Population pharmacokinetics of fentanyl in the critically ill. *Critical Care Medicine*. **44**: 64–72.

29 Durnin C *et al.* (2001) Pharmacokinetics of oral immediate-release hydromorphone (Dilaudid IR) in subjects with moderate hepatic impairment. *Proceedings of the Western Pharmacology Society*. **44**: 83–84.

30 Tallgren M *et al.* (1997) Pharmacokinetics and ventilatory effects of oxycodone before and after liver transplantation. *Clinical Pharmacology and Therapeutics*. **61**: 655–661.

31 Taylor D, Barnes, T. and Young, A (eds) (2018) *The Maudsley Prescribing Guidelines in Psychiatry* (13th edn): Wiley Blackwell. pp. 635–643.

32 Albani F *et al.* (1991) Kinetics of intravenous metoclopramide in patients with hepatic cirrhosis. *European Journal of Clinical Pharmacology*. **40**: 423–425.

33 Magueur E *et al.* (1991) Pharmacokinetics of metoclopramide in patients with liver cirrhosis. *British Journal of Clinical Pharmacology*. **31**: 185–187.

34 Figg WD *et al.* (1996) Pharmacokinetics of ondansetron in patients with hepatic insufficiency. *Journal of Clinical Pharmacology*. **36**: 206–215.

35 North-Lewis P (ed.) (2008) *Drugs and the Liver*. Pharmaceutical Press, London. pp. 211.

36 Alvin J *et al.* (1975) The effect of liver disease in man on the disposition of phenobarbital. *Journal of Pharmacology and Experimental Therapeutics*. **192**: 224–235.

37 Marwick KF *et al.* (2012) Antipsychotics and abnormal liver function tests: Systematic review. *Clinical Neuropharmacology*. **35**: 244–253.

38 Shull HJ *et al.* (1976) Normal disposition of oxazepam in acute viral hepatitis and cirrhosis. *Annals of internal medicine*. **84**: 420–425.

39 Kraus JW *et al.* (1978) Effects of aging and liver disease on disposition of lorazepam. *Clinical Pharmacology and Therapeutics*. **24**: 411–419.

40 Ghabrial H *et al.* (1986) The effects of age and chronic liver disease on the elimination of temazepam. *European Journal of Clinical Pharmacology*. **30**: 93–97.

41 Klotz U *et al.* (1975) The effects of age and liver disease on the disposition and elimination of diazepam in adult man. *Journal of Clinical Investigation*. **55**: 347–359.

42 Parker G and Roberts CJ (1983) Plasma concentrations and central nervous system effects of the new hypnotic agent zopiclone in patients with chronic liver disease. *British Journal of Clinical Pharmacology*. **16**: 259–265.

43 NICE (2018) Acute alcohol withdrawal. *NICE Pathways*. www.nice.org.uk.

44 Weersink RA *et al.* (2018) Safe use of proton pump inhibitors in patients with cirrhosis. *British Journal of Clinical Pharmacology* **84**: 1806–1820.

45 Tripathi D *et al.* (2015) UK guidelines on the management of variceal haemorrhage in cirrhotic patients. *Gut*. **64**: 1680–1704.

46 Sungaila I *et al.* (1992) Spironolactone pharmacokinetics and pharmacodynamics in patients with cirrhotic ascites. *Gastroenterology*. **102**: 1680–1685.

47 Potosek J *et al.* (2014) Integration of palliative care in end-stage liver disease and liver transplantation. *Journal of Palliative Medicine*. **17**: 1271–1277.

Updated (minor change) February 2022

19: VARIABILITY IN RESPONSE TO DRUGS

19

VARIABILITY IN RESPONSE TO DRUGS

There is great inter-individual variability in the way people respond to a drug (Box A). Some of this variability is predictable in the presence of clinical factors known to impact upon the pharmacokinetics and/or pharmacodynamics of a drug. For example, an age-related decrease in overall metabolic capacity of the liver, because of reductions in liver mass, liver enzyme activity and hepatic blood flow, results in the elderly being at a significantly higher risk of toxicity from drugs metabolized in the liver. Similarly, an age-related decline in renal function can reduce the excretion of active drugs and metabolites, e.g., morphine-6-glucuronide and morphine-3-glucuronide, increasing the risk of toxicity from morphine (see Chapter 17, p.731).

Genetic variations also contribute towards differences in drug response. Clinically, these are less predictable, although some may be detected with specific testing. They are particularly important for drugs metabolized by cytochrome P450 (CYP450), with the rate of metabolism either reduced or increased. Examples of how these manifest include:

- reduced or no response because of:
  - ▷ the failure to convert a pro-drug to its active form
  - ▷ increased metabolism of an active drug to an inactive metabolite
- increased toxicity because of:
  - ▷ more rapid conversion to the active form or to a metabolite which is more active than the parent drug
  - ▷ failure to metabolize an active drug to inactive metabolite(s).

Other genetic variations, such as genes coding for receptors or drug transporters, also can influence overall response, e.g., the μ-opioid receptor or P-glycoprotein transporter and the response to opioids. Induction or inhibition of CYP450 activity also can result from a drug–drug or drug–food interaction, causing similar manifestations to those resulting from genetic variation. Each of these factors is considered in more detail below.

VARIABILITY IN RESPONSE TO OPIOIDS

Many factors contribute to the inter-individual variation in response to opioids.[1-5]

μ-Opioid receptor

This is the key receptor mediating opioid analgesia.[6] Genetic variation in the μ-opioid receptor gene has been associated with variation in opioid response in acute post-operative pain,[7] chronic non-cancer pain,[8,9] and cancer pain.[10,11] However, meta-analysis of opioid pain studies showed no overall association with pain and only weak associations with **morphine** dose or undesirable effects.[12]

Box A Common factors affecting response to drugs

Adherence
Whether drug regimen adhered to or not

Genetic variation/polymorphism
Sequence variation, including single nucleotide polymorphisms, gene deletions, gene duplications resulting in altered protein function, e.g. of receptors, enzymes, drug transporters

Pharmacokinetics
Absorption
Distribution
Metabolism
Drug–drug and drug–food interactions
Excretion

Pharmacodynamics
Receptor–drug interaction and effect
Drug–drug and drug–food interactions
Decreased/increased receptor affinity due to concurrent disease state

Physiological factors
Sex
Age
Ethnicity
Hormonal changes
Circadian and seasonal factors

Environmental factors
Diet
Environmental toxins
Alcohol and recreational drugs
Smoking

Potential specific associations/concomitant disease
Diabetes mellitus
GI microbiology
Hypoalbuminaemia
Liver failure
Malabsorption
Malnutrition
Obesity
Renal failure

P-glycoprotein

The membrane-bound drug transporter P-glycoprotein influences drug absorption and drug excretion.[13,14] It limits the uptake of compounds from the GI tract, regulates the transfer of various drugs across the blood–brain barrier,[15] and influences drug excretion by the liver and kidneys. It is encoded by the ATP-binding cassette subfamily B member 1 (ABCB1) gene.

P-glycoprotein modulation of opioid CNS concentrations varies substantially between opioids, with **morphine**, **fentanyl** and **methadone** being among those most affected.[16,17] In animals, removal (in 'knockout' mice) or inhibition (by **ciclosporin**) of P-glycoprotein activity enhances absorption and increases CNS concentrations of **fentanyl** and **morphine**, resulting in prolonged analgesia.[18] Thus, inhibitors of P-glycoprotein (e.g. **ciclosporin**, **clarithromycin**, **erythromycin**, **itraconazole**, **ketoconazole**, **quinidine** (not UK), **verapamil**) could increase CNS effects of opioids.

Variation in ABCB1 has been associated with increased pain relief with **morphine** in cancer pain[10] and decreased opioid requirements in mixed chronic pain.[9] Studies have shown conflicting results in relation to opioid-induced nausea and vomiting and other undesirable effects.[19-21]

Catechol-O-methyltransferase

Catechol-O-methyltransferase (COMT) is an enzyme which has a significant impact on the metabolism of several important neurotransmitters: dopamine, adrenaline (epinephrine) and noradrenaline (norepinephrine). The COMT gene is polymorphic, and <25% of Caucasians have low-activity variants.

One common variant in which the amino acid valine is substituted for methionine results in a 3–4 times decrease in COMT activity. It has been associated with increased pain sensitivity and higher μ-opioid system activation in experimental pain,[22,23] and increased **morphine** dose requirements in cancer patients.[24] Other variants of the COMT gene are associated with increased undesirable opioid effects, e.g. nausea and vomiting.[19,25,26]

Hepatic metabolism

Opioid metabolism takes place primarily in the liver. Opioids are metabolized via two main pathways, CYP450 and uridine diphosphate glucuronosyltransferase (UGT; Table 1). Two phases of metabolism are generally described: phase 1 metabolism (modification reactions) and phase 2 metabolism (conjugation reactions).

The most important phase 1 reaction is oxidation, catalysed by CYP450. The most important phase 2 reaction is glucuronidation, catalysed by UGT. Glucuronidation produces molecules which are highly hydrophilic and thus easily excreted by the kidneys.[27] Drug–drug interactions can occur from changes in CYP450 (see below) or UGT activity, although the latter are less well documented.[28]

Table 1 Major opioid enzyme pathways

Drug	*Pathway*[a]			
	CYP2D6	*CYP3A4/5*	*CYP2B6*	*UGT*
Alfentanil		++		
Buprenorphine		++		+
Codeine	++			+
Dihydrocodeine	+			+
Fentanyl		++		
Hydrocodone	+			
Hydromorphone				++
Methadone		++	++	
Morphine				++
Oxycodone	+	++		
Oxymorphone		+		+
Sufentanil		++		
Tapentadol				++
Tramadol	++	++		

a. ++ for CYP pathways may result in clinically important drug–drug interactions (Table 8).

GENETIC POLYMORPHISM IN CYTOCHROME P450 (CYP450)

About 75% of all drugs are metabolized partly or completely by CYP450 (Box B). Thus, variation in activity of the CYP450 system can have a major impact on drug action.

Box B Cytochrome P450 (CYP450)[29,30]

CYP450 is a super-family of numerous enzymic proteins responsible for the oxidative metabolism of many drugs and some endogenous substances (e.g. fatty acids, eicosanoids, steroids, bile acids).

The root symbol used in naming the individual enzymes is CYP, followed by:
- a number designating the enzyme family (18 in humans)
- a capital letter designating the subfamily (44 in humans)
- a number designating the individual enzyme.

CYP450 enzymes exist in virtually all tissues, but their highest concentration is in the liver.

The enzymes concerned with drug metabolism are mostly CYP1–CYP3; these account for about 70% of the total CYP450 content of the liver.

The most important enzyme is CYP3A4, followed by CYP2D6 and CYP2C9.

The presence of CYP3A4 in the wall of the GI tract is important; it probably acts in conjunction with P-glycoprotein, and to determine the extent of the intestinal metabolism of CYP3A4 substrates.

Some 20–25% of drugs are affected by genetic variants of drug-metabolizing enzymes.[31] The bulk of the population will manifest a normal distribution in terms of the rate of drug metabolism, with activity ranging from well below average to well above average, but generally lumped together as extensive metabolizers (EM).[32] In addition, there are discrete genetic populations of individuals who fall beyond the ends of the spectrum. These are designated poor (PM) and ultra-rapid metabolizers (URM). More recently, intermediate metabolizers have been identified for some enzymes (Table 2).[29]

Table 2 Metabolizer status[33]

Category	*Description*	*Possible impact*
Poor (PM) *or* slow	Lacks functional enzyme (deletion of gene or non-functional variant)	Increased toxicity due to slower drug metabolism (e.g. flecainide, phenytoin) *or* Therapeutic failure due to poor metabolism of a pro-drug to its active form (e.g. codeine) or a parent drug to an active metabolite (e.g. tamoxifen, tramadol)
Intermediate	Has two decreased-function enzymes or one decreased, one non-functional	Comparable to slow metabolizer but less marked
Extensive (EM) *or* rapid	Has at least one fully functional enzyme	This is the norm
Ultra-rapid (URM)	Increased enzyme activity (duplication of gene or other mutation); relatively rare	Therapeutic failure due to faster drug metabolism *or* Increased toxicity due to faster conversion of parent drug to more active metabolite (e.g. tramadol) *or* pro-drug to active form (e.g. codeine)

As a general rule, a URM may need a higher dose to obtain a therapeutic effect, and a PM a lower dose to prevent increased undesirable effects (Table 3).[31] Exceptions are pro-drugs where metabolites are mainly responsible for the effect of the drug (see below). The effects of such genetic variations can be further modified by the co-administration of the relevant CYP450 inhibitor or inducer.

Table 3 Genetic polymorphism and PM/URM status[a,27,29,34-36]

Pathway	*A selection of affected drugs*	*Population affected*
CYP2C9	NSAIDs Phenytoin Sulfonylureas (glipizide, tolbutamide) Warfarin	Caucasians 35% Asian/African <1%
CYP2C19	Antidepressants (amitriptyline, imipramine, sertraline) Clopidogrel[b] Diazepam PPIs	Asians 10–35% Africans 15% Caucasians 2–5%
CYP2D6 (debrisoquine hydroxylase)	β-Blockers (metoprolol)[c] Codeine[b] Oxycodone SSRIs (some, e.g. paroxetine) Tamoxifen[b] TCAs (amitriptyline, imipramine, nortriptyline)[b,d] Tramadol[b]	Africans 0–34% Caucasians 5–10% Asians ≤1%

a. there are a roughly similar number URM and PM
b. enzyme conversion produces active or more-active metabolite
c. 70% dose reduction recommended in PM; note also that co-administration with paroxetine (2D6 inhibitor) increases plasma concentrations 4 times
d. TCAs most likely to need a lower dose.

Of particular note is **codeine**, for which most of its analgesic effect results from partial conversion to **morphine** by O-demethylation catalysed by CYP2D6 (see p.378).[37,38] Compared with the general population (EM), a PM produces little or no **morphine** from **codeine** and obtains little or no pain relief. On the other hand, undesirable effects are comparable in both categories.[39,40] At the other extreme, URM produce more **morphine**; this can lead to life-threatening opioid toxicity which, rarely, has been fatal in children (e.g. following adenoidectomy/tonsillectomy; a contributing factor included altered respiratory drive due to obstructive sleep apnoea).[41-45]

Genetic variation involving CYP2D6 is also important in relation to **tramadol**, for which the (+) O-desmethyltramadol metabolite is responsible for the opioid analgesic effect. A PM produces little or none and thus obtains little or no analgesic benefit;[46] conversely, a URM produces higher levels with a potential to cause opioid toxicity (see p.383).[47]

Polymorphism in CYP3A4/5 may be of less clinical significance when considering opioid response.[48] Nonetheless, CYP3A4 activity varies up to 10 times and could be partly responsible for different dose requirements.[49] Opioids potentially affected are the fentanils, **methadone**, **oxycodone** and, to a lesser extent, **buprenorphine**.

Although genetic variation can result in serious consequences, pharmacogenetic testing is not routine, partly because it is not cost-effective.[50,51] Thus, generally, close clinical monitoring is recommended for drugs with a major metabolic enzyme pathway affected by genetic polymorphism (Table 3 and Table 8). However, in some settings, e.g. oncology, testing has been used to determine if an individual is likely to respond to a specific drug, e.g. **cetuximab** (colorectal cancer), **trastuzumab** (breast cancer) and **dasatinib** (acute lymphoblastic leukaemia).

CYP450 DRUG–DRUG INTERACTIONS

Pharmacokinetic drug–drug interactions mediated through increased or decreased activity of CYP450 enzymes are common, but the resultant clinical impact is difficult to predict.[29,52-54] Some drugs (inducers) increase the activity of specific CYP450 enzymes, and others (inhibitors) decrease enzyme activity (Table 7 and Table 8).

When CYP450 inhibitors or inducers are co-administered with drugs that are already affected by genetic polymorphisms, they will either augment or mitigate the clinical effects of the genetic variation.

CYP3A4 enzymes are also present in the wall of the GI tract. Thus, the impact of the concurrent use of CYP3A4 inducers or inhibitors with CYP3A4 substrates may be greater when the latter are taken PO compared with parenterally, e.g. the use of **rifampicin** with PO or parenteral **oxycodone**.[55]

Induction

Onset and offset of enzyme induction is gradual, possibly 2–3 weeks, because:

- onset depends on drug-induced synthesis of new enzyme
- offset depends on elimination of the enzyme-inducing drug and the decay of the increased enzyme stores.

Induction of the rate of drug biotransformation generally leads to a decrease in the parent drug plasma concentration, and thus a *decreased effect*. However, if the substrate drug is an inactive pro-drug or metabolism produces a more active metabolite, induction will result in an *increased effect* and possible toxicity.

The impact of enzyme induction depends on the relative importance of the induced pathway to the substrate's metabolism, whether active metabolites are present, and on the concentration (dose) of the inducer. Sequential dose adjustments, either up or down, may be necessary to maintain the desired clinical effect of the affected drug.[29] Converse dose adjustments may be required if the inducer is discontinued, e.g. **methadone** toxicity has occurred following discontinuation of **carbamazepine**, an inducer.[56]

Some anti-epileptics (e.g. **carbamazepine**, **phenobarbital**, **phenytoin**) and some other drugs (e.g. **rifampicin**, **St John's wort**) induce members of the CYP3A subfamily (Table 4). **Rifampicin** is the most potent clinically used inducer of cytochrome CYP3A. Some oestrogens are metabolized by CYP3A4/5, and induction by **rifampicin** (or another enzyme inducer) can cause oral contraceptive failure.

Particular care should be taken if initiating an enzyme inducer, e.g. **carbamazepine** or **rifampicin**, with opioids, because this may result in increased opioid metabolism and loss of analgesia.

Chronic alcohol consumption can induce CYP450 enzymes, mostly CYP2E1 and possibly CYP3A. However, in cirrhosis, overall enzyme activity is reduced. Smoking tobacco can induce CYP1A2.

Table 4 Examples of drug interactions based on enzyme induction of CYP3A4/5

Substrate	*Inducers*	*Outcome*
Carbamazepine	Phenytoin	Metabolism ↑, effect ↓
Fentanyl IV	Carbamazepine	↑ fentanyl doses needed in those taking carbamazepine[57]
Fentanyl TD	Rifampicin	Metabolism ↑, effect ↓[58-60]
Methadone	Carbamazepine, phenobarbital, phenytoin, rifampicin, St John's wort	Metabolism ↑, effect ↓ (possible recurrence of pain ± withdrawal symptoms)[61]
Midazolam	Carbamazepine, phenytoin	Metabolism ↑, effect ↓[62]
Oxycodone	Rifampicin, St John's wort	Metabolism ↑, effect ↓[55,63]
Phenytoin	Rifampicin	Metabolism ↑, halflife halved, effect ↓[64]
Protease inhibitors (for HIV)	St John's wort	Metabolism ↑, treatment failure[65-67]

Inhibition

Inhibition of drug biotransformation begins *within a few hours* of the administration of the inhibitor drug. For most drugs, inhibition leads to an increase in the plasma concentration and effect of the substrate drug, and increased risk of toxicity. However, the converse is true with *pro-drugs*, e.g.

clopidogrel, where the plasma concentration of the active metabolite is reduced, increasing the risk of therapeutic failure. Table 5 gives examples of altered drug effects resulting from enzyme inhibition.

Table 5 Examples of drug interactions based on enzyme inhibition

Substrate	*Inhibitors*	*Outcome*
Codeine	Quinidine (not UK) (CYP2D6)	Biotransformation to morphine ↓, analgesic effect ↓[68]
Clopidogrel	Esomeprazole, omeprazole (CYP2C19)	Biotransformation to active metabolite ↓, antithrombotic effect ↓[69-72]
Diazepam	Cimetidine (multiple CYP)	Metabolism ↓, effect ↑[73]
Lovastatin (not UK), simvastatin	Clarithromycin, erythromycin (CYP3A4/5)	Metabolism ↓, risk of undesirable effects ↑ (e.g. raised creatinine kinase plasma concentration, muscle pain, rhabdomyolysis)
Theophylline	Ciprofloxacin (CYP1A2)	Metabolism ↓ (18–113%), effect ↑[74]
TCAs	SSRIs (multiple CYP)	Metabolism ↓ (plasma concentrations ↑ 50–350%), effect ↑[75-77]
Warfarin	Fluvoxamine (multiple CYP)	Metabolism ↓ (plasma concentration ↑ 65%), effect ↑[78]

The mechanism of enzymatic inhibition is either reversible or irreversible. In reversible inhibition, the inhibitor drug (e.g. azole antifungal) binds to the P450 enzyme and prevents the metabolism of the substrate drug.[79,80] The extent of inhibition of one drug by another depends on the drugs' relative affinities for the P450 enzyme and the respective doses. In irreversible inhibition, the enzyme is destroyed or inactivated by the inhibitor drug or its metabolites (e.g. **clarithromycin, erythromycin**).

CYP450 DRUG–DRUG INTERACTIONS IN PALLIATIVE CARE

It can be challenging to determine the likelihood of a clinically relevant drug–drug interaction in practice. Many patients receiving palliative care are elderly and have several chronic conditions, resulting in the use of numerous drugs, typically 7–8 (range 1–20), that may undergo frequent change.[81,82] This polypharmacy increases the likelihood of drug interactions involving CYP450, with possibly 10–20% of patients receiving a combination likely to produce a clinically relevant CYP-mediated interaction (Table 6).[81,82]

It is also important to consider the effects of stopping a CYP450 inducer or inhibitor on a substrate drug, such as an opioid; e.g. stopping **rifampicin** (a potent inducer) in a patient taking **fentanyl** or **oxycodone** can result in opioid toxicity; conversely, stopping **clarithromycin** (a potent inhibitor) in a patient taking **oxycodone** may result in a reduced effect. Patients who smoke and take opioids, particularly **methadone,** may also be at risk of opioid toxicity if they discontinue smoking due to progressive illness.[83]

For a longer list of commonly used drugs which are moderate to potent enzyme inhibitors or inducers, also see Table 8.

Table 6 Common drug combinations likely to produce clinically important CYP-mediated interactions in palliative care patients[81,82]

Drug combination	*Likely outcome of the interaction*[a]
Benzodiazepines[b] + CYP3A4 inhibitor e.g. diazepam + itraconazole	Diazepam ↑
Benzodiazepines[b] + CYP3A4 inducer e.g. midazolam + carbamazepine	Midazolam ↓
Corticosteroids + CYP3A4 inhibitor e.g. dexamethasone + clarithromycin	Dexamethasone ↑
Corticosteroids + CYP3A4 inducer e.g. dexamethasone + phenytoin	Dexamethasone ↓
Diazepam + omeprazole[c]	Diazepam ↑
Opioids[b] + CYP3A4 inhibitor e.g. oxycodone + fluconazole	Oxycodone ↑
Opioids[b] + CYP3A4 inducer e.g. fentanyl + carbamazepine	Fentanyl ↓

a. ↑ = drug effect increased, ↓ = effect decreased
b. which are full or part substrates of CYP3A4 (Table 8)
c. inhibitor of CYP2C19 (Table 8).

In one series, about 50% of the interactions involved corticosteroids, and 25% analgesics.[81] In a second series, the most frequently used inducers or inhibitors of CYP450 (and/or P-glycoprotein, or UGT) were **dexamethasone**, **esomeprazole**, **omeprazole**, **fluconazole**, **ciprofloxacin**, **carbamazepine**, **carvedilol** and **verapamil** (also see Table 8).[82] Interactions may be missed, e.g. recurrence of pain may be interpreted as disease progression rather than altered analgesic metabolism. The *BNF* has a comprehensive list of drug interactions and their significance.

Serotonin toxicity (see Antidepressants, Box A, p.217) is generally a pharmacodynamic interaction resulting from the combination of two or more serotonergic drugs. However, in some circumstances, a pharmacokinetic interaction may contribute to an increase in serotonergic transmission, e.g. **fluoxetine** (a CYP2D6 and CYP2C19 inhibitor) and **amitriptyline**.

The addition of a CYP450 inhibitor to a drug known to prolong the QT interval may result in increased plasma levels, QT prolongation and risk of *torsade de pointes*, e.g. **itraconazole** (a CYP3A4 inhibitor) with **methadone**.

CYP450 DRUG–FOOD INTERACTIONS

An important interaction associated with CYP450 inhibition is a food–drug interaction involving grapefruit juice and CYP3A substrates administered PO, including some benzodiazepines (**diazepam**, **midazolam**, **triazolam** (not UK)), some statins (**atorvastatin**, **lovastatin** (not UK), **simvastatin**), **buspirone**, **ciclosporin**, **felodipine**, **nifedipine** and **saquinavir**.[29,84-86]

Grapefruit juice contains several bioflavonoids (naringenin, naringin, kaempferol and quercetin) and furanocoumarins (bergamottin) which non-competitively inhibit oxidation reactions mediated by CYP3A enzymes in the wall of the GI tract.[85,87,88] The effect is unpredictable, because the quantity of these components in grapefruit products varies considerably.[89,90]

The effect is maximal when grapefruit juice is ingested 30–60min before the drug. A single 250mL glass of grapefruit juice can inhibit CYP3A for 24–48h, and regular intake continually suppresses GI CYP3A.[29,85] Thus, patients taking drugs metabolized by CYP3A are warned to avoid grapefruit juice, particularly if the drug has a narrow therapeutic index, e.g. **ciclosporin**. Pomelo, Seville orange and lime juices may also inhibit CYP3A;[91,92] apple juice has not been implicated.

Besides inhibiting CYP3A, naringin (and thus grapefruit juice) inhibits organic anion-transporting polypeptide 1A2 (OATP1A2), a carrier protein in the wall of the GI tract which is responsible for the uptake of several drugs. Orange juice (through its major flavonoid, hesperidin) has a similar effect,[93] and possibly apple juice.[94] Drugs which may have their absorption reduced by this inhibition include some β-blockers (**atenolol**, **celiprolol**), **ciclosporin**, **etoposide**, **fexofenadine**, **itraconazole** and quinolone antibacterials (**ciprofloxacin**, **levofloxacin**).[93,94]

Case reports of serious adverse events related to grapefruit–drug interactions include:

- **amiodarone** → *torsade de pointes*
- **atorvastatin** and **simvastatin** → rhabdomyolysis.

Other drugs which may be affected by grapefruit include novel oral anticoagulants (**apixaban**, **rivaroxaban**), calcium channel blockers (**amlodipine**, **felodipine**, **verapamil**), CNS drugs (**quetiapine**, **buspirone**), cytotoxics (**nilotinib**, **lapatinib**) and immunosuppressants (**ciclosporin**, **tacrolimus**, **sirolimus**).[95] Interactions are generally drug-specific, not a class effect, and the *BNF* or SPC should be referred to for more information.

There is also concern that ingestion of cranberry juice may also modify drug action, mediated through flavonoids which specifically inhibit CYP2C9 (see Urinary tract infections, Box C, p.526). **Warfarin** is an example of a drug that might be affected by this interaction and, indeed, early reports linked cranberry juice with adverse events associated with **warfarin**.[96-99] However, recent reports suggest that this interaction is unlikely to occur with the amounts of cranberry juice recommended for prophylaxis against UTIs.[100-103]

Nonetheless, an interaction with **warfarin** cannot be ruled out, particularly when large volumes of cranberry juice are drunk regularly, or when cranberry products other than juice are taken.[100,101,104] Thus, the INR should be monitored more closely in patients on **warfarin** if they consume large amounts of cranberry juice or take other cranberry supplements for prophylaxis against UTIs.[100]

QUANTIFYING THE EFFECTS OF CYP450 INHIBITION AND INDUCTION

Quantification of the effects of CYP450 inhibitors and inducers is still evolving. The more important enzymes for drug metabolism have generally accepted probe substrates and potent inhibitors and inducers (Table 7), and these are used to determine reliable results, e.g. for new drugs in development. Increasingly, data are becoming available which predict the clinical importance of drug–drug interactions. However, there is still much to be determined and, in palliative care where polypharmacy is the norm, in addition to understanding the pharmacokinetics of any drug used, a general awareness of potential interactions is important (Table 8).

Table 7 Examples of *in vivo* probe substrates and potent inhibitors and inducers used for evaluation (all PO)[105]

Enzyme	*Substrate*	*Inhibitor*	*Inducers*
CYP1A2	Caffeine Theophylline Tizanidine	Fluvoxamine	Tobacco smoking
CYP2B6	Efavirenz		Rifampicin
CYP2C8	Repaglinide	Clopidogrel Gemfibrozil	Rifampicin
CYP2C9	Tolbutamide Warfarin	Fluconazole	Rifampicin
CYP2C19	Esomeprazole Lansoprazole Omeprazole Pantoprazole	Fluvoxamine	Rifampicin
CYP2D6	Dextromethorphan	Fluoxetine Paroxetine Quinidine (not UK)	None known
CYP3A4	Midazolam	Clarithromycin Fluconazole Itraconazole Ketoconazole Ritonavir	Rifampicin

Table 8 Examples of enzyme or transporter protein substrates, inhibitors and inducers that may result in clinically significant drug interactions[a,28,82,105]

Enzyme or transporter protein	*Substrates*	*Moderate or potent inhibitors*	*Moderate or potent inducers*
CYP1A2	Amitriptyline Clomipramine Clozapine Duloxetine Flecainide Imipramine Melatonin Mirtazapine Olanzapine Propranolol Ramelteon (not UK) Theophylline Tizanidine Trimipramine	Cimetidine[b] Ciprofloxacin Fluvoxamine	Phenytoin Rifampicin Tobacco smoking
CYP2B6	Methadone		Rifampicin
CYP2C8	Loperamide Pioglitazone Repaglinide Rosiglitazone (not UK)	Clopidogrel	Rifampicin
CYP2C9[c]	Celecoxib Chlorpropamide (not UK) Diclofenac Flurbiprofen Fluvastatin Glibenclamide (glyburide) Gliclazide Glimepiride Glipizide Ibuprofen Irbesartan Losartan Nateglinide Phenytoin Tolbutamide Torasemide (torsemide) Warfarin	Amiodarone Fluconazole	Carbamazepine Enzalutamide Rifampicin
CYP2C19[c]	Amitriptyline Citalopram Clomipramine Clopidogrel Diazepam Fluoxetine Imipramine Lansoprazole Omeprazole Pantoprazole Phenytoin Sertraline	Esomeprazole Fluconazole Fluoxetine Fluvoxamine Omeprazole Ticlopidine Voriconazole	Apalutamide Enzalutamide Rifampicin

continued

Table 8 Continued

Enzyme or transporter protein	*Substrates*	*Moderate or potent inhibitors*	*Moderate or potent inducers*
CYP2D6[c]	Amitriptyline Carvedilol Codeine Desipramine (not UK) Dextromethorphan Dihydrocodeine Duloxetine Flecainide Fluoxetine Hydrocodone (not UK) Imipramine Metoprolol Mirtazapine Nebivolol Nortriptyline Ondansetron Oxycodone Paracetamol Paroxetine Pindolol Propranolol Risperidone Sertraline Tamoxifen Timolol Tolterodine Tramadol Trazodone Trimipramine Venlafaxine	Cimetidine[b] Duloxetine Fluoxetine Paroxetine	
CYP3A4/5[d,e]	Alfentanil Alprazolam Amiodarone Aprepitant Atorvastatin Budesonide (PO) Buprenorphine Carbamazepine Clarithromycin Clorazepate Codeine Dexamethasone Diazepam Diltiazem Domperidone Erythromycin Estradiol Eszopiclone (not UK) Felodipine Fentanyl Haloperidol Imipramine Itraconazole	Aprepitant Cimetidine[b] Ciprofloxacin Clarithromycin Diltiazem Erythromycin Fluconazole Grapefruit juice Itraconazole Verapamil Voriconazole	Apalutamide Carbamazepine Enzalutamide Modafinil Phenobarbital (and other barbiturates) Phenytoin Rifampicin St John's wort

continued

Table 8 Continued

Enzyme or transporter protein	*Substrates*	*Moderate or potent inhibitors*	*Moderate or potent inducers*
CYP3A4/5[d,e] (continued)	Ketamine Loperamide Losartan Lovastatin (not UK) Methadone Methylprednisolone Midazolam Mirtazapine Naldemedine Naloxegol Nifedipine Omeprazole Oxybutynin Oxycodone Paracetamol (acetaminophen) Phenytoin Quetiapine Risperidone Rivaroxaban Sertraline Simvastatin Tamoxifen Tolterodine Tolvaptan Toremifene Tramadol Trazodone Venlafaxine Verapamil Voriconazole Warfarin Zolpidem Zopiclone		
P-glycoprotein[e]	Dabigatran Digoxin Edoxaban Loperamide	Amiodarone Carvedilol Ciclosporin Clarithromycin Erythromycin Felodipine Itraconazole Verapamil	Carbamazepine Rifampicin St John's wort

a. *not* an exhaustive list; limited to drugs most likely to be encountered in palliative care and *excludes* anticancer, HIV and immunosuppressive drugs (seek specialist advice)

b. cimetidine is classified as a weak inhibitor of multiple CYP enzymes

c. enzyme can also be subject to genetic polymorphism; see Table 3

d. CYP3A enzyme is also expressed in the GI mucosa, resulting in substantial first-pass metabolism of some drugs during absorption

e. there is a large overlap between the substrates, inhibitors and inducers of P-glycoprotein and CYP3A.

1 Droney J *et al.* (2011) Evolving knowledge of opioid genetics in cancer pain. *Clinical Oncology*. **23**: 418–428.
2 Lloyd RA *et al.* (2016) Pharmacogenomics and patient treatment parameters to opioid treatment in chronic pain: a focus on morphine, oxycodone, tramadol and fentanyl. *Pain Medicine*. **0**: 1–19.
3 Ross JR *et al.* (2006) Clinical pharmacology and pharmacotherapy of opioid switching in cancer patients. *Oncologist*. **11**: 765–773.
4 Somogyi AA *et al.* (2007) Pharmacogenetics of opioids. *Clinical Pharmacology & Therapeutics*. **81**: 429–444.
5 Solhaug V and Molden E (2017) Individual variability in clinical effect and tolerability of opioid analgesics - Importance of drug interactions and pharmacogenetics. *Scandinavian Journal of Pain*. **17**: 193–200.
6 Matthes H *et al.* (1996) Loss of morphine-induced analgesia, reward effect and withdrawal symptoms in mice lacking the mu-opioid-receptor gene. *Nature*. **383**: 819–823.
7 Hwang IC *et al.* (2014) OPRM1 A118G gene variant and postoperative opioid requirement: a systematic review and meta-analysis. *Anesthesiology*. **121**: 825–834.
8 Janicki PK *et al.* (2006) A genetic association study of the functional A118G polymorphism of the human mu-opioid receptor gene in patients with acute and chronic pain. *Anesthesia & Analgesia*. **103**: 1011–1017.
9 Lotsch J *et al.* (2009) Cross-sectional analysis of the influence of currently known pharmacogenetic modulators on opioid therapy in outpatient pain centers. *Pharmacogenetics and Genomics*. **19**: 429–436.
10 Campa D *et al.* (2008) Association of ABCB1/MDR1 and OPRM1 gene polymorphisms with morphine pain relief. *Clinical Pharmacology & Therapeutics*. **83**: 559–566.
11 Klepstad P *et al.* (2004) The 118A > G polymorphism in the human mu-opioid receptor gene may increase morphine requirements in patients with pain caused by malignant disease. *Acta Anaesthesiologica Scandinavica*. **48**: 1232–1239.
12 Walter C and Lotsch J (2009) Meta-analysis of the relevance of the OPRM1 118A>G genetic variant for pain treatment. *Pain*. **146**: 270–275.
13 Schinkel AH (1997) The physiological function of drug-transporting P-glycoproteins. *Seminars in Cancer Biology*. **8**: 161–170.
14 Marzolini C *et al.* (2004) Polymorphisms in human MDR1 (P-glycoprotein): recent advances and clinical relevance. *Clinical Pharmacology & Therapeutics*. **75**: 13–33.
15 Davis MP *et al.* (eds) (2009) Pharmacogenetics and opioids. *Opioids in Cancer Pain* (2nd edn) OUP, Oxford, pp. 287–299.
16 Dagenais C *et al.* (2004) Variable modulation of opioid brain uptake by P-glycoprotein in mice. *Biochemical Pharmacology*. **67**: 269–276.
17 Barratt DT *et al.* (2012) ABCB1 haplotype and OPRM1 118A > G genotype interaction in methadone maintenance treatment pharmacogenetics. *Pharmacogenomics and Personalized Medicine*. **5**: 53–62.
18 Thompson SJ *et al.* (2000) Opiate-induced analgesia is increased and prolonged in mice lacking P-glycoprotein. *Anesthesiology*. **92**: 1392–1399.
19 Ross JR *et al.* (2008) Genetic variation and response to morphine in cancer patients: catechol-O-methyltransferase and multidrug resistance-1 gene polymorphisms are associated with central side effects. *Cancer*. **112**: 1390–1403.
20 Zwisler ST *et al.* (2010) The antinociceptive effect and adverse drug reactions of oxycodone in human experimental pain in relation to genetic variations in the OPRM1 and ABCB1 genes. *Fundamental & Clinical Pharmacology*. **24**: 517–524.
21 Coulbault L *et al.* (2006) Environmental and genetic factors associated with morphine response in the postoperative period. *Clinical Pharmacology & Therapeutics*. **79**: 316–324.
22 Kim H *et al.* (2006) Genetic polymorphisms in monoamine neurotransmitter systems show only weak association with acute post-surgical pain in humans. *Molecular Pain*. **2**: 24.
23 Zubieta JK *et al.* (2003) COMT val158met genotype affects mu-opioid neurotransmitter responses to a pain stressor. *Science*. **299**: 1240–1243.
24 Rakvag TT *et al.* (2005) The Val158Met polymorphism of the human catechol-O-methyltransferase (COMT) gene may influence morphine requirements in cancer pain patients. *Pain*. **116**: 73–78.
25 Laugsand EA *et al.* (2011) Clinical and genetic factors associated with nausea and vomiting in cancer patients receiving opioids. *European Journal of Cancer*. **47**: 1682–1691.
26 Kolesnikov Y *et al.* (2011) Combined catechol-O-methyltransferase and mu-opioid receptor gene polymorphisms affect morphine postoperative analgesia and central side effects. *Anesthesia & Analgesia*. **112**: 448–453.
27 Smith HS (2009) Opioid metabolism. *Mayo Clinic Proceedings*. **84**: 613–624.
28 Baxter K, Preston CL *Stockley's Drug Interactions*. London: Pharmaceutical Press. www.medicinescomplete.com (accessed December 2019).
29 Wilkinson GR (2005) Drug metabolism and variability among patients in drug response. *New England Journal of Medicine*. **352**: 2211–2221.
30 Sim SC (2005) Human Cytochrome P450 (CYP). Allele Nomenclature Committee. Available from: www.CYPalleles.ki.se.
31 Stamer UM *et al.* (2010) Personalized therapy in pain management: where do we stand? *Pharmacogenomics*. **11**: 843–864.
32 Meyer U (1991) Genotype or phenotype: the definition of a pharmacogenetic polymorphism. *Pharmacogenetics*. **1**: 66–67.
33 Sajantila A *et al.* (2010) Pharmacogenetics in medico-legal context. *Forensic Science International*. **203**: 44–52.
34 Poulsen L *et al.* (1996) The hypoalgesic effect of tramadol in relation to CYP2D6. *Clinical Pharmacology and Therapeutics*. **60**: 636–644.
35 Riddick D (1997) Drug biotransformation. In: Kalant H, Roschlau W (eds) *Principles of Medical Pharmacology*, 6th edn. New York: Oxford University Press.
36 Williams DG *et al.* (2002) Pharmacogenetics of codeine metabolism in an urban population of children and its implications for analgesic reliability. *British Journal of Anaesthesia*. **89**: 839–845.
37 Persson K *et al.* (1992) The postoperative pharmacokinetics of codeine. *European Journal of Clinical Pharmacology*. **42**: 663–666.
38 Findlay JWA *et al.* (1978) Plasma codeine and morphine concentrations after therapeutic oral doses of codeine-containing analgesics. *Clinical Pharmacology and Therapeutics*. **24**: 60–68.
39 Eckhardt K *et al.* (1998) Same incidence of adverse drug events after codeine administration irrespective of the genetically determined differences in morphine formation. *Pain*. **76**: 27–33.
40 Susce MT *et al.* (2006) Response to hydrocodone, codeine and oxycodone in a CYP2D6 poor metabolizer. *Progress in Neuropsychopharmacology and Biological Psychiatry*. **30**: 1356–1358.
41 Gasche Y *et al.* (2004) Codeine intoxication associated with ultrarapid CYP2D6 metabolism. *New England Journal of Medicine*. **351**: 2827–2831.
42 Koren G *et al.* (2006) Pharmacogenetics of morphine poisoning in a breastfed neonate of a codeine-prescribed mother. *Lancet*. **368**: 704.
43 Kirchheiner J *et al.* (2007) Pharmacokinetics of codeine and its metabolite morphine in ultra-rapid metabolizers due to CYP2D6 duplication. *Pharmacogenomics Journal*. **7**: 257–265.

44 Racoosin JA *et al.* (2013) New evidence about an old drug - risk with codeine after adenotonsillectomy. *New England Journal of Medicine*. **368**: 2155–2157.

45 MHRA (2013) Codeine: restricted use as an analgesic in children and adolescents after European safety review. *Drug Safety Update*. www.gov.uk/drug-safety-update.

46 Stamer UM *et al.* (2007) Concentrations of tramadol and O-desmethyltramadol enantiomers in different CYP2D6 genotypes. *Clinical Pharmacology and Therapeutics*. **82**: 41–47.

47 Stamer UM *et al.* (2008) Respiratory depression with tramadol in a patient with renal impairment and CYP2D6 gene duplication. *Anesthesia and Analgesia*. **107**: 926–929.

48 Pirmohamed M and Park BK (2003) Cytochrome P450 enzyme polymorphisms and adverse drug reactions. *Toxicology*. **192**: 23–32.

49 Haddad A *et al.* (2007) The pharmacological importance of cytochrome CYP3A4 in the palliation of symptoms: review and recommendations for avoiding adverse drug interactions. *Supportive Care in Cancer*. **15**: 251–257.

50 Kimmel SE *et al.* (2013) A pharmacogenetic versus a clinical algorithm for warfarin dosing. *New England Journal of Medicine*. **369**: 2283–2293.

51 Pirmohamed M *et al.* (2013) A randomized trial of genotype-guided dosing of warfarin. *New England Journal of Medicine*. **369**: 2294–2303.

52 Aeschlimann J and Tyler L (1996) Drug interactions associated with cytochrome P-450 enzymes. *Journal of Pharmaceutical Care in Pain and Symptom Control*. **4**: 35–54.

53 Johnson MD *et al.* (1999) Clinically significant drug interactions. *Postgraduate Medicine*. **105**: 193–222.

54 Samer CF *et al.* (2013) Applications of CYP450 testing in the clinical setting. *Molecular Diagnosis & Therapy*. **17**: 165–184.

55 Nieminen TH *et al.* (2009) Rifampin greatly reduces the plasma concentrations of intravenous and oral oxycodone. *Anesthesiology*. **110**: 1371–1378.

56 Benitez-Rosario MA *et al.* (2006) Methadone-induced respiratory depression after discontinuing carbamazepine administration. *Journal of Pain and Symptom Management*. **32**: 99–100.

57 Tempelhoff R *et al.* (1990) Anticonvulsant therapy increases fentanyl requirements during anaesthesia for craniotomy. *Canadian Journal of Anaesthesiology*. **37**: 327–332.

58 Takane H *et al.* (2005) Rifampin reduces the analgesic effect of transdermal fentanyl. *Annals of Pharmacotherapy*. **39**: 2139–2140.

59 Sasson M and Shvartzman P (2006) Fentanyl patch sufficient analgesia for only one day. *Journal of Pain and Symptom Management*. **31**: 389–391.

60 Morii H *et al.* (2007) Failure of pain control using transdermal fentanyl during rifampicin treatment. *Journal of Pain and Symptom Management*. **33**: 5–6.

61 Kreek MJ *et al.* (1976) Rifampin-induced methadone withdrawal. *New England Journal of Medicine*. **294**: 1104–1106.

62 Backman J *et al.* (1996) Concentrations and effects of oral midazolam are greatly reduced in patients treated with carbamazepine or phenytoin. *Epilepsia*. **37**: 253–257.

63 Nieminen TH *et al.* (2010) St John's wort greatly reduces the concentrations of oral oxycodone. *European Journal of Pain*. **14**: 854–859.

64 Kay L *et al.* (1985) Influence of rifampicin and isoniazid on the kinetics of phenytoin. *British Journal of Clinical Pharmacology*. **20**: 323–326.

65 Piscitelli SC *et al.* (2000) Indinavir concentrations and St John's wort. *Lancet*. **355**: 547–548.

66 Henderson L *et al.* (2002) St John's wort (*Hypericum perforatum*): drug interactions and clinical outcomes. *British Journal of Clinical Pharmacology*. **54**: 349–356.

67 Flexner C (2000) Dual protease inhibitor therapy in HIV-infected patients: pharmacologic rationale and clinical benefits. *Annual Review of Pharmacology and Toxicology*. **40**: 649–674.

68 Sindrup S *et al.* (1992) The effect of quinidine on the analgesic effect of codeine. *European Journal of Clinical Pharmacology*. **42**: 587–591.

69 MHRA (2010) Clopidogrel and proton pump inhibitors: interaction – updated advice. *Drug Safety Update*. www.gov.uk/drug-safety-update.

70 Society for Cardiovascular Angiography and Interventions (2009) A national study of the effect of individual proton pump inhibitors on cardiovascular outcomes in patients treated with clopidogrel following coronary stenting: the clopidogrel Medco outcomes study. Available from: www.scai.org.

71 Juurlink DN *et al.* (2009) A population-based study of the drug interaction between proton pump inhibitors and clopidogrel. *Canadian Medical Association Journal*. **180**: 713–718.

72 Ho PM *et al.* (2009) Risk of adverse outcomes associated with concomitant use of clopidogrel and proton pump inhibitors following acute coronary syndrome. *JAMA*. **301**: 937–944.

73 Klotz U and Reimann I (1980) Delayed clearance of diazepam due to cimetidine. *New England Journal of Medicine*. **302**: 1012–1014.

74 Nix D *et al.* (1987) Effect of multiple dose oral ciprofloxacin on the pharmacokinetics of theophylline and indocyanine green. *Journal of Antimicrobial Chemotherapy*. **19**: 263–269.

75 Vandel S *et al.* (1992) Tricyclic antidepressant plasma levels after fluoxetine addition. *Neuropsychobiology*. **25**: 202–207.

76 Finley P (1994) Selective serotonin reuptake inhibitors: pharmacologic profiles and potential therapeutic distinctions. *Annals of Pharmacotherapy*. **28**: 1359–1369.

77 Pollock B (1994) Recent developments in drug metabolism of relevance to psychiatrists. *Harvard Reviews of Psychiatry*. **2**: 204–213.

78 Tatro D (1995) Fluvoxamine drug interactions. *Drug Newsletter*. **14**: 20.

79 Monaham B (1990) Torsades de pointes occurring in association with terfenadine. *Journal of the American Medical Association*. **264**: 2788–2790.

80 Honig P *et al.* (1993) Terfenadine-ketoconazole interaction. Pharmacokinetic and electrocardiographic consequences. *Journal of the American Medical Association*. **269**: 1513–1518.

81 Wilcock A *et al.* (2005) Potential for drug interactions involving cytochrome P450 in patients attending palliative day care centres: a multicentre audit. *British Journal of Clinical Pharmacology*. **60**: 326–329.

82 Kotlinska-Lemieszek A *et al.* (2014) Polypharmacy in patients with advanced cancer and pain: a European cross-sectional study of 2282 patients. *Journal of Pain and Symptom Management*. **48**: 1145–1159.

83 Wahawisan J *et al.* (2011) Methadone toxicity due to smoking cessation–a case report on the drug-drug interaction involving cytochrome P450 isoenzyme 1A2. *Annals of Pharmacotherapy*. **45**: e34.

84 Maskalyk J (2002) Grapefruit juice: potential drug interactions. *Canadian Medical Association Journal*. **167**: 279–280.

85 Dahan A and Altman H (2004) Food-drug interaction: grapefruit juice augments drug bioavailability-mechanism, extent and relevance. *European Journal of Clinical Nutrition*. **58**: 1–9.

86 MHRA (2008) Statins: interactions, and updated advice for atorvastatin. *Drug Safety Update*. www.gov.uk/drug-safety-update.

87 Rouseff RL (1988) Liquid chromatographic determination of naringin and neohesperidin as a detector of grapefruit juice in orange juice. *Journal – Association of Official Analytical Chemists*. **71**: 798–802.

88 Gibaldi M (1992) Drug interactions. Part II. *Annals of Pharmacotherapy*. **26**: 829–834.
89 Tailor S *et al.* (1996) Peripheral edema due to nifedipine-itraconazole interaction: a case report. *Archives of Dermatology*. **132**: 350–352.
90 Fukuda K *et al.* (2000) Amounts and variation in grapefruit juice of the main components causing grapefruit-drug interaction. *Journal of Chromatography B, Biomedical Sciences and Applications*. **741**: 195–203.
91 Savage I (2008) Forbidden fruit: interactions between medicines, foods and herbal products *Pharmaceutical Journal* **281**: f17.
92 Baxter K (2008) Drug interactions and fruit juices. *Pharmaceutical Journal*. **281**: 333.
93 Bailey DG *et al.* (2007) Naringin is a major and selective clinical inhibitor of organic anion-transporting polypeptide 1A2 (OATP1A2) in grapefruit juice. *Clinical Pharmacology and Therapeutics*. **81**: 495–502.
94 Sampson M (2008) New reasons to avoid grapefruit and other juices when taking certain drugs. Report from the 236th National Meeting of the American Chemical Society. Philadelphia, August 19th 2008.; www.eurekalert.org/pub_releases/2008-08/acs-nrt072308.php.
95 Bailey DG *et al.* (2013) Grapefruit-medication interactions: forbidden fruit or avoidable consequences? *Canadian Medical Association Journal*. **185**: 309–316.
96 Grant P (2004) Warfarin and cranberry juice: an interaction? *Journal of Heart Valve Disease*. **13**: 25–26.
97 MHRA (2004) Interaction between warfarin and cranberry juice: new advice. *Current Problems in Pharmacovigilance*. **30**: 10 (Archived).
98 MHRA (2003) Possible interaction between warfarin and cranberry juice. *Current Problems in Pharmacovigilance*. **29**: 8
99 Suvarna R *et al.* (2003) Possible interaction between warfarin and cranberry juice. *BMJ*. **327**: 1454.
100 O'Mara N (2007) Does a cranberry juice-warfarin interaction really exist? *Pharmacist's Letter/Prescriber's Letter*. **23**: 1–3.
101 Aston JL *et al.* (2006) Interaction between warfarin and cranberry juice. *Pharmacotherapy*. **26**: 1314–1319.
102 Lilja JJ *et al.* (2007) Effects of daily ingestion of cranberry juice on the pharmacokinetics of warfarin, tizanidine, and midazolam--probes of CYP2C9, CYP1A2, and CYP3A4. *Clinical Pharmacology and Therapeutics*. **81**: 833–839.
103 Li Z *et al.* (2006) Cranberry does not affect prothrombin time in male subjects on warfarin. *Journal of the American Dietetic Society*. **106**: 2057–2061.
104 Welch J and Forster K (2007) Probable elevation in international normalized ratio from cranberry juice. *Journal of Pharmacy Technology*. **23**: 104–107.
105 FDA (2006) Drug development and drug interactions: table of substrates, inhibitors and inducers. www.fda.gov (accessed June 2019).

Updated December 2019

20: PROLONGATION OF THE QT INTERVAL IN PALLIATIVE CARE

20

The QT interval has attained greater clinical significance since it became apparent that various factors which prolong the QT interval, particularly drugs, predispose to a potentially fatal ventricular arrhythmia, *torsade de pointes*.

An accurate diagnosis of *torsade de pointes* is important, because its management differs from other forms of ventricular tachycardia. Indeed, conventional drug treatments for ventricular tachycardia can exacerbate the underlying electrochemical derangement and perpetuate *torsade de pointes*.

Palliative care clinicians caring for patients with cardiac disease, HIV infection, or using **methadone** need to be particularly aware of this phenomenon.

The QT interval lies on the electrocardiograph (ECG) between the beginning of the QRS complex (which marks the start of ventricular depolarization) and the end of the T wave (which marks the end of ventricular repolarization) (Figure 1).

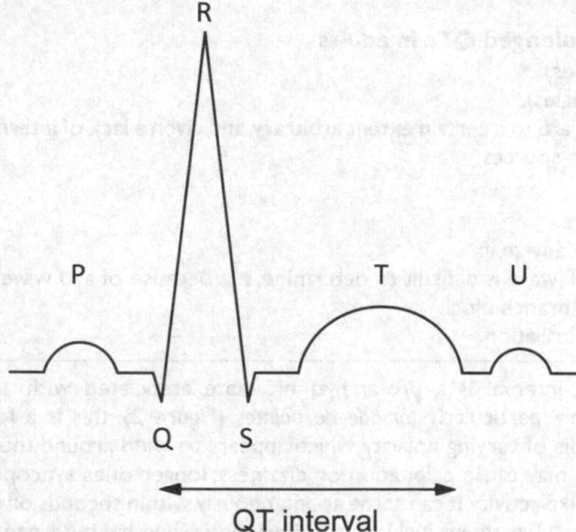

Figure 1 The QT interval.

The QT interval tends to be longer with slower heart rates. For comparative purposes, it is important to adjust ('correct') the observed QT interval to take account of this. The corrected value is designated QTc. Some ECG machines automatically calculate QTc, and this is a useful guide. However, automatic calculations can be inaccurate, particularly in the presence of atrial fibrillation, frequent ventricular ectopics, or a noisy trace. Thus, manual calculation of QTc is more accurate (Box A).[1,2] There are several ways of doing this, and local practice varies.

Box A Measuring the QT interval and calculating QTc[1,3-5]

ECG

A 12-lead ECG at 25mm/sec at 10mm/mV amplitude is generally adequate, taken after the patient has rested supine for about 5min.

Measure the QT interval together with the preceding RR interval in 3–5 heartbeats from leads II and V5/V6.

Calculate the mean QT and RR interval from these 3–5 measurements.

Calculate QTc. Multiple formulae exist and there is no gold standard; commonly used ones include:

- Bazett's (exponential square root):

$$QTc = \frac{QT\,(sec)}{\sqrt{RR}\,(sec)}$$

- Fridericia's (exponential cube root):

$$QTc = \frac{QT\,(sec)}{\sqrt[3]{RR}\,(sec)}$$

- Framingham (linear):

$$QTc = QT + 0.154\,(1–RR)$$

Generally, Fridericia's and Framingham perform better than Bazett's, which has a tendency to overestimate QTc, particularly at heart rates ≥100 beats/min.

Definition of prolonged QTc in adults

- >450msec (males)
- >460msec (females).

Note. These limits are to a certain extent arbitrary, and given a lack of international consensus, they vary between sources.

Obtain advice

Obtain cardiology advice if:

- the end of the T wave is difficult to determine, e.g. because of a U wave
- there is bundle branch block
- there is atrial fibrillation.

A prolonged QT interval is a pro-arrhythmic state associated with an increased risk of ventricular arrhythmia, particularly *torsade de pointes* (Figure 2); this is a form of polymorphic ventricular tachycardia of varying polarity which appears to wind around the baseline, and hence its name. Short runs may cause palpitation or dizziness; longer ones syncope (generally without warning) or seizure-like activity. It can settle spontaneously within seconds or degenerate into fatal ventricular fibrillation.[6] Treatment includes cardioversion when haemodynamically compromised, **magnesium sulfate** IV (e.g. 2g over 10–15min) to stabilize the myocardium, and interventions to increase heart rate (e.g. cardiac pacing).[6,7]

Additional premonitory ECG signs of *torsade de pointes* include T-U wave distortion (more exaggerated in a beat after a pause), T-wave alternans (marked alternate variation in size), new ventricular ectopics or couplets, and nonsustained polymorphic ventricular tachycardia initiated in the beat after a pause.[8]

The risk of *torsade de pointes* grows as the QTc interval increases, particularly >500msec. A drug which leads to an increase in QTc interval of 30–60msec should also raise concern and, if by >60msec, serious concern about the risk of arrhythmia.[9]

Drugs prolong the QT interval mainly through potassium-channel blockade (particularly I_{Kr} 'rapid' subtype) by interfering with potassium currents in (enhanced) and out (reduced) of the cardiac myocytes, modifying their repolarization and prolonging the duration of the action potential.[10] The resulting dispersion of intramural repolarization may promote triggered activity and re-entry, the electrophysiological substrate for *torsade de pointes*. Several drugs have been definitely linked with *torsade de pointes* (Box B). The incidence of *torsade de pointes* is greatest with cardiac anti-arrhythmics, particularly those with class Ia or III activity. Concerns about safety have resulted in some drugs either having dose restrictions applied, e.g. **domperidone** (p.271), **citalopram/escitalopram** (p.232) and **ondansetron** (p.277), or being withdrawn completely from the UK market, e.g. **astemizole, cisapride, sertindole, terfenadine, thioridazine.**

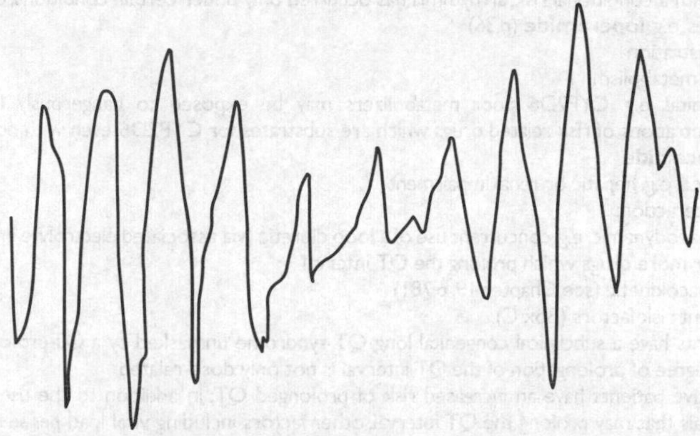

Figure 2 *Torsade de pointes.* Twisting complexes of ventricular tachycardia.

Box B Drugs available in the UK with a known risk of prolonged QT interval and *torsade de pointes*[a]

Anti-arrhythmic drugs
Amiodarone
Disopyramide
Dronedarone
Flecainide
Sotalol

Antidepressant drugs
Citalopram
Escitalopram

Antimicrobial drugs
Fluconazole
Macrolides: azithromycin, clarithromycin, erythromycin
Quinolones: ciprofloxacin, levofloxacin, moxifloxacin
Pentamidine

Antimalarial drugs
Chloroquine

Psychotropic drugs
Chlorpromazine
Droperidol
Haloperidol
Levomepromazine
Pimozide
Sulpiride

Miscellaneous
Anagrelide
Arsenic trioxide
Cilostazol
Cocaine
Domperidone
Donepezil
Methadone
Ondansetron
Oxaliplatin
Propofol
Saquinavir
Sevoflurane
Terlipressin
Toremifene
Vandetanib

a. for a full list, including those considered a possible or conditional risk, see www.crediblemeds.org

The website www.crediblemeds.org identifies drugs:

- with a *known risk* of prolonged QT interval and *torsade de pointes* (Box B)
- with a *possible risk*; insufficient evidence that authorized use causes arrhythmia
- with a *conditional risk;* see below
- to be avoided by patients with congenital long QT syndrome.

For drugs with a conditional risk, arrhythmia has occurred only under certain conditions, e.g. with:[11-13]

- high doses, e.g. **loperamide** (p.36)
- IV administration
- impaired metabolism:
  - ▷ congenital, e.g. CYP2D6 poor metabolizers may be exposed to dangerously high plasma concentrations of risk-related drugs which are substrates for CYP2D6, even with normal doses, e.g. **flecainide**
  - ▷ acquired, e.g. hepatic or renal impairment
- a drug interaction:
  - ▷ pharmacodynamic, e.g. concurrent use of a loop diuretic (via associated electrolyte imbalance) or two or more drugs which prolong the QT interval
  - ▷ pharmacokinetic (see Chapter 19, p.781)
- concurrent risk factors (Box C).

Some patients have a subclinical congenital long QT syndrome unmasked by a QT-prolonging drug.[6] Thus, the degree of prolongation of the QT interval is not only dose-related.

HIV-positive patients have an increased risk of prolonged QT; in addition to the use of multiple antiretrovirals that may prolong the QT interval, other factors including viral load *per se* increase the risk.[14]

An additional contributory factor may be central sleep apnoea, which is associated with bradycardia and QT prolongation, and is reported to occur in 30% of patients on **methadone** maintenance.[15]

Box C Main additional risk factors in drug-induced *torsade de pointes*

Increasing age (particularly >70 years)

Female sex

Congenital long QT syndrome

Baseline prolonged QT interval

Electrolyte imbalance:

- hypocalcaemia
- hypokalaemia
- hypomagnesaemia

Cardiac disease, e.g.:

- bradycardia <50 beats/min
- left ventricular hypertrophy
- heart failure
- recent conversion from atrial fibrillation
- ventricular arrhythmia

Implications for practice

General recommendations to guide practice are given in Box D.[16] A QT risk assessment tool is available to guide decision making (www.medsafetyscan.org).

Palliative care patients in general may be at higher risk of a prolonged QT interval given the high prevalence of multiple drug use and metabolic disturbance. Polypharmacy is the norm in palliative care,[17] and using more than one drug concurrently increases the risk of drug interactions.[18-20] However, of 300 patients referred to a specialist palliative care unit who were not imminently dying, although 48 (16%) had a prolonged QT interval, only 2 (0.7%) had a severely prolonged uncorrected QT interval of >500msec (Figure 3).[9,21] Both patients had ischaemic heart disease and, if being considered for a QT-prolonging drug such as **methadone**, would have been identified by following the guidance to undertake an ECG in patients with one or more risk factors.

Nonetheless, a common sense approach should prevail, and the benefit of certain drugs used in the last days of life, e.g. **haloperidol**, **levomepromazine**, is likely to far outweigh any risk, and an ECG is not required.[22]

Methadone

There have been longstanding concerns relating to the occurrence of serious adverse events with **methadone**, including deaths, from apparent unintentional overdose, particularly in the first 2 weeks of administration. As the use of **methadone** increased, for both **methadone** maintenance and chronic pain, so did the number of deaths, disproportionately more than with

Box D A clinical approach to drug-induced QT prolongation

When using drugs known to prolong the QT interval, a prescriber needs to:

- understand the pharmacology of the drug, in particular factors which may lead to accumulation, e.g. drug–drug interaction, impaired elimination
- whenever possible, avoid the concurrent use of more than one drug which prolongs the QT interval
- use the lowest effective dose of the QT-prolonging drug
- evaluate and balance the potential benefit against the potential risk, taking into account the specific circumstances of the patient and the presence of other risk factors (Box C), e.g.:
  - ▷ in patients with a known (pre-existing) prolonged QT interval, avoid the use of all QT-prolonging drugs except under specialist guidance (Box B)
  - ▷ in patients with cardiac disease, drugs which prolong the QT interval should generally be avoided unless no suitable alternative exists
  - ▷ in patients with cardiac disease, if a cardiac anti-arrhythmic known to prolong the QT interval is prescribed, consider undertaking an ECG before starting the drug and once steady-state is achieved (generally 5 times the drug halflife), together with regular monitoring of plasma potassium, calcium and magnesium concentrations to ensure these remain well within their normal ranges
  - ▷ in patients without cardiac disease but with other risk factors, consider similar monitoring to above when using a QT-prolonging drug
  - ▷ for advice about patients at the end of life, and also methadone, see below
- explain to the patient (and family) the risk involved and the reasons for using the drug in question, to allow an informed decision to be made
- a drug which increases QTc interval by 30–60msec should raise concern and, if by >60msec, serious concern about the risk of *torsade de pointes* (particularly when the resultant QTc interval exceeds 500msec)
- report instances of drug-related QT prolongation to the MHRA through the yellow card scheme at www.mhra.gov.uk/index.htm
- consider *torsade de pointes* as a possible cause of palpitations, syncope or seizure-like activity.

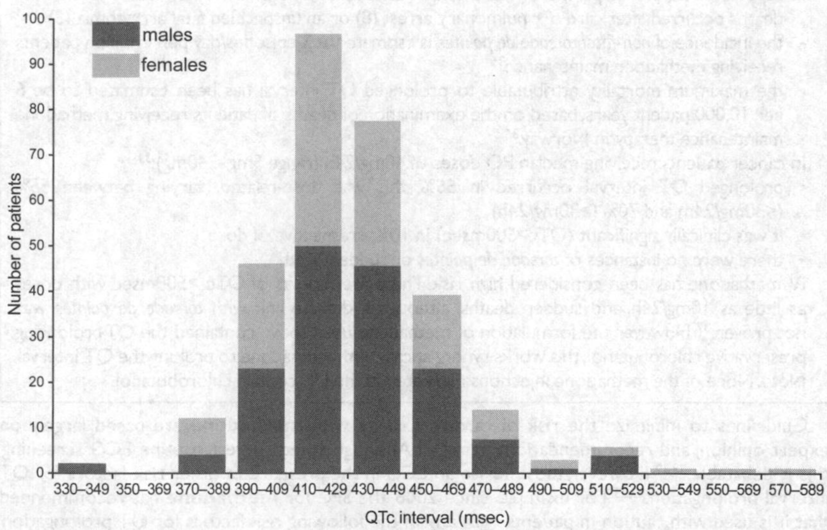

Figure 3 Distribution of the QT interval in 300 palliative care patients.[21]

other opioids, resulting in the US FDA issuing an alert to health professionals in 2006.[15] A major factor is considered to be a lack of knowledge among clinicians about the need to carefully monitor the use of **methadone**, particularly during the first 2–4 weeks (see p.469). Although many of these deaths are likely to be a result of respiratory depression, *torsade de pointes* may be a contributing factor (Box E).

Box E Methadone, prolonged QT interval and *torsade de pointes*

The association between methadone and a prolonged QT interval was first reported in 1973.[23] The link with *torsade de pointes* was made in 2002, when it was described in 17 patients receiving a median dose of methadone of 330mg/24h PO; all had QT interval >500msec, and most had other risk factors.[24]

Subsequently, methadone has been found to block ion channels associated with QT prolongation, and to increase the QT interval and the risk of *torsade de pointes*, generally in a dose-dependent manner.[25]

However, although some found QTc unaltered by doses <100mg/24h PO,[26] QTc >500msec and *torsade de pointes* have been reported with daily doses as low as 30–40mg PO.[27] A review of 21 patients on methadone with confirmed prolonged QT interval and *torsade de pointes* found generally higher daily doses (median 130mg, range 40–700mg). However, multiple risk factors were common, including female sex, heart disease, hypokalaemia, hypomagnesaemia, drug interaction, multiple QT-prolonging drugs, hepatic impairment, sinus bradycardia and cocaine misuse.[28] The frequent co-existence of other risk factors makes it difficult to quantify the risk from methadone alone and may explain the inconsistent dose relationship seen between methadone and QT prolongation.

Although slight prolongation of the QT interval by methadone appears to be common, the clinical significance of this is unclear. A marked increase in QTc to >500msec is seen in a small proportion of patients given methadone (generally about ≤5%, but 16% in one report).[25,27-33] The incidence of *torsade de pointes* and of *fatal torsade de pointes* is hard to quantify, but both are likely to be rare, e.g.:

- of the 2,009 adverse drug events for methadone reported to the MHRA between 1964 and September 2021, 47 (11 fatal) were classified as cardiac arrhythmias; these included 6 and 3 reports of *torsade de pointes* or ventricular fibrillation respectively, all non-fatal. Most of the deaths occurred after cardio ± pulmonary arrest (8) or an unspecified fatal arrhythmia (3)[34]
- the incidence of *non-fatal torsade de pointes* is estimated at 3 episodes/day per 1 million patients receiving methadone maintenance[35]
- the maximum mortality attributable to prolonged QT interval has been estimated to be 6 per 10,000 patient years, based on the examination of deaths of patients receiving methadone maintenance therapy in Norway.[36]

In cancer patients receiving median PO doses of 40mg/24h (range 5mg–240mg):[33]

- prolonged QT interval occurred in 65%; this was dose-related, varying between 55% (<30mg/24h) and 70% (>30mg/24h)
- it was clinically significant (QTc>500msec) in 10%, irrespective of dose
- there were no instances of *torsade de pointes* or sudden death.

IV methadone has been considered high risk. There are reports of QTc >500msec with doses as little as 10mg/24h, and sudden deaths, although a definite link with *torsade de pointes* was not proven.[37] However, the formulation of methadone used above contained the QT-prolonging preservative chlorobutanol; this works synergistically with methadone to prolong the QT interval. Note. None of the methadone injections marketed in the UK contain chlorobutanol.

Guidelines to minimize the risk of cardiac toxicity with **methadone** are based largely on expert opinion, and recommendations vary.[22,25] Although some suggest routine ECG screening, this is debatable.[38,39] However, most advise an ECG in the presence of other risk factors for QT interval prolongation.[22,25] For example, since 2006, the SPC for **methadone** has recommended that it is used with caution in patients with any of the following risk factors for QT prolongation:

- a history of cardiac conduction abnormalities
- advanced heart disease or ischaemic heart disease
- liver disease

- a family history of sudden death
- electrolyte abnormalities
- concurrent treatment with drugs which:
  - ▷ may cause electrolyte abnormalities
  - ▷ have a potential to prolong the QT interval
  - ▷ inhibit CYP3A4 (see p.781).

ECG monitoring is recommended in such patients before starting **methadone** and repeated when the dose is stabilized. Some guidelines suggest an annual ECG thereafter.[25] ECG monitoring is also recommended in patients without recognized risk factors for QT prolongation, before dose titration above 100mg/24h PO, and 1 week after such up-titration (an arbitrary dose, based on expert opinion; others suggest 120mg/24h PO).[25] Monitoring of serum electrolytes, e.g. potassium, magnesium, is generally recommended in patients taking diuretics or at risk of hypokalaemia, e.g. because of vomiting or diarrhoea.

Other guidelines also recommend an ECG if other risk factors or cardiac symptoms (e.g. palpitation, dizziness, fainting spells, seizures) develop during treatment, and highlight the importance of educating patients taking **methadone** to avoid where possible the use of other drugs which can prolong the QT interval or inhibit **methadone** metabolism, and to urgently report cardiac symptoms.[40]

Guidance specific for palliative care is limited.[41,42] In the USA, an expert group has developed a guideline for the use of *parenteral* **methadone** for chronic pain and in the palliative/hospice setting. Partly because of the increased risk presented by the preservative chlorobutanol (Box E), an ECG is recommended:

- before starting IV therapy and after 1 and 4 days of treatment
- when the dose is significantly increased
- if an additional risk factor for QT prolongation develops.[41]

Monitoring serum electrolytes in high risk patients and discussing the potential risks of prolonged QT interval and *torsade de pointes* with the patient and carers are also recommended. Consideration of burden vs. benefit is paramount and, in those with life-limiting illness, the potential benefit of controlling otherwise refractory pain may far outweigh the risks, even when monitoring for arrhythmia is impractical.[41]

One North American guideline covering methadone given by any route, links recommended levels of ECG monitoring with goals of care.[42] Such a common sense approach should prevail: ECG monitoring is generally irrelevant in the last days of life.[22] On the other hand, for a patient with a reasonable prognosis, it may be appropriate to identify any risk factors for QT prolongation and consider ECG monitoring as recommended in the SPC. Nonetheless, research is required to establish the magnitude of the risk of *torsade de pointes* with **methadone** and the overall value of adopting the above approaches in the palliative care setting.

If the baseline QT is prolonged, an alternative opioid should be considered. Further, if the QT interval increases to >500msec when on **methadone**, generally it should be discontinued and an alternative used, e.g. SL **buprenorphine**. However, there has been a report of the successful use of parenteral **methadone** for analgesia in a patient with a prolonged QT interval.[43] Implantable cardioverter defibrillators have also been used in addicts with *torsade de pointes* who needed to remain on **methadone**.[44]

Generally, **methadone** is available as a racemic mixture. *S*–**methadone** is a more potent blocker of the potassium channels in the cardiac myocytes than *R*–**methadone** (commercially available as **levomethadone**). CYP2B6 also displays stereoselectivity for the metabolism of *S*–**methadone**, and initial findings suggest that CYP2B6 poor metabolizers (found in about 6% of Caucasians and African-Americans) have higher levels of *S*–**methadone** and may thus be at greater risk of prolonged QTc.[45] The use of **levomethadone** may thus be safer in this respect but, at present, availability is limited to a few countries (not UK).[46,47]

1 Goldenberg I *et al.* (2006) QT interval: how to measure it and what is "normal". *Journal of Cardiovascular Electrophysiology*. **17**: 333–336.

2 Talebi S *et al.* (2015) Underestimated and unreported prolonged QTc by automated ECG analysis in patients on methadone: can we rely on computer reading? *Acta Cardiologica*. **70**: 211–216.

3 Rautaharju PM *et al.* (2009) AHA/ACCF/HRS recommendations for the standardization and interpretation of the electrocardiogram: part IV: the ST segment, T and U waves, and the QT interval. *Journal of the American College of Cardiology*. **53**: 982–991.

4 Vandenberk B *et al.* (2016) Which QT correction formulae to use for QT monitoring? *Journal of the American Heart Association*. **5**: e003264.

5 Patel PJ *et al.* (2016) Optimal QT interval correction formula in sinus tachycardia for identifying cardiovascular and mortality risk: findings from the Penn Atrial Fibrillation Free study. *Heart Rhythm*. **13**: 527–535.

6 Schwartz PJ and Woosley RL (2016) Predicting the unpredictable: drug-Induced QT prolongation and torsades de pointes. *Journal of the American College of Cardiology*. **67**: 1639–1650.

7 Thomas SH and Behr ER (2016) Pharmacological treatment of acquired QT prolongation and torsades de pointes. *British Journal of Clinical Pharmacology*. **81**: 420–427.
8 Drew BJ *et al.* (2010) Prevention of torsade de pointes in hospital settings: a scientific statement from the American Heart Association and the American College of Cardiology Foundation. *Circulation*. **121**: 1047–1060.
9 European Medicines Agency (2005) The clinical evaluation of QT/QTc interval prolongation and proarrhythmic potential for non-antiarrhythmic drugs. CPMP/ICH/2/04.
10 Haverkamp W *et al.* (2000) The potential for QT prolongation and proarrhythmia by non-antiarrhythmic drugs: clinical and regulatory implications. Report on a policy conference of the European Society of Cardiology. *European Heart Journal*. **21**: 1216–1231.
11 Idle JR (2000) The heart of psychotropic drug therapy. *Lancet*. **355**: 1824–1825.
12 Zipes DP *et al.* (2006) ACC/AHA/ESC 2006 guidelines for management of patients with ventricular arrhythmias and the prevention of sudden cardiac death. *Europace*. **8**: 746–837.
13 Heemskerk CPM *et al.* (2018) Risk factors for QTc interval prolongation. *European Journal of Clinical Pharmacology*. **74**: 183–191.
14 Liu J *et al.* (2019) QT prolongation in HIV-positive patients: review article. *Indian Heart Journal*. **71**: 434–439.
15 Andrews CM *et al.* (2009) Methadone-induced mortality in the treatment of chronic pain: role of QT prolongation. *Cardiology Journal*. **16**: 210–217.
16 Al-Khatib SM *et al.* (2003) What clinicians should know about the QT interval. *Journal of the American Medical Association*. **289**: 2120–2127.
17 Twycross RG *et al.* (1994) Monitoring drug use in palliative care. *Palliative Medicine*. **8**: 137–143.
18 Bernard SA and Bruera E (2000) Drug interactions in palliative care. *Journal of Clinical Oncology*. **18**: 1780–1799.
19 Davies SJ *et al.* (2004) Potential for drug interactions involving cytochromes P450 2D6 and 3A4 on general adult psychiatric and functional elderly psychiatric wards. *British journal of clinical pharmacology*. **57**: 464–472.
20 Wilcock A *et al.* (2005) Potential for drug interactions involving cytochrome P450 in patients attending palliative day care centres: a multicentre audit. *British journal of clinical pharmacology*. **60**: 326–329.
21 Walker G *et al.* (2003) Prolongation of the QT interval in palliative care patients. *Journal of Pain and Symptom Management*. **26**: 855–859.
22 Wilcock A and Beattie JM (2009) Prolonged QT interval and methadone: implications for palliative care. *Current Opinion in Supportive and Palliative Care*. **3**: 252–257.
23 Stimmel B *et al.* (1973) Electrocardiographic changes in heroin, methadone and multiple drug abuse: a postulated mechanism of sudden death in narcotic addicts. *Proceedings of the National Conference on Methadone Treatment*. **1**: 706–710.
24 Krantz MJ *et al.* (2002) Torsade de pointes associated with very-high-dose methadone. *Annals of Internal Medicine*. **137**: 501–504.
25 Martin JA *et al.* (2011) QT interval screening in methadone maintenance treatment: report of a SAMHSA expert panel. *Journal of Addictive Diseases*. **30**: 283–306.
26 Stallvik M *et al.* (2013) Corrected QT interval during treatment with methadone and buprenorphine--relation to doses and serum concentrations. *Drug and Alcohol Dependence*. **129**: 88–93.
27 Stringer J *et al.* (2009) Methadone-associated QT interval prolongation and torsades de pointes. *American Journal of Health System Pharmacy*. **66**: 825–833.
28 Vieweg WVR *et al.* (2013) Methadone, QTc interval prolongation and torsade de pointes: Case reports offer the best understanding of this problem. *Therapeutic advances in psychopharmacology*. **3**: 219–232.
29 Reddy S *et al.* (2010) The effect of oral methadone on the QTc interval in advanced cancer patients: a prospective pilot study. *Journal of Palliative Medicine*. **13**: 33–38.
30 Price LC *et al.* (2014) Methadone for pain and the risk of adverse cardiac outcomes. *Journal of Pain and Symptom Management*. **48**: 333–342.
31 Huh B and Park CH (2010) Retrospective analysis of low-dose methadone and QTc prolongation in chronic pain patients. *Korean Journal Anesthesiology*. **58**: 338–343.
32 van den Beuken-van Everdingen MH *et al.* (2013) Prolonged QT interval by methadone: relevance for daily practice? A prospective study in patients with cancer and noncancer pain. *Journal of Opioid Management*. **9**: 263–267.
33 Lovell AG *et al.* (2019) Evaluation of QTc interval prolongation among patients with cancer using enteral methadone. *American Journal of Hospice & Palliative Medicine*. **36**: 177–184.
34 MHRA (2021) Methadone. Interactive drug analysis profile. https://info.mhra.gov.uk/drug-analysis-profiles (accessed 9th September 2021).
35 Hanon S *et al.* (2010) Ventricular arrhythmias in patients treated with methadone for opioid dependence. *Journal of Interventional Cardiac Electrophysiology*. **28**: 19–22.
36 Anchersen K *et al.* (2009) Prevalence and clinical relevance of corrected QT interval prolongation during methadone and buprenorphine treatment: a mortality assessment study. *Addiction*. **104**: 993 999.37 Kornick CA *et al.* (2003) QTc interval prolongation associated with intravenous methadone. *Pain*. **105**: 499–506.
38 Haigney MC (2011) First, do no harm: QT interval screening in methadone maintenance treatment. *Journal of Addictive Diseases*. **30**: 309–312.
39 Bart G (2011) CSAT's QT interval screening in methadone report: outrageous fortune or sea of troubles? *Journal of Addictive Diseases*. **30**: 313–317.
40 Office of Alcoholism and Substance Abuse Services (2009 March) Medical advisory panel positon on QTc interval screening in methadone treatment. www.oasas.ny.gov.
41 Shaiova L *et al.* (2008) Consensus guideline on parenteral methadone use in pain and palliative care. *Palliative and Supportive Care*. **6**: 165–176.
42 McPherson ML *et al.* (2019) Safe and appropriate use of methadone in hospice and palliative care: expert consensus white paper. *Journal of Pain and Symptom Management*. **57**: 635–645.
43 Sekine R *et al.* (2007) The successful use of parenteral methadone in a patient with a prolonged QTc interval. *Journal of Pain and Symptom Management*. **34**: 566–569.
44 Patel AM *et al.* (2008) Role of implantable cardioverter-defibrillators in patients with methadone-induced long QT syndrome. *American Journal of Cardiology*. **101**: 209–211.
45 Eap CB *et al.* (2007) Stereoselective block of hERG channel by (S)-methadone and QT interval prolongation in CYP2B6 slow metabolizers. *Clinical Pharmacology & Therapeutics*. **81**: 719–728.
46 Gaertner J *et al.* (2008) Methadone: a closer look at the controversy. *Journal of Pain and Symptom Management*. **36**: e4–7.
47 Ansermot N *et al.* (2010) Substitution of (R,S)-methadone by (R)-methadone: Impact on QTc interval. *JAMA Internal Medicine*. **170**: 529–536.

Updated September 2021

21: DRUG-INDUCED MOVEMENT DISORDERS

Drug-induced movement disorders (DIMD) include:
- extrapyramidal reactions
  - ▷ onset ≤weeks: acute akathisia, dystonia and parkinsonism (Box A)
  - ▷ onset ≥months: tardive akathisia, dyskinesia and dystonia (Box B)
- catatonia (see Benzodiazepines and Z-drugs, Box C, p.173)
- cerebellar ataxia (Box C)
- postural (essential) tremor (Box D)
- disorders with concurrent non-motor symptoms
  - ▷ acute dopamine depletion (neuroleptic/antipsychotic malignant syndrome; see Antipsychotics, Box A, p.192)
  - ▷ serotonin toxicity (see Antidepressants, Box A, p.217)
  - ▷ antidepressant withdrawal syndrome (see Antidepressants, Box B, p.224).

The risk is associated with dose, pre-existing neurological disease and a genetic predisposition.[1-3]

Most DIMDs develop within days or weeks of starting or increasing one of the drugs described below. However, many other drugs are implicated, and symptom onset can be delayed by months or even years, or arise as a result of a drug interaction. Thus, DIMD should be considered in any unexplained movement disorder; if in doubt, seek advice from a clinical pharmacist.

Pharmacology

Most extrapyramidal reactions are caused by drugs that block dopamine receptors in the CNS; these include all antipsychotics and **metoclopramide**. Antipsychotics differ in their propensity for causing extrapyramidal reactions. A lower risk is associated with lower affinity for the D_2-receptor, D_2-receptor partial agonism, $5HT_{1A}$-receptor partial agonism and/or $5HT_2$-receptor antagonism (see p.184). Thus, the risk is a spectrum (in descending order):
- **haloperidol** (the highest risk)
- phenothiazines (e.g. **levomepromazine**)
- **risperidone**
- **olanzapine**
- **quetiapine**, **clozapine** (the lowest risk).[4]

However, the overall tolerability of different antipsychotics is comparable, because lower rates of extrapyramidal reactions are offset by increased rates of sedation and/or undesirable metabolic effects (see p.184).[5]

With atypical antipsychotics, although the above risk spectrum still applies, akathisia remains a more common problem than dystonia and parkinsonism.

Serotonin-modulating drugs affect both the extrapyramidal system and spinal motor neurones. Extrapyramidal dopaminergic neurones are inhibited by $5HT_{2A}$- and $5HT_{2C}$-receptors.[6] Spinal serotonin release correlates with motor activity, stimulating spinal motor neurones at low levels and inhibiting them at higher levels.[7]

Box A Acute extrapyramidal reactions[1,8-15]

Causes
- dopamine modulators (antipsychotics, metoclopramide, levodopa)
- serotonin modulators (SSRIs, $5HT_3$ antagonists, 5-hydroxytryptophan)
- anti-epileptics (carbamazepine, valproate)
- miscellaneous (diltiazem, lithium).

Classification

Parkinsonism

Generally occurs within weeks of starting the causal drug:
- resting tremor (suppressed during voluntary movements)
- muscular rigidity
- bradykinesia (e.g. shuffling gait, expressionless face).

Acute dystonia

Abnormal positioning or spasm of one or more muscle group, occurring within days of starting the causal drug:
- dysphagia
- dysphonia
- jaw (trismus, gaping, grimacing)
- tongue (dysarthria, protrusion)
- head and neck (retrocollis, torticollis)
- laryngopharyngeal spasm
- limbs or trunk
- fixed direction of gaze (oculogyric crisis).

Acute akathisia

Motor restlessness, occurring within days–weeks of starting the causal drug:
- pacing to relieve restlessness
- inability to sit or stand still
- fidgety movements or swinging of legs
- rocking from foot to foot when standing.

Treatment

Reduce or stop causal drug, or switch to an alternative with a lower risk, e.g.:
- metoclopramide → domperidone
- antipsychotic → quetiapine (see text above).

If patient is distressed, treat symptomatically while waiting for the causal drug to be cleared:
- *parkinsonism:* start an antimuscarinic, e.g. procyclidine 2.5–5mg PO t.d.s. or 5–10mg IV/IM
- *dystonia:* start an antimuscarinic (as above); if ineffective or contra-indicated, benzodiazepines are an alternative (e.g. diazepam 5mg IV then PO)
- *akathisia:* start propranolol[a] 10mg PO t.d.s.; increase if necessary every few days to a maximum dose of 120mg/24h; further benefit above this level is unlikely. Alternatives include:
  - ▷ mirtazapine 15mg PO at bedtime
  - ▷ antimuscarinics, particularly if concurrent parkinsonism
  - ▷ benzodiazepines (as above).

a. selective β_1 antagonists, e.g. atenolol, are *less* effective for akathisia, because they penetrate the blood–brain barrier less readily than non-selective β antagonists.

Box B Tardive (delayed onset) extrapyramidal reactions[1,13-16]

Causes

Long-term (>3 months) treatment with antipsychotics or metoclopramide, particularly in the elderly, those on high doses and those receiving 'typical' antipsychotics (see p.184). Also seen after reduction or cessation of treatment (withdrawal-emergent dyskinesia).

Clinical features (may co-exist)

- *tardive dyskinesia:* involuntary athetoid (writhing) and choreiform movements of the tongue, jaw and extremities, exacerbated by anxiety and reduced by drowsiness and during sleep
- *tardive dystonia:* abnormal positioning of the limbs and tonic contractions of the neck and trunk muscles causing torticollis, lordosis or scoliosis
- *tardive akathisia:* motor restlessness.

Treatment

- reduce or stop causal drug, or switch to an alternative with a lower risk, e.g.:
  - ▷ metoclopramide → domperidone
  - ▷ antipsychotic → quetiapine (see text above)
- withdraw antimuscarinics (these exacerbate tardive dyskinesia)
- seek specialist advice before initiating other drug treatments (e.g. tetrabenazine).

Box C Drug-induced cerebellar ataxia[2]

Causes

Generally occurs within days or weeks of starting the causal drug; occasionally seen after using causal drug for months–years (particularly lithium, phenytoin, valproate). Typically resolves but can persist indefinitely, particularly when caused by lithium, phenytoin or cytarabine.

- anti-epileptics
- benzodiazepines
- cytotoxics (cytarabine, irinotecan)
- immunosuppressants (cyclosporine, tacrolimus)
- miscellaneous (lithium, metronidazole).

Clinical features

- intention tremor, past pointing
- clumsy, poorly co-ordinated movements (dysdiadochokinesis)
- nystagmus.

Treatment

Reduce or stop causal drug.

Box D Drug-induced postural tremor[1,17]

Causes

- anti-epileptics (valproate)
- antidepressants
- antipsychotics
- bronchodilators (salbutamol, theophylline)
- psychostimulants (caffeine, methylphenidate)
- lithium.

Clinical features

Tremor with frequency of 8–12 cycles per second, best observed with hands held outstretched.

Treatment

Reduce or stop causal drug.

1 DSM-5 (Desk Reference to the Diagnostic Criteria from DSM-5). The American Psychiatric Association.
2 van Gaalen J *et al.* (2014) Drug-induced cerebellar ataxia: a systematic review. *CNS Drugs*. **28**: 1139–1153.
3 Barnes TR (2011) Evidence-based guidelines for the pharmacological treatment of schizophrenia: recommendations from the British Association for Psychopharmacology. *Journal of Psychopharmacology*. **25**: 567–620.
4 Rummel-Kluge C *et al.* (2012) Second-generation antipsychotic drugs and extrapyramidal side effects: a systematic review and meta-analysis of head-to-head comparisons. *Schizophrenia Bulletin*. **38**: 167-177.
5 Lieberman JA *et al.* (2005) Effectiveness of antipsychotic drugs in patients with chronic schizophrenia. *New England Journal of Medicine*. **353**: 1209–1223.
6 Stahl SM (2013) Chapter 4: Psychosis and schizophrenia. *Essential Psychopharmacology: Neuroscientific Basis and Practical Applications*, 4th edn. USA: Cambridge University Press. pp. 79–128
7 Perrier JF and Cotel F (2015) Serotonergic modulation of spinal motor control. *Current Opinion in Neurobiology*. **33**: 1–7.
8 Poyurovsky M (2010) Acute antipsychotic-induced akathisia revisited. *British Journal of Psychiatry*. **196**: 89–91.
9 Laoutidis ZG and Luckhaus C (2014) 5-HT2A receptor antagonists for the treatment of neuroleptic-induced akathisia: a systematic review and meta-analysis. *International Journal of Neuropsychopharmacology*. **17**: 823-832.
10 Lima AR *et al.* (2002) Benzodiazepines for neuroleptic-induced acute akathisia. *Cochrane Database of Systematic Reviews*. **1**: CD001950. www.thecochranelibrary.com.
11 Gagrat D *et al.* (1978) Intravenous diazepam in the treatment of neuroleptic-induced acute dystonia and akathisia. *American Journal of Psychiatry*. **135**: 1232–1233.
12 Bondon-Guitton E *et al.* (2011) Drug-induced parkinsonism: a review of 17 years' experience in a regional pharmacovigilance center in France. *Movement Disorders*. **26**: 2226–2231.
13 World Health Organization. The ICD-10 classification of mental and behavioural disorders. http://apps.who.int/classifications/icd10/.
14 Taylor D *et al.* (2018) Chapter 2: Schizophrenia. *The Maudsley Prescribing Guidelines in Psychiatry*, 13th edn. Wiley-Blackwell. pp. 3–230.
15 Anderson I and McAllister-Williams H (2016) Chapter 3: Antipsychotics. *Fundamentals of Clinical Psychopharmacology*, 4th edn. CRC Press. pp 47–76.
16 Bhidayasiri R *et al.* (2013) Evidence-based guideline: treatment of tardive syndromes: report of the Guideline Development Subcommittee of the American Academy of Neurology. *Neurology*. **81**: 463–469.
17 Morgan JC and Sethi KD (2005) Drug-induced tremors. *Lancet Neurolology*. **4**: 866–876.

Updated September 2019

22: DRUGS AND FITNESS TO DRIVE

This chapter summarizes the evidence regarding the effect of centrally acting drugs of most relevance to palliative care, e.g. opioids, anti-epileptics, antidepressants, benzodiazepines, cannabinoids, on driving performance and the risk of a road traffic accident.

Although impaired driving performance from stable doses of centrally acting drugs is not inevitable, prescribers have a duty of care to inform patients of the risk of impairment, particularly during initial titration, and advise them appropriately. As a minimum, patients should be informed that:

- it is their legal responsibility to drive only if they feel 100% safe to do so
- drugs should be taken in accordance with the advice of the PIL or a health professional; this has specific implications relating to the use of certain drugs and the potential for prosecution (see below).

The presence of other factors which can impair driving performance must also be taken into account, e.g. pain, depression, insomnia, anxiety, frailty, visual disturbance. Conversely, treatment of some of these factors, e.g. pain, depression, with an appropriate centrally acting drug can reverse the impaired driving performance. Thus, the advice given must be tailored to the individual circumstances of the patient.[1,2]

In relation to underlying diagnoses, particularly the risk of seizures, see the DVLA fitness to drive advice.[2]

22

Evaluating the effect of drugs on driving performance

The evidence relating to the impact of centrally acting drugs on driving can be conflicting and difficult to interpret. For example, although epidemiological studies of road traffic accidents generally find higher rates of use of centrally acting drugs, the underlying conditions requiring their use can also impair driving performance.[3-5] Such confounding factors can be controlled for by studying actual or simulated driving, or surrogate laboratory markers of such skills, before and after drug administration. However, this approach may not capture all influences on driving performance, from altered attention and reaction time to impaired judgement and risk taking.[3,4,6] Thus, in this chapter, the methodology underlying the evidence is indicated for each drug class.

Guidance for patients

In the UK, drivers are liable to prosecution if driving or attempting to drive while impaired by drugs, *whether prescribed or illicit.*[7] Thus, it is important to remind patients of this when prescribing drugs which could impair their driving performance (Box A).

Further, an amendment to the Road Traffic Act[8] for England, Wales and Scotland specifies levels for certain drugs (Box B) above which drivers are liable to prosecution, *even when driving is not impaired*, unless following the directions of a PIL or health professional. The main focus of this law is the *illicit* use of drugs.

The evidence for sedative drugs most relevant to palliative care practice, summarized in Table 1, suggests that patients should be warned not to drive after starting and when titrating potentially sedating medication, or after taking a dose for break-through pain. They should be warned that sedation will be increased by the concurrent use of alcohol (even within normal alcohol driving limits) or other sedating medication, whether obtained by prescription, over the counter or illicitly.

More specifically, patients receiving opioids, anti-epileptics and antidepressants can consider driving once a stable dose is achieved if they are not affected by drowsiness and not impaired by the disease itself. If possible, use a less sedating drug, e.g. consider the use of an SSRI rather than a TCA when treating depression.[2] For benzodiazepines, particularly if taken in the daytime and/or those with a long halflife, the risk is more persistent, and consideration should be given to using a less sedating alternative, e.g. an SSRI for anxiety, or not driving. The risk with stable doses of prescribed cannabinoids is unclear.

Providing the patient with written information also helps (Box A). Other examples of information leaflets are available on the www.palliativedrugs.com Document library under Prescribing issues (Driving on medication).

Box A Example of a patient advice leaflet: medicines, drowsiness and driving (based on references[8-11])

The medicines you are taking do not automatically disqualify you from driving in the UK. *However, it is illegal to drive if medicines are reducing the speed of your reactions or general alertness.* Both the label and the PIL will warn you about possible drowsiness. If so, it is important that you take the following precautions:

Do not drive

- unless you feel 100% safe to do so
- after starting or increasing the dose of any drug that may make you drowsy (whether prescribed for you or bought from a pharmacist); wait until the drowsiness fully wears off (for painkillers this takes about 5 days, sometimes longer)
- after taking an extra dose of a sedative medicine, e.g. for at least 3 hours after a 'rescue' dose of morphine for pain
- if you feel drowsy or dizzy, or if your thinking, reactions, co-ordination or eyesight are impaired
- after drinking alcohol (even a small amount increases the effect of other drugs).

Restarting driving

You may try driving when you feel 100% safe to do so and you no longer feel drowsy. Begin by making a short trip:

- on roads that are quiet and familiar
- at a quiet time of day when the light is good
- with a companion who may take over driving if required.

If you and your companion are happy with your attentiveness, reactions and general ability, then you may start to drive.

Do not exhaust yourself by driving long distances. If in doubt, discuss with your doctor or other health professional.

Who to inform if you are planning to drive

- *your doctor*, who can warn you about medicines which might affect your general alertness or the speed of your reactions
- *your insurance company*, to be sure that you are covered. (Note. It may help if you send the company a copy of this leaflet.)

Although you do not automatically need to inform the DVLA that you are taking regular painkillers, in practice insurance companies generally advise this.

In relation to cancer, you must inform the DVLA if you have a brain tumour, a secondary tumour in your brain or if you have had a fit or problems with eyesight.

If in doubt, discuss with your doctor or the DVLA medical advisory helpline (0300 790 6806, and have your driving licence number ready).

Be prepared!

If you are taking any of the following medicines, it is recommended that, when driving, you carry evidence to confirm that they have been prescribed for you, e.g. a repeat prescription together with your doctor's contact details:

- *benzodiazepines:* clonazepam, diazepam, lorazepam, oxazepam, temazepam
- *opioids:* diamorphine, methadone, morphine
- *others:* amfetamine, cannabis-based medicines, ketamine.

The police use roadside tests to look for illicit use of these medicines. Carrying evidence that you are taking legitimately supplied medicines is not a legal requirement, but may minimize inconvenience if stopped.

However, it *is* a legal requirement that you are taking them *as advised*; do not change the dose without first discussing it with your doctor or other health professional.

Box B Drugs relevant to palliative care with specific limits set for prosecution under Section 5a of the Road Traffic Act[8,a]

Benzodiazepines	**Psychostimulants**
Clonazepam	Amfetamine
Diazepam	
Lorazepam	**Miscellaneous**
Oxazepam	Δ[9]-tetrahydrocannabinol
Temazepam	Ketamine
Opioids	
Diamorphine	
Methadone	
Morphine	

a. cocaine, Ecstasy, flunitrazepam (not UK), lysergic acid diethylamide (LSD) and methylamfetamine are also included on the full Department for Transport list, which is based on commonly misused drugs.

22

Table 1 Drugs and driving: a summary of the evidence available for sedative drugs relevant to palliative care practice

Class of drug	*Impact on risk of road traffic accidents*	*Comments*[a]
Opioids	With chronic use of a stable dose carefully titrated to avoid drowsiness and cognitive impairment, increased risk unlikely[12]	Multiple factors confound studies of road traffic collisions (see text), but on-the-road and simulator studies find that impaired cognition and driving performance generally subside 1 week after the start of treatment or after dose increments. The risk is shared by weak opioids.[12] Additional transient impairment occurs with doses for break-through pain
Anti-epileptics	With chronic use of a stable dose carefully titrated to avoid drowsiness and cognitive impairment, no increased risk[13]	Cognition impaired by multiple high-dose anti-epileptics; marginally less with newer drugs (e.g. gabapentin) compared with older drugs (e.g. carbamazepine)[14,15]
Antidepressants	Possible increased risk; unclear if related to the drug or underlying reason for their use, e.g. depression[16]	In simulator studies, sedative antidepressants impair performance for 1–2 weeks after the start of treatment, whereas SSRIs cause less impairment[5]
Benzodiazepines and Z-drugs	Increased risk[17]	Risk only partially decreases with time and is related to dose, halflife and concurrent alcohol. Risk from nocturnal use of shorter-halflife hypnotic benzodiazepines and Z-drugs is unclear[17,18]
Cannabinoids	Risk increased initially. The degree of tolerance to chronic use of stable doses of prescribed cannabinoids is uncertain	Most studies deal with illicit use, frequently confounded by alcohol consumption and risk-taking behaviours[19-21]

a. advice should also take into account the presence of any co-morbid conditions known to impair driving performance, e.g. pain, depression, insomnia.

Risk from specific drug classes

Opioids

In epidemiological studies, ≤10% of drivers responsible for road traffic accidents have consumed opioid analgesics.[22-25] However, these data do not distinguish between the risk associated with stable and tolerable doses of opioids versus the risk from impairment due to:

- newly started opioids
- inappropriately high-dose opioids
- other psychotropics taken concurrently
- illicit opioid use
- the pain itself.

In simulator and on-the-road tests, driving performance does not appear to be affected by stable doses of appropriately titrated strong opioids:[6,12,26]

- cognition returns to normal about 1 week after the start of treatment or after dose increments
- long-term opioid analgesia for cancer pain and non-cancer pain has little or no impact on surrogate laboratory measures of driving performance compared with:
  - ▷ healthy volunteers
  - ▷ cancer patients not taking opioids
  - ▷ patients with various causes of cerebral impairment who have passed a standardized fitness-to-drive test
- patients with non-cancer pain taking opioids at stable doses for ≥1 week do not differ from those not taking opioids or from healthy volunteers in tests of actual driving performance.

The effects of opioids on cognition are mixed. Although some studies found that opioids improve cognition (possibly as a consequence of reducing pain-related impairment), others found worsening cognition, particularly with higher doses (equivalent to 120–190mg/24h of PO morphine).[27]

The optimal interval between dose initiation or increase and returning to driving is unclear and may vary between individuals and formulation used, e.g. steady-state plasma concentrations of TD **fentanyl** are generally achieved after 36–48h but, according to the manufacturers, this is sometimes achieved only after 6 days (p.440).

Anti-epileptics

Epidemiological studies examining **carbamazepine**, **phenytoin** and **valproate** do not find an increased risk of road traffic accidents.[25] However, the use of multiple or high-dose anti-epileptics, particularly **phenobarbital**, is associated with marked cognitive impairment. Newer drugs, e.g. **gabapentin**, may cause marginally less impairment than older drugs, e.g. **carbamazepine**, **valproate**.[14,15] Patients with epilepsy who adhere strictly to their anti-epileptic regimen are less likely to have road traffic accidents than those patients who do not.[1]

Antidepressants

In driving simulation studies and standard on-the-road tests, sedating antidepressants (e.g. **amitriptyline**, **mirtazapine**) initially impair driving performance. However, performance generally returns to baseline within 1–2 weeks. In similar studies, driving performance is unaffected by non-sedating antidepressants (e.g. SSRIs, **venlafaxine**),[5] and on this basis they are the preferred choice in patients wanting to drive. However, results of epidemiological studies suggest that both sedating and non-sedating antidepressants are associated with an increased risk of road traffic accidents.[16] Depression *per se* impairs driving performance and may help explain these findings.[28] Nonetheless, caution appears necessary regardless of age and choice of antidepressant.

Benzodiazepines and Z-drugs

Both simulated driving tests and epidemiological studies find benzodiazepines increase the risk of road traffic accidents. The risk is highest in those taking higher doses, drugs with a longer halflife, or concurrent alcohol. The risk only partially decreases with time.[17]

The risk from a bedtime dose of a Z-drug or hypnotic benzodiazepine with a short halflife is unclear; findings of both driving simulator and epidemiological studies are conflicting.[17,18]

Cannabinoids

Recreational cannabis use causes dose-dependent impairment of driving ability.[29] The risk is synergistically increased by concurrent alcohol consumption.[19] In the USA, states decriminalizing recreational access have seen an increase in cannabis-related road traffic accidents.[21]

On the other hand, the risk associated with the use of stable doses of *prescribed* cannabinoids appears to be different (p.251). USA states legalizing access for medicinal, but not recreational, use have *not* experienced an increase in road traffic accidents.[21] Patients with multiple sclerosis and painful spasticity showed no change in surrogate markers of driving ability after receiving **nabilone** 2mg/day for 4 weeks (n=6)[30] or Sativex® for 6 weeks (n=31).[31] Patients with chronic pain taking stable doses of cannabinoids do not differ from those not taking cannabinoids in tests of cognition and reaction time.[32] Thus, similar to other psychotropics, stable doses of cannabinoids may allow tolerance to impairment to develop.

However, caution remains necessary. Advise against driving during initial dose titration. Once a patient is on a stable dose and the degree of psychomotor impairment caused by cannabinoids has been evaluated, restarting driving can be discussed. As with all medications, the impact of the underlying condition should also be taken into account; e.g. in one study, half of participants with multiple sclerosis had evidence of driving impairment before commencing cannabinoids.[31]

1 Hetland A and Carr DB (2014) Medications and impaired driving. *Annals of Pharmacotherapy*. **48**: 494–506.
2 DVLA (2021) Assessing fitness to drive – a guide for medical professionals. *UK Government*. www.gov.uk/dvla/fitnesstodrive.
3 Mailis-Gagnon A *et al.* (2012) Systematic review of the quality and generalizability of studies on the effects of opioids on driving and cognitive/psychomotor performance. *Clinical Journal of Pain*. **28**: 542–555.
4 Dassanayake T *et al.* (2011) Effects of benzodiazepines, antidepressants and opioids on driving: a systematic review and meta-analysis of epidemiological and experimental evidence. *Drug Safety*. **34**: 125–156.
5 Brunnauer A and Laux G (2017) Driving under the influence of antidepressants: a systematic review and update of the evidence of experimental and controlled clinical studies. *Pharmacopsychiatry*. **50**: 173–181.
6 Verster JC and Roth T (2012) Predicting psychopharmacological drug effects on actual driving performance (SDLP) from psychometric tests measuring driving-related skills. *Psychopharmacology*. **220**: 293–301.
7 Carter T (2006) Fitness to Drive: A Guide for Health Professionals. Royal Society of Medicine Press, London.
8 Department for Transport (2014) Guidance for healthcare professionals on drug driving. www.gov.uk.
9 Pease N *et al.* (2004) Driving advice for palliative care patients taking strong opioid medication. *Palliative Medicine*. **18**: 663–665.
10 Twycross RG (1997) Oral Morphine in Advanced Cancer. (3e). Beaconsfield Publishers, Beaconsfield.
11 MHRA (2014) New law on driving having taken certain drugs. Information leaflet to give to patients. www.gov.uk.
12 Ferreira D *et al.* (2018) The impact of therapeutic opioid agonists on driving-related psychomotor skills assessed by a driving simulator or an on-road driving task: A systematic review. *Palliative Medicine*. **32**: 786–803.
13 Neutel I (1998) Benzodiazepine-related traffic accidents in young and elderly drivers. *Human Psychopharmacology*. **13 (suppl)**: s115–s123.
14 Aldenkamp AP *et al.* (2003) Newer antiepileptic drugs and cognitive issues. *Epilepsia*. **44 (suppl 4)**: 21–29.
15 Brunbech L and Sabers A (2002) Effect of antiepileptic drugs on cognitive function in individuals with epilepsy: a comparative review of newer versus older agents. *Drugs*. **62**: 593–604.
16 Hill L *et al.* (2017) Depression, antidepressants and driving safety. *Injury Epidemiology*. **4**: 10.
17 Brandt J and Leong C (2017) Benzodiazepines and Z-Drugs: an updated review of major adverse outcomes reported on in epidemiologic research. *Drugs in R&D*. **17**: 493–507.
18 Nevriana A *et al.* (2017) New, occasional, and frequent use of zolpidem or zopiclone (alone and in combination) and the risk of injurious road traffic crashes in older adult drivers: a population-based case control and case-crossover study. *CNS Drugs*. **31**: 711–722.
19 Bondallaz P *et al.* (2016) Cannabis and its effects on driving skills. *Forensic Science International*. **268**: 92–102.
20 Neavyn M *et al.* (2014) Medical marijuana and driving: a review. *Journal of Medical Toxicology*. **10**: 269–279.
21 Lee J *et al.* (2018) Investigation of associations between marijuana law changes and marijuana-involved fatal traffic crashes: A state-level analysis. *Journal of Transport and Health*. **10**: 194–202.
22 Chihuri S and Li G (2017) Use of prescription opioids and motor vehicle crashes: A meta analysis. *Accident analysis and prevention*. **109**: 123–131.
23 Chihuri S and Li G (2019) Use of prescription opioids and initiation of fatal 2-vehicle crashes. *JAMA Network Open*. **2**: e188081.
24 Li G and Chihuri S (2019) Prescription opioids, alcohol and fatal motor vehicle crashes: a population-based case-control study. *Injury Epidemiology*. **2**: e188081.
25 Rudisill T *et al.* (2016) Medication use and the risk of motor vehicle collisions among licensed drivers: A systematic review. *Accident analysis and prevention*. **96**: 255–270.
26 Schumacher M *et al.* (2017) Effect of chronic opioid therapy on actual driving performance in non-cancer pain patients. *Psychopharmacology (Berl)*. **234**: 989–999.
27 Pask S *et al.* (2020) The effects of opioids on cognition in older adults with cancer and chronic noncancer pain: a systematic review. *Journal of Pain and Symptom Management*. **59**: 871–893.
28 Brunnauer A *et al.* (2016) Mobility behaviour and driving status of patients with mental disorders - an exploratory study. *International Journal of Psychiatry in Clinical Practice*. **20**: 40–46.
29 Department for Transport (2010) A review of evidence related to drug driving in the UK: A report submitted to the North Review Team by P. G. Jackson and C. J. Hilditch. Currently available from http://webarchive.nationalarchives.gov.uk.
30 Kurzthaler I *et al.* (2005) The effect of nabilone on neuropsychological functions related to driving ability: an extended case series. *Human Psychopharmacology*. **20**: 291–293.
31 Freidel M *et al.* (2015) Drug-resistant MS spasticity treatment with Sativex® add-on and driving ability. *Acta Neurologica Scandinavica*. **131**: 9–16.
32 Sznitman S *et al.* (2021) Medical cannabis and cognitive performance in middle to old adults treated for chronic pain. *Drug and Alcohol Review*. **40**: 272–280.

Updated June 2021

23: TAKING CONTROLLED AND PRESCRIPTION DRUGS TO OTHER COUNTRIES

Some patients receiving palliative care travel to other countries and need to take medicinal products with them. Two sets of laws need to be considered, those of the country that they are leaving and those of the country or countries to which they are travelling. Detailed advice can be obtained from the regulatory authorities, embassies or consulates in the relevant countries.[1]

23

UK customs regulations

It is advisable to check for the latest guidance by contacting the Home Office directly or visiting its website:

The Home Office
Drugs and Firearms Licensing Unit
5th Floor, Fry Building
2 Marsham Street
London SW1P 4DF
Tel: 020 7035 6330
e-mail: dflu.ie@homeoffice.gov.uk
https://www.gov.uk/controlled-drugs-licences-fees-and-returns

The UK customs regulations for travelling with prescribed medicinal products are the same for leaving or entering the UK. For UK residents, the main limitation is likely to be the legislation of the country/countries to which they are travelling (see below).

Although not a legal requirement, when patients are travelling with *any* prescribed medicinal product, the UK Home Office advises that patients carry a covering letter from a doctor, because it provides good supporting evidence that the medicinal products are for the patient's own use and in quantities necessary for that period of travel.[2] The letter should state:

- the patient's name, address and date of birth
- the destination(s) and dates of outward and return travel
- the names, forms, strengths, doses and total amounts of the drugs being carried.

All prescribed medicinal products should be kept in their original packaging and carried in the patient's hand luggage, together with the covering letter ± import/export licence that may be required for controlled drugs (see below) in case customs wants to examine them.

In the UK, a covering letter is sufficient to permit air passengers to carry >100mL of a liquid/gel medicine in their hand luggage. The liquid/gel medicines must be carried in containers that permit examination by airport staff.[3] Note. Countries outside the EU may have different rules on carrying liquids as a transit or transfer passenger.

In the UK, a covering letter is also sufficient to permit essential medical equipment to be carried in hand luggage, e.g. hypodermic syringes, inhalers, cooling gel packs, TENS machine. Such equipment must be presented at security to be screened separately.[3] Note. If oxygen is required, patients must contact the airline in advance to order a supply, as they cannot take their own cylinders on board.[3,4] (Note. Reference 4 contains additional useful information on the practicalities of international travel.)

Controlled drugs

If travelling for ≥3 months *and* carrying ≥3 months' supply of Schedule 2, 3 and 4 part I and part II controlled drugs for personal use into or out of the UK, a personal import/export licence is required. A licence application form can be downloaded from the website above. Once completed, it must be e-mailed to the Home Office Drugs and Firearms Licensing Unit along with a letter (on headed notepaper) from a doctor confirming the patient's name, travel itinerary, names of prescribed controlled drugs, dosages and total amounts of each to be carried. At least 2 weeks should be allowed for processing.[4] Applications from patients who are abroad, to import drugs into the UK, take longer.

If patients are carrying ≤3 months' supply of Schedule 2, 3 and 4 part I and part II controlled drugs for personal use, a personal import/export licence is *not* needed and a covering letter is sufficient. Thus, for some patients travelling ≥3 months, one option may be to carry ≤3 months' supply and seek further supplies from a doctor in the country in which they will be staying.

A list of controlled drug schedules is included in the *BNF* and on the UK government website.[5,6] The amount being carried must not exceed what is required for personal use for the duration of the travel as specified in the covering letter ± personal import/export licence.

Customs regulations in other countries

It is important to fulfil the prescription and controlled drug import/export requirements for *all* the countries in which the patient will pass through customs, otherwise entry may be refused.

The International Narcotics Control Board has produced a list of *suggested* maximum quantities of internationally controlled substances beyond which a traveller would require an import/export licence (Table 1). *However, patients should check the exact legal details and the quantities they are allowed to take into the country or countries, before travelling, with the relevant embassies or consulates, and the procedure for declaration at customs.* For example, **codeine, dihydrocodeine** or **diamorphine** are not allowed in certain countries. A contact list of foreign embassies in the UK is available.[7] It is also advisable to carry a duplicate copy of the prescription, preferably stamped by the pharmacy from which the drugs were obtained.

Table 1 Suggested maximum quantities of controlled substances for international travellers[a,8]

Drug	*Quantity*
Buprenorphine	300mg
Codeine	12g
Diazepam	300mg
Dihydrocodeine	12g
Dronabinol	1g
Fentanyl transdermal patches[b]	100mg
Fentanyl (other formulations)	20mg
Hydromorphone	300mg
Lorazepam	75mg
Methadone	2g
Methylphenidate	2g
Morphine	3g
Oxycodone	1g
Temazepam	600mg

a. this is not a complete list; see referenced source for more details

b. approximately, this adds up to 6 fentanyl 100microgram/h patches, and 8, 12, 24 and 48 of the 75, 50, 25 and 12microgram/h patches, respectively.

1 Foreign and Commonwealth Office (2019) London diplomatic list: foreign embassies in the UK. www.gov.uk

2 UK government. Controlled drugs: personal licences. www.gov.uk (accessed November 2019).

3 UK government. Hand luggage restrictions at UK airports. www.gov.uk (accessed November 2019).

4 Myers K (2017) Flying home: helping patients to arrange international travel. *Hospice UK*. www.hospiceuk.org

5 British National Formulary. Controlled drugs and drug dependence. London: BMJ Group and Pharmaceutical Press. www.medicinescomplete.com (accessed November 2019).

6 UK government. List of the most commonly encountered drugs controlled under the misuse of drugs legislation. www.gov.uk (accessed November 2019).

7 Foreign and Commonwealth Office (2016) London diplomatic list: foreign embassies in the UK. www.gov.uk

8 International Narcotics Control Board (2012) International guidelines for national regulations concerning travellers under treatment with internationally controlled drugs. www.incb.org

Updated November 2019

24: OBTAINING SPECIALS

For a full explanation of the authorization process, definitions and general details related to prescribing of medicinal products without a marketing authorization (unauthorized) in the UK, see p.xix.

'Specials' encompass special-order manufactured formulations (Box A) and products that require importation, e.g. **metolazone** tablets. They do not have a marketing authorization in the UK and are thus unauthorized.

The MHRA maintains a register of manufacturing sites which includes special-order manufacturers, NHS manufacturing units and specialist importing companies (updated monthly).[1] Contact details for NHS manufacturing units are also listed in the *BNF*, and the Association of Pharmaceutical Specials Manufacturers lists information about commercial companies and their services.[2,3]

MHRA guidance is available for the supply of specials;[4] specific guidance is also available for the supply, manufacture, importation and distribution of unauthorized cannabis-based medicinal products.[5]

Box A Special-order manufactured formulations

A special-order manufactured formulation includes the following:

- a bespoke formulation made by a specials manufacturer holding a manufacturer's specials licence (MS) for an individual patient, *without* end-product analytical testing, e.g. a specific strength of an oral solution for a child
- a commonly requested formulation manufactured by a specials manufacturer holding an MS, produced in multiple quantities (batches), *with* end-product analytical testing, e.g. some prefilled opioid syringes, ketamine oral solution, alfentanil nasal/buccal spray.

To ensure the quality of the product, the Royal Pharmaceutical Society advises that a certificate of conformity (bespoke products) or a certificate of analysis (batch-manufactured specials) should be requested by pharmacists with every product.

A certificate of conformity is a signed statement by the manufacturer that it believes the product complies with the purchaser's specification.

A certificate of analysis is evidence that critical parameters have been confirmed by retrospective physical, chemical or microbiological assay of a sample of the final product.

An MS guarantees that the sourcing of ingredients, product development, packaging and labelling, manufacturing and ex-factory supply processes are to regulatory standards. Unlike an MA, *it does not include formal evaluation of safety or efficacy of the product, and therefore there is no SPC.*

Issues to consider when prescribing and supplying a special[6,7]

Prescribers need to know (or be made aware) if a product is unauthorized.[4] This includes readily available batch-made specials for local 'routine' specialist use, e.g. **ketamine** oral solution. Pharmacists have a professional duty to liaise with the prescriber regarding the supply of a special. Royal Pharmaceutical Society guidance is available for both prescribers and pharmacists, underpinned by five principles (Box B).[6,7]

24

Box B Principles for the prescribing, procurement and supply of a special[6,7]
1 Establish a clinical need.
2 Understand the patient's experience and make a shared decision.
3 Identify medicines and preparations.
4 Monitor and review.
5 Ensure effective prescribing governance.

Product specification

Specials are supplied according to the specification agreed between the purchaser and the manufacturer. Thus, it is important to understand the patient's exact requirements and to specify details relating to dosage, strength or concentration, and formulation, e.g.:

- *tablets:* scored/non-scored, e.g. scored **levomepromazine** 6mg tablets
- *oral liquid:*
  - ▷ consistency, e.g. solutions rather than suspensions for administration via EFT
  - ▷ alcohol content, sugar content, flavouring, e.g. for children
- *injections/nasal or buccal sprays/eye drops:*
  - ▷ drug salt, e.g. for imported injections when there are UK supply issues
  - ▷ racemic mix or enantiomer, e.g. for **ketamine** vs. **S-ketamine** injection
  - ▷ excipients, e.g. propylene glycol content which may not be suitable for all routes of administration
- *creams/ointments:*
  - ▷ type of base and excipients, e.g. to avoid allergens or to prolong shelf-life.

Because the quality and bio-equivalence of the product can vary between manufacturers or imported products, whenever possible the same supplier should be used.

Availability and shelf-life

Practical issues such as availability and shelf-life can influence the choice of the product, formulation and supplier. Shelf-lives may be short, particularly for preservative-free formulations, which will have implications for quantities prescribed, cost and ordering of repeat prescriptions. Some commonly requested batch-made specials, e.g. **ketamine** oral solution, are kept as stock in some specialist units. However, in the community a supply may not be so readily available and may require several days to organise.

Cost

Generally, costs for specials are higher than for authorized products. Some commonly prescribed specials are listed in part VIIIB of the Drug Tariff (Arrangements for payment of specials and imported unlicensed medicines). This standardizes the cost to the prescriber for that product. However, for products not listed in this section, the price can vary significantly depending on which supply route and/or manufacturer is used by the hospital/community pharmacy.

Transfer of care

Close collaboration between primary and secondary care health professionals is essential to ensure continuity of supply and product consistency for the patient.[6-8] In the community there may be less familiarity with specials, and they may take longer to obtain and cost more. The new prescriber and dispensing pharmacist need to understand the clinical need for the special, the specific formulation details and the practical implications of taking over the prescribing and supply of the special.

Further, the patient/carer should be informed that they have been prescribed a special and given appropriate information about use, product specification and implications for follow-up supply.

Record keeping

Pharmacists should keep records of the source, quantity obtained, batch numbers and the quantity supplied of the unauthorized product, along with prescriber and patient details. They must also record and report any adverse reactions associated with their use.[4,6] Although pharmacists should record patient details (hence the commonly used term 'named patient supply'), there is no legal requirement to provide special-order manufacturers or specialist importing companies with this information.[4] When ordering, most companies require confirmation that the product is being supplied for a definite individual clinical need that cannot be satisfied by an existing authorized product.

In hospitals, some specials, e.g. **ketamine** oral solution, are used as standard supplies and kept as stock at ward level. Thus, they may be used without obtaining patient details; however, this is considered acceptable as long as the hospital formulary committee takes responsibility and appropriate governance is in place, e.g. a risk stratification and management plan.[2,9]

1 MHRA (2018) Human and veterinary medicines: register of licensed manufacturing sites. Available from: www.gov.uk (accessed December 2019).
2 British National Formulary Special order manufacturers. London: BMJ Group and Pharmaceutical Press. www.medicinescomplete.com (accessed December 2019).
3 Association of Pharmaceutical Specials Manufacturers Find a supplier. https://apsm-uk.com/find-a-supplier.php (accessed December 2019).
4 MHRA (2014) The supply of unlicensed relevant medicinal products ("specials"). *MHRA Guidance Note 14*. Available from: www.gov.uk
5 MHRA (2018) The supply of unlicensed cannabis-based products for medicinal use in humans. Available from: www.gov.uk.
6 Royal Pharmaceutical Society (2015) Professional guidance for the procurement and supply of specials. www.rpharms.com.
7 Royal Pharmaceutical Society (2016) Prescribing specials. Guidance for the prescribers of specials. www.rpharms.com.
8 Royal Pharmaceutical Society (2012) Keeping patients safe when they transfer between care providers - getting the medicines right. www.rpharms.com.
9 Royal Pharmaceutical Society (2016) Personal communication. *Professional Support department*. www.rpharms.com.

Updated January 2020

25: MANAGEMENT OF POSTOPERATIVE PAIN IN OPIOID-DEPENDENT PATIENTS

Opioid-dependent patients include those using long-term opioids for:

- pain relief (mostly cancer but also non-cancer pain)
- long-term opioid maintenance for opioid dependence
- current substance misuse.

All such patients will require *additional opioids* to relieve *additional pain*. It is thus crucially important that pre-operative, peri-operative and postoperative doses take this into account, and that *extra amounts* of a strong opioid are prescribed. Generally, these will be larger than the typical doses used by non-opioid-dependent patients in these circumstances.[1] For example, if only typical postoperative doses are prescribed (e.g. **morphine** 2.5–10mg IV/SC q1h p.r.n.), patients who are tolerant to higher doses may experience little or no pain relief. However, opioid requirements vary widely and close monitoring is essential.

Because tolerance to undesirable effects, e.g. respiratory depression, develops more rapidly than to analgesia (often within days or 1–2 weeks at most), opioids can be safely titrated to the higher doses required in opioid-dependent patients.

Further, a sudden significant reduction in overall opioid dose may precipitate an opioid withdrawal syndrome, possibly accompanied by *hyperalgesia*. This will magnify the postoperative pain and any other underlying pain. Thus, under-prescribing can lead to devastating overwhelming pain.

As far as possible, a multidisciplinary approach should be adopted, e.g. pre-operative consultation with the patient's substance misuse team, the anaesthetist and the acute pain team to develop a pain management plan, which should include intra-operative and postoperative monitoring, with dose adjustments made by an experienced anaesthetist. There are no uniform recommendations, but Box A outlines the general approach.[2-10] Addicts receiving maintenance therapy with **methadone**, high-dose SL **buprenorphine** or **naltrexone** require additional considerations (see below).

Other classes of drugs used for analgesia, e.g. antidepressants, anti-epileptics, should also be continued with as little interruption as possible.[11]

Addicts receiving methadone maintenance therapy

Generally, **methadone** maintenance therapy is administered once daily, which is adequate to prevent opioid withdrawal symptoms, but not pain, for 24h. In acute pain, the maintenance dose should be continued at the same dose but, by giving half the daily dose b.d., it contributes better towards analgesia (e.g. 40mg once daily → 20mg b.d.).[8] When the PO route cannot be used, SC or CSCI are alternative routes of administration (see p.469).

Addicts receiving high-dose SL buprenorphine maintenance therapy

Buprenorphine acts as a partial agonist at the μ-opioid receptor, to which it binds with a higher affinity than other μ-opioid receptor agonists. Thus, when **buprenorphine** is present in sufficient amounts, it will antagonize the analgesic effects of other μ-opioid receptor agonists. This is probable only with the higher doses used SL for opioid maintenance, i.e. ≥16mg/24h (see p.428). This has led some to advocate discontinuing high-dose SL **buprenorphine** 5–7 days before elective surgery to avoid compromising postoperative pain relief, and to manage withdrawal symptoms with **methadone** instead.[13] On the other hand, various μ-opioid receptor agonists have been successfully used for postoperative pain in patients on SL **buprenorphine** 2–32mg/24h, although higher doses than usual may be required.[14-16]

25

Box A Management of postoperative pain in opioid-dependent patients

1 Consider local anaesthetic or multimodal approaches to analgesia, e.g. regional blocks, paracetamol, NSAIDs, ketamine, dexmedetomidine, clonidine, etc.

2 Identify the baseline opioid dose: in patients misusing opioids, this may mean a best-guess estimate.

3 Generally, the baseline opioid dose should be continued as a regular prescription.

4 Reduce the baseline dose if:
- the surgery will improve the pre-operative pain
- the baseline opioid needs to be replaced by an alternative opioid; because of possible incomplete cross-tolerance, reduce the dose calculated from equipotency tables by at least a third, particularly when dealing with large doses, e.g. morphine ≥1g PO/24h or equivalent (see Strong opioids, Table 3, p.401).

5 Patients on m/r opioids PO can take them (and other analgesics) on the day of surgery, even if fasting, unless there is a specific contra-indication.[8]

6 If PO is not possible pre- or immediately postoperatively, an alternative route, e.g. CSCI or CIVI, should be used to deliver the baseline dose. This can also be done via IV patient-controlled analgesia (PCA; see point 12).

7 Before restarting m/r opioids PO, ensure that GI function has returned to normal. Gastric stasis can lead to delayed dissolution and drug absorption, followed by 'dose dumping' when motility improves, with consequential overdose. Conversely, surgery that shortens GI transit time (e.g. small bowel resection) may render the use of m/r products inappropriate.

8 If the surgery is unlikely to lead to major changes in skin perfusion, and the ongoing opioid requirements are unlikely to change, it is best to leave TD fentanyl patches in place and give additional p.r.n. opioid.

9 If TD patches are removed, pain relief will persist for several hours, because fentanyl is distributed widely throughout the body, particularly in adipose tissue (see p.440). Note. In postoperative patients, after a patch has been removed, the mean time for the plasma fentanyl concentration to drop below the minimum effective level is 16h, with a range of 2–23h.[12]

10 Continue long-term ED or IT pumps unchanged unless the surgery is expected to reduce the pain for which these are being used.

11 Prescribe an appropriate dose of a strong opioid for p.r.n. use; typically equivalent to 1/10–1/6 of the total daily dose.

12 With IV PCA, a larger bolus dose is generally necessary compared with the typical bolus dose of morphine 1mg. PCA can also be used to continuously deliver part or all of the baseline opioid dose.

Example
Patient on long-term morphine 300mg/24h PO = 100mg/24h IV = 4mg/h IV.
PCA background infusion = 2–3mg/h IV.
PCA bolus dose = 2mg IV with a 5min lockout period between doses.

With addicts, if there is considerable uncertainty about their opioid intake, it may be safer to underestimate both the background infusion dose and bolus dose required.

13 Close monitoring is required to:
- identify inadequate dosing (unrelieved pain, withdrawal phenomena)
- ensure rapid dose titration
- prevent excessive dosing (sedation, respiratory depression)
- ensure that bolus doses are not being misused.

For someone on high-dose SL **buprenorphine** who experiences acute pain unexpectedly, options include:

- regional anaesthesia
- optimizing the use of non-opioid analgesics (Box A)
- prescribing a μ-opioid receptor agonist, e.g. IV **morphine**, **fentanyl**; higher doses than usual may be required
- progressively increasing the SL **buprenorphine** dose up to 24–32mg/24h, and giving in divided doses t.d.s.–q.d.s.[13,15]

Addicts receiving long-term naltrexone therapy

The opioid antagonist **naltrexone** is used to prevent relapse in opioid ex-addicts (by blocking the opioid 'high') and in the treatment of alcohol dependence. It blocks all types of opioid receptor and is long-acting. It thus prevents/blocks opioid analgesia. Analgesia for these patients is even more challenging (see Opioid antagonists (therapeutic target within the CNS), Box A, p.494).[17]

1 Rapp SE *et al.* (1995) Acute pain management in patients with prior opioid consumption: a case-controlled retrospective review. *Pain.* **61**: 195–201.

2 Macintyre PE (2001) Safety and efficacy of patient-controlled analgesia. *British Journal of Anaesthesia.* **87**: 36–46.

3 Roberts DM and Meyer-Witting M (2005) High-dose buprenorphine: perioperative precautions and management strategies. *Anaesthesia and Intensive Care.* **33**: 17–25.

4 Alford DP *et al.* (2006) Acute pain management for patients receiving maintenance methadone or buprenorphine therapy. *Annals of Internal Medicine.* **144**: 127–134.

5 British Pain Society (2007) *Pain and Substance Misuse: Improving the Patient Experience.* London: British Pain Society. www.britishpainsociety.org

6 Macintyre PE and Ready LB (2006) *Acute Pain Management – A Practical Guide*, 2nd edn. Saunders Ltd. pp 272.

7 Mehta V and Langford RM (2006) Acute pain management for opioid dependent patients. *Anaesthesia.* **61**: 269–276.

8 Huxtable CA *et al.* (2011) Acute pain management in opioid-tolerant patients: a growing challenge. *Anaesthesia and Intensive Care.* **39**: 804–823.

9 British Pain Society (2010) Cancer pain management. London: British Pain Society. Available from: www.britishpainsociety.org

10 Schwenk ES *et al.* (2018) Consensus guidelines on the use of intravenous ketamine infusions for acute pain management from the American Society of Regional Anesthesia and Pain Medicine, the American Academy of Pain Medicine, and the American Society of Anesthesiologists. *Regional Anesthesia and Pain Medicine.* **43**: 456–466.

11 Farrell C and McConaghy P (2012) Perioperative management of patients taking treatment for chronic pain. *British Medical Journal.* **345**: e4148.

12 Grond S *et al.* (2000) Clinical pharmacokinetics of transdermal opioids: focus on transdermal fentanyl. *Clinical Pharmacokinetics.* **38**: 59–89.

13 Savage SR *et al.* (2008) Challenges in using opioids to treat pain in persons with substance use disorders. *Addiction Science and Clinical Practice.* **4**: 4–25.

14 Kornfield H and Manfredi L (2010) Effectiveness of full agonist opioids in patients stablized on buprenorphine undergoing major surgery: a case series. *American Journal of Therapeutics.* **17**: 523–528.

15 Heit HA and Gourlay DL (2008) Buprenorphine: new tricks with an old molecule for pain management. *Clinical Journal of Pain.* **24**: 93–97.

16 Macintyre PE *et al.* (2013) Pain relief and opioid requirements in the first 24 hours after surgery in patients taking buprenorphine and methadone opioid substitution therapy. *Anaesthesia and Intensive Care.* **41**: 222–230.

17 Vickers AP and Jolly A (2006) Naltrexone and problems in pain management. *British Medical Journal.* **332**: 132–133.

Updated (minor change) June 2019

26: DRUGS FOR PRURITUS

Pathophysiology

Pruritus is a common symptom, which can be severe and distressing. It is considered chronic when persisting >6 weeks. Although pruritus is limited to skin, conjunctivae or a mucous membrane (including the upper respiratory tract), the cause is not always peripheral (Box A).

Box A A neuro-anatomical classification of pruritus	
Peripheral causes	**Central causes**
Cutaneous ('pruritoceptive'), e.g.	Neuropathic, e.g.
skin diseases	brain injury[1]
urticaria (most)	brain abscess
stinging nettle rash	brain tumour[1]
insect bite reactions	multiple sclerosis
drug (± rash)	Neurogenic, e.g.
cutaneous mastocytosis (rare)	opioid
Neuropathic, e.g.	cholestasis
post-herpetic neuralgia	paraneoplastic
	Psychogenic
	Mixed peripheral and central causes
	Uraemia

Pruritogens

The afferent nerve fibres mostly associated with peripheral causes of pruritus are a subset of C-fibres.[2,3] Their terminals are more superficial than the nociceptive C-fibres, close to the junction between epidermis and dermis, and are stimulated by a wide range of pruritogens (Box B).

Box B Chemical mediators of pruritus (pruritogens)	
Amines, e.g.	Growth factors, e.g.
histamine	nerve growth factor (NGF)
serotonin	Vasoconstrictors, e.g.
Opioids	endothelin-1 (ET-1)
Eicosanoids[a], e.g.	Neuropeptides, e.g.
leukotriene B4 (LB4)	substance P
thromboxane A2	calcitonin gene-related peptide (CGRP)
Cytokines, e.g.	bradykinin
interleukin-31 (IL-31)	somatostatin
tumour necrosis factor alpha (TNF-α)	vasoactive intestinal peptide (VIP)
Proteases, e.g.	
tryptase	

a. collective term for metabolites of arachidonic acid, including prostanoids and leukotrienes.

Some types of pruritus do not respond, or respond only weakly, to H_1 antihistamines. This is explained by most of the pruritus-sensitive C-fibres being histamine independent (90%) rather than histamine dependent. These form two distinct populations of neurones and peripheral pathways for pruritus,[4] one activated by histamine and the other by alternative pruritogens.[5]

There is a complex interaction between various skin and immune cells and sensory neurones which relay signals to the thalamus via the contralateral spinothalamic tract. Subsequently, multiple higher centres are engaged in generating the sensation of itch and the response to it. Various inhibitory pathways exist, e.g. from the periaqueductal gray matter to the thalamus and dorsal horn; activation of the pain pathway also inhibits pruritic signal transmission at the dorsal horn.

Some of the more important pruritogens and receptors are highlighted below. For a more detailed review, see Brennan (2016).[4]

Histamine

Histamine is an important chemical mediator of pruritus of cutaneous origin (along with the wheal and flare of urticaria). Endogenous histamine released in the skin is mostly from mast cells and mediates pruritus via H_1-, H_4-[6,7] and possibly H_3-receptors.[8] Further, histamine probably also stimulates the formation of other pruritogens.[9]

H_4-receptors are also found in the spinal cord and brain.[10] Thus, histamine may be involved in some forms of central pruritus. H_4 antihistamines are in development.

Proteases

Proteases, e.g. tryptase, are released from mast cells and keratinocytes and act on PAR2 receptors expressed on afferent neurones and keratinocytes.[11,12]

Serotonin/5HT

Serotonin/5HT is a weaker pruritogen than histamine.[13] SSRIs relieve pruritus associated with primary biliary cholangitis,[14,15] cancer[16] and uraemia.[17] **Ondansetron** relieves pruritus related to spinal **morphine**,[18] but *not* cholestatic or uraemic pruritus.[19]

Eicosanoids

These are produced from the essential fatty acid arachidonic acid. Leukotriene B4 is highly pruritogenic, activating TRPV1 channels on pruritus-sensitive neurones. It also enhances the release of serotonin from mast cells.[4]

Other eicosanoids may help reduce pruritus, e.g. the anti-inflammatory prostaglandin E1, levels of which may be enhanced by gamma-linolenic acid (GLA), a component of evening primrose oil. In uraemic pruritus, benefit is reported from GLA 2.2% cream (applied to the whole body after a daily bath, and to pruritic sites t.d.s.) and PO evening primrose oil capsules containing GLA 45mg (dosed at 90mg b.d.).[20,21]

Cytokines

Interleukin-31 is a pruritogen produced by mast cells, keratinocytes and lymphocytes in the skin; it is also present in the dorsal root ganglion. It acts directly on peripheral pruritus-sensitive neurones and also by inducing leukotriene B4 production in keratinocytes.[22]

TNF-α also plays a role in pruritus and explains the benefit of thalidomide, which inhibits its formation (see Commentary).

Substance P

Substance P is released from mast cells and mediates pruritus via NK_1-receptors. The expression of these receptors is increased on keratinocytes in pruritic skin disease.[23] **Aprepitant**, an NK_1 antagonist, relieves pruritus in cancer patients receiving targeted anti-cancer drugs.[24] **Capsaicin** cream (p.685) depletes substance P from sensory nerve endings in the skin and is of benefit in pruritus, particularly uraemic.

Pruritus in systemic disease

Pruritus occurs in many systemic conditions (Box C), and may be caused by peripheral or central mechanisms, or both (Box D).

Drugs

All drugs have the potential to cause an allergic reaction which can cause pruritus, with or without a rash (Box E). The mechanism involves the release of histamine from mast cells. The pruritus responds to H_1 antihistamines (and stopping the offending drug).

Box C Systemic disease associated with pruritus[25]

Endocrine
Carcinoid syndrome
Diabetes mellitus (associated with genital candidosis)
Hyperparathyroidism (secondary to chronic renal failure)[a]
Hyperthyroidism
Hypothyroidism

Haematological
Leukaemia
Lymphoma
Mastocytosis
Multiple myeloma
Polycythaemia rubra vera

Hepatic
Cholestasis
Hepatitis
Primary biliary cholangitis

Renal
Chronic renal failure

Other
AIDS
Cancer
Multiple sclerosis

a. correction of hypercalcaemia leads to the rapid relief; in other circumstances, hypercalcaemia is *not* associated with pruritus.

Box D Some of the causal factors in pruritus[a]

Cholestasis
Endogenous opioids ↑
Autotaxin and LPA[b] ↑
Serotonin release ↑

Old age
Dry skin
Mast cell degranulation[26] ↑
Skin sensitivity to histamine[26] ↑

Paraneoplastic
Histamine release from basophils
Serotonin release ↑
Immune response

Renal failure
Cytokines
Substance P release ↑
Skin divalent ions (Ca^{2+}, Mg^{2+}, PO_4^{2-}) ↑
Skin vitamin A ↑
Mast cell proliferation
μ- and κ-opioid receptor imbalance
Peripheral neuropathy

Targeted treatment with anti-EGFR drugs or tyrosine kinase inhibitors
Secretion of stem cell factors ↑ and accumulation of dermal mast cells in areas of skin rash
NK_1-receptors in mast cells and keratinocytes in inflamed areas[27] ↑

a. dry skin is often an important concurrent factor
b. plasma concentrations of autotaxin and lysophosphatidic acid (LPA) correlate with pruritus and are reduced by antipruritic treatments, e.g. rifampicin (p.518).[28]

Box E Common allergic drug skin reactions

Rashes
Cephalosporins
Penicillins
Phenytoin
Sulfonamides

Urticaria
Cephalosporins
Penicillins
Radio-opaque dyes
Sulfonamides

Opioid-induced pruritus

There are two types of opioid-induced pruritus. One is an allergic reaction related to cutaneous histamine release, and possibly occurs in only ~1% of patients receiving an opioid systemically. It responds to H_1 antihistamines and a switch in opioid.

Histamine is also released after an *intradermal* injection of an opioid (and responds to H_1 antihistamines). However, this is probably irrelevant in relation to pruritus associated with systemic opioids, because *in vitro* studies indicate that the dose of **morphine** or **methadone** needed to release histamine from mast cells is 10,000 times greater than the dose needed for μ agonist effects.[29]

The second type is a central reaction to opioids, and is less histamine-dependent.[30–32] In surgical (opioid-naïve) patients who receive spinal opioids pre-operatively, the incidence is ≤80%, but in patients with chronic pain already taking opioids by another route, only 10–15%.[33–35] The incidence also depends on the opioid used; for example, with caesarean section, pruritus is more common with epidural **morphine** than epidural **hydromorphone**.[36]

However, anecdotally in cancer patients receiving palliative care, the incidence of pruritus in such patients appears to be virtually zero,[37] possibly because of the concurrent use of **bupivacaine**.[38,39]

Several hours after spinal injection, pruritus typically spreads rostrally through the thorax from the level of the injection, and is typically maximal in the face, but may be limited to the nose (more likely when **bupivacaine** is given concurrently).[40]

Although pruritus induced by either systemic or spinal **morphine** is relieved by **naloxone** or **naltrexone**, this risks reversal of analgesia.[41] Other options are discussed in Chapter 32, p.908.

Management

Correct the correctable

Consider and treat:
- dry skin: very common in advanced cancer. Even when there is a probable endogenous cause, rehydration of the skin may obviate the need for specific measures (see Emollients, p.677)
- review the patient's medication: if a drug is the likely cause (Box E), it should be stopped and an alternative prescribed if necessary (for opioids, see Table 1). With **penicillins**, the pruritic rash may not appear until several days after the antibacterial has been stopped
- atopic dermatitis: topical corticosteroid and an emollient (p.677)
- contact dermatitis: topical corticosteroid, identify causal substance, avoid further contact
- scabies: topical **permethrin** or **malathion** (see respective SPCs)
- cholestatic pruritus secondary to obstruction of the common bile duct: this resolves if the jaundice is relieved by inserting an intraductal stent via ERCP or other drainage procedure
- uraemic pruritus in haemodialysis patients: optimize renal support, correct hyperphosphataemia, iron deficiency
- Hodgkin's lymphoma: radiotherapy and/or chemotherapy.

Non-drug treatment

Non-drug treatment includes the following measures:
- avoid soap; use moisturizing soap substitutes
- apply emollient b.d.–t.d.s.
- discourage scratching: file fingernails, allow gentle rubbing
- avoid prolonged hot baths
- dry the skin by patting gently with a soft towel or use a hair dryer *on a cool setting*
- avoid overheating and sweating, particularly in bed at night
- increase air humidity in the bedroom to avoid skin drying.

Drug treatment

Topical applications

Traditional topical antipruritics include **phenol** 0.5–3%, **levomenthol (menthol)** 0.5–2% and **camphor** 0.5–3% (see p.685). Although not practical to apply topical products over the whole body, some patients with generalized pruritus have areas of greater intensity and obtain benefit from the more selective application of a topical antipruritic.

In uraemic pruritus, **capsaicin** cream 0.025–0.075% once daily–q.d.s. may help.[42] Some patients find the burning sensation after application unacceptable (see p.651 and p.685). Transdermal high-dose **capsaicin** has been reported to be of benefit in localized pruritus, e.g. brachioradial pruritus[43] and notalgia paresthetica.[44]

Although **doxepin** has also been used topically in various conditions, it has several disadvantages which limit such use (see p.685).

Table 1 Suggested treatment for specific causes of pruritus (UK)[a,b]

Condition	*Step 1*	*Step 2*	*Step 3*
Cholestasis[c]	Sertraline 25–100mg once daily **A**[d,15,55]	Rifampicin 150mg once daily–300mg b.d. **A**[55–57]	Naltrexone 12.5–250mg once daily **A**[e,57,58]
Uraemia	If localized, capsaicin cream 0.025–0.075% once daily–q.d.s. **A**[42]	Gabapentin 100–400mg or pregabalin 25–75mg after haemodialysis **A**[f,42]	Doxepin 10mg once daily–b.d. **A**[49–51] *or* Nalfurafine (not UK) 5microgram IV after haemodialysis **A**[42]
Systemic opioids (for spinal opioids, see Chapter 32, p.908)	Stat dose of H_1-antihistamine, e.g. chlorphenamine 4–12mg; if after 2–3h there is definite benefit, prescribe 4mg t.d.s. (for alternatives, see main text below) *or* a less sedative second generation H_1-antihistamine, e.g. cetirizine 10mg once daily/at bedtime[59]	Switch opioid, e.g. morphine → oxycodone[32,60]	Ondansetron 8mg b.d.
Hodgkin's lymphoma	Prednisolone 30–60mg once daily	Cimetidine 800mg/24h[g,61]	Carbamazepine 200mg b.d.[62]
Paraneoplastic, other causes, idiopathic	Sertraline 50–100mg once daily *or* Paroxetine 5–20mg once daily **A**[16]	Mirtazapine 15–30mg at bedtime[63]	Thalidomide (see When all else fails, below)

a. strength of recommendations: grade **A** is based on evidence from ≥1 RCTs, and grade **B** on well-designed non-randomized studies; where no grade is given, the recommendation is based on case reports and/or expert opinion

b. given PO unless stated otherwise

c. in biliary obstruction due to cancer, where bile duct stenting is impossible or unwanted

d. compared with **rifampicin** there are less RCT data for **sertraline**, but efficacy appears similar (see Commentary below); given its tolerability, familiarity and fewer interactions, *PCF* recommends **sertraline** is generally tried first

e. unsuitable for patients who need opioids for pain relief (see Opioid antagonists (therapeutic target within CNS), p.492); for the use of **methylnaltrexone** in cholestasis, see Other options below.

f. although some studies started at the upper end of these dose ranges, to reduce the risk of CNS undesirable effects, it is generally advisable to start at the lower end

g. in various haematological cancers, there are anecdotal reports of enhanced benefit when an H_1 antagonist and an H_2 antagonist are used in combination.

Systemic treatment

If the skin is inflamed as a result of scratching (but not infected), consider a corticosteroid, e.g. **dexamethasone** 2–4mg PO each morning or **prednisolone** 10–20mg PO each morning for 1 week.

Unless specific treatment is indicated, consider a trial of a sedative antihistamine either at bedtime (pruritus is generally worse at bedtime and through the night) or round-the-clock, depending on circumstances. Either an H_1-receptor antagonist or a phenothiazine with antihistaminic properties can be used:

- **chlorphenamine** 4mg PO at bedtime *or* 4mg q4h p.r.n.; useful for rapid dose escalation to determine if an antihistamine is of benefit
- **promethazine** *hydrochloride* 25–50mg PO at bedtime *or* 10–20mg b.d.–t.d.s.
- **hydroxyzine** 25mg PO at bedtime *or* 25mg b.d.–q.d.s.
- **alimemazine (trimeprazine)** 10–30mg PO at bedtime *or* 10mg b.d.–t.d.s.
- **levomepromazine** 6.25–25mg PO at bedtime.[45] Note. Although 6mg tablets are available, they are more expensive; their use should be reserved for when the splitting of tablets is impractical (see p.201).

For some patients, a benzodiazepine is as effective as a sedative antihistamine.[46]

Doxepin, a TCA and potent H_1- and H_2-receptor antagonist, is a further alternative. Although most TCAs have antihistaminic properties, **doxepin** is the most potent in this respect, but it is expensive.[47] Some patients with chronic urticaria unresponsive to conventional H_1 antihistamines obtain relief from **doxepin** 10–75mg PO at bedtime (in the UK 25mg capsules are the smallest dose available).[48] **Doxepin** 10mg PO once daily–b.d. is effective in patients with uraemic pruritus,[49] but less so than a dose of either **gabapentin** 100–300mg PO or **pregabalin** 50mg PO after each session of haemodialysis.[50,51]

Table 1 provides clinicians with a synopsis of possible treatments of choice. Some are supported by evidence from RCTs but, for others, the evidence is low level (opinions and/or clinical experiences of respected authorities). Further information is available elsewhere.[52–54]

Commentary

There appear to be similarities between neuropathic pain, pruritus and cough, the common theme being peripheral and central sensitization of the sensory nervous system. This may explain why a range of anti-epileptics and antidepressants have been reported as effective treatments for these very different symptoms. The persistence of pruritus in patients with myeloproliferative disorders despite disease control suggests central sensitization.

The inclusion of **carbamazepine** as an option for the treatment of pruritus with lymphoma or cancer is based on its successful use in just four patients (three with B-cell lymphoma and one with myeloma).[62] It had previously been used with good effect in three patients with multiple sclerosis.[64]

Although potentially a class effect, it is unknown if other SSRIs are as equally effective as **fluvoxamine, paroxetine** and **sertraline**, which improve pruritus in various situations including solid cancers, haematological cancers, non-cancer disorders, idiopathic pruritus and possibly also uraemia.[17,65] **Sertraline** is a good choice because of a lower risk of drug interactions and discontinuation reactions. In a pilot study of uraemic pruritus, the antidepressant **mirtazapine**, an H_1-, $5HT_2$-, $5HT_3$-receptor antagonist, (15mg PO at night) was as effective as **gabapentin** (100mg PO at night);[66] anecdotally **mirtazapine** is also effective in pruritus associated with cancer and lymphoma.[63] Anecdotally, patients who fail to respond to an SSRI may respond to **mirtazapine**, and sometimes vice versa.

Although **ondansetron**, a $5HT_3$ antagonist, relieves pruritus induced by spinal **morphine**,[18] it does *not* relieve cholestatic or uraemic pruritus.[67]

The classic hepatic enzyme inducer **rifampicin** (p.518), in a dose of 300–600mg PO once daily, has been shown to be of benefit in two RCTs lasting 1–2 weeks in patients with cholestatic pruritus.[56,57] Because of rare reports of severe hepatotoxicity with **rifampicin** and because of intolerance in cachectic patients, a lower starting dose of 150mg PO once daily is advisable, see p.518. **Sertraline** may also benefit cholestatic pruritus, but because of comparatively less RCT experience, specialty guidelines generally position it below **rifampicin**.[68,69] However, in a small RCT (n=36), sertraline (100mg PO once daily) and **rifampicin** (300mg PO once daily) provided similar benefit when first assessed after 4 weeks of use.[55] Thus, given its tolerability, familiarity and limited interactions compared with **rifampicin**, *PCF* recommends **sertraline** is generally tried first.

An imbalance in peripheral opioid receptors in nerve, skin and immune cells may contribute to uraemic pruritus, specifically a reduced expression/activation of κ-opioid (pruritus-suppressing) receptors relative to μ-opioid (pruritus-inducing) receptors. Thus, both κ *agonists*, e.g. **nalfurafine** (not UK) and μ *antagonists*, e.g. **naltrexone**, have been explored in this setting. Only the former provide consistent benefit, although to a lesser degree than that achieved with gabapentinoids.[42,70] Peripherally selective κ agonists are in development, e.g. **difelikefalin**.[71]

Some patients with liver metastases and cholestasis produce endogenous opioids which may cause both pruritus and analgesia.[72] Anecdotally, although pain-free and not requiring opioids beforehand, some patients with cancer and cholestatic pruritus experience pain after treatment with **naltrexone**. Further, transient opioid withdrawal effects can occur when opioid antagonists are used for cholestatic pruritus; in this setting, **naltrexone** is less effective than **rifampicin** and is generally considered a third-line treatment.[71] Although PO **nalfurafine** 2.5–5microgram/24h (not UK) also reduces cholestatic pruritus, the clinical relevance has been questioned.[71,73] The benefit reported with **buprenorphine** has *not* been confirmed in an RCT (p.428).

For the management of pruritus in polycythaemia vera, see the latest British Society for Haematology guidelines.[74]

Other options

In *en cuirasse* breast cancer complicated by inflammation, local pruritus and pain, an NSAID may reduce both pruritus and pain.[75] An NSAID can also be helpful whenever there is inflammation present, either primary or secondary to scratching.

Specialist guidelines recommend **colestyramine** for cholestatic pruritus in *incomplete* biliary obstruction, e.g. primary biliary cholangitis.[68,69] However, the two RCTs which showed benefit with **colestyramine** (4g PO once or twice daily) were methodologically poor.[57] Further, many patients find **colestyramine** unpalatable, and it may cause nausea, vomiting and diarrhoea. Because it binds bile salts within the gut, it is ineffective in *complete* biliary obstruction. Although the peroxisome proliferator-activated receptor (PPAR) agonist **bezafibrate** (400mg PO once daily) is of benefit in cholestatic pruritus, its place in palliative care, if any, is uncertain.[76,77]

It has long been known that 17-α alkyl androgens relieve pruritus associated with cholestasis.[78,79] However, because they can be hepatotoxic, cholestasis (and thus the accompanying jaundice) may worsen. In patients with primary biliary cholangitis, this may be unwelcome. Over the decades, several of this class of androgens have been withdrawn from the market for commercial reasons. Where available, **danazol** (not UK) 200mg PO once daily–t.d.s. or **methyltestosterone** (not UK) 25mg SL once daily can be used fourth-line when **sertraline**, **rifampicin** and **naltrexone** are ineffective.[78–80]

Some recommendations are more or less specific to one particular disease. For example, **gabapentin** (and **pregabalin**) is effective in uraemic pruritus,[42] whereas in an RCT in cholestasis **gabapentin** was less effective than placebo.[81] However, there are anecdotal reports of benefit of **gabapentin** in neuropathic pruritus and in pruritus of unknown origin.[82,83] Dose as for neuropathic pain (see p.300).

Montelukast 10mg PO once daily, a leukotriene receptor antagonist, may benefit uraemic pruritus.[84]

Case reports suggest **methylnaltrexone**, a peripherally acting opioid antagonist (see p.500), may be of benefit in cholestatic pruritus. In two jaundiced patients with cancer, pruritus resolved completely 30min–12h after a dose of **methylnaltrexone**, with a duration of benefit ranging from 24h to 3 weeks.[85] This avoids the risk of opioid withdrawal and/or reversal of opioid analgesia, making it a reasonable option to try in patients receiving opioids.

Aprepitant, a neurokinin-1 (NK-1) receptor antagonist, has been used successfully for the management of severe pruritus related to targeted biological cancer treatment with anti-EGFR antibodies and tyrosine kinase inhibitors.[24] There are also case reports of benefit in other patients with pruritus of various causes, e.g. paraneoplastic, cutaneous lymphoma.[86,87] Various NK-1 antagonists are in development, mostly for pruritus associated with skin diseases.[71]

When all else fails

The treatments suggested for pruritus associated with 'other causes or idiopathic' (Table 1, bottom row) should be considered in all cases of intractable pruritus if the more specific options have failed to relieve.

Thalidomide 100–200mg PO at bedtime has been used successfully in paraneoplastic, Hodgkin's lymphoma and uraemic pruritus.[88–90] However, its cost is prohibitive, and it may cause severe neuropathy when used long-term (see p.603).

Midazolam may be of benefit in intractable central pruritus.[91,92] In one patient with cancer of the pancreas and cholestatic pruritus, CSCI **midazolam** was effective 'within a few hours' (a 2mg bolus followed by 1mg/h, increasing by 1mg/h every 15min p.r.n.), whereas **lorazepam** 1mg PO q6h or 2mg at bedtime (and several other psychotropic drugs) was ineffective.[92]

Lidocaine 0.5mg/kg/h CSCI has been used successfully in a patient with cutaneous T-cell lymphoma in the last days of life.[93] No loading dose was given, and the patient was not monitored as per the general norm, e.g. blood pressure, ECG (see p.77). The pruritus settled in 3–4h and the patient died 3 days later. Previously well controlled on **gabapentin** 100mg PO at bedtime, **lidocaine** was introduced when the patient could no longer swallow. A case series of 19 patients with cutaneous T-cell lymphoma and intractable pruritus (mean of four other treatments) reported complete or partial response for most days of treatment with **lidocaine** CSCI (starting dose 0.1–0.9mg/kg/h) over a median (range) duration of use of 6 (1–70) days.[94]

1 Dey DD *et al.* (2005) Central neuropathic itch from spinal-cord cavernous hemangioma: a human case, a possible animal model, and hypotheses about pathogenesis. *Pain.* **113**: 233–237.

2 Schmelz M *et al.* (1997) Specific C-receptors for itch in human skin. *Journal of Neuroscience.* **17**: 8003–8008.

3 Schmelz M *et al.* (2000) Which nerve fibers mediate the axon reflex flare in human skin? *Neuroreport.* **11**: 645–648.

4 Brennan F (2016) The pathophysiology of pruritus – A review for clinicians. *Progress in Palliative Care.* **24**: 133–146.

5 Namer B *et al.* (2008) Separate peripheral pathways for pruritus in man. *Journal of Neurophysiology.* **100**: 2062–2069.

6 Cowden JM *et al.* (2010) The histamine H4 receptor mediates inflammation and pruritus in Th2-dependent dermal inflammation. *Journal of Investigative Dermatology.* **130**: 1023–1033.

7 Dunford PJ *et al.* (2007) Histamine H4 receptor antagonists are superior to traditional antihistamines in the attenuation of experimental pruritus. *Journal of Allergy and Clinical Immunolgy.* **119**: 176–183.

8 Sugimoto Y *et al.* (2004) Pruritus-associated response mediated by cutaneous histamine H3 receptors. *Clinical and Experimental Allergy.* **34**: 456–459.

9 Yao G *et al.* (1992) Histamine-caused itch induces Fos-like immunoreactivity in dorsal horn neurons: effect of morphine pretreatment. *Brain Research.* **599**: 333–337.

10 Strakhova MI *et al.* (2009) Localization of histamine H4 receptors in the central nervous system of human and rat. *Brain Research.* **1250**: 41–48.

11 Steinhoff M *et al.* (2003) Proteinase-activated receptor-2 mediates itch: a novel pathway for pruritus in human skin. *Journal of Neuroscience.* **23**: 6176–6180.

12 Reddy VB *et al.* (2008) Cowhage-evoked itch is mediated by a novel cysteine protease: a ligand of protease-activated receptors. *Journal of Neuroscience.* **28**: 4331–4335.

13 Lowitt M and Bernhard J (1992) Pruritus. *Seminars in Neurology.* **12**: 374–384.

14 Browning J *et al.* (2003) Long-term efficacy of sertraline as a treatment for cholestatic pruritus in patients with primary biliary cirrhosis. *American Journal of Gastroenterology.* **98**: 2736–2741.

15 Mayo MJ *et al.* (2007) Sertraline as a first-line treatment for cholestatic pruritus. *Hepatology.* **45**: 666–674.

16 Zylicz Z *et al.* (2003) Paroxetine in the treatment of severe non-dermatological pruritus: a randomized, controlled trial. *Journal of Pain and Symptom Management.* **26**: 1105–1112.

17 Shakiba M *et al.* (2012) Effect of sertraline on uremic pruritus improvement in ESRD patients. *International Journal of Nephrology.* **2012**: 363901.

18 Borgeat A and Stirnemann H-R (1999) Ondansetron is effective to treat spinal or epidural morphine-induced pruritus. *Anesthesiology.* **90**: 432–436.

19 Weisshaar E *et al.* (1997) Can a serotonin type 3 (5-HT3) receptor antagonist reduce experimentally-induced itch? *Inflammation Research.* **46**: 412–416.

20 Chen YC *et al.* (2006) Therapeutic effect of topical gamma-linolenic acid on refractory uremic pruritus. *American Journal of Kidney Diseases.* **48**: 69–76.

21 Yoshimoto-Furuie K *et al.* (1999) Effects of oral supplementation with evening primrose oil for six weeks on plasma essential fatty acids and uremic skin symptoms in hemodialysis patients. *Nephron.* **81**: 151–159.

22 Andoh T *et al.* (2017) Involvement of leukotriene B4 released from keratinocytes in itch-associated response to intradermal interleukin-31 in mice. *Acta Dermato-Venereologica.* **97**: 922–927.

23 Chang SE *et al.* (2007) Neuropeptides and their receptors in psoriatic skin in relation to pruritus. *British Journal of Dermatology.* **156**: 1272–1277.

24 Santini D *et al.* (2012) Aprepitant for management of severe pruritus related to biological cancer treatments: a pilot study. *Lancet Oncology.* **13**: 1020–1024.

25 Greaves M (1992) Itching-research has barely scratched the surface. *New England Journal of Medicine.* **326**: 1016–1017.

26 Guillet G *et al.* (2000) Increased histamine release and skin hypersensitivity to histamine in senile pruritus: study of 60 patients. *European Academy of Dermatology and Venerology.* **14**: 65–68.

27 Gerber PA *et al.* (2010) Preliminary evidence for a role of mast cells in epidermal growth factor receptor inhibitor-induced pruritus. *Journal of the American Academy of Dermatology.* **63**: 163–165.

28 Kremer AE *et al.* (2012) Serum autotaxin is increased in pruritus of cholestasis, but not of other origin, and responds to therapeutic interventions. *Hepatology.* **56**: 1391–1400.

29 Barke K and Hough L (1993) Opiates, mast cells and histamine release. *Life Sciences.* **53**: 1391–1399.

30 Reisine T and Pasternak G (1996) Opioid analgesics and antagonists. In: Hardman J et al. (eds). *Goodman and Gilman's The Pharmacological Basis of Therapeutics*. 9 ed. London: McGraw-Hill. 521–555.
31 Krajnik M. Opioid-induced pruritus. In: Zylicz Z *et al.*, editors. *Pruritus in Advanced Disease*. London: Oxford University Press. 84–96.
32 Tarcatu D *et al.* (2007) Are we still scratching the surface? A case of intractable pruritus following systemic opioid analgesia. *Journal of Opioid Management*. **3**: 167–170.
33 Paice JA *et al.* (1996) Intraspinal morphine for chronic pain: a retrospective, multicenter study. *Journal of Pain and Symptom Management*. **11**: 71–80.
34 Winkelmuller W *et al.* (1999) Intrathecal opioid therapy for pain: efficacy and outcomes. *Neuromodulation*. **2**: 67–76.
35 Smith TJ *et al.* (2002) Randomized clinical trial of an implantable drug delivery system compared with comprehensive medical management for refractory cancer pain: impact on pain, drug-related toxicity, and survival. *Journal of Clinical Oncology*. **20**: 4040–4049.
36 Chaplan SR *et al.* (1992) Morphine and hydromorphone epidural analgesia. *Anesthesiology*. **77**: 1090–1094.
37 Lynch L (2014) Personal communication.
38 Asokumar B *et al.* (1998) Intrathecal bupivacaine reduces pruritus and prolongs duration of fentanyl analgesia during labor: a prospective, randomized, controlled trial. *Anaesthesia and Analgesia*. **87**: 1309–1315.
39 Reich A and Szepietowski JC (2010) Opioid-induced pruritus: an update. *Clinical Experimental Dermatology*. **35**: 2–6.
40 Ballantyne J *et al.* (1988) Itching after epidural and spinal opiates. *Pain*. **33**: 149–160.
41 Kjellberg F and Tramer M (2001) Pharmacological control of opioid-induced pruritus: a quantitative systematic review of randomized trials. *European Journal of Anaesthesiology*. **18**: 346–357.
42 Hercz D *et al.* (2020) Interventions for itch in people with advanced chronic kidney disease. *Cochrane Database Systematic Reviews*. **12**: CD011393. www.cochranelibrary.com.
43 Zeidler C *et al.* (2013) A capsaicin 8% patch for the treatment of brachioradial pruritus. *Acta Dermato-venereologica*. **93**: 599–640.
44 Metz M *et al.* (2011) Treatment of notalgia paraesthetica with an 8% capsaicin patch. *British Journal of Dermatology*. **165**: 1359–1361.
45 Closs S (1997) Pruritus and methotrimeprazine. Personal communication.
46 Muston H *et al.* (1979) Differential effect of hypnotics and anxiolytics on itch and scratch. *Journal of Investigative Dermatology*. **72**: 283.
47 Figge J *et al.* (1979) Tricyclic antidepressants: potent blockade of histamine H_1 receptors of guinea pig ileum. *European Journal of Pharmacology*. **58**: 479–483.
48 Figueiredo A *et al.* (1990) Mechanism of action of doxepin in the treatment of chronic urticaria. *Fundamental and Clinical Pharmacology*. **4**: 147–158.
49 Pour-Reza-Gholi F *et al.* (2007) Low-dose doxepin for treatment of pruritus in patients on hemodialysis. *Iranian Journal of Kidney Diseases*. **1**: 34–37.
50 Haber R *et al.* (2020) Comparison of gabapentin and doxepin in the management of uremic pruritus: A randomized crossover clinical trial. *Dermatologic Therapy*. **33**: e14522.
51 Foroutan N *et al.* (2017) Comparison of pregabalin with doxepin in the management of uremic pruritus: a randomized single blind clinical trial. *Hemodialysis International*. **21**: 63–71.
52 Misery L *et al.* (eds) (2016) *Pruritus*. London: Springer.
53 Siemens W *et al.* (2016) Pharmacological interventions for pruritus in adult palliative care patients. *Cochrane Database of Systematic Reviews*. **11**: CD008320. www.cochranelibrary.com.
54 Millington G *et al.* (2018) British Association of Dermatologists' guidelines for the investigation and management of generalized pruritus in adults without an underlying dermatosis, 2018. *British Journal of Dermatology*. **178**: 34–60.
55 Ataei S *et al.* (2019) Comparison of sertraline with rifampin in the treatment of cholestatic pruritus: a randomized clinical trial. *Reviews on Recent Clinical Trials*. **14**: 217–223.
56 Ghent C and Carruthers S (1988) Treatment of pruritus in primary biliary cirrhosis with rifampin. Results of a double-blind crossover randomized trial. *Gastroenterology*. **94**: 488–493.
57 Tandon P *et al.* (2007) The efficacy and safety of bile acid binding agents, opioid antagonists, or rifampin in the treatment of cholestasis-associated pruritus. *American Journal of Gastroenterology*. **102**: 1528–1536.
58 Wolfhagen F *et al.* (1997) Oral naltrexone treatment for cholestatic pruritus: a double-blind, placebo-controlled study. *Gastroenterology*. **113**: 1264–1269.
59 Gaudy-Marqueste C (ed) (2016) Antihistamines. In: *Pruritus*. Springer, London. 363–377.
60 Hassenbusch SJ *et al.* (2004) Polyanalgesic Consensus Conference 2003: an update on the management of pain by intraspinal drug delivery-- report of an expert panel. *Journal of Pain and Symptom Management*. **27**: 540–563.
61 Aymard J *et al.* (1980) Cimetidine for pruritus in Hodgkin's disease. *British Medical Journal*. **280**: 151–152.
62 Korfitis C and Trafalis DT (2008) Carbamazepine can be effective in alleviating tormenting pruritus in patients with hematologic malignancy. *Journal of Pain and Symptom Management*. **35**: 571–572.
63 Davis M *et al.* (2003) Mirtazapine for pruritus. *Journal of Pain and Symptom Management*. **25**: 288–291.
64 Osterman PO (1976) Paroxysmal itching in multiple sclerosis. *British Journal of Dermatology*. **95**: 555–558.
65 Pakfetrat M *et al.* (2018) Sertraline can reduce the uremic pruritus in hemodialysis patient: a double blind randomized clinical trial from Southern Iran. *Hemodialysis International*. **22**: 103–109.
66 Gholyaf M *et al.* (2020) Effect of mirtazapine on pruritus in patients on hemodialysis: a cross-over pilot study. *International Urology and Nephrology*. **52**: 1155–1165.
67 To TH *et al.* (2012) The role of ondansetron in the management of cholestatic or uremic pruritus--a systematic review. *Journal of Pain and Symptom Management*. **44**: 725–730.
68 Hirschfield GM *et al.* (2018) The British Society of Gastroenterology/UK-PBC primary biliary cholangitis treatment and management guidelines. *Gut*. **67**: 1568–1594.
69 Lindor KD *et al.* (2019) Primary biliary cholangitis: 2018 practice guidance from the American Association for the Study of Liver Diseases. *Hepatology*. **69**: 394–419.
70 Fishbane S *et al.* (2020) A Phase 3 Trial of Difelikefalin in Hemodialysis Patients with Pruritus. *New England Journal of Medicine*. **382**: 222–232.
71 Kremer A (2019) What are new treatment concepts in systemic itch? *Experimental Dermatology*. **28**: 1485–1492.
72 Bergasa NV *et al.* (1994) Cholestasis in the male rat is associated with naloxone-reversible antinociception. *Journal of Hepatology*. **20**: 85–90.
73 Kumada H *et al.* (2017) Efficacy of nalfurafine hydrochloride in patients with chronic liver disease with refractory pruritus: A randomized, double-blind trial. *Hepatology Research*. **47**: 972–982.
74 McMullin M *et al.* (2019) A guideline for the diagnosis and management of polycythaemia vera. A British Society for Haematology Guideline. *British Journal Haematology*. **184**: 176–191.

75 Twycross RG (1981) Pruritus and pain on en cuirass breast cancer. *Lancet.* **2**: 696.
76 de Vries E *et al.* (2021) Fibrates for Itch (FITCH) in fibrosing cholangiopathies: a double-blind, randomized, placebo-controlled trial. *Gastroenterology.* **160**: 734–743.
77 Dyson J and Jones D (2021) Bezafibrate for the treatment of cholestatic pruritus: time for a change in management? *Gastroenterology.* **160**: 649–651.
78 Ahrens E *et al.* (1950) Primary biliary cirrhosis. *Medicine.* **29**: 299–364.
79 Lloyd-Thomas H and Sherlock S (1952) Testosterone therapy for the pruritus of obstructive jaundice. *British Medical Journal.* **2**: 1289–1291.
80 Twycross RG and Zylicz Z (2004) Systemic therapy: Making rational choices. In: Zylicz Z *et al.* (eds.) *Pruritus in advanced disease.* Oxford University Press, London, pp. 161–178.
81 Bergasa NV *et al.* (2006) Gabapentin in patients with the pruritus of cholestasis: a double-blind, randomized, placebo-controlled trial. *Hepatology.* **44**: 1317–1323.
82 Kanitakis J (2006) Brachioradial pruritus: report of a new case responding to gabapentin. *European Journal of Dermatology.* **16**: 311–312.
83 Yesudian PD and Wilson NJ (2005) Efficacy of gabapentin in the management of pruritus of unknown origin. *Archives of Dermatology.* **141**: 1507–1509.
84 Mahmudpour M *et al.* (2017) Therapeutic effect of montelukast for treatment of uremic pruritus in hemodialysis patients. *Iranian Journal of Kidney Diseases.* **11**: 50–55.
85 Hohl CM *et al.* (2015) Methylnaltrexone to palliate pruritus in terminal hepatic disease. *Journal of Palliative Care.* **31**: 124–126.
86 Vincenzi B *et al.* (2010) Aprepitant against pruritus in patients with solid tumours. *Supportive Care in Cancer.* **18**: 1229–1230.
87 Torres T *et al.* (2012) Aprepitant: Evidence of its effectiveness in patients with refractory pruritus continues. *Journal of the American Academy of Dermatology.* **66**: e14–e15.
88 Silva S *et al.* (1994) Thalidomide for the treatment of uremic pruritus: a crossover randomized double-blind trial. *Nephron.* **67**: 270–273.
89 Goncalves F (2010) Thalidomide for the control of severe paraneoplastic pruritus associated with Hodgkin's disease. *American Journal of Hospice and Palliative Care.* **27**: 486–487.
90 Lowney AC *et al.* (2014) Thalidomide therapy for pruritus in the palliative setting--a distinct subset of patients in whom the benefit may outweigh the risk. *Journal of Pain and Symptom Management.* **48**: e3–e5.
91 Thomsen JS *et al.* (2002) Suppression of spontaneous scratching in hairless rats by sedatives but not by antipruritics. *Skin Pharmacology and Applied Skin Physiology.* **15**: 218–224.
92 Prieto LN (2004) The use of midazolam to treat itching in a terminally ill patient with biliary obstruction. *Journal of Pain and Symptom Management.* **28**: 531–532.
93 McDonald JC *et al.* (2015) Control of intractable pruritus in a patient with cutaneous T-cell lymphoma using a continuous subcutaneous infusion of lidocaine. *Journal of Pain and Symptom Management.* **49**: e1–e3.
94 Norris J *et al.* (2019) Does continuous subcutaneous infusion of lignocaine relieve intractable pruritus associated with advanced cutaneous T-cell lymphoma? A retrospective case series review. *Palliative Medicine.* **33**: 552–556.

Updated (minor change) October 2021

27: ORAL NUTRITIONAL SUPPLEMENTS

This section provides an overview of cachexia and the use of oral nutritional supplements in adults with cancer. It does not address nutritional supplements in children, patients with renal or hepatic failure, tube feeding or parenteral nutrition, but indicates where these may be required.

Introduction

Weight loss is a common adverse feature of cancer, associated with increased morbidity, poorer treatment tolerability and outcomes, and reduced survival. It generally occurs in the context of cancer cachexia, a multifactorial syndrome characterized by an ongoing loss of *skeletal muscle* mass (± fat), leading to progressive functional impairment.[1] There is negative protein and energy balance driven by a variable combination of reduced food intake and abnormal metabolism, with no standard treatment available for the latter.[2]

Screening

Whatever the cause of malnutrition, early detection and intervention is preferable and requires a multiprofessional pro-active approach. NICE guidance suggests that all patients should be screened for malnutrition when:

- admitted to hospital, and weekly thereafter
- admitted to care homes, and repeated if there is clinical concern
- first seen in outpatients, and repeated if there is clinical concern
- registering with a general practice.

As a minimum, screening should evaluate:

- the body mass index (BMI):

$$\text{BMI} = \frac{\text{weight (kg)}}{\text{height}^2\text{ (m)}}$$

- percentage unintentional weight loss
- time over which nutrient intake has been unintentionally reduced and/or the likelihood of future impaired intake.[3]

Screening tools include the Malnutrition Universal Screening Tool (MUST) and the Nutritional Risk Screening Tool 2002.[4,5] Although they are easy to complete, only the latter has been validated specifically for use in patients with cancer.[5,6] The Patient Generated Subjective Global Assessment is a specific tool for patients with cancer, but requires more training and takes longer to complete.[7,8]

NICE guidance suggests nutritional support should be considered for patients with:

- BMI <18.5kg/m^2
- unintentional weight loss of >10% in the last 3–6 months
- BMI <20kg/m^2 and unintentional weight loss of >5%
- inadequate oral intake for >5 days
- malabsorption, increased nutrient losses, increased catabolism.[3]

Using these criteria, 30% and 60% of patients with thoracic or upper GI cancers respectively are malnourished even at the time of diagnosis.[9,10] Further, it could be argued that the remainder are at risk of malnutrition because of increased catabolism.

Recent cancer-specific recommendations have suggested lower thresholds for the diagnosis of cachexia, i.e. *any* of the following:

- weight loss >5% over past 6 months
- BMI <20kg/m^2 and weight loss >2%
- sarcopenia and weight loss >2%.[1]

Ideally, patients identified as at risk by the screening process should then have their nutritional status assessed by an appropriately trained health professional (typically a dietitian) in order to produce an individualized nutrition care plan, which includes monitoring.[6,11] The assessment would take into account the patient's physical condition and prognosis, state of hydration, dietary intake, estimation of nutritional requirements, identification of underlying symptoms contributing to malnutrition (e.g. poor oral health or dentition, nausea, early satiety), and other psychosocial and dietary considerations.

Assessment and management

Box A is mostly based on the European Society for Clinical Nutrition and Metabolism (ESPEN) guidelines on nutrition in cancer patients.[2]

Box A Guidelines on nutrition in cancer patients

Nutritional assessment should be performed and nutritional support started when:

- malnutrition exists *or*
- a patient has inadequate nutritional intake, i.e.:
  - ▷ unable to eat for >1 week *or*
  - ▷ estimated energy intake <60% of requirement for >1–2 weeks.

Daily energy requirement

When energy expenditure cannot be measured, a reasonable estimate of daily total energy expenditure (TEE) is 25–30Kcal/kg/day.

Note. This estimate is less accurate in patients who are severely underweight (underestimates TEE) or obese (overestimates TEE).

Daily protein requirement

Generally 1–1.5g/kg/day; limit to 1 and 1.2g/kg/day in acute and chronic renal failure respectively.

Daily fluid requirement

Generally 30–35mL/kg/day; 30mL/kg/day in patients with cachexia, because of changes in extracellular fluid volumes and reduced fluid clearance.

In addition, account for losses caused by pyrexia, malabsorption, fistulas, high-output stomas.

Aims of nutrition therapy

- identify, prevent and treat reversible elements of malnutrition
- maintain/improve food intake and mitigate derangements in protein, carbohydrate and lipid metabolism
- maintain skeletal muscle and physical performance
- improve tolerability of anticancer treatments
- improve quality of life.

General approach

With the exception of patients at the end of life, the aim is to meet a patient's energy and substrate requirements by offering interventions step by step, i.e.:

- dietary fortification
- oral nutritional supplements
- artificial enteral or parenteral nutrition.

Nutrition should be introduced slowly over several days when there is a risk of refeeding syndrome (see p.850).

Physical therapy (activities of daily living, resistance and aerobic training) should be encouraged to prevent muscle deconditioning and promote muscle anabolism, mass and strength.

Drugs are used in specific circumstances (see below).

Route

In a patient with a functioning GI tract, the enteral route (PO, or tube feeding when PO insufficient/not feasible) is preferred to the parenteral route.

Tube feeding can be delivered via transnasal or percutaneous (e.g. gastrostomy, jejunostomy) routes; percutaneous is preferred for long-term use (>30 days).

continued

Box A Continued

Tube feeding is preferable in patients with head and neck or oesophageal cancers causing dysphagia, or when severe radiation-therapy-induced oral or oesophageal mucositis is anticipated (when the percutaneous route may need to be used). Patients should be taught how to manage the dysphagia and maintain their swallowing function.

The parenteral route is preferred when there is an increased risk of bleeding or infections from tube placement, e.g. in neutropenic or thrombocytopenic patients, or when the GI tract is not functioning. Generally, it should be avoided in patients with a prognosis of <2 months, when the burden is considered to outweigh the benefit.

Formula

Standard nutrient composition formulas (1–1.5kcal/mL) should generally be used.

For patients with early satiety or increased nutritional requirements, high-energy high-protein formulas may be preferable.

In weight-losing patients with insulin resistance, it is recommended to increase the proportion of energy intake from fat rather than carbohydrate.

Peri-operatively, for upper GI cancer, formulas which provide immune-modulating substrates, e.g. arginine, n-3 fatty acids, nucleotides, are recommended.

Drug treatment

In patients with advanced cancer and anorexia, corticosteroids and progestogens can enhance appetite, with inconsistent effects on body weight and quality of life. They should be used for short periods only, e.g. 1–3 weeks, weighing their benefits against their undesirable effects, particularly the risk of thrombosis with progestogens (p.599).

In patients with advanced cancer undergoing chemotherapy at risk of weight loss or who are malnourished, supplementation with long-chain n-3 fatty acids (e.g. eicosapentaenoic acid (EPA)) or fish oil can stabilize or improve appetite, lean body mass and body weight. Typical doses are 1–2g n-3 fatty acids/day and 4–6g fish oil/day.

In patients with early satiety due to delayed gastric emptying, the prokinetic drugs domperidone (p.271) and metoclopramide (p.268) can be considered, taking their respective risks of undesirable cardiovascular and CNS effects into account.

There is insufficient evidence to recommend the use of androgens, cannabinoids or NSAIDs.

Peri-operative

Patients receiving curative or palliative surgery at risk of malnutrition should receive nutritional support as part of a programme of enhanced recovery after surgery. This should extend to ongoing nutritional support following discharge from hospital.

GI cancer patients undergoing surgical resection should receive peri-operative immune-modulating nutrition (see Formula above).

Radiation therapy

Adequate nutritional intake should be maintained during radiation therapy, particularly to the head and neck, thorax and GI tract, using the general approach. Tube feeding is recommended when severe dysphagia is present or anticipated (see Route above).

Anticancer drug treatment

Adequate nutritional intake and physical activity should be maintained. In those receiving potentially curative drug treatments, including stem cell transplant, consider enteral nutrition when counselling + oral nutritional supplements are inadequate. The parenteral route can be considered when there is severe mucositis, intractable vomiting, ileus, severe malabsorption, protracted diarrhoea or symptomatic graft versus host disease affecting the GI tract.

Cancer survivors

A healthy lifestyle is recommended, which includes maintaining a healthy weight (BMI 18.5–25kg/m^2), being physically active, and having a diet high in vegetables, fruits and whole grains and low in saturated fat, red meat and alcohol.

continued

Box A Continued

Patients with advanced cancer on no anticancer treatment

Those malnourished or at risk should be assessed with a particular focus on improving symptoms impacting on nutrition, together with eating- or weight-loss-associated psychosocial distress.

Nutritional interventions should be offered only after considering (together with the patient) the likely prognosis, the potential benefit to quality of life and survival, and associated burdens.

Patients with dysphagia should be assessed by a speech and language therapist (SALT).

End of life

Generally, hunger and the urge to eat are much diminished or absent in the last weeks/days of life.[12,13] There is little or no benefit from nutritional support in this setting, and the focus of care is on providing symptom relief, addressing patient and family-eating-related distress, and the use of appetite stimulants when appropriate.[1] Small amounts of food can be offered as desired by the patient to alleviate hunger, and for pleasure and social purposes.[14]

Routine artificial hydration has little or no benefit in the imminently dying. It may have a limited role in selected circumstances, e.g. to improve delirium or symptomatic dehydration, and a short trial (e.g. 24h) may be appropriate. It should *not* be used for the palliation of dry mouth or thirst, for which regular oral care measures are effective.

Provision of oral nutrition support

Correct the correctable

If oral intake is to be improved, attention must be paid to:

- the ability to obtain and prepare food
- oral problems, e.g. xerostomia, mucositis, oral candidosis
- uncontrolled symptoms that may impact on nutrition, e.g. nausea and vomiting
- dysphagia.

Generally, patients with neurogenic dysphagia or swallowing difficulties which put them at risk of aspiration should be assessed by a speech and language therapist (SALT). Certain consistencies of fluid or food may be safer in these circumstances. The International Dysphagia Diet Standardisation Initiative (https://iddsi.org) provides a common terminology that describes fluid and food thickness, ranging from stages 0 (thin liquid) to 7 (regular food), along with resources for patients. A dietitian or SALT can advise on which nutritional supplements have a consistency/stage appropriate for a patient's needs.

General advice

This includes:

- meal patterns, e.g. eat small amounts frequently
- substitute water-based drinks with milk-based drinks, e.g. hot chocolate, malted drinks, milky coffee or fortified milk-free alternatives
- encourage intake of some protein at each meal
- encourage high-energy foods where possible, e.g. use full-fat dairy products, margarine, olive or rapeseed oil (fats are the most concentrated source of energy)
- consider relaxing pre-imposed dietary restrictions, e.g. diabetic diet; if necessary, adjust drugs for diabetes to maintain adequate glycaemic control
- making use of microwave meals and convenience foods; quick and easy to prepare, often small portions
- avoiding dry foods when taste impaired; encourage flavouring foods with, e.g., herbs and sauces.

Generally, weight gain is more likely with both dietary advice and nutritional supplements than with dietary advice alone in patients with Illness-related malnutrition.[15]

Appetite stimulants

See Progestogens (p.599) and Systemic corticosteroids (p.556).

Oral nutritional supplements

Oral nutritional supplements should be considered when a patient is unable to improve their nutritional intake by diet alone. Generally, they should supplement existing intake rather than replace it, e.g. 1–2 cartons/day of a 1.5kcal/mL milk-based nutritional supplement. However, some products are nutritionally complete and, if ingested in sufficient quantities, can be used as a sole source of nutrition (e.g. see Table 2).

Oral nutritional supplements are available in liquid, semi-solid or powder formulations. General prescribing guidelines are in Box B and product details in Tables 1–13, including for thickeners and thickened drinks for use in patients with dysphagia. Generally, the supplements are ordered within the tables according to their energy density and protein content per unit measure, e.g. per bottle, sachet or grams of powdered product.

Box B Guidelines for prescribing oral nutritional supplements

1 Ensure correctable underlying problems are addressed and general nutritional advice has been given (see text).

2 Exclude any food allergies. Advisory Committee on Borderline Substances approved products list potential allergens. If necessary, seek advice from a dietitian.

3 To aid adherence, be guided by the patient's preferences and provide a variety of locally available formulations and flavours, either separately or in commercially available starter packs, e.g.:
- Abbott: Ensure Plus Commence®
- Nutricia: Complan® Shake, Fortijuce®, Fortisip® Compact, Fortisip® Extra and Fortisip® Range (contains Fortisip®, Fortijuce® and Fortisip® Yoghurt Style).

4 Provide information on how to use the supplements, together with any special instructions, e.g.:
- keep supplements chilled to improve palatability
- use the straw provided with supplement to minimize unpleasant odour
- use supplement as a between-meal snack, not as a meal replacement
- maintain good oral hygiene
- once opened, supplements can be stored in a refrigerator for up to 24h.

5 Review patient after 1 week:
- prescribe the required number of cartons/units per day of the formulation and flavour(s) which are acceptable to the patient
- if none are acceptable, try an alternative, e.g. juice-based or milkshake powder.

6 Review patient after 4 weeks of supplement use. If weight loss continues, seek advice from a dietitian. Monitoring should continue on a monthly basis until supplements are no longer required.

Patients with renal or hepatic failure, malabsorption, dysphagia, or at risk of refeeding syndrome (p.850) should be referred to a dietitian.

Energy content is given per unit and per mL, and the protein content per unit. For other supplements, the nutritional content is given per 100mL or 100g as appropriate. Flavours frequently alter; check availability with the manufacturer. Unless otherwise stated, all products listed are Advisory Committee on Borderline Substances (ACBS) approved for patients with disease-related malnutrition.

The oral nutritional supplements listed are gluten-free and most are suitable for vegetarians. Those containing fish oils (e.g. EPA), micronutrients or colourings derived from animal sources may not be acceptable to strict vegetarians, vegans or patients of certain religious and ethnic groups. If uncertain with patients who have specific dietary restrictions, consult a dietitian or the manufacturers for advice.

Ingesting sufficient quantities orally may be difficult for patients with anorexia or taste changes, and various strategies, including recipes suggested by the manufacturers, can be tried to aid compliance (Box C).

Box C Aiding compliance with milk- and juice-based supplements

Milk-based	**Juice-based**
Serve chilled ± ice	Serve chilled ± ice
Add extra full-fat milk	Add extra fruit juice
Make a smoothie by adding fresh fruit and ice cream	Make a spritzer by adding soda water/ lemonade/carbonated water
Make into a jelly	Make into a jelly
Use instead of milk on cereals and in puddings (unflavoured)	Pour over fresh or tinned fruit
Use to make custard/rice pudding (vanilla flavour)	Freeze to make an ice lolly or ice cubes

Further recipes are available from:
www.abbottnutrition.co.uk
www.fresenius-kabi.co.uk
www.nestlehealthscience.co.uk
www.nutricia.co.uk

Table 1 Milkshake-style nutritional supplements (suitable as a sole source of nutrition)[a,b]
Included for completeness: generally, supplements with higher energy and protein content should be used.

Product	*Unit size*	*Energy content*	*Protein content*	*Flavours/comments*
Ensure® (Abbott)	250mL can	250kcal (1kcal/mL)	10g	Chocolate, coffee, vanilla
Fresubin® Original Drink (Fresenius)	200mL bottle	200kcal (1kcal/mL)	9g	Blackcurrant, chocolate, mocha, nut, peach, vanilla

a. avoid acidic citrus/tangy flavours in patients with a sore mouth
b. best served chilled.

Table 2 High-energy milkshake-style nutritional supplements (suitable as a sole source of nutrition)[a,b]

Product	*Unit size*	*Energy content*	*Protein content*	*Flavours/comments*
Ensure® Compact (Abbott)	125mL bottle	300kcal (2.4kcal/mL)	13g	Banana, strawberry, vanilla
Fortisip® Compact (Nutricia)	125mL bottle	300kcal (2.4kcal/mL)	12g	Apricot, banana, chocolate, forest fruit, mocha, strawberry, vanilla
Ensure® Plus Milkshake Style (Abbott)	200mL bottle	300kcal (1.5kcal/mL)	13g	Banana, chocolate, coffee, fruits of the forest, neutral, peach, raspberry, strawberry, vanilla
Fortisip® Bottle (Nutricia)	200mL bottle	300kcal (1.5kcal/mL)	12g	Banana, caramel, chocolate, neutral, orange, strawberry, tropical fruit, vanilla
Fresubin® Energy Drink (Fresenius)	200mL bottle	300kcal (1.5kcal/mL)	11g	Banana, blackcurrant, cappuccino, chocolate, lemon, strawberry, tropical fruit, vanilla, unflavoured
Resource® Energy (Nestle Health Science)	200mL bottle	300kcal (1.5kcal/mL)	11g	Apricot, banana, chocolate, coffee, strawberry–raspberry, vanilla

a. avoid acidic citrus/tangy flavours in patients with a sore mouth
b. best served chilled.

Table 3 Savoury-style nutritional supplements[a,b]

Product	*Unit size*	*Energy content*	*Protein content*	*Flavours/comments*
Ensure® Plus Savoury (Abbott)	200mL bottle	300kcal (1.5kcal/mL)	13g	Suitable as a sole source of nutrition; chicken
Vitasavoury® (Vitaflo)	50g sachet	309kcal (6kcal/g)	6g	375kcal and 9g protein when reconstituted with full-fat milk (100mL); not for use as a sole source of nutrition; chicken, golden vegetable
Meritene® Energis Soup (Nestle Health Science)	50g sachet	207kcal (4.1kcal/g)	7g	300kcal and 12g protein when reconstituted with full-fat milk (150mL); contains 3.7g fibre; chicken, vegetable

a. best served warm, do not boil; sachets can be reconstituted with warm water or full-fat milk
b. vitamin and mineral content varies between products.

Table 4 Milkshake-style nutritional supplements with fibre (suitable as a sole source of nutrition)[a,b]

Product	*Unit size*	*Energy content*	*Protein content*	*Flavours/comments*
Fortisip® Compact Fibre (Nutricia)	125mL bottle	300kcal (2.4kcal/mL)	12g	Contains 4.5g fibre; mocha, strawberry, vanilla
Resource® 2.0 Fibre (Nestle Health Science)	200mL bottle	400kcal (2.0kcal/mL)	18g	Contains 5g soluble fibre (50:50 FOS:GOS), do not exceed 4 bottles/ day; apricot, coffee, strawberry, summer fruit, vanilla, unflavoured
Ensure® Plus Fibre (Abbott)	200mL bottle	310kcal (1.6kcal/mL)	13g	Contains 5g fibre and FOS; banana, chocolate, raspberry, strawberry, vanilla
Fresubin® Energy Fibre Drink (Fresenius)	200mL bottle	300kcal (1.5kcal/mL)	11g	Contains 4g mixed fibre blend; banana, caramel, cherry, chocolate, strawberry, vanilla

FOS = fructooligosaccharide, GOS = galactooligosaccharide

a. useful for patients with constipation

b. shake well before use.

Table 5 Yoghurt-style nutritional supplements (suitable as a sole source of nutrition)[a,b]

Product	*Unit size*	*Energy content*	*Protein content*	*Flavours/comments*
Ensure® Plus Yoghurt Style (Abbott)	200mL bottle	300kcal (1.5kcal/mL)	13g	Peach, strawberry
Fortisip® Yoghurt Style (Nutricia)	200mL bottle	300kcal (1.5kcal/mL)	12g	Peach-orange, raspberry, vanilla–lemon

a. can be more palatable in patients with taste change (citrus/tangy flavours vs. sweet)

b. avoid acidic citrus/tangy flavours in patients with a sore mouth.

Table 6 Fruit juice-style nutritional supplements (not suitable as a sole source of nutrition)[a,b]

Product	*Unit size*	*Energy content*	*Protein content*	*Flavours/comments*
Ensure® Plus Juce (Abbott)	220mL bottle	330kcal (1.5kcal/mL)	11g	Apple, fruit punch, lemon and lime, orange, peach, strawberry
Fortijuce® (Nutricia)	200mL bottle	300kcal (1.5kcal/mL)	8g	Apple, blackcurrant, forest fruit, lemon, orange, strawberry, tropical
Fresubin® Jucy Drink (Fresenius)	200mL bottle	300kcal (1.5kcal/mL)	8g	Apple, blackcurrant, cherry, orange, pineapple

a. may be preferable for patients with a dry mouth

b. avoid acidic citrus/tangy flavours in patients with a sore mouth.

Table 7 High-protein milkshake-style nutritional supplements (not suitable as a sole source of nutrition)[a]

Product	*Unit size*	*Energy content*	*Protein content*	*Flavours/comments*
Altraplen® Compact (Nualtra)	125mL bottle	300kcal (2.4kcal/mL)	12g	Banana, hazel chocolate, strawberry, vanilla
Altraplen® Protein (Nualtra)	200mL bottle	300kcal (2.4kcal/mL)	20g	Strawberry, vanilla
Fortisip® Compact Protein (Nutricia)	125mL bottle	300kcal (2.4kcal/mL)	18g	Banana, berries, cool red fruits, hot tropical ginger, mocha, peach–mango, strawberry, unflavoured, vanilla
Fresubin® 2kcal Drink (Fresenius)	200mL bottle	400kcal (2kcal/mL)	20g	Apricot–peach, cappuccino, fruits of the forest, toffee, unflavoured, vanilla
Fresubin® 2kcal Fibre Drink (Fresenius)	200mL bottle	400kcal (2kcal/mL)	20g	Contains 3g fibre; apricot–peach, cappuccino, chocolate, lemon, unflavoured, vanilla
Ensure® TwoCal (Abbott)	200mL bottle	400kcal (2kcal/mL)	17g	Contains 2g FOS; banana, strawberry, vanilla, unflavoured
Fortisip® Extra (Nutricia)	200mL bottle	320kcal (1.6kcal/mL)	20g	Strawberry, vanilla
Fresubin® Protein Energy Drink (Fresenius)	200mL bottle	300kcal (1.5kcal/mL)	20g	Cappuccino, chocolate, wild strawberry, tropical fruits, vanilla

FOS = fructooligosaccharide, a soluble fibre

a. consider in patients with high protein loss or wounds when overall energy intake is adequate.

Table 8 Semi-solid nutritional supplements (suitable as a sole source of nutrition)[a]

Product	*Unit size*	*Energy content*	*Protein content*	*Flavours/comments*
Fresubin® Creme (Fresenius)	125g pot	230kcal (1.8kcal/g)	13g	Cappuccino, chocolate, praline, strawberry, vanilla
Forticreme® Complete (Nutricia)	125g pot	200kcal (1.6kcal/g)	12g	Banana, chocolate, forest fruit, vanilla
Fresubin® YOcreme (Fresenius)	125g pot	187kcal (1.5kcal/g)	9g	Apricot–peach, biscuit, lemon, raspberry, unflavoured
Nutricrem (Nualtra)	125g pot	225kcal	13g	Vanilla, strawberry, mint chocolate and chocolate orange
Ensure® Plus Creme (Abbott)	125g pot	171kcal (1.4kcal/g)	7g	Banana, chocolate, vanilla, unflavoured
Nutilis® Fruit Stage 3 (Nutricia)	150g pot	206kcal (1.4kcal/g)	11g	Contains 4g fibre; apple, strawberry
ProSource® Jelly (Nutrinovo)	118mL pot	90kcal (0.75kcal/mL)	20g	Blackcurrant, fruit punch, lime, orange

a. useful for patients with dysphagia. However, because product consistencies can vary (e.g. with storage, temperature), seek SALT team advice on the most appropriate to use.

Table 9 Powdered milkshake-style nutritional supplements (not suitable as a sole source of nutrition)[a,b,c]

Product	*Unit size*	*Energy content*	*Protein content*	*Flavours/comments*
Calshake® (Fresenius)	87g sachet	431kcal (5kcal/g)	4g	600kcal and 12g protein when reconstituted with full-fat milk (240mL); banana, chocolate, strawberry, unflavoured, vanilla; in boxes of 7
Scandishake Mix® (Nutricia)	85g sachet	425kcal (5kcal/g)	3g	588kcal and 12g protein when reconstituted with full-fat milk (240mL); banana, caramel, chocolate, strawberry, vanilla, unflavoured; in boxes of 6
Enshake® (Abbott)	97g sachet	437kcal (8.5kcal/g)	8g	600kcal and 16g protein when reconstituted with full-fat milk (240mL); banana, chocolate, strawberry, vanilla; in boxes of 6
Ensure® Shake (Abbott)	57g sachet	253kcal (4kcal/g)	10g	389kcal and 17g protein when reconstituted with full-fat milk (200mL); banana, chocolate, strawberry, vanilla; in boxes of 7
Foodlink® Complete (Nualtra)	450g box	245kcal (4kcal/g)	12g	1 serving = 4 heaped dessert spoons. 383kcal, 17g protein when reconstituted with full-fat milk (200mL); banana, chocolate, strawberry, vanilla, unflavoured
Foodlink® Complete with fibre (Nualtra)	57g sachet	245kcal (4kcal/g)	12g	4.5g fibre per sachet. 383kcal and 17g protein when reconstituted with full-fat milk (200ml); strawberry, chocolate, banana, natural and vanilla. Can be reconstituted with fruit juice
Aymes® Shake (Aymes)	57g sachet	252kcal (1.6kcal/mL)	9g	388kcal and 16g protein when reconstituted with 200mL full-fat milk; with added vitamins and minerals; banana, chocolate, neutral, strawberry, vanilla
Fresubin® Powder Extra (Fresenius)	62g sachet	260kcal (4kcal/g)	11g	397kcal and 18g protein when reconstituted with full-fat milk (200mL); with added vitamins and minerals; chocolate, strawberry, vanilla, unflavoured
Complan® Shake (Nutricia)	57g sachet	250kcal (4kcal/g)	9g	385kcal and 16g protein when reconstituted with full-fat milk (200mL); with added vitamins and minerals; banana, chocolate, strawberry, vanilla, unflavoured

a. high palatability
b. some products are lower in vitamins and minerals compared with other supplements
c. milkshake-style should be reconstituted using full-fat milk to optimize energy content.

Table 10 OTC nutritional supplements (not suitable as a sole source of nutrition)

Product	*Unit size*	*Energy content*[a]	*Protein content*	*Comments*
Meritene® Energis® Shakes (Nestle Health Science)	30g sachet	107kcal (3.6 kcal/g)	9g	243kcal and 16g protein when reconstituted with 200mL full-fat milk; chocolate, strawberry, vanilla

a. unconstituted.

Table 11 Special application nutritional products[a,b]

Product	*Unit size*	*Energy content*	*Protein content*	*Flavours/comments*
Ensure® Plus Advance (Abbott)	220mL bottle	330kcal (1.5kcal/mL)	20g	For use in patients over 65 years who have, or are at risk of, malnutrition; contains 13microgram vitamin D and 499mg calcium; banana, chocolate, coffee, strawberry, vanilla
Forticare® (Nutricia)	125mL bottle	204kcal (1.6kcal/mL)	11g	For use in patients with cachexia (pancreatic cancer and lung cancer undergoing chemotherapy). Contains EPA, DHA, fibre and antioxidants. Recommended dose 3 bottles/day (providing 2.2g EPA and 1.1g DHA); not nutritionally complete at this dose; cappuccino, orange–lemon, peach–ginger
Supportan® Drink (Fresenius)	200mL bottle	300kcal (1.5kcal/mL)	20g	For use in patients with cachexia (pancreatic cancer and lung cancer undergoing chemotherapy). Contains EPA and DHA, antioxidants and fibre. Recommended dose 2 bottles/day (providing 2.85g EPA and DHA); cappuccino, tropical fruits
ProSure® (Abbott)	240mL Tetra Pak	305kcal (1.3kcal/mL)	16g	For use in patients with cachexia (pancreatic cancer and lung cancer undergoing chemotherapy). Contains EPA and antioxidants. An intake of 1.5–2 cartons/day is required for benefit; not nutritionally complete at this dose; vanilla
Oral Impact® (Nestle Health Science)	74g sachet	309kcal	18g	Contains immune-modulating substrates and soluble fibre (e.g. n-3 fatty acids, arginine, nucleotides). Pre-operatively, 2–4 sachets a day (dissolved in 250mL of cool boiled water) recommended for 5–7 days; not nutritionally complete at this dose; citrus, coffee, tropical
Respifor® (Nutricia)	125mL bottle	188kcal (1.5kcal/mL)	9g	For early-intervention use in patients with COPD. Recommended dose 125mL t.d.s. in combination with activity plan for 3 months; chocolate, strawberry, vanilla

continued

Table 11 Continued

Product	*Unit size*	*Energy content*	*Protein content*	*Flavours/comments*
Elemental E028 Extra Liquid® (Nutricia)	250mL carton	215kcal (0.9kcal/mL)	6g	A liquid elemental feed for patients with intractable malabsorption or radiation enteritis. Protein source is a mixture of essential and non-essential amino acids. Nutritionally complete; grapefruit, orange and pineapple, summer fruits
Elemental E028 Extra Powder® (Nutricia)	100g sachet	427kcal/100g	13g/ 100g	An elemental feed for patients with intractable malabsorption or radiation enteritis. Protein source is a mixture of essential and non-essential amino acids. Nutritionally complete. Reconstitute with 100g powder in 500mL water; banana, orange, unflavoured
Vital® 1.5kcal (Abbott)	200mL bottle	300kcal (1.5kcal/mL)	14g	A peptide-based sip feed for patients with malabsorption: nutritionally complete; vanilla, café latte, mixed berry
Survimed® OPD Drink (Fresenius)	200mL bottle	200kcal (1kcal/mL)	9g	A peptide-based sip feed for patients with malabsorption; nutritionally complete; vanilla
Peptamen® Vanilla Bottle (Nestle Health Science)	200mL bottle	200kcal (1kcal/mL)	8g	For patients with impaired GI function. Contains protein source as peptides, and fat is 70% MCT to improve digestion and absorption. Nutritionally complete. Can be flavoured with 2 scoops of Nestle Nutrition Flavour Mix/100mL to improve palatability; banana, chocolate, coffee, lemon and lime, strawberry
Resource® OptiFibre® (Nestle Health Science)	250g tub (5g per scoop) 10g sachet	–	–	For use with patients who have constipation. Each scoop contains 4.3g and each sachet 6g of soluble fibre (partially hydrolysed guar gum) and is mixed into hot or cold liquids and foods. Introduce gradually; begin with 1 scoop or half a sachet and increase by 1 scoop or half a sachet every 3 days. Recommended dose is 2 sachets/3 scoops/day, maximum 32g/day
Forceval® Capsules (Alliance)	15, 30 and 90 cap pack	–	–	Multivitamin, mineral and trace element supplement given as 1 capsule daily. Capsule can be opened and contents mixed, e.g. with a teaspoon of jam

EPA = eicosapentaenoic acid, DHA = docosahexaenoic acid, MCT = medium-chain triglyceride

a. use with dietetic supervision

b. listed according to type.

Table 12 Modular carbohydrate, protein and fat supplements (not suitable as a sole source of nutrition)[a,b]

Product	*Unit size*	*Energy source*	*Energy content*	*Comments*
Polycal® Powder (Nutricia)	400g tub	Carbohydrate	384kcal/100g (19kcal/5g)	Glucose polymer powder to add to food and drinks; unflavoured
Maxijul® Super Soluble Powder (SHS)	132g sachet, 200g, 25kg tub	Carbohydrate	380kcal/100g	Glucose polymer powder to add to food and drinks; recommended dilution 1:2; unflavoured
Vitajoule® (Vitaflo)	500g tub	Carbohydrate	380kcal/100g	Glucose syrup powder to add to food and drinks; unflavoured
Polycal® Liquid (Nutricia)	200mL bottle (30mL shot)	Carbohydrate	334kcal/100mL 7g protein/100mL (100kcal/30mL 2g protein/30mL)	Glucose polymer solution; can be used undiluted or diluted in drinks; orange, unflavoured
Protifar® (Nutricia)	225g tub (2.5g/scoop)	Protein	368kcal/100g 87g protein/100g	High-protein powder to add to food and drinks; unflavoured
Fresubin® 5kcal SHOT (Fresenius)	120mL bottle	Fat	500kcal/100mL	LCT and MCT fat emulsion. Recommended dose 30mL t.d.s.–q.d.s.; lemon, unflavoured
Liquigen® (Nutricia)	250mL bottle	Fat	450kcal/100mL	MCT fat emulsion; unflavoured
Calogen® (Nutricia)	200mL, 500mL bottle	Fat	450kcal/100mL	LCT fat emulsion. Recommended dose 30mL t.d.s.; banana, strawberry, unflavoured
Calogen® Extra (Nutricia)	200mL bottle, 40mL shot	Fat, carbohydrate	400kcal/100mL 5g protein/100mL	High-energy fat emulsion with protein, carbohydrate, vitamins and minerals. Recommended dose 40mL t.d.s.; strawberry, unflavoured
Super Soluble Duocal® (Nutricia)	400g tub	Fat, carbohydrate	492kcal/100g	Fat and glucose polymer powder to add to food and drinks; unflavoured
ProSource® Liquid (Nutrinovo)	100 x 30mL sachet	Protein and carbohydrate	333kcal/100mL 33g protein/100mL (30mL sachet: 100kcal, 10g protein)	Protein and energy liquid to drink as a 'shot' or add to food and drinks; citrus–berry, lemon, orange, unflavoured

continued

Table 12 Continued

Product	*Unit size*	*Energy source*	*Energy content*	*Comments*
ProSource® Plus (Nutrinovo)	100 x 30mL sachet	Protein and carbohydrate	333kcal/100mL 50g protein/100mL (30mL sachet: 100kcal, 15g protein)	Protein and energy liquid to drink as a 'shot' or add to food and drinks; berry, citrus, orange crème, unflavoured
Pro-Cal® Powder (Vitaflo)	15g sachet 510g, 1.5kg, 12.5kg tub	Protein, fat, carbohydrate	667kcal/100g 14g protein /100g (15g sachet: 100kcal, 2g protein)	Energy and protein powder to add to food and drinks; unflavoured
MCTprocal® (Vitaflo)	480g (30 x 16g sachet)	Protein, MCT, carbohydrate	700kcal/100g 12g protein/100g 60g MCT (16g sachet: 112kcal, 2g protein, 10g MCT)	Energy, protein and MCT powder to add to food and drinks; unflavoured
Pro-Cal Shot® (Vitaflo)	120mL (30mL shot)	Protein, fat, carbohydrate	334kcal/100mL 7g protein/100mL	Fat, protein and carbohydrate emulsion; banana, strawberry, unflavoured
Pro-Cal® Shot (Vitaflo)	720mL (6 x 120mL) (30mL shot)	Protein, fat, carbohydrate	333kcal/100mL 7g protein/100mL (30mL shot: 100kcal, 2g protein)	Fat, protein and carbohydrate emulsion; strawberry, unflavoured

MCT = medium-chain triglyceride, LCT = long-chain triglyceride

a. use with dietetic supervision

b. listed according to type.

Table 13 Thickened drinks and thickeners[a,b]

Product	*Unit size*	*Energy content*	*Comments*
Thickened drinks			
Fresubin® Thickened (Fresenius)	200mL bottle	150kcal/100mL 10g protein/100mL	Texture-modified supplement drink of stage 1 and stage 2 consistency; strawberry, vanilla
Resource® Thickened Drinks (Nestle Health Science)	114mL cup	89kcal/100mL 0.1–0.4g protein	Ready to use, available in syrup (stage 1) and custard (stage 2) consistencies; apple, orange
Nutilis Complete Drink Level 2	125mL bottle	250kcal 12g protein	2kcal/mL; strawberry, vanilla
Nutilis Complete Drink Level 3	125mL bottle	306kcal 12g protein	2.45kcal/mL; chocolate, lemon tea, mango and passion fruit, strawberry, vanilla
Nutilis Complete Crème Level 3	125g pot	306kcal 12g protein	2.45kcal/mL; chocolate, strawberry, vanilla
Nutilis Fruit Level 4	150g pot	206kcal 11g protein	1.37kcal/g; apple, strawberry
Thickeners			
Multi-thick® (Abbott)	250g can	366kcal/100g	Modified maize starch. Can be used to thicken fluids and food
Nutilis® Clear (Nutricia)	175g can (1.25g sachets/ scoop)	290kcal/100g	Maltodextrin, xanthan gum and guar gum. Can be used to thicken foods and fluids. Fluids remain clear
Nutilis® Powder (Nutricia)	300g can 12g sachet	363kcal/100g	Modified maize starch. Can be used to thicken fluids and food
Resource® Thicken Up® (Nestle Health Science)	4.5g sachet 227g can	365kcal/100g	Modified maize starch. Can be used to thicken fluids and food
Resource® Thicken Up Clear™ (Nestle Health Science)	1.2g sachet 125g can	306kcal/100g	Maltodextrin, xanthan gum and potassium chloride. Can be used to thicken fluids and food. Fluids remain clear
Thick and Easy® Instant Food Thickener (Fresenius)	9g sachet 225g, 4.5kg tub	373kcal/100g	Modified maize starch. Can be used to thicken fluids and food

a. for patients with dysphagia. However, because product consistencies can vary (e.g. with storage, temperature), seek SALT team advice on the most appropriate to use

b. listed according to type.

Cautions

Patients with renal or hepatic failure, malabsorption, dysphagia, or at risk of refeeding syndrome (see below) should be referred to a dietitian.

The high sugar content and acidity of some nutritional supplement drinks can encourage dental caries, and patients should be advised on good oral hygiene. However, sipping the supplement over a prolonged period may be unavoidable in patients with early satiety.

Generally, patients with diabetes can use nutritional supplements without problem. However, monitoring of blood sugars may be required when using supplements with a high carbohydrate content, e.g. carbohydrate modular supplements. Rarely, and generally in patients already taking large doses of additional vitamins, nutritional supplements have contributed to ingestion of harmful amounts of vitamins, e.g. vitamin B6 leading to sensory neuropathy. Drug–nutrient interactions may occur with:

- vitamin K, present in significant quantities in the nutritional supplement drinks, and **warfarin** → reduced anticoagulation
- eicosapentaenoic acid, in Forticare®, Oral Impact®, Prosure® and Supportan®, and **warfarin** → enhanced anticoagulation.[16,17]

Also see drug interactions and complications with enteral feeding tubes (Chapter 28, p.853).

Refeeding syndrome

Refeeding syndrome is a potentially fatal condition caused by major shifts in fluids and electrolytes in malnourished patients who are started too rapidly on enteral or parenteral nutrition.[18,19] Biochemically, refeeding syndrome is characterized primarily by hypophosphataemia.

During a period of starvation, the body adapts in various ways to cope with the lack of readily available carbohydrate, and switches to using fat and protein as the main source of energy. If malnutrition is prolonged, there are further hormonal and metabolic changes aimed at preventing protein and muscle breakdown. Several intracellular minerals become severely depleted (although plasma concentrations may remain normal).

During refeeding, glycaemia leads to increased insulin secretion and a series of sequential effects, including decreases in the plasma concentrations of phosphate, potassium, magnesium and thiamine. If unrecognized and untreated, refeeding syndrome can result in life-threatening complications, including cardiac arrhythmia and multi-organ failure.[19] It is thus important that high-risk patients should be managed by appropriately trained health professionals.

Although a regimen of rapid refeeding is unlikely in patients with advanced cancer and chronic oligophagia and/or cachexia, palliative care clinicians should be aware of the syndrome and have a basic understanding of its management (Box D).

Box D Risk factors for and management of refeeding syndrome[20,21]

Patients who have had very little or no nutritional intake for >5 days are at risk of refeeding syndrome. It is associated with high morbidity and mortality and should be managed by appropriately trained health professionals.

High-risk patients

Those with one or more of the following:

- BMI <16kg/m^2
- unintentional weight loss of >15% in the last 3–6 months
- little or no nutritional intake for >10 days
- low plasma concentrations of PO_4^-, K^+, Mg^{2+} before restarting feeding.

Or two or more of the following:

- BMI <18.5kg/m^2
- unintentional weight loss >10% within the last 3–6 months
- little or no nutritional intake for >5 days
- a history of alcohol abuse
- use of insulin, chemotherapy, antacids or diuretics.

Management

If not high risk: For the first 2 days, patients who have had little or nothing to eat for ≥5 days should only be offered/given nutritional support estimated to meet ≤50% of their ideal requirements. After this, if biochemical parameters are satisfactory, it is safe to provide full nutrition.

continued

Box D Continued

If high risk:

- ensure adequate hydration
- before feeding and for the next 10 days, administer:
  - ▷ thiamine 200–300mg PO once daily
  - ▷ strong compound vitamin B 1–2 tablets t.d.s. (or IV vitamin B once daily)
  - ▷ multivitamin and mineral supplement PO once daily
- start nutritional support at ≤10kcal/kg/day
- increase intake progressively to achieve full nutritional requirements after 3–4 days
- if pre-feeding plasma concentrations are low, prescribe biochemical supplements:
  - ▷ magnesium (e.g. 0.2mmol/kg/day IV, 0.4mmol/kg/day PO)
  - ▷ phosphate (e.g. 0.3–0.6mmol/kg/day)
  - ▷ potassium (e.g. 2–4mmol/kg/day).

Monitoring

Daily until stable, and then 2–3 times weekly: fluid balance, nutritional intake, biochemical parameters, and general physical and psychological condition.

1 Fearon K *et al.* (2011) Definition and classification of cancer cachexia: an international consensus. *Lancet Oncology*. **12**: 489–495.
2 Arends J *et al.* (2016) ESPEN guidelines on nutrition in cancer patients. *Clinical Nutrition*. **36**: 11–48.
3 National Collaborating Centre for Acute Care (2006) Nutrition support in adults: oral nutrition support, enteral tube feeding and parenteral nutrition. Clinical guidelines. London: National Institute for Clinical Excellence.
4 Malnutrition Advisory Group (2003) The Malnutrition Universal Screening Tool (MUST). BAPEN, UK. www.bapen.org.uk
5 Kyle UG *et al.* (2006) Comparison of tools for nutritional assessment and screening at hospital admission: a population study. *Clinical Nutrition*. **25**: 409–417.
6 Davies M (2005) Nutritional screening and assessment in cancer-associated malnutrition. *European Journal of Oncology Nursing*. **9 (Suppl 2)**: S64–73.
7 Ottery FD (1996) Definition of standardized nutritional assessment and interventional pathways in oncology. *Nutrition*. **12**: S15–19.
8 Bauer J *et al.* (2002) Use of the scored Patient-Generated Subjective Global Assessment (PG-SGA) as a nutrition assessment tool in patients with cancer. *European Journal of Clinical Nutrition*. **56**: 779–785.
9 Chauhan A *et al.* (2007) NICE guidance for screening for malnutrition: implications for lung cancer services. *Thorax*. **62**: 835.
10 Halliday V *et al.* (2010) Screening for malnutrition: implications for upper gastrointestinal cancer services. *Journal of Surgical Oncology*. **102**: 543–544.
11 Thoresen L and de Soysa AK (2006) The nutritional aspects of palliative care. *European Journal of Palliative Care*. **13**: 194–197.
12 McCann RM *et al.* (1994) A comfort care for terminally ill patients: the appropriate use of nutrition and hydration. *Journal of the American Medical Association*. **272**: 179–181.
13 Sarhill N *et al.* (2003) Evaluation of nutritional status in advanced metastatic cancer. *Supportive Care in Cancer*. **11**: 652–659.
14 Antoun S *et al.* (2006) Artificial nutrition at the end of life: is it justified? *European Journal of Palliative Care*. **13**: 194–197.
15 Baldwin C and Weekes C (2008) Dietary advice for illness-related malnutrition in adults. *Cochrane Database of Systematic Reviews*. **1**: CD002008. www.thecochranelibrary.com
16 Baxter K and Preston CL *Stockley's Drug Interactions*. London: Pharmaceutical Press. www.medicinescomplete.com (accessed December 2017).
17 Holbrook AM *et al.* (2005) Systematic overview of warfarin and its drug and food interactions. *Archives of Internal Medicine*. **165**: 1095–1106.
18 Mehanna HM *et al.* (2008) Refeeding syndrome: what it is, and how to prevent and treat it. *British Medical Journal*. **336**: 1495–1498.
19 Boateng AA *et al.* (2010) Refeeding syndrome: treatment considerations based on collective analysis of literature case reports. *Nutrition*. **26**: 156–167.
20 NICE (2006) Nutrition support in adults. Clinical guidelines CG32. www.nice.org.uk
21 Todorovic VE and Mafrici B (2018) *A Pocket Guide to Clinical Nutrition*, 5th edn. Parenteral and Enteral Nutrition Specialist Group, British Dietetic Association. www.peng.org.uk

Updated December 2019

28: DRUG ADMINISTRATION TO PATIENTS WITH SWALLOWING DIFFICULTIES OR ENTERAL FEEDING TUBES

GENERAL PRINCIPLES

Where possible, PO is the preferred method of drug administration. For patients who have swallowing difficulties, an important first step is to reduce the number of drugs and frequency of administration. For the essential drugs remaining, alternative formulations and routes of administration can then be considered (Figure 1).

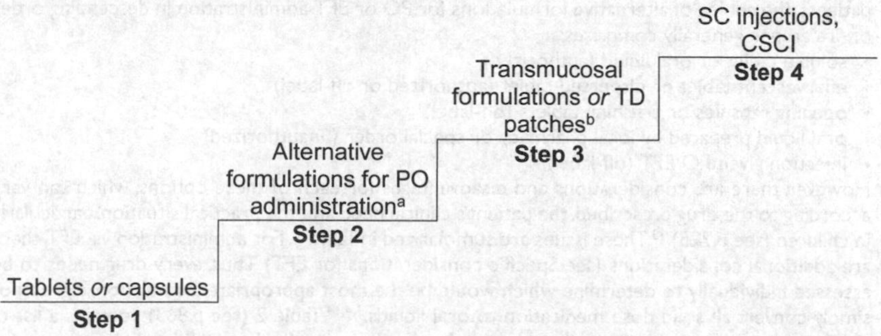

Figure 1 Common alternative formulations used in palliative care.

a. options include soluble, effervescent, dispersible or orodispersible tablets, oral solutions, suspensions or syrups, and modifying tablets/capsules; some may be suitable for administration via an existing EFT (see Choosing a suitable formulation)

b. transmucosal includes buccal, SL, nasal and rectal formulations; generally, Step 3 products are used less when SC injections/CSCI are readily available.

Generally, authorized approaches are preferred. Thus, for essential drugs, first consider:

- an alternative authorized PO formulation of the drug(s), e.g. using a soluble tablet or an oral liquid instead of a capsule
- swapping to an alternative drug with a more suitable PO formulation.

For some patients, swapping to an authorized non-oral route of administration, e.g. TD patches, may be preferable.[1]

Modifying or administering a product in a way not specified in the manufacturer's SPC results in either off-label use (e.g. emptying out the contents of a capsule, giving a drug by EFT) or an unauthorized product (e.g. mixing drugs in a syringe driver). Ultimately, practice is influenced by availability, experience and patient choice.

Drug therapy, the formulations used, and swallowing ability should be kept under review, particularly before inpatient discharge. Training and detailed written instructions regarding the supply, preparation and administration of each drug should be given to the patient and/or carer and primary care team.[2–5]

Wrong-route errors occurring with drugs intended for PO or other enteral routes are considered by NHS England as 'never events'.[6] Guidance on minimizing wrong-route errors has been published by the UK National Patient Safety Agency (NPSA).[7] Only enteral syringes should be used to draw up and administer oral liquids. Many local guidelines stipulate once-only use. The NPSA has also produced guidance on testing the position of NG tubes and highlighted the risks of their misplacement (also a 'never event').[6,8,9]

The administration of drugs by EFT is considered a level 3 skill for care workers in care homes. Staff must be adequately trained.[5,9,10] General guidance for the administration of drugs by EFT is given in QCG: Administration of drugs by enteral feeding tube (see p.861). Also see Specific considerations for EFT below.

CHOOSING A SUITABLE FORMULATION FOR PO OR EFT ADMINISTRATION

When planning to change to an alternative formulation or administer a drug by EFT, guidance should be obtained from a pharmacist. For those with impaired swallowing, a speech and language therapist (SALT) should also be consulted, in order to understand the degree of swallowing impairment and perform a risk assessment.[11,12]

The use of a drug off-label has implications for the prescriber and those administering it (see p.xix). Written instructions on the correct administration should be provided.

Taking into account the balance of risks and uncertainties for drug administration to these patients, the choice of alternative formulations for PO or EFT administration in descending order of preference generally comprises:

- soluble tablet or oral liquid (authorized)
- effervescent tablet or dispersed tablet (authorized or off-label)
- opening capsules or crushing tablets (off-label)
- oral liquid prepared by local pharmacy or special order (unauthorized)
- injection given PO/EFT (off-label).

However, there are considerations and disadvantages for each of these options, which can vary according to the drug prescribed, the patient's clinical need and the practical situation, particularly in children (see p.725).[13] These issues are summarized in Table 1. For administration via EFT, there are additional considerations (see Specific considerations for EFT). Thus, every drug needs to be assessed individually to determine which would be the most appropriate formulation, e.g. do not simply convert all solid dose medication to oral liquids.[1,4,14] Table 2 (see p.863) contains a list of the formulations available for palliative care drugs with authorized and off-label alternatives for patients with swallowing difficulties and EFT.

Option 1: Authorized soluble tablet or oral liquid

If available, soluble tablets are generally the preferred option. Soluble tablets dissolve *completely* when placed in 10mL water, to give a solution of the drug, in contrast to effervescent, dispersible or orodispersible tablets, which disperse in water or in the mouth to give particles (see Option 2 below).

Liquid formulations may be available as solutions, suspensions or syrups and are not always suitable as direct substitutes for solid dosage forms for several reasons:

- *excipients, e.g. sorbitol, ethanol, glycerol, propylene glycol, causing undesirable effects:* many oral liquid formulations contain excipients, which, in large volumes, can cause osmotic diarrhoea, particularly with jejunal administration, e.g. sorbitol ≥15g/24h. The normal osmolality of GI secretions is 100–400mosm/kg, but many liquid formulations are >1,000mosm/kg.[15,16] Reduce osmolality by diluting with as much water as is practical. Some liquid formulations contain alcohol, e.g. Oramorph®, **loperamide, phenobarbital, ranitidine**. The quantities and types of excipients are particularly important to consider for children[13]

Table 1 Summary of the issues to consider when choosing a suitable formulation[a]

Formulation	*Considerations / disadvantages*
Soluble tablet (authorized)	Availability Sodium content, may be high Cost
Oral liquid (authorized)	Excipients causing undesirable effects Bio-availability and dosing frequency Viscosity and particle size Volume and palatability Storage Cost
Effervescent tablet, dispersible tablet (authorized) *or* Dispersed tablet (off-label)	Sodium content, may be high Particle size Practicality Cost of authorized formulations
Opening capsules (off-label)[b] *or* Crushing tablets (off-label)[b]	Occupational exposure Particle size Practicality, e.g. manual dexterity Reduced dose (≤20% lost with crushing) Risk of using an inappropriate formulation, e.g. m/r (see text)
Locally prepared or special order oral liquid (unauthorized)	As for authorized oral liquid *plus*: shelf-life/expiry storage conditions continuity of supply reduced quality assurance variable formulations between special order manufacturers higher cost than authorized oral liquid
Injection given PO or by EFT (off-label)	Osmolality/hypertonicity/unsuitable pH Excipients unsuitable for PO administration Risk of wrong-route error Continuity of supply in the community Cost

a. see text for full details, and also see Specific considerations for EFT

b. generally off-label; some specific products may be authorized, see individual SPCs.

- *altered bio-availability and/or dosing frequency:* an oral liquid formulation may have a different bio-availability from the corresponding solid formulation, e.g. **citalopram**, **fusidic acid**, **itraconazole**, **phenytoin**, necessitating a different dose. When converting from an m/r formulation to an immediate-release oral liquid, the dose and/or frequency may need to be changed
- *viscosity and particle size of suspensions:* patients may be unable to swallow a highly viscous formulation or particulate suspension. EFTs are easily blocked by a highly viscous formulation, e.g. **amoxicillin–clavulanate**, liquid paraffin, syrups or by particles from a suspension, e.g. **ciprofloxacin**, **clarithromycin**. Viscosity may be reduced by diluting with 30–50mL water if practical.[16] Conversely, some patients cannot swallow thin liquids; commercially available thickeners are not compatible with all liquid medicines, and thickening liquid medicines is discouraged[17–19]
- *large volumes:* caused by, e.g. high doses, multiple drugs, may be impractical, unpalatable and costly.

Option 2: Effervescent tablet or dispersed tablet (authorized or off-label)

Do not administer a formulation by EFT if it has failed to disperse into small, barely visible particles or has an oily residue. Sediment and oily films increase the risk of blocking EFTs.[16,20]

Do not confuse *orodispersible* formulations with *oromucosal* buccal/SL formulations. The latter are designed to be absorbed by the oral mucosa and not the GI tract. This also makes them unsuitable for EFT administration.

Effervescent tablets and authorized dispersible tablets disintegrate in water to particle/granule form. Many standard tablets will also disperse or dissolve within 5min when mixed with 10mL water, even if not marketed as dispersible/soluble (see Table 2 for those commonly used in palliative care). Although off-label, this is often the most practical option both for patients with swallowing difficulties and those with an EFT (see QCG: Administration of drugs by enteral feeding tube, p.861). However, for any tablets dispersed in water, the following should be noted:

- the resulting particles/granules may be too large for administration by fine-bore EFT
- fractional dosing from effervescent or dispersed tablets is not recommended, due to inaccuracy
- ensure the whole dose is taken by administering rinsings from the container
- this option is *not* suitable for:
  - ▷ patients unable to swallow biphasic preparations, i.e. solids and liquids together
  - ▷ modified-release, e/c or film-coated tablets
  - ▷ antibacterials, cytotoxics, prostaglandin analogues or hormone antagonists, unless a specific closed-system procedure is used to prevent topical or inhaled exposure (seek advice from a pharmacist).

Orodispersible tablets are designed to disperse on the tongue and are generally swallowed with the saliva without water. Some orodispersible formulations may be more suitable than others for patients with swallowing difficulties and suitability may depend on the extent of dysphagia. The formulations, dose equivalences and administration of orodispersible tablets vary depending on the drug concerned. Individual product details should be consulted before using by EFT.

Option 3: Opening capsules or crushing tablets

It is sometimes feasible to open capsules and add the contents to soft food, fruit juice or other liquids to aid those with swallowing difficulties or to disperse the contents in water for administration by EFT. Small quantities of soft food or liquids, e.g. a tablespoon (15mL), should be used to ensure that the entire dose is administered.

Opening capsules is authorized for some products, e.g. Losec® capsules, Zomorph® capsules, (see SPCs for specific details). However, this is generally off-label and advice should be obtained from a pharmacist to ensure that this will not cause undesirable effects or problems with absorption, e.g. interference with the delivery mechanism (e.g. for **dabigatran**, opening increases bio-availability) or interaction with milk in yoghurt/custard (reduces bio-availability).

Opening capsules is *not* recommended for certain drugs, e.g. antibacterials, cytotoxics, prostaglandin analogues or hormone antagonists, because it puts the administrator at risk of topical and inhaled exposure to the contents. There are also risks to the patient if unsuitable formulations are used, e.g. m/r formulations may be harmful if accidentally chewed or crushed, or if the contents are irritant, e.g. **demeclocycline**.[21]

A few capsules contain liquid contents, e.g. **nifedipine**. Because of the small volume of the contents (which varies between brands), it is *not* recommended that these are used as a source of a drug for patients with swallowing difficulties or for EFT administration.

Crushing tablet/capsule contents to facilitate dispersion is *not* generally necessary, as many tablets and capsule contents will disperse sufficiently in water without crushing (see Option 2). Only a few tablets are authorized to be crushed. Care must be taken to ensure that crushing is undertaken correctly (Box A), because:[21,22]

- incorrect crushing is a common source of medication error
- crushing certain formulations is dangerous
- there is a risk of loss of dose or subsequent cross-contamination.

Thus, crushing should generally be considered a last resort and avoided unless specifically recommended by a pharmacist.[1,5]

Box A Crushing oral tablets[10,16,20,23–26]

General principles for crushing

Crushing should be considered a last resort and avoided unless specifically recommended by a pharmacist. For products *unsuitable* for crushing, see below.

For medicines that are suitable for crushing, use a tablet crusher, a closed-system crushing syringe, or pestle and mortar.

Crush each drug separately to an even, fine powder and administer immediately, e.g. by mixing with 10mL water and drawing into an enteral syringe, or with a spoon of soft food (see text).

Ensure the whole dose is administered, including rinsings.

Do not crush

M/r formulations (including m/r capsule contents), because this will destroy the m/r mechanism and result in dangerous dose peaks and troughs.

E/c (gastro-resistant) formulations (including e/c capsule contents), because this will destroy the e/c properties of the formulation, may alter bio-availability, and may block an EFT.

Film-coated formulations, because they can be difficult to effectively crush and/or may have an unpleasant taste or anaesthetic effect on the tongue.

Antibacterials, cytotoxics, prostaglandin analogues or hormone antagonists, because there are risks to the administrator through inhalation and/or topical absorption. However, closed-system crushing syringes may be an option in certain situations; seek advice from a pharmacist.

Buccal or sublingual formulations, because their bio-availability may be dramatically reduced if swallowed and absorbed by the GI tract rather than by the oral mucosa.

Option 4: Locally prepared or special order oral liquid

An oral liquid formulation prepared locally or by special order (see Chapter 24, p.817) may be an alternative if an authorized product is not available or not suitable.[27] The same issues as for authorized oral liquids need to be considered (Table 1). However, it may be possible for an experienced pharmacist to alter a formulation with careful consideration of quality, storage and shelf-life, and thus make it more suitable.[27] In addition, continuity of supply after a patient has returned home, short shelf-life, storage conditions (e.g. refrigeration), differences in formulation between manufacturers, and higher cost need to be considered;[4] these may make this option impractical.

Option 5: Injection (given PO or by EFT)

Formulations for injection are often unsuitable for enteral administration. This may be for one or more reasons:

- high osmolality or hypertonicity; the high solute concentration can cause osmotic diarrhoea
- unsuitable pH of the formulation or acidic conditions of the stomach chemically degrading the drug, e.g. **omeprazole**
- formulation with a different salt of unknown bio-availability
- an additive which is irritant to the GI tract, e.g. polysorbate 80 (Tween® 80) in **amiodarone**[1]
- risk of wrong-route administration, e.g. IV administration by mistake[6,7]
- cost.

Nonetheless, when possible, this off-label use of an injectable drug may occasionally be useful; however, because of the risks, it should only be used if specifically recommended by a pharmacist.

Generally, all injections suitable for enteral administration should be diluted before administration, e.g. with 30–50mL water by EFT. Bio-availability between the solid dose form and the injection solution may be different and alter clinical response, e.g. more rapid absorption and higher peak levels may occur.

SPECIFIC CONSIDERATIONS FOR EFT

There is a high risk of medication errors associated with administering drugs by EFT.[28] Specific additional considerations are needed before considering this route, along with those highlighted above for choosing a suitable formulation. In palliative care, this route of administration is generally only used for patients with an existing EFT. However, some patients who have an EFT may still be able to take certain medicines/formulations PO. Thus it is important to be aware of the type and function of the EFT and discuss medicines administration with the multi-disciplinary team.[5]

Testing of tube position before drug administration

Fatalities from aspiration have occurred as a result of incorrect placement of NG tubes.[9,29] Thus, even when placement devices are used, it is essential that correct NG tube position is confirmed *before anything is administered via the tube*. This includes water for activating lubricant to facilitate removal of the placement device.

Staff must be trained and competent in confirming NG tube placement.[30] Specific CE marked pH paper for testing gastric contents must be used to confirm pH is within the 'safe' range of 1–5.5.[8] Radiographic confirmation in accordance with specific NPSA guidance is necessary only when there is doubt.[31]

Correct NG tube position should be confirmed before each feed, before each drug administration and at least once daily. A break in feeding of 1h is required before testing. However, for patients on continuous feeding, multiple drug administration times, or acid-suppressing drugs (e.g. antacids, H_2 antagonists and PPIs), this is impractical. Providing initial tube placement has been correctly confirmed and there is no reason to suspect displacement, tube position should be confirmed by observation of the external tube length and positioning in accordance with NPSA guidelines.[8]

Nasoduodenal and nasojejunal tubes are usually inserted under some form of guidance (e.g. endoscopic, radiological) to ensure correct tube placement. Initial confirmation of position should be undertaken as per local guidelines. Subsequent confirmation of tube position should be undertaken by observation of the external tube length (see above); testing with pH paper is not appropriate.

Note. Semi-permanent and permanent devices, e.g. gastrostomy tubes, do not require repeated confirmation of position.

Site of drug delivery

The position of the tube may alter the bio-availability of a drug, e.g. with jejunal tubes, absorption may be unpredictable because of the effects of pH or because the tube may extend beyond the main site of absorption of the drug, e.g. **cephalexin, metronidazole benzoate**.[1,15] Care should also be taken with drugs that have a narrow therapeutic range, e.g. **digoxin, warfarin, phenytoin** and other anti-epileptics.[15] Drugs which undergo extensive first-pass hepatic metabolism may have greater systemic effects because of increased absorption from direct delivery to the jejunum, e.g. opioids, TCAs.[32] Undesirable effects may also be increased, because of rapid delivery into the jejunum. The acid barrier of the stomach is bypassed with jejunal tubes; some centres use aseptic technique for drug administration, to reduce the risk of infective diarrhoea.

Function of the tube

Drugs should not be administered if the tube is on free drainage or suction.[16]

Number of lumens

Ensure the correct lumen is used with multi-lumen tubes; some tubes have one lumen terminating in the stomach and another in the jejunum. *Do not use an aspiration gastric decompression port for drug administration.*

Lumen size

The outer diameter of an EFT is measured by the French gauge (1 French unit = 0.33mm).[32] However, the internal diameter of equivalent French gauge tubes varies between manufacturers.

The tube material also affects the internal lumen size, e.g. silicone and latex tubes have thicker walls and therefore narrower internal lumens. Narrow lumen, e.g. 5–12 French, or long tubes, e.g. NJ, are more likely to block, particularly with thick oral syrups and suspensions with large particles. Wide bore tubes require larger flush volumes.

Flushing the tube

This is essential to minimize drug interactions with the feeds. Water is the standard flush; use sterile water for jejunal tubes or immunocompromised patients, because the acid barrier in the stomach is bypassed.[1] Tubes should be flushed before drug administration, in between drugs, and after drug administration, ideally with 30mL water.[1,33] Use a 50mL enteral syringe to reduce the risk of tube rupture, which can be caused by smaller syringes. Flush slowly with a push-pause technique to prevent leaving a coating of feed on the internal tube surface. Record the total flush and drug volume administered when fluid balance is being monitored.

Feeding regimen

With continuous feeding and multiple drug administration periods, it may be necessary to adjust the feeding rate to compensate for the breaks in feed administration. If possible, the drug schedule should be rationalized, aiming for once daily drug administration to allow time for adequate nutrition.[32] Liaison between dietician and pharmacist will help to produce an optimal schedule.

Drug interactions and complications with EFT drug administration

Drugs should *never* be added to enteral feeds, because this increases the risk of incompatibility, microbial contamination, tube blockage and underdosing or overdosing if the feed rate is altered.[34]

Drugs can interact with food in many ways.[35,36] Because enteral feeds are in liquid form, the content, consistency and pH are different to those of a normal diet and are variable between brands. Thus, enteral feeds can cause different problems, associated with bio-availability, physical compatibility and chemical interactions. In addition, complications can also arise from:

- *binding of drugs to the internal surface of the tube, reducing absorption*, e.g. **carbamazepine**,[37] **clonazepam**, **diazepam**, **phenytoin**
- *physical interaction with the feed, causing coagulation*, particularly if the drug formulation is acidic, i.e. pH<4.[16] This applies to many syrups,[32] and risks tube blockage and reduced drug absorption. Abdominal distension caused by excessive gas production from effervescence has been reported when sodium bicarbonate solutions, used to deliver PPI formulations, have come into contact with the feed[38]
- *chemical interaction between the drug and the feed, resulting in reduced drug available for absorption*, e.g. **carbamazepine**, **ciprofloxacin**, **digoxin**, **penicillins**, **phenytoin**, **theophylline**, **warfarin**[39]
- *chemical interaction between the drug and feed, causing a non-absorbable drug–feed complex*, e.g. bezoar (insoluble concretion) formation with **sucralfate**, in the tube or in the stomach[35,40]
- *indirect drug or nutrient interactions*, e.g. the **vitamin K** or **eicosapentaenoic acid** content of a feed affecting the action of **warfarin**[35] (also see p.849)
- *the effects of malnutrition on drug pharmacokinetics*
- *properties of certain drugs*, e.g. bulk-forming laxatives may block the tube; use an enteral feed with a high fibre content instead.[16]

Usual considerations for physical and chemical drug–drug interactions must also be taken into consideration, particularly if rationalizing drug administration to once or twice a day.

Flushing the tube effectively, diluting potentially problematic formulations, inserting a feed break as outlined in the QCG: Administration of drugs by enteral feeding tube (p.861) and choosing an appropriate formulation will reduce the risk of dangerous interactions. Clinically, the most important interactions are those drugs with a narrow therapeutic range, e.g. **digoxin**, **theophylline**, **warfarin**, **phenytoin** and other anti-epileptics; these may warrant monitoring plasma concentrations. Clinical response should also be monitored closely. Appropriate precautionary measures may need to be taken if the feed is discontinued, particularly if dose adjustments were made because of an interaction.

Administration of e/c (gastro-resistant) and m/r formulations by EFT

Generally, these products should *not* be administered by EFT, because of the risk of blocking the tube. However, some capsules/granules/compressed tablets contain e/c or m/r granules for which specific procedures have been developed to allow administration of the coated granules by EFT, e.g. **esomeprazole** gastro-resistant tablets and gastro-resistant granules for oral suspension (Nexium®), **lansoprazole** orodispersible tablets (Zoton FasTab®), certain m/r **morphine** formulations (Zomorph® capsules) and **omeprazole** capsules (Losec®). See the manufacturer's SPC and/or specialist information for details (Table 2).[1] In order to avoid dangerous dose peaks and troughs or tube blockage, it is essential that:

- the recommended procedure is strictly adhered to and is used only for that *specific* formulation and brand
- the correct tube size and type are used
- extreme care is taken to avoid crushing the coated granules, thereby destroying the coating
- clinical response is monitored closely.

Unblocking EFTs

Care is required when unblocking an EFT, as this may result in bolus drug administration from residual drug in the tube. The tube may also become dislodged, and confirmation of correct positioning is recommended (see Testing of tube position).

Tube blockage may be caused by the feed, e.g. stagnant or contaminated feed, incorrect drug administration, e.g. particle blockage, inadequate flushing regimens or interaction between the feed and drug. It can be minimized by effective flushing and choosing an appropriate formulation. It is more likely with narrow lumens (35% of 8Fr tubes vs. 20% of PEG tubes).[41,42] Many tubes can be unblocked using 15–30mL water in a 50mL enteral syringe and a push-pull action, although this may take 20–30min. Excessive force must not be used to unblock a tube, because of the danger of perforation.

Various other agents have anecdotally been used to unblock tubes, e.g. carbonated drinks or cranberry juice. However, these are acidic solutions and can make the situation worse by causing feed coagulation,[16] and are no longer recommended.[1] Pancreatic enzymes, e.g. **pancreatin** (p.63), help only if the blockage is caused by the feed. Sodium bicarbonate needs to be added to activate the enzymes, which may not be practical. Re-insertion of guide wires is not advisable unless under specialist supervision.[1]

For blockages which do not resolve with water, consult a specialist nutrition nurse if available.

ALTERNATIVE ENTERAL FORMULATIONS IN PALLIATIVE CARE

Table 2 (see p.863) contains collated information on alternative formulations that can be considered for patients with swallowing difficulties or for EFT administration for drugs featured in *PCF* and selected commonly used drugs.

Quick Clinical Guide: Administration of drugs by enteral feeding tube

Do not add drugs to enteral feeds, because this increases the risk of incompatibility, microbial contamination, tube blockage and underdosing or overdosing if the feed rate is altered.

Before drug administration

1 The administration of drugs by an enteral feeding tube (EFT) is considered a level 3 skill for care workers in care homes. Staff must be adequately trained.

2 Drug charts should state the specific route of administration, e.g. nasogastric (NG), nasojejunal (NJ), and specify the lumen to be used to prevent wrong-route errors.

3 Check that there is documented confirmation that the EFT was correctly positioned following insertion. For NG tubes, use CE marked pH paper intended for testing human gastric contents (safe range pH1–5.5 after a 1h break in feeding) or, when there is doubt, by approved radiographic confirmation in accordance with NPSA guidelines.

4 If practical, reconfirm correct NG tube position before each drug administration. For patients on continuous feeding, multiple drug administration times or on acid-suppressants (antacids, H_2 antagonists, PPIs), if correct tube placement confirmed initially and there is no reason to suspect displacement, confirm tube position by observation of the external tube length (in accordance with NPSA guidelines); likewise for NJ tubes.

5 The patient should be in a sitting position to prevent regurgitation and pulmonary aspiration.

6 All EFT lumens should be clearly labelled.

7 To prevent accidental parenteral administration, only use dedicated enteral syringes and connectors.

Drug administration

8 Stop the feed and ensure any other ports are closed and airtight.

9 Flush the EFT using a **push-pause** action with 15–30mL of water (*use sterile water throughout if jejunal tube or immunocompromised patient*). This helps to clear the tube and prevent physical interactions with the feed, which could result in coagulation and blockage of the tube.

10 Check if time off the feed is necessary before and/or after drug administration to optimize drug absorption and/or reduce the risk of chemical interactions.

11 Choose the most suitable formulation of each drug (see Choosing a suitable formulation, p.854, and Table 2, p.863); see Box A (p.862) for guidelines on how to prepare dispersed formulations, if needed.

12 Administer each drug separately:

- a 50mL enteral syringe reduces the risk of rupture of the EFT; a 2mL or smaller enteral syringe can be used for very small quantities to accurately measure the dose
- flush between each drug with 15–30mL of water using a **push-pause** action.

13 After drug administration, flush the EFT using a **push-pause** action with 15–30mL of water.

14 Resume feeding after any necessary feed break (see point 10).

continued

Box A Guidelines for preparation of dispersed formulations for EFT administration

Information about the preparation of each medication should be documented on the prescription and in the patient's notes.

Prepare each drug separately.

Place the tablet(s) or capsule contents into the barrel of a 50mL enteral syringe (do not crush); use a large container/drug pot for effervescent formulations.

Add 10mL cold tap water (50mL for effervescent formulations), allow to disperse, then mix well:

- *use sterile water for jejunal tubes or immunocompromised patients*
- if using a drug pot or other container, once dispersed, draw up the contents using a 50mL enteral syringe; this reduces the risk of rupture of the EFT.

Inspect the contents of the enteral syringe to ensure that there are no large particles that might block the EFT.

If using a drug pot or other container, rinse with water, draw up with the same enteral syringe, and administer the rinsings through the tube.

To ensure the patient receives the whole dose, use the same enteral syringe to draw up and administer the flush.

Thoroughly clean any equipment with hot soapy water according to local policy to avoid cross-contamination.

Important considerations

- generally, this approach is *not* suitable for modified-release, e/c or film-coated tablets; use an appropriate alternative product
- for antibacterials, cytotoxics, prostaglandin analogues and hormone antagonists, consult a pharmacist; a specific closed system procedure must be used to prevent topical or inhaled exposure.

After drug administration

15 Document the total volume of fluid given (including flushes) on a fluid balance chart.

16 Monitor the clinical response, particularly if:
- changing from m/r to immediate-release formulations
- the drug has a narrow therapeutic range
- the bio-availability of the drug differs between solid dose form and liquid.

Updated December 2021

Table 2 Information on alternative enteral formulations available for administering drugs to patients with swallowing difficulties or by EFT[1,10,43–45]

Drug	*Authorized soluble tablet or oral liquid available*	*Tablet/capsule contents may disperse sufficiently for 8Fr NG tube*[a,b]	*Oral liquid can be prepared by local pharmacy or special order*	*Injection available and can be diluted and administered PO or by EFT*	*Comments*
Acetylcysteine	Yes	Yes (effervescent)	Yes	Yes	Use effervescent tablets
Amiloride	Yes	No data	Yes	No	Sugar- and sorbitol-free oral solutions available
Aminophylline[a]	No	No	Yes	Yes	Consider discontinuing therapy due to dosing complexities Give aminophylline injection orally as a diluted oral solution;[1] take care converting from m/r to immediate-release or convert oral aminophylline total daily dose to oral *unauthorized* theophylline liquid (aminophylline 250mg PO = theophylline 200mg PO) and split into t.d.s. regimen (see theophylline below). Monitor blood levels
Amiodarone	No	No	Yes[c]	No	Unauthorized 50mg/5mL and 100mg/5mL oral suspension can be obtained via special order A 25mg/5mL suspension or 200mg/5mL suspension can be prepared.[44] Injection contains irritant Tween 80
Amitriptyline	Yes	No	Yes	No	Sugar- and sorbitol-free oral solutions available
Amlodipine	Yes	Yes	Yes[d]	No	The Rosemont oral solutions are authorized for EFT use. A 1mg/mL suspension can be prepared (90 day shelf-life)[d,1] or with 1% methylcellulose in syrup (56 day shelf-life).[1] Disperse tablet for intrajejunal administration
Amoxicillin	Yes	No data	No data	Yes	Dilute oral suspensions with an equal volume of water to reduce viscosity for EFT use; dispersible tablets and powder sachets available
Antacids	Yes	No data	Yes[c]	No	Not recommended by EFT, as can coagulate with feed; not needed with jejunal tube. Antacid with oxetacaine oral suspension is available[c]

continued

Table 2 Continued

Drug	*Authorized soluble tablet or oral liquid available*	*Tablet/capsule contents may disperse sufficiently for 8Fr NG tube*[a,b]	*Oral liquid can be prepared by local pharmacy or special order*	*Injection available and can be diluted and administered PO or by EFT*	*Comments*
Apixaban	No	See comments	Yes	No	Tablets may be crushed and mixed with 60mL water for EFT use; a 0.25mg/mL suspension (7 day shelf-life) can be prepared with Ora-Plus:water 50:50[46]
Ascorbic acid	No	Yes (effervescent)	Yes	No	Add effervescent tablets (only available OTC) to 50mL water
Aspirin	No	Yes (dispersible)	Yes	No	Use dispersible tablet
Atenolol	Yes	No data	Yes	No data	
Baclofen	Yes	Yes (Teva)	Yes	No data	Authorized oral liquids are viscous and contain sorbitol (2.75g/5mL Lioresal®); dilute with an equal volume of water for EFT use Dispersing tablets is preferable, particularly for intrajejunal administration
Bendroflumethiazide	No	No data	Yes[c]	No	Unauthorized 2.5mg/5mL oral suspension can be obtained via special order; viscous liquid; no information on suitability for EFT
Bethanechol	No	No data	Yes[d]	No	A 5mg/mL suspension with cherry syrup can be prepared (60 day shelf-life)[1]
Bisacodyl[a]	No	No	Yes[c]	No	Unauthorized 2.5mg/5mL oral suspension can be obtained via special order
Calcium & vitamin D	No	Yes (effervescent)	No data	No	Use effervescent granules or effervescent tablet and add to 50mL water. The solution can crystallize, and calcium can bind to phosphate in enteral feed. Flush EFT well to avoid
Carbamazepine[a]	Yes	No data	Yes	No	Oral liquid contains sorbitol (1.25g/5mL Tegretol®) Dilute with an equal volume of water to reduce adherence to EFT. Monitor for increased undesirable effects, particularly with intrajejunal administration

continued

Table 2 Continued

Drug	*Authorized soluble tablet or oral liquid available*	*Tablet/capsule contents may disperse sufficiently for 8Fr NG tube*[a,b]	*Oral liquid can be prepared by local pharmacy or special order*	*Injection available and can be diluted and administered PO or by EFT*	*Comments*
Carbocisteine	Yes	No data	No data	No	
Cefalexin	Yes	No data	No data	No	Dilute oral suspensions with equal volume of water to reduce viscosity for EFT use. May be reduced absorption with intrajejunal administration. Avoid opening capsules/crushing tablets due to risk of cephalosporin sensitization
Cefradine	No	No data	No data	No	Avoid opening capsules/crushing tablets due to risk of cephalosporin sensitization
Celecoxib	No	Yes	Yes	No	Capsule contents are authorized to be sprinkled onto apple sauce, yoghurt or mashed banana
Chlorphenamine	Yes	No data	Yes	Yes	Dilute oral syrups with equal volume of water to reduce viscosity for EFT use; may contain ethanol
Chlorpromazine	Yes	No	Yes	No data	Some oral liquids contain sorbitol Handle with care to avoid contact sensitization; do not crush tablets
Cimetidine	Yes	Yes (effervescent)	Yes	No	Some oral liquids contain sorbitol (Tagamet® negligible). Use effervescent tablet added to 30mL water, or diluted liquid for intrajejunal administration
Cinnarizine	No	Yes	Yes	No	
Ciprofloxacin	Yes	Yes (Ranbaxy, Generics)	Yes	No data	Authorized oral suspension not recommended for EFT, because too viscous and granular. Disperse tablet with 30–50mL sterile water, *not tap water* (to avoid ion chelation). Stop feed for 1h before and 1–2h after dose. Do not administer with iron or zinc. May be reduced absorption with intrajejunal administration

continued

Table 2 Continued

Drug	*Authorized soluble tablet or oral liquid available*	*Tablet/capsule contents may disperse sufficiently for 8Fr NG tube*[a,b]	*Oral liquid can be prepared by local pharmacy or special order*	*Injection available and can be diluted and administered PO or by EFT*	*Comments*
Citalopram	Yes	Yes (Generics)	Yes	No	10mg of tablet equivalent to 8mg of oral liquid (4 drops). Oral liquid should be mixed with water for EFT, or water/orange/apple juice for PO use; contains alcohol (0.01units/mL)
Clarithromycin[a]	Yes	No data	No data	No	Dilute oral liquid with an equal volume of water for EFT. Do not use EFT less than 9Fr gauge
Clindamycin	No	Yes (capsules); see comments	Yes[c]	No data	Unauthorized 75mg/5mL oral suspension can be obtained via special order Avoid inhalation of the capsule contents
Clomipramine[a]	No	Yes	Yes[c]	No	Unauthorized 50mg/5mL oral suspension can be obtained via special order
Clonazepam	Yes	No data	Yes[c,d]	Yes	Authorized oral solutions 500microgram/5mL and 2mg/5mL contain alcohol (0.01 units/5mL) and must *not* be diluted. No information on suitability via EFT Dilute all other formulations with 30–50mL water to reduce risk of binding to the tube. Disperse tablets for intrajejunal administration. Injection contains alcohol and other excipients Unauthorized 2.5mg/mL oral drops and 0.5mg orodispersible tablets can be imported
Clonidine	Yes	Yes (100microgram Catapres®)	Yes	Yes (Catapres®)	A 100microgram/mL formulation with simple syrup can be prepared (1 month shelf-life).[1] Injection only available via special order
Co-amoxiclav	Yes	No	No data	No data	Oral liquid not recommended for EFT, because too viscous
Co-beneldopa[a] (benserazide with levodopa)	No	Yes (dispersible)	Yes	No	Use dispersible tablets for EFT use

continued

Table 2 Continued

Drug	*Authorized soluble tablet or oral liquid available*	*Tablet/capsule contents may disperse sufficiently for 8Fr NG tube*[a,b]	*Oral liquid can be prepared by local pharmacy or special order*	*Injection available and can be diluted and administered PO or by EFT*	*Comments*
Co-careldopa[a] (carbidopa with levodopa)	No	Yes (Sinemet®)	Yes[c,d]	No	Unauthorized 12.5mg/50mg/5mL and 25mg/100mg/5mL oral suspensions available Disperse tablets for EFT use. An intestinal gel for EFT use is available (specialist use only)
Codeine phosphate	Yes	No data	Yes	No data	Dilute authorized oral liquid with an equal volume of water to reduce viscosity for EFT use. Tablets disperse, but no information on suitability by EFT Some dispersible or effervescent formulations contain 20mmol sodium per tablet
Codeine with aspirin (co-codaprin)	No	Yes (dispersible)	No data	No	Add dispersible tablet to 50mL water
Codeine with paracetamol (co-codamol)	No	Yes (effervescent or dispersible)	Yes	No	Add effervescent or dispersible tablet to 50mL water
Co-trimoxazole	Yes	No	No data	No	Oral liquid (Septrin®) contains sorbitol and needs diluting 3 times to reduce viscosity for EFT use
Cyclizine	No	No data	Yes[c]	Yes	Unauthorized 50mg/5mL oral solution and suspension can be obtained via special order
Cyproheptadine	No	Yes	Yes	No	
Cyproterone	No	Yes	Yes	No	Tablets disperse, but no information on suitability by EFT
Dabigatran etexilate	No	No	No	No	Do not open capsules, as this increases the bio-availability
Dantrolene	No	Yes	Yes[c]	No	Injection formulation may hydrolyse in the stomach Unauthorized 10mg/5mL, 25mg/5mL or 100mg/5mL oral suspension can be obtained via special order

continued

Table 2 Continued

Drug	*Authorized soluble tablet or oral liquid available*	*Tablet/capsule contents may disperse sufficiently for 8Fr NG tube*[a,b]	*Oral liquid can be prepared by local pharmacy or special order*	*Injection available and can be diluted and administered PO or by EFT*	*Comments*
Demeclocycline	No	No	Yes	No	Capsule contents are irritant and only sparingly soluble. Absorption is reduced by calcium
Desmopressin	Yes	Yes (Desmotabs, DDAVP®)	Yes	No data	DesmoMelt®, DDAVP Melt®, Noqdirna® and generic desmopressin oral lyophilisates are for SL use only, not for EFT administration
Dexamethasone	Yes	Yes (Aspen)	Yes	Yes	Authorized oral liquid contains sorbitol 500microgram/5mL
Dexamfetamine[a]	Yes	No data	Yes	No	
Diamorphine	No	No data	Yes	No data	
Diazepam	Yes	Yes (Teva)	Yes	Yes	Dilute authorized oral liquid with an equal volume of water to reduce viscosity and risk of binding to the EFT. Disperse tablets for intrajejunal administration. Anecdotal evidence of using injection enterally; drug loss may occur due to binding to tube
Diclofenac *sodium*[a]	No	Yes (dispersible)	Yes[c]	No	Use authorized dispersible tablet for EFT Unauthorized 50mg/5mL oral suspension can be obtained via special order
Dicycloverine	Yes	No data	No data	No	Dilute oral liquid with an equal volume of water for EFT use
Digoxin	Yes	No data	Yes	Yes	In theory, 50microgram Lanoxin® oral liquid = 62.5microgram tablet; however, in practice, unlikely to be clinically important; monitor plasma concentrations if changing formulation or using a high-fibre feed. Do not dilute the oral liquid. May cause diarrhoea Lanoxin® tablets disperse, but no information on suitability by EFT Bio-availability of the injection PO or EFT is unpredictable and not recommended

continued

Table 2 Continued

Drug	*Authorized soluble tablet or oral liquid available*	*Tablet/capsule contents may disperse sufficiently for 8Fr NG tube*[a,b]	*Oral liquid can be prepared by local pharmacy or special order*	*Injection available and can be diluted and administered PO or by EFT*	*Comments*
Dihydrocodeine[a]	No	No data	Yes	No	
Dihydrocodeine with paracetamol (co-dydramol)	No	No data	Yes[c]	No	Unauthorized 10mg/500mg/5mL oral suspension can be obtained via special order
Docusate sodium	Yes	No	No data	No	Dilute oral liquid with an equal volume of water for EFT use
Domperidone	Yes	No data	Yes	No	Dilute oral liquid with an equal volume of water for EFT use. Contains sorbitol 2.3g/5mL. Consider dispersing tablets for intrajejunal administration
Doxepin	No	Yes (Marlborough)	Yes	No	
Doxycycline	No	Yes (dispersible)	Yes	No data	Use dispersible tablets; do not open capsules, as contents are irritant
Edoxaban	No	See comments	No data	No	Tablets may be crushed and mixed with water (for EFT) or apple sauce
Erythromycin[a]	Yes	No	No data	No data	Dilute oral liquid with an equal volume of water for EFT use. Some brands contain sorbitol. Tablets and capsule contents are e/c, therefore not suitable for EFT
Eslicarbazepine acetate	Yes	No data	No data	No	
Esomeprazole	No	Yes (Nexium®)	Yes	No data	Nexium® tablets and granules for suspension are authorized for administration via a gastric tube. The tablet contains a compressed core of e/c microgranules which can be dispersed and flushed via an 8Fr gauge NG tube. Do not crush. Strictly follow the procedure in the SPC to prevent tube blockage

continued

Table 2 Continued

Drug	*Authorized soluble tablet or oral liquid available*	*Tablet/capsule contents may disperse sufficiently for 8Fr NG tube*[a,b]	*Oral liquid can be prepared by local pharmacy or special order*	*Injection available and can be diluted and administered PO or by EFT*	*Comments*
Famotidine	No	Yes	Yes[d]	No	A 40mg/5mL oral suspension can be prepared (1 month shelf-life)[d]
Ferrous sulfate	Yes	No	Yes[c]	No	Ironorm® 625mg/5mL oral drops available Unauthorized 60mg/5mL oral solution or suspension can be obtained via special order Convert to an alternative iron salt oral liquid preparation Ferrous sulfate 200mg = 7mL Galfer® *or* 12mL Sytron® (contains sorbitol 2g/5mL); dilute with an equal volume of water for EFT use
Flecainide	No	Yes (Generics)	Yes[c,d]	Yes	Use de-ionized/sterile water, *not tap water.* Note crushed tablets have a local anaesthetic effect. *Do not* dilute the injection or mix with alkaline solutions, e.g. chlorides, phosphates, sulfates Unauthorized 10mg/5mL oral suspension and 25mg/5mL oral solution and suspension can be obtained via special order
Flucloxacillin	Yes	No	No data	Yes	Dilute oral liquid with an equal volume of water for EFT use. Stop feed for 1h before and after dose. Avoid opening capsules, due to risk of sensitization
Fluconazole	Yes	Yes (50mg capsule)	No data	No	Do not use the 150mg capsule contents
Fludrocortisone	No	No data	Yes[c]	No	Unauthorized 50microgram/5mL and 100microgram/5mL oral suspension can be obtained via special order
Fluoxetine	Yes	No data	Yes	No	Capsule contents can be dispersed, and dispersible tablet available, but no information on suitability via EFT
Fosfomycin	Yes (granules)	Yes (granules)	No data	No data	Granules can be dispersed in 50mL water for EFT; stop feed for 2h before and 1h after each dose

continued

Table 2 Continued

Drug	*Authorized soluble tablet or oral liquid available*	*Tablet/capsule contents may disperse sufficiently for 8Fr NG tube*[a,b]	*Oral liquid can be prepared by local pharmacy or special order*	*Injection available and can be diluted and administered PO or by EFT*	*Comments*
Furosemide	Yes	No data	Yes	No data	Frusol® oral solutions are authorized for NG and PEG administration; see SPC for details Oral liquids may be alkaline and may coagulate with other acidic preparations. Flush EFT well to avoid
Gabapentin	Yes	Yes (Neurontin®)	Yes[c]	No	The authorized oral solution contains propylene glycol and other excipients which, in high doses, may exceed WHO daily intake limits Gabapentin Rosemont 50mg/mL oral solution is authorized for NG and PEG administration; see SPC for details
Gliclazide[a]	No	No data	Yes[c]	No	Unauthorized 40mg/5mL and 80mg/5mL oral suspension can be obtained via special order
Glycopyrronium	Yes	No	Yes[c]	Yes	Unauthorized tablets disperse coarsely and may leave sediment. Unauthorized oral formulations can be obtained via special order or can be made locally from glycopyrronium powder or injection (see p.12). Cost of bulk powder may be prohibitive
Granisetron	No	Yes (Kytril®)	Yes[d]	Yes	250microgram/5mL suspension can be prepared.[d] TD patch available
Haloperidol	Yes	No data	Yes	No data	
Hydrocortisone	Yes	Yes (MSD)	Yes[c]	Yes	Injection contains significant amounts of phosphate. Unauthorized 5mg/5mL or 10mg/5mL oral suspension can be obtained via special order
Hydromorphone[a]	No	No	Yes	No data	Do not administer contents of m/r capsules by EFT, due to high risk of blockage

continued

Table 2 Continued

Drug	*Authorized soluble tablet or oral liquid available*	*Tablet/capsule contents may disperse sufficiently for 8Fr NG tube*[a,b]	*Oral liquid can be prepared by local pharmacy or special order*	*Injection available and can be diluted and administered PO or by EFT*	*Comments*
Hyoscine *butylbromide*	No	No	Yes[c]	Yes	Injection may be stored for 24h in a refrigerator once opened. Unauthorized 10mg/5mL oral solution and suspension can be obtained via special order
Hyoscine *hydrobromide*	No	Yes	Yes[c]	Yes	Unauthorized 300microgram/5mL or 500microgram/5mL oral solution and suspension can be obtained via special order. TD patch available Tablets may be dispersed but absorption may be variable
Ibandronic acid	No	No	No data	No data	Consider alternative route of administration
Ibuprofen[a]	Yes	No	Yes	No	Oral liquid contains sorbitol 500microgram/5mL; dilute with an equal volume of water (more for intrajejunal administration) to reduce viscosity for EFT use
Imipramine	Yes	No	Yes	No	Dilute commercially available oral solution with an equal volume of water to reduce viscosity for EFT use
Ispaghula husk	No	No	No data	No	Do not administer via EFT due to high risk of blockage; consider using a high-fibre feed
Itraconazole	Yes	No	Yes	No data	Stop the feed for 2h before and after dose. Oral liquid contains sorbitol and is acidic. Flush EFT well to avoid coagulation. Absorption via jejunum may be reduced
Ketamine	No	No	Yes[c]	Yes	A 50mg/5mL oral solution using the injection formulation can be prepared by pharmacy; 7 day shelf-life (see p.691). Unauthorized 50mg/5mL oral solution and suspension can be obtained via special order
Lactulose	Yes	No	No data	No	Dilute oral liquid with 2–3 times volume of water for EFT use
Lamotrigine	No	Yes (dispersible)	Yes[c,d]	No	Use authorized dispersible tablet Unauthorized 50mg/5mL oral suspension can be obtained via special order. A 5mg/5mL suspension can be prepared[d]

continued

Table 2 Continued

Drug	*Authorized soluble tablet or oral liquid available*	*Tablet/capsule contents may disperse sufficiently for 8Fr NG tube*[a,b]	*Oral liquid can be prepared by local pharmacy or special order*	*Injection available and can be diluted and administered PO or by EFT*	*Comments*
Lansoprazole	No	Yes (FasTab®), and capsules	Yes[c]	No	Add orodispersible tablet (FasTab®) to 10mL of water and administer by EFT using a push-pull technique to keep the granules suspended. *Do not crush* For tubes smaller than 8Fr, open capsules and mix e/c granules with 10mL of 8.4% sodium bicarbonate (14 day shelf-life in a refrigerator if locally prepared by pharmacy)[1] Unauthorized 5mg/5mL, 15mg/5mL and 30mg/5mL oral suspension can be obtained via special order
Levetiracetam	Yes	Yes (500mg Keppra®)	Yes	No data	Use the oral liquid for EFT
Levomepromazine	No	Yes (Nozinan®)	Yes[c]	Yes	Tablet dispersion is coarse and may block tubes smaller than 8Fr Unauthorized 2.5mg/5mL and 6mg/5mL oral suspensions can be obtained via special order
Lofepramine	Yes	No	Yes	No	Oral liquid is viscous and contains sorbitol 1.4g/5mL, but diluting is not recommended; thus, not suitable for EFT. Bio-availability may be increased with intrajejunal administration
Loperamide	Yes	No	Yes[c]	No	Oral solution contains alcohol. Do not dilute Unauthorized 25mg/5mL oral solution and suspension (both alcohol free) can be obtained via special order
Loratadine	Yes	No data	No data	No	Dilute oral liquid with an equal volume of water for intrajejunal administration to reduce osmolarity
Lorazepam	Yes	No	Yes[c]	No data	Tablets do not disperse easily. Tablets (Genus brand) and injection can be used sublingually
Macrogols	Yes	See comments	No data	No	Generally, not suitable for EFT use due to the large volume required to dissolve the powder and potential for interaction with feeds; however, some anecdotal experience

continued

Table 2 Continued

Drug	*Authorized soluble tablet or oral liquid available*	*Tablet/capsule contents may disperse sufficiently for 8Fr NG tube*[a,b]	*Oral liquid can be prepared by local pharmacy or special order*	*Injection available and can be diluted and administered PO or by EFT*	*Comments*
Magnesium glycerophosphate	Yes	No data	Yes[c]	No	Unauthorized 4mmol/5mL oral solution and suspension can be obtained via special order[c] Various unauthorized tablets available; some will disperse, but no information on suitability by EFT
Mebeverine[a]	Yes	No data	Yes	No	135mg tablet = 15mL oral liquid 50mg/5mL. Most effective when given 20min before food
Medroxyprogesterone acetate	No	Yes (Provera® 5mg, 100mg)	Yes	Yes (Depo-Provera®)	
Megestrol acetate	No	Yes (Megace®)	Yes	No	Unauthorized 40mg/mL oral suspension can be imported
Melatonin[a]	Yes	No data	Yes[c]	No	
Menadiol sodium phosphate	No	No data	Yes[c]	No	Tablets disperse, but no information on suitability by EFT. Unauthorized 5mg/5mL oral suspension can be obtained via special order
Metformin[a]	Yes	Yes (powder for solution)	Yes	No	Sachets disperse fully in 20mL of water for EFT (manufacturer recommends 150mL for PO use)
Methadone	Yes	No data	Yes	No data	Methadone oral liquid has been used by EFT
Methenamine	No	No data	No data	No	Tablets are authorized to be crushed and mixed with milk or fruit juice for swallowing difficulties. No information on suitability by EFT
Methylphenidate[a]	No	No data	Yes[c]	No	Unauthorized 5mg/5mL oral suspension can be obtained via special order

continued

Table 2 Continued

Drug	*Authorized soluble tablet or oral liquid available*	*Tablet/capsule contents may disperse sufficiently for 8Fr NG tube*[a,b]	*Oral liquid can be prepared by local pharmacy or special order*	*Injection available and can be diluted and administered PO or by EFT*	*Comments*
Methylprednisolone	No	Yes (Medrone®)	Yes	Yes (Solu-Medrone®)	
Metoclopramide[a]	Yes	No data	Yes	Yes	Some liquids may contain sorbitol. Maxolon® tablets disperse, but no information on suitability by EFT
Metronidazole	Yes	No	Yes	No data	Dilute authorized oral liquid with an equal volume of water for NG use and stop feed for 1h before the dose to allow gastric pH to recover to metabolize the benzoate salt. The benzoate salt is metabolized in the stomach, therefore *not* suitable for intrajejunal administration. A 50mg/mL suspension with cherry syrup can be prepared (60 day shelf-life);[1] it does not require a break in feeding and is more suitable for intrajejunal administration
Midazolam	No	No	Yes	Yes	Authorized 5mg/mL and 10mg/mL oromucosal solution for *buccal* use available as unit-dose preparations Injection can be used via PO, buccal, intranasal and PR routes; injection can be diluted with apple/blackcurrant juice, chocolate sauce or cola for PO administration Unauthorized 2.5mg/mL oral liquid available via special order
Mirtazapine	Yes	Yes (orodispersible)	Yes	No	Use oral liquid or orodispersible tablets; intrajejunal administration not recommended due to reduced absorption
Moclobemide	No	No data	Yes	No	
Modafinil	No	No data	Yes	No	Unauthorized 100mg/5mL oral suspension available via special order

continued

Table 2 Continued

Drug	*Authorized soluble tablet or oral liquid available*	*Tablet/capsule contents may disperse sufficiently for 8Fr NG tube*[a,b]	*Oral liquid can be prepared by local pharmacy or special order*	*Injection available and can be diluted and administered PO or by EFT*	*Comments*
Morphine[a]	Yes	No data (immediate-release)	Yes	No data	Oral liquid can be used; 10mg/5mL contains alcohol (0.05 units/5mL). Dilute with an equal volume of water for intrajejunal administration, to reduce osmolarity Unauthorized 10mg/5mL oral solution (alcohol free) available via special order M/r granules in Zomorph® capsules are authorized for gastric administration via a 16Fr tube (internal diameter 2.5mm) with an open distal end or lateral pores (see SPC). Certain tubes cause problems[e]. The m/r granules should be mixed (*do not crush*) with 30mL water. Ensure the m/r granules are not crushed by the syringe plunger and that all are administered; add extra water if necessary. There is some anecdotal data on using 8Fr tubes[1] The m/r granules in MXL® capsules are *not* suitable for EFT administration Some feeds interact with morphine; a feed break of 2h before and 1h after each dose is recommended Intrajejunal use may *increase* absorption
Nabilone	No	Yes	No data	No	
Naltrexone	No	No data	Yes[c]	No	Unauthorized 5mg/5mL oral solution and suspension can be obtained via special order
Naproxen[a]	Yes	Yes	Yes[c]	No	
Nefopam	No	No	Yes	No	
Nifedipine[a]	No	See comments	Yes[c,d]	No	Consider an alternative product, e.g. amlodipine. Drawing up contents of liquid capsules *not* recommended; volumes vary between manufacturers, liquid is light sensitive, and risk of profound hypotension, particularly if converting from m/r preparation. Unauthorized 5mg/5mL and 10mg/5mL oral suspension or 20mg/mL oral drops can be obtained via special order A 20mg/5mL suspension can be prepared using capsule contents[d,44]

Table 2 Continued

Drug	*Authorized soluble tablet or oral liquid available*	*Tablet/capsule contents may disperse sufficiently for 8Fr NG tube*[a,b]	*Oral liquid can be prepared by local pharmacy or special order*	*Injection available and can be diluted and administered PO or by EFT*	*Comments*
Nitrazepam	Yes	No data	Yes[c]	No	Dilute authorized oral liquid to reduce osmolality for intrajejunal use Unauthorized 5mg/5mL oral suspension can be obtained via special order
Nitrofurantoin[a]	Yes	Yes	Yes	No	Dilute authorized oral liquid with an equal volume of water for EFT use
Olanzapine	No	Yes (Zyprexa Velotab®)	Yes[c]	No	Unauthorized 2.5mg/5mL oral suspension can be obtained via special order
Omeprazole	Yes	Yes (Dexcel); Losec MUPS®, Mezzopram dispersible	Yes[c]	Yes	Authorized 2mg/mL and 4mg/mL powder for oral suspension is available but expensive; for EFT a feed break of 30min before and after each dose is recommended A 2mg/mL formulation with 20mg capsule contents and 10mL sodium bicarbonate 8.4% can be prepared by pharmacy (45 day shelf-life in a refrigerator)[1] Unauthorized 5mg/5mL and 40mg/5mL oral suspensions can be obtained via special order Orodispersible tablet (Losec MUPS®) can be added to 25mL of water and administered by EFT using a push-pull technique to keep the granules suspended. *Do not crush.* Suitable for 8Fr gauge. A similar technique can be used for Mezzopram dispersible tablets (see SPC) *Tablets* (Dexcel) disperse; larger doses may be required in gastric administration, as this method destroys the e/c coating Contact manufacturer for details of use of injection or infusion via EFT

continued

Table 2 Continued

Drug	*Authorized soluble tablet or oral liquid available*	*Tablet/capsule contents may disperse sufficiently for 8Fr NG tube*[a,b]	*Oral liquid can be prepared by local pharmacy or special order*	*Injection available and can be diluted and administered PO or by EFT*	*Comments*
Ondansetron	Yes	No data	Yes	Yes	Oral liquid contains sorbitol 3g/5mL. Zofran® tablets disperse, but no information on suitability by EFT or of the orodispersible tablet (Zofran Melt®). The injection is acidic; flush well to avoid coagulation with feed
Oxcarbazepine[a]	Yes	Yes (Trileptal®)	Yes	No	Oral suspension is preferred for EFT use; contains ethanol, propylene glycol and sorbitol. Dilute with water before use Tablets are film-coated but will disperse sufficiently if agitated
Oxybutynin[a]	Yes	Yes (Tillomed)	Yes	No	Authorized oral liquid contains sorbitol 1.3g/5mL. Ditropan® may disperse, but no information on suitability by EFT. TD patch available
Oxycodone[a]	Yes	No data	Yes	No data	Anecdotal reports of use of liquid preparation by EFT
Pantoprazole	No	No data	Yes	No data	A 10mg/5mL formulation with 40mg tablet and 20mL sodium bicarbonate 4.2% can be prepared by pharmacy (14 day shelf-life in a refrigerator)
Paracetamol	Yes	Yes (dispersible or effervescent)	Yes	No data	Add dispersible tablet to 50mL of water; consider sodium content
Paroxetine	Yes	No data	Yes	No	Dilute oral liquid with an equal volume of water for EFT use; contains sorbitol
Phenobarbital	Yes	No data	Yes[c,d]	No data	Authorized elixir contains alcohol (0.38units/10mL dose). An unauthorized 50mg/5mL alcohol-free suspension can be obtained via special order or locally prepared Dilute oral liquids with an equal volume of water for intrajejunal administration to reduce osmolarity Tablets may disperse, but no information on suitability by EFT

continued

Table 2 Continued

Drug	*Authorized soluble tablet or oral liquid available*	*Tablet/capsule contents may disperse sufficiently for 8Fr NG tube*[a,b]	*Oral liquid can be prepared by local pharmacy or special order*	*Injection available and can be diluted and administered PO or by EFT*	*Comments*
Phenoxymethyl-penicillin	Yes	No data	No data	No	Stop feed for 2h before and 1h after dose
Phenytoin	Yes	Yes (Flynn; capsules)	Yes[c]	No data	Not recommended due to significant problems. If unavoidable, stop feed for 2h before and after dose and flush tube with 50mL water to minimize interaction with feed. Convert to once daily dose. Phenytoin *base* 30mg/5mL oral suspension (Epanutin®); 90mg (15mL) = 100mg phenytoin *sodium* tablet/capsule; shake liquid well then dilute dose with 30–50mL water, administer and flush Unauthorized concentrated oral liquid 90mg/5mL can be obtained via special order Flynn hard capsule contents will disperse Monitor plasma levels and adhere to a consistent protocol Jejunal absorption is poor
Phytomenadione	No	No	Yes	Yes (Konakion MM®)	The injection is incompatible with certain types of siliconized syringes. Braun syringes are known to be compatible
Pilocarpine	No	No data	Yes	No	Eyedrops 4% can be used orally (see p.668)
Piroxicam	No	Yes (dispersible)	No data	No	Add dispersible tablet (Feldene Melt®) to 50mL water, as it is irritant
Potassium supplements[a]	Yes	Yes (effervescent)	Yes	No data	Flush EFT well to prevent physical interaction with feed. Add effervescent tablets to 50mL water. Oral liquid contains sorbitol 2g/5mL and may cause diarrhoea; dilute with 50–100mL water; not recommended for intrajejunal administration
Prednisolone[a]	Yes	Yes	Yes	No	

continued

Table 2 Continued

Drug	*Authorized soluble tablet or oral liquid available*	*Tablet/capsule contents may disperse sufficiently for 8Fr NG tube*[a,b]	*Oral liquid can be prepared by local pharmacy or special order*	*Injection available and can be diluted and administered PO or by EFT*	*Comments*
Pregabalin	Yes	Yes (Lyrica® capsules)	Yes[c]	No	Unauthorized 75mg/5mL oral suspension can be obtained via special order
Prochlorperazine	Yes	Yes	No data	No data	Dilute oral liquid with an equal volume of water. Disperse tablets for intrajejunal administration; *buccal* tablets are an alternative route
Promethazine *hydrochloride*	Yes	Yes (Phenergan®)	Yes	No data	Dilute oral liquid with an equal volume of water
Propantheline	No	No data	Yes	No	A feed break of 2h before and 1h after each dose is recommended
Propranolol[a]	Yes	No data	Yes	Yes	Dilute oral liquid with an equal volume of water for EFT use
Quetiapine[a]	Yes	No data	Yes[c]	No	
Ranitidine	Yes	Yes (effervescent)	Yes[c]	Yes	Add effervescent tablets to 30mL water; consider sodium content. Authorized oral liquid contains alcohol (0.04units/5mL) and sorbitol An unauthorized 5mg/5mL oral solution (alcohol free) can be obtained via special order
Rifampicin	Yes	No data	Yes[d]	No data	Stop feed for 2h before and 30min after dose. Dilute authorized oral liquid with equal volume of water. Do not open capsules; risk of contact sensitization. A 125mg/5mL suspension can be prepared (7 day shelf-life)[d]
Risperidone	Yes	Yes (Risperdal®) or orodispersible	Yes	No	

continued

Table 2 Continued

Drug	*Authorized soluble tablet or oral liquid available*	*Tablet/capsule contents may disperse sufficiently for 8Fr NG tube*[a,b]	*Oral liquid can be prepared by local pharmacy or special order*	*Injection available and can be diluted and administered PO or by EFT*	*Comments*
Rivaroxaban	No	See comments	No data	No	Tablets may be crushed and mixed with water (for EFT) or apple sauce; not suitable for intrajejunal administration due to reduced absorption
Ropinirole[a]	No	Yes (Requip®)	Yes	No	Disperse tablets in 10mL water for EFT use
Senna	Yes	No data	No data	No	
Sertraline	No	Yes (Lustral®)	Yes[c]	No	Coarse tablet dispersion may block tube; consider alternative drug Note crushed tablets have a local anaesthetic effect Unauthorized 25mg/5mL, 50mg/5mL and 100mg/5mL oral suspension can be obtained via special order
Sodium fusidate	Yes	No data	No data	No data	Sodium fusidate tablets 500mg = 750mg oral suspension. Oral liquid contains sorbitol; not suitable for intrajejunal administration due to decreased absorption
Sodium valproate[a]	Yes	Yes (Epilim® Crushable)	Yes	No	Dilute oral liquid with an equal volume of water for EFT use. Some formulations contain sorbitol. Consider dispersing crushable tablets for intrajejunal administration or dilute oral liquid 3–4 times. Chronosphere® m/r granules suspended in 10mL water can be administered via 10Fr NG tubes or 9Fr PEG tubes
Spironolactone	No	Yes (Most generics, Aldactone®)	Yes[c,d]	No	Unauthorized oral formulations can be obtained via special order; dilute with an equal volume of water for EFT use Disperse tablet for intrajejunal administration A 125mg/5mL suspension can be prepared[d]. Other suspension formulae are also available[44]

continued

Table 2 Continued

Drug	*Authorized soluble tablet or oral liquid available*	*Tablet/capsule contents may disperse sufficiently for 8Fr NG tube*[a,b]	*Oral liquid can be prepared by local pharmacy or special order*	*Injection available and can be diluted and administered PO or by EFT*	*Comments*
Sucralfate	Yes	No	Yes	No	Do not use sucralfate via EFT. Oral liquid *not* recommended, due to high viscosity, bezoar formation and binding with feed; likely to block tube. Need to stop feed for 1h before and after dose; impractical for q4h schedule
Tamsulosin[a]	No	No	Yes[c]	No	Unauthorized 400microgram/5mL oral solution and suspension can be obtained via special order
Tapentadol[a]	Yes	No data	No data	No	
Temazepam	Yes	No	Yes	No	Oral liquid contains sorbitol and may contain ethanol; do not dilute. May be less effective for jejunal use
Tetracycline	No	No data	Yes[d]	No	A 125mg/5mL suspension can be prepared (7 day shelf-life).[d] Significant interaction with enteral feed makes four times a day dosing difficult by EFT
Theophylline[a]	No	No	Yes[c,d]	No	Unauthorized 50mg/5mL oral solution and suspension can be obtained via special order. Convert total daily dose of m/r preparations to oral *unauthorized* liquid and split into t.d.s. regimen. Stop feed for 1h before and 1h after dose. Dilute oral liquid with an equal volume of water. Monitor plasma levels closely There is some information on giving aminophylline injection orally[l]
Tizanidine	No	Yes (Teva)	Yes[c]	No	Unauthorized 2mg/5mL oral solution and suspension can be obtained via special order
Tolbutamide	No	No	Yes	No	

continued

Table 2 Continued

Drug	*Authorized soluble tablet or oral liquid available*	*Tablet/capsule contents may disperse sufficiently for 8Fr NG tube*[a,b]	*Oral liquid can be prepared by local pharmacy or special order*	*Injection available and can be diluted and administered PO or by EFT*	*Comments*
Topiramate	Yes	Yes (Topamax® tablets)	Yes[c]	No	Do not use Topamax® Sprinkle capsules by EFT, as the beads stick to the tube causing blockage Not recommended for intrajejunal administration, due to risk of reduced absorption
Tramadol[a]	Yes	Yes (Ranbaxy capsules, Zydol® soluble, Zamadol Melt®)	Yes[d]	No data	Use authorized dispersible tablets. Oral drops 100mg/mL available; further dilute with water. Zydol® capsule contents may disperse, but no information on suitability by EFT A 25mg/5mL suspension can be prepared
Tranexamic acid	No	Yes (Cyklokapron®, Manx)	Yes[c]	Yes	Unauthorized 250mg/5mL and 500mg/5mL oral solution and suspension can be obtained via special order
Trazodone	Yes	Yes (Molipaxin 50mg capsules)	Yes	No	Dilute oral liquid with an equal volume of water.
Trimethoprim	Yes	No data	Yes	No	Administer the dose during a break in feeding if practical. Dilute authorized oral liquid with an equal volume of water; some formulations contain sorbitol
Vancomycin	No	No	Yes	Yes	The reconstituted injection is authorized for oral and NG tube use (24h shelf-life in fridge for enteral use); flavouring syrups may be added immediately prior to use
Venlafaxine[a]	Yes	Yes (Teva)	Yes	No	
Warfarin	Yes	Yes	Yes	No	Stop feed for 1h before and 1–2h after dose. INR may be affected by the varying content of vitamin K in feeds

continued

Table 2 Continued

Drug	*Authorized soluble tablet or oral liquid available*	*Tablet/capsule contents may disperse sufficiently for 8Fr NG tube*[a,b]	*Oral liquid can be prepared by local pharmacy or special order*	*Injection available and can be diluted and administered PO or by EFT*	*Comments*
Zinc sulfate	No	Yes (effervescent)	Yes	No	Add effervescent tablet to 10mL water. Jejunal administration may reduce bio-availability
Zolpidem	No	Yes (Ratiopharm)	Yes	No	
Zopiclone	No	No	Yes[c]	No	Unauthorized 3.75mg/5mL and 7.5mg/5mL oral solution and suspension can be obtained via special order

a. do not use m/r or e/c preparations unless specifically indicated. Take care if converting from m/r to immediate-release preparations, because dose, frequency and clinical effect may be different

b. use the brand or manufacturer if specified; different brands may not disperse sufficiently for 8Fr NG tube administration; dispersion time may take up to 5min and require agitation

c. unauthorized product listed in part VIIIB of the NHS Drug Tariff, available from specials manufacturers or imported (see Chapter 24, p.817)

d. a simple suspension using 1:1 mixture of Ora-Plus and Ora-Sweet as a vehicle can be prepared by some local pharmacies; 28 day shelf-life unless otherwise stated[44]

e. tubes that should *not* be used for administration of Zomorph® capsules include Mallinkrodt enral 205-09-1, Bioser 1147221, Vygon 39110 and Vygon 2395.09. Tubes known to be successful in administering Zomorph® capsules include Pharma Plast LEVIN CH/FG 18, Vygon 391.16, Ventrol 15016IT 85753, Ventrol 82316 16A, Bioser 1147239 and Sherwood 90L100A.

1 White R and Bradnam V. *Handbook of Drug Administration via Enteral Feeding Tubes*. London: Pharmaceutical Press. www.medicinescomplete.com (accessed November 2021).
2 BAPEN (British Association of Parenteral and Enteral Nutrition) (2004) Administering drugs via enteral feeding tubes. A practical guide. BAPEN. Available from: www.bapen.org.uk.
3 Royal Pharmaceutical Society (2012) Keeping patients safe when they transfer between care providers – getting the medicines right. www.rpharms.com.
4 Royal Pharmaceutical Society (2016) Prescribing specials. Guidance for the prescribers of specials. www.rpharms.com.
5 Care Quality Commission (2020) Enteral feeding and medicines administration. www.cqc.org.uk (accessed July 2021).
6 NHS England (2018) Never Events List (updated February 2021). www.england.nhs.uk.
7 National Patient Safety Agency (2007) Promoting safer measurement and administration of liquid medicines via oral and other enteral routes. *Patient Safety Alert*. NPSA/2007/19 (archived).
8 National Patient Safety Agency (2011) Reducing the harm caused by misplaced nasogastric feeding tubes in adults, children and infants. *Patient Safety Alert and Supporting Information*. NPSA/2011/PSA2002 (archived).
9 National Patient Safety Agency (2012) Harm from flushing of nasogastric tubes before confirmation of placement. *Rapid Response Report*. NPSA/2012/RRR001 (archived).
10 UK Medicines Information (2019) What are the therapeutic options for patients unable to take solid oral dosage forms. *Medicines Q&A*. www.sps.nhs.uk.
11 Jackson LD *et al.* (2008) Safe medication swallowing in dysphagia: a collaborative improvement project. *Healthcare Quarterly*. **11**: 110–116.
12 Wright D (2011) How to help if a patient can't swallow. *Pharmaceutical Journal*. **286**: 272–274.
13 NPPG & RCPCH (2020) Choosing an oral liquid medicine for children. Position statement. www.nppg.org.uk.
14 Mc Gillicuddy A *et al.* (2017) The knowledge, attitudes and beliefs of patients and their healthcare professionals around oral dosage form modification: A systematic review of the qualitative literature. *Research in Social and Administrative Pharmacy*. **13**: 717–726.
15 Adams D (1994) Administration of drugs through a jejunostomy tube. *British Journal of Intensive Care*. **4**: 10–17.
16 Thomson F et *al.* (2000) Enteral and parenteral nutrition. *Hospital Pharmacist*. **7**: 155–164.
17 Prescqipp (2017) Care homes – Assisting people with swallowing difficulties. *Bulletin 188*. www.prescqipp.info.
18 Institute for Safe Medication Practices Canada (2019) Potentially harmful interaction between polyethylene glycol laxative and starch-based thickeners. Bulletin 19 (7). www.ismp-canada.org.
19 UK Medicines Information (2020) Thickening agents and thickened fluids: do they interact with medicines? *Medicines Q&A*. www.sps.nhs.uk.
20 Gilbar P (1999) A guide to drug administration in palliative care. *Journal of Pain and Symptom Management*. **17**: 197–207.
21 Royal Pharmaceutical Society (2011) Pharmaceutical issues when crushing, opening or splitting oral dosage forms. www.rpharms.com.
22 Centre for Policy on Ageing (2012) Safety of medicines in care homes: Managing and administering medication in care homes for older people. www.careengland.org.uk.
23 Schier JG *et al.* (2003) Fatality from administration of labetalol and crushed extended-release nifedipine. *Annals of Pharmacotherapy*. **37**: 1420–1423.
24 Cornish P (2005) "Avoid the crush": hazards of medication administration in patients with dysphagia or a feeding tube. *Canadian Medical Association Journal*. **172**: 871–872.
25 Wright DN et *al.* (2017) Medication management of adults with swallowing difficulties. *Guidelines*. MGP Ltd. www.guidelines.co.uk.
26 UK Medicines Information (2020) What are considerations when crushing tablets or opening capsules in a care home setting? *Medicines Q&A*. www.sps.nhs.uk.
27 Royal Pharmaceutical Society of Great Britain (2015) Professional guidance for the procurement and supply of pharmaceutical specials. www.rpharms.com.
28 Sohrevardi SM *et al.* (2017) Medication errors in patients with enteral feeding tubes in the intensive care unit. *Journal of Research in Pharmacy Practice*. **6**: 100–105.
29 NHS England (2013) Placement devices for nasogastric tube insertion DO NOT replace initial position checks. *Patient Safety Alert*. NHS/PSA/W/2013/. www.england.nhs.uk/patient-safety.
30 NHS England (2016) Nasogastric tube misplacement: continuing risk of death and severe harm. *Patient Safety Alert*. NHS/PSA/RE/2016/006. www.england.nhs.uk.
31 McFarland A (2017) A cost utility analysis of the clinical algorithm for nasogastric tube placement confirmation in adult hospital patients. *Journal of Advanced Nursing*. **73**: 201–216.
32 Williams NT (2008) Medication administration through enteral feeding tubes. *American Journal of Health-System Pharmacy*. **65**: 2347–2357.
33 Phillips NM and Nay R (2008) A systematic review of nursing administration of medication via enteral tubes in adults. *Journal of Clinical Nursing*. **17**: 2257–2265.
34 Engle KK and Hannawa TE (1999) Techniques for administering oral medications to critical care patients receiving continuous enteral nutrition. *American Journal of Health System Pharmacy*. **56**: 1441–1444.
35 Preston CL. *Stockley's Drug Interactions*. London: Pharmaceutical Press. www.medicinescomplete.com (accessed November 2021).
36 Schmidt LE and Dalhoff K (2002) Food-drug interactions. *Drugs*. **62**: 1481–1502.
37 Clark-Schmidt AL et *al.* (1990) Loss of carbamazepine suspension through nasogastric feeding tubes. *American Journal of Hospital Pharmacy*. **47**: 2034–2037.
38 Freeman KL and Trezevant MS (2009) Interaction between liquid protein solution and omeprazole suspension. *American Journal of Health System Pharmacy*. **66**: 1901–1902.
39 Wohlt PD et *al.* (2009) Recommendations for the use of medications with continuous enteral nutrition. *American Journal of Health System Pharmacy*. **66**: 1458–1467.
40 Garcia-Luna PP et *al.* (1997) Esophageal obstruction by solidification of the enteral feed: a complication to be prevented. *Intensive Care Medicine*. **23**: 790–792.
41 Marcuard SP and Stegall KS (1990) Unclogging feeding tubes with pancreatic enzyme. *Journal of Parenteral Enteral Nutrition*. **14**: 198–200.

42 McClave SA and Neff RL (2006) Care and long-term maintenance of percutaneous endoscopic gastrostomy tubes. *Journal of Parenteral and Enteral Nutrition*. **30 (Suppl 1)**: S27–S38.
43 Palliativedrugs.com (2003) July Newsletter. Available from: www.palliativedrugs.com.
44 Smyth J (2021) *The NEWT guidelines for administration of medication to patients with enteral feeding tubes or swallowing difficulties* (4e). Pharmacy Department, Wrexham Maelor Hospital, Betsi Cadwaladr University Local Health Board (east), Wales.
45 UK Medicines Information (2020) Which injections can be given orally or via enteral feeding tubes? *Medicines Q&A*. www.sps.nhs.uk.
46 Caraballo M *et al.* (2017) Compounded Apixaban suspensions for enteral feeding tubes. *Hospital Pharmacy*. **52**: 478–482.

Updated December 2021

29: CONTINUOUS SUBCUTANEOUS DRUG INFUSIONS

29

CSCI IN CLINICAL PRACTICE

The administration of drugs by continuous subcutaneous infusion (CSCI) is common in palliative care in the UK, particularly in patients for whom swallowing medication has become increasingly difficult or impossible.[1-3]

Ambulatory battery-powered infusion devices are generally used to administer the CSCI.[2] CSCI is as effective as continuous IV infusion (CIVI),[4] and at least as good as intermittent bolus injections.[5] In settings where it is difficult to be certain that intermittent regular injections will be administered on time, CSCI is likely to provide better round-the-clock comfort.

Indications for CSCI

CSCI is *not* 'step 4' on the analgesic ladder; it is a useful alternative route of administration in various circumstances,[6] including:

- persistent nausea and vomiting
- dysphagia
- bowel obstruction
- coma
- poor absorption of oral drugs (rare)
- patient preference.

Before setting up a CSCI, it is important to explain to the patient and family:

- the reason(s) for using this route
- how the infusion device works
- the advantages and possible disadvantages of CSCI for the patient (Box A).

Drugs used by CSCI

For most drugs, this route of administration is off-label (see p.xix).[7] However, there is extensive documented clinical experience of CSCI with many drugs used in palliative care.[3,8] In addition, there are reports of other drugs given less frequently by this route, e.g. **diclofenac** (p.362), **furosemide** (p.67), **levetiracetam** (p.312), **olanzapine** (p.203), **paracetamol** (p.331), **parecoxib** (p.373), **ranitidine** (p.29), **valproate** (p.307).

For CSCI, the injectable formulation must be of a suitable concentration to deliver the required dose in a relatively small volume, and also be relatively non-irritant (see Infusion site problems, below).

Although often administered by CSCI, several drugs with a long duration of action, e.g. **dexamethasone**, **levomepromazine**, **olanzapine**, **parecoxib**, can be given as a bolus injection or short infusion, SC or IV, once daily or b.d. (Table 1).[1]

Bolus SC injections should be given via a separate SC butterfly needle/cannula and *not* via a side arm or port of a CSCI cannula or infusion line. This avoids potential problems with drug incompatibility or loss of symptom control caused by the flush replacing the CSCI contents of the infusion tubing.

Box A Advantages and disadvantages of CSCI

Advantages

Saving nurses' time.

Round-the-clock comfort, because plasma drug concentrations are maintained without peaks and troughs.

Less need for repeated injections.

Generally needs to be loaded once daily.

Control of multiple symptoms with a combination of drugs.

Independence and mobility maintained, because the infusion device is lightweight and can be worn in a holster.

Patient preference.

Disadvantages

Initial cost of infusion devices.

Training of staff, together with need to maintain competency.

Lack of flexibility if more than one drug is being administered.

Lack of reliable compatibility data for some mixtures.

Possible inflammation and pain at the infusion site.

Although uncommon, problems with the infusion device can lead to break-through pain (or other symptom) if the problem is not resolved quickly.

Table 1 Drugs which can be given by bolus injection or short infusion once daily or b.d. instead of by CSCI

Drug	*Plasma halflife (h)*	*Duration of action (h)*
Clonazepam[a] (not UK)	20–60	≤12–24
Dexamethasone	3–4.5	36–54
Esomeprazole	1.3	>24
Famotidine	3	6–10
Furosemide	0.5–2	6–8
Granisetron	10–11	≤24
Haloperidol	13–35	≤24
Levetiracetam	6–8	24
Levomepromazine[b]	15–30	≤24
Methadone[b]	8–75	≤12
Olanzapine (not UK)	34–52	12–48
Omeprazole	0.5–3	>24
Pantoprazole	1	>24
Parecoxib	8[c]	6–12
Tranexamic acid	2–3	24

a. for SC/IV bolus doses, dilute each 1mg/mL amp with 1mL WFI

b. relatively irritant SC

c. active metabolite valdecoxib.

PRESCRIBING CSCI

CSCI must be prescribed in the relevant section of the patient's drug chart. Some specialist units have separate CSCI drug charts (examples are available in the Document library of www.palliativedrugs.com); these must be linked or referred to in the patient's main drug chart. The prescription should specify:[9]

- the dose of each drug to be administered over the infusion period (generally 24h)
- the diluent
- the final volume of the infusion.

Compatibility of the drug(s) and the diluent should be confirmed before the CSCI is set up (see Mixing drugs, below); if it is not a routine combination, ideally this should be documented in the patient's notes (see p.xix).

If symptoms are controlled, start the CSCI 2–4h before the next dose of PO opioid would have been given. If symptoms are uncontrolled, set up the CSCI immediately with stat doses of the same drugs.

Rescue medication

Appropriate doses of p.r.n. medication must also be prescribed. These are given via a separate SC needle/cannula (left *in situ* for this purpose) and flushed with compatible diluent (see Diluent, below). The side arm or port of the CSCI infusion line must *not* be used, because of potential problems with drug incompatibility or loss of symptom control caused by the flush replacing the CSCI contents of the infusion tubing.

Converting from PO to CSCI

Drugs are generally *more* bio-available by injection than PO. This means that the dose of a drug given by CSCI will be *less* than the dose previously given PO, generally between 1/3 and 2/3 of the PO dose. The bio-availability data given at the end of the pharmacology section in the individual drug monographs serve as a guide to the appropriate reduction. Thus, the dose of a drug with oral bio-availability of 75% should be reduced by a quarter when given SC, halved if 50% bio-available, and so on. Particular care should be taken with strong opioids (see Appendix 2, Table 3, p.931).

Converting from CSCI to PO

Some patients are able to revert from CSCI to PO medication, e.g. those being treated for nausea and vomiting. When this seems possible, convert the drugs sequentially rather than all at once. For example, convert the anti-emetic medication first and, if the nausea and vomiting do not recur, change the other medication 1–2 days later.

Remember: just as drug doses were reduced when starting CSCI, doses will generally need to be increased when reverting to PO. This is particularly the case with strong opioid analgesics; e.g., **morphine** 15mg/24h CSCI will need to be increased to **morphine** 30mg/24h PO.

The CSCI is generally discontinued when the first dose of the PO medication is administered. It is important to review p.r.n. medication and to adjust it appropriately.

Converting from TD patches to CSCI (or vice versa)

The TD and CSCI routes are considered equipotent in terms of total daily dose (see Appendix 2, p.925).

As a general rule, TD **buprenorphine** or **fentanyl** patches should be continued when the need for supplemental opioid via CSCI is short-term, e.g. in the last days of life. It is simpler to supplement the patch with a CSCI of **morphine** or other opioid than to convert completely to a single alternative opioid. See the respective Quick Clinical Guides for **buprenorphine** or **fentanyl** for more information, including the conversion of a CSCI opioid to a TD patch (p.438 and p.448).

DILUENT

PCF recommends that generally WFI is used as the standard diluent of choice. However, sodium chloride 0.9% should be considered if there is a potential or actual problem with inflammatory reactions at the skin injection site (see Infusion site problems, p.895).

The main purpose of diluents is to help reduce site irritation and enable drug delivery over a prescribed time. It is essential that the diluent is compatible with the drug(s) in the syringe. The SPC may indicate compatible diluents, particularly if a drug is authorized for CSCI. However, the information may not be comprehensive, and is unlikely to cover compatibility when drugs are mixed. Generally, either WFI or sodium chloride 0.9% can be used. They both have advantages and disadvantages (Table 2).

Table 2 Comparison of diluents

WFI	*Sodium chloride 0.9%*[10]
Advantages	**Advantages**
Less chance of incompatibility	Isotonic. Preferable for diluting irritant drugs (potentially less infusion site-reaction)
Generally more compatibility data available for commonly used drugs	
Disadvantages	**Disadvantages**
Large volumes are hypotonic, which may cause infusion site pain or skin reaction (generally not a problem in practice, because infusion rates are so slow)	Incompatible with some drugs, e.g. cyclizine; higher concentrations of diamorphine >40mg/mL or haloperidol >1mg/mL
	Generally less compatibility data available for commonly used drugs

In the UK, WFI is widely used as the first-line diluent, because it can be used to dilute all commonly used drugs in palliative care, including **cyclizine *lactate*** (p.273) and higher concentrations of **diamorphine *hydrochloride*** (>40mg/mL) or **haloperidol** (>1mg/mL). There is also a wealth of supporting compatibility data and clinical experience for WFI (see Appendix 3, p.933).

For some drugs, e.g. **granisetron**, **hydromorphone**, **ketamine**, **ketorolac**, **octreotide** and **ondansetron**, more compatibility data exist with sodium chloride 0.9%, and some prefer to use this as the diluent. Further, sodium chloride 0.9% would be a reasonable first-line diluent in those countries where **cyclizine *lactate*** or **diamorphine** are unavailable or not used.

Some centres in the USA use glucose 5% in water as the first-line diluent. However, this is acidic and unsuitable for very alkaline drugs, e.g. **dexamethasone**, **furosemide**, **ketorolac**, **phenobarbital**.

To avoid confusion, consistency of practice within individual units is important.[11]

INFUSION VOLUME

Factors influencing the final volume of the CSCI include the total volume of the drugs, the infusion device being used, the maximum rate of delivery, the intended infusion time and local guidelines. Greater dilution reduces:

- the risk of incompatibility
- the impact of priming a line (less drug in the 'dead space')
- injection site skin reactions from the drug.

For these reasons, 20mL syringes are now generally recommended as the minimum standard size to be used.

In deciding how much diluent to use, one approach is to dilute the contents to a standard volume; generally, this is at or close to the maximum fill volume for the size of syringe being used, e.g.:

- for a total drug volume <10mL, dilute to 17mL in a 20mL Luer Lock syringe
- for a total drug volume >10mL, dilute to 22mL in a 30mL Luer Lock syringe.

Particular care will be required when mixing drugs where compatibility depends on the final drug concentrations, e.g. **cyclizine**, **dexamethasone**, **haloperidol**, **ketorolac** (see Drug compatibility, below, and Appendix 3, footnotes of Charts 1–7, p.936–p.949).

In some situations, the total volume of drugs may exceed the maximum volume/24h that an infusion device can deliver, i.e. about 23mL or 35mL in a 30mL or 50mL BD Plastipak Luer Lock syringe, respectively, for a BD BodyGuard™ T syringe pump. This is most likely with combinations that include higher doses of **fentanyl**, **metoclopramide**, **midazolam**, **morphine** or **oxycodone**. This problem can generally be circumvented by:

- using a more concentrated formulation (see below)
- switching from:
  - ▷ **morphine** to **diamorphine** or **hydromorphone**
  - ▷ **fentanyl** to **alfentanil**
- changing the contents of the syringe driver more frequently, e.g. every 12h
- using a different infusion device with a larger capacity.[12]

When a cartridge/cassette/bag infusion system is used, a larger final volume is possible. Even so, some centres standardize to 50mL volume with a maximum rate of 2mL/h.

Caution is required when using a more concentrated formulation, e.g. **fentanyl** 5mg/mL, **oxycodone** 50mg/mL or **midazolam** 5mg/mL, because compatibility can differ from the normal strength formulation (Box B). Further, confusion between the normal and the more concentrated formulations has resulted in overdoses. Consequently, some organizations restrict the availability of the more concentrated formulations.[13]

INFUSION DURATION

In the UK, CSCI syringes are generally timed to empty over 24h.[3,14] The main reasons for this are:

- extrapolation of sterility guidelines from CIVI
- availability of stability and compatibility data
- standardization of practice (for safety reasons)
- tradition, based on the limitations of older syringe drivers.

Generally, 24h is satisfactory in terms of sterility, stability and practicality.[15,16]

For certain infusion devices, e.g. CADD pumps and elastomeric devices, stability and compatibility data may exist for a longer duration of infusion, e.g. 48–72h.[14] Generally, these solutions are made up in aseptically controlled environments, e.g. pharmacy aseptic units, to ensure sterility.

Infusion stability

Drug stability and compatibility are closely related. 'Stability' describes how much of the drug remains in its original form in a given period of time. 'Compatibility' describes whether the addition of a diluent or a drug causes a physical or chemical interaction. Various factors affect the stability of the drug in the CSCI and potentially could lead to incompatibility and impaired symptom control (Box B).

Box B Factors affecting CSCI drug stability or compatibility[17-20]

Diluent (see above).

Final concentration of drug

The *concentration* of the drug in the solution (the *quantity* of the drug divided by the *total final volume*) should be checked against stability and compatibility data (see Appendix 3, p.933).

Order of mixing

This is particularly important when compatibility is concentration dependent; e.g. dexamethasone and ranitidine should always be the last drug added to an already diluted and mixed syringe to reduce the risk of incompatibility.

Brand/formulation/strength of the drug

Injections contain various excipients, e.g. preservatives, diluents and stabilizing compounds, which can differ between brands, countries and even between different strengths of the same drug, e.g. oxycodone (see Appendix 3, Table 1, p.950).

Duration of infusion (see above)

Note. The rate at which drugs degrade can be increased by:

Higher temperature: patients should not wear the infusion device under clothes

Exposure to light: e.g. levomepromazine turns purple/pink/yellow; cover the infusion.

Adsorption onto delivery system material

E.g. ≤50% of a dose of clonazepam onto PVC tubing

MIXING DRUGS

The combination of two or more authorized (licensed) drugs results in a new unauthorized (unlicensed) product being formed. Doctors and other independent prescribers (nurses, pharmacists) can mix, and direct others to mix, drugs (including controlled drugs) for administration to a particular patient. Supplementary prescribers can mix and direct others to mix when part of a clinical management plan (also see p.xxi).[21]

In the UK, it is common practice to administer two or three different drugs in the same infusion device.[1,2,22] Some centres mix four or more drugs. However, the greater the number of drugs mixed, the greater the probability of compatibility problems. Accordingly, *PCF* recommends that generally no more than three drugs should be mixed in one syringe.

Drug compatibility

When mixing drugs, it is essential to consider drug compatibility (Box C). Physical and/or chemical changes can occur, which could lead to reduced efficacy.[23]

Box C Drug compatibility data

Physical compatibility

If mixing two or more drugs does not result in a physical change, e.g. discolouration, clouding or crystallization, they are said to be physically compatible.

Observational data

Data from many palliative care services about the visual appearance of various drug mixtures over the infusion period (generally 24h) have been collated for use in the www.palliativedrugs.com Syringe Driver Survey Database (SDSD). However, observational data are subjective and imprecise; generally, only major incompatibilities can be identified in this way.

Laboratory data

These are generally derived from microscopic examination of a drug mixture under polarized light at specified concentrations and several time points when kept under controlled conditions. Although more robust, these are not definitive; a solution may remain physically clear even when there is chemical incompatibility.[24]

Chemical compatibility

If mixing two or more drugs does not result in a chemical change leading to loss or degradation of one or more of the drugs, the mixture is said to be chemically compatible. Chemical compatibility data are generally obtained by analysing the drug mixture by high-performance liquid chromatography (HPLC) at specified concentrations and several time points when kept under controlled conditions.

Occasionally, a drug combination has been shown to be chemically compatible but physically incompatible.

Ideally both physical and chemical compatibility data should be known. However, because of the infinite number of possible drug combinations and a dearth of published chemical compatibility studies, generally decisions are taken on the basis of physical compatibility, based on observational data and clinical experience.

Information sources

Information on CSCI compatibility can be obtained from several sources:

- *for infusions with WFI as a diluent:* Charts 1–7 (see Appendix 3, p.933) summarize the compatibility data for the more commonly used 2- and 3-drug combinations. They have been compiled from clinical observations in palliative care services in the UK, New Zealand and Australia, and from published compatibility data
- *for infusions with sodium chloride 0.9% as a diluent:* Charts 8–14 (available in the extended appendix section of the on-line *PCF* on www.medicinescomplete.com) summarize the compatibility data for the more commonly used 2- and 3-drug combinations. They have been compiled from

clinical observations in palliative care services in the UK, New Zealand and Australia, and from published compatibility data
- *Syringe Driver Survey Database* (SDSD) on www.palliativedrugs.com. This is a continually updated resource and contains observational compatibility data on mixing combinations of drugs reported by health professionals. For this to be of maximum benefit, members are urged to donate information about both *successful* and *unsuccessful* combinations for which there are no previously published data
- *The Syringe Driver: Continuous Subcutaneous Infusions in Palliative Care*[22]
- *Palliative Care Matters* www.pallcare.info
- *Handbook on Injectable Drugs.*[17]

Generally, these sources can only indicate if a drug combination is likely to be stable and compatible. Many factors affect drug compatibility and/or stability (Box B), which helps explain conflicting reports. If there is doubt about the relevance of the compatibility data to the situation in which a given drug combination is to be used, advice should be obtained from a clinical pharmacist. Regular checks of the CSCI together with the patient's condition should always be undertaken (see Checks in use, below).

General principles for compatibility

When there is a lack of robust compatibility data for the prescribed drugs, the following general principles should be noted:
- generally, drugs with a similar pH are more likely to be compatible than those with widely differing ones (Table 3)
- most drugs are acidic in solution; however, **dexamethasone**, **diclofenac**, **esomeprazole**, **furosemide**, **ketorolac**, **omeprazole** and **phenobarbital** are alkaline in solution and often cause compatibility problems (Table 3); as a result, **diclofenac**, **esomeprazole**, **furosemide**, **omeprazole** and **phenobarbital** should be administered separately and not be mixed with other drugs
- dilute to the maximum volume possible
- compatibility with **cyclizine** or **haloperidol** is often concentration dependent, and these drugs are more likely to cause problems at higher concentrations
- the risk of precipitation with **dexamethasone** is reduced if it is added last to an already dilute drug mixture. On the other hand, as already noted, **dexamethasone** has a long duration of action. Thus, except when it is being given to reduce the risk of skin reactions (see Infusion site problems, below), there is no real need to give it by CSCI (Table 1)
- the risk of precipitation of some combinations of **ranitidine** can be reduced by adding it last to an already dilute drug mixture (see p.29)
- occasionally, initial cloudiness or separation (precipitation) may occur, which resolves on full mixing; however, ensure it fully resolves and monitor the infusion closely. (Note. Delayed cloudiness can be caused by chemicals from the syringe or tubing leaching out)
- protect from direct sunlight (particularly **levomepromazine**) and heat
- the more drugs combined, the greater the risk of incompatibility; generally, *PCF* recommends a maximum of three drugs in one syringe
- checks in use should be undertaken more regularly (see Checks in use, below), monitoring both the infusion and expected clinical outcome. Where incompatibilities are found, e.g. crystal formation, details should be submitted to the SDSD, to help build a database of evidence for drug combinations.

Table 3 Approximate pH values of parenteral drug formulations[17,25]

Drug[a]	*pH*	*Drug*[a]	*pH*
Alfentanil	4–6	Lacosamide	3.5–5
Buprenorphine	4–6	Levetiracetam	5–7
Clonazepam	3.6	Levomepromazine	4.5
Clonidine	4–4.5	Lidocaine	5–7
Cyclizine *lactate*	3.3–3.7	Methadone	3–6.5
Dexamethasone *sodium phosphate*	7–10.5	Metoclopramide	4.5–6.5
Diamorphine[b]		Midazolam	3
Diclofenac	7.8–9	Morphine *sulfate*	2.5–6.5
Esomeprazole[c]	9–11	Octreotide	3.9–4.5
Famotidine	5–6.4	Olanzapine (not UK)	5.4–5.9
Fentanyl	4–7.5	Omeprazole[c]	8.8–10.3
Furosemide	8–9.3	Ondansetron	3.3–4
Glycopyrronium	2–3	Oxycodone	4.5–5.5
Granisetron	4.7–7.3	Pantoprazole[c]	9–11.5
Haloperidol	3–3.8	Paracetamol	5.5
Hydromorphone	4–5.5	Parecoxib[c]	7.5–8.5
Hyoscine *butylbromide*	3.7–5.5	Phenobarbital	9.2–10.2
Hyoscine *hydrobromide*	5–7	Ranitidine	6.7–7.3
Ketamine	3.5–5.5	Tranexamic acid	6.5–8
Ketorolac	6.9–7.9	Valproate *sodium*[c]	7.6

a. pH values may vary between each strength and different brands

b. powder for reconstitution; most stable when reconstituted so that the pH is 3.8–4.5

c. powder for reconstitution.

SITE OF CSCI

See Box D. Plastic/Teflon cannulae are preferred to metal cannulae, because they reduce the risk of site reactions and needle stick injury.[26-28] A 20mm 21-gauge cannula is used for a patient of average build, but a smaller 25-gauge is more appropriate for smaller or emaciated patients.[29] Insert at an angle of approximately 45° and ensure placement into SC tissue.

Where possible, use fine-bore tubing with a small priming volume (preferably <0.3mL) and secure the tubing to the skin with a transparent semipermeable adhesive dressing (e.g.Tegaderm®), with a loop to reduce the likelihood of needle/cannula displacement.

An infusion site may be satisfactory for ≥1 week (and occasionally 2–3 weeks).[27,30] However, generally prophylactic site rotation is advised, e.g. every 3–5 days, with the exact duration varying between centres.

Box D Siting a CSCI[8]

Preferred sites	**Areas to avoid**
Anterior chest wall[a]	Oedematous areas
Anterolateral aspects of upper arms[b]	Skin folds
Supra- or interscapular area[c]	Breast
	Broken, inflamed or infected skin
Alternative sites	Recently irradiated skin sites
Anterior abdominal wall	Cutaneous tumour sites
Anterior surface of the thighs	Bony prominences
	Near a joint
	Scarring

a. ideally avoid in cachectic patients

b. ideally avoid in ambulatory patients or bedbound patients who need turning

c. useful when risk of inadvertent removal, e.g. patient with terminal agitation.

Infusion site problems

These occur in ≤25% of patients (Box E).[1,27] The risk of local irritation is increased when injectable formulations have an osmolality of >600mOsmol/kg, a pH <4 or >11, or contain excipients that may be irritant, e.g. ethanol, glycerin, propylene glycol.[8,31]

Apart from discomfort, local inflammation may impair drug absorption and thereby symptom control.

Box E Causes of infusion site problems[22,32,33]
Anatomical site Local bruising (caused by needle/cannula) Irritant drug(s) Tonicity/osmolality of the solution pH of the solution Incompatible drug–diluent mixture Allergy to nickel needle Glass particles from ampoules Sterile abscess Infection Infrequent resiting

Site reactions can be reduced by:

- using a less irritant parenteral drug formulation, e.g. **haloperidol** instead of **prochlorperazine** (Box F)
- considering the use of sodium chloride 0.9% as a diluent, when compatibility data exist (see Diluent, above)
- diluting the solution as much as practical; this may include changing the syringe q12h instead of q24h to permit further dilution
- using a plastic cannula instead of a butterfly needle (always use in patients with a known metal allergy)
- changing the site prophylactically every 2–3 days, particularly if using irritant drugs
- applying **hydrocortisone** 1% cream to the skin around the needle entry site, and covering it with an occlusive dressing
- adding **dexamethasone** (e.g. 0.66mg) to the solution if compatibility data permit.[30]

Although the routine addition of **dexamethasone** has been recommended on the grounds that it extends the life of an infusion site by about 50%, the fact that some sites have lasted 2–3 weeks without **dexamethasone** means that routine use cannot be recommended.[30]

Box F Parenteral drug formulations which are irritant CSCI
Strongly irritant; do *not* give by CSCI Chlorpromazine Diazepam Prochlorperazine (sometimes given by SC bolus)
Relatively irritant by CSCI; precautions may be necessary[a] Cyclizine Diclofenac Ketamine Ketorolac Levomepromazine Methadone Octreotide[b] Ondansetron Phenobarbital[c] Promethazine[c]

a. see text and respective monographs

b. painful if given as SC bolus; this is reduced if warmed to body temperature before injection

c. strongly irritant with risk of tissue necrosis if given by SC bolus injection.

INFUSION DEVICES

In the UK, ambulatory syringe pumps (also called syringe drivers) are the most commonly used infusion devices for delivering drugs by CSCI. The use of other infusion devices, e.g. cartridges/cassettes/elastomeric devices prepared by a pharmacist adds significantly to the cost.

Until recently, the CME/McKinley T34™ has been the most frequently used syringe pump.[34,35] However, several safety issues have arisen.[36-38] Subsequently, older editions of the CME/McKinley T34™ pumps or versions running older software are no longer recommended and are being replaced with the BD BodyGuard™ T version by the manufacturer.[39] However, some CME T34™ 3rd edition pumps with updated software are still in use. Thus, *PCF* provides information on the BD BodyGuard™ T, which is also relevant to the CME T34™ 3rd edition with updated software, see QCG: Setting up a BD BodyGuard™ T syringe pump (p.897).

Setting up the infusion device

Full instructions can be found in the manufacturer's user guides. In addition, relevant general issues include:

- *priming of the infusion line; PCF* recommends priming the infusion line before loading the syringe into the pump. This uses approx. 0.3mL volume depending on the type of infusion line. This means that a small proportion of the dose drawn up for the patient will be lost in the 'dead space' when a new infusion is first set up. The final volume in the syringe should be noted and used to check the infusion rate (automatically calculated by some syringe drivers/pumps). Subsequent infusions given by the same line will not need priming, therefore the final volume and thus the infusion rate will be slightly different
- *protection from light*; the syringe and pump should be covered if using in direct sunlight, to minimize the risk of stability problems, particularly for **levomepromazine** (see Box B), and/or pump malfunctions[36]
- *protection from heat*; the syringe and pump should also be protected from excessive heat, e.g. avoid covering with excessive layers of clothes/bedclothes
- *battery connection*; ensure there is a tight battery connection. Pumps have failed because of battery connection problems
- *cleaning;* clean using only disposable wipes impregnated with isopropyl alcohol 70%. Pumps have failed because of exposure to excessive quantities of liquids from cleaning procedures.[38]

Also see QCG: Setting up a BD BodyGuard™ T syringe pump (p.897).

Checks in use

Specific record charts should be used for checking a CSCI; examples are available in the Document library of www.palliativedrugs.com. These record charts should be used in addition to the prescription chart. Checks should be documented within 1h of setting up the CSCI and then q4h:

- is the device still working?
- is the correct rate still infusing?
- amount of time and volume of solution left, and whether the infusion is running to time (based on the preceding 4h)
- appearance of the solution in the tubing and syringe/cartridge/bag
- condition of the skin site
- battery status.

Do not remove the syringe/cartridge/bag from the infusion device to perform these checks. If checking indicates a problem, action should be taken and then documented; e.g. if the infusion needs to be resited (and hence reprimed), the time, the new site and the new infusion volume/syringe length should be recorded. Other comments might include details of incompatibility and mention of any mishaps, e.g. the delivery device found disconnected.

Quick Clinical Guide: Setting up a BD BodyGuard™ T syringe pump for CSCI

For full instructions, see the manufacturer's user guide and local guidelines. This QCG is also applicable to the CME T34™ syringe pump 3rd edition with updated software.

PCF recommends the default settings of:
- 'Locked' program
- 'Duration' mode set to an infusion duration of 24h
- manual priming before loading the syringe in the pump.

For use with any other settings, see manufacturer's user guide.

PCF does *not* recommend the use of the automatic purge. Although designed to reduce the slack in the pump mechanism and achieve the correct flow rate more quickly (about 20min vs. 2h), it is more complex to set up and the clinical relevance of the time difference is unknown. Further, patients should have access to p.r.n. medication for the relief of any symptoms.

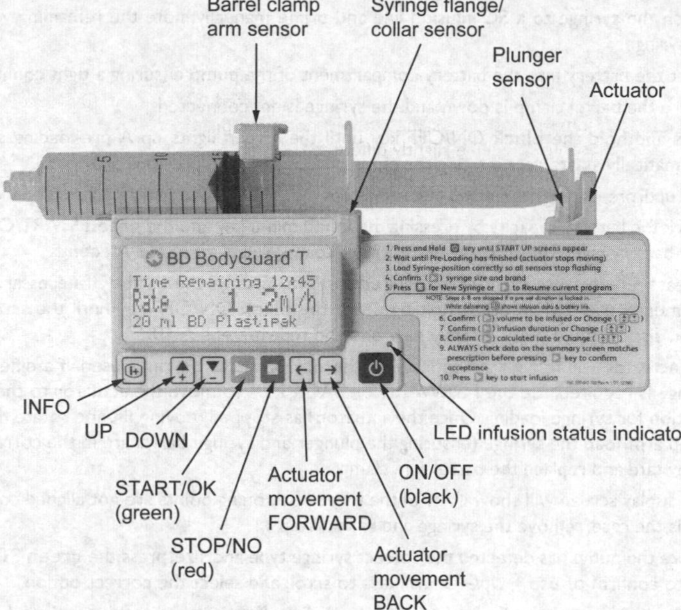

Figure The BD BodyGuard™ T syringe pump
Courtesy and © Becton, Dickinson and Company; adapted with permission

Additional equipment

- 9V (6LR61) alkaline battery + spare battery (each lasts about 2–3 days)
- 20mL, 30mL or 50mL Luer Lock syringe
- syringe extension set (SC infusion line) with a Luer Lock connector; manufacturer recommends a BD line with an integrated anti-free-flow and anti-siphon valve
- lock box and key; a larger one is available to accommodate a 50mL syringe
- transparent adhesive dressing.

1 A CSCI may take several hours to provide effective symptom control. SC bolus doses of the appropriate rescue medication should be available to relieve any symptoms.

2 Fill a Luer Lock syringe with the drugs and dilute the contents to a standard volume; e.g. at, or close to, the maximum fill volume, see table below. Particular care will be required when mixing drugs where compatibility depends on the final drug concentrations.

Syringe size	*Maximum fill volume*[a]
20mL syringe	17mL
30mL syringe	23mL
50mL syringe	35mL

a. for a BD Plastipak Luer Lock syringe, rounded to the nearest possible whole mL; volumes can vary between manufacturers.

Note. Dexamethasone should be the last drug added to an already dilute combination of drugs in order to reduce the risk of incompatibility.

3 The syringe should be made up immediately before use, using strict aseptic technique. Ensure adequate mixing has occurred; the solution should be clear and free from discoloration, crystals or precipitate.

4 Label the syringe, taking care to avoid completely obscuring the solution or covering the point at which the barrel clamp is applied, as this can lead to errors in syringe identification.

5 Attach the syringe to a SC infusion line and prime manually; note the remaining volume in the syringe.

6 Insert the battery into the battery compartment of the pump ensuring a tight connection.

7 Ensure the barrel clamp is down and the syringe is *not* connected.

8 Press and hold the **black** ON/OFF key until the screen lights up. A pre-loading sequence automatically starts, recalibrating the pump and clearing the previous program.

9 Wait until pre-loading has finished (actuator stops moving and 'Load syringe' appears on the screen).

10 Check the battery capacity by pressing the INFO menu key and the **green** START/OK key to view battery level. The screen will return to 'Load syringe' after a few seconds.

At least 40% battery capacity is required for 24h. Change the battery if necessary, e.g. for community use. Switch off by holding down the **black** ON/OFF key until the screen goes blank, discard the battery, insert a new one and repeat steps 7–10.

11 The actuator will move automatically to the size of the last syringe used. If a different size syringe is required, use the FORWARD or BACK keys to move the actuator to the correct position for syringe loading. Once the actuator has stopped moving, lift and rotate the barrel clamp arm, load the syringe (ensuring the plunger and syringe barrel are in the correct slots) and rotate and replace the barrel arm clamp.

12 The display screen will show if any of the three positioning points are not aligned correctly. If this is the case, remove the syringe and repeat step 11.

13 Ensure the pump has detected the correct syringe type and size; press the **green** START/OK key to confirm or use + Up/– Down keys to scroll and select the correct option.

14 A new programme *must* be set for each new syringe. If the pump gives the option of resuming a previous programme, it has been set up incorrectly. Do *not* take this option (press **red** STOP/NO key). Turn off the pump, remove the syringe and start again.

15 The screen will display the infusion summary. Check that the correct infusion volume (as documented after priming) and duration (24h) is shown on the display. Although the rate is automatically calculated, it is good practice to double check this by dividing the volume by the time. Press the **green** START/OK key if settings are correct.

16 Insert the cannula subcutaneously in the patient in a suitable position; secure and attach the syringe and infusion line to the cannula.

17 Press the **green** START/OK key to start the infusion.

The screen will continually show the time remaining for the infusion and the rate (mL/h), along with the syringe selected alternating with 'Pump delivering'. A green flashing LED light above the **black** ON/OFF key will indicate the infusion is running.

18 Lock the keypad by pressing and holding the INFO menu key for about 5 secs until the display shows Keypad LOCK ON (to unlock, do the same until the display shows Keypad LOCK OFF).

19 Secure the pump in the lock box provided.

20 Protect the syringe from excessive sunlight and heat, e.g. electric blankets.

21 Regular checks on the progress, the visual appearance of the infusion and administration site should be performed and documented during the infusion. Do *not* remove the syringe from the pump to perform these checks. If checking indicates a problem, action should be taken and then documented. An infusion progress summary can be obtained while infusing by pressing the INFO menu key.

22 If there is a problem, an audible alarm will sound until the pump is paused or the problem rectified. The screen will display the cause of the alarm. With high priority alarms, a red flashing LED light appears above the **black** ON/OFF key and the infusion will stop; with low priority alarms, the LED light is a steady yellow and the infusion continues. *For implications and actions, see the Troubleshooting section in the manufacturer's user guide.*

23 Do not add drugs to a syringe or infusion line once the infusion has been commenced. Additional bolus drugs needed should be administered by a separate cannula.

24 The infusion may sometimes need to be temporarily stopped (e.g. to change the battery) or disconnected (e.g. when the patient bathes/showers), see Box A.

Box A Temporarily stopping and disconnecting the infusion

- Unlock the keypad
- press the **red** STOP/NO key to stop the infusion
- press and hold the **black** ON/OFF key to switch the pump off; leave the syringe attached to the pump
- *when temporarily disconnecting the infusion:* disconnect the infusion line at the cannula end; cap off both the infusion line and the cannula
- store pump, syringe and infusion line safely; lock in a CD cupboard if it contains a CD.

After interruption:

- check patient details and prescription are correct
- turn on the pump by pressing and holding the **black** ON/OFF key
- when prompted, confirm the syringe size and brand by pressing the **green** START/OK key
- confirm you want to resume the infusion by pressing the **green** START/OK key again
- check and confirm the volume, duration and rate
- if the details are correct, reconnect the infusion line to the cannula
- press the **green** START/OK key to start the infusion
- Lock the keypad.

25 A near end of infusion alarm will sound for 15min before the infusion is completed, accompanied by a steady yellow LED light above the **black** ON/OFF key. Unlock the keypad. If the infusion, has not quite finished, press the INFO menu key and record the volume infused, followed by the **red** STOP/NO key. If the infusion has completely finished, press the **green** START/OK key to confirm the end of the infusion. In both cases press and hold the **black** ON/OFF key to switch the pump off.

26 *If the next prescription is to be repeated exactly*, the same infusion line may be re-used as per local policy. Clamp the infusion line and remove the completed syringe from the pump, *but leave it temporarily connected to the patient*. Follow the guidance from step 1 to set up the new syringe; (at step 5, priming is not needed). At step 16, remove the old syringe from the infusion line and reconnect the infusion line to the new syringe on the pump; complete the remaining steps in the set-up as before.

27 *If the next prescription is different (or changed mid infusion)*, stop the infusion as in step 25; disconnect the infusion line from the patient *before* removing the syringe from the pump. Set up the next prescription from step 1 of the guidance, using a new syringe and new infusion line.

28 Limit cleaning to wiping the external pump surface with disposable wipes impregnated with isopropyl alcohol 70%, *with the pump turned off.*

Updated February 2022

1 Wilcock A *et al.* (2006) Drugs given by a syringe driver: a prospective multicentre survey of palliative care services in the UK. *Palliative Medicine*. **20**: 661–664.
2 O'Doherty CA *et al.* (2001) Drugs and syringe drivers: a survey of adult specialist palliative care practice in the United Kingdom and Eire. *Palliative Medicine*. **15**: 149–154.
3 Dickman A *et al.* (2017) Identification of drug combinations administered by continuous subcutaneous infusion that require analysis for compatibility and stability. *BMC Palliative Care*. **16**: 22.
4 Nelson KA *et al.* (1997) A prospective within-patient crossover study of continuous intravenous and subcutaneous morphine for chronic cancer pain. *Journal of Pain and Symptom Management*. **13**: 262–267.
5 Watanabe S *et al.* (2008) A randomized double-blind crossover comparison of continuous and intermittent subcutaneous administration of opioid for cancer pain. *Journal of Palliative Medicine*. **11**: 570–574.
6 Anderson SL and Shreve ST (2004) Continuous subcutaneous infusion of opiates at end-of-life. *Annals of Pharmacotherapy*. **38**: 1015–1023.
7 Fonzo-Christe C *et al.* (2005) Subcutaneous administration of drugs in the elderly: survey of practice and systematic literature review. *Palliative Medicine*. **19**: 208–219.
8 Duems-Noriega O and Arino-Blasco (2015) Subcutaneous fluid and drug delivery: safe, efficient and inexpensive. *Reviews in Clinical Gerontology*. **25**: 117–146.
9 National Patient Safety Agency (2010) Safer ambulatory syringe drivers. In: Rapid Reponse Report RRR019. www.nrls.npsa.uk.
10 Schneider J *et al.* (1997) A study of the osmolality and pH of subcutaneous drug infusion solutions. *Australian Journal of Hospital Pharmacy*. **27**: 29–31.
11 Flowers C and McLeod F (2005) Diluent choice for subcutaneous infusion: a survey of the literature and Australian practice. *International Journal of Palliative Nursing*. **11**: 54–60.
12 Fudin J *et al.* (2000) Use of continuous ambulatory infusions of concentrated subcutaneous (s.q.) hydromorphone versus intravenous (i.v.) morphine: cost implications for palliative care. *American Journal of Hospice and Palliative Care*. **17**: 347–353.
13 Department of Health (2015) Never events list for 2015/2016. www.gov.uk.
14 Baker J *et al.* (2018) The current evidence base for the feasibility of 48-hour continuous subcutaneous infusions (CSCIs): a systematically-structured review. *PLoS One*. **13**: E0194236.
15 BNF Prescribing in palliative care and guidance on intravenous infusions. London: BMJ Group and Pharmaceutical Press. www.medicinescomplete.com (accessed March 2017).
16 National Patient Safety Agency (2007) Promoting safer use of injectable medicines. Patient safety alert. NPSA/2007/20. www.npsa.nhs.uk.
17 Trissel LA. *Handbook on Injectable Drugs*. Maryland, USA: American Society of Health System Pharmacists (accessed March 2022).
18 Kohut J, 3rd *et al.* (1996) Don't ignore details of drug-compatibility reports. *American Journal of Health System Pharmacy*. **53**: 2339.
19 Vermeire A and Remon JP (1999) Stability and compatibility of morphine. *International Journal of Pharmacology*. **187**: 17–51.
20 Schneider JJ *et al.* (2006) Effect of tubing on loss of clonazepam administered by continuous subcutaneous infusion. *Journal of Pain and Symptom Management*. **31**: 563–567.
21 UK Government (2012) The Human Medicines Regulations. SI 2012/1916. London. www.legislation.gov.uk.
22 Dickman A and Schneider J (2016) *The Syringe Driver: Continuous Subcutaneous Infusions in Palliative Care*, 4th edn. Oxford: Oxford University Press.
23 Foinard A *et al.* (2012) Impact of physical incompatibility on drug mass flow rates: example of furosemide-midazolam incompatibility. *Annals of Intensive Care*. **2**: 28.
24 Good PD *et al.* (2004) The compatibility and stability of midazolam and dexamethasone in infusion solutions. *Journal of Pain and Symptom Management*. **27**: 471–475.
25 Gray A *et al. Injectable Drugs Guide*. London: Pharmaceutical Press. www.medicinescomplete.com (accessed March 2022).
26 Dawkins L *et al.* (2000) A randomized trial of winged Vialon cannulae and metal butterfly needles. *International Journal of Palliative Nursing*. **6**: 110–116.
27 Mitchell K *et al.* (2012) Incidence and causes for syringe driver site reactions in palliative care: A prospective hospice-based study. *Palliative Medicine*. **26**: 979–985.
28 Ross JR *et al.* (2002) A prospective, within-patient comparison between metal butterfly needles and Teflon cannulae in subcutaneous infusion of drugs to terminally ill hospice patients. *Palliative Medicine*. **16**: 13–16.
29 Khan M and Younger G (2007) Promoting safe administration of subcutaneous infusions. *Nursing Standard*. **21**: 50–58.
30 Reymond L *et al.* (2003) The effect of dexamethasone on the longevity of syringe driver subcutaneous sites in palliative care patients. *Medical Journal of Australia*. **178**: 486–489.
31 Wang W (2015) Tolerability of hypertonic injectables. *International Journal of Pharmaceutics*. **490**: 308–315.
32 Oliver D (1991) The tonicity of solutions used in continuous subcutaneous infusions. The cause of skin reactions? *Hospital Pharmacy Practice*. **Sept**: 158–164.
33 Graham F (2006) Syringe drivers and subcutaneous sites: a review. *European Journal of Palliative Care*. **13**: 138–141.
34 Palliativedrugs.com (2014) Which syringe driver do you use? *Latest additions (March)*. www.palliativedrugs.com.
35 Freemantle A *et al.* (2011) Safer ambulatory syringe drivers: experiences of one acute hospital trust. *International Journal of Palliative Nursing*. **17**: 86–91.
36 Field Safety Notice (2016) CME Medical: CME ambulatory syringe pumps - T34, T60 and TPCA. FSN2016-004. www.gov.uk.
37 MHRA (2019) All T34 ambulatory syringe pumps need a sponge pad fitted to the battery compartment to prevent battery connection issues. MDA/2019/2013 www.gov.uk/drug-device-alerts.
38 MHRA (2019) All models of T34 ambulatory syringe pumps – updated cleaning advice and maintenance requirements due to the risk of fluid ingress. MDA/2019/2030 www.gov.uk/drug-device-alerts.
39 MHRA (2021) Infusion pumps: T34 syringe drivers. *Guidance*. www.gov.uk.

Updated (minor change) February 2022

30: TRANSDERMAL PATCHES

Transdermal (TD) patches can be used to administer highly lipid-soluble drugs. Conventional TD patches come in one of two formulations:

- *reservoir:* drug in a reservoir with a rate-limiting membrane to control release
- *matrix:* drug embedded in an adhesive matrix, with the release rate determined by the physical properties of the matrix.

The high concentration of drug in the patch relative to the skin provides a concentration gradient that maintains the relatively constant drug release rate over the application period.

Conventional TD patches are *not* suitable for use when a rapid effect is needed, e.g. acute or uncontrolled pain requiring rapid titration, because of the time taken for the drug to reach the systemic circulation (hours) and steady state (days). When removing the patch, significant plasma concentrations may exist for ≤24h because of the reservoir of drug within the skin.

Cautions

After reports of serious adverse events (overdoses and deaths), regulatory authorities in the UK, USA and Canada have issued safety warnings about the use of TD **fentanyl** that are also applicable to TD **buprenorphine**. For full details, see p.440 and p.428 respectively.[1-5] However, contributing factors include:

- inappropriate use for short-term (e.g. postoperative) pain
- lack of patient education about safe use, storage and disposal, leading to accidental exposure and deaths of others, particularly children
- lack of awareness of the impact of increased temperature or direct external heat
- failure to remove old patches when applying new ones.

External heat sources and/or increase in body temperature

The rate of drug absorption can increase if the skin under the patch becomes vasodilated, e.g. in febrile patients, at high ambient temperatures,[6] when sunbathing or when using an external heat source (e.g. electric blanket, hot water bottle, heat/tanning lamp, sauna, hot tub). For **buprenorphine** and **fentanyl**, this has resulted in fatal overdoses.

Note. Patients may swim or shower with a patch, but should avoid soaking in a hot bath.

TD patches and MRI

National and specialty guidance advises that patches known to contain or possibly contain metal and/or affected by heat should be removed before the patient enters the scan room and replaced afterwards.[7,8] Patients should be advised to bring a replacement patch with them to facilitate this.

The two main risks from wearing TD patches during MRI are skin burns and drug toxicity (Box A).

Although some patches are safe, confirmation of this is difficult because:

- the SPC may not contain comprehensive information on excipients
- limited testing means that manufacturers are generally unwilling to comment on patch safety during MRI
- visual inspection of a patch to see if it contains metal can be deceptive; clear patches may contain metal ions.[10]

Because of these difficulties and recent guidance,[7,8] most MRI units have a policy of removing all TD patches before MRI.

Box A Risks from wearing TD patches during MRI

Direct contact burn to the skin underneath the TD patch

Some patches contain metal:

- in the backing, e.g. aluminium (Hapoctasin®) *or*
- as metal salts in other parts of the patch, e.g. aluminium acetylacetonate in the adhesive layer (BuTrans®, Transtec®).

The magnetic field from the scanner heats up the metal, and burns have been reported to the MHRA and FDA.[7,9]

Drug toxicity due to increase in body temperature ± direct heating

As well as heating up the patch, MRI can also increase body temperature via the absorption of energy from the magnetic field. Generally, the increase in body temperature is limited to 0.5–1°C, depending on the type of scan. However, for certain applications with small or surface coils, local temperature can rise to ≤39°C for the trunk and ≤40°C for limbs. Increased absorption can lead to a serious overdose for buprenorphine or fentanyl patches.[4,7,8]

Use of TD patches

Prescribing

TD **buprenorphine** and TD **fentanyl** are available for analgesia. Their use is summarized in the respective individual monographs (see p.428 and p.440) and Quick Clinical Guides (see p.438 and p.448).

Further information on dose conversion ratios from PO opioids to TD **buprenorphine** and **fentanyl** can also be found in Appendix 2, p.925.

For **buprenorphine** and **fentanyl** patches, various branded and generic products are available. As well as differences in appearance, there are also differences between products in the length of time the patch should be applied. Prescribing by brand is recommended to avoid confusion.[1]

Application and disposal

Under *no* circumstances should a *reservoir* patch be cut in an attempt to reduce the dose. Leakage from the cut reservoir could result in either the patient receiving minimal or no drug or an overdose from the rapid absorption of drug through the surrounding skin.

PCF does not generally recommend cutting *matrix* patches, because of similar concerns. The increased range of available strengths has made the need for this less likely. However, in a few situations it may be necessary, e.g. when using **hyoscine *hydrobromide*** patches in children.[11]

Patches should be inspected before application and not used if they are damaged in any way. A new site of application should be used each time a patch is changed. Application should be to dry, non-inflamed, non-irradiated, clean, hairless skin on the upper trunk or arm (unless otherwise specified in the SPC; e.g. **hyoscine *hydrobromide*** patches are applied behind the ear), avoiding areas with large scars.

Application to the upper back may be preferable in a confused patient, to reduce the risk of unintended patch removal.

Body hair may be clipped with scissors (*not* shaved). If the skin is washed beforehand, only water should be used; soap, oils, creams or ointments should *not* be applied, because they may interfere with drug absorption. The patch should be pressed firmly in place for at least 30 seconds; adhesive tape (e.g. Micropore®) can be applied to the edges to aid adherence. The date of application and/or date of renewal should be written on the patch, if possible. When necessary, more than one patch can be applied to the same area of the body, as long as the edges do not touch.

Careful removal of the patch helps to minimize local skin irritation. It should be noted that used patches still contain some drug and must be disposed of carefully. Patches should be folded in half with the adhesive side inwards and discarded in a sharps container (hospital) or a dustbin (home), and hands washed. In hospital, disposal of controlled drugs should be witnessed and documented.

For patients undergoing MRI, adequate arrangements should be in place for safe disposal of the removed patches, particularly controlled drugs. Rescue medication should be available (where necessary) and a new patch applied as soon as possible after the scan.

Monitoring

Monitoring is essential to ensure:

- the patches remain firmly attached to the skin to prevent loss of efficacy
- old patches are removed before new patches are applied
- re-application to the same area of skin is avoided for the necessary duration (see SPC); some inpatient units use body maps to facilitate site rotation.

The date and time the patch was applied, the strength, brand, number of patches and the site of application should be recorded and monitored at least twice daily. The date and time of removal and destruction should also be recorded.

For strong opioids, palliativedrugs.com has developed a specific TD patch monitoring chart, which can be downloaded from the Document library (Topic: Pain, Strong opioids).

1 Care Quality Commission and NHS England (2013) Safer use of controlled drugs — preventing harms from fentanyl and buprenorphine transdermal patches. *Use of controlled drugs supporting information*. www.cqc.org.uk (archived).
2 Health Canada (2008) Fentanyl transdermal patch and fatal adverse reactions. *Canadian Adverse Reaction Newsletter*. **18(3)**: 1–2.
3 FDA (2015) Fentanyl transdermal system (marketed as Duragesic) information. *Post Market Drug Safety Information for Patients and Providers*. www.fda.gov/drugs/drug-safety-and-availability
4 MHRA (2008) Fentanyl patches: serious and fatal overdose from dosing errors, accidental exposure, and inappropriate use. *Drug Safety Update*. www.gov.uk/drug-safety-update
5 Jumbelic MI (2010) Deaths with transdermal fentanyl patches. *American Journal of Forensic Medicine and Pathology*. **31**: 18–21.
6 Sindali K *et al.* (2012) Life-threatening coma and full-thickness sunburn in a patient treated with transdermal fentanyl patches: a case report. *Journal of Medical Case Reports*. **6**: 220.
7 MHRA (2015) Safety guidelines for magnetic resonance imaging equipment in clinical use. www.gov.uk
8 Society of Radiographers (2019) Safety in magnetic resonance imaging. www.sor.org
9 Kantorovich A (2016) Transdermal patches that must be removed before MRI. *Pharmacy Times*. www.pharmacytimes.com
10 Anderton D and Cary P (2009) Medicated patches and MRI imaging — a burning issue. Poster presentation 20. *35th UKMI Practice Development Seminar*.
11 Jassal S and Aindow A (2017) *APPM Master Formulary*, 4th edn. Association of Paediatric Palliative Medicine. www.appm.org.uk

Updated October 2019

31: NEBULIZED DRUGS

Nebulizers are used in asthma and COPD for both acute exacerbations and long-term prophylaxis (see Bronchodilators, p.121).[1-3] Other uses include the pulmonary delivery of antimicrobial drugs for cystic fibrosis, bronchiectasis and AIDS-related pneumonia. For the supplementary role of nebulized bronchodilators in anaphylaxis, see Appendix 1, Box C, p.922.

Nebulizers are also used in palliative care (see below). The aim is to deliver a therapeutic dose of a drug as an aerosol in particles small enough to be inspired within 5–10min. A nebulizer is preferable to a hand-held inhaler when:

- a large drug dose is needed
- co-ordinated breathing is difficult
- pressurized metered-dose inhaler (pMDI) + a spacer is ineffective
- a drug is unavailable in an inhaler.

In these circumstances, by improving drug delivery, a nebulizer can result in better symptom relief.[4] However, nebulizers are noisy, more expensive and less convenient than hand-held inhalers; they are also ineffective in patients with shallow breathing and in those unable to sit up to at least 45°, i.e. semi-upright or more. The higher doses administered can also increase the risk of undesirable effects, and their use should be carefully monitored to ensure ongoing efficacy and tolerability.

Commonly used nebulizers are:

Jet: the aerosol is generated by a flow of gas from, e.g., an electrical compressor or piped air. At least 50% of the aerosol produced at the recommended driving gas flow should be particles small enough to inhale.

Ultrasonic: the aerosol is generated by ultrasonic vibrations of a piezo-electric crystal.

Aerosol output (the mass of particles in aerosol form produced/min) is not necessarily the same as drug output (the mass of drug produced/min as an aerosol). Ideally, the drug output of a nebulizer should be known for each of the different drugs given. Various factors affect the drug output and deposition:

- gas flow rate; the optimum is 6–8L/min of air or oxygen (see below)
- chamber design
- volume (commonly 2–2.5mL, up to 4mL)
- residual volume (commonly 0.5mL)
- physical properties of the drug in solution
- breathing pattern of the patient.

The choice of gas can be crucial. Air via an electrical compressor or piped air is generally used, and *always* in a patient at risk of hypercapnia; if they are dependent on low concentration oxygen, give this simultaneously via a nasal cannula. Oxygen is *always* used when treating acute asthma, delivered via piped oxygen or a large oxygen cylinder.

The choice of nebulizer can also be crucial, particularly when trying to produce an aerosol small enough to deliver a drug to the alveoli. Services that provide nebulizers will generally offer information, education and support for patients and their families (Box A). Information should include:

- a description of the equipment and its use
- drugs used, doses and frequencies
- equipment maintenance/cleaning
- action to take if treatment becomes less effective
- action to take and emergency telephone number to use if equipment breaks down.

Patients should be instructed to take steady normal breaths (interspersed with occasional deep ones), and nebulization time should be less than 10min or 'to dryness'. Because there is always a residual volume, 'dryness' should be taken as 1min after spluttering starts.

Whereas a mask can be used for bronchodilators, *a mouthpiece should generally be used for other drugs, to limit environmental contamination and/or contact with the patient's eyes.* However, a mask may be preferable in patients who are acutely ill, fatigued or very young, regardless of the nature of the drug. Patients' nebulizer technique should be checked periodically.[5]

Nebulizers can also be used in patients with long-term tracheostomies (via a tracheostomy mask or T-piece circuit) or receiving non-invasive ventilation (via the ventilator tubing). However, for patients not completely dependent on non-invasive ventilation, nebulized bronchodilators are more effective when given during breaks from ventilation.[6]

Portable battery-operated nebulizers may be used in aircraft at the discretion of the cabin crew, but the airline must be notified in advance (also see Oxygen, p.144). The British Lung Foundation (03000 030 555) can provide patients with travel advice.

Although nebulizers and electrical compressors are generally not available on the NHS (but are VAT free), many respiratory services do loan equipment, including that suitable for travel.

Box A Example advice about using a nebulizer at home

To help your breathing, your doctor has prescribed a drug to be used with a nebulizer. The nebulizer converts the drug into a fine mist which you inhale.

The apparatus

Your nebulizer system consists of the following parts:

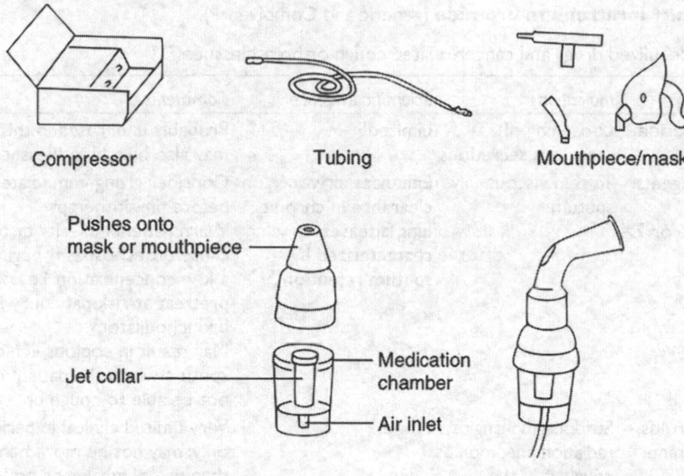

The compressor is the portable pump which pumps air along the tubing into the nebulizer. The nebulizer is a small chamber for the liquid medicine, through which air is blown to make a mist.

The nebulizer has a screw-on top onto which the mask or mouthpiece is attached.

How to use your nebulizer

Place the medication in the nebulizer, replace the screw-on top and turn the compressor on. Inhale by mouthpiece or mask while breathing at a normal rate. Stop 1 minute after the nebulizer contents start spluttering or after a maximum of 10 minutes.

General advice

If you have a cough, the nebulizer may help you to expectorate, so have some tissues nearby.

You may wish to use the nebulizer before attempting an activity which makes you feel out of breath.

If the effects of the nebulizer wear off or you have any questions or concerns about it, please speak to your doctor or nurse.

Cleaning

Wash the mouthpiece/mask and nebulizer in warm water and detergent, then rinse and dry well. Ideally this should be done after every use, but *once a day as a minimum*. Attach the tube and run the nebulizer empty for a few moments after cleaning it to make sure the equipment is dry. Once a week, unplug and wipe the compressor and tubing with a damp cloth.

Nebulizers in palliative care

For the use of nebulized **tranexamic acid** in haemoptysis, see Haemostatics, p.114.

Various drugs have been given by nebulizer to ease cough and breathlessness in advanced cancer (Table 1 and Table 2). However, apart from the use of bronchodilators for reversible airflow obstruction, there is often little evidence to support their use. Thus, some are *not* recommended by *PCF* for routine use (Table 1). The remainder should be considered only when other avenues have failed (Table 2) and reviewed after 2 days to check effectiveness.

In patients with asthma, when using **lidocaine** or **bupivacaine** for a dry cough (not recommended for breathlessness), consider pretreating with **salbutamol** because of the risk of initial bronchospasm.[7] After nebulized local anaesthetic, patients should be advised not to eat or drink for 1h, because the reduced gag/cough reflex increases the risk of aspiration (also see Antitussives, p.158).

Because of lack of data about physico-chemical compatibility and aerodynamic properties, manufacturers generally do not recommend mixing nebulizer solutions. Further, when mixing products in this way, the combination is considered an unauthorized product (see Chapter 24, Box A, p.817). However, some ready-mixed combinations are commercially available, e.g. **salbutamol + ipratropium bromide** (generic and Combivent®).

Table 1 Nebulized drugs and cancer-related cough or breathlessness[2,14]

Class of drug[a]	*Indications*	*Scientific evidence*	*Comments*
Sodium chloride 0.9%	Loosening of tenacious secretions	Limited[15]	Probably underused in this setting; may also help breathlessness
Mucolytic agents, e.g. sodium chloride 3% or 7%	To thin viscous sputum	Enhances airway clearance in chronic lung diseases characterized by sputum retention[16,17]	Consider giving immediately before physiotherapy Warn patients of salty taste. May cause bronchospasm; begin with a low concentration, i.e. 3% and pretreat at-risk patients with a bronchodilator[16] May result in copious liquid sputum which the patient may still not be able to cough up
Corticosteroids, e.g. budesonide	Stridor, lymphangitis, radiation pneumonitis, cough after the insertion of a stent	None	Very limited clinical experience only; may not be more beneficial than use of inhaler or oral routes
†Local anaesthetics, e.g. lidocaine, bupivacaine	Cough, particularly if caused by lymphangitis carcinomatosa	Conflicting evidence for both breathlessness[18,19] and cough[20]	May cause bronchospasm; consider pretreating at-risk patients with a bronchodilator.[20] Reduces gag reflex; risk of aspiration immediately after treatment
†Opioids, e.g. morphine, fentanyl	Breathlessness associated with diffuse lung disease	Despite anecdotal reports of benefit, the evidence does not support routine use[21]	Not recommended; risk of bronchospasm
Bronchodilators, e.g. salbutamol	Treatment of severe reversible airway obstruction	Extrapolated from patients with asthma and COPD	Try pMDI + spacer first.[22,23] Use nebulizers only if trial of therapy shows real benefit
†Furosemide	Breathlessness	Despite anecdotal reports of benefit, the evidence does not support routine use (see Furosemide, p.67)	Not recommended

a. a mask can be used for bronchodilators; a mouthpiece should be used for all other drugs to limit environmental contamination and/or contact with the patient's eyes. However, a mask may be unavoidable in those incapable of using a mouthpiece, e.g. when acutely ill, fatigued or very young.

Table 2 Recommended uses of nebulized drugs in palliative care

Indication	*Drug*	*Initial regimen*	*Dose titration*	*Comments*
Tenacious secretions	Sodium chloride 0.9%	5mL p.r.n.	Up to q2h	
	Sodium chloride 3%	4mL p.r.n.	Up to q.d.s.	Risk of bronchospasm
	Sodium Chloride 7%	4mL p.r.n.	Up to b.d.	
Reversible airway obstruction	Salbutamol	2.5mg q4–6h	Up to 5mg q4h	Risk of sensitivity to cardiac stimulant effects
Cough	*†Lidocaine 2%	5mL p.r.n.	Up to q.d.s.	Risk of bronchospasm
	*†Bupivacaine 0.25%	5mL p.r.n.	Up to q.d.s.	Loss of gag reflex; nil by mouth for 1h after nebulization

There are limited data indicating that 2-drug mixtures comprising one drug from any two of the classes below will be physically and/or chemically compatible (for all strengths):

- *β_2-adrenergic receptor agonists (β_2 agonists):* **salbutamol** or **terbutaline** (Bricanyl®)
- *antimuscarinic:* **ipratropium bromide**
- *corticosteroids:* **budesonide** (Pulmicort®) or **fluticasone** (Flixotide®).[8-13]

Solutions should be mixed immediately before use, using aseptic technique. If the colour changes or cloudiness/precipitation occurs, the mixture should be discarded. If dilution is necessary, sterile sodium chloride 0.9% is generally best. There is no information on 3-drug mixtures, and these cannot be recommended.

1 The Nebulizer Project Group of the British Thoracic Society Standards of Care Committee (1997) Current best practice for nebuliser treatment. *Thorax.* **52 (Suppl 2)**: S1–3.

2 European Respiratory Society (2001) Guidelines on the use of nebulizers. *European Respiratory Journal.* **18**: 228–242.

3 NICE (2018) Chronic obstructive pulmonary disease in over 16s: diagnosis and management. *Clinical Guideline.* NG115. Updated July 2019. www.nice.org.uk

4 Tashkin DP *et al.* (2007) Comparing COPD treatment: nebulizer, metered dose inhaler, and concomitant therapy. *American Journal of Medicine.* **120**: 435–441.

5 Ari A and Restrepo RD (2012) Aerosol delivery device selection for spontaneously breathing patients: 2012. *Respiratory Care.* **57**: 613–626.

6 Davidson AC *et al.* (2016) BTS/ICS guideline for the ventilatory management of acute hypercapnic respiratory failure in adults. *Thorax.* **71 (Suppl 2)**: ii1–35.

7 Slaton RM *et al.* (2013) Evidence for therapeutic uses of nebulized lidocaine in the treatment of intractable cough and asthma. *Annals of Pharmacotherpy.* **47**: 578–585.

8 Roberts G and Rossi S (1993) Compatibility of nebuliser solutions. *Australian Journal of Hospital Pharmacy.* **23**: 35–37.

9 McKenzie JE and Cruz-Rivera M (2004) Compatibility of budesonide inhalation suspension with four nebulizing solutions. *Annals of Pharmacotherapy.* **38**: 967–972.

10 Burchett DK *et al.* (2010) Mixing and compatibility guide for commonly used aerosolized medications. *American Journal of Health System Pharmacy.* **67**: 227–230.

11 Joseph JC (1997) Compatibility of nebulizer solution admixtures. *Annals of Pharmacotherapy.* **31**: 487–489.

12 Harriman A-M *et al.* (1996) Can we mix nebuliser solutions? Stability of drug admixtures in solutions for nebulisation. *Pharmacy in Practice.* 347–348.

13 UK Medicines Information (2018) Which commonly used nebuliser solutions are compatible? *Medicines Q&A.* www.evidence.nhs.uk

14 Ahmedzai S and Davis C (1997) Nebulised drugs in palliative care. *Thorax.* **52 (Suppl 2)**: s75–77.

15 Tarrant BJ *et al.* (2017) Mucoactive agents for chronic, non-cystic fibrosis lung disease: a systematic review and meta-analysis. *Respirology.* **22**: 1084–1092.

16 Hill AT *et al.* (2019) British Thoracic Society Guideline for bronchiectasis in adults. *Thorax.* **74 (Suppl 1)**: 1–69.

17 Wark P and McDonald VM (2018) Nebulised hypertonic saline for cystic fibrosis. *Cochrane Database of Systematic Reviews.* **9**: CD001506. www.thecochranelibrary.com

18 Winning A *et al.* (1988) Ventilation and breathlessness on maximal exercise in patients with interstitial lung disease after local anaesthetic aerosol inhalation. *Clinical Science.* **74**: 275–281.

19 Wilcock A *et al.* (1994) Safety and efficacy of nebulized lignocaine in patients with cancer and breathlessness. *Palliative Medicine.* **8**: 35–38.

20 Slaton RM *et al.* (2013) Evidence for therapeutic uses of nebulized lidocaine in the treatment of intractable cough and asthma. *Annals of Pharmacotherapy.* **47**: 578-585.

21 Barnes H *et al.* (2016) Opioids for the palliation of refractory breathlessness in adults with advanced disease and terminal illness. *Cochrane Database of Systematic Reviews.* **3**: CD011008. www.thecochranelibrary.com

22 Congleton J and Muers MF (1995) The incidence of airflow obstruction in bronchial carcinoma, its relation to breathlessness, and response to bronchodilator therapy. *Respiratory Medicine.* **89**: 291–296.

23 Colacone A *et al.* (1993) A comparison of albuterol administered by metered dose inhaler (and holding chamber) or wet nebulizer in acute asthma. *Chest.* **104**: 835–841.

Updated November 2019

32: SPINAL ANALGESIA

INDICATIONS

Spinal analgesia is used extensively for obstetric or peri-operative pain relief, but is uncommon in palliative care.[1] Only 2–4% of cancer patients receiving specialist palliative care proceed to spinal analgesia because of inadequate relief with systemic analgesia.[2,3] Spinal analgesia is effective in >50% of patients. Good communication between the palliative care, pain and primary care teams is essential. Typical indications for spinal analgesia include:

- systemic opioid intolerance (an unacceptable balance between efficacy and toxicity)
- refractory neuropathic pain (e.g. lumbosacral plexopathy, visceral neuropathic pain)
- refractory nociceptive pain from progressive tumour or bone metastases.

The aim is to provide optimum pain relief in a patient with a short life expectancy. Rapid disease progression and a changing pain picture is typical, and the combination of drugs used and/or their doses may need to be changed frequently.[4]

CONTRA-INDICATIONS

Uncorrected coagulopathy, systemic or local infection, and raised intracranial pressure. Extra caution is necessary with:

- spinal deformity
- incipient spinal cord compression
- myelosuppressive chemotherapy
- intracranial metastases.

ROUTE, PLACEMENT AND DELIVERY DEVICE CONSIDERATIONS

Before insertion of a spinal catheter, baseline blood tests help to evaluate renal, hepatic, bone marrow and metabolic function and exclude coagulopathies and any significant infection. Neurological and cardiopulmonary examination provide a baseline for future reference, and a spinal MRI provides useful anatomical information.

A shared decision to proceed with an intervention should be based on an individualized assessment of the risks and benefits and a discussion involving the patient, carers and wider multidisciplinary team.

Clinical services caring for patients receiving spinal analgesia need clear procedures to be in place to minimize risk at all stages of treatment. Maintaining the necessary level of competence is challenging when such approaches are used infrequently.[5] Guidelines and refresher training are both important.

Analgesics are delivered to the intrathecal (IT) or epidural (ED) space via an indwelling catheter placed by an anaesthetist (or spinal or neurosurgeon in some centres). Options include:

- 'blind' (without radiological screening) sited catheters
- catheters tunnelled subcutaneously away from the spine
- fully implanted systems (IT only).

Tunnelled and fully implanted systems reduce the risk of displacement and infection. Fluoroscopically screened catheter placement ensures drug placement at the optimal dermatome level. Simple placement under local anaesthetic, without tunnelling or radiological screening, can be satisfactory for external pumps.

The preferred route and delivery device are influenced by local custom and the likely duration of use (Table 1). Although ED catheters are sometimes left in place for several months, the preferred route is IT for spinal analgesia expected to be needed for more than a few weeks. Devices vary in relation to fixed vs. variable delivery rates, patient-controlled boluses, and cost.

Table 1 Suggested route and delivery device

Likely duration of use	*Route and device*	*Comments*
≤3 weeks	External ED device (re-usable)	Fewer initial complications than IT (8% vs. 25%); less headache from CSF leakage[6]
3 weeks–3 months	External IT device (re-usable)	Fewer later complications than ED (5% vs. 55%); less catheter occlusion or migration[6]
≥3 months	Implantable IT device	More expensive initially, lower running costs; more cost-effective long-term

There is a relative underuse of implanted IT pumps in the UK, in part because availability is limited to a few regional centres.[7] There will be at least one responsible treating physician at each centre, with 24h access to advice and a clear plan for emergency admissions. *Inexperienced staff should never make significant changes to a patient's infusion without advice and support from a senior experienced clinician.*

Opioids administered IT act locally on opioid receptors in the superficial laminae of the dorsal horn of the spinal cord. Thus, compared with the ED route, lower doses are needed, e.g. a woman having a caesarean section might be given ED **diamorphine** 3mg compared with IT 300microgram. Smaller doses permit the use of smaller devices and/or reducing the frequency of refilling (see below). IT administration generally also provides better pain relief than the ED route.

For *implanted IT systems*, because of the slow infusion rate and the tiny volumes used, drugs delivered into the CSF do *not* diffuse rostrally to the brain stem, whether given by infusion or as a bolus. CSF flow is pulsatile with oscillatory displacements, but no net bulk flow.[8-10] CSF samples from points progressively further away from the catheter tip demonstrate a steeply reducing concentration gradient for **morphine**.[11]

Studies of porcine IT drug delivery (ITDD) using **bupivacaine** at rates reflecting human implanted ITDD (20–1,000microL/h, and boluses of 1,000microL over 5min every hour) also showed that most of the drug is recovered <1cm from the site of administration.[12] Drug diffusion within the spinal cord parenchyma was higher with boluses and with higher rates of infusion.[13]

Thus, the area of analgesia is completely dependent on the site of the catheter, which must be at or above the dermatomal level of the patient's pain and posterior in the spinal canal. For bilateral pain, it is best positioned in the midline and, for unilateral pain, slightly to the same side as the pain.

On the other hand, IT drugs from an *external pump* use high volumes and infusion rates, and there is more potential for rostral spread in the CSF. Additional rostral and caudal areas of pain can be covered, and a blindly sited catheter (without fluoroscopy) can be effective.

In contrast, drugs administered as a single IT *bolus* as part of an anaesthetic technique involve relatively large volumes and forces of injection, and often barbotage, to facilitate drug spread either rostrally or caudally. The fluid mechanics here are completely different from those at work in an implanted system. On occasion, opioids have reached the brain stem with consequent adverse effects (see Undesirable effects). However, this does *not* happen with implanted systems, even at the maximum rate of infusion. *For a SynchroMed® II pump, this is 1mL/h compared with an anaesthetic bolus of up to 3.5mL in a few seconds.*

Drugs delivered to the ED space must diffuse through the meninges in order to reach the spinal cord and adjacent nerve roots. The level of the spinal cord at which the catheter is sited determines the area over which maximal analgesia is obtained. Because an ED dose is much higher than an IT one, migration or misplacement of ED catheters into the IT space (a rare event) will deliver an excessive dose resulting in significant toxicity, including potentially respiratory arrest and death; thus it must be recognized and treated urgently.

Although, theoretically, the same delivery devices can be used for SC, IV and spinal infusion, the use of a device specifically designed for spinal delivery is recommended. Further, following accidental wrong route administration of drugs, e.g. IT/ED instead of IV and vice versa, a dedicated NRFit™ connector, incompatible with Luer connectors, is recommended for IT, ED and regional block devices.[14,15] Distinct pumps and connectors will reduce the potential for confusion in a patient receiving concurrent spinal and SC/IV infusions. However, such recommendations must be weighed against the considerable advantage of staff using a delivery device with which they are familiar from frequent SC/IV use.

BOLUS VS. CONTINUOUS INFUSION

Bolus-based regimens are best for break-through pain, and pain not responsive to opioids. Most implanted IT pumps for cancer pain will contain both an opioid and a local anaesthetic. The development of tolerance seen with *continuous* infusions is delayed or prevented by a bolus-based regimen.

Personal Therapy Manager®

This is a hand-held device for a patient to self-administer boluses from the Medtronic SynchroMed® II pump (the only implanted pump currently available with this facility). It can be used for opioid, local anaesthetic and mixed regimens. The device is wirelessly linked to the pump, i.e. it will work only with the pump to which it was first bonded. The physician programmes the pump, detailing the dose of the primary drug, the duration of the infusion, the lock-out interval and the maximum activations/24h.

CHOICE OF DRUGS FOR IT USE

Parenteral formulations of the same drug vary between manufacturers, and it is essential to confirm that a specific brand is suitable for IT use. This requires the formulation to meet a more stringent endotoxin limit and it must *not*:

- be irritant or toxic to the CNS
- contain anti-microbial preservatives
- be at extremes of pH or osmotic strength
- contain other excipients unless accepted for IT use, e.g. some pH adjusters.

For some drugs, no commercially available formulations are suitable, and unauthorized products for IT administration have to be obtained via special order (see Chapter 24, p.817). Seek specialist pharmacist advice.

Opioids (**morphine** or **hydromorphone** for implanted IT pumps and the option of **diamorphine** for external systems), local anaesthetics (**bupivacaine**) and α_2 agonists (**clonidine**) are the most commonly used drugs. A solo opioid infusion may be appropriate for someone with stable pain, e.g. from stable bone metastases, but *most patients with progressive cancer pain need either a combination of drugs or a local anaesthetic alone.*

Health professionals and pharmacists should familiarize themselves with the guidance and supporting material about the legal implications of mixing medicines before administration,[16,17] together with any local policy and practice.

In the UK, specific brands of **baclofen**, **bupivacaine**, **levobupivacaine** and **ziconotide** are authorized for IT use. Other drugs are used off-label in accordance with the recommendations of the Polyanalgesic Consensus Conference (PACC).[3] It is essential that the parenteral formulation of the drug used is suitable for IT administration (see above).

Because each patient's complex pain is different, drug regimens have to be individualized. There is little or no place for predetermined (slow-moving) algorithms. For example, to manage worsening pain, a previously stable continuous opioid infusion may need to be up-titrated (± the addition of **clonidine**), followed by a decision to add in or switch to **bupivacaine**, with a low background infusion and boluses for break-through pain.

For opioid-naïve patients, recommended IT starting doses are shown in Table 2. Recommended maximum opioid concentrations and daily doses are shown in Table 3. The maximum opioid doses aim to minimize the risk of catheter tip granuloma formation (see p.916); this is less relevant with relatively short-term use, although granulomas have been reported after 4 weeks.[18]

Table 2 Opioid-naïve patients: recommended IT starting doses[3]

Drug	*Starting doses/24h*
Bupivacaine	10microgram–4mg
Clonidine	20–100microgram
Hydromorphone	10–150microgram
Morphine	100–500microgram
Ziconotide	0.5–1.2microgram

Table 3 Recommended maximum IT concentrations and doses[3]

Drug	*Maximum concentration (mg/mL)*	*Maximum daily dose (mg)*
Bupivacaine	30[a]	15–20[a]
Clonidine	1	600*microgram*
Hydromorphone	15	10
Morphine	20	15
Ziconotide	100*microgram/mL*	19.2*microgram*

a. may be exceeded in end-of-life care and in complicated cases.

Opioids

In the UK, **morphine**, **hydromorphone** and **diamorphine** are widely used, the latter because of its solubility and lack of preservatives. However, because of a risk of precipitation, **diamorphine** should *not* be used in Medtronic SynchroMed® pumps (see Drug Compatibility, below), but can be used in Flowonix Prometra® pumps.

The advantages of IT administration are greatest with hydrophilic opioids, e.g. **diamorphine**, **morphine** and **hydromorphone**, because they remain for longer in the CSF.[19] In contrast, **fentanyl** is highly lipid-soluble and has minimal effect at the spinal cord level because it is rapidly absorbed and redistributed systemically. Thus, spinal administration has no advantages over systemic use, and should be discouraged.[19]

There is much uncertainty about dose equivalents between routes. Most centres have their own conversion tables based on the oral morphine equivalent (OME) dose in mg/24h, which is then converted to an IT dose.

Experience at one centre suggests, for example, that an appropriate starting dose for someone who has been receiving:

- OME 300mg/24h is about IT **morphine** 1mg/24h
- OME 200mg/24h is about IT **hydromorphone** 1mg/24h.[4]

Note. These are recommended *starting doses* and should *not* be confused with 'equivalent doses' recommended when switching PO to SC/IV or vice versa (see Appendix 2, p.925).

Local anaesthetics

Bupivacaine is the most widely used local anaesthetic for spinal analgesia. It has inherent bactericidal properties, which theoretically reduces the risk of infection. Alternatives include **levobupivacaine**. Motor weakness can be a limiting undesirable effect; predisposing factors include pre-existing neurological damage.

Self-administered boluses of **bupivacaine** IT using a Personal Therapy Manager® can be particularly effective for progressive cancer pain. The maximum bolus dose is 20mg, but doses as little as 0.5–2mg may be effective.

The motor and sensory changes can be predicted according to the level of the catheter. For example, a bolus through a catheter sited at:

- S2 (the bottom of the dural sac): will cause perineal and buttock numbness, but is unlikely to cause leg weakness
- T12: leg weakness is expected
- T6: there may be some leg weakness, but not as profound as at T12
- T4 (or thereabouts): may affect cardiac nerves, with resultant bradycardia and hypotension (opioids can also do this).

Hypotension can occur with both infusions and boluses, and relates to vasodilation caused by the drug's impact on the sympathetic nervous system. It is more likely:

- with higher catheters (above the lumbar sympathetic chain at L2–4)
- with higher bolus doses (e.g. 5–20mg)
- if the patient is septic, hypovolaemic or generally unwell.

The patient should be sitting or lying and monitored when they first use the bolus facility. Downward dose adjustments may be necessary during episodes of infection, sepsis, bleeding and hypovolaemia.

Numbness and weakness can last for ≤3h, but there is generally a period of usable pain-free time after that before the local anaesthetic wears off altogether. It is possible to adjust doses and duration of infusion to a certain extent in an attempt to reduce undesirable effects. However, often numbness = pain relief, and the patient has to learn to time their boluses to minimize functional limitations.

A starting bolus dose would be **bupivacaine** 1–2mg IT, which can be given by the single bolus facility on the pump and, depending on the response, can be titrated up or down. This dose is unlikely to cause any cardiovascular effect or profound numbness or weakness, although it can significantly augment pre-existing weakness in the frail.

α-Adrenergic receptor agonists

IT **clonidine** (typical regimen 50–150microgram/24h) is generally given concurrently with an opioid and a local anaesthetic. Because of systemic absorption, there is a dose-dependent risk of hypotension and bradycardia (see p.82).[2]

Benefit is seen particularly in neuropathic pain. Abrupt cessation (e.g. because of pump failure) may cause severe rebound hypertension. Administer oral **clonidine** while seeking specialist advice.

Ziconotide

Ziconotide is an intrathecal calcium channel blocker, acting on presynaptic N-type calcium channels in the dorsal horn of the spinal cord.[20,21] Consequently, it is useful for opioid-tolerant patients. It is recommended as first-line therapy for both nociceptive and neuropathic pain, and there is good evidence to support its use in cancer pain.[22,23] It is a big, highly ionized protein molecule and, unlike the other spinally applied drugs, distributes widely throughout central neural tissue independent of the site of the catheter.

However, undesirable effects are common, and can be both dose- and treatment-limiting. Thus, in practice, a slow titration schedule is used, with increases ranging from 0.5–1.2microgram/day *every 1–2 weeks* or longer. Consequently, it may take several months to reach an effective dose. **Ziconotide** is only available in the UK with an authorized individual funding request.

Other drugs

Ketamine is a non-competitive NMDA-receptor-channel blocker (see p.691), but has been shown to be neurotoxic in both animal IT infusion models and in humans.[24,25] Nonetheless, it may have a role if all else has failed in the last days–weeks of life, although sourcing a suitable product for IT use may be difficult.

A **baclofen** (p.658) product is authorized for IT use for spasticity, but not for pain. The spinal use of several other drugs has been reported, but are not recommended either because of toxicity (e.g. **dexmedetomidine, droperidol, methadone, methylprednisolone, midazolam, ondansetron, pethidine, tramadol, tetracaine**) or inefficacy (e.g. **gabapentin, octreotide, ropivacaine**).

DRUG COMPATIBILITY

Combinations of **morphine** or **diamorphine** with **bupivacaine ± clonidine** are widely used, particularly with external devices. Long-term compatibility data for drug combinations in both external devices (at room temperature) and implanted pump reservoirs (at body temperature) are limited.[2] Several factors can affect drug stability and compatibility (see Chapter 29, Box B, p.891). It is important to check with a pharmacist that the compatibility data are relevant to spinal use, and to confirm the appropriate diluent.

When mixing drugs for long periods it is important to consider the material the delivery device is made of, because this can affect drug stability; e.g. **diamorphine** should not be used in SynchroMed® pumps, because of reports of precipitation.

Compatibility data at room temperature

There are compatibility data on the following combinations at *room temperature*:

- **diamorphine** with **bupivacaine**, 4 weeks[26]
- **morphine sulfate** with **bupivacaine** or **clonidine**, 2 months[27,28]
- **hydromorphone** with **bupivacaine**, 3 days[29]
- **clonidine** with **bupivacaine**, 2 weeks.[30]

Compatibility data at body temperature

There are compatibility data on the following combinations at *body temperature*:

- **morphine sulfate** with **clonidine ± bupivacaine**, ≤3 months in a SynchroMed® pump[31,32]
- **hydromorphone**, 4 months in a SynchroMed® pump[33]
- **clonidine** with **hydromorphone**, 1.5 months (only **clonidine** evaluated).[34]

Delivery devices with mixtures for administration over >24h should be prepared in a sterile environment, e.g. a licensed pharmacy. Drugs should be preservative-free.[2]

UNDESIRABLE EFFECTS AND COMPLICATIONS OF SPINAL ANALGESIA

These relate to:

- the drugs (Table 4)
- medical complications, e.g. bleeding, infection (Table 5)
- the delivery system (Table 5).[35]

Respiratory failure is either the result of central depression of respiratory drive (opioids) or impaired motor output to the respiratory muscles at the spinal level (**bupivacaine**). Rate of onset varies: systemic redistribution of the spinally administered opioid causes respiratory depression within minutes or hours, whereas diffusion through the CSF causes delayed onset, occurring after 6–48h.

Table 4 Drug-related undesirable effects

Drug	*Undesirable effect*	*Comment*
Withdrawal of systemic opioids	Diarrhoea and intestinal colic	Partly avoidable if laxatives stopped and then re-titrated after switch to spinal route
Opioids	Nausea and vomiting	Uncommon in patients previously on systemic opioids
Opioids	Pruritus	Rare when given to patients who are switching from systemic opioids, and when spinal opioid combined with bupivacaine
Bupivacaine	Motor or sensory disturbance; dose-dependent	Persistent motor impairment 5–10%
Opioids, bupivacaine	Urinary retention	Removal of the urinary catheter after 3–4 days is successful in most patients; if persistent, may relate to underlying pathology
Opioids, bupivacaine	Respiratory depression	Rare
Opioids, bupivacaine, clonidine	Hypotension	Site dependent, see text. Clonidine also causes bradycardia
Opioids[a]	Catheter tip granulomas	Seen in about 3% of long-term IT infusions; mostly asymptomatic;[36] more common with ED infusions
Opioids	Decreased libido ± disturbed menstruation	Seen in most patients with IT opioids given for >1 year, but can occur sooner.[37] Measure testosterone and LH at baseline and annually in men; estradiol, progesterone, LH, FSH in women[2]
Opioids	Hypocorticalism or growth hormone deficiency	Seen in about 15%[37]
Opioids	Oedema	Common; possibly 10–20%
Opioids	Immunomodulation	Frequency and significance uncertain. May be more pronounced with systemic opioids[38]

a. less common with non-opioids.

Table 5 Non-drug complications of spinal analgesia[39]

Undesirable effect	*Comment*
Traumatic catheter placement	
CSF leakage headache	Uncommon
ED haematoma	Rare
Neurological tissue damage	Rare
Infection[40]	
Exit site infection	Occasional
ED abscess	Occasional
Meningitis	Occasional
Delivery system	
Device-related complications	E.g. catheter-related (fracture, kinking, displacement or withdrawal); pump failure (battery failure, mechanical failure, programming or refilling error)

When using an implanted IT system, because the drugs do not spread rostrally, respiratory depression is likely to be the result of opioid given by another route, e.g. PO/SL opioid before using an IT bolus for break-through pain.

MRI will cause programmable implanted pumps to malfunction. The rotor arm of the Medtronic SynchroMed® II pump is inactivated by a magnetic field but should restart when removed from it.[41,42] The Flowonix Prometra® pump[43] needs to be emptied, filled with sodium chloride 0.9% and turned off, because there is a risk that the contents of the pump reservoir will be rapidly emptied into the CSF. Guidance for the radiologist is available from the manufacturers; this includes safe MRI tesla ranges and pump orientation. The Medtronic pump will need to be interrogated after a scan to check that it has restarted, and the Flowonix refilled and restarted.

MANAGEMENT OF LIFE-THREATENING COMPLICATIONS

Clinicians caring for patients with spinal analgesia should be aware of potential life-threatening drug-related complications. Clinical areas should have resuscitation equipment, including IV fluids, **naloxone** and **ephedrine** (Box A). However, hypotension and collapse in terminally ill patients with implantable IT pumps is more likely to be caused by other conditions, e.g. sepsis, CVS events.

Box A Emergency management of life-threatening complications

Stop spinal infusion.
Administer oxygen.
Obtain IV access.
If patient arrests, follow local resuscitation procedures.

Respiratory depression (sedation often precedes bradypnoea)
Sit the patient up.
If respiratory rate ≤8 breaths/min, the patient is barely rousable, and/or cyanosed, administer 100microgram boluses of IV naloxone every 2min until respiratory status is satisfactory (see p.498).
Further boluses may be necessary, because naloxone is shorter acting than morphine and other spinal opioids.

Hypotesion (systolic <80mmHg)
Lay patient flat (not head down).
Check heart rate: if <40 beats/min, treat bradycardia (below) *or*
If no evidence of fluid overload, give an IV fluid challenge, e.g. 500mL of a colloidal plasma expander over 30min.
Examine for alternative causes such as bleeding.
If no response to fluids, give ephedrine 6mg IV.

Bradycardia
ECG monitoring, if available.
Administer atropine (0.6mg boluses IV, up to total 3mg).
If atropine ineffective, give ephedrine 6mg IV.

MANAGEMENT OF UNDESIRABLE OPIOID EFFECTS

The transient undesirable effects seen when starting systemic opioids are also seen when starting spinal opioids *de novo* (see Strong opioids, Box B, p.394).[44] However, some undesirable effects are particularly associated with starting spinal opioid analgesia either *de novo* or after switching from a more traditional route.

Opioid discontinuation (diarrhoea, colic, sweating, restlessness)

Spinal delivery results in a massive reduction in the patient's total opioid dose. Laxatives should be discontinued and re-titrated. If peripheral withdrawal symptoms occur, approximately 25% of the pre-spinal systemic opioid should be given p.r.n.

Opioid-induced pruritus

This is generally a central reaction to opioids, and largely histamine-independent.[45] In surgical (opioid-naïve) patients who receive spinal opioids pre-operatively, the incidence is ≤80%, but it is uncommon in patients with cancer pain.

If spinal opioid-induced pruritus occurs in a palliative care patient, consider:

- **ondansetron** 8mg IV stat and p.r.n. (or 8mg b.d. PO for 2 days)
- switching to an alternative opioid
- if all else fails, ultra-low dose **naloxone**:
  - ▷ titrate to effect using repeat IV bolus doses of 40microgram
  - ▷ if pruritus recurs, give 0.25–1microgram/kg/h by IVI.[45,46]

Note. Ondansetron appears effective for pruritus associated with **morphine**, but not **fentanyl** or **sufentanil**.[47,48]

OTHER COMPLICATIONS

Suspected infection

Catheter-related infections can occur, often with coagulase positive or negative staphylococci.

Exit site infection: transparent dressings allow the early identification of exit site erythema. Systemic and topical antibacterials should be started promptly; this reduces the incidence of deeper infection/meningitis. However, prophylactic antibacterials should *not* be routinely used.

ED abscesses: present with fever, escalating pain (this is invariable; either the original pain or back pain at the ED site, or both) and new neurological impairment. Evaluation includes blood cultures, aspiration of fluid from the spinal catheter for microscopy and culture, neurological examination, identification of other potential sources of fever, and MRI (see warning about MRI in Undesirable effects). Seek early advice from a microbiologist and spinal or neurosurgeon. The risk increases with time. Distant non-healing wounds may be a risk factor.

Meningitis: presents with fever and/or meningeal irritation (neck stiffness, stretch signs). Evaluation includes blood and line microscopy and cultures, WBC, neurological examination, and identification of other potential sources of fever. Also consider MRI, particularly if new neurological impairment is present (but see warning about MRI in Undesirable effects). Spinal catheters need not be automatically removed, and allow a means of obtaining CSF for culture. Mild meningeal irritation can be a normal phenomenon post-procedure, and patients can be safely observed while awaiting CSF cultures if they are systemically well and the above evaluations reveal no evidence of infection. A prolonged operation time when placing the catheter is a risk factor for serious catheter-related infection.

New neurological impairment

It can be difficult to distinguish between new neurological signs and symptoms caused by complications of spinal analgesia and those caused by disease progression (Box B). Disease-related neurological impairment is common: spinal cord compression occurs in ≤6% of patients receiving spinal analgesia. ED metastases are present in ≤70% of patients with refractory cancer pain. They are associated with motor impairment, and higher **morphine** and **bupivacaine** dose requirements (although not higher pain scores). Those with spinal canal stenosis (>50%) also have higher IT insertion complication rates.[49]

Catheter tip granulomas are lumps of inflammatory tissue formed in the lining of the thecal sac as a reaction to opioids. Granulomas may present as catheter occlusion (manifesting as renewed and increasing pain) or local mass effects (spinal cord or cauda equina compression with associated pain).[51] They generally occur several months–years after starting a spinal infusion, with the risk increasing over time.[52] Pain typically precedes neurological impairment, which develops gradually over days–weeks.[53]

Box B Differential diagnosis of new neurological impairment in patients receiving spinal analgesia

Neurological damage caused by insertion of the catheter.

Bupivacaine-induced; dose-dependent, generally seen only when IT doses exceed 15mg/day, but unmasking of incipient spinal cord compression can occur with lower doses.[2,50]

Disease progression, e.g. cauda equina or spinal cord compression.

Catheter complication, e.g. ED abscess or haematoma, catheter tip granuloma.

Evaluation

Neurological examination: to confirm the location of the problem: is it related to the catheter or could it be a separate second phenomenon?

Time of onset (after starting infusion):

- immediate: spinal medication, 'unmasking' of subclinical impairment, or neurological damage at insertion
- after days–weeks or longer: ED abscess, haematoma, or disease progression
- after several months–years: catheter tip granuloma.

Investigation: MRI = optimum (but see warning in Undesirable effects on p.913).

Granulomas are more common with ED infusions, and occur particularly with (less lipid-soluble) **morphine** or **hydromorphone** at higher concentrations.[18] Animal studies indicate that using the *lowest concentration* of opioid and the *highest infusion rate* reduces the chance of granuloma formation. Granulomas often resolve spontaneously within a few weeks of stopping an infusion.

The risk of a granuloma may also be lowered by using:

- a bolus-based regimen
- **clonidine** as an opioid-sparing agent.

In the absence of neurological impairment, treatment options include catheter tip relocation, opioid dose reduction and/or considering a non-opioid. Surgical excision may be necessary if symptoms persist or there is neurological impairment.[18]

Exacerbation of pain

A sudden increase in pain should be initially treated with p.r.n. opioid medication PO/SC while the cause is investigated. Possibilities include:

- worsening of the original pain
- development of a new pain because of:
  - ▷ disease progression or co-morbidity
  - ▷ spinal catheter-related abscess, haematoma or granuloma
- reduced effect of the infusion
  - ▷ catheter dislodgement or disconnection
  - ▷ delivery device malfunction
  - ▷ tolerance developing to the drugs; seen with both opioids and **bupivacaine** when given as continuous infusions.

Plain radiographs may show a kinked, dislodged or disconnected catheter. Catheter position and patency can be confirmed by injection of a radiological contrast agent after first aspirating the catheter dead space to avoid delivery of the dead-space contents as a bolus. The contrast agent must be appropriate for CSF use; *IT delivery of inappropriate radiological contrast agents can cause arachnoiditis and death.*

Delivery device malfunction may involve:

- a problem with the catheter (kinking, fracture, displacement, occlusion)
- an empty syringe (problem with last refill, altered delivery rate, calendar error about next refill date)
- a problem with the pump itself (battery failure, mechanical failure).

The function of the rotor arm of the Medtronic SynchroMed® II pump can be checked using fluoroscopy. After a static image is taken, the pump is programmed to deliver at the maximum rate of infusion, and another static image is taken a few minutes later. If the rotor arm is turning, then it will be in a different position on the second image. It moves too slowly to be visible on a continuous screening mode. The infusion can then be reprogrammed to the rate intended.

RECORD KEEPING

It is recommended that monitoring charts are used with spinal infusions, comparable with those widely used for checking CSCI (see p.896). The use of a spinal chart should be cross-referenced on the patient's main prescription chart and should list the drugs being infused.

The National Neuromodulation Registry for record keeping with implanted IT pumps includes patient demographics, drug doses, outcome data (global perceived effect with standardized measures of pain and quality of life), complications and revisions. The Quality Improvement Compendium produced by the Royal College of Anaesthetists includes suggested data to collect for IT drug delivery in the management of cancer-related pain.[54]

1 Kurita GP *et al.* (2011) Spinal opioids in adult patients with cancer pain: a systematic review: a European Palliative Care Research Collaborative (EPCRC) opioid guidelines project. *Palliative Medicine*. **25**: 560–577.

2 Duarte R *et al.* (2016) Intrathecal drug delivery for the management of pain and spasticity in adults: an executive summary of the British Pain Society's recommendations for best clinical practice. *British Journal of Pain*. **10**: 67–69.

3 Deer TR *et al.* (2017) The Polyanalgesic Consensus Conference (PACC): Recommendations on intrathecal drug infusion systems best practices and guidelines. *Neuromodulation*. **20**: 96–132.

4 Lynch L (2014) Intrathecal drug delivery for cancer pain. In: *Practical Management of Complex Cancer Pain*. Eds. Manohar Sharma, Karen Simpson, Michael Bennett, and Sanjeeva Gupta. Oxford, Oxford University Press, pp. 197–225.

5 Faculty of Pain Medicine of the Royal College of Anaesthetists (2016) Guidance on competencies for intrathecal drug delivery. www.fpm.ac.uk.

6 Crul BJP and Delhaas EM (1991) Technical complications during long term subarachnoid or epidural administration of morphine in terminally ill cancer patients: A review of 140 cases. *Regional Anesthesia*. **16**: 209–213.

7 Duarte R *et al.* (2020) The unmet need for intrathecal drug delivery pumps for the treatment of cancer pain in England: an assessment of the hospital episode statistics database. *Neuromodulation*. **23**: 1029–1033.

8 Hsu Y *et al.* (2012) The frequency and magnitude of cerebrospinal fluid pulsations influence intrathecal drug distribution: key factors for interpatient variability. *Anesthesia and Analgesia*. **115**: 386–394.

9 Tagen KM (2015) CNS wide simulation of low resistance and drug transport due to spinal microanatomy. *Journal Biomechanics*. **48**: 2144–2154.

10 Hettiarachchi HD *et al.* (2011) The effect of pulsatile flow on intrathecal drug delivery in the spinal canal. *Annals of Biomedical Engineering*. **39**: 2592–2602.

11 Wallace M and Yaksh TL (2012) Characteristics of distribution of morphine and metabolites in cerebrospinal fluid and plasma with chronic intrathecal morphine infusion in humans. *Anesthesia and Analgesia*. **115**: 797–804.

12 Bernards CM (2006) Cerebrospinal fluid and spinal cord distribution of baclofen and bupivacaine during slow intrathecal infusion in pigs. *Anesthesiology*. **105**: 169–178.

13 Flack SH *et al.* (2011) Morphine distribution in the spinal cord after chronic infusion in pigs. *Anesthesia and Analgesia*. **112**: 460–464.

14 NPSA (National Patient Safety Agency) (2011) Safer spinal (intrathecal), epidural and regional devices. In: Patient Safety Alert Update PSA001. www.nrls.npsa.uk

15 NHS Improvement (2017) Supporting information for Patient Safety Alert: connector to NRFitTM for intrathecal and epidural procedures, and delivery of regional blocks. www.england.nhs.uk.

16 Department of Health (2010) Mixing of medicines prior to administration in clinical practice: medical and non-medical prescribing. HMSO, London. www.gov.uk

17 National Prescribing Centre (2010) Mixing of medicines prior to administration in clinical practice - responding to legislative changes. Liverpool. Available from: www.npc.nhs.uk (archive website).

18 Deer TR *et al.* (2012) Polyanalgesic Consensus Conference--2012: consensus on diagnosis, detection, and treatment of catheter-tip granulomas (inflammatory masses). *Neuromodulation*. **15**: 483–495.

19 Bujedo BM (2014) Spinal opioid bioavailability in postoperative pain. *Pain Practice*. **14**: 350–364.

20 Zamponi GW *et al.* (2015) The physiology, pathology, and pharmacology of voltage-gated calcium channels and their future therapeutic potential. *Pharmacological Reviews*. **67**: 821–870.

21 Takasusuki T and Yaksh TL (2011) Regulation of spinal substance P release by intrathecal calcium channel blockade. *Anesthesiology*. **115**: 153–164.

22 Smith TJ et *al.* (2002) Randomized clinical trial of an implantable drug delivery system compared with comprehensive medical management for refractory cancer pain: impact on pain, drug-related toxicity, and survival. *Journal of Clinical Oncology*. **20**: 4040–4049.

23 Staats PS et *al.* (2004) Intrathecal ziconotide in the treatment of refractory pain in patients with cancer or AIDS: a randomized controlled trial. *JAMA*. **291**: 63–70.

24 Vranken JH *et al.* (2005) Neuropathological findings after continuous intrathecal administration of S(+)-ketamine for the management of neuropathic cancer pain. *Pain*. **117**: 231–235.

25 Vranken JH et *al.* (2006) Severe toxic damage to the rabbit spinal cord after intrathecal administration of preservative-free S(+)-ketamine. *Anesthesiology*. **105**: 813–818.

26 Mehta A and Kay E (1996) Admixtures' storage is extended. *Pharmacy in Practice*. **6**: 113–118.

27 Trissel LA *et al.* (2002) Physical and chemical stability of low and high concentrations of morphine sulfate with bupivacaine hydrochloride packaged in plastic syringes. *International Journal of Pharmaceutical Compounding*. Jan-Feb: 70–73.

28 Xu Quanyun A et *al.* (2002) Physical and chemical stability of low and high concentrations of morphine sulfate with clonidine hydrochloride packaged in plastic syringes. *International Journal of Pharmaceutical Compounding*. Jan-Feb: 66–69.

29 Christen C et *al.* (1996) Stability of bupivacaine hydrochloride and hydromorphone hydrochloride during simulated epidural coadministration. *American Journal of Health System Pharmacy*. **53**: 170–173.

30 Trissel LA. *Handbook on Injectable Drugs*. Maryland, USA: American Society of Health System Pharmacists (accessed March 2017).

31 Hildebrand KR *et al.* (2003) Stability and compatibility of morphine-clonidine admixtures in an implantable infusion system. *Journal of Pain and Symptom Management.* **25**: 464–471.

32 Classen AM *et al.* (2004) Stability of admixture containing morphine sulfate, bupivacaine hydrochloride, and clonidine hydrochloride in an implantable infusion system. *Journal of Pain and Symptom Management.* **28**: 603–611.

33 Hildebrand KR *et al.* (2001) Stability and compatibility of hydromorphone hydrochloride in an implantable infusion system. *Journal of Pain and Symptom Management.* **22**: 1042–1047.

34 Rudich Z *et al.* (2004) Stability of clonidine in clonidine-hydromorphone mixture from implanted intrathecal infusion pumps in chronic pain patients. *Journal of Pain and Symptom Management.* **28**: 599–602.

35 Naumann C (1999) Drug adverse events and system complications of intrathecal opioid delivery for pain: origins, detection, manifestations and management. *Neuromodulation.* **2**: 92–107.

36 Paice JA *et al.* (1996) Intraspinal morphine for chronic pain: a retrospective, multicenter study. *Journal of Pain and Symptom Management.* **11**: 71–80.

37 Abs R *et al.* (2000) Endocrine consequences of long-term intrathecal administration of opioids. *Journal of Clinical Endocrinology and Metabolism.* **85**: 2215–2222.

38 Budd K and Shipton E (2004) Acute pain and the immune system and opioimmunosuppression. *Acute Pain.* **6**: 123–135.

39 Cook TM *et al.* (2009) Major complications of central neuraxial block: report on the Third National Audit Project of the Royal College of Anaesthetists. *British Journal of Anaesthesia.* **102**: 179–190.

40 Holmfred A *et al.* (2006) Intrathecal catheters with subcutaneous port systems in patients with severe cancer-related pain managed out of hospital: the risk of infection. *Journal of Pain and Symptom Management.* **31**: 568–572.

41 Nitescu P *et al.* (1995) Complications of intrathecal opioids and bupivacaine in the treatment of "refractory" cancer pain. *Clinical Journal of Pain.* **11**: 45–62.

42 MHRA (2008) Implantable drug pumps manufactured by Medtronic - Synchro EL models 8626 and 8627 and SynchroMed II model 8637. *Medical Device Alert.* MDA/2008/2087. www.gov.uk/drug-device-alerts.

43 MHRA (2009) Effects of MRI on implantable drug pumps. *Drug Safety Update.* www.gov.uk/drug-safety-update.

44 Rawal N *et al.* (1987) Present state of extradural and intrathecal opioid analgesia in Sweden. A nationwide follow-up survey. *British Journal of Anaesthesia.* **59**: 791–799.

45 Reich A and Szepietowski JC (2010) Opioid-induced pruritus: an update. *Clinical Experimental Dermatology.* **35**: 2–6.

46 Kumar K and Singh S (2013) Neuroaxial opioid-induced pruritus: an update. *Journal of Anaesthesiology Clinical Pharmacology.* **29**: 303–307.

47 Borgeat A and Stimemann H-R (1999) Ondansetron is effective to treat spinal or epidural morphine-induced pruritus. *Anesthesiology.* **90**: 432–436.

48 Prin M *et al.* (2016) Prophylactic ondansetron for the prevention of intrathecal fentanyl- or sufentanil-mediated pruritus: a meta-analysis of randomized trials. *Anesthesia and Analgesia.* **122**: 402–409.

49 Appelgren L *et al.* (1997) Spinal epidural metastasis: implications for spinal analgesia to treat "refractory" cancer pain. *Journal of Pain and Symptom Management.* **13**: 25–42.

50 van Dongen RTM *et al.* (1997) Neurological impairment during long-term intrathecal infusion of bupivacaine in cancer patients: a sign of spinal cord compression. *Pain.* **69**: 205–209.

51 MHRA (2008) Implantable drug pumps for intrathecal therapy - risk of temporary or permanent neurological impairment. *Drug Device Alerts.* www.gov.uk/drug-device-alerts.

52 Deer TR (2004) A prospective analysis of intrathecal granulomas in chronic pain patients: a review of the literature and report of a surveillance study. *Pain Physician.* **7**: 225–228.

53 Miele VJ *et al.* (2006) A review of intrathecal morphine therapy related granulomas. *European Journal of Pain.* **10**: 251–261.

54 Royal College of Anaesthetists (2020) Raising the Standards: RCoA quality improvement compendium. www.rcoa.ac.uk.

Updated July 2021

Appendix 1: Anaphylaxis

Anaphylaxis is an acute, life-threatening, systemic allergic or hypersensitivity reaction. It develops rapidly in minutes or, at most, a few hours. It manifests as potentially life-threatening compromise in airway/breathing and/or circulation. It may occur without typical changes or circulatory shock.[1]

Pathophysiology

Anaphylaxis is caused by the sudden release of numerous inflammatory mediators from mast cells and basophils into the systemic circulation. This results in:

- vasodilation, hypotension, capillary leakage (leading to cardiovascular collapse)
- mucosal and laryngeal oedema, bronchoconstriction (leading to respiratory difficulty).[1]

Most commonly, the allergic reaction results from the interaction of an allergen with specific IgE antibodies bound to mast cells and basophils, leading to the release of:

- preformed chemical mediators, e.g. chymase, histamine, tryptase
- newly synthesized mediators, e.g. cytokines, leukotrienes, platelet activating factor, prostaglandins.

Anaphylaxis may also be caused by other immunological mechanisms, e.g. IgG–antigen complexes, complement activation (anaphylatoxins C3a and C5a). Some drugs, e.g. NSAIDs, can cause direct activation of mast cells. Other non-immunological triggers of anaphylaxis include exercise and cold.[1] In terms of management, it is *not* necessary to identify the precise trigger; the difference is relevant only when investigations are being considered.[2]

Anaphylaxis is:

- specific to a given drug or chemically related class of drugs
- more likely after parenteral drug administration
- more frequent in patients taking β-blockers (see below), ACE inhibitors or in those who have **aspirin**-induced asthma or systemic lupus erythematosus
- more severe in patients >65 years and those with concurrent illness, particularly upper respiratory tract infection and chronic respiratory or cardiovascular disease.[3]

Anaphylaxis is rare in palliative care. When it occurs, it is generally associated with antibacterials (see p.507) or an NSAID (see p.350). Although refined **arachis (peanut) oil**, which is present in some medicinal products, is unlikely to cause an allergic reaction, **arachis oil** enemas are contra-indicated in patients with peanut or soya allergies. **Chlorhexidine** has also been implicated, including after the use of a **chlorhexidine** skin wipe.[4]

Clinical features

Anaphylaxis is likely when the following criteria are met after exposure to a possible trigger:

- sudden onset and rapid progression (minutes–few hours)
- life-threatening circulatory or respiratory problems
- skin and/or mucosal changes (subtle or absent in 10–20%) (Box A).[1,5]

Before progressing to life-threatening respiratory or circulatory problems, patients with a history of anaphylaxis may present with:

- sudden onset and rapidly progressing skin and/or mucosal changes plus GI symptoms (abdominal pain, colic, vomiting) *or*
- hypotension alone.[1]

The differential diagnosis of anaphylaxis is extensive but includes:

- life-threatening conditions, e.g. choking, severe asthma, shock, seizure
- non-life-threatening conditions, e.g. urticaria or angioedema, vasovagal episode, panic attack.

Lack of a complete history or definite diagnosis should not delay initial treatment; if in doubt, give IM **adrenaline** and call an ambulance.

Box A Clinical features of anaphylaxis

Essential

Sudden onset of life-threatening circulatory *and/or* respiratory problems, e.g.:

Circulatory problems	***Respiratory problems***
Tachycardia	Airway
Hypotension	pharyngeal/laryngeal oedema
Shock	hoarse voice
Decreased consciousness	stridor
Cardiac arrest	Breathing
	breathlessness
	wheeze/bronchospasm (10%)
	cyanosis
	respiratory arrest

Probable	**Possible**
Skin/mucosal changes (80%):	Agitation
flushing or pallor	Confusion
erythema of skin	Incontinence
itching	Tingling of the extremities
urticaria	Rhinitis
angioedema[a], mostly face, hands, feet	Conjunctivitis
	Gastrointestinal symptoms
	abdominal pain
	diarrhoea
	vomiting

a. angioedema is swelling in the dermis, subcutaneous and submucosal tissues.

Management

National guidelines vary; the advice here is based on guidance published by the Resuscitation Council UK[5] and NICE.[6] Drugs and basic resuscitation equipment for treatment of anaphylaxis must be available in all clinical settings, either as part of a resuscitation kit or in an 'anaphylaxis box'.

Adrenaline (epinephrine), a direct-acting sympathomimetic, is effective in attenuating anaphylaxis if given promptly and in sufficient dose.[5] Through its α_1-receptor agonist effects, it causes vasoconstriction, increases peripheral vascular resistance and reduces mucosal oedema. As a β_1 agonist, it increases the rate and force of myocardial contraction. As a β_2 agonist, it dilates bronchial airways, increases glycogenolysis and suppresses activity of mast cells, reducing the release of histamine and other inflammatory mediators.

Adrenaline *is given by IM injection (Box B), and this is the preferred route.* Most episodes of anaphylaxis respond to one dose of IM **adrenaline**, with 10% requiring two doses and 2% requiring three doses (anaphylaxis that does not respond to two doses of IM **adrenaline** is considered 'refractory').

Adrenaline (epinephrine) auto-injector should only be used to treat anaphylaxis when no other form of **adrenaline** is available; give 300microgram or 500microgram IM (brand dependent) and repeat after 5min p.r.n.

Patients taking β-blockers, TCAs or MAOIs

Patients taking β-blockers, particularly non-cardioselective ones, are at increased risk of severe anaphylaxis because the β-receptor-mediated effects of **adrenaline** are blunted. Further, unopposed stimulation of α-receptors, with reflex vagotonic effects, may lead to bradycardia, coronary artery constriction, *hypertension* and intracerebral haemorrhage. TCAs and MAOIs potentiate **adrenaline** and increase the risk of cardiac arrhythmias.

Previous UK anaphylaxis guidelines recommended halving the dose of **adrenaline** given to patients on β-blockers, TCAs and MAOIs. However, current guidelines note the large interindividual variation in response to **adrenaline**, and this recommendation has been withdrawn. Patients on these drugs should be given a full initial dose of **adrenaline**, with further doses titrated according to the initial response.[5]

For patients taking β-blockers and unresponsive to **adrenaline**, give **glucagon**. **Glucagon** has β-receptor-independent inotropic, chronotropic and vasoactive effects (Box C).[5]

Box B Management of anaphylaxis in adults[5]

Patients should be treated using the **A**irway, **B**reathing, **C**irculation, **D**isability, **E**xposure (ABCDE) approach.

1. Call for help and an ambulance (in non-hospital settings).
2. Remove trigger if possible, e.g. stop IV antibacterial or blood product.
3. Position patient on back, with or without legs elevated:
   - position semi-recumbent if breathless or vomiting
   - do *not* attempt to stand or sit the patient upright; this increases the risk of cardiovascular arrest
   - unconscious patients should be placed in the recovery position.
4. Give **adrenaline (epinephrine)** IM into the anterolateral aspect of the middle third of the thigh:
   - use 1:1,000 (1mg/1mL); give 500microgram (0.5mL).
5. Establish airway and give high-flow oxygen (>10L/min); target saturations 94–98% (88–92% if risk of hypercapnic respiratory failure). Monitor heart rate, blood pressure, oxygen saturations, ECG.
6. If there is no response within 5min:
   - repeat IM **adrenaline** 500microgram *and*
   - insert IV cannula and give sodium chloride 0.9% 500mL–1L IV fluid bolus over 10min.
7. Repeat IM **adrenaline** 500microgram every 5min until blood pressure, pulse and breathing are satisfactory or until ambulance arrives.
8. If cardiorespiratory arrest occurs, start cardiopulmonary resuscitation if appropriate to the patient's circumstances, e.g. taking prognosis, stated wishes into consideration. IV adrenaline (*not* IM) is recommended after a cardiac arrest; give only in a hospital setting (Box C).

Box C Supplementary measures for refractory anaphylaxis[5]

Refractory anaphylaxis is defined as no improvement in circulatory and respiratory symptoms after two doses of IM adrenaline.

Airway: obstruction (stridor)

- give *nebulized* adrenaline 5mg (5mL of 1mg/mL).

Breathing: severe bronchospasm

- give *nebulized* bronchodilator through oxygen every 5min p.r.n.:
  - ▷ start with salbutamol 5mg; if wheeze persists, switch to ipratropium bromide 500microgram, *or*
- give a slow IV injection of salbutamol 250microgram diluted to 5mL with WFI.

Circulation: hypotension

- repeat sodium chloride 0.9% 500mL–1L IV fluid bolus over 10min; up to 3–5L may be required.

Other drug measures

Corticosteroids

- hydrocortisone 200mg IV.

In patients taking a β-blocker

Both IM adrenaline and *nebulized* salbutamol may be less effective:

- give glucagon 1mg IV every 5min p.r.n. *or* give as IVI 1–2mg/h
- switch sooner to *nebulized* ipratropium bromide or IV salbutamol (see above).

Peripheral IVI adrenaline

IVI adrenaline can cause ventricular arrhythmias, cardiac ischaemia and hypertension; give only if experienced in its use and where full intensive care facilities are available.

- use 1:1,000 (1mg/1mL); dilute 1mg (1mL) in 100mL sodium chloride 0.9% and connect using an infusion pump via a dedicated line
- start at 0.5–1mL/kg/h and titrate according to response.

Additional drug treatment once the patient is stable

When the patient has recovered, additional measures can be considered. These are no longer part of initial emergency treatment of anaphylaxis, as they have no benefit in treating the life-threatening feature of anaphylaxis and may delay administration of IM adrenaline.

Antihistamines

These may be helpful in treating urticaria or angioedema. A non-sedating antihistamine is preferred, e.g. **cetirizine** 10mg–20mg PO once daily.[5] If PO is not possible, give **chlorphenamine** 10mg IM (or 10mg IV over 1min) and up to 40mg/24h.

Corticosteroids

The routine use of a corticosteroid is no longer recommended in anaphylaxis because of the lack of definite benefit and the possibility of harm (greater risk of ICU admission). Thus, corticosteroids are used only in refractory anaphylaxis (Box C) or where other indications co-exist, e.g. an acute asthma exacerbation. Give in the usual dose for the indication, preferably PO.

Monitoring following recovery from anaphylaxis

Monitor pulse, blood pressure, pulse oximetry and ECG tracings, ideally in a clinical area with full resuscitation facilities. In 5% of patients there is a biphasic anaphylactic episode, on average recurring within 12h. Thus a stratified approach to monitoring duration is recommended:[6]

- minimum 2h observation if good response (within 5–10min) to single dose of adrenaline given within 30min of onset of anaphylaxis *and* complete resolution of symptoms *and* patient already has adrenaline auto-injector *and* has adequate supervision following discharge
- minimum 6h observation if 2 doses IM adrenaline given or previous biphasic reaction
- minimum 12h observation if >2 doses adrenaline required *or* severe asthma/respiratory compromise *or* ongoing allergen absorption (e.g. modified-release medication) *or* patient unable to respond to deterioration.

A registry (anaphylaxie.net) has been established, and health professionals are encouraged to report all episodes of anaphylaxis.

Follow-up

After the successful treatment of the acute event, other measures need to be considered (Box D).

Box D Follow-up[5,6]

If the patient's prognosis is months rather than weeks, take three timed blood samples for mast cell tryptase:

- the first as soon as possible after starting emergency treatment (but do not delay treatment)
- the second 1–2h (but no later than 4h) after onset of anaphylaxis
- the third at least 24h after recovery, or at follow-up allergy clinic (for baseline tryptase values).

If three timed samples are not possible, take one sample within 2h and no later than 4h after onset of anaphylaxis. Tryptase levels are elevated in only about 60% of adults with clinically confirmed anaphylaxis.

Advise patients to avoid the suspected environmental, dietary or drug trigger.

Provide information about recognizing and managing an anaphylactic reaction.

Unless anaphylaxis is definitely caused by a drug or blood product, supply the patient with two adrenaline auto-injectors, e.g. EpiPens, and show how to use them.[6–8]

Adrenaline auto-injectors are device-specific in terms of injection technique; thus the patient should continue to use the same brand.

Refer to an allergy clinic before discharge.

1 Cardona V *et al.* (2020) World allergy organization anaphylaxis guidance 2020. *World Allergy Organization Journal.* **13**: 100472.
2 Khan BQ and Kemp SF (2011) Pathophysiology of anaphylaxis. *Current Opinion in Allergy and Clinical Immunology.* **11**: 319–325.
3 NICE (2016) Surveillance report – Anaphylaxis: assessment and referral after emergency treatment (2011). *Clinical Guideline.* CG134 www.nice.org.uk.
4 MHRA (2012) All medical devices and medicinal products containing chlorhexidine. Risk of anaphylactic reaction due to chlorhexidine allergy. *Medical Devices Alert.* MDA/2012/2075 www.gov.uk/drug-device-alerts.
5 Resuscitation Council UK (2021) Emergency treatment of anaphylaxis. *Guidelines for healthcare providers.* www.resus.org.uk.
6 NICE (2011) Anaphylaxis. Assessment to confirm an anaphylactic episode and the decision to refer after emergency treatment for a suspected anaphylactic episode (Updated August 2020). *Clinical Guideline.* CG134 www.nice.org.uk.
7 MHRA (2021) Adrenaline auto-injectors: reminder for prescribers to support safe and effective use. www.gov.uk/drug-safety-update.
8 Ewan P *et al.* (2016) British Society for Allergy and Clinical Immunology Guideline: prescribing an adrenaline auto-injector. *Clinical and Experimental Allergy.* **46**: 1258–1280.

Updated January 2022

A2

Appendix 2: Opioid dose conversion ratios

General approach

It is crucial to appreciate that conversion ratios are *never* more than an approximate guide. Thus, careful monitoring during conversion is necessary to avoid both underdosing and excessive dosing. Also see Opioid switching ('rotation'), p.400.

This chapter provides a summary of selected opioid dose conversion ratios. These can be used to calculate equivalent doses of opioids when switching from a weak opioid to **morphine**, or from one strong opioid to another. Caution is always necessary. Conversion ratios are *never* more than an approximate guide, because of:

- wide interindividual variation in opioid pharmacokinetics; influencing factors include age, ethnicity, renal or hepatic impairment
- other variables including dose and duration of opioid treatment, direction of switch in opioid, nutritional status and concurrent medications
- their method of derivation, e.g. single dose rather than chronic dose studies using a range of clinical doses.

Careful monitoring is particularly necessary when:

- switching at high doses
- there has been a recent rapid escalation of the first opioid
- switching to **methadone**.

Explicit guidance on switching opioids is difficult because both the reasons for switching and the patients' circumstances differ. One guideline, based on expert consensus, recommends routinely reducing the calculated equivalent dose of the new opioid by 25–50% (see p.400). Various patient factors are then taken into account to modify the rule, e.g. no reduction in a young patient in severe pain switching at low dose, or an even bigger reduction in an older delirious patient in moderate pain switching at high dose.

Certainly, a dose reduction of at least 50% would seem prudent when switching at high doses (e.g. **morphine** or equivalent doses of ≥1g/24h), in elderly or frail patients, because of intolerable undesirable effects (e.g. delirium), or when there has been a recent rapid escalation of the first opioid (possibly due to opioid-induced hyperalgesia). In such circumstances, p.r.n. doses can be relied on to make up any deficit while re-titrating to a satisfactory dose of the new opioid.

A separate strategy is necessary for **methadone** (p.469).

Determining the dose of the second opioid

Select the appropriate table based on the routes of administration:

Route	*Table*	*Page*
PO to PO	1	927
PO to TD	2	928
PO to SC/IV	3	931
SC/IV to SC/IV	4	932

The tables relate mainly to switching to or from **morphine**. If switching from an opioid other than **morphine** to another opioid, it will be necessary to convert the dose of the first opioid to **morphine** equivalents, and then use that quantity to determine the dose of the second opioid. With any switch:

- round the calculated dose up or down to the nearest convenient dose of the formulation concerned, e.g. tablet, TD patch, ampoule
- decide on an appropriate p.r.n. dose.

The conversion ratios in this chapter are based on referenced sources given in the various individual opioid monographs. Where these differ significantly from the manufacturers' recommended ratios, the latter are included for comparison.

Table 1 *PCF* recommended dose conversion ratios: PO to PO. Before use, see General approach (p.925)

Conversion	*Ratio*	*Calculation*	*Example*	*Monograph*
Codeine to morphine	10:1	Divide 24h codeine dose by 10	Codeine 240mg/24h PO → morphine 24mg/24h PO	Codeine, p.378
Dihydrocodeine to morphine	10:1	Divide 24h dihydrocodeine dose by 10	Dihydrocodeine 240mg/24h PO → morphine 24mg/24h PO	Dihydrocodeine, p.381
Hydrocodone to morphine	1.5:1	Divide 24h hydrocodone dose by 1.5 (i.e. decrease dose by 1/3)	Hydrocodone 60mg/24h PO → morphine 40mg/24h PO	Not UK
Tramadol to morphine	10:1	Divide 24h tramadol dose by 10	Tramadol 400mg/24h PO → morphine 40mg/24h PO	Tramadol, p.383
Morphine to hydromorphone	5:1	Divide 24h morphine dose by 5	Morphine 60mg/24h PO → hydromorphone 12mg/24h PO	Hydromorphone, p.466
	7.5:1[a]	*Divide 24h morphine dose by 7.5*	*Morphine 60mg/24h PO → hydromorphone 8mg/24h PO*	Hydromorphone, p.466
Morphine to methadone	Variable	See methadone, p.469		
Morphine to oxycodone	1.5:1	Divide 24h morphine dose by 1.5 (i.e. decrease dose by 1/3)	Morphine 60mg/24h PO → oxycodone 40mg/24h PO	Oxycodone, p.480
	2:1[a]	*Divide 24h morphine dose by 2*	*Morphine 60mg/24h PO → oxycodone 30mg/24h PO*	Oxycodone, p.480

a. italicized entries = manufacturers' recommendations.

Table 2 *PCF* recommended dose conversion ratios: PO to TD. Before use, see General approach (p.925)

Conversion	*Ratio*	*Calculation*	*Example*	*Monograph*
Morphine to buprenorphine	100:1	Multiply 24h morphine dose in mg by 10 to obtain 24h buprenorphine dose in microgram; divide answer by 24 to obtain microgram/h patch strength	Morphine 300mg/24h PO → buprenorphine 3,000microgram/24h → 125microgram/h; *round up* to 70microgram/h x 2 or *round down* to 70 + 35microgram/h patches	Buprenorphine, p.428
	75–115:1[a]	*Use the manufacturer's guidelines in SPC, summarized in Box A, p.929*		Buprenorphine, p.428
Morphine to fentanyl	100:1	Multiply 24h morphine dose in mg by 10 to obtain 24h fentanyl dose in microgram; divide answer by 24 to obtain microgram/h patch strength	Morphine 300mg/24h PO → fentanyl 3,000microgram/24h → 125microgram/h; give as 100 + 25microgram/h patches	Fentanyl, p.440
	100:1 or 150:1[a,b]	*Use the manufacturer's guidelines in SPC, summarized in Box B, p.930*	*For 150:1, the fentanyl dose will be smaller than that obtained with 100:1*	Fentanyl, p.440

a. italicized entries = manufacturers' recommendations

b. recommended ratio varies according to the duration of use of the previous strong opioid; see Box B, p.930.

For determining the appropriate p.r.n. morphine dose for patients receiving TD buprenorphine or TD fentanyl, see p.438 and 448 respectively.

Box A Summary of manufacturers' recommendations for starting TD buprenorphine (for full details, see specific SPC)[a]

BuTrans® 5, 10, 15 and 20microgram/h TD buprenorphine patch

Patients aged 18 years and over

The lowest BuTrans® dose (BuTrans® 5microgram/h TD patch) should be used as the initial dose. Consideration should be given to the previous opioid history of the patient as well as to the current general condition and medical status of the patient.

Conversion from opioids

BuTrans® can be used as an alternative to treatment with other opioids. Such patients should be started on the lowest available dose (BuTrans® 5microgram/h TD patch) and continue taking short-acting supplemental analgesics during titration, as required.

Transtec® 35, 52.5 and 70microgram/h TD buprenorphine patch

Patients over 18 years of age

The dose should be adapted to the condition of the individual patient (pain intensity, suffering, individual reaction). The lowest possible dose providing adequate pain relief should be given.

Conversion from opioids

Patients on a step II (weak opioid) analgesic should begin with buprenorphine 35microgram/h TD. The administration of a non-opioid analgesic can be continued, depending on the patient's overall medical condition.

When switching from a step III (strong opioid) analgesic to buprenorphine TD, the nature of the previous medication, administration and the mean daily dose should be taken into account in order to avoid the recurrence of pain. It is generally advisable to titrate the dose individually, starting with the lowest TD patch strength (35microgram/h). Clinical experience has shown that patients who were previously treated with higher doses of a strong opioid (approximately 120mg oral morphine per day) may start therapy with the next-highest TD patch strength (i.e. 52.5microgram/h).

Sufficient supplementary immediate-release analgesics should be made available during dose titration.

The necessary strength of buprenorphine TD must be adapted to the requirements of the individual patient and checked at regular intervals.

After application of the first buprenorphine TD patch, the buprenorphine serum concentrations rise slowly and there is unlikely to be a rapid onset of effect. Consequently, a first evaluation of the analgesic effect should only be made after 24h.

The previous analgesic medication (with the exception of transdermal opioids) should be given in the same dose during the first 12h after switching to TD, and appropriate rescue medication given on demand in the following 12h.

a. several branded generic products are available which follow the same recommendations; see individual SPC.

Box B Summary of manufacturer's recommendations for starting Durogesic DTrans® (for full details see SPC)[a]

Durogesic DTrans® 12/25/50/75/100microgram/h TD fentanyl patch

Adults:

Initial dose selection

The initial Durogesic DTrans® dose should be based on the patient's current opioid use, degree of opioid tolerance and the stability of their clinical status.

In opioid-naïve patients, generally the TD route is not recommended, and patients should be titrated with an immediate-release opioid to a dose equivalent to Durogesic DTrans® 12–25microgram/h before switching to Durogesic DTrans®. When this is not possible, use an initial dose of 12microgram/h.

In opioid-tolerant patients, the initial dose of Durogesic DTrans® should be based on the previous 24h opioid analgesic requirement, expressed as the oral 24h morphine equivalent. The dose of Durogesic DTrans® is then derived from Tables 1 and 2 according to the patient's clinical status:

Table 1 Adults who need opioid rotation (e.g. because of undesirable effects) or who are less clinically stable (conversion ratio of morphine PO to fentanyl TD of about 150:1)

Oral 24h morphine (mg/24h)	*Durogesic DTrans® (microgram/h)*
<90	12
90–134	25
135–224	50
225–314	75
315–404	100
405–494	125
495–584	150
585–674	175
675–764	200
765–854	225
855–944	250
945–1034	275
1035–1124	300

Table 2 Adults on a stable and well-tolerated opioid regimen (conversion ratio of morphine PO to fentanyl TD of about 100:1)

Oral 24h morphine (mg/24h)	*Durogesic DTrans® (microgram/h)*
≤44	12
45–89	25
90–149	50
150–209	75
210–269	100
270–329	125
330–389	150
390–449	175
450–509	200
510–569	225
570–629	250
630–689	275
690–749	300

Previous analgesic therapy should be phased out gradually from the time of the first patch application until analgesic efficacy with Durogesic DTrans® is attained. The initial evaluation of the analgesic effect of Durogesic DTrans® should not be made until the patch has been worn for 24h, due to the gradual increase in serum fentanyl concentrations up to this time.

a. several branded generic products are available which follow the same recommendations; see individual SPC.

Table 3 *PCF* recommended dose conversion ratios; PO to SC/IV. Before use, see General approach (p.925)

Conversion	*Ratio*	*Calculation*	*Example*	*Monograph*
Hydromorphone to hydromorphone	2:1[a]	Divide 24h hydromorphone dose by 2	Hydromorphone 32mg/24h PO → hydromorphone 16mg/24h SC/IV	Hydromorphone, p.466
	3:1[b]	*Divide 24h hydromorphone dose by 3*	*Hydromorphone 32mg/24h PO → hydromorphone 10mg/24h SC/IV*	Hydromorphone, p.466
Methadone to methadone	2:1[c]	Divide 24h methadone dose by 2	Methadone 30mg/24h PO → methadone 15mg/24h SC/IV	Methadone, p.469
Morphine to alfentanil	30:1	Divide 24h morphine dose by 30	Morphine 60mg/24h PO → alfentanil 2mg/24h SC/IV	Alfentanil, p.420
Morphine to diamorphine	3:1	Divide 24h morphine dose by 3	Morphine 60mg/24h PO → diamorphine 20mg/24h SC/IV	Diamorphine, p.417
Morphine to fentanyl	Variable[d,e]	Divide 24h morphine dose in mg by 100–150	Morphine 60mg/24h PO → fentanyl 400microgram/24h SC/IV	Fentanyl, p.440
Morphine to hydromorphone	10:1	Divide 24h morphine dose by 10	Morphine 60mg/24h PO → hydromorphone 6mg/24h SC/IV	Hydromorphone, p.466
Morphine to methadone	Variable	See methadone, p.469		
Morphine to morphine	2:1	Divide 24h morphine dose by 2	Morphine 60mg/24h PO →morphine 30mg/24h SC/IV	Morphine, p.404
Morphine to oxycodone	2:1	Divide 24h morphine dose by 2	Morphine 60mg/24h PO → oxycodone 30mg/24h SC/IV	Oxycodone, p.480
Oxycodone to oxycodone	1.5:1[f]	Divide 24h oxycodone dose by 1.5 (i.e. decrease dose by 1/3)	Oxycodone 30mg/24h PO → oxycodone 20mg/24h SC/IV	Oxycodone, p.480
	2:1[b]	*Divide 24h oxycodone dose by 2*	*Oxycodone 30mg/24h PO → oxycodone 15mg/24h SC/IV*	Oxycodone, p.480

a. because mean oral bio-availability is 50% (range 35–60%), some centres use a conversion ratio of 2:1 rather than 3:1
b. italicized entries = manufacturer's recommendation
c. because mean oral bio-availability is 80% (range 40–100%), some centres use 1:1, e.g. methadone 30mg/24h PO → methadone 30mg/24h SC/IV; see p.469
d. the same conversion ratios as for morphine PO to fentanyl TD can be used for morphine PO to fentanyl SC/IV; see Table 2
e. volume constraints for a syringe driver may prevent doses >500microgram/24h being used; alfentanil is an alternative
f. because mean oral bio-availability is 75% (range 60–87%), some centres use a conversion ratio of 1.5:1 rather than 2:1.

Table 4 *PCF* recommended dose conversion ratios; SC/IV to SC/IV. Before use, see General approach (p.925)

Conversion	*Ratio*	*Calculation*	*Example*	*Monograph*
Morphine to alfentanil	15:1	Divide 24h morphine dose by 15	Morphine 30mg/24h SC/IV → alfentanil 2mg/24h SC/IV	Alfentanil, p.420
Morphine to buprenorphine	30–40:1	Divide 24h morphine dose in mg by 30–40	Morphine 40mg/24h SC/IV → buprenorphine 1mg/24h SC/IV	Buprenorphine, p.428
Morphine to diamorphine	1.5:1	Divide 24h morphine dose by 1.5 (i.e. decrease dose by 1/3)	Morphine 30mg/24h SC/IV → diamorphine 20mg/24h SC/IV	Diamorphine, p.417
Morphine to fentanyl	50–75:1[a,b]	Divide 24h morphine dose in mg by 50–75	Morphine 30mg/24h SC/IV → fentanyl 400microgram/24h SC/IV	Fentanyl, p.440
Morphine to hydromorphone	5:1	Divide 24h morphine dose by 5	Morphine 30mg/24h SC/IV → hydromorphone 6mg/24h SC/IV	Hydromorphone, p.466
Morphine to methadone	Variable	See methadone, p.469		
Morphine to oxycodone	1:1	Use same dose as 24h morphine dose	Morphine 30mg/24h SC/IV → oxycodone 30mg/24h SC/IV	Oxycodone, p.480

a. extrapolated from the manufacturer's recommended ratio for morphine PO to fentanyl TD, which varies according to the duration of use of the previous strong opioid; see Table 2 and Box B

b. volume constraints for a syringe driver may prevent doses >500microgram/24h being used; alfentanil is an alternative.

Updated (minor change) February 2022

Appendix 3: Compatibility charts

A3

PCF recommends that generally water for injection (WFI) is used as the standard diluent of choice because there is less likelihood of incompatibility. However, sodium chloride 0.9% should be considered when there is actual or potential for inflammation at the injection site (see Chapter 29, p.889).

Charts 1–7 and Table 1 summarize the compatibility data available for the more commonly used 2-drug and 3-drug combinations given by CSCI in WFI. Charts summarizing the compatibility data available for the more commonly used 2-drug and 3-drug combinations given by CSCI in sodium chloride 0.9% can be found in the extended appendix section of the on-line *PCF* on www.medicinescomplete.com. For compatibility information for drugs given less frequently by this route, e.g. **fentanyl** (p.444), **levetiracetam** (p.313), **ranitidine** (p.29), see individual drug monographs.

The charts have been compiled from clinical observations in palliative care services submitted to the www.palliativedrugs.com Syringe Driver Survey Database (SDSD) from the UK, New Zealand and Australia, and from published compatibility data (see reference list). The SDSD is a continually updated resource and contains more detailed observational compatibility data on mixing up to 4 drugs in either WFI or sodium chloride 0.9%.

A traffic-light system has been devised for use in the clinical setting as a practical summary of the data available:

- *red* = do not use (available information indicates a compatibility problem)
- *amber* = proceed with caution (possible compatibility problem, depending on the order of mixing or drug concentrations)
- *green* = reported compatible (data may be observational, physical or chemical, i.e. may be practice- or evidence-based).

Multiple factors affect drug stability and compatibility, including drug concentration, brand/formulation of the drug (e.g. compatibility for **oxycodone** 10mg/mL and 50mg/mL formulations differs), diluent, infusion time, exposure to light, ambient temperature, order of mixing and delivery system material (see Chapter 29, Box B, p.891). These factors probably explain why conflicting reports occur. *Regular monitoring of all CSCI drug combinations is essential*, even for those coded green. If there is doubt about the relevance of the compatibility data in any particular situation, e.g. at the extremes of dose and concentration, advice should be obtained from a clinical pharmacist.

Dexamethasone often causes compatibility problems. It should always be the last drug to be added to an already dilute combination of drugs, thus reducing the risk of precipitation. However, because **dexamethasone** has a long duration of action, it can generally be given as a bolus SC injection once daily.

Health professionals are urged to contact hq@palliativedrugs.com if their experience indicates that the code for a combination should be changed. Submissions to the SDSD of details of successful combinations for which there are no published data are also welcome.

Most of the information in these charts relates to the use of drugs outside the scope of their marketing authorization, and health professionals using this information must satisfy themselves as to its appropriateness in any given clinical situation (also see p.xix). Further, health professionals should familiarize themselves with the guidance and supporting material relating to the legal implications of mixing medicines before administration (Department of Health, 2010) together with any local policy and practice (also see p.xix).

Allwood M (1984) Diamorphine mixed with antiemetic drugs in plastic syringes. *British Journal of Pharmaceutical Practice*. **6**: 88–90.

Allwood M (1991) The stability of diamorphine alone and in combination with anti-emetics in plastic syringes. *Palliative Medicine*. **5**: 330–333.

Allwood M *et al.* (1994) Stability of injections containing diamorphine and midazolam in plastic syringes. *International Journal of Pharmacy Practice*. **3**: 57–59.

Al-Tannak NF *et al.* (2012) A stability indicating assay for a combination of morphine sulphate with levomepromazine hydrochloride used in palliative care. *Journal Clinical Pharmacy and Therapeutics*. **37**: 71-73.

Ambados F (1995) Compatibility of morphine and ketamine for subcutaneous infusion. *Australian Journal of Hospital Pharmacy*. **25**: 352.

Back I *Syringe driver database*. www.pallcare.info (accessed May 2013).

Barcia E *et al.* (2003) Compatibility of haloperidol and Hyoscine-N-butylbromide in mixtures for subcutaneous infusion to cancer patients in palliative care. *Supportive Care in Cancer*. **11**: 107-113.

Chin A *et al.* (1996) Stability of Granisetron hydrochloride with dexamethasone sodium phosphate for 14 days. *American Journal of Health-System Pharmacy*. **53**: 1174-1176.

Department of Health (2010) Mixing of medicines prior to administration in clinical practice: medical and non-medical prescribing. Department of Health Gateway reference **14330**. www.gov.uk

Dickman A and Schneider J (2016) *The Syringe Driver: Continuous Subcutaneous Infusions in Palliative Care*, 4th edn. Oxford: Oxford University Press.

Fawcett J *et al.* (1994) Compatibility of cyclizine lactate and haloperidol lactate. *American Journal of Hospital Pharmacy*. **51**: 2292–2294.

Fielding H *et al.* (2000) The compatibility and stability of octreotide acetate in the presence of diamorphine hydrochloride in polypropylene syringes. *Palliative Medicine*. **14**: 205–207.

Frimley Park Hospital NHS Trust (1998) *Personal communication.*

Gardiner P (2003) Compatibility of an injectable oxycodone formulation with typical diluents, syringes, tubings, infusion bags and drugs for potential co-administration. *Hospital Pharmacist*. **10**: 354–361.

Good PD *et al.* (2004) The compatibility and stability of midazolam and dexamethasone in infusion solutions. *Journal of Pain and Symptom Management*. **27**: 471–475.

Grassby P and Hutchings L (1997) Drug combinations in syringe drivers: the compatibility and stability of diamorphine with cyclizine and haloperidol. *Palliative Medicine*. **11**: 217–224.

Grassby PF (1995) *UK stability database (Apr 1995 and Jul 1997)*. Welsh Pharmaceutical Services, St. Mary's Pharmaceutical Unit, Corbett Road, Penarth, South Glamorgan.

Hagan R *et al.* (1996) Stability of ondansetron hydrochloride and dexamethasone sodium phosphate in infusion bags and syringes for 32 days. American *Journal of Health-System Pharmacy*. **53**: 1431-1435.

Hines S and Pleasance S (2009) Compatibility of an injectable high strength oxycodone formulation with typical diluents, syringes, tubings, infusion bags and drugs for potential co-administration. *European Journal of Hospital Pharmacy Practice* **15**: 32–38.

Hines S and Pleasance S (2011) Compatibility of injectable hydromorphone formulations with typical diluents, components of giving sets and drugs for potential co-administration. *European Journal of Hospital Pharmacy Practice*. **17**: 47-53.

Huang E and Anderson RP (1994) Compatibility of hydromorphone hydrochloride with haloperidol lactate and ketorolac tromethamine. *American Journal of Hospital Pharmacy*. **51**: 2963.

Hughes A *et al.* (1997) Ketorolac: continuous subcutaneous infusion for cancer pain. *Journal of Pain and Symptom Management*. **13**: 315–317.

Ingallinera TS *et al.* (1979) Compatibility of glycopyrrolate injection with commonly used infusion solutions and additives. *American Journal of Hospital Pharmacy*. **36**: 508–510.

Lau M-H *et al.* (1998) Compatibility of ketamine and morphine injections. *Pain*. **75**: 389–390.

Lawson WA *et al.* (1991) Stability of hyoscine in mixtures with morphine for continuous subcutaneous administration. *Australian Journal of Hospital Pharmacy*. **21**: 395–396.

LeBelle MJ *et al.* (1995) Compatibility of morphine and midazolam or haloperidol in parenteral admixtures. *Canadian Journal of Hospital Pharmacy*. **48**: 155–160.

Mehta AC and Kay EA (1997) Storage time can be extended: A stability study of alfentanil and midazolam admixture stored in plastic syringes. *Pharmacy in Practice*. **7**: 305-308.

Mendenhall A and Hoyt DB (1994) Incompatibility of ketorolac tromethamine with haloperidol lactate and thiethylperazine maleate. *American Journal of Hospital Pharmacy*. **51**: 2964.

Middleton M and Reilly CS (1994) Do morphine and ketamine keep? The stability of morphine and ketamine separately and combined for use as an infusion. *Hospital Pharmacy Practice*. **4**: 57-58.

Napp (2010) *Personal communication.*

Napp (2014) OxyNorm 10mg/mL solution for injection or infusion. *SPC*. Available at www.medicines.org.uk.

Negro S *et al.* (2002) Physical compatibility and in vivo evaluation of drug mixtures for subcutaneous infusion to cancer patients in palliative care. *Supportive Care in Cancer*. **10**: 65-70.

NHS Argyll and Clyde (2005) Syringe driver guidelines for Graseby MS26 (mm/24h). *Document Library: Syringe drivers and infusion pumps (syringe driver guidelines)*. Available at www.palliativedrugs.com

NUH (Nottingham University Hospitals) NHS Trust (2002) *Data on file.* Hayward House, Nottingham.

Palliativedrugs.com (2006) Syringe Driver Survey Results. *Newsletter archive (June/July)*. www.palliativedrugs.com

Palliativedrugs.com *Syringe Driver Survey Database*. www.palliativedrugs.com (accessed January 2014).

Pesko LJ *et al.* (1988) Physical compatibility and stability of metoclopramide injection. *Parenterals*. **5**: 1–3, 6–8.

Peterson G *et al.* (1991) A preliminary study of the stability of midazolam in polypropylene syringes, *Australian Journal of Hospital Pharmacy*. **21**: 115-118.

Pinguet F *et al.* (1995) Compatibility and stability of granisetron, dexamethasone, and methylprednisolone in injectable solutions. *Journal of Pharmaceutical Sciences*. **84**: 267–268.

Regnard C *et al.* (1986) Antiemetics/diamorphine mixture compatibility in infusion pumps. *British Journal of Pharmaceutical Practice*. **8**: 218–220.

Riley and Fallon (1994) Octreotide in terminal malignant obstruction of the gastrointestinal tract. *European Journal of Palliative Care*. **1**: 23-25.

Sample E (2001) *Personal communication*. Burnaby Hospital, British Columbia, Canada.

Sanofi (2014) Nozinan injection. *SPC*. Available at www.medicines.org.uk

Schneider JJ (2001) *Personal communication*. Pharmacy Department, University of Newcastle, Callaghan, Australia.

Smith JC *et al.* (2000) The stability of diamorphine and glycopyrrolate in PCA syringes. *Pharmaceutical Journal*. **265 (Suppl. R69)**.

Stewart JT *et al.* (1998) Stability of ondansetron hydrochloride and 12 medications in plastic syringes. *American Journal of the Health-System Pharmacy*. **55**: 2630-2634.

Storey P *et al.* (1990) Subcutaneous infusions for control of cancer symptoms. *Journal of Pain and Symptom Management*. **5**: 33–41.

Thomas B (2011) *Personal communication*. Pharmacist, LOROS (Leicestershire and Rutland Organisation for the Relief of Suffering) Hospice, UK.

Trissel LA *Handbook on Injectable Drugs*. Maryland, USA: American Society of Health-System Pharmacists. www.medicinescomplete.com (accessed May 2013).

Trissel LA *et al.* (1994) Compatibility and stability of ondansetron hydrochloride with morphine sulphate and with hydromorphone hydrochloride in 0.9% sodium chloride injection at 4,22 and 32 degrees C. *American Journal of Hospital Pharmacy*. **51**: 2138-2142.

Virdee H *et al.* (1997) The chemical stability of diamorphine and ketorolac in 0.9% sodium chloride stored in plastic syringes. *Pharmacy in Practice*. February: 82-83.
Walker SE *et al.* (1991) Compatibility of dexamethasone sodium phosphate with hydromorphone hydrochloride or diphenhydramine hydrochloride. *American Journal of Hospital Pharmacy*. **48**: 2161-2166.
Watson DG et al. (2005) Compatibility and stability of dexamethasone sodium phosphate and ketamine hydrochloride subcutaneous infusions in polypropylene syringes. *Journal of Pain and Symptom Management*. **31**: 80-86.

General key for charts

(black box)	Do *not* use; *incompatible* at usual concentrations
(light grey box)	Use with caution; compatibility may depend on order of mixing or drug concentrations
a,b,c, etc.	Some reports of *incompatibility*, but may be compatible at other concentrations (see footnotes)
(mid grey box)	Reported compatible (data may be observational, physical or chemical, i.e. practice- or evidence-based)
?	No data. Please provide information on this combination to the Syringe Driver Survey Database (SDSD), www.palliativedrugs.com
(dark box)	Not applicable or not generally recommended, e.g. seek specialist advice when combining multiple anti-emetics
#	Use non-PVC tubing; up to 50% of a dose of clonazepam is adsorbed by PVC tubing
##	Dexamethasone sodium phosphate can generally be given once daily by SC bolus injection. If given by CSCI, to minimize the risk of incompatibility, always add it last to a maximally diluted syringe
###	Compatibility data for oxycodone 10mg/mL formulation only; for 50mg/mL formulation, see Table 1,

Alf	Alfentanil
Clzm	Clonazepam (not UK)
Cyc	Cyclizine
Dex/Dexamethasone	Dexamethasone *sodium phosphate*
Dia	Diamorphine
Gly	Glycopyrronium
Gra	Granisetron
Hal	Haloperidol
HBBr	Hyoscine *butylbromide*
HHBr	Hyoscine *hydrobromide*
Hyd	Hydromorphone
Keta	Ketamine
Ketor	Ketorolac
Levo	Levomepromazine
Meto	Metoclopramide
Mid	Midazolam
MS	Morphine *sulfate*
MT	Morphine *tartrate* (not UK)
Oct	Octreotide
Ond	Ondansetron
Oxy	Oxycodone 10mg/mL

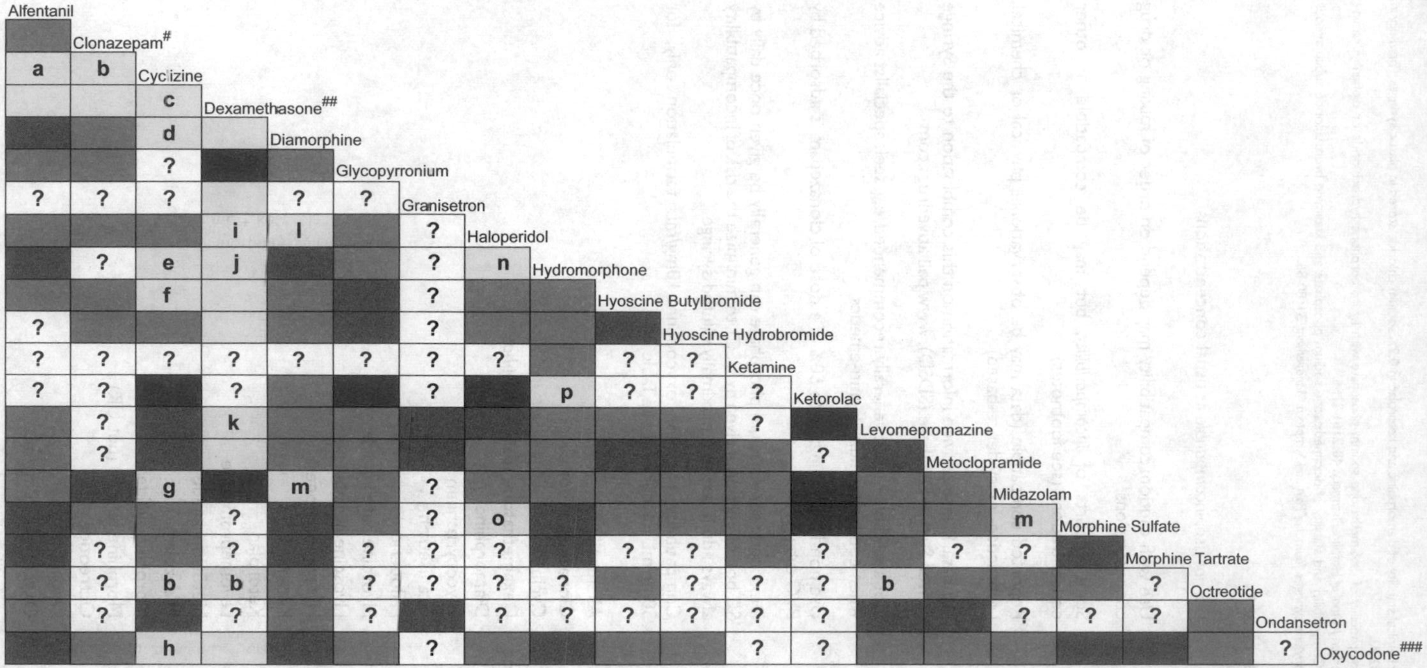

	Alfentanil	Clonazepam#	Cyclizine	Dexamethasone##	Diamorphine	Glycopyrronium	Granisetron	Haloperidol	Hydromorphone	Hyoscine Butylbromide	Hyoscine Hydrobromide	Ketamine	Ketorolac	Levomepromazine	Metoclopramide	Midazolam	Morphine Sulfate	Morphine Tartrate	Octreotide	Ondansetron
Clonazepam#																				
Cyclizine	a	b																		
Dexamethasone##			c																	
Diamorphine			d																	
Glycopyrronium			?																	
Granisetron	?	?	?		?	?														
Haloperidol				i	l		?													
Hydromorphone		?	e	j			?	n												
Hyoscine Butylbromide			f				?													
Hyoscine Hydrobromide	?						?													
Ketamine	?	?	?	?	?	?	?	?		?	?									
Ketorolac	?	?		?			?		p	?	?	?								
Levomepromazine		?		k								?								
Metoclopramide		?											?							
Midazolam			g		m		?													
Morphine Sulfate				?			?	o								m				
Morphine Tartrate		?		?		?	?	?		?	?		?		?	?				
Octreotide		?	b	b		?	?	?	?		?	?	?	b				?		
Ondansetron		?		?		?		?	?	?	?	?	?			?	?	?		
Oxycodone###			h				?					?	?							?

Note. This chart summarizes the compatibility information available for drug combinations in **WFI** used for CSCI over 24h in palliative care units and the literature (see p.933). It includes compatibility data for oxycodone 10mg/mL formulation only; for 50mg/mL, see Table 1. It should be used in conjunction with the key and the footnotes. Further information about each combination may be found on the www.palliativedrugs.com Syringe Driver Survey Database (SDSD). Charts with drug combinations diluted in sodium chloride 0.9% can be found in the extended appendix section of the on-line *PCF*.

Chart 1 Compatibility chart for *two* drugs in ***WFI.***

Chart 1 footnotes

All drug concentration values (mg/mL) specified below are the maximum *final* concentrations of each drug in the syringe after mixing and dilution reported compatible; at higher concentrations *incompatibility* has either been reported or may occur. For full reference details, see p.933.

a. alfentanil 0.24mg/mL + cyclizine 8.8mg/mL (Dickman *et al.* 2011, palliativedrugs.com 2014)
b. some observational reports of *incompatibility* from miscellaneous sources
c. cyclizine 8.33mg/mL + dexamethasone sodium phosphate 0.33mg/mL (Dickman *et al.* 2011, palliativedrugs.com 2014)
d. cyclizine up to 20mg/mL + diamorphine up to 20mg/mL, or cyclizine maximum 10mg/mL + diamorphine >20mg/mL, or cyclizine >20mg/mL + diamorphine maximum 15mg/mL (Grassby and Hutchings 1997)
e. cyclizine 8.82mg/mL + hydromorphone 5.8mg/mL(Hines and Pleasance 2011); one report of *incompatibility* at *lower* concentrations (Back 2013)
f. generally regarded as *incompatible*; one report of compatibility of low concentrations for a *12h* infusion of cyclizine 3.7mg/mL + hyoscine *butylbromide* 1.5mg/mL (palliativedrugs.com 2014)
g. cyclizine 8.82mg/mL + midazolam 0.88mg/mL (Back 2013, palliativedrugs.com 2014)
h. cyclizine 3mg/mL + oxycodone 9mg/mL; cyclizine concentrations between 3mg/mL and 8mg/mL may be used as long as the oxycodone concentration is reduced to below 3mg/mL by diluting with WFI (Napp 2010, Napp 2014)
i. dexamethasone sodium phosphate 0.15mg/mL + haloperidol 0.38mg/mL (Dickman *et al.* 2011, palliativedrugs.com 2014)
j. dexamethasone sodium phosphate 2mg/mL + hydromorphone 20mg/mL, or dexamethasone sodium phosphate >2mg/mL + hydromorphone 10mg/mL (Walker *et al.* 1991, Hines and Pleasance 2011)
k. dexamethasone sodium phosphate 0.11mg/mL + levomepromazine 2.78mg/mL (Dickman *et al.* 2011, palliativedrugs.com 2014)
l. diamorphine up to 50mg/mL + haloperidol 4mg/mL, or diamorphine 50–100mg/mL + haloperidol 3mg/mL (Grassby and Hutchings 1997)
m. diamorphine or morphine sulfate + midazolam generally regarded as compatible (palliativedrugs.com 2014, Dickman *et al.* 2011); one report *of incompatibility* for diamorphine (palliativedrugs.com 2014); microscopic precipitation may occur with morphine (LeBelle *et al.* 1995)
n. variable reports at higher concentrations, e.g. haloperidol 2.5mg/mL + hydromorphone 5mg/mL compatible (Huang and Anderson 1994), haloperidol 3mg/mL + hydromorphone 20mg/mL compatible (Hines and Pleasance 2011), but haloperidol 2mg/mL + hydromorphone 10mg/mL *incompatible* (Storey *et al.* 1990)
o. haloperidol <1mg/mL + morphine sulfate <10mg/mL (palliativedrugs.com 2014, Storey *et al.* 1990, Trissel 2006, LeBelle *et al.* 1995)
p. hydromorphone 0.5mg/mL + ketorolac 15mg/mL (Huang and Anderson 1994).

	Alf + Clzm#	Alf + Cyc	Alf + Dex##	Alf + Gly	Alf + Gra	Alf + Hal	Alf + HBBr	Alf + HHBr	Alf + Keta	Alf + Ketor	Alf + Levo	Alf + Meto	Alf + Mid	Alf + Oct
Cyclizine	a													
Dexamethasone##	?	?												
Glycopyrronium		?	?											
Granisetron	?	?	?	?										
Haloperidol		b	?		?									
Hyoscine Butylbromide	?	?	?		?									
Hyoscine Hydrobromide		?	?		?	?								
Ketamine	?	?	?	?	?	?	?	?						
Ketorolac	?	?	?	?	?	?	?	?	?					
Levomepromazine	?		?					?	?	?				
Metoclopramide	?		?			?			?	?				
Midazolam		c	?		?				?	?				
Octreotide	?	?	?	?	?	?	?	?	?	?			?	
Ondansetron	?	?	?	?		?	?	?	?	?			?	?

Note. This chart summarizes the compatibility information available for drug combinations in **WFI** used for CSCI over 24h in palliative care units and the literature (see p.933). It should be used in conjunction with the key and the footnotes. Further information about each combination may be found on the www.palliativedrugs.com Syringe Driver Survey Database (SDSD). Charts with drug combinations diluted in sodium chloride 0.9% can be found in the extended appendix section of the on-line *PCF*.

Chart 2 Compatibility chart for alfentanil: *three* drugs in ***WFI***.

Chart 2 footnotes

All drug concentration values (mg/mL) specified below are the maximum *final* concentrations of each drug in the syringe after mixing and dilution reported compatible; at higher concentrations, *incompatibility* has either been reported or may occur. For full reference details, see p.933.

Concentration-dependent *incompatibility* reported with 2-drug combinations of **alfentanil** + **cyclizine** (see Chart 1, p.936).

a. alfentanil 0.53mg/mL + clonazepam 0.24mg/mL + cyclizine 8.82mg/mL (Dickman *et al.* 2011)
b. one report of *incompatibility* (Back 2013), but several other reports of compatibility (Dickman *et al.* 2011, palliativedrugs.com 2014)
c. alfentanil 3mg/mL + cyclizine 6mg/mL + midazolam 1.2mg/mL (Dickman et al. 2011).

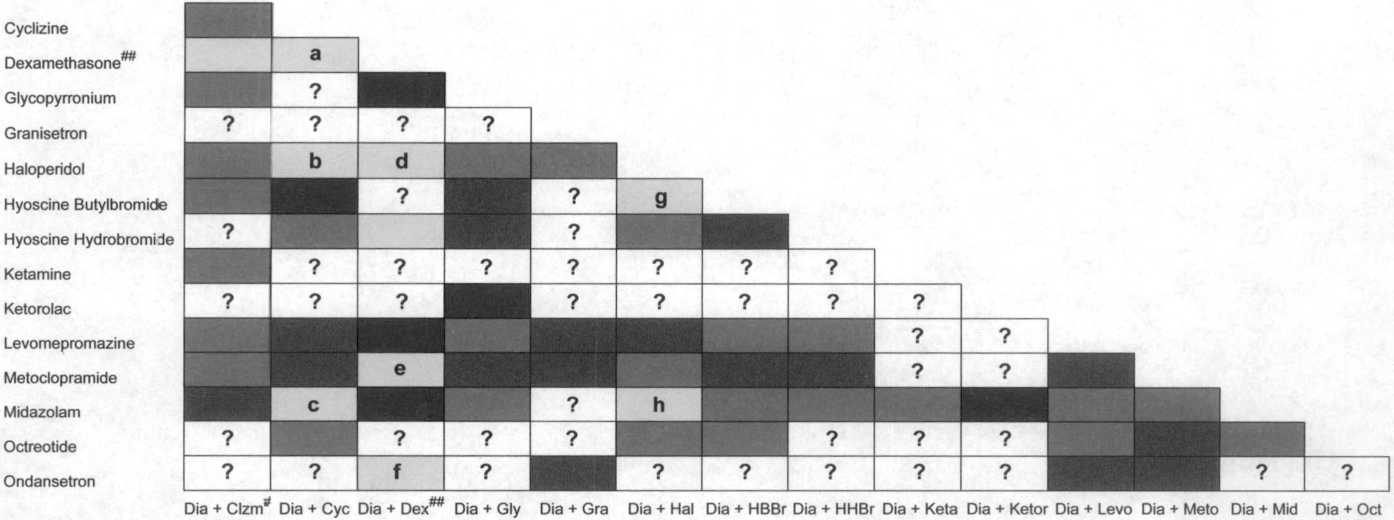

	Dia + Clzm[#]	Dia + Cyc	Dia + Dex[##]	Dia + Gly	Dia + Gra	Dia + Hal	Dia + HBBr	Dia + HHBr	Dia + Keta	Dia + Ketor	Dia + Levo	Dia + Meto	Dia + Mid	Dia + Oct
Cyclizine														
Dexamethasone[##]		a												
Glycopyrronium		?												
Granisetron	?	?	?	?										
Haloperidol		b	d											
Hyoscine Butylbromide			?		?	g								
Hyoscine Hydrobromide	?				?									
Ketamine		?	?	?	?	?	?	?						
Ketorolac	?	?	?		?	?	?	?	?					
Levomepromazine									?	?				
Metoclopramide			e						?	?				
Midazolam		c			?	h								
Octreotide	?		?	?	?			?	?	?				
Ondansetron	?	?	f	?		?	?	?	?	?			?	?

Note. This chart summarizes the compatibility information available for drug combinations in **WFI** used for CSCI over 24h in palliative care units and the literature (see p.933). It should be used in conjunction with the key and the footnotes. Further information about each combination may be found on the www.palliativedrugs.com Syringe Driver Survey Database (SDSD). Charts with drug combinations diluted in sodium chloride 0.9% can be found in the extended appendix section of the on-line *PCF*.

Chart 3 Compatibility chart for diamorphine: *three* drugs in ***WFI***.

Chart 3 footnotes

All drug concentration values (mg/mL) specified below are the maximum *final* concentrations of each drug in the syringe after mixing and dilution reported compatible; at higher concentrations, *incompatibility* has either been reported or may occur. For full reference details, see p.933.

Concentration-dependent *incompatibility* reported with 2-drug combinations of **diamorphine** + **cyclizine** or **haloperidol** (see Chart 1, p.936).

a. diamorphine 5.88mg/mL + cyclizine 8.82mg/mL + dexamethasone sodium phosphate 0.71mg/mL (Dickman *et al.* 2011, palliativedrugs.com 2014)
b. diamorphine 56mg/mL + cyclizine 13mg/mL + haloperidol 2.1mg/mL (Grassby 1995, palliativedrugs.com 2014)
c. diamorphine 37mg/mL + cyclizine 8.82mg/mL + midazolam 2.35mg/mL (palliativedrugs.com 2014)
d. diamorphine 25mg/mL + dexamethasone sodium phosphate 0.35mg/mL + haloperidol 0.59mg/mL (Dickman *et al.* 2011)
e. diamorphine 3.53mg/mL + dexamethasone sodium phosphate 0.59mg/mL + metoclopramide 2.35mg/mL (Dickman *et al.* 2011)
f. diamorphine 35mg/mL + dexamethasone sodium phosphate 0.06mg/mL + ondansetron 1.41mg/mL (Dickman *et al.* 2011)
g. diamorphine 117.7mg/mL + haloperidol 0.59mg/mL + hyoscine *butylbromide* 3.53mg/mL (palliativedrugs.com 2014)
h. diamorphine 28mg/mL+ haloperidol 2mg/mL + midazolam 1mg/mL (palliativedrugs.com 2014).

	Hyd + Clzm[#]	Hyd + Cyc	Hyd + Dex[##]	Hyd + Gly	Hyd + Gra	Hyd + Hal	Hyd + HBBr	Hyd + HHBr	Hyd + Keta	Hyd + Ketor	Hyd + Levo	Hyd + Meto	Hyd + Mid	Hyd + Oct
Cyclizine	?													
Dexamethasone[##]	?	?												
Glycopyrronium	?	?	?											
Granisetron	?	?	?	?										
Haloperidol	?	?	?	?	?									
Hyoscine Butylbromide	?	?	?		?	?								
Hyoscine Hydrobromide	?	?	?		?	?								
Ketamine	?	?	?	?	?	c	?	?						
Ketorolac	?	?	?	?	?		?	?	?					
Levomepromazine	?		?	?			?	?	?	?				
Metoclopramide	?		?			?			?	?				
Midazolam		?	b	?	?	d	?	?	?	?				
Octreotide	?	a	?	?	?	?	?	?	?	?	?		?	
Ondansetron	?	?	?	?		?	?	?	?	?			?	?

Note. This chart summarizes the compatibility information available for drug combinations in **WFI** used for CSCI over 24h in palliative care units and the literature (see p.933). It should be used in conjunction with the key and the footnotes. Further information about each combination may be found on the www.palliativedrugs.com Syringe Driver Survey Database (SDSD). Charts with drug combinations diluted in sodium chloride 0.9% can be found in the extended appendix section of the on-line *PCF*.

Chart 4 Compatibility chart for hydromorphone: *three* drugs in ***WFI***.

Chart 4 footnotes

All drug concentration values (mg/mL) specified below are the maximum *final* concentrations of each drug in the syringe after mixing and dilution reported compatible; at higher concentrations, *incompatibility* has either been reported or may occur. For full reference details, see p.933.

Concentration-dependent *incompatibility* reported with 2-drug combinations of **hydromorphone + cyclizine, dexamethasone, haloperidol** or **ketorolac** (see Chart 1, p.936).

a. hydromorphone 1.67mg/mL + cyclizine 16.67mg/mL + octreotide 0.02mg/mL; *incompatibility* has been reported with cyclizine and octreotide; see 2-drug chart (Dickman 2011)
b. generally regarded as *incompatible*, despite observational reports of compatibility, as dexamethasone + midazolam 2-drug combination are *incompatible* although may be visually clear, see Chapter 29, Box C, p.892 (Good 2004)
c. hydromorphone 3.75mg/mL + haloperidol 0.16mg/mL + ketamine 31.25mg/mL (palliativedrugs.com 2014)
d. hydromorphone 0.35mg/mL + haloperidol 0.06mg/mL + midazolam 0.23mg/mL (palliativedrugs.com 2014).

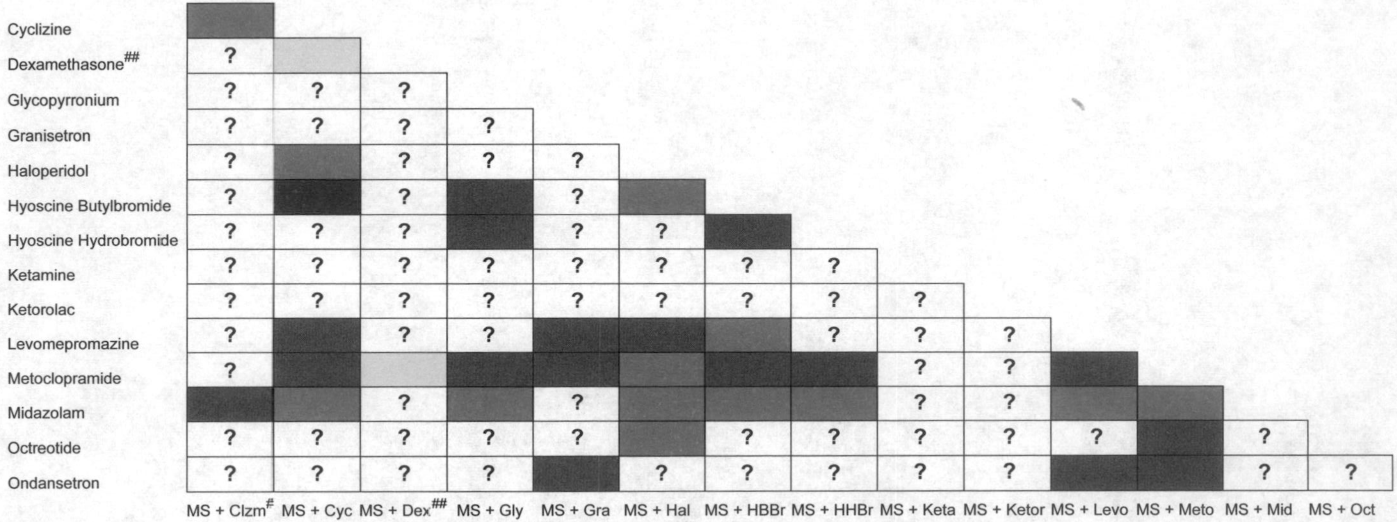

	MS + Clzm[#]	MS + Cyc	MS + Dex[##]	MS + Gly	MS + Gra	MS + Hal	MS + HBBr	MS + HHBr	MS + Keta	MS + Ketor	MS + Levo	MS + Meto	MS + Mid	MS + Oct
Cyclizine														
Dexamethasone[##]	?													
Glycopyrronium	?	?	?											
Granisetron	?	?	?	?										
Haloperidol	?		?	?	?									
Hyoscine Butylbromide	?		?		?									
Hyoscine Hydrobromide	?	?	?		?	?								
Ketamine	?	?	?	?	?	?	?	?						
Ketorolac	?	?	?	?	?	?	?	?	?					
Levomepromazine	?		?	?				?	?	?				
Metoclopramide	?								?	?				
Midazolam			?		?				?	?				
Octreotide	?	?	?	?	?		?	?	?	?	?		?	
Ondansetron	?	?	?	?		?	?	?	?	?			?	?

Note. This chart summarizes the compatibility information available for drug combinations in **WFI** used for CSCI over 24h in palliative care units and the literature (see p.933). It should be used in conjunction with the key and the footnotes. Further information about each combination may be found on the www.palliativedrugs.com Syringe Driver Survey Database (SDSD). Charts with drug combinations diluted in sodium chloride 0.9% can be found in the extended appendix section of the on-line *PCF*.

Chart 5 Compatibility chart for morphine sulfate: *three* drugs in ***WFI***.

Chart 5 footnote

Concentration-dependent *incompatibility* reported with 2-drug combinations of **morphine sulfate + haloperidol** (see Chart 1, p.936).

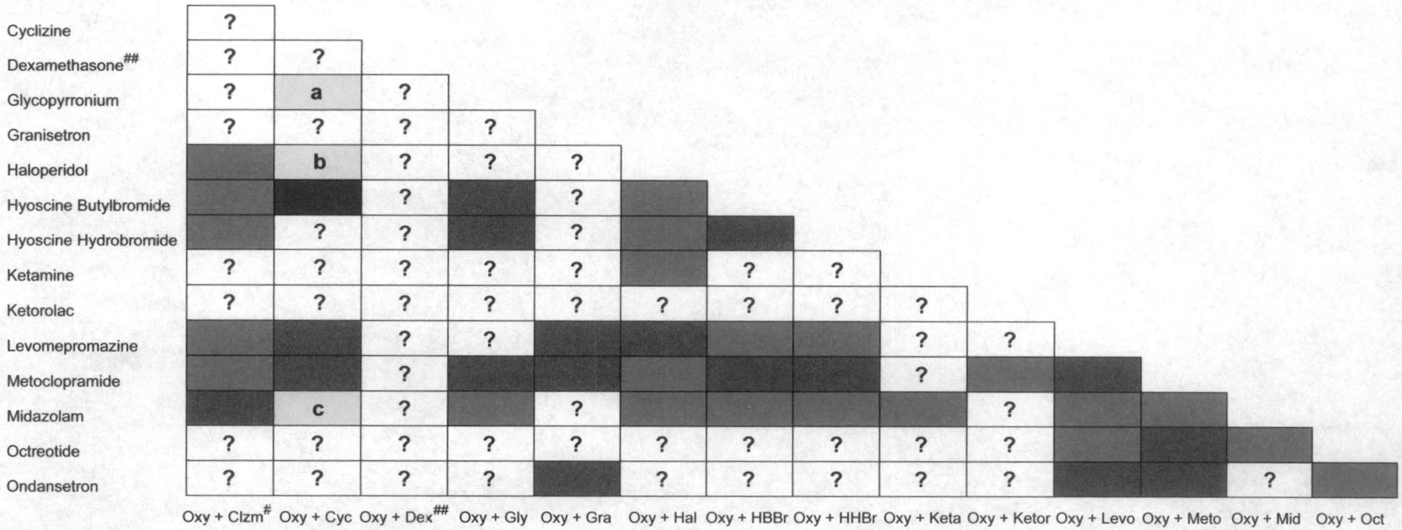

	Oxy + Clzm#	Oxy + Cyc	Oxy + Dex##	Oxy + Gly	Oxy + Gra	Oxy + Hal	Oxy + HBBr	Oxy + HHBr	Oxy + Keta	Oxy + Ketor	Oxy + Levo	Oxy + Meto	Oxy + Mid	Oxy + Oct
Cyclizine	?													
Dexamethasone##	?	?												
Glycopyrronium	?	a	?											
Granisetron	?	?	?	?										
Haloperidol		b	?	?	?									
Hyoscine Butylbromide			?		?									
Hyoscine Hydrobromide		?	?		?									
Ketamine	?	?	?	?	?		?	?						
Ketorolac	?	?	?	?	?	?	?	?	?					
Levomepromazine			?	?					?	?				
Metoclopramide			?						?					
Midazolam		c	?		?					?				
Octreotide	?	?	?	?	?	?	?	?	?	?				
Ondansetron	?	?	?	?		?	?	?	?	?			?	

Note. Compatibility data for oxycodone 10mg/mL formulation only; for 50mg/mL formulation, see Table 1. This chart summarizes the compatibility information available for drug combinations in **WFI** used for CSCI over 24h in palliative care units and the literature (see p.933). It should be used in conjunction with the key and the footnotes. Further information about each combination may be found on the www.palliativedrugs.com Syringe Driver Survey Database (SDSD). Charts with drug combinations diluted in sodium chloride 0.9% can be found in the extended appendix section of the on-line *PCF*.

Chart 6 Compatibility chart for oxycodone 10mg/mL formulation: *three* drugs in ***WFI***.

Chart 6 footnotes

All drug concentration values (mg/mL) specified below are the maximum *final* concentrations of each drug in the syringe after mixing and dilution reported compatible; at higher concentrations *incompatibility* has either been reported or may occur. For full reference details, see p.933.

Concentration-dependent *incompatibility* reported with 2-drug combinations of **oxycodone + cyclizine** (see Chart 1, p.936).

a. oxycodone 3.5mg/mL + cyclizine 7.5mg/mL + glycopyrronium 0.06mg/mL (Dickman *et al.* 2011, Napp 2010)

b. oxycodone 1.9mg/mL + cyclizine 7.14mg/mL + haloperidol 0.95mg/mL; higher concentrations have been reported compatible, but it is unclear whether the higher strength oxycodone formulation has been used (50mg/mL), which has a different compatibility profile (palliativedrugs.com 2014, Dickman *et al.* 2011, Napp 2010)

c. oxycodone 2.22mg/mL + cyclizine 8.33mg/mL + midazolam 0.28mg/mL; *incompatibility* with some 2-drug combinations of cyclizine + midazolam (Back 2013, palliativedrugs.com 2014, Napp 2010).

	Clzm[#] + Meto	Cyc + Dex[##]	Cyc + Hal	Cyc + HBBr	Dex[##] + Mid	Gly + Keta	Gly + Levo	Hal + Mid	HBBr + Ketor	Levo + Mid
Haloperidol		?		b	d	?				
Hyoscine Butylbromide		a	b							
Hyoscine Hydrobromide		?	?		?					
Ketamine	?	?	?	?	?		?		?	?
Ketorolac	?	?	?	?	?	?	?			?
Metoclopramide					?	?			?	
Midazolam		?		c			?			
Octreotide	?	?	?	?	?	?		?	?	?

Note. This chart summarizes the compatibility information available for drug combinations in **WFI** used for CSCI over 24h in palliative care units and the literature (see p.933). It should be used in conjunction with the key and the footnotes. Further information about each combination may be found on the www.palliativedrugs.com Syringe Driver Survey Database (SDSD). Charts with drug combinations diluted in sodium chloride 0.9% can be found in the extended appendix section of the on-line *PCF*.

Chart 7 Compatibility chart for non-opioids: *three* drugs in ***WFI***.

Chart 7 footnotes

All drug concentration values (mg/mL) specified below are the maximum *final* concentrations of each drug in the syringe after mixing and dilution reported compatible; at higher concentrations *incompatibility* has either been reported or may occur. For full reference details, see p.933.

a. cyclizine 8.82mg/mL + dexamethasone sodium phosphate 0.71mg/mL + hyoscine *butylbromide* 2.35mg/mL (Dickman *et al.* 2011)
b. generally regarded as *incompatible* (NUH 2002); one report of compatibility (Back 2013)
c. generally regarded as *incompatible*; *incompatibility* reported with 2-drug combinations of cyclizine + hyoscine *butylbromide* and some 2-drug combinations of cyclizine + midazolam (NUH 2002, palliativedrugs.com 2014)
d. generally regarded as *incompatible* despite observational reports of compatibility, as dexamethasone + midazolam 2-drug combination are *incompatible* although may be visually clear; see Chapter 29, Box C, p.892 (Good 2004).

Compatibility information for oxycodone 50mg/mL formulation

When mixed with other drugs, some differences in compatibility have been demonstrated for the 10mg/mL and 50mg/mL formulations of oxycodone solution for injection, e.g. with cyclizine (Gardiner 2003, Hines and Pleasance 2009). This may be due to the different ratios of excipients in each formulation. The manufacturer recommends that the compatibility information for each formulation is considered separately and not extrapolated from one formulation to another.

Chemical compatibility data between oxycodone 50mg/mL solution for injection and other drugs over 24h at room temperature are summarized in Table 1. Full details are available on the SDSD on www.palliativedrugs.com. Please submit details to the SDSD of successful combinations containing oxycodone 50mg/mL and, more importantly, details of combinations that were incompatible.

Table 1 Oxycodone 50mg/mL formulation compatibility with other drugs (Hines and Pleasance 2009)

	Oxycodone 250mg diluted[a]		*Oxycodone 500mg undiluted*	
	Dose (mg)	*Concentration (mg/mL)*	*Dose (mg)*	*Concentration (mg/mL)*
Cyclizine[b,c,d]	150	8.8	50	4.5
Dexamethasone *sodium phosphate*	20	1.2	40	2
Glycopyrronium	1.2	0.07	2.4	0.1
Haloperidol	7.5	0.4	15	1.2
Hyoscine *butylbromide*	30	1.8	60	4.6
Hyoscine *hydrobromide*	1.2	0.07	2.4	0.15
Ketamine	400	23.5	800	44.4
Levomepromazine	100	5.9	200	11.1
Metoclopramide	50	2.9	100	3.3
Midazolam	50	2.9	100	3.3

a. oxycodone 50mg/mL formulation, 5mL (250mg) mixed with the drug and diluted to 17mL with WFI or sodium chloride 0.9%; oxycodone final concentration 14mg/mL

b. use WFI only; *incompatible* with sodium chloride 0.9%

c. maximum concentrations found compatible for cyclizine and oxycodone 50mg/mL formulation; concentration-dependent *incompatibility* found above this

d. for practical purposes, a cyclizine concentration of >4mg/mL to a maximum of 8mg/mL may be used if the oxycodone concentration is kept ≤14mg/mL by diluting with WFI (Napp, 2010).

Updated May 2017

Drug Index

Note. Main references are in **bold**.

Supplementary Topic Index

A textbook on pain and symptom management should be consulted for a full discussion on these topics.

Note:
1. **Words** in **bold type** indicate a chapter or an appendix.
2. **Numbers** in **bold type** indicate the main entry for that topic.